Nursing Care Plans

Transitional Patient & Family Centered Care

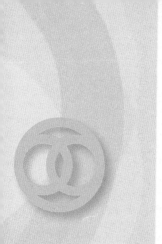

Nursing Care Plans

Transitional Patient & Family Centered Care

7TH EDITION

LYNDA JUALL CARPENITO, RN, MSN, CRNP, FIN

Family Nurse Practitioner
ChesPenn Health Services
Chester, Pennsylvania

Nursing Consultant
Mullica Hill, New Jersey

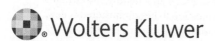

. Wolters Kluwer

Philadelphia • Baltimore • New York • London
Buenos Aires • Hong Kong • Sydney • Tokyo

Acquisitions Editor: Natasha McIntyre
Director of Product Development: Jennifer Forestieri
Development Editor: Annette Ferran
Editorial Coordinator: Emily Buccieri
Editorial Assistant: Dan Reilly
Production Project Manager: Marian Bellus
Design Coordinator: Terry Mallon
Manufacturing Coordinator: Karin Duffield
Prepress Vendor: S4Carlisle Publishing Services

Seventh Edition

9 8 7 6 5 4 3 2 1

Printed in China

Library of Congress Cataloging-in-Publication Data

Names: Carpenito, Lynda Juall, author.
Title: Nursing care plans: transitional patient & family centered care /
   Lynda Juall Carpenito.
Description: Seventh edition. | Philadelphia: Wolters Kluwer Health, [2017]
   | Includes bibliographical references and index.
Identifiers: LCCN 2016036749 | ISBN 9781496349262
Subjects: | MESH: Patient Care Planning | Nursing Process | Family Nursing |
   Transitional Care | Nursing Records
Classification: LCC RT49 | NLM WY 100.1 | DDC 610.73—dc23 LC record available at
   https://lccn.loc.gov/2016036749

LWW.com

To My Mother: Elizabeth Julia Juall

Every year brought me a new appreciation and admiration for this woman. In her 90s there is not much she did not do. To honor her fierce independence, every effort was taken so she could live in her home. The goal was to keep her happy and as safe as possible.

She role-modeled respect for all, forgiveness, and independence.

She was determined she could, and she did!—gardening, water aerobics, casino blackjack. . .

After a sudden illness at 96, she declined, but kept her spirit and was determined to recover.

I knew she would not. I promised her a good death in her home, and so I moved into her home for 4 months. It was a special time for us. Witnessing her decline was painful, but it was a privilege to return the gift she gave me all my life: unconditional love.

One night I sat with her and told her that her will was strong but her heart was failing. I asked her to stop fighting and to allow herself to drift away and to meet her God, her mom and her sisters. She looked at me and made the sign of the cross and folded her hands in prayer. She did decline and died one-and-a-half days later.

She is one generation of my family's Hungarian Woman Warriors, and I proudly walk in their footprints, carry their swords to battle injustice, and cherish deeply our loved ones.

> *Love your daughter*
>
> *Lynda*

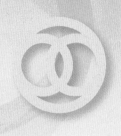

Contributors

Deborah H. Brooks, MSN, ANP-BC, CNN-NP
Nurse Practitioner
Division of Nephrology
Medical Center University of South Carolina
Charleston, South Carolina
(*RC of Acute Urinary Retention, RC of Renal Insufficiency, RC of Renal Calculi, Hemodialysis, Peritoneal Dialysis Acute Kidney Failure [Injury], Chronic Kidney Disease, Nephrectomy*)

Heather R. Carpenito, RN, BSN
FNP student
Wilmington University
Wilmington, Delaware
Clinician, Cardiac Monitor Unit
Inspira Medical System
Woodbury, New Jersey
(*Acute Coronary Syndrome*)

Helen I. de Graaf-Waar, RN, MSc
Staff Advisor/Consultant
Erasmus MC
Rotterdam, The Netherlands
(*Palliative Care with LJ Carpenito*)

Patricia Golato, MSN, CRNP, FNP-C
Advanced Practice Nurse
HIV Early Intervention Program
Cooper University Hospital
Camden, New Jersey
(*Diabetes Mellitus*)

Elizabeth Kroll, RN, MSN, CMSRN
Nursing Faculty
Department of Nursing
Muskegon Community College
Muskegon, Michigan
(*Myasthenia Gravis, Guillain-Barré Syndrome*)

Lisa Wallen, RN, ANP-BC
Certified Wound Specialist
Senior Wound Specialist
Strong Hyperbaric and Wound Center
University of Rochester
Rochester, New York
(*Pressure Ulcers co-authored with LJ Carpenito*)

Susan Johnson Warner, RN, CPNP, MPH, EdD
Founding Director and Professor
Nursing Department
St. Cloud State University
St. Cloud, Minnesota
(*Generic Medical Care Plan for Hospitalized Infants/ Children/Adolescents*)

Teresa Wilson, MS, APRNC-OB, CNS, BC
Nurse Home Visitor
Casa de los Niños, Nurse–Family Partnership
Tucson, Arizona
(*Generic Newborn Care Plan; Generic Care Plan for Woman/ Support Persons during Prenatal Period; Generic Care Plan for Woman/Support Persons during Postpartum Period*)

6th-Edition Contributors

Carie Bilicki, RE, MSN, ACNS-BC, OCN
Clinical Nurse Specialist
Froedtert Health
Milwaukee, Wisconsin
(*Initial Cancer Diagnosis, Breast Surgery, Chemotherapy, Radiation*)

Kimberly Dupree Harrelson, BSN, RN, CRRN, DNP
Senior Study Research Coordinator (RN) for the
Blood Pressure in Dialysis Study (BID Study)
The Medical University of South Carolina (MUSC)
Charleston, South Carolina
(*Laminectomy*)

Suzanne Pach, RN, MSN, FNP-C
Stroke Nurse Practitioner
University of South Carolina
Charleston, South Carolina
(*Parkinson's Disease, Cerebrovascular Accident*)

Amy Salgado, RN, MSN
Clinical Coordinator–Carondelet-PCOA Transitional
Care Navigation Program
Carondelet Health Network
Tucson, Arizona
(*RC of Bleeding, RC of Decreased Cardiac Output, RC of Dysrhythmias, RC of Hypovolemia, RC of Pulmonary Edema, Heart Failure, Hypertension, Acute Coronary Syndrome, Peripheral Arterial Disease [Atherosclerosis]*)

Preface

Nursing is primarily assisting individuals, sick or well, in activities that contribute to health or its recovery, or to a peaceful death so that they perform unaided when they have the necessary strength, will, or knowledge. Nursing also helps individuals carry out prescribed therapy and to be independent of assistance as soon as possible (Henderson & Nite, 1960).

Historically, nurses have represented the core of the health care delivery system (including acute, long-term, and community agencies), but their image continues to be one of individuals whose actions are dependent on physician supervision. Unfortunately, what Donna Diers wrote over 15 years ago is still relevant today:

> *Nursing is exceedingly complicated work since it involves technical skill, a great deal of formal knowledge, communication ability, use of self, timing, emotional investment, and any number of other qualities. What it also involves—and what is hidden from the public—is the complex process of thinking that leads from the knowledge to the skill, from the perception to the action, from the decision to the touch, from the observation to the diagnosis. Yet it is this process of nursing care, which is at the center of nursing's work, that is so little described. . .* (Diers, 1981, p. 1, emphasis supplied)

Physicians regularly and openly explain their management plans to the public, especially to clients and their families. Nurses, however, often fail to explain the nursing care plan to clients and family. This book provides both a framework for nurses to provide responsible nursing care and guidelines for them to document and communicate that care. These care plans should not be handwritten. They must be reference documents for practicing nurses. Write or free text the different care the client needs in addition to the standard.

The focus of this 7th edition of *Nursing Care Plans* is transitional nursing care for individuals and their families in an acute care facility. In order for transitions to home or a community care facility to be timely, appropriate, and safe, many factors must be considered. In every care plan, the following elements have been highlighted to enhance the transition process:

- **Transitional Risk Assessment Plan** to begin at admission to assess individual's vulnerability for infection, pressure ulcers, falls, and delayed transition. Evidence-based risk assessment tools for each potential hospital-acquired condition are illustrated on the inside back cover.
- **Clinical Alerts** are placed in the plans to advise the clinical or student nurse of a serious event that requires immediate action.
- **Clinical Alert Reports** are a list of clinical observations or findings that are communicated to the novice or student nurses and/or medical assistants before they begin care that needs to be monitored for. Changes in status need to be reported in a timely and sometimes urgent fashion.
- **Carp's Cues** notes from the author to emphasize a certain principle of care.
- **STAR** is an acronym for Stop, Think, Act, Review. This is a process to be utilized "when something just is not right."
- **SBAR** is an acronym (Situation, Background, Assessment, Recommendation) for the method of concisely organizing a communication to another professional regarding a concern about a client/family status or situation.
- **Transition to Home/Community Care** is an element in each care plan placed before the last diagnosis, Risk for Ineffective Self-Health Management, that focuses the nurse on evaluating for the presence of risk factors that can delay transition.

Unit II contains frequently occurring nursing diagnoses* and collaborative problems that supplement the care plans in Unit III. For example, if an individual is admitted for Acute Coronary Syndrome and has also recently lost his sister to cancer, the nurse can refer to Unit II to the Grieving nursing diagnosis. In another situation, an individual had a total knee replacement and also has type II diabetes mellitus. In Unit II, the collaborative problem Risk for Complications of Hypo/Hyperglycemia would be added to the problem list. The entire care plan for Diabetes Mellitus would not be indicated because the priorities of care would be in the Total Knee Replacement Care Plan. Risk for Complications of Hyper/Hypoglycemia would be added to monitor blood glucose levels.

This book also incorporates the findings of a validation study, a description of which (method, subjects, instrument findings) is presented in the section titled Validation Project, following the Preface. These findings should be very useful for practicing nurses, students of nursing, and departments of nursing.

The Bifocal Clinical Practice Model underpins this book and serves to organize the nursing care plans in Unit I. Chapter 1 describes and discusses the Bifocal Clinical Practice Model, which differentiates nursing diagnoses from other problems that nurses treat. In this chapter, nursing diagnoses and collaborative problems are explained and differentiated. The relationship of the type of diagnosis to outcome criteria and nursing interventions is also emphasized.

Communication is emphasized as the critical key to preventing adverse events in Chapter 2. The imperative of timely, clinically pertinent communication is emphasized with SBAR and reducing the barriers to "speaking up." Chapter 3 focuses on early identification of high-risk individuals and/or family. The eight hospital-acquired conditions that are deemed preventable by the Centers for Medicare and Medicaid Services are presented. Nurses' unique role in their prevention is discussed.

The preparation of individual/family for care at home or transition to a community care facility is the focus of Chapter 4. The assessment of risk factors in the individual and his or her support system and home environment is presented for early identification of potential barriers to a timely, safe transition. Chapter 5 gives an overview of the 10 steps in care planning and takes the student nurse through each phase of this process. The purpose is to reduce writing of care plans but instead for the student to use the care plan as a reference and then to add or delete on the basis of other comorbidities and/or their clinical assessments. The process of identification of priority diagnoses is described.

What is the most important thing to do for this individual right now is the focus of Chapter 6. Moral distress in nurses is described with preventive strategies. Professional nursing practice must represent the art and the science of the profession. The care plans in this book represent the science of nursing. A nurse who is a scientist but has not incorporated the art of this profession into his or her practice is providing care but is not caring. This chapter will emphasize caring as a critical component of our profession.

Unit III presents care plans that represent a compilation of the complex work of nursing in caring for individuals (and their families) experiencing medical disorders or surgical interventions or undergoing diagnostic or therapeutic procedures. It uses the nursing process to present the type of nursing care that is expected to be necessary for clients experiencing similar situations. The plans provide the nurse with a framework for providing initial, or essential, care. The intent of this book is to assist the nurse to identify the responsible care that nurses are accountable to provide. The incorporation of recent research findings further enhances the applicability of the care plans. By using the Bifocal Clinical Practice Model, the book clearly defines the scope of independent and collaborative practice.

Section 4 contains five specialty care plans for newborns, children, adolescents, the family in the postpartum period, and individuals with mental health disorders.

Additional Resources

Additional resources to accompany this edition such as printable individual information guides like "Getting Started to Quitting Smoking" can be accessed at thePoint at http://thePoint.lww.com/Carpenito6e

The author invites comments and suggestions from readers. Correspondence can be directed to the publisher or to the author's email at juall46@msn.com.

References

Diers, D. (1981). *Why write? Why publish? Image*, 13, 991–997.
Henderson, V., & Nite, G. (1960). *Principles and practice of nursing* (5th ed., p. 14). New York, NY: Macmillan.

*Nursing diagnoses contain definitions designated as NANDA-I and characteristics and factors identified with a blue asterisk from Herdman, T. H., and Kamitsuru, S. (Eds.). Nursing Diagnoses: Definitions and Classification 2015-2017. Copyright © 2014, 1994 -2014 by NANDA International. Used by arrangement with John Wiley & Sons Limited.

Validation Project

Background

In 1984, this author published diagnostic clusters under medical and surgical conditions (Carpenito, 1984). These diagnostic clusters represented nursing diagnoses and collaborative problems described in the literature for a medical or surgical population. After the initial diagnostic clusters were created, they were reviewed by clinicians who practiced with specific corresponding populations.

Since 1984, numerous other authors (Doenges, 1991; Holloway, 1988; Sparks, 1993; Ulrich, 1994) have generated similar groupings. Before 1993, none of the clusters have been studied to determine their frequency of occurrence. In other words, are some diagnoses in the diagnostic cluster treated more frequently than others? To this date in 2013, this validation study by this author remains to be the only research with this clinical focus.

Reasons for Study

In the past 10 years, the health care delivery system has experienced numerous changes. Specifically, clients are in the acute care setting for shorter periods. These client populations all share a high acuity. This acuity is represented with multiple nursing diagnoses and collaborative problems. However, do all these diagnoses have the same priority? Which diagnoses necessitate nursing interventions during the length of stay?

Care planning books report a varied number of diagnoses to treat under a specific condition. For example, in reviewing a care plan for a client with a myocardial infarction, this author found the following number of diagnoses reported: Ulrich, 16; Carpenito, 11; Doenges, 7; Holloway, 4. When students review these references, how helpful are lists ranging from 4 to 16 diagnoses? How many diagnoses can nurses be accountable for during an individual's length of stay?

The identification of nursing diagnoses and collaborative problems that nurses treat more frequently than others in certain populations can be very useful data to:

- Assist nurses with decision making
- Determine the cost of nursing services for population sets
- Plan for resources needed
- Describe the specific responsibilities of nursing

Novice nurses and students can use these data to anticipate the initial care needed. They can benefit from data reported by nurses experienced in caring for clients in specific populations.

These data should not eliminate an assessment of an individual client to evaluate if additional nursing diagnoses or collaborative problems are present and establish priority for treatment during the hospital stay. This individual assessment will also provide information to delete or supplement the care plans found in this book. The researched data will provide a beginning focus for care.

By identifying frequently treated nursing diagnoses and collaborative problems in client populations, institutions can determine nursing costs on the basis of nursing care provided. Nurse administrators and managers can plan for effective use of staff and resources. Knowledge of types of nursing diagnoses needing nursing interventions will also assist with matching the level of preparation of nurses with appropriate diagnoses.

To date, the nursing care of clients with medical conditions or postsurgical procedures has centered on the physician-prescribed orders. The data from this study would assist departments of nursing to emphasize the primary reason why clients stay in the acute care setting—for treatment of nursing diagnoses and collaborative problems. The purpose of this study is to identify which nursing diagnoses and collaborative problems are most frequently treated when a person is hospitalized with a specific condition.

Method

Settings and Subjects

The findings presented are based on data collected from August 1993 to March 1994. The research population consisted of registered nurses with over two years' experience in health care agencies in the United States and Canada. A convenience sample of 18 institutions represented five U.S. geographical regions (Northeast, Southeast, North-Midwest, Northwest, Southwest) and Ontario province in Canada. The display lists the participating institutions. The target number of R responses was 10 per condition from each institution. The accompanying table illustrates the demographics of the subjects.

Instrument

A graphic rating scale was developed and pilot-tested to measure self-reported frequencies of interventions provided to clients with a specific condition. Each collaborative problem listed under the condition was accompanied by the question "When you care for clients with this condition, how often do you monitor for this problem?"

Each nursing diagnosis listed under the condition was accompanied by the question "When you care for clients with this condition, how often do you provide interventions for this nursing diagnosis?"

The respondent was asked to make an X on a frequency scale of 0% to 100%. Scoring was tabulated by summing the scores for each question and calculating the median.

PARTICIPATING INSTITUTIONS

Allen Memorial Hospital
1825 Logan Avenue
Waterloo, Iowa 50703

Carondelet St. Joseph's Hospital
350 N. Wilmont Road
Tucson, Arizona 85711-2678

The Evanston Hospital
Burch Building
2650 Ridge Avenue
Evanston, Illinois 60201

Huron Valley Hospital
1601 East Commerce Road
Milford, Michigan 48382-9900

Lehigh Valley Hospital
Cedar Crest & I-78
Allentown, Pennsylvania 18105-1556

Memorial Medical Center of Jacksonville
3625 University Blvd., South
Jacksonville, Florida 32216

Presbyterian Hospital
200 Hawthorne Lane
Charlotte, North Carolina 28233-3549

St. Francis Medical Center
211 St. Francis Drive
Cape Girardeau, Missouri 63701

St. Joseph Hospital
601 N. 30th Street
Omaha, Nebraska 68131

St. Peter Community Hospital
2475 Broadway
Helena, Montana 39601

San Bernardino County Medical Center
780 E. Gilbert Street
San Bernardino, California 92415-0935

Sioux Valley Hospital
1100 South Euclid Avenue
Sioux Falls, South Dakota 57117-5039

University of Minnesota Hospital
420 Delaware Street, S.E.
Minneapolis, Minnesota 55455

University of New Mexico Hospital
2211 Lomas Blvd., N.E.
Albuquerque, New Mexico 87131

Victoria Hospital
800 Commissioners Road, East
London, Canada N6A 4G5

Wills Eye Hospital
900 Walnut Street
Philadelphia, Pennsylvania 19107

Wilmer Ophthalmological Institute
Johns Hopkins Hospital
Baltimore, Maryland 21287-9054

Winthrop-University Hospital
259 First Street
Mineola, New York 11501

Data Collection

Before data collection, the researcher addressed the requirements for research in the institution. These requirements varied from a review by the nursing department's research committee to a review by the institutional review board (IRB).

After the approval process was completed, each department of nursing was sent a list of the 72 conditions to be studied and asked to select only those conditions that were regularly treated in their institution. Only those questionnaires were sent to the respective institutions. Study institutions received a packet for those selected conditions containing 10 questionnaires for each condition. Completed questionnaires were returned by the nurse respondent to the envelope, and the envelope sealed by the designated distributor. Nurse respondents were given the option of putting their questionnaire in a sealed envelope before placing it in the larger envelope.

Since two of the study institutions did not treat ophthalmic conditions, questionnaires related to these conditions were sent to two institutions specializing in these conditions.

Findings

Of the 19 institutions that agreed to participate, 18 (including the two ophthalmic institutions) returned the questionnaires. The target return was 160 questionnaires for each condition. The range of return was 29% to 70%, with the average rate of return of 52.5%.

Each condition has a set of nursing diagnoses and collaborative problems with its own frequency score. The diagnoses were grouped into three ranges of frequency: 75% to 100%—frequent; 50% to 74%—often; <50%—infrequent. Each of the 72 conditions included in the study and this book has the nursing diagnoses and collaborative problems grouped according to the study findings.

Future Work

This study represents the initial step in the validation of the nursing care predicted to be needed when a client is hospitalized for a medical or surgical condition. It is important to validate which nursing diagnoses and collaborative problems necessitate nursing interventions. Future work should focus on the identification of nursing interventions that have priority in treating a diagnosis, clarification of outcomes realistic for the length of stay, and evaluation and review by national groups of nurses.

DEMOGRAPHICS OF RESPONDENTS

Questionnaires	
Sent	9,920
Returned	5,299
% returned	53.4%
Average Age	39
Average Years in Nursing	15
Level of Nursing Preparation	
Diploma	22.7%
AD	25.7%
BSN	36.5%
MSN	12.4%
PhD	1.5%
No indication	1.2%

References

Carpenito, L. J. (1984). *Handbook of nursing diagnosis*. Philadelphia, PA: J. B. Lippincott.

Carpenito, L. J. (1991). *Nursing care plans and documentation*. Philadelphia, PA: J. B. Lippincott.

Doenges, M., & Moorhouse, M. (1991). *Nurse's pocket guide: Nursing diagnoses with interventions*. Philadelphia, PA: F. A. Davis.

Holloway, N. M. (1988). *Medical surgical care plans*. Springhouse, PA: Springhouse.

Sparks, S. M., & Taylor, C. M. (1993). *Nursing diagnoses reference manual*. Springhouse, PA: Springhouse.

Ulrich, S., Canale, S., & Wendell, S. (1994). *Medical-surgical nursing: Care planning guide*. Philadelphia, PA: W. B. Saunders.

Acknowledgments

The Validation Project could not have been completed without the support of the following nurses who coordinated the data collection in their institutions:

Tammy Spier, RN, MSN
Department of Nursing Services
Department of Staff Development
Allen Memorial Hospital
Waterloo, Iowa

Donna Dickinson, RN, MS
Carol Mangold, RN, MSN
Carondelet St. Joseph's Hospital
Tucson, Arizona

Kathy Killman, RN, MSN
Liz Nelson, RN, MSN
The Evanston Hospital
Evanston, Illinois

Margaret Price, RN, MSN
Lynn Bobel Turbin, RN, MSN
Nancy DiJanni, RN, MSN
Huron Valley Hospital
Milford, Michigan

Pat Vaccaro, RN, BSN, CCRN
Deborah Stroh, RN
Mary Jean Potylycki, RN
Carolyn Peters, RN
Sue DeSanto, RN
Christine Niznik, RN
Carol Saxman, RN
Kelly Brown, RN
Judy Bailey, RN
Nancy Root, RN
Cheryl Bitting, RN
Carol Sorrentino, RN
Lehigh Valley Hospital
Allentown, Pennsylvania

Loretta Baldwin, RN, BSN
Karin Prussak, RN, MSN, CCRN
Bess Cullen, RN
Debra Goetz, RN, MSN
Susan Goucher, RN
Sandra Brackett, RN, BSN

Barbara Johnston, RN, CCRN
Lisa Lauderdale, RN
Randy Shoemaker, RN, CCRN
Memorial Medical Center of Jacksonville
Jacksonville, Florida

Karen Stiefel, RN, PhD
Jerre Jones, RN, MSN, CS
Lise Heidenreich, RN, MSN, FNP, CS
Christiana Redwood-Sawyer, RN, MSN
Presbyterian Hospital
Charlotte, North Carolina

Pauline Elliott, RN, BSN
St. Francis Medical Center
Cape Girardeau, Missouri

Dena Belfiore, RN, PhD

Dianne Hayko, MSRN, CNS
St. Joseph Hospital
Omaha, Nebraska

Jennie Nemec, RN, MSN
St. Peter Community Hospital
Helena, Montana

Eleanor Borkowski, RN
Tina Buchanan, RN
Jill Posadas, RN
Deanna Stover, RN
Margie Bracken, RN
Barbara Upton, RN
Kathleen Powers, RN
Jeanie Goodwin, RN
San Bernardino County Medical Center
San Bernardino, California

Kathy Karpiuk, RN, MNE
Monica Mauer, RN
Susan Fey, RN

Joan Reisdorfer, RN

Cheryl Wilson, Health Unit Coordinator
Gail Sundet, RN
Pat Halverson, RN
Ellie Baker, RN
Jackie Kisecker, RN
Cheri Dore-Paulson, RN
Kay Gartner, RN
Vicki Tigner, RN
Jan Burnette, RN
Maggie Scherff, RN
Sioux Valley Hospital
Sioux Falls, South Dakota

Keith Hampton, RN, MSN
University of Minnesota Hospital
Minneapolis, Minnesota

Eva Adler, RN, MSN
Jean Giddens, RN, MSN, CS
Dawn Roseberry, RN, BSN
University of New Mexico Hospital
Albuquerque, New Mexico

Carol Wong, RN, MScN
Cheryl Simpson, RN
Victoria Hospital
London, Canada

Heather Boyd-Monk, RN, MSN
Wills Eye Hospital
Philadelphia, Pennsylvania

Fran Tolley, RN, BSN
Vicky Navarro, RN, MAS
Wilmer Ophthalmological Institute
Johns Hopkins Hospital
Baltimore, Maryland

Joan Crosley, RN, PhD
Winthrop-University Hospital
Mineola, New York

My gratitude also extends to each of the nurses who gave their time to complete the questionnaires. A sincere thank-you to Dr. Ginny Arcangelo, who at the time of the research was the Director of the Family Nurse Practitioner Program at Thomas Jefferson University in Philadelphia, for her work as the methodology consultant to the project.

A study of this magnitude required over 9,000 questionnaires to be produced, duplicated, and distributed. Over 100,000 data entries were made, yielding the findings found throughout this edition.

Gracias to my patient friends, who understood the chaos of the last year that held me absent from doing other things: Maureen, Ginny, Judy, Karen, Bob, and Donna.

On a personal level, my son Olen Juall Carpenito and his wife, Heather, have given me two special gifts—my grandsons Olen, Jr. and Aiden. They light up my world every day. Love, Ona.

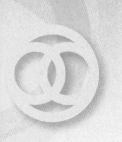

Contents

Section 2   Individual Collaborative Problems   197

Unit III Individual and Family-Centered Care Plans 275

Section I Medical Conditions 281

Section 2 Surgical Procedures 602

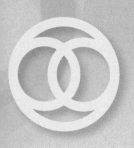

Unit I

Introduction to Individual and Family-Centered Care

"Continuum of Care is a concept involving an integrated system of care that guides and tracks client care over time through a comprehensive array of health services spanning all levels of intensity and all phases of illness from diagnosis to the end of life" (Zazworsky, Personal Communication).

All health care facilities are in this rapidly changing environment from the acute care hospital to the primary care medical home. Community care also provides skilled care facilities and home health agencies.

Principles of Individual and Family-Centered Care

* Competent, trustworthy staff
* Care is respectful
* Dignity is protected
* All care processes are explained clearly and understood
* Family/support persons are involved
* Physical and emotional comfort are priorities
* Decisions are made collaboratively and differences respected
* Transition process begins on admission
* Preparation for safe and comfortable transition to home

The focus of this book is to:

* Provide evidence-based, caring care that is a priority for the condition and length of stay.
* Guide the student nurse or clinician to identify high-risk individuals for adverse events.
* Emphasize elements to address for timely and safe transition from the acute care setting.

In order for the individual and family to be prepared to assume care that is safe and correct at home, five components must be addressed in an ongoing process beginning on admission to transition to home care and follow-up in a medical home. All of these components are integrated in all the care plans in this edition.

Components of Effective, Safe Transition

1. On admission, identification of individuals/support persons who have barriers to a timely, effective transition
2. On admission, identification of individuals who are high risk for an adverse outcome/event during hospitalization
3. Early identification of support persons or absence of (or unavailable) and their ability to continue care in the home setting
4. Deliberate, ongoing preparation to provide care in the home settings and teaching of when to seek advice
5. Identification of follow-up care: When? Where? etc.

The motives for preventing adverse events (falls, infections, readmissions) may for some in health care be primarily financial. The Centers of Medicare and Medicaid have clearly set forward financial penalties for adverse event occurrences which are deemed preventable.

These reforms are long overdue. Clerical nurses would benefit from viewing these critical changes not as burdens but instead as opportunities to integrate them into the core of every interaction with an individual and family. As you provide care explain why you do what you are doing and, if indicated, what will need to be done at home. For example, as you change a dressing, have the individual and family member view the incision. Point out how it is healing and advise what needs to be reported when at home. Make each moment a teachable moment.

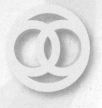

Chapter 1

The Bifocal Clinical Practice Model

The classification activities of the North American Nursing Diagnosis Association International (NANDA-I) have been instrumental in defining nursing's unique body of knowledge. This unified system of terminology:

- Defines the accountability of nursing and differentiates this profession from other health care professions
- Provides consistent language for oral, written, and electronic communication
- Stimulates nurses to examine new knowledge
- Establishes a system for automation and reimbursement
- Provides an educational framework
- Allows efficient information retrieval for research and quality assurance
- Provides a consistent structure for literature presentation of nursing knowledge
- Clarifies nursing as an art and a science for its members and society
- Establishes standards to which nurses are held accountable

Appendix A of this text provides a list of nursing diagnoses grouped under Functional Health Patterns.

Clearly, nursing diagnosis has influenced the nursing profession positively. Integration of nursing diagnosis into nursing practice, however, has proved problematic. Although references to nursing diagnosis in the literature have increased exponentially since the first meeting, in 1973, of the National Group for the Classification of Nursing Diagnoses (which later became NANDA-I), nurses have not seen efficient and representative applications. For example, nurses have been directed to use nursing diagnoses exclusively to describe their clinical focus. Nevertheless, nurses who strongly support nursing diagnosis often become frustrated when they try to attach a nursing diagnosis label to every facet of nursing practice. Some of the dilemmas that result from the attempt to label as nursing diagnoses all situations in which nurses intervene are as follows:

1. *Using nursing diagnoses without validation.* When the nursing diagnoses are the only labels or diagnostic statements the nurse can use, the nurse is encouraged to "change the data to fit the label." For example, using the Imbalanced Nutrition category for all who are given nothing-by-mouth status. Risk for Injury also frequently serves as a "wastebasket" diagnosis because all potentially injurious situations (e.g., bleeding) can be captured within a Risk for Injury diagnosis.

2. *Renaming medical diagnoses.* Clinical nurses know that an important component of their practice is monitoring for the onset and status of physiologic complications and initiating both nurse-prescribed and physician-prescribed interventions. Morbidity and mortality are reduced and prevented because of nursing's expert monitoring and management.

    If nursing diagnoses are to describe all situations in which nurses intervene, then clearly a vast number must be developed to describe the situations identified in the International Code of Diseases (ICD-10). Table 1.1 represents examples of misuse of nursing diagnoses and the renaming of medical diagnoses. Examination of the substitution of nursing diagnosis terminology for medical diagnoses or pathophysiology in Table 1.1 gives rise to several questions:

    - Should nursing diagnoses describe all situations in which nurses intervene?
    - If a situation is not called a nursing diagnosis, is it then less important or scientific?

Table 1.1 Diagnostic Errors: Renaming Medical Diagnoses With Nursing Diagnosis Terminology

Medical Diagnosis	Nursing Diagnosis
Acute Coronary Syndrome	Decreased Cardiac Output
Shock	Decreased Cardiac Output
Adult Respiratory Distress	Impaired Gas Exchange
Chronic Obstructive Lung Disease	Impaired Gas Exchange
Asthma	Impaired Gas Exchange
Alzheimer's Disease	Impaired Cerebral Tissue Perfusion
Increased Intracranial Pressure	Impaired Cerebral Tissue Perfusion
Retinal Detachment	Disturbed Sensory Perception: Visual
Thermal Burns	Impaired Tissue Integrity
Incisions, Lacerations	Impaired Skin Integrity
Hemorrhage	Deficient Fluid Volume
Heart Failure	Excess Fluid Volume
Paralytic Ileus	Gastrointestinal Dysfunction

- How will it serve the profession to rename medical diagnoses as nursing diagnoses?
- Will using the examples in Table 1.1 improve communication and clarify nursing?

3. *Omitting problem situations in documentation.* If a documentation system requires the use of nursing diagnosis exclusively, and if the nurse does not choose to "change the data to fit a category" or "to rename medical diagnoses," then the nurse has no terminology to describe a critical component of nursing practice. Failure to describe these situations can seriously jeopardize nursing's effort to justify and affirm the need for professional nurses in all health care settings (Carpenito, 1986).

Bifocal Clinical Practice Model

Nursing's theoretical knowledge derives from the natural, physical, and behavioral sciences, as well as the humanities and nursing research. Nurses can use various theories in practice, including family systems, loss, growth and development, crisis intervention, and general systems theories.

The difference between nursing and the other health care disciplines is nursing's depth and breadth of focus. Certainly, the nutritionist has more expertise in the field of nutrition, and the pharmacist in the field of therapeutic pharmacology than any nurse. Every nurse, however, brings a knowledge of nutrition and pharmacology to interactions. The depth of this knowledge is sufficient for many clinical situations; when it is insufficient, consultation is required. No other discipline has this varied knowledge, and this explains why attempts to substitute other disciplines for nursing have proved costly and ultimately unsuccessful. Figure 1.1 illustrates this varied expertise.

The Bifocal Clinical Practice Model (Carpenito, 1986) represents situations that influence individuals, groups, and communities as well as the classification of these responses from a nursing perspective. The situations are organized into five broad categories: pathophysiologic, treatment-related, personal, environmental, and maturational (Fig. 1.2). Without an understanding of such situations, the nurse will be unable to diagnose responses and intervene appropriately.

Clinically, these situations are important to nurses. Thus, as nursing diagnoses evolved, nurses sought to substitute nursing terminology for these situations; for example, Impaired Tissue Integrity for burns and High Risk for Injury for dialysis. Nurses do not prescribe for and treat these situations (e.g., burns and dialysis). Rather, they prescribe for and treat the *responses* to these situations in individuals.

The practice focus for clinical nursing is at the response level, not at the situation level. For example, an individual who has sustained burns may exhibit a wide variety of responses to the burns and the treatments. Some responses may be predicted, such as High Risk for Infection; others, such as fear of losing a job, may not be predictable. In the past, nurses focused on the nursing interventions associated with treating

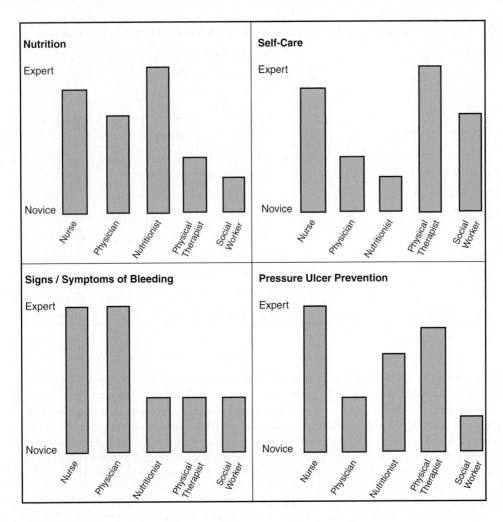

FIGURE 1.1 Knowledge of multidisciplines of selected topics.

burns rather than on those associated with the individual's responses. *This resulted in nurses being described as "doers" rather than "knowers"; as technicians rather than scientists.*

Nursing Diagnoses and Collaborative Problems

The Bifocal Clinical Practice Model describes the two foci of clinical nursing: nursing diagnoses and collaborative problems.

Pathophysiologic
Myocardial infarction
Borderline personality disorder
Burns

Treatment-related
Anticoagulants
Dialysis
Arteriogram

Personal
Dying
Divorce
Relocation

Environmental
Overcrowded school
No handrails on stairs
Rodents

Maturational
Peer pressure
Parenthood
Aging

FIGURE 1.2 Examples of pathophysiologic, treatment-related, personal, environmental, and maturational situations.

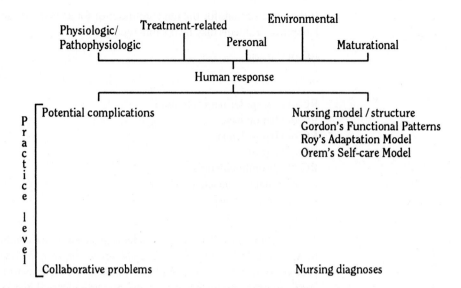

FIGURE 1.3 Bifocal clinical practice model. (© 1987, Lynda Juall Carpenito.)

A nursing diagnosis is a clinical judgment about individual, family, or community responses to actual or potential health problems/life processes. Nursing diagnosis provides the basis for selection of nursing interventions to achieve outcomes for which the nurse has accountability (NANDA, 2009).

Collaborative problems are certain physiologic complications that nurses monitor to detect onset or changes of status. Nurses manage collaborative problems using physician/NP/PA–prescribed and nursing-prescribed interventions to minimize the complications of the events (Carpenito, 1999).

Figure 1.3 illustrates the Bifocal Clinical Practice Model.

The nurse makes independent decisions for both collaborative problems and nursing diagnoses. The difference is that in nursing diagnoses, nursing prescribes the definitive treatment to achieve the desired outcome, whereas in collaborative problems, prescription for definitive treatment comes from both nursing and physicians/nurse practitioners (NPs). Some physiologic complications (such as Risk for Infection and Risk for Pressure Ulcers) are nursing diagnoses because nurses can order the definitive treatment. In a collaborative problem, the nurse uses surveillance to monitor for the onset and change in status of physiologic complications, and manages these changes to prevent morbidity and mortality. These physiologic complications are usually related to disease, trauma, treatments, medications, or diagnostic studies. Thus, collaborative problems can be labeled Risk for Complications of (specify),[1] for example, Risk for Complications of Hemorrhage or Risk for Complications of Renal Failure.

Monitoring, however, is not the sole nursing responsibility for collaborative problems. For example, in addition to monitoring an individual with increased intracranial pressure, the nurse also restricts certain activities, maintains head elevation, implements the medical regimen, and continually addresses the individual's psychosocial and educational needs.

The following are some collaborative problems that commonly apply to certain situations:

Situation	Collaborative Problem
Myocardial Infarction	Risk for Complications (RC) of Arrhythmias
Craniotomy	RC of Increased Intracranial Pressure
Hemodialysis	RC of Fluid/Electrolyte Imbalance
Surgery	RC of Hemorrhage
Cardiac Catheterization	RC of Arrhythmias

[1]Previously labeled Potential Complications: (specify)

If the situation calls for the nurse to monitor for a cluster or group of physiologic complications, the collaborative problems may be documented as

RC of Cardiac

or

RC of Postop: Urinary retention
RC of Hemorrhage
RC of Hypovolemia
RC of Hypoxia
RC of Thrombophlebitis
RC of Renal insufficiency
RC of Paralytic ileus
RC of Evisceration

A list of common collaborative problems grouped under conditions that necessitate nursing care appears in Appendix A. *Not all physiologic complications, however, are collaborative problems.* Nurses themselves can prevent some physiologic complications such as infections from external sources (e.g., wounds and catheters), contractures, incontinence, and pressure ulcers. Thus, such complications fall into the category of nursing diagnosis.

Nursing Interventions

Nursing interventions are treatments or actions that benefit an individual by presenting a problem, reducing or eliminating a problem, or promoting a healthier response. Nursing interventions can be classified as either of two types: nurse-prescribed or physician/physician assistant (PA)/NP[2]–prescribed. Independent interventions are nurse-prescribed; delegated interventions are physician/PA/NP–prescribed. Both types of interventions, however, require independent nursing judgment. By law, the nurse must determine whether it is appropriate to initiate an intervention regardless of whether it is independent or delegated (Carpenito, 1999).

Carpenito (1986) stated that the relationship of diagnosis to interventions is a critical element in defining nursing diagnoses. Many definitions of nursing diagnoses focus on the relationship of selected interventions to the diagnoses. A certain type of intervention appears to distinguish a nursing diagnosis from a medical diagnosis or other problems that nurses treat. The type of intervention distinguishes a nursing diagnosis from a collaborative problem and also differentiates between problem risk/high risk and possible nursing diagnoses. Table 1.2 outlines definitions of each type and the corresponding intervention

Table 1.2 Differentiation Among Types of Diagnoses		
Diagnostic Statement	**Corresponding Individual Outcome or Nursing Goals**	**Focus of Intervention**
Actual Diagnosis Three-part statement, including nursing diagnostic label, etiology, and signs/symptoms	Change in individual behavior moving toward resolution of the diagnosis or improved status	Reduce or eliminate problem
Risk/High-Risk Diagnosis Two-part statement, including nursing diagnostic label and risk factors	Maintenance of present conditions	Reduce risk factors to prevent an actual problem
Possible Diagnosis Two-part statement, including nursing diagnostic label and unconfirmed etiology or unconfirmed defining characteristics	Undetermined until problem is validated	Collect additional data to confirm or rule out signs/symptoms or risk factors
Collaborative Problems Potential or actual physiologic complication	Nursing goals	Determine onset or status of the problem; manage change in status

---

[2]NP/PAs have the legal authority to prescribe medical interventions and can thus diagnose and treat collaborative problems.

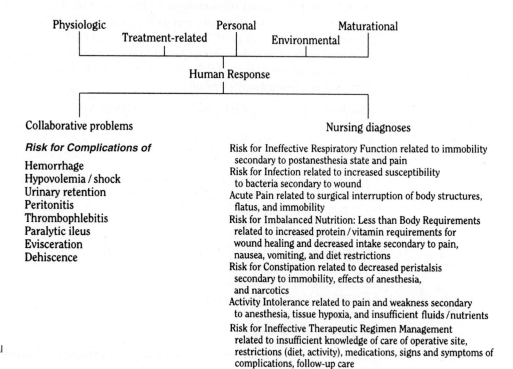

Abdominal surgery (postoperative)

Physiologic   Personal   Maturational
          Treatment-related   Environmental

Human Response

Collaborative problems   Nursing diagnoses

Risk for Complications of

Hemorrhage
Hypovolemia / shock
Urinary retention
Peritonitis
Thrombophlebitis
Paralytic ileus
Evisceration
Dehiscence

Risk for Ineffective Respiratory Function related to immobility
     secondary to postanesthesia state and pain
Risk for Infection related to increased susceptibility
     to bacteria secondary to wound
Acute Pain related to surgical interruption of body structures,
     flatus, and immobility
Risk for Imbalanced Nutrition: Less than Body Requirements
     related to increased protein / vitamin requirements for
     wound healing and decreased intake secondary to pain,
     nausea, vomiting, and diet restrictions
Risk for Constipation related to decreased peristalsis
     secondary to immobility, effects of anesthesia,
     and narcotics
Activity Intolerance related to pain and weakness secondary
     to anesthesia, tissue hypoxia, and insufficient fluids / nutrients
Risk for Ineffective Therapeutic Regimen Management
     related to insufficient knowledge of care of operative site,
     restrictions (diet, activity), medications, signs and symptoms of
     complications, follow-up care

FIGURE 1.4 Diagnostic cluster for individual recovering from abdominal surgery.

focus. For example, for a nursing diagnosis of Pressure Ulcer related to immobility as manifested by a 2-cm epidermal lesion on the individual's left heel, the nurse would order interventions to monitor the lesion and to heal it. In another individual with a surgical wound, the nurse would focus on prevention of infection and promotion of healing.

Risk for Infection would better describe the situation than Impaired Tissue Integrity. *Nursing diagnoses are not more important than collaborative problems, and collaborative problems are not more important than nursing diagnoses.*

Priorities are determined by the individual's situation, not by whether it is a nursing diagnosis or a collaborative problem.

A *diagnostic cluster* represents those nursing diagnoses and collaborative problems that have a high likelihood of occurring in an individual population. The nurse validates their presence in the individual. Figure 1.4 represents the diagnostic cluster for an individual after abdominal surgery. Unit III contains diagnostic clusters for medical and surgical conditions or goals.

Goals/Outcome Criteria

In a nursing care plan, goals (outcome criteria) are "statements describing a measurable behavior of individual/family that denote a favorable status (changed or maintained) after nursing care has been delivered" (Alfaro-LeFevre, 2014). Outcome criteria help to determine the success or appropriateness of the nursing care plan. If the nursing care plan does not achieve a favorable status even though the diagnosis is correct, the nurse must change the goal or the plan. If neither option is indicated, the nurse confers with the physician/NP/PA for delegated orders. Nursing diagnoses should *not* represent situations that require physician/NP orders for treatment. Otherwise, how can nurses assume accountability for diagnosis and treatment? For example, consider an individual with a nursing diagnosis, Risk for Impaired Cerebral Tissue Perfusion related to effects of recent head injury and these goals. The individual will demonstrate continued optimal cerebral pressure as evidenced by:

• Pupils equally reactive to light and accommodation
• No change in orientation or consciousness

If this individual were to exhibit evidence of increased intracranial pressure, would it be appropriate for the nurse to change the goals? What changes in the nursing care plan would the nurse make to stop the cranial pressure from increasing? Actually, neither action is warranted. Rather, the nurse should confer with the physician/NP/PA for delegated orders to treat increased intracranial pressure. When the nurse formulates individual goals or outcomes that require delegated medical orders for goal achievement, the situation is not a nursing diagnosis but a collaborative problem. In this case, the individual's problem would be better described as a collaborative problem:

Risk for Complications of Increased Intracranial Pressure

Collaborative Outcomes

The individual will be monitored for early signs and symptoms of increased intracranial pressure and will receive interventions to achieve physiologic stability.

Indicators of physiologic stability:

- Alert, oriented, calm
- Pupils, equal, reactive to light and accommodation
- Pulse 60 to 100 bpm
- Respirations 16 to 20 bpm
- BP >90/60, <140/90 mm Hg
- No nausea/vomiting
- Mild to no headache

These collaborative goals represent the nursing accountability for monitoring for physiologic instability and providing interventions (nursing and medical) to maintain or restore stability.

SUMMARY   The Bifocal Clinical Practice Model provides nurses with a framework to diagnose the unique responses of an individual and significant others to various situations. Clear definition of the two dimensions of nursing enhances the use and minimizes the misuse of nursing diagnoses. The Bifocal Clinical Practice Model describes the unique knowledge and focus of professional nursing.

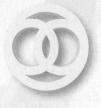

Chapter 2

Communication: The Critical Key to Preventing Adverse Events

The literature identifies that clinical mistakes and adverse events are caused by human error, at-risk behavior, or reckless behavior. In this chapter, root causes for errors creating adverse events in a safe culture will be discussed.

Sentinel Events

The Joint Commission recommends, "Careful investigation and analysis of Patient Safety Events (events not primarily related to the natural course of the patient's illness or underlying condition), as well as evaluation of corrective actions, is essential to reduce risk and prevent patient harm" (The Joint Commission, 2016). These event are known as sentinel events.

Since 2008, the Joint Commission has compiled a report of sentinel events and root causes. Reporting is voluntary and represents only a small portion of actual events (The Joint Commission, 2016). The principle of root cause is that clinical adverse events are not caused by a single human error "but by a combination of factors relating to organizational practices, structured by which errors are missed and adverse incidents are not prevented" (Nicolini, Mengis, & Swan 2012). The Joint Commission identified the most frequent root causes of sentinel events. Inadequate communication appears as the third most frequent cause of these events since 2009 (The Joint Commission, 2016).

Examples of Failure to Communicate

Incident 1

When a student performs a catheterization, contaminates the catheter, and inserts it anyway.
Cause: Failure to communicate the need for assistance or the need to stop and start the procedure again. This event increases the risk of infection for the individual.

Incident 2

An individual's condition is declining and the physician/NP does not respond to the nurse's assessment and need for evaluation. The individual's further decline is the result of the nurse's not notifying the next in the chain of command (manager, chief of staff).

Incident 3

A nurse observes a protocol violation that will increase the risk of infection (e.g., contamination of venous access during dressing change). Does the nurse stop the person or ignore it? Would it matter if it was the surgeon or a nurse breaking protocol?

Incident 4

An individual falls while trying to access the bathroom. Was the person's risk factors for fall clearly communicated during the "hand-off" report?

Incident 5

During "hand-off," staff are engaging in personal discussions instead of pertinent clinical information, does someone acknowledge that this time must be reserved for pertinent clinical information?

Incident 6

The emergency room (ER) nurse calls to advise the nurse a new admission is on his way to the unit. Does the nurse alert the ER nurse that she or he needs to hold the person there for a half hour more or does she or he rush through some treatments instead?

Barriers to "Speaking Up"

What prevents a nurse from calling a physician/NP when needed, reporting on negligent staff members, asking for help, discussing poor prognoses with a family, or providing responsible end-of-life care?

- Fear
- Inexperience
- Not taken seriously
- Retaliation
- Intimidation
- Disruptive response

In 2008, the Joint Commission issued a sentinel event alert regarding behaviors that undermine a culture of safety (The Joint Commission, 2016). "Reporting raises the level of transparency in the organization and promotes a culture of safety" (The Joint Commission, 2016).

Intimidating and disruptive behaviors can foster medical errors, contribute to poor individual satisfaction and to preventable adverse outcomes, increase the cost of care, and cause qualified clinicians, administrators, and managers to seek new positions in more professional environments. Safety and quality of individual care is dependent on teamwork, communication, and a collaborative work environment. To assure quality and to promote a culture of safety, health care organizations must address the problem of behaviors that threaten the performance of the health care team.

Intimidating and disruptive behaviors include overt actions such as verbal outbursts and physical threats, as well as passive activities such as refusing to perform assigned tasks or quietly exhibiting uncooperative attitudes during routine activities. Intimidating and disruptive behaviors are often manifested by health care professionals in positions of power. Such behaviors include reluctance or refusal to answer questions or return phone calls or pages; condescending language or voice intonation; and impatience with questions. Overt and passive behaviors undermine team effectiveness and can compromise the safety of individuals. All intimidating and disruptive behaviors are unprofessional and should not be tolerated.

 Carp's Cues

Institute of Safe Medication Practices reported that 17% of respondents had felt pressured to accept a medication order despite concerns about its safety on at least three occasions in the previous year, 13% had refrained from contacting a specific prescriber to clarify the safety of an order on at least 10 occasions, and 7% said that in the previous year they had been involved in a medication error where intimidation played a part.

Most nurses can relate numerous incidents, wherein during morning report (hand-offs), the nurse reports a change in an individual's condition during the night that was not reported to the physician because of "fear of the response."

Disruptive Behavior

Hospitals are mandated to have a policy that (The Joint Commission, 2016):

* Defines disruptive and inappropriate behavior
* Outlines a process for managing disruptive and inappropriate behaviors.

Everyone is entitled to having a "bad day" on occasion within limits. Disruptive behavior is a pattern of inappropriate, abusive conduct that harms and intimidates others. In health care settings, this behavior compromises the quality care and/or individual safety.

Any member of the health care team can be disruptive (a nurse, manager, administrator, medical assistant, physician, nurse practitioner, etc.). It is unacceptable at any level and there needs to be a culture of zero tolerance. Even in an atmosphere where disruptive behavior is expected and tolerated, individual nurses can choose to speak up.

Everyone can develop the skills to communicate effectively and also preserve his or her dignity.

Carp's Cues

"So for most nurses, the first step in addressing disruptive behavior is internal. It starts with an absolute belief that nobody deserves to be yelled at for making or witnessing a mistake, much less while doing their job correctly and competently" (Lyndon et al., 2012).

Effective Communication

"Communication failures are the leading cause of inadvertent patient harm" (Leonard, Graham, & Bonacum, 2004, p. i86). "Analysis of 2455 sentinel events reported to the Joint Commission for Hospital Accreditation revealed that the primary root cause in over 70% was communication failure" (The Joint Commission, 2004, quoted in Leonard et al., 2004, p. i86).

> Effective communication and teamwork is essential for the delivery of high quality, safe patient care. Communication failures are an extremely common cause of inadvertent patient harm. The complexity of medical care, coupled with the inherent limitations of human performance, make it critically important that clinicians have standardized communication tools, create an environment in which individuals can speak up and express concerns, and share common "critical language." (Leonard et al., 2004, p. i85)

As described earlier in this chapter, it is "equally important . . . creating an environment that feels 'safe' to team members so they will speak up when they have safety concerns" (Leonard et al., 2004, p. i86).

SBAR

The Situation, Background, Assessment, and Recommendation (SBAR) technique has become the Joint Commission's stated industry best practice for standardized communication in health care (The Joint Commission, 2012). Nurses are taught to use detailed, narrative form in reports in contrast to physicians, who are taught to communicate using only the key information. SBAR serves to bridge the communication gap. SBA was used in the US military, aviation, and law enforcement to improve communication during emergencies. Leonard et al. (2004) developed SBAR for use in health care centers. SBAR is a framework for communicating pertinent information among health care professionals clearly and consistently. SBAR quickly organize the briefing information in your mind or on paper using, before calling a physician/ NP/ PA.

This format is useful in hand-offs (shift report) when an urgent response is needed and in conflict situations (Leonard et al., 2004). SBAR examples are found throughout the plans. The following is from the collaborative problem *Risk for Complications of Deep Vein Thrombosis* (Unit II, Section 2).

> Briefly and concisely, critically important pieces of information can be transmitted in a predictable structure. Not only is there familiarity in how people communicated, but the SBAR structure helps develop desired critical thinking skills. The person initiating the communication knows that before they pick up the telephone that they need to provide an assessment of the problem and what they think an appropriate solution is. (Leonard et al., 2004, p. i86)

Table 2.1   SBAR Guidelines

When calling the physician/nurse practitioner, follow the SBAR process:

(S) Situation: What is the situation you are calling about? What is going on with the individual?

- Indicate the identity of yourself, unit, and the individual room number.
- Briefly state the problem/situation, what it is, when it happened or started, and how severe it is.

(B) Background: Pertinent background information related to the situation could include the following:

The admitting diagnosis and date of admission

List of current medications, allergies, IV fluids, and labs

Most recent vital signs

Lab results: provide the date and time test was done and results of previous tests for comparison

Other clinical information

Code status

(A) Assessment: What is your assessment of the situation? What do you think the problem is?

(R) Recommendation: What is your recommendation or what do you want?

Examples:

- "I need you to come now and see the individual."
- Order change
- Notification that their assigned individual has been admitted
- Need to transfer to ICU
- Any tests needed?
- Need to talk to individual family about code status

Thus, a nurse at the bedside may not be able to put a concise label or description on what is clinically unfolding, but very probably knows "something is wrong, and I need your help." Lowering the threshold to obtain help, and treating the request respectfully and legitimately creates a much safer system. (Leonard et al., 2004, p. i86)

Table 2.1 outlines the format of SBAR with examples.

STAR

When confronted with a change in an individual's condition, utilize the STAR approach:

STAR		
Stop		
Think	What is wrong with this situation? How does this individual's condition change for the worse?
Act	If unsure, consult with an experienced nurse.
Recommend	State what your next action is (e.g., reassess or implement SBAR).

If one is reluctant to act, prior to notifying or discussing an individual with a physician/NP/PA, discuss the situation with the manager or coordinator.

Carp's Cues

Avoid having experienced colleagues call instead of yourself, which will only continue your fears and inexperience. Students can be assisted with a clinical nurse or faculty listening while the student talks. The faculty person can add data if needed. This is an invaluable lesson that must be practiced as a student.

- Consider the following before making the call:
  - Selecting the appropriate physician/NP/PA
  - Assess the person yourself before calling
  - Open the electronic health record of the person
  - Relate allergies, pertinent medications, p.o. status, fluids, lab results
  - Report vital signs and focus on changes
  - Clarify code status or if it is unknown

Unit II and the care plans contain numerous examples of SBAR.

Medical care is extremely complex, and this complexity coupled with inherent human performance limitations, even in skilled, experienced, highly motivated individuals, ensures there will be mistakes. (Leonard et al., 2004, p. i86)

Effective teamwork and communication can help prevent these inevitable mistakes from becoming consequential, and harming patients and providers. (Leonard et al., 2004, p. i86)

The Hand-Off Process

Hand-off is a term used to describe the transfer of information (along with authority and responsibility) during transitions in care across the continuum (Friesen, White, & Byers, 2008). Also known as shift report, transfer report, or sign over, hand-off is utilized at:

- Change of shift on a unit
- Transfer to the care of another facility
- Discharge to a community agency

Effective hand-offs support the transition of critical information and specifically identifies high-risk and clinically unstable individuals. Unfortunately, the literature describes adverse events and safety risks occurring when the hand-off process is compromised, incomplete, and/or missing.

All health care facilities have a format/process for hand-offs; however, the quality and accuracy of the hand-off is primarily dependent on the involved clinicians. Nurses engaged in hand-offs can increase the accuracy and clarity of the dialogue. Refer to Table 2.2 for strategies to increase the effectiveness of the hand-off. The usual data, name, room, age, medical diagnoses, meds, and treatment will also be presented.

 Carp's Cues

Nursing care is 24 hours/7 days a week. Care of an individual is not completed when a shift is over. The care continues and thus it is a "hand-off."

Sometimes, a treatment may have to be handed over to the next nurse. Work as a 24-hour team and less frustration will occur. Nursing is a difficult profession with huge responsibilities. Lend a hand to your nursing colleague because it is the right thing to do.

Note: Nurses who habitually hand-off incomplete care without cause is a management problem.

Table 2.2 Tips to Increase the Effectiveness of Hand-Offs

1. Establish that the dialogue will be limited to that which will improve the care to individuals.
   - Avoid negative discussions of family, visitors, and individuals
   - Avoid socialization
   - Avoid criticizing staff, personnel, etc.
2. Relate to the priorities of care for the individual.
   - Frequency of vital signs
   - Changes in condition
   - Physician/NP/PA involvement
   - Last prn medication dose, time
   - Risk status for falls, pressure ulcers
3. Report what has been done or needs to be addressed to prepare for transition.
   - Teaching, referrals
   - Individual/family involvement
   - Individuals'/families' understanding of condition, home care

SUMMARY

Despite the explosion of technology as electronic medical records, invasive lines with alarms, bed alarms, cardiac alarms, and PCA pumps, the safety and comfort of individuals and their families depend primarily on the expertise of the bedside nurse.

The nurse's personal sense of authority applies the same standard of care to the president of the local bank as to the man addicted to prescription pain medications who is complaining of pain post abdominal surgery. The expert nurse knows when "something is not right" or when "wrong is wrong" and must speak up.

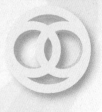

Chapter 3

Early Identification of High-Risk Individuals and/or Families

On admission, all individuals will have a nursing assessment of vital signs, functional health patterns, and body systems (e.g., skin, respiratory, cardiac) using the Nursing Admission Data Base. Refer to Appendix B for an example.

After the initial assessment, the nurse needs to determine the likelihood that the individual will have an uncomplicated complex transition. For the majority of individuals, the transition will be uncomplicated as described below:

- Will usually return to their own home or someone else's for a short stay
- Have care needs that can be managed by the individual or support system and do not require complex planning, teaching, or referrals

To differentiate between a predicted uncomplicated or complex transition, the following assessments are indicated:

 Carp's Cues

Individuals/families that were providing good care at home for long-term chronic conditions may be able to resume this care with little help. Keep in mind that a change in the individual's status or support system situation can change a transition process from complex to uncomplicated.

- Medication reconciliation and barriers to adherence
- Factors that are barriers to effective transition to home care
- Factors that increase the individual's risk for injury, falls, pressure ulcers, and/or infection during hospitalization

Medication Reconciliation and Barriers to Adherence

When it comes to administering drugs, there's a lot that can go wrong: Wrong drug. Wrong dose. Wrong patient. Wrong time. Wrong route of administration. Each year, these types of medication errors harm an estimated 1.5 million patients in the United States, including 400,000 in hospitals and 800,000 in long-term care settings. (Institute of Medicine, 2006)

Medication errors occur 46% of the time during transitions, admission, transfer, or discharge from a clinical unit/hospital. Almost 60% of individuals have at least one discrepancy in their medication history completed on admission (Cornish et al., 2005). "The most common error (46.4%) was omission of a regularly used medication. Most (61.4%) of the discrepancies were judged to have no potential to cause serious harm.

However, 38.6% of the discrepancies had the potential to cause moderate to severe discomfort or clinical deterioration" (Cornish et al., 2005, p. 424).

Medication reconciliation on admission to the health care facilities often entails:

- Name of medication (prescribed, over the counter)
- Prescribed dose
- Frequency (daily, bid, tid, as needed)

> **CLINICAL ALERT:** A list of medications that have been prescribed by a provider does not represent a process of medication reconciliation. A family member recently took an older relative to the ER with chest pain. A typed list of her medications was given to the ER nurse. No discussion occurred about her medication.
>
> Unfortunately, one of the two hypertension medications she regularly took was not entered in the electronic health record. Since her blood pressure was elevated on admission and persisted, another antihypertensive medication was ordered. After two days, another medication was added with good results.
>
> The first medication that was added was the medication she was already taking before admission. So essentially, no new medication was added as a result of the error. She spent three unnecessary days in the hospital, with increased costs to Medicare, and would have definitely rather been home eating her own food and having a good night's sleep in her own bed.

According to the Joint Commission (2015),

> Medication reconciliation is the process of comparing an individual's medication orders to all of the medications that the patient has been taking. This reconciliation is done to avoid medication errors such as omissions, duplications, dosing errors, or drug interactions. It should be done at every transition of care in which new medications are ordered or existing orders are rewritten. Transitions in care include changes in setting, service, practitioner, or level of care. The process comprises five steps: (1) develop a list of current medications; (2) develop a list of medications to be prescribed; (3) compare the medications on the two lists; (4) make clinical decisions based on the comparison; and (5) communicate the new list to appropriate caregivers to the patient. (p. 1)

Table 3.1 outlines a list of sources of medications to review during medication reconciliations.

Critical to acquiring a list of medications authorized in Table 3.1 are the additional assessment questions, which are the defining elements for medication reconciliation: "versus a list of medications reported to be taking."

Table 3.1   Sources of Medication History

The medication history can be obtained from a variety of sources:
• The individual
• A list the individual may have from primary care provider[a]
• The medications themselves, if brought in from home
• A friend or family member
• A medical record
• The individual's pharmacy

[a]Optimal source, which is then verified with individual/family.

For each medication reported, the individual/family member is asked the following:

- What is the reason you are taking each medication?
- Are you taking the medication as prescribed? Specify once a day, twice a day, etc.
- Are you skipping any doses? Do you sometimes run out of medications?
- How often are you taking the medication prescribed "if needed as a pain medication"?
- Have you stopped taking any of these medications?
- How much does it cost you to take your medications?
- Are you taking anybody else's medication?

Factors That Increase Are Barriers to Effectively Transition to Home

Individuals, on admission to an acute care setting, necessitate an assessment to determine the presence of barriers to a timely transition to home care (or a community health setting).

Barriers that effectively transition from acute care setting are:

- Personal
- Support system
- Home environment

Personal Barriers

Determine if any of these barriers to self-care are responsible for this admission. Access the appropriate resource in the institution as early as possible to initiate resolving or reducing barriers (e.g., social service, home care).

Individuals are assessed for disabilities and compromised functioning at admission. Assess if the individual:

- Is homeless
- Has no medical insurance
- Unable to live alone
- Physically impaired
- Mentally compromised
- Can read, level of comprehension
- Can understand English
- Is abusing drugs, alcohol

Support System Barriers

Preparing family members/support persons for home care is addressed in each care plan in Unit III. If a support system is not present, nonexistent, or incapable to providing home care, refer to the appropriate resource in the institution as early as possible (e.g., social service, home care agency).

Determine the present status of a support system. Assess:

- What kind of assistance is needed for homecare 24/7 (e.g., daily visits, phone calls, etc.)?
- Is there a support system? Who?
- Are they willing/available to provide assistance?
- Will they arrange for assistance from others?
- Are they capable of providing needed care at home (e.g., elderly spouse)?

Home Environment

If there are barriers to home care due to the environment, refer to the appropriate resource in the institution as early as possible (e.g., social service, home health nursing agency).

Determine the status of the home environment. Assess:

- Where does the person live? Home alone? Shelter? Homeless? With others?
- Can equipment for home care be accessed? Insurance coverage? Home barriers?
- Is the person capable of accessing home/apartment? Stairs?

- Is there access to a bathroom without using stairs?
- Is there a temporary alternative (e.g., family member's home)?

Hospital-Acquired Conditions

Factors That Increase the Individual's Risk of Injury, Falls, Pressure Ulcers and/or Infection During Hospitalization and Preventable Hospital-Acquired Conditions

In 2008, the Centers for Medicare and Medicaid Services (CMS) published "Roadmap for Implementing Value-Driven Healthcare in the Traditional Medicare Fee-for-Service Program." The CMS's objective is "to improve the accuracy of Medicare's payment under the acute care hospital inpatient prospective payment system . . . while providing additional incentives for hospitals to engage in quality improvement efforts" (CMS, 2008a).

Of equal importance is that additional payments will be denied for the treatment of the following 14 hospital-acquired conditions (CMS, 2008a, 2015):

- Stage II and IV pressure ulcers
- Falls and trauma such as fractures, dislocations, intracranial injuries, crushing injuries, burns, and other injuries
- Manifestations of poor glycemic control (e.g., ketoacidosis, hyperosmolar coma, hypoglycemic coma, secondary diabetes with ketoacidosis, or hyperosmolarity)
- Catheter-associated urinary tract infections (UTIs)
- Vascular catheter-associated infections
- Surgical-site infection, mediastinitis, following coronary artery bypass graft (CABG)
- Surgical-site infection following bariatric surgery for obesity (laparoscopic gastric bypass, gastroenterostomy, laparoscopic gastric restrictive surgery)
- Surgical-site infection following certain orthopedic procedures (spine, neck, shoulder, elbow)
- Surgical-site infection following cardiac implantable electronic device (CIED)
- Foreign objects retained after surgery
- Deep vein thrombosis (DVT) pulmonary embolism (PE) following certain orthopedic procedures (total knee replacement, hip replacement)
- Iatrogenic puemothorax with venous catheterization
- Air embolism
- Blood incompatibility

Buerhaus and Kurtzman (2008) wrote,

> Most hospital nurses are salaried; hospitals consider those salaries a cost of doing business. In most hospitals, nurses represent about 40% of the direct-care budget. By contrast, physicians are revenue generators because hospitals charge the CMS and other payers for the costs of the resources used to produce medical care provided by or ordered by physicians. Until now, there hasn't been a mechanism under Medicare payment policies for measuring nurses' specific economic contribution to hospitals. CMS-1533-FC offers a mechanism for doing so; to the degree that nursing care prevents costly complications, hospitals will not lose money. In this way, the new Medicare payment rule has the potential to more clearly demonstrate nurses' economic value to hospitals. (p. 30)

A white paper[1] on Preventing Never Events/Evidence-Based Practice reported the following (Leonardi, Faller, & Siroky, 2011, p. 8):

- 1 in 25 individuals suffer injury at a cost of $17 to $29 billion/year (Agency for Healthcare Research and Quality [AHRQ], 2010).
- 1.5 million injuries occurred in 2008 from medical errors at an average cost of $13,000/injury or a total of $19.5 billion (Shreve et al., 2010).
- 7% of admissions had some type of medical injury according to inpatient billing records (Shreve et al., 2010).

---

[1]A white paper in nursing is an authoritative report of research or expert opinion to understand an issue, solve a problem, or make a decision.

Table 3.2   Examples of Prevention of Hospital-Acquired Conditions or Detection of Complications
Unit II Section 1: Nursing Diagnoses • Risk for surgical site infection • Risk for catheter site infection • Risk for pressure ulcers Section 2: Collaborative Problems • Risk for complication of deep vein thrombosis • Risk for complications of fat embolism • Risk for complications of sepsis **Unit III: Medical/Surgical/Treatment Plans** • Seizure disorders • Risk for aspiration • Total hip replacement • Risk for complication of dislocation • Long-term access devices • Risk for complication of an embolism

- 42,243 individuals (0.2% of inpatients) developed a hospital-acquired infection (HAI).
- There were an estimated 722,000 HAIs in US acute care hospitals in 2011. About 75,000 individuals with HAIs died during their hospitalizations. More than half of all HAIs occurred outside of the intensive care unit (Centers for Disease Control and Prevention [CDC], 2015a).

Studies have demonstrated a correlation of lowered rates of complication, nurse-to-individual ratios, and high-quality nursing care (Aiken et al., 2010; Kane, Shamliyan, Mueller, Duval, & Wilt, 2007; Leonardi et al., 2011; Moore et al., 2010; Unruh & Fottler, 2006). The white paper concluded that the number of nurses on a unit strengthens safety (Leonardi et al., 2011). In addition to adequate nursing staffing, the following were noted to enhance quality (Leonardi et al., 2011, p. 15; Savitz, Jones, & Bernard, 2005):

- Unfinished or incomplete care
- Use of standardized technique, such as hand washing, skin preparation, and wound dressings
- Prudent monitoring of invasive medical devices, such as catheters, chest tubes, and IVs
- Systematic skin inspection, cleaning, and positioning
- Adherence to care pathways/protocols
- Other measure that reflect communications, collaboration, documentation, and teamwork

High-Risk Nursing Diagnoses for Preventable Hospital-Acquired Conditions

This edition has identified the importance of prevention of eight conditions identified by CMS. Using evidence-based guidelines, the following can be accessed:

- Nursing diagnoses that represent prevention of infection, falls, pressure ulcers, and delayed discharge
- Collaborative problems that identify individuals at high risk for air emboli, deep vein thrombosis, sepsis
- Medical condition, postsurgical care, and treatment plan specifically identify adverse events that are associated with clinical diagnoses or situations
- Standardized risk assessment tools for falls, infection, and pressure ulcers that are incorporated in every care plan

Table 3.2 illustrates examples of prevention of hospital-acquired conditions or detection of complications.

SUMMARY

Nurses have been the primary health care professionals in all health care facilities for decades. Unfortunately, the impact of scientific, caring nursing has eluded measurement and thus has been invisible. Individuals are admitted to hospitals for medical or surgical care that requires professional nursing. If professional nursing was not indicated, their medical condition would be managed by the primary care provider or specialist in an ambulatory setting. If professional nursing care is not indicated past a surgical procedure, it is completed as a same-day surgery. *The reason an individual is admitted to an intensive care unit is for specialized nursing care. The reason individuals are transitioned to their homes is that they no longer need professional nursing care in the hospital. The reason an individual is transferred to a skilled care facility is that he or she needs a type of professional and skilled nursing care. The assumption that individuals are admitted to hospitals primarily for medical care is erroneous. They need professional nursing expertise in order for medical management to be successful.*

As a profession, nurses have rights and responsibilities. This author has addressed the responsibilities of nursing associated with medical and surgical conditions and treatments. In addition, the rights of clinicians are addressed with multiple strategies so that other members of the health care team stop and listen when the nurse "speaks up."

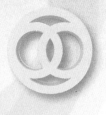

Chapter 4

Preparation of Individual/ Family for Care at Home

In recent years, the Center for Medicare and Medicaid and other third-party payers, for example, health care insurance companies, have created structure for reimbursement that has incentives to prevent adverse events as falls and to enable a timely transition from the hospital (Centers for Medicare and Medicaid Services, 2008b; The Joint Commission, 2008a).

Nurses may view this new emphasis on a safe, timely transition as only a means "to save finances" for the health care institution on the third-party payer, when in fact this shift in emphasis has enhanced the respect for expert nursing care, which traditionally has been undervalued and invisible. The economic contribution that expert nursing lend has dramatically improved their regard in health care settings (Iuga & McGuire, 2014).

Preventing adverse events as falls, pressure ulcers, and infections and reducing length of stay are most beneficial to individuals and their families.

Each day an individual stays in the hospital, the risk of the following consequences is increased:

- Sleep deprivation
- Deconditioning
- Hospital-acquired infections
- Hospital-acquired injuries
- Family disruption
- Sensory overload
- Nutritional deficits
- Complications of immobility (e.g., pressure ulcer)
- Multiple stressors resulting in pain, fear, or anxiety

In order for an individual to effectively transition from the hospital/skilled care to home, new behaviors and skills are needed. For successful outcomes and prevention of complications, the individual/family has to engage in learning these new behaviors and skills.

Engagement versus Compliance

In the NANDA-I classification system, the nursing diagnosis *Noncompliance* was accepted in 1973 and last revised in 1998. The label *Noncompliance* has never reflected a proactive approach to an individual/family who was not participating in recommended treatments or lifestyle changes. It implies the individual is ignoring the health care provider's advice. Recently health care literature is full of alternative strategies directed for health care professional to improve health outcomes with individual/families.

This author has chosen to retire this nursing diagnosis and replace it with *Compromised Engagement* and *Risk for Compromised Engagement*. Refer to Unit II, Section 1 for the new diagnosis of *Compromised Engagement* and *Risk for Compromised Engagement*.

Engagement (compliance) depends on various factors, including motivation, perception of vulnerability, beliefs about controlling or preventing illness, environment, quality of health instruction, and ability to access resources (cost and accessibility). "An important aspect of adherence is recognizing the patient's right to choose whether or not to follow treatment recommendations" (Robinson, Callister, Berry, & Dearing, 2008).

The presence of nurses across most settings provide the profession the strategic leverage not only to change the profession's own practices, but also to transform health care delivery in the direction of individual engagement and care centered around them. Nursing takes on tremendous responsibility within the health care environment on behalf of the ill individual. Yet nursing must become even more focused on the individual and family as the center of the world in which health and health care are provided (Sofaer & Schumann, 2013, p. 5).

 Carp's Cues

When in the "patient role," it is easy to become intimidated by the health care system and health care professionals. Frosch et al. (2011) cited that many people identified certain behaviors that they perceived as challenging to their physicians' or nurses' authority, for example, as asking questions, seeking additional opinions on diagnoses and treatment, questioning the treatment plans, and discussing with their physicians treatment information found online or on TV (Frosch et al., 2011). These individuals can be labeled "difficult" and uncooperative.

Types of Literacy

Functional Illiteracy

Functional illiteracy refers to the capacity of someone, who has reading and writing skills yet incapable of managing ordinary everyday needs and requirements of most employments.

Illiterate individuals, who cannot read or write, are easier to identify than someone who is functionally illiterate.

Health Literacy

Health literacy is the capacity to obtain, process, and understand basic health information and services needed to make appropriate health decisions (Ratzan & Parker, 2000) and to follow instructions for treatment (AMA, 2007). In 2003, the National Assessment of Adult Literacy (NAAL) reported that 14% of English speaking adults in the United States had below basic health literacy, (Kutner, Greenberg, Jin, & Paulsen, 2006). A large study on the scope of health literacy at two public hospitals (Williams et al., 1995) found the following:

- One-half of English speaking individuals could not read and understand basic health education material.
- 60% could not understand a routine consent form.
- 26% could not understand the appointment card.
- 42% failed to understand directions for taking their medications.

The AMA's Committee of Health Literacy found inadequate health literacy was most prevalent in the elderly and individuals who report poor overall health (AMA, 1999). The report concluded that individuals who reported "the worse health status and have less understanding about their medical conditions and treatment had the lowest level of health literacy" (AMA, 1999, p. 57).

 Carp's Cues

"Social and educational levels have little relationship to health literacy" (Speros, 2004, p. 638). Individuals will hide the literacy problems if allowed. Many individuals are at risk of misunderstanding, but it is hard to identify them (DeWalt et al., 2010).

Table 4.1 illustrates the red flags of low literacy.

The Evolving and Complex Health Care System

The Patient Protections and Affordable Care Act of 2010 affirms and supports a new era of health care delivery in the United States (Frosch & Elwyn, 2014). The law references individual centeredness, individual satisfaction, individual experiences, individuals engaged in shared decision making, and health

Table 4.1 Red Flags for Low Literacy

- Frequently missed appointments
- Incomplete registration forms
- Noncompliance with medication
- Unable to name medications, or explain purpose or dosing
- Identifies pills by looking at them, not reading label
- Unable to give coherent, sequential history
- Asks fewer questions
- Lack of follow-through on tests or referrals

Source: DeWalt, D. A. & McNeill, J. (2013). Integrating health literacy with health care performance management. *Institute of Medicine.* Retrieved from http://www.orpca.org/files/BPH_Integrating_Health_Literacy_Measures.pdf

literacy throughout the document (Frosch & Elwyn, 2014). The health care system is increasingly expecting individuals to self-manage their conditions and this continues to increase in the following areas (DeWalt et al., 2010):

- Self-assessment of health status (e.g., peak flow meters, glucose testing)
- Self-treatment (act on information) (e.g., insulin adjustments, wound care)
- Prevention (e.g., nutrition, exercise, dental care, cancer screenings)
- Access to health care system (e.g., decisions to go to emergency room [ER], when to call primary care, referral process, follow-up instructions, navigation of insurance/Medicare coverage)

As expectations and standards increase, the nurse is faced with decreasing time to achieve outcomes with, say, for example, same-day surgery and decreased length of stay.

In order to be successful in this complex process, individuals must be literate in managing daily life *and* their health.

Strategies to Improve Comprehension

Principles of Health Care Teaching

For comprehension to occur, the nurse must accept that there is limited time and that the use of this time is enhanced by:

- Using every contact time to teach something
- Creating a relaxed encounter
- Appropriate eye contact
- Slowing down—break it down into short statements
- Limited content—focus on two or three concepts
- Using plain language (Refer to Box 4.1)
- Engaging individual/family into discussion
- Using graphics
- Explaining what you are doing to the individual/family and why
- Asking them to tell you about what you taught (Tell them to use their own words.)

> **CLINICAL ALERT:**
> - Research shows that individuals remember and understand less than half of what clinicians explain to them (Rost & Roter, 1987; Willliams et al., 1995).

Use the Teach-Back Method (Refer to Fig. 4.1)

- Explain/demonstrate
  - Explain one concept (e.g., medication, condition, when to call primary care provider [PCP])
  - Demonstrate one procedure (e.g., dressing charge, use of inhaler)
- Assess for understanding
  - I want to make sure I explained _____ clearly. Can you tell me _____?

Box 4.1 REPLACING MEDICAL JARGON/WORDS WITH PLAIN WORDS

Medical Jargon/Words	Plain Words
Hepatic	Livers
Pulmonary function	Lungs
Medications	Pills
Nutrition	Food
Beverages	Drinks
Dermatologist	Skin doctor
Ophthalmologist	Eye doctor
Dermatitis	Rash
Conjunctivitis	Eye infection
Gastrointestinal specialist	Stomach doctor
Antihypertensive medicine	Blood pressure medications
Anticoagulant	Blood thinner
Enlarge	Bigger infection
Lesion	Sore
Lipids	Fats
Menses	Period
Osteoporosis	Decrease in the inside of the bone
Depression	Feeling sad
Normal range	Good
Toxic	High levels
Anti-inflammatory	Helps swelling and irritation go away
Dose	How much medicine you should take
Contraception	Helps you not get pregnant
Generic	Does not have a brand name—same drug or _____
Oral	By mouth
Monitor	Keep track of
Referral	See another doctor/nurse practitioner

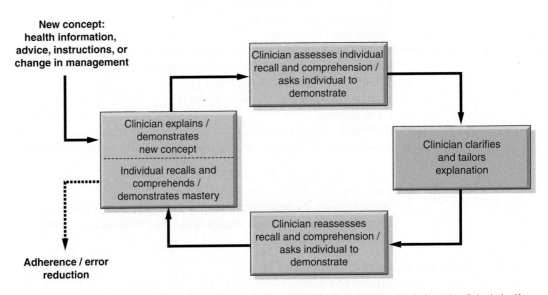

FIGURE 4.1 The Teach-Back Process. (Source: Berkman, N. D., DeWalt, D. A., Pignone, M. P., Sheridan, S. L., Lohr, K. N., Lux, L., ... Bonito, A. J. (2004). Literacy and health outcomes. (Evidence report/technology assessment #87.) (AHRQ Publication No. 04-E007-2). Rockville, MD: Agency for Healthcare Research and Quality.)

- Tell me what I told you
- Show me how to _____
- Avoid asking "Do you understand?"
- Clarify
  - Add more explanation if you are not satisfied that the person understood or can perform the activity.
  - If the person cannot report the information, do not repeat the same explanation; rephrase it.

 Carp's Cues

Be careful the persons/families do not think you are testing them. Assure them it is important that you help them to understand that the teach method can help you teach and also diagnose educational needs. When individuals/families do not understand what was said or demonstrated, the Teach-Back needs to be revised in a manner that will improve understanding. Teach-Back has the potential to improve health outcomes because if done correctly, it forces the nurse to limit the information the individual needs to know. The likelihood of success is increased when the individual is not overwhelmed.

- Teach-Back sample questions
  - When should you call your PCP?
  - How do you know your incision is healing?
  - What foods should you avoid?
  - How often should you test your blood sugar?
  - What should you do for low blood sugar?
  - What weight gain should you call your PCP to report?
  - Which inhaler is your rescue inhaler?
  - Is there something you have been told to do that you do not understand?
  - What should you bring to your PCP office?
  - Is there something you have a question about?

 Carp's Cues

Use every opportunity to explain a treatment, a medication, the condition, and/or restrictions. For example, as you change a dressing:
- Explain and ask the individual/family member to re-dress the wound
- Point out how the wound is healing and what would indicate signs of infection

Elements to Address for Optional Self-Care or Care at Home

The Condition

- Medical conditions
  - What do you know about your condition?
  - How do you think this condition will affect you after you leave the hospital?
  - What do you want to know about your condition?
- Surgical procedure
  - What do you know about the surgery you had?
  - Do you have any questions about your surgery?
  - How will surgery affect you after you leave the hospital?

Medications

- Renew all the medications that they will continue to take at home
- Explain what over the counter (OTC) drugs not to take
- Finish all the meds like antibiotics
- Do not take any medications home unless approved by PCP
- Bring all your medications during the next visit to your PCP (e.g., prescribed, OTC, vitamins, herbal medicines)

Name: Sarah Smith Pharmacy phone number: 123-456-7890					Date Created: 12/15/07		
Name	**Used For**	**Instructions**	**Morning**	**Afternoon**	**Evening**	**Night**
Simvastatin 20mg	Cholesterol	Take 1 pill at night				⬤
Furosemide 20mg	Fluid	Take 2 pills in the morning and 2 pills in the evening	⬭ ⬭		⬭ ⬭	
Insulin 70/30	Diabetes (Sugar)	Inject 24 units before breakfast and 12 units before dinner	24 units		12 units	

FIGURE 4.2 Example of a Pill Card. (Source: DeWalt, D. A., Callahan, L. F., Hawk, V. H., Broucksou, K. A., Hink, A., Rudd, R., & Brach, C. (2010, April). *Health Literacy Universal Precautions Toolkit* (Prepared by North Carolina Network Consortium, The Cecil G. Sheps Center for Health Services Research, The University of North Carolina at Chapel Hill, under Contract No. HHSA290200710014.) (AHRQ Publication No. 10-0046-EF). Rockville, MD: Agency for Healthcare Research and Quality.)

- Depending on the literacy level of the individual/family, provide
  - A list of each medication, their use, times to take, with food or without food
  - Create a pill card with columns
    - Pictures of pill
    - Simple terms for what they are used for
    - Time using symbols with pictures of pills in spaces
  - Fill a weekly pill box

Figure 4.2 illustrates a pill card. For a printable pill card to use with individuals, refer to thePoint*.

CLINICAL ALERT:
- Warn individuals/families if a pill looks different, and check with pharmacy.
- Emphasize not to take any other medications except those on list unless approved by PCP.
- In the author's practice, the hospital pharmacy does not cover certain beta-blockers for hypertension, and hence the individuals' medication is charged. When they have a follow-up visit, during medication reconciliation, it is discovered he or she is taking back beta-blockers.

Financial Implications of Prescribed Medication

- Does the person have insured medication coverage? If yes, does it cover the medication ordered? If yes, what is the co-pay? Can the person afford this?
- If there is no _____ or no medication coverage, how will the person access these medications?
- Is there an inexpensive generic(s) available?
- Which medications are critical?

CLINICAL ALERT:
- Most pharmaceutical companies provide free branded medications (not generic) through individual-assisted programs, which can be accessed via the pharmaceutical's website.
- Social service departments can also assist with this process.
- Some medications can be acquired for no cost or low cost, such as certain diabetic medications and antibiotics (e.g., at Target, ShopRite).
- Advise individuals/families to call PCP office if they do not want to continue a medication before they stop, to discuss why (e.g., side effects).
- Some medication prescriptions can be acquired for no cost or low cost.

Diet

- Ask individual/family to report if there are any dietary limitations
- Ensure there are written directions
- Explain why some foods/beverages are to be avoided (e.g., in a low-salt diet, avoid olives, pickles)
- Consider accessing a nutritional consult

Activities

Provide instructions on the following:
- Activities permitted and restrictions
- When they can drive
- When they can return to work; what kind of job they have

Treatments

- Explain each treatment to be continued at home
- Have the individual/family demonstrate the procedure
- Write down what signs/symptoms should be reported (e.g., decrease in output for catheter)

Evaluation

- Can this treatment be provided safely by the individual or caregiver?
- If not, consult with the transition specialist in the health care agency for a home health nurse assessment

SUMMARY

The positive outcomes achieved in the acute care setting will quickly evaporate if the individual/family is not prepared to continue care at home. Teach-Back is an effective strategy to focus on "need to know" rather than overwhelming everyone, leading them to be confused and stressed. Fear and uncertainty are a very common reason individuals return to the ER and are often readmitted.

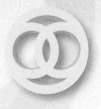

Chapter 5

10 Steps to Care Planning (Or What Are the Most Important Care Needed for an Individual/ Family at This Time?)

Care plans have one primary purpose: to provide directions for the nursing staff for a particular individual. Abbreviated care plans are usually in the electronic health record. For students and nurses inexperienced in caring for an individual with a particular condition or after a certain surgical procedure, these directions (care plan) need to be detailed.

For example, an individual who has diabetes mellitus is having abdominal surgery. An inexperienced nurse or student will need to refer to the generic care plan for a surgical individual and to the single collaborative problems *Risk for Complications of Hypo/Hyperglycemia* (low or high blood glucose). An experienced nurse will not need to read a care plan for abdominal surgery but will need to know that the individual also has diabetes and will need blood glucose monitoring.

Step 1: Assessment

If you interview your assigned individual before you write your care plan, complete your assessment using the form recommended by your faculty (e.g., Functional Health Assessment). If you need to write a care plan before you interview the individual, go to Step 2. For students, after you complete your assessment, circle all information that points to the individual's strengths. You can write all the strengths on an index card.

Strengths are factors that will help the individual recover, cope with stressors, and progress to his or her original health before hospitalization, illness, or surgery. Examples of strengths include the following:

- Being optimistic and motivated
- Having a healthy lifestyle
- Positive spiritual framework
- Positive support system
- Ability to perform self-care
- No eating difficulties
- Effective sleep habits
- Alert, good memory
- Financial stability, good health insurance
- Relaxed most of the time

Risk factors are situations, personal characteristics, disabilities, or medical conditions that can hinder the individual's ability to heal, cope with stressors, and progress to his or her original health before hospitalization, illness, or surgery. Examples of risk factors include the following:

- No or unavailable support system
- Pattern of nonengagement (e.g., missed appointments, erratic medication use)
- Obesity
- Unhealthy life style
- Limited ability to speak or understand English
- Limited literacy
- Memory problems
- Hearing problems
- Self-care problems before hospitalization
- Difficulty walking
- Financial problems, inadequate health insurance
- Tobacco use, substance abuse
- Alcohol problem
- Moderate to high anxiety most of the time
- Frail, elderly
- Presence of chronic diseases
  - Arthritis
  - Diabetes mellitus
  - HIV
  - Multiple sclerosis
  - Depression
  - Cardiac disorder
  - Pulmonary disease
  - Chronic pain

Step 2: Same-Day Assessment

As a student, if you have not completed a screening assessment of your assigned individual, determine the following as soon as possible by asking the individual, family, or the nurse assigned to your assigned individual:

- Before hospitalization, could or did the individual. . .
  - perform self-care?
  - need assistance?
  - walk unassisted?
  - have memory problems?
  - have hearing problems?
  - smoke cigarettes?
- What conditions or diseases, and risk factors are preset that make him or her more vulnerable to:
  - Falling
  - Infection
  - Nutrition/fluid imbalances
  - Pressure ulcers
  - Severe or panic anxiety
  - Physiological instability (e.g., electrolytes, blood glucose, blood pressure, respiratory function, healing problems)
- When you assess the assigned individual, determine if any of the following risk factors are present:
  - Impaired ability to speak/understand English
  - Communication difficulties, limited literacy
  - Moderate to high anxiety

Write significant data on the index card. Go to Step 3.

In some nursing programs, students do not have the opportunity to see or assess their assigned individual before the clinical day. Therefore, they must assess the individual on their first clinical day.

Step 3: Create Your Initial Care Plan

Why is the individual in the hospital? Go to the index in this book and look up the medical condition or surgical procedure that applies to your assigned individual. If you find the condition or surgical procedure, go to Step 4.

If the condition the individual is hospitalized for is not in the index, refer to the generic medical care plan at the beginning of Section 1. If the individual had surgery, refer to the generic surgical or ambulatory care plan at the beginning of Section 2.

Step 4: Additional Problems

If the medical condition or risk factor puts the individual at high risk for a physiological complication such as electrolyte imbalances or increased intracranial pressure or for nursing diagnoses such as *Impaired Skin Integrity*, *Risk for Infection Transmission*, or *Self-Care Deficit*, go to the individual indexes for collaborative problems and/or nursing diagnoses. You will find the problem or nursing diagnoses there. Go to Step 5.

Author's Note

These individual indexes provide numerous options when your assigned individual has risk factors and medical conditions in addition to the primary reason he or she is hospitalized.

Step 5: Initiate the Transitional Risk Assessment Plan (TRAP)

- Initiate the TRAP on your assigned individual to identify his or her level of risk for adverse events. Timely, effective transition requires close coordination of care during all stages of the hospitalization. Beginning on admission, include planning transition follow-up care with the primary care provider, enhanced education and self-management training, proactive end-of-life counseling, and extending the resources and clinical expertise into the home or another health care facility (see Box 5.1).

Step 6: Review the Collaborative Problems on Standard Plan

- Review the collaborative problems listed. These are the physiological complications that you need to monitor. Do not delete any because they all relate to the condition or procedure that the individual has had. You will need to add how often you should take vital signs, record intake and output, change dressings, and so forth. Ask the nurse you are assigned with for prescribed frequencies for monitoring and treatment or where this information is noted.
- Review each intervention for collaborative problems. Are any interventions unsafe or contraindicated for the individual? For example, if the individual has edema and renal problems, the fluid requirements may be too high for him or her.

Step 7: Review the Nursing Diagnoses on the Standard Plan

- Review each nursing diagnosis on the plan.
  - Does it apply to your assigned individual?
  - Does your assigned individual have any risk factors (see your index card) that could make this diagnosis worse or increase the risk? If yes, add them to the related factors as:
    - Anxiety related to unexpected hospitalization, unknown diagnosis, and recent loss of job.

Box 5.1   TRANSITIONAL RISK ASSESSMENT PLAN

- Implement on admission the Transitional Risk Assessment Plan (TRAP):
  - Refer to inside back cover.
  - Add each validated risk diagnosis to individual's problem list with the risk code in parentheses.
- Refer to Unit II for the individual risk nursing diagnoses/collaborative problems for outcomes and interventions.
- Analyze your assessment of the individual's risk factors, and determine if the individual is:
  - High Risk for Injury
  - High Risk for Infection
  - High Risk for Falls
  - High Risk for Ineffective Health Management (delayed transition)
- Add identified high-risk diagnoses to the problem list and/or care plan. Refer to Unit II, Section 1 for specifics.

Interventions

Review the intervention for each nursing diagnosis:
- Are they relevant for the individual?
- Are any interventions not appropriate or contraindicated for your assigned individual?
- Can you add any specific interventions?
- Do you need to modify any interventions because of risk factors (see index card)?

Author's Note

Remember that you cannot individualize a care plan for an individual until you spend time with him or her, but you can add and delete any inappropriate interventions on the basis of your preclinical knowledge of this individual (e.g., medical diagnosis, coexisting medical conditions).

Goals/Outcome Criteria

Review the goals listed for the nursing diagnosis:
- Are they pertinent to your assigned individual?
- Delete goals that are inappropriate for your assigned individual.
- Assume the goals are targeted to be achieved by transition.
- Evaluate after caring for this individual if there has been progress to achieve the goal by transition.

Step 8: Prepare the Care Plan (Written or Printed)

If agreed upon by the instructor, you can prepare the care plan by:

- Selecting the care plan from this book
- Creating a problem list for your assigned individual using the nursing diagnoses and collaborative problems from the care plan your selected
- Adding additional nursing diagnoses and/or collaborative problems as indicated
- Being prepared to provide rationales for why some interventions are not relevant or contraindicated

Now that you have a care plan of the collaborative problems and nursing diagnoses, find out which are associated with the primary condition for which the individual was admitted. If your assigned individual is a healthy adult undergoing surgery or was admitted for an acute medical problem and you have not assessed any significant risk factors in Step 1, you have completed the initial care plan. Go to Step 10.

Step 9: Additional Priority Nursing Diagnoses and Collaborative Problems

So far, the care plan contains the priority care that is predicated to be needed because of the person's medical or surgical condition. In addition, high-risk diagnoses have been added as *High Risk for Falls*. Often nurses attempt to define priorities by exclusively using a physiologic model such as accuracy, circulation, and so forth. Of course, physiologic instability when a new onset or increasing is a priority. However, other physiologic dysfunctions such as constipation, infections, unstable gait, or confusion can also be priorities. In addition, an emotional crisis or disruptive behavior can be priorities. Thus, it is more useful clinically to view priorities as a group of nursing diagnoses/collaborative problem selected for an individual/family.

Priority of Set Diagnoses

Carp's Cues

Priority identification is a very important but difficult concept. Because of shortened hospital stays and because individuals have several chronic diseases, nurses cannot address most of the nursing diagnoses and collaborative problems for each individual. Nurses must focus on those for which the individual would be harmed, more stressed, or not progress to a timely, successful transition.

Table 5.1   Differentiate the Types of Clinical Priorities

- Urgent priorities
  - New changes or worsening of an individual's condition or a potential for violent situations that requires immediate action (e.g., contact physician/nurse practitioner for immediate action, access Rapid Response team or Code team, security alert)
- Priority set of diagnoses
  - Are a group of nursing diagnoses or collaborative problems that, if not managed, will deter progress to achieve positive outcomes and to a timely, successful transition
  - Are associated with their primary medical or surgical condition
  - May contain additional necessary diagnoses or collaborative problems if indicated by medical or personal problems
- Stressful or disruptive response priorities
  - Stressful responses
    - Moderate anxiety or fear
    - Family crisis
  - Disruptive responses*a*
    - Protocol/rule violations (e.g., smoking, equipment tampering)
    - Anger (perceived as nonthreatening)
    - Repetitive, unreasonable demands

*a*Discussed in Chapter 6.

Table 5.2   Example of an Individual's Priority Set of Diagnoses

An individual's priority set includes primary condition necessitating admission, coexisting medical conditions with related collaborative problems, and personal risks factors as a nursing diagnosis.

Admitting diagnosis: pneumonia	Insert diagnostic cluster from Unit III, Section 1
Coexisting medical condition: diabetes mellitus	*Risk for Complications of Hypo/Hyperglycemia* from Unit II, Section 2
Personal stressors/barriers (e.g., cannot read)	*Risk for Nonengagement Related to Low Literacy*, refer to Unit II, Section 1

Initially, it is important to differentiate between priority and nonpriority diagnoses. A priority set of nursing diagnoses is described in Table 5.1.

> **CLINICAL ALERT:**
> - Of the three types of priorities, urgent priorities acquire immediate attention. In Unit III, care plans are clinical alerts to advise the clinician or student nurse that a clinical situation necessitates immediate action.

Fundamentally, the set contains (refer to Table 5.2 for an example of an Individual's Priority Set of Diagnoses):

- All of the nursing diagnoses and collaborative problems identified in the diagnostic cluster for the individual's medical condition or surgical procedure that necessitated admission
- Additional collaborative problems associated with coexisting medical conditions that require monitoring as *Risk for Complications of Hypo/Hyperglycemia* in an individual having surgery, who also has diabetes mellitus
- Additional nursing diagnoses that, if not managed or prevented now, will deter recovery, negatively affect the person's/family's functional states, and/or delay a timely, successful transition (e.g., *Grieving for a Deceased Friend, Chronic Confusion*)

Carp's Cues

When someone with diabetes mellitus is admitted for a medical condition as pneumonia or surgical procedure as total hip replacement, do not activate the care plan for diabetes mellitus in Unit III. Some critical deficits in knowledge about diabetes mellitus such as differentiation of high versus low glucose levels and what to do must be addressed during hospitalization. Other teaching that is needed for management of diabetes mellitus can be done post transition in the primary care setting or in individual or group classes. A home health nursing consult may be indicated.

The following questions can help to determine if the individual or family has additional nursing diagnoses/collaborative problems that need nursing interventions:

- Are additional collaborative problems associated with coexisting medical conditions that require monitoring (e.g., hypoglycemia)?
- Are there additional nursing diagnoses that, if not managed or prevented now, will deter recovery or affect the individual's functional status (e.g., *High Risk for Constipation*)?
- What problem does the individual perceive as priority?
- What nursing diagnoses are important but treatment for them can be delayed without compromising functional status?

You can address nursing diagnoses not on the priority list by referring the individual for assistance after discharge (e.g., counseling, weight loss program).

 Carp's Cues

Priority identification is a very important but difficult concept. Because of shortened hospital stays and because many individuals have several chronic diseases at once, nurses cannot address all nursing diagnoses that are present in every individual. Nurses must focus on those for which the individual would be harmed physically or emotionally or may not make progress if they were not addressed. Ask your clinical faculty to review your list. Be prepared to provide rationales for your selections.

Step 10: Evaluate the Status of Your Assigned Individual (After You Provide Care)

Collaborative Problems

Review the collaborative outcomes for the collaborative problems:

- Assess the individual's status.
- Compare the data to established norms (indicators).
- Judge if the data fall within acceptable ranges.
- Conclude if the individual is stable, improved, unimproved, or worse.

Is the individual stable or improved?

- If yes, continue to monitor the individual and to provide interventions indicated.
- If not, has there been a dramatic change (e.g., elevated blood pressure, decreased urinary output)? Have you consulted with an experienced nurse or notified the prescribing physician, advanced practice nurse, or physician assistance? Have you increased your monitoring of the individual?

Nursing Diagnosis

Review the goals or outcome criteria for each nursing diagnosis. Did the individual demonstrate or state the activity defined in the goal? If yes, then communicate (document) the achievement on your plan. If not note if there is any progress and evaluate reasons why the individual did not achieve the goal. Was the goal:

- Not realistic because of other priorities?
- Not acceptable to the individual?

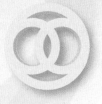

Chapter 6

Barriers to Providing Concerned, Compassionate Professional Care

Principles of Individual and Family-Centered Care

When practicing in a hospital or other health care facility, the following principles of individual and family-centered care are obiligatory:

- Staff are competent and trustworthy.
- Care is respectful.
- Dignity is protected.
- All care processes are explained clearly and understood.
- Family/support persons are involved.
- Physical and emotional comforts are priorities.
- Decisions are made collaboratively and differences are respected.
- Transition process begins on admission.
- Preparation for safe and comfortable transition to home is made.

Values Clarification

Nurses are individuals that come to the clinical setting as a sum total of their life experiences, which have formed their own preferences, bias, and expectations from others. Likewise, individuals and their families, too, come to the clinical setting as a sum total of their life experiences, which have formed their own preferences, bias, and expectations from others. Sometimes the nurse and the ill person have similar values. Frequently, they are not the same, however. The responsibility to bridge the gap rests on the professional nurse.

Values clarification is a process to find out how you feel about something and how it can affect your responses to others. Values are learned through observation and experience. Therefore, they are influenced greatly by cultural, ethnic, and religious background and by family and peer groups.

"People are often unaware of what some of their values consist of because values are so entrenched into how a person thinks and behaves. Subsequently, values are frequently acted upon in an automatic fashion. When a nurse is not aware of their values, especially when it comes to precarious subject matter, they may inadvertently impose their point of view onto others" (Stephany & Murkowski, 2015, p. 58). Or the nurse's negative bias can interfere with having a therapeutic relationship.

Try the following value-clarification exercises:

Situation 1: You board a bus, and there are three seats available, all next to someone already seated. You need to sit down. In one seat is an older man in dirty clothes who is poorly groomed. In another seat is a young woman with multiple tattoos, sobbing quietly. In the third seat is a very obese women, covering one-third of the seat next to her. Which seat would you choose to take?

What are the reasons for your choice?

What surprised you about your reaction?

Situation 2: During the hand-off (shift report), three new admissions are reported on. The first person is a 28-year-old pregnant woman from a motor vehicle accident who was legally drunk. Her pregnancy history is G 4 P0 with a history of three terminations. The second person is a 42-year-old man admitted for chest pain. He has had multiple admissions for chest pain, with cardiac disease ruled out. He uses cocaine, barbiturates, and alcohol daily. The third person is a 37-year-old woman with chronic leg ulcers. She is obese with a body mass index (BMI) of 45. She smokes cigarettes.

Which individual would you choose to take on?

Why?

Why did you not choose one of the other two?

What if you are assigned to the person you most do not want to take care of?

What in your life has influenced your attitudes in caring for obese individuals, substance abusing individuals, or individuals who habitually make bad decisions, such as not using birth control?

Do your values and attitudes affect how you nurse?

As nurses, we encounter individual and families with the best and worse behaviors. We do not like some individuals for what they have done. As professional nurses, we have ethical obligations to provide the standard of care to all individual's we encounter.

However, we are humans with prejudices and biases. So how do we bridge giving compassionate, competent care with our gut impulse of aversion?

Consider the following:

- Can you completely judge each of these people with the limited information you have?
- How much do you know about this person?
- Make an attempt to relate to the person as a human being who is ill, not on the basis of the poor choices they have made.
- Are all your decisions in your personal life well thought out, good for you, or good for those who love you?
- There is nothing wrong with having bad thoughts. However, it is profoundly damaging to speak cruel words or provide incomplete or substandard care.
- Avoid engaging in group discussions that promote stereotyping and will further discourage the individual from receiving compassionate, competent care.
- You may be the first person in a health care setting that has been kind and respectful to this individual. This does mean you approve of their behavior but can still be caring and professional.

 ## Carp's Cues

Sometimes, because you are human, you will find caring for someone to be very problematic. It may be wise to ask another nurse to take your place for the sake of the person, not yours. When we are uncomfortable with an individual or family member, we tend to avoid the room. This may seem benign but denying an ill individual your presence is the most malevolent action you can choose.

Stressors/Barriers

All hospitalized individuals/families have stressors. The key is, are they interfering with the person's ability to recover and progress to transition to home care? In addition, some stressors need acknowledgment and dialog because "it just is right." When someone is admitted with injuries from a car accident, the nurse should allow the person an opportunity to share. Opening an opportunity to share never means "we have the solution," but only that we are willing to listen to the pain of others.

Stressful or Disruptive Behavior Response Priorities

 ## Carp's Cues

This is a new addition to the author's defining of priorities of care. This is a result of numerous accounts of nurses' experiences with disrespectful, repetitive, unrealistic, demanding, and/or threatening behavior of individuals and/or families. It also represents some personal experiences as a nurse practitioner in primary care.

Zero-Tolerance Clinical Situations

All individuals and their support systems in health care settings are in a high-stress situation. Inappropriate or rude incidents need to be treated as an incident unless they are on a zero-tolerance list (refer to Table 6.1).

The Joint Commission and other organizations have identified disruptive behaviors of a nurse, manager, physician, or nurse practitioner that can or have caused adverse events to occur. When nurses are recipients of threatening, demanding or unrealistic, rude demands by individuals/families, care is compromised. Abusive individuals and families will receive the standard of care, but it will create barriers that may delay a response to a request and avoidance of the individual's room.

Table 6.1	Zero-Tolerance Clinical Situations

- "Personal" insults (e.g., racial, gender)
- Deliberate violation of infection prevention
- Tampering of equipment (e.g., patient-controlled anesthesia pump)
- Repetitive, deliberate vulgar language/actions (e.g., inappropriate exposing of genitals)
- Throwing any object at personnel
- Deliberate contamination of bodily fluids (e.g., urinating or spitting on floor or in garbage can)

Some mentally impaired/confused individuals may be unaware of their behaviors.

Health systems have evolved from an environment that tolerated disruptive and disrespectful behavior from some physicians and administrators to one with policies to support an environment of respect and true colleagueship. Unfortunately, this has not occurred when the nurse is a recipient of disruptive, abusive behavior by individuals and families. Frequently, the reports of the behavior are ignored and nurse's attempts to reduce the behavior are criticized. The "customer" is not always right. Nurses must be assured that administration will protect them and preserve their dignity.

Carp's Cues

In an environment where administrative support is lacking, let the most competent, experienced nurse have the assignment. This may increase the likelihood of successful outcomes. In addition, do not change personnel. Consistent, experienced nurses can set rules of behavior, with a likelihood that the individuals/families may improve their behavior.

"Stress-full" Behavior

Illness by its nature is disruptive to one's life. Hospitalization compounds these disruptions. Stressors experienced by all individuals and their families are:

- Fear of the unknown
- Isolation
- Loss of privacy
- Exposure of body parts
- Sleep disruption
- Invasive procedures by "strangers"
- Painful procedure

Additional stressors for some may be:

- Financial burden of situation
- Preexisting coping problems
- Language barriers
- Literacy barriers
- Cultural barriers
- Withdrawal from alcohol/drug dependence
- Family conflicts
- Unavailable or lack of support systems

"Stress-full" individuals and their families may not behave as desired. Actually, nurses should expect their behavior to be heightened responses to the stressors of impatience, anger, or unrealistic requests. When experiencing disruptive behavior not identified as zero-tolerance behavior, the nurse needs to implement STAR.

STAR   **Stop**

  Think • Am I looking at the "whole picture" or just the incident?
        • What do I know about this person?
        • What do I not know?

  Act   • Nurses cannot read individual's or family members' minds, but one can ask:
          • "What are you most worried about?"
          • "How can I help you? This situation must be very hard."
          • When someone is abrupt, rude, or angry, lower your voice and ask:
            • "You sound upset, is there something I can help you with?"
            • "Is there something that I said or did that was disrespectful to you?"
            • Gently suggest another solution that is more acceptable.
            • Explain why their requests are unreasonable and offer an alternative option.

  Review • Did you learn something you did not know that enhanced your understanding?

Barriers to Caring

Nurses daily encounter individuals and their families who are facing devastating illness or injuries. In addition to the above individuals and families, nurses will be caring for individuals who have conditions that could have been prevented. Some causes of health problems and even fatal disorders are:

- Smoking
- Obesity
- Drug abuse
- Alcohol abuse
- Medication nonchalance (e.g., seeing disorder, hypertension, diabetes mellitus)

STAR   **Stop**

Think
- Is the care I am providing this person respectful and caring?
- Do I or someone I love have a lifestyle that is unhealthy?
- If my lifestyle is healthy, does that mean everyone can make the same choices as I do?

Carp's Cues

All behavior is meaningful, and one is responsible for one's choice; however, not everyone has been supported, loved, and cared for. Obesity, addictions (tobacco, alcohol, drug), and adherence to medical advice are very complex conditions and require more intervention than just believing "they can stop."

Act
- Give yourself a gift by getting to know the person who is addicted, obese, or nonadherent. You may be surprised.

Review
- Nurses are human, too, so do your best, do no harm, and take care of yourself.

The Power of One Nurse

Every day, most nurses are faced with unspeakable horrors and suffering. Students seek desperately to learn what to say or do when faced with these situations. Some nurses never learn because they want to solve the situation and take away the suffering. This suffering of individuals or families is theirs to the core of their being. Nurses cannot take this suffering away, but they can choose to be present in the midst of the suffering. They cannot answer why, but they can:

- Stand/sit quietly for a moment and listen
- Touch an arm
- Offer an embrace

Say:

- I am sorry
- How can I help you?

These words and actions are as therapeutic as any medications or treatment.

Carp's Cues

Years ago, my father had cranial surgery. Postoperatively, he became delirious and paranoid. When they called me to come to the hospital, I found my dad alone and tied down, with fear in his eyes. He recognized me, but became acutely distressed that I was also in danger. Needless to say, the care was horrific.

Two years later, he needed the same cranial surgery. He was on the same unit, and postoperatively as I was visiting him, he became acutely confused and was afraid. Of course, I was upset seeing my dad in this state. The nurses quickly moved him into a private room. As a nurse quickly wheeled by, she stopped and touched my arm and said, "How are you?" There was no answer, but she sent me a powerful caring message. My dad had a 24-hour sitter and did recover.

P.S. One year before my dad's second surgery, this hospital had received Magnet Recognition from the American Nurses Association. Well done ANA, well done!

SUMMARY

- Know the power of one nurse.
- Use your power to care, not to harm.
- Know that when you avoid a room, you are doing harm.
- Expect respect.

- Tolerate unpleasant behavior that is fueled by anxiety and fear.
- Learn to be comfortable with suffering individuals. This means *you can sit in a dark cave with me and not talk about the light.*
- Report zero-tolerance behaviors immediately.
- Provide the same care to the janitor as you would to the bank president.
- Defend the right of all individuals and their families to receive the same care you would expect for your children, partner, parent, or dear friend.

Unit II

Manual of Nursing Diagnoses

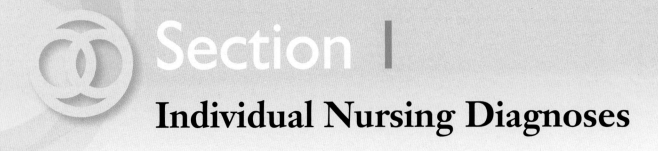

Section I

Individual Nursing Diagnoses

INDIVIDUAL AND FAMILY-CENTERED CARE

ACTIVITY INTOLERANCE

NANDA-I Definition

Insufficient physiologic or psychological energy to endure or complete required or desired daily activities

Defining Characteristics

An altered physiologic response to activity

Respiratory

Exertional dyspnea*

Shortness of breath

Excessively increased rate

Decreased rate

Pulse

Weak

Decreased

Excessively increased

Failure to return to preactivity level after 3 minutes

Rhythm change

EKG changes reflecting arrhythmias or ischemia

Blood Pressure

Abnormal blood pressure response to activity

Increased diastolic pressure greater than 15 mm Hg

Failure to increase with activity

Verbal report of weakness

Pallor or cyanosis

Verbal reports of vertigo

Verbal report of fatigue*

Confusion

---

*Nursing diagnoses contain definitions designated as NANDA-I and characteristics and factors identified with a blue asterisk from Herdman, T. H., & Kamitsuru, S. (Eds.). *Nursing Diagnoses: Definitions and Classification 2015–2017.* Copyright © 2014, 1994–2014 by NANDA International. Used by arrangement with John Wiley & Sons Limited. Companion website: www.wiley.com/go/nursingdiagnoses

Related Factors

Any factors that compromise oxygen transport, physical conditioning, or create excessive energy demands that outstrip the individual's physical and psychological abilities can cause activity intolerance. Some common factors follow.

Pathophysiologic

Related to deconditioning secondary to prolonged immobilization and pain related to imbalance between oxygen supply/demand

Related to compromised oxygen transport system secondary to:

Cardiac

Cardiomyopathies

Arrhythmias

Myocardial infarction (MI)

Congenital heart disease

Congestive heart failure

Angina

Valvular disease

Respiratory

Chronic obstructive pulmonary disease (COPD)

Bronchopulmonary dysplasia

Atelectasis

Circulatory

Anemia

Hypovolemia

Peripheral arterial disease

Related to increased metabolic demands secondary to:

Acute or Chronic Infections

Viral infection

Endocrine or metabolic disorders

Mononucleosis

Hepatitis

Chronic Diseases

Renal

Inflammatory

Neurologic

Hepatic

Musculoskeletal

Related to inadequate energy sources secondary to:

Obesity

Malnourishment

Inadequate diet

Treatment Related

Related to inactivity secondary to assistive equipment (e.g., walkers, crutches, braces)

Related to increased metabolic demands secondary to:

Malignancies

Diagnostic studies

Surgery

Treatment schedule/frequency

Related to compromised oxygen transport secondary to:

Hypovolemia

Bed rest

Immobility

Situational (Personal, Environmental)

Related to inactivity secondary to:

Depression

Inadequate social support

Sedentary lifestyle

Related to increased metabolic demands secondary to:

Environmental barriers (e.g., stairs)
Climate extremes (especially hot, humid climates)
Air pollution (e.g., smog)
Atmospheric pressure (e.g., recent relocation to high-altitude living)

Related to inadequate motivation secondary to:

Fear of falling   Pain
Depression   Dyspnea
Obesity   Generalized weakness

Maturational

Older adults may have decreased muscle strength and flexibility, as well as sensory deficits. These factors can undermine body confidence and may contribute directly or indirectly to activity intolerance.

Author's Note

Activity Intolerance is a diagnostic judgment that describes an individual with compromised physical conditioning. This individual can engage in therapies to increase strength and endurance. *Activity Intolerance* is different than *Fatigue*; *fatigue* is a pervasive, subjective draining feeling. Rest does treat *Fatigue*, but it can also cause tiredness. Moreover, in *Activity Intolerance*, the goal is to increase tolerance and endurance to activity; in *Fatigue*, the goal is to assist the individual to adapt to the fatigue, not to increase endurance.

Goals

NOC
Activity Intolerance

The individual will progress activity to (specify level of activity desired), evidenced by these indicators:

* Identify factors that aggravate activity intolerance.
* Identify methods to reduce activity intolerance.
* Maintain blood pressure within normal limits 3 minutes after activity.

Interventions

NIC
Activity Tolerance,
Energy Management,
Exercise Promotion,
Sleep Enhancement,
Mutual Goal Setting

Explain the Risks of Inactivity

* Overweight
* Obesity
* Increased risk of numerous health conditions: hypertension, heart disease, coronary heart disease, diabetes, type 2 diabetes, high cholesterol

    R: Mobilization is prescribed to exploit the benefits on the cardiovascular, respiratory, hematologic, renal, as well as the musculoskeletal and neurologic systems to support increasing levels of physiologic work demands (Grossman & Porth, 2014).

Monitor the Individual's Response to Activity and Record Response

* Take resting pulse, blood pressure, and respirations.
* Consider rate, rhythm, and quality (if signs are abnormal—e.g., pulse above 100—consult with physician/nurse practitioner/physician assistant about advisability of increasing activity).
* If indicated, have the individual perform the activity.
* Take vital signs immediately after activity.
* Ask the individual to rest for 3 minutes; take vital signs again.
* Discontinue the activity if there is/are:
  * Complaints of chest pain, vertigo, or confusion
  * Decreased pulse rate
  * Failure of systolic blood pressure to increase
  * Decreased systolic blood pressure
  * Increased diastolic blood pressure by 15 mm Hg
  * Decreased respiratory response

    R: Clinical responses that require discontinuation or reduction in the activity level are evidence of compromised cardiac or respiratory ability (Grossman & Porth, 2014).

- Reduce the intensity or duration of the activity if:
  - The pulse takes longer than 3 to 4 minutes to return to within 6 beats of the resting pulse.
  - The respiratory rate increase is excessive after the activity.

    R: The cardiopulmonary responses to activity involve the circulatory functions of the heart and blood vessels and the gas exchanges in the respiratory system (Grossman & Porth, 2014). Response to activity can be evaluated by comparing preactivity blood pressure, pulse, and respiration with postactivity results. These, in turn, are compared with recovery time.

> **CLINICAL ALERT:**
> - If the individual cannot stand without buckling the knees, he or she is not ready for ambulation; help to practice standing in place with assistance.

Increase the Activity Gradually

- Increase tolerance for activity by having the individual perform the activity more slowly, for a shorter time, with more rest pauses, or with more assistance.
- Minimize the deconditioning effects of prolonged bed rest and imposed immobility:
  - Begin active range of motion (ROM) at least twice a day. For the individual who is unable, the nurse should perform passive ROM.
  - Encourage isometric exercise.
  - Encourage the individual to turn and lift self actively unless contraindicated.
  - Gradually increase tolerance by starting with 15 minutes the first time out of bed.
  - Choose a safe gait. (If the gait appears awkward but stable, continue; stay close by and give clear coaching messages, e.g., "Look straight ahead, not down.")
  - Allow the individual to gauge the rate of ambulation.
  - Provide sufficient support to ensure safety and prevent falling.
  - Encourage to wear comfortable walking shoes (slippers do not support the feet properly).

    R: Activity tolerance develops cyclically through adjusting frequency, duration, and intensity of activity until the desired level is achieved. Increasing activity frequency precedes increasing duration and intensity (work demand). Increased intensity is offset by reduced duration and frequency. As tolerance for more intensive activity of short duration develops, frequency is once again increased (Grossman & Porth, 2014).

- Plan rest periods according to the person's daily schedule.

    R: They should occur throughout the day and between activities to allow time for recovery.

Promote a Sincere "Can-Do" Attitude

- Allow the individual to set the activity schedule and functional activity goals. If the goal is too low, negotiate (e.g., "Walking 25 feet seems low. Let's increase it to 50 feet. I'll walk with you.").
- Plan a purpose for the activity, such as sitting up in a chair to eat lunch, walking to a window to see the view, or walking to the kitchen to get some juice.
- Praise the individual for progress, no matter how small.

    R: Do not underestimate the value of praise and encouragement as effective motivational techniques.

Interventions for Individuals With Chronic Pulmonary Insufficiency (COPD Foundation, 2015)

- Encourage conscious controlled-breathing techniques during increased activity and times of emotional and physical stress (techniques include pursed-lip and diaphragmatic breathing).
- Teach pursed-lip breathing. The person should breathe in through the nose, then breathe out slowly through partially closed lips while counting to seven and making a "pu" sound. (Often, people with progressive lung disease learn this naturally.)

    R: Pursed-lip breathing slows breathing down, thus keeping airways open longer so trapped air can be exhaled. This improves the exchange of oxygen and carbon dioxide (COPD Foundation, 2015).

- Teach diaphragmatic breathing (COPD Foundation, 2015).
  - Place your hands on the individual's abdomen below the base of the ribs and keep them there while he or she inhales.
  - To inhale, the individual relaxes the shoulders, breathes in through the nose, and pushes the stomach outward against your hands. The individual holds the breath for 1 to 2 seconds to keep the alveoli open, then exhales.
  - To exhale, the individual breathes out slowly through the mouth while you apply slight pressure at the base of the ribs.
  - Have the person practice this breathing technique several times with you; then, the individual should place his or her own hands at the base of the ribs to practice alone.
  - Once the technique has been learned, have the individual practice it a few times each hour.
  - Encourage the use of adaptive breathing techniques to decrease the work of breathing.

    R: The diaphragm is the main muscle of breathing. In individuals with COPD, when the diaphragm weakens, the muscles in the neck, shoulders, and back are used instead (COPD Foundation, 2015).

- "Explain that the tripod position, in which the patient sits or stands leaning forward with the arms supported, forces the diaphragm down and forward and stabilizes the chest while reducing the work of breathing. Point out that this reduces competing demands of the arm, chest, and neck muscles needed for breathing" (Bauldoff, 2015; *Bauldoff, Hoffman, Sciurba, & Zullo, 1996; *Breslin, 1992).

- Providing arm support (e.g., resting elbows on a tabletop while shaving or eating) may enhance independence and improve functional capacity.

    *R: Research has shown that arm support during performance of arm tasks reduces diaphragmatic recruitment, increases respiratory endurance (*Bauldoff et al., 1996, Bauldoff, 2015), and increases arm exercise endurance.*

- While in the hospital, discuss the effects of smoking with a focus on the specific health problems of the individual, e.g., frequent infections, leg cramps, worsening of COPD, cardiac problems.

    R: A Cochrane review 5 of over 50 clinical trials has found that high-intensity behavioral interventions that begin during a hospital stay and include at least one month of supportive contact after discharge promote smoking cessation among hospitalized individuals (Rigotti, Clair, Munafò, & Stead, 2012).

IMPAIRED COMMUNICATION[1]

Definition

The state in which a person experiences, or is at risk to experience, difficulty exchanging thoughts, ideas, wants, or needs with others

Defining Characteristics

Inappropriate or absent speech or response
Impaired ability to speak or hear
Incongruence between verbal and nonverbal messages
Stuttering
Slurring
Word-finding problems
Weak or absent voice
Statements of being misunderstood or not understanding
Dysarthria
Aphasia
Language barrier

---

[1]This diagnosis is not presently on the NANDA-I list, but has been added for clarity and usefulness.

Related Factors

Pathophysiologic

Related to disordered, unrealistic thinking secondary to:

Schizophrenic disorder   Delusional disorder
Psychotic disorder   Paranoid disorder

Related to impaired motor function of muscles of speech secondary to:

Cerebrovascular accident ("Brain attack")
Oral or facial trauma
Brain damage (e.g., birth/head trauma)
Central nervous system (CNS) depression/increased intracranial pressure
Tumor (of the head, neck, or spinal cord)
Chronic hypoxia/decreased cerebral blood flow
Nervous system diseases (e.g., myasthenia gravis, multiple sclerosis, muscular dystrophy, Alzheimer's disease)
Vocal cord paralysis/quadriplegia

Related to impaired ability to produce speech secondary to:

Respiratory impairment (e.g., shortness of breath)   Malocclusion or fractured jaw
Laryngeal edema/infection   Missing teeth
Oral deformities   Dysarthria
Cleft lip or palate

Related to auditory impairment

Treatment Related

Related to impaired ability to produce speech secondary to:

Endotracheal intubation
Surgery of the head, face, neck, or mouth
CNS depressants
Tracheostomy/tracheotomy/laryngectomy
Pain (especially of the mouth or throat)

Situational (Personal, Environmental)

Related to decreased attention secondary to fatigue, anger, anxiety, or pain
Related to no access to or malfunction of hearing aid
Related to psychological barrier (e.g., fear, shyness)
Related to lack of privacy
Related to unavailable interpreter

Maturational

Infant/Child
Related to inadequate sensory stimulation

Older Adult (Auditory Losses)
Related to hearing impairment
Related to cognitive impairments secondary to (specify)

Author's Note

Impaired Communication is clinically useful with individuals with communication-receptive deficits and language barriers.

Impaired Communication may not be useful to describe communication problems that are a manifestation of psychiatric illness or coping problems. If nursing interventions focus on reducing hallucinations, fear, or anxiety, Confusion, Fear, or Anxiety would be more appropriate.

Goals

NOC
Communication

The person will report improved satisfaction with ability to communicate as evidenced by the following indicators:

- Demonstrates increased ability to understand.
- Demonstrates improved ability to express self.
- Uses alternative methods of communication, as indicated.

Interventions

NIC
Communication
Enhancement: Speech,
Communication
Enhancement:
Hearing Active
Listening, Socialization
Enhancement

> **CLINICAL ALERT:**
> - Low health literacy, cultural barriers, and limited English proficiency have been termed the "triple threat" to effective health communication by The Joint Commission (Schyve, 2007).

Identify a Method to Communicate Basic Needs

- Assess ability to comprehend, speak, read, and write
- Provide alternative methods of communication
  - Use a computer, pad and pencil, hand signals, eye blinks, head nods, and bell signals.
  - Make flash cards with pictures or words depicting frequently used phrases (e.g., "Wet my lips," "Move my foot," "I need a glass of water," or "I need a bedpan").
  - Encourage the person to point, use gestures, and pantomime.

    R: Using alternative forms of communication can help decrease anxiety, isolation, and alienation; promote a sense of control; and enhance safety (*Iezzoni, O'Day, Keleen, & Harker, 2004).

Practice "Listening to Understand Rather Than Listening to Respond"
(Procter, Hamer, McGarry, Wilson, & Froggatt, 2014, p. 93) **by Quieting Your Mind**

R: When one listens to respond, one is thinking of their response. "Withholding one's reactions to what is being said, hearing what is being said, and then exploring the person's perspective with curious questioning, rather than launching into one's own agenda, leads one to develop a more balance and inclusive appraisal of the person's situation"(Procter et al., 2014, p. 93).

Identify Factors That Promote Communication

R: Communication is the core of all human relations. Impaired ability to communicate spontaneously is frustrating and embarrassing. Nursing actions should focus on decreasing tension and conveying understanding of how difficult the situation must be for the individual (Miller, 2015).

- Create atmosphere of acceptance and privacy.
- Face the individual and establish eye contact if possible. Avoid standing over person; sit down.
- Use uncomplicated one-step commands and directives.
- Match words with actions; use pictures.
- If low literacy is present, refer to Appendix C.

    R: Establishing an alternative form of communication is imperative for all individuals to prevent heightened anxiety, isolation, and alienation; which will promote a sense of control; and enhance a sense of security (Boyd, 2014; Miller, 2015).

If the Person Can Speech-Read, Do Not Call It Lip-Reading
(*Bauman & Gell, 2000; Office of Student Disabilities Services, 2014)

R: Studies show that only 23% of people who are hard of hearing become effective speech readers (Office of Student Disabilities Services, 2014).

- Look directly at the person; even a slight turn of your head can obscure the speech reading view and:
  - Speak slowly and clearly.
  - Do not yell, exaggerate, or overenunciate.

    R: It is estimated that only 3 out of 10 spoken words are visible on the lips. Overemphasis of words distorts lip movements and makes speech reading more difficult.

- Try to enunciate each word without force or tension. Short sentences are easier to understand than long ones.
- Do not place anything in your mouth when speaking.
- Mustaches that obscure the lips, and putting your hands in front of your face can make lip reading difficult.
- Avoid standing in front of light—have the light on your face so the person can see your lips.
- If the person looks surprised/perplexed/bemused, stop and clarify.
- Use open-ended questions, which must be answered by more than "yes" or "no."

  R: Open-ended questions ensure that your information has been communicated (Office of Student Disabilities Services, 2014).

- Reinforce important communications by writing them down.

  R: "Only 40% of the English language is visible. Speech reading is difficult and fatiguing in the hospital. Unfamiliar terminology, anxiety, and poor lighting can contribute to errors." "Even the best speech reader only catches about 25%–30% of what is said. However, be aware that about 10% of the population move their lips in such a way that it is absolutely impossible to speech-read even one word they say" (Office of Student Disabilities Services, 2014).

- Assess ability to communicate in English, determine language the individual speaks best.

  R: Studies have shown that individuals with limited English proficiency have less access to care, poorer adherence to treatment regimens, and consequently contribute to increased health disparities. A majority of nurses reported that language barriers are a significant impediment to quality care and a source of stress in the workplace. Incomplete nursing assessments, misunderstood medical information, and the lack of therapeutic relationships between providers and individual/families are problems encountered (Houle, 2010).

- Do not evaluate understanding based on "yes" or "no" responses.
- Assess the individual's ability to read, write, speak, and comprehend English and for red flags for lack of comprehension as (DeWalt et al., 2010):
  - Frequently missed appointments
  - Incomplete registration forms
  - Noncompliance with medication
  - Unable to name medications, explain purpose, or dosing
  - Identifies pills by looking at them, not reading label
  - Unable to give coherent, sequential history
  - Asks fewer questions
  - Lack of follow-through on tests or referrals
- Use a fluent translator when discussing important matters (e.g., taking a health history, signing an operation permit). Reinforce communications through the translator with written information. (Many hospitals require a "Certified Translator" to be used at least once per day. This should be documented in the medical record per hospital policy.)
- Use a telephone translating system when necessary.

  R: Effective communication is critical and must be ensured with persons who do not speak or understand English.

Initiate Health Teaching and Referrals, if Needed

- Seek consultation with a speech or audiology specialist.

Geriatric Interventions

CLINICAL ALERT:
- Approximately one in three people between the ages of 65 and 74 has hearing loss, and nearly half of those older than 75 have difficulty hearing (National Institute on Deafness and Other Communication Disorders, 2013).

Implement Interventions to Improve Communication

- If the person can hear with a hearing aid, make sure that it is on and functioning.
- If the person can hear with one ear, speak slowly and clearly into the good ear. It is more important to speak distinctly than to speak loudly.
- If the person can read and write, provide pad and pencil at all times (even when going to another department).
- If the person can understand only sign language, have an interpreter with him or her as much as possible.
- Write and speak all important messages.
- Validate the person's understanding by asking questions that require more than "yes" or "no" answers. Avoid asking, "Do you understand?"

R: Many older adults with hearing impairments do not wear hearing aids. Those who wear them must be encouraged to use them consistently, clean and maintain them, and replace batteries. Encourage the person to be assertive in letting others know about situations and environmental areas in which they experience difficulty because of background noise (Miller, 2015).

IMPAIRED VERBAL COMMUNICATION

NANDA-I Definition

Decreased, delayed, or absent ability to receive, process, transmit, and/or use a system of symbols

Defining Characteristics

Difficulty or inability to speak words but can understand others
Articulation or motor planning deficits

Related Factors

See *Impaired Communication.*

Goals

Communication:
Expressive Ability

The person will demonstrate improved ability to express self as evidenced by the following indicators:

- Relate decreased frustration with communication.
- Use alternative methods as indicated.

Interventions

Active Listening,
Communication
Enhancement: Speech
Deficit

Identify a Method for Communicating Basic Needs

- See *Impaired Communication* for general interventions.

Identify Factors That Promote Communication

For Individuals With Dysarthria (Slurred or Slow Speech)

R: Dysarthria is caused by paralysis, weakness, or inability to coordinate the muscles of the mouth (Grossman & Porth, 2014).

- Do not alter your speech or messages, because the comprehension is not affected; speak on an adult level.

- Encourage the individual to make a conscious effort to slow down speech and to speak louder (e.g., "Take a deep breath between sentences.").
- Ask the individual to repeat unclear words; observe for nonverbal cues to help understanding.
- If the individual is tired, ask questions that require only short answers.
- If speech is unintelligible, teach use of gestures, written messages, and communication cards.

For Those Who Cannot Speak (e.g., Endotracheal Intubation, Tracheostomy)

R: Research reported that individuals treated with mechanical ventilation experience a moderate to extreme level of psychoemotional distress because they cannot speak and communicate their needs (Khalaila, Zbidat, Anwar, Bayya, Linton, & Sviri, 2011).

- Reassure that speech will return, if it will. If not, explain available alternatives (e.g., esophageal speech, sign language).
- Do not alter your speech, tone, or type of message; speak on an adult level.
  - Use gestures, head nods, mouthing of words, writing, use of letter/picture boards and common words or phrases tailored to meet individualized patients' needs (Grossbach, Stranberg, & Chlan, 2011).

    R: Every attempt must be made for successful communication. Each individual uses about three modes of communication while unable to speak, including squeezing hands (92%), shaking or nodding the head (86%), lip reading (83%), facial expressions (83%), pen and paper (57%), word or picture charts (17%), alphabet boards (6%), and electronic voice output (5%) (Grossbach et al., 2011).

Utilize Stress-Reducing and Comfort Intervention With Every Encounter

R: Research has supported that interventions to prevent emotional distress among individuals with mechanical ventilation should target those with communication difficulties (Khalaila et al., 2011).

- Touch
- "It must be frightening to be in your situation. Is there anything I can do to make you feel better, safer?"
- Ensure the call bell system is always visible and available.

Promote Continuity of Care to Reduce Frustration

Observe for Signs of Frustration or Withdrawal
- Verbally address frustration over inability to communicate.
- Maintain a calm, positive attitude (e.g., "I can understand you if we work at it.").
- Allow tears (e.g., "It's OK. I know it's frustrating. Crying can let it all out.").
- For the individual with limited speaking ability (e.g., can make simple requests, but not lengthy statements), encourage letter writing or keeping a diary to express feelings and share concerns.
- Anticipate needs, and ask questions that need a simple "yes" or "no" answer.

    R: After survival, perhaps the most basic human need is to communicate with others. Communication provides security by reinforcing that individuals are not alone and that others will listen. Researchers have reported that "difficulty in communication was a positive predictor of patients' psychological distress, and length of anesthesia was a negative predictor. Fear and anger were also positively related to difficulty in communication" (Khalaila et al., 2011).

Maintain a Specific Care Plan

- Document the method of communication that is used (e.g., "Uses word cards," "Points for bedpan" alphabet board, picture board writing materials).
- Record directions for specific measures (e.g., allow him to keep a urinal in bed).

ACUTE CONFUSION

NANDA-I Definition

Abrupt onset of reversible disturbances of consciousness, attention, cognition, and perception that develop over a short period of time

Defining Characteristics

Abrupt onset of:

Fluctuation in cognition[*]
Fluctuation in level of consciousness[*]
Fluctuation in psychomotor activity*
Increased agitation*
Reduced ability to focus
Disorientation
Increased restlessness*
Hypervigilance
Incoherence
Fear
Anxiety
Excitement

Symptoms are worse at night or when fatigued or in new situations.

Illusions
Hallucinations[*]
Delusions
Misperceptions[*]

Related Factors

Pathophysiologic

Related to abrupt onset of cerebral hypoxia or disturbance in cerebral metabolism secondary to (Miller, 2015):

Fluid and Electrolyte Disturbances

Dehydration
Acidosis/alkalosis
Hypercalcemia/hypocalcemia

Hypokalemia
Hyponatremia/hypernatremia
Hypoglycemia/hyperglycemia

Nutritional Deficiencies

Folate or vitamin B_{12} deficiency
Anemia

Niacin deficiency
Magnesium deficiency

Cardiovascular Disturbances

Acute coronary syndrome
Congestive heart failure
Arrhythmias

Heart block
Temporal arteritis
Subdural hematoma

Respiratory Disorders

Chronic obstructive pulmonary disease: Tuberculosis and pneumonia
Pulmonary embolism

Infections

Sepsis   Urinary tract infection (especially elderly)   Meningitis, encephalitis

Metabolic and Endocrine Disorders

Thyroid disorders   Postural hypotension
Adrenal disorders   Hypothermia/hyperthermia
Pituitary disorders   Hepatic or renal failure
Parathyroid disorders

Central Nervous System (CNS) Disorders

Cerebral vascular accident   Normal-pressure hydrocephalus
Multiple infarctions   Head trauma
Tumors   Seizures and postconvulsive states

Treatment Related

Related to a disturbance in cerebral metabolism secondary to:
Surgery
Side effects of certain medication:

Diuretics	Barbiturates, Opioids	Sulfa drugs
Digitalis	Methyldopa	Ciprofloxacin
Propranolol	Disulfiram	Metronidazole
Atropine	Lithium	Acyclovir
Oral hypoglycemic	Phenytoin	H2 receptor antagonists
Anti-inflammatories	Benzodiazepines	Anticholinergic
Antianxiety agents	Phenothiazines	

Over-the-counter cold, cough, and sleeping preparations

Situational (Personal, Environmental)

Related to disturbance in cerebral metabolism secondary to:

Withdrawal from alcohol, opioids, sedatives, hypnotics
Heavy metal or carbon monoxide intoxication

Related to:

Pain   Immobility
Depression   Unfamiliar situations

Goals

NOC
Cognition, Cognitive
Orientation, Distorted
Thought Self-Control

The person will have diminished episodes of delirium as evidenced by the following indicators:

- Be less agitated
- Participate in ADLs
- Be less combative

Interventions

NIC
Delirium Management,
Calming Technique,
Reality Orientation,
Environmental
Management: Safety

> **CLINICAL ALERT:**
> - Delirium is a distressing but preventable condition that is common in older people (Heaven et al., 2014).
> - It is associated with increased morbidity, mortality, functional decline, hospitalization, and significant health care costs (Heaven et al., 2014).

- Assess for causative and contributing factors, by referring to related factors above.

  R: "Delirium may be present when admitted to hospital, any care setting, or may develop during a stay. It usually develops over 1–2 days" (Cook & Lloyd, 2010).

- Identify whether the individual's behavior is (Cook & Lloyd, 2010):
  - Hyperactive (fast/loud speech, impatient, anger, restlessness, uncooperative, nightmares, wandering, persistent thoughts, easily startled)
  - Hypoactive (unawareness, lethargy, decreased alertness, slow/sparse speech, apathy, staring, decreased motor activity)

- Mixed responses

   R: Delirium can present with hyperactive, hypoactive, or mixed signs and symptoms. Hypoactive behavior is often unrecognized as manifestations of acute confusion (Cook & Lloyd, 2010).

> **CLINICAL ALERT:**
> - Implement falls prevention protocol with *Risk for Falls*.

- If individual is not confused, assess for the presence of prehospitalization risk factors (Cook & Lloyd, 2010).

  - Severe illness
  - Visual/hearing impairments
  - Physically frail
  - Medication side effects
  - Fracture of neck of femur
  - Dehydration/sepsis
  - Excess alcohol use
  - Some cognitive impairment

- If confusion is present, use *Risk for Acute Confusion*.

   R: Old age is not a risk factor for acute confusion. Avoid accepting old age as a cause of acute confusion.

Implement Interventions to Modify Risk Factors (Francis, 2015)

- Orientation protocols—Provision of clocks, calendars, windows with outside views, and verbally reorienting

   R: Persistent reorientation may mitigate confusion that results from disorientation in unfamiliar environments.

- Cognitive stimulation

   R: Cognitive stimulation, for example, visitors, engaging in previously enjoyable activities, such as games, help to reduce confusion.

- Facilitation of physiologic sleep

   R: Sleep protocols reduce unnecessary awakenings and environmental noise. Refer to Disturbed Sleep Patterns for specifics. One randomized trial reported that the use of earplugs at night was associated with a lower incidence of confusion in ICU individuals (Van Rompaey, Elseviers, Van Drom, Fromont, & Jorens, 2012).

- Early mobilization
- Use adaptive devices (e.g., focused lighting, glasses, and hearing aids).

   *R: One study found that early institution of physical and occupational therapy in mechanically ventilated, critically ill individuals along with consequent interruption in use of sedatives resulted in a lower rate of hospital days with delirium (*Schweickert et al., 2009).*

   R: Adaptive devices can diminish confusing sensory input.

- Educate family, significant others, and caregivers about the situation and coping methods (Cook & Lloyd, 2010; *Young, 2001).
- Explain the cause of acute confusion.
- Explain that the individual does not realize the situation.
- Explain the need to remain patient, flexible, and calm.
- Stress the need to respond to the individual as an adult.
- Explain that the behavior is part of a disorder and is not voluntary.

   R: Differentiating between acute (reversible) and chronic (irreversible) confusion is important for family and caregivers (Miller, 2015).

- Maintain standards of empathic, respectful care.
- Be an advocate. Function as a role model with coworkers.
- Expect empathic, respectful care, and monitor its administration.
- Attempt to obtain information for conversation (likes, dislikes; interests, hobbies; work history). Interview early in the day.
- Encourage significant others and caregivers to speak slowly with a low voice pitch and at an average volume (unless hearing deficits are present), with eye contact, and as if expecting the individual to understand.

   R: Communication can be enhanced with useful and meaningful topics as one adult to another.

- Assess for nonverbal signs of pain (e.g., grimacing, moaning when repositioned).

   R: Communication difficulties prevent usual assessment foci.

- Provide respect and promote sharing.
- Pick out meaningful comments and continue talking.
- Call the individual by name, and introduce yourself each time you make contact; use touch if welcomed.

- Use the name the individual prefers; avoid "Pops" or "Mom," which is unacceptable and can increase confusion.
- Convey to the individual that you are concerned and friendly (through smiles, an unhurried pace, humor, and praise; do not argue; use light touch if comforting).

   R: This demonstrates unconditional positive regard and communicates acceptance and affection to a person who has difficulty interpreting the environment (*Hall, 1991).

- Do not endorse confusion.
- Do not argue with the individual.
- Determine the best response to confused statements.
- Sometimes the confused individual may be comforted by a response that reduces his or her fear; for example, "I want to see my mother," when his or her mother has been dead for 20 years. The nurse may respond with, "I know that your mother loved you."
- Direct the individual back to reality; do not allow him or her to ramble.
- Remember to acknowledge your entrance with a greeting and your exit with a closure (e.g., "I will be back in 10 minutes").

   R: Unconditional positive regard communicates acceptance and affection to a person who has difficulty interpreting the environment.

- Encourage the family to bring in familiar objects from home (e.g., photographs, afghan).
- Ask the individual to tell you about the picture.
- Focus on familiar topics.
- Discuss current events, seasonal events (e.g., snow, water activities); share your interests (e.g., travel, crafts).

   R: Strategies that emphasize normalcy can contribute to positive self-esteem and reduce confusion.

- Prevent injury to the individual by referring to *Risk for Injury* for strategies for assessing and manipulating the environment for hazards.

> ***Clinical Alert Report***
> - Advise ancillary staff/student to report an increase in anxiety and/or confusion.

CHRONIC CONFUSION

NANDA-I Definition

Irreversible, long-standing, and/or progressive deterioration of intellect and personality characterized by decreased ability to interpret environmental stimuli; decreased capacity for intellectual thought processes; and manifested by disturbances of memory, orientation, and behavior

Defining Characteristics

Progressive or long-standing:

Cognitive or intellectual losses
Altered perceptions
Poor judgment
Loss of language abilities
Affective or personality losses
Progressively lowered stress threshold
Purposeless behavior
Violent, agitated, or anxious behavior
Compulsive repetitive behavior
Withdrawal or avoidance behavior

Related Factors

Pathophysiologic (Hall, 1991)

Related to progressive degeneration of the cerebral cortex secondary to:

Alzheimer's disease*   Multi-infarct dementia (MID)*
Combination

Related to disturbance in cerebral metabolism, structure, or integrity secondary to:

Pick's disease   Creutzfeldt–Jakob disease
Toxic substance injection   Degenerative neurologic disease
Brain tumors   Huntington's chorea
Multiple sclerosis   Psychiatric disorders
End-stage diseases (AIDS, cirrhosis, cancer, renal failure, cardiac failure, and chronic
    obstructive pulmonary disease)

Goals

NOC

Cognitive Ability, Cognitive Orientation, Distorted Thought Self-Control, Surveillance: Safety, Emotional Support, Environmental Management, Fall Prevention, Calming Technique

The person will participate to the maximum level of independence in a therapeutic milieu as evidenced by the following indicators:

- Decreased frustration
- Diminished episodes of combativeness, sexual disinhibition
- Increased hours of sleep at night
- Stabilized or increased weight

Interventions

NIC

Dementia Management: Multisensory Therapy, Cognitive Stimulation, Calming Technique, Reality Orientation, Environmental Management: Safety

Refer to Interventions Under *Acute Confusion*

Promote the Individual's Safety

- Refer to *Risk for Falls*.
    R: Confused persons are at high risk for injury.

Implement Falls Prevention Protocol With *Risk for Falls*.

> **CLINICAL ALERT:**
> - "One important element of maintaining a connection with a patient with dementia is fostering greater engagement by facilitating family interaction with the patient" (Epstein & Street, 2011).
> - "Isolation can quickly become a way of life for a patient with dementia when family members become exhausted, which further hinders their ability to support the patient" (Volland & Fisher, 2014).

Assess Who the Person Was Before the Onset of Confusion

- Educational level, career
- Hobbies, lifestyle
- Coping styles
    *R: Assessing the individual's personal history can provide insight into current behavior patterns and communicates the nurse's interest. Specific personal data can improve individualization of care (*Hall, 1991).*

Observe the Individual to Determine Baseline Behaviors

- Best time of day
- Response time to a simple question
- Amount of distraction tolerated
- Judgment
- Insight into disability
- Signs/symptoms of depression
- Routine

R: Baseline behavior can be used to develop a plan for activities and daily care routines.

Address Disruptive Behaviors by Focusing on the Underlying Unmet Need (*Cohen-Mansfield, 2000)

- For aggression triggered by pain or discomfort, address for sources of pain (e.g., constipation, UTI).
- For pacing triggered by boredom, plan opportunities to engage individual in an activity.
- For repetitive questioning or statements triggered by a need to communicate, increase meaningful dialogue during all caregiving encounters.

  *R: The focus on the individual's needs rather than on behavior helps to target more appropriate interventions (*Cohen-Mansfield, 2000).*

Promote the Individual's Sense of Integrity (Miller, 2015)

- Adapt communication to individual's level.
  - Avoid "baby talk" and a condescending tone of voice.
  - Use simple sentences and present one idea at a time.
  - If the individual does not understand, repeat the sentence using the same words.
- Use positive statements; avoid "don'ts."
- Unless a safety issue is involved, do not argue.
- Avoid general questions such as "What would you like to do?" Instead, ask, "Do you want to go for a walk or work on your rug?"
- Be sensitive to the feelings the individual is trying to express.
- Avoid questions you know the individual cannot answer.
- If possible, demonstrate to reinforce verbal communication.
- Use touch to gain attention or show concern unless a negative response is elicited.
- Maintain good eye contact and pleasant facial expressions.
- Determine which sense dominates the individual's perception of the world (e.g., auditory, kinesthetic, olfactory, or gustatory). Communicate through the preferred sense.

  R: Alzheimer's disease-related dementia affects communication abilities (i.e., receptive and expressive).

Confused Individuals are Very Vulnerable to Abuse

Monitor for and Address Unacceptable Staff Behavior Toward Individual

Consult With Physician/Nurse Practitioner/Physician Assistant Regarding Whether Certain Treatments are Needed

- Discontinue or reduce dosage of medications that increase disturbances of cognition (e.g., sedatives, analgesics).
- Avoid cauterizations/intravenous lines if possible.
- Consider an intermittent access device instead of continuous IV therapy.

  R: Tethering lines are restrictive, confusing, and pose an increased risk of infection and trauma.

- If catheter is necessary, place urinary collection bag at the end of the bed with catheter between rather than draped over legs. Velcro bands can hold the catheter against the leg.

Assess for Nonverbal Signs of Pain (e.g., Grimacing, Moaning When Repositioned)

R: Communication difficulties prevent usual assessment foci.

- Allow an opportunity to draw using colored pencils.

  R: Drawing allows self-expression and opportunities to make choices (e.g., what to draw, what colors).

- Ask the family to bring in recordings of the individual's favorite music.

  R: Studies have shown that playing favorite music improves social interactions, memories, and reduces abnormal vocalizations (Miller 2015).

If Combative, Determine the Source of Fear and Frustration

- Fatigue
- Misleading or inappropriate stimuli
- Change in routine, environment, caregiver
- Pressure to exceed functional capacity
- Physical stress, pain, infection, acute illness, discomfort

R: Fatigue is the most frequent cause of dysfunctional episodes. Physical stressors can precipitate a dysfunctional episode (e.g., urinary tract infections, caffeine, constipation).

If an Aggressive Episode Occurs

* Address the individual by surname. Assume a dependent position relative to the individual.
* Distract the individual with cues that require automatic social behavior (e.g., "Mrs. Smith, would you like some juice now?").
* Document antecedents, behavior observed, and consequences.

R: With careful recording of the episode, these strategies can reduce aggression and may prevent future episodes.

Implement Techniques to Lower the Stress Threshold
(*Hall & Buckwalter, 1987; Miller, 2015)

* Reduce competing or excessive stimuli.
  * Keep the environment simple and uncluttered.
  * Use simple written cues to clarify directions for use of radio and television.
  * Eliminate or minimize unnecessary noise.

    *R: Overstimulation, understimulation, or misleading stimuli can cause dysfunctional episodes because of impaired sensory interpretation (*Hall, 1994).*

Initiate Health Teaching and Referrals as Needed

* Support groups
* Community-based programs (e.g., day care, respite care)
* Alzheimer's association (www.alz.org)
* Long-term care facilities

Clinical Alert Report

* Advise ancillary staff/student to report an increase in anxiety and/or confusion.

CONSTIPATION

NANDA-I Definition

Decrease in normal frequency of defecation accompanied by difficult or incomplete passage of stool and/or passage of excessively hard, dry stool

Defining Characteristics

Hard, formed stool*	Defecation fewer than two times a week
Prolonged and difficult evacuation	Distended abdomen*
Generalized fatigue*	Decreased bowel sounds
Straining on defecation	Palpable rectal mass*
Feeling of inadequate emptying*	

Related Factors

Pathophysiologic

Related to defective nerve stimulation, weak pelvic floor muscles, and immobility secondary to:

Spinal cord lesions	Cerebrovascular accident (CVA, stroke)
Spinal cord injury	Neurologic diseases (multiple sclerosis, Parkinson's)
Spina bifida	Dementia

Related to decreased metabolic rate secondary to:

Obesity	Diabetic neuropathy
Uremia	Hypothyroidism

Related to decreased response and an urge to defecate secondary to:
Cognitive/affective disorders
Related to painful defecation
Related to decreased peristalsis secondary to hypoxia (cardiac, pulmonary)
Related to motility disturbances secondary to irritable bowel syndrome

Treatment Related

Related to side effects of (specify):

Iron	Anticholinergics
Diuretics	Phenothiazines
Narcotics (codeine, morphine)	Antidepressants

Related to effects of anesthesia and surgical manipulation on peristalsis
Related to habitual laxative use
Related to mucositis secondary to radiation

Situational (Personal, Environmental)

Related to decreased peristalsis secondary to:

Immobility	Pregnancy
Stress	Insufficient exercise

Related to irregular evacuation patterns
Related to inadequate diet (lack of roughage, fiber, thiamine) or fluid intake

Goals

NOC
Bowel Elimination,
Hydration, Knowledge:
Diet

The individual will report bowel movements at least every 2 to 3 days as evidenced by the following indicators:

- Describe components for effective bowel movements.
- Explain rationale for lifestyle change(s).

Author's Note

- Yearly, more than 2.5 million Americans see their health care provider for relief from constipation (Wald, 2015). Constipation occurs in 15% to 30 % of older adults living in the community and 75% to 80% living in institutional settings (Miller, 2015).
- *Constipation* results from delayed passage of food residue in the bowel because of factors that the nurse can treat and teach the individual (e.g., dehydration, insufficient dietary roughage, immobility). Often, constipation is reported, and with further assessment, it is the person's misunderstanding of normal defecation patterns (Erichsén, Milberg, Jaarsma, &Friedrichsen, 2015). *Perceived Constipation* refers to a faulty perception of constipation with self-prescribed overuse of laxatives, enemas, and/or suppositories. NANDA-I added a new diagnosis of Chronic Functional Constipation.

Interventions

Assess Contributing Factors

- Refer to *Related Factors.*

> **CLINICAL ALERT:**
> - Constipation is often viewed as expected and benign.
> - Constipation can be responsible for undiagnosed pain and exacerbating confusion in individuals who cannot communicate.
> - Mostly all episodes of constipation can be prevented.

- If fecal impaction is present:
  - If fecal impaction is suspected, perform a digital rectal examination (DRE). Remove fecal impaction. Refer to procedure manual as needed.

R: Caution regarding producing the Valsalva maneuver, which can cause hypotension.

NIC
Bowel Management,
Fluid Management,
Constipation/Impaction
Management, Nutrition
Therapy

Consult With Physician/Nurse Practitioner/Physician Assistant for Stool Softener

R: Stool softeners do not treat constipation, but can prevent dry, hard stools by chemically drawing fluid into intestines.

Promote Corrective Measures

- Regular time for elimination
  - Review daily routine.
  - Provide a stimulus to defecation (e.g., coffee, prune juice).
  - Advise the individual to attempt to defecate about 1 hour or so after meals and that remaining in the bathroom for a suitable length of time may be necessary.

    R: The gastrocolic and duodenocolic reflexes stimulate mass peristalsis two or three times a day, most often after meals.
- Reduce immobility. Provide frequent ambulation of hospitalized individual when tolerable.
- Refer to Impaired Physical Mobility for a progressive ambulation program, for example, sitting upright in bed > sitting on side of bed > sitting in chair > walking.

  R: Regular physical mobility promotes muscle tonicity needed for fecal expulsion. It also increases circulation to the digestive system, which promotes peristalsis and easier feces evacuation.
- Balanced diet
  - Avoid food low in fiber (e.g., starches, white bread, pasta, white rice, dairy products, processed foods). Review list of foods high in fiber: for example, fresh fruits, fruit juices, and vegetables with skins, beans (navy, kidney, lima), nuts, and seeds, whole-grain breads, cereal, and bran.

    R: Diets high in unrefined fibrous food produce large, soft stools that decrease the colon's susceptibility to disease. Diets low in fiber and high in concentrated refined foods produce small, hard stools that increase the colon's susceptibility to disease. An increase in fiber without optimal hydration will worsen constipation.
- Adequate fluid intake
  - Encourage fluid intake of at least 2 L (8 to 10 glasses) unless contraindicated.
  - Discuss fluid preferences.

    R: Sufficient fluid intake, at least 2 L daily unless contraindicated, is necessary to maintain bowel patterns and to promote proper stool consistency.
- Use the bathroom instead of a bedpan if possible. Allow suitable position (sitting and leaning forward, if not contraindicated).

  R: Flexing the hip pulls the anal canal open, which decreases resistance of feces movement. An upright position uses gravity to promote feces movement. Elevating the legs can increase intra-abdominal pressure.

Initiate Health Teaching and Referrals as Indicated

- Explain the relationship of lifestyle changes to constipation. Emphasize that constipation can be prevented.

  R: Sedentary lifestyle, inadequate fluid intake, inadequate dietary fiber, and stress can contribute to constipation.
- Go to thePoint and print Getting Started to Prevent Constipation.

> ### *Clinical Alert Report*
> - Advise ancillary staff/student to report early signs of constipation (e.g., difficulty in passing stools) and if individual reports more than 2 days have passed without a bowel movement.

RISK FOR CORNEAL INJURY

NANDA-I Definition

Vulnerable to Infection or inflammatory lesion in the corneal tissue that can affect superficial or deep layers, which may compromise health.

NANDA-I Risk Factors

Blinking <5 times/min
Exposure of the eyeball
Glasgow Coma Scale <7
Intubation
Mechanical ventilation
Periorbital edema
Pharmaceutical agent
Prolonged hospitalization
Tracheostomy
Use of supplemental oxygen

Goals

NOC
Knowledge: Illness
Care, Infection Control,
Symptom Control,
Hydration

The individual/family will:

- Be instructed to report eye pain or blurring (if able) immediately
- Be monitored for redness and watery eyes, white to gray area on cornea (late sign)
- Demonstrate methods to prevent infection such as:
  - Wash hands before eye care.
  - Gently pull lower lid, and instill drops or a line of ointment in pocket of the lid.
  - Avoid any contamination of eye care products. Never touch dropper or tube tip to eyelid.

Interventions

NIC
Eye Care Infection
Protection; Medication
Administration:
Eye, Comfort Level,
Hydration, Anxiety
Reduction (family)

Identify High-Risk Individuals

- Unconscious
- Sedated for >48 hours
- Paralyzed
- Ventilatory support

> **CLINICAL ALERT:**
> - The above conditions prevent eye closure, lack of random eye movements, and diminished or loss of blink reflex. The exposure and drying of the eye can result in superficial keratopathy. This can compromise the integrity of the surface of the cornea, resulting in ulceration, perforation, and scarring. The effects of mechanical ventilation increase intraocular pressure, resulting in edema (*Joyce, 2002).

Monitor:
- Every 8 hours for eye comfort loss of blink reflex, incomplete eyelid closure, unconscious or heavily sedated mechanically intubate (Leadingham, 2014).

  R: The inability to actively maintain appropriate eyelid alignment and closure puts the individual at an increased risk for eye complications (Leadingham, 2014).

- For red and watery eyes
- For pain in the eye (if can report)
- For white to gray area on cornea (late sign)

Report Any Changes in the Eye Appearance or Report of Eye Pain or Blurring (if Able) Immediately

*R: Keratitis is an inflammation of the cornea caused by corneal exposure and a compromise in the normal tear film and/or bacterial or viral infections (Leadingham, 2014; *Joyce, 2002).*

Initiate Eye Care Protocol

R: Dryness and disruption of corneal epithelium can lead to blurring of vision, and it can also place the corneal tissue at risk for infection, which can complicate with considerable visual loss. Cornea drying can occur quickly in high-risk individuals after 48 hours (Leadingham, 2014).

Provide Eye Care as Prescribed

- Eye drops, lubricants, antibiotics
- If eyelid closure cannot be passively maintained, mechanical eye closure application should be applied (Leadingham, 2014).

    R: The application of a mechanical eye closure device prevents eye complications (dry eye, infection, and corneal abrasion), for example, patches, gauze, eye shields, polyethylene covers (Leadingham, 2014).

Provide Eye Care for Unconscious, Heavily Sedated, or Individuals Who Cannot Maintain Complete Eye Closure

- Moisture chambers, saline-soaked gauze, and the instillation of a lubricant.
- If no eye care protocol has been prescribed, consult with physician/immediately.

Prevent Infection

- Wear gloves with all eye care.
- Instruct family not to touch or wipe the eye area of an individual.
- Gently pull lower lid, and instill drops or a line of ointment in pocket of the lid.
- Avoid any contamination of eye care products. Never touch dropper or tube tip to eyelid. If this occurs, discard the medicine.
- Offer to demonstrate to a new nurse or student nurse.

    *R: Studies have reported the effectiveness of these preventive practices. The use of polyethylene covers has been found to be most effective (*Joyce, 2002; Leadingham, 2014; Rosenberg & Eisen, 2008). Every attempt is made to prevent contamination of the eye. Eye drops can become contaminated when the container's tip touches the eyelid and is exposed to bacteria.*

Evaluate Hydration Status Frequently

R: Mild dehydration can make dry eyes worse (Rosenberg et al. 2008).

Explain to Individual and/or Significant Others the Reason for the Eye Care Treatments (e.g., Use of Shields, Polyethylene Covers [Plastic Wrap]).

R: The individual's appearance with eye patches or polyethylene covers can be very disturbing to significant others for the individual. Compromised vision is frightening.

Initiate Health Teaching/Referrals as Indicated

- Advise to see primary care provider or an eye specialist if there are signs and symptoms of dry eyes, infection, and eye pain.
- If person wears contacts, refer to Internet for prevention of infection. Here are the best ways to prevent eye infections if you wear contacts. Access at http://www.techtimes.com/articles/20235/20141114/prevent-against-eye-infections-contacts.htm

    R: Prolonged dry eyes can cause eye infections, scarring of the cornea surface, and vision problems. Eye complaints must be addressed immediately.

> **Clinical Alert Report**
> - Advise ancillary staff/student to report any complaints of eye pain.

DIARRHEA

NANDA-I Definition

Passage of loose, unformed stools

Defining Characteristics*

At least three loose, liquid stools per day
Urgency
Cramping/abdominal pain
Hyperactive bowel sounds

Related Factors

Pathophysiologic

Related to malabsorption or inflammation* secondary to (specify):*

Colon cancer	Crohn's disease	Gastritis
Diverticulitis	Peptic ulcer	Spastic colon
Irritable bowel	Celiac disease (sprue)	Ulcerative colitis

Related to lactose deficiency, dumping syndrome
Related to increased peristalsis secondary to increased metabolic rate (hyperthyroidism)
Related to infectious process secondary to:*

Trichinosis	Shigellosis	Dysentery
Typhoid fever	Cholera	Infectious hepatitis
Malaria	Microsporidia	Cryptosporidium

Related to excessive secretion of fats in stool secondary to liver dysfunction
Related to inflammation and ulceration of gastrointestinal mucosa secondary to high levels of nitrogenous wastes (renal failure)

Treatment Related

Related to malabsorption or inflammation secondary to surgical intervention of the bowel
Related to side effects of (specify) (e.g., diuretics, antibiotics)*
Related to tube feedings

Situational (Personal, Environmental)

Related to stress or anxiety

Goals

NOC
Bowel Elimination, Electrolyte & Acid–Base Balance, Fluid Balance, Hydration, Symptom Control

The individual/parent will report less diarrhea as evidenced by the following indicators:

- Describe contributing factors when known.
- Explain rationale for interventions.

Interventions

NIC
Bowel Management, Diarrhea Management, Fluid/Electrolyte Management, Nutrition Management, Enteral Tube Feeding

Monitor for Dehydration

- Hourly output less than 0.5 mL/kg/hr
- Dark-colored urine
- Low serum potassium, low serum sodium
- Dizziness, headache

R: Undetected hypovolemia can cause electrolyte imbalances and decreased blood flow to heart, brain, and kidneys.

Closely Monitor the Elderly for Dehydration

R: The body compensates for fluid losses by concentrating urine and increasing the thirst response. As one ages, these mechanisms are less effective; thus dehydration can occur more rapidly with severe complications of arrhythmias and decreased cardiac output (Grossman & Porth, 2014).

- Monitor perianal tissue for redness/excoriation. Use a barrier cream.

    R: Gastric enzymes can irritate and excoriate perianal tissue.

> **CLINICAL ALERT:**
> - Early signs of dehydration in the elderly require interventions.

Advise to (Wanke, 2015)

- Ingest boiled starches and cereals (e.g., potatoes, noodles, rice, wheat, and oat) with salt; crackers, bananas, soup, and boiled vegetables may also be consumed.
- Avoid foods with high fat content.
- Avoid milk (lactose) products, fat, whole grains, fried and spicy foods, and fresh fruits and vegetables.
- Avoid alcohol and caffeine drinks.
- Avoid artificial sweeteners (e.g., diet beverages).
- Gradually add semisolids and solids (e.g., crackers, yogurt, rice, bananas, and applesauce).

    R: Foods with complex carbohydrates (e.g., rice, toast, and cereal) facilitate fluid absorption into the intestinal mucosa. Drinks with caffeine act like diuretics, thus increasing dehydration. Artificial sweeteners can have a laxative effect on the digestive system.

- Encourage liquids (e.g., tea, water, apple juice, flat ginger ale).
- Caution against the use of very hot or cold liquids.
- See *Deficient Fluid Volume* for additional interventions.

    R: Soft drinks (nondietetic or dietetic) and sport drinks are unsatisfactory for fluid replacement for moderate or severe fluid loss because of their high sugar and salt content (*Bennett, 2000).

- Reduce GI side effects of tube feeding. Refer to Care Plan: "Enteral Nutrition" in Unit III.

Conduct Health Teaching as Indicated

- Explain safe food handling (e.g., required temperature storage, washing of food preparation objects after use with raw food, and frequent hand washing).
- Instruct the individual to call primary care provider if diarrhea lasts more than 24 hours.
- Instruct the individual to seek *immediate* medical care if blood and mucus are in stool and if fever is present.

    R: Acute bloody diarrhea (dysentery) has certain causative pathogens (e.g., campylobacter jejuni, shigella, and salmonella) that require antibiotic therapy (Wanke, 2015).

> ***Clinical Alert Report***
> - Advise ancillary staff/student to report an increase in diarrhea and/or decrease in urinary output.

RISK FOR DISUSE SYNDROME

NANDA-I Definition

At risk for deterioration of body systems as the result of prescribed or unavoidable musculoskeletal inactivity

Defining Characteristics

Presence of a cluster of actual or risk nursing diagnoses related to inactivity:

Risk for Pressure Ulcer
Risk for Constipation

Risk for Altered Respiratory Function
Risk for Ineffective Peripheral Tissue Perfusion
Risk for Infection
Risk for Activity Intolerance
Risk for Impaired Physical Mobility
Risk for Injury
Powerlessness
Disturbed Body Image

Related Factors

Pathophysiologic

Related to decreased sensorium/unconsciousness
Related to neuromuscular impairment secondary to (specify)

Treatment Related

Related to:

Surgery (amputation, skeletal)   Mechanical ventilation
Traction/casts/splints   Invasive vascular lines
Prescribed immobility

Situational (Personal, Environmental)

Related to:

Depression   Debilitated state
Fatigue   Pain

Author's Note

Risk for Disuse Syndrome describes an individual at risk for the adverse effects of immobility. *Risk for Disuse Syndrome* identifies vulnerability to certain complications and also altered functioning in a health pattern. As a syndrome diagnosis, its etiology or contributing factor is within the diagnostic label (*Disuse*); a "related to" statement is not necessary.

Goals

NOC
Endurance, Immobility
Consequences:
Physiologic, Immobility
Consequences: Psycho-
Cognitive, Mobility, Joint
Movement

The individual will not experience complications of immobility as evidenced by the following indicators:

- Intact skin/tissue integrity
- Maximum pulmonary function
- Maximum peripheral blood flow
- Full range of motion
- Bowel, bladder, and renal functioning within normal limits
- Uses of social contacts and activities when possible
- Make decisions regarding care when possible
- Share feelings regarding immobile state

Interventions

> **CLINICAL ALERT:**
> - "Observation of 45 hospitalised medical patients indicated that, on average, 83% of the hospital stay was spent lying in bed. The amount of time spent standing or walked ranged from 0.2–21%" (Kalisch, Lee, & Dabney, 2013).

Identify Causative and Contributing Factors

- Pain; refer also to *Impaired Comfort.*
- Fatigue; refer also to *Fatigue.*

NIC
Bed Rest Care,
Bowel Management,
Activity Therapy,
Energy Management,
Mutual Goal Settings,
Exercise Therapy, Fall
Prevention, Pressure
Ulcer Prevention, Body
Mechanics Correction,
Self-Care Assistance,
Skin Surveillance,
Positioning, Coping
Enhancement, Decision
Making, Support
Therapeutic Play

- Decreased motivation; refer also to *Activity Intolerance*.
- Depression; refer also to *Ineffective Coping*.
- Immobility; refer to *Impaired Physical Mobility*
- Consult with physical therapy for a mobilization plan.

Promote Optimal Respiratory Function

- Vary the position of the bed, thus gradually changing the horizontal and vertical positions of the thorax, unless contraindicated.
- Assist individual to reposition, turning frequently from side to side (hourly if possible).
- Encourage deep breathing and controlled coughing exercises five times every hour.

  R: Bed rest decreases chest expansion and cilia activity and increases mucus retention, increasing risks of pneumonia (Zomorodi, Topley, & McAnaw, 2012).

Maintain Usual Pattern of Bowel Elimination

- Refer to *Constipation* for specific interventions.

Prevent Pressure Ulcers

- Refer to *Risk for Pressure Ulcer*.

  R: Principles of pressure ulcer prevention include reducing or rotating pressure on soft tissue. If pressure exceeds intra-capillary pressure (approximately 32 mm Hg), capillary occlusion causes tissue damage (Grossman & Porth, 2014).

Promote Factors That Improve Venous Blood Flow

- Elevate extremity above the level of the heart (may be contraindicated in cases of severe cardiac or respiratory disease).
- Ensure that the individual avoids standing or sitting with legs dependent for long periods.
- Avoid pillows behind the knees, or suggest a bed that is elevated at the knees.
- Tell the individual to avoid crossing the legs.
- Remind the individual to change positions, move extremities, or wiggle fingers and toes every hour.
- Ensure that the individual avoids garters and tight elastic stockings above the knees.
- Monitor legs for edema, tissue warmth, and redness daily.

  R: Increased serum calcium resulting from bone destruction caused by lack of motion and weight-bearing increases blood coagulability. This, in addition to circulatory stasis, makes the individual vulnerable to thrombosis formation (Grossman & Porth, 2014).

> **CLINICAL ALERT:**
> - Any change in peripheral circulation, onset of edema, tissue warm, or c/o of leg aches/pains need immediate attention to rule out thrombosis.

Maintain Limb Mobility and Prevent Contractures

- Increase limb mobility.
  - Perform range-of-motion exercises (frequency to be determined by individual's condition).
- Position the individual in alignment to prevent complications.
  - Point toes and knees toward ceiling when the individual is supine. Keep them flat when in a chair.
  - Use footboard.
  - Instruct the individual to wiggle toes, point them up and downward, rotate ankles inward and outward every hour.

    R: These strategies prevent foot drop, a serious complication of immobility.
- Prevent urinary stasis and calculi formation.
  - Provide a daily fluid intake of 2,000 mL or more (unless contraindicated).

    R: The peristaltic contractions of the ureters are insufficient when in a reclining position; thus, there is stasis of urine in the renal pelvis. Interventions to maintain hydration prevent hypercoagulability and clot formation and urine concentration of stone-forming elements (Grossman & Porth, 2014).

Reduce and Monitor Bone Demineralization

- Promote weight-bearing when possible (tilt-table).
- Maintain vigorous hydration.

    R: The upright position improves bone strength, increases circulation, and prevents postural hypotension (Grossman & Porth, 2014).

Promote Sharing and a Sense of Well-Being

- Encourage the individual to share feelings and fears regarding restricted movement.
- Encourage the individual to wear own clothes, rather than pajamas, and unique adornments (e.g., baseball caps, colorful socks) to express individuality.
- Be creative; vary the physical environment and daily routine when possible.
    - Update bulletin boards, change pictures on the walls, and move furniture within the room.
    - Maintain a pleasant, cheerful environment (e.g., plenty of light, flowers).
    - Place the individual near a window, if possible.
    - Provide reading material (print or audio), radio, and television.
    - Plan an activity daily to give the individual something to look forward to; always keep promises.
    - Discourage the use of television as the primary source of recreation unless it is highly desired.
    - Consider using a volunteer to spend time reading to the individual or helping with an activity.
    - Encourage suggestions and new ideas (e.g., "Can you think of things you might like to do?").

    R: Decreased activity reduces social contacts, reduces problem-solving ability, and decreases coping ability and orientation to time. Strategies are focused on increasing visual and auditory stimuli, engaging in decision making and activities to reduce monotony (Miller, 2015).

Initiate health teaching and referrals as needed

- Refer to community health nurse for a home evaluation.

> ### *Clinical Alert Report*
> - Advise ancillary staff/student to report changes in mobility, respirations, bowel movements, and skin condition and any complaints of leg pain.

RISK FOR FALLS

NANDA-I Definition

Vulnerable to increased susceptibility to falling that may cause physical harm and compromised health.

Risk Factors

Pathophysiologic

Related to altered cerebral function secondary to hypoxia
Related to syncope, vertigo, or dizziness
Related to impaired mobility secondary to:

Cerebrovascular accident   Parkinsonism
Arthritis

Related to loss of limb
Related to impaired vision
Related to hearing impairment
Related to fatigue
Related to orthostatic hypotension

Treatment Related

Related to lack of awareness of environmental hazards secondary to confusion
Related to improper use of aids (e.g., crutches, canes, walkers, wheelchairs)
Related to tethering devices (e.g., IV, Foley, compression therapy, telemetry)
Related to prolonged bed rest
Related to side effects of medication(s)

Situational (Personal, Environmental)

Related to history of falls
Related to improper footwear
Related to unstable gait

Older Adult

Related to faulty judgments, secondary cognitive deficits
Related to sedentary lifestyle and loss of muscle strength
Related to fear of falling and the resulting physiologic deconditioning

Author's Note

All individuals in health care facilities are at risk for falls because of factors such as medication side effects, unfamiliar environment, and equipment; thus, routine fall prevention strategies are initiated for all individuals in the facility. However, some individuals are at high risk for falls, such as frail elderly, individuals with cognitive or mobility impairments. Additional Interventions are indicated, and these individuals are identified as High Risk for Falls.

Goals

NOC
Risk Control, Fall Occurrence, Fall Prevention Behavior, Personal Safety Behavior, Safe Home Environment

The individual will not injure himself or herself during hospital stay as evidenced by the following indicators:

- Identify factors that increase risk of injury.
- Describe appropriate safety measures.
- Will agree to ask for help when needed.

Interventions

NIC
Fall Prevention; Environmental Management: Safety, Health Education; Surveillance: Safety, Risk Identification; Technology Management; Medication Management; Family Involvement Promotion; Environmental Management: Home Preparation

> **CLINICAL ALERT:**
> - The Centers of Disease Control and Prevention (CDC) (2015b) reports:
>   - One out of three older adults (those aged 65 or older) falls each year, but less than half talk to their health care providers about it.
>   - Among older adults, falls are the leading cause of both fatal and nonfatal injuries.
>   - In 2013, 2.5 million nonfatal falls among older adults were treated in emergency departments, and more than 734,000 of these individuals were hospitalized.
>   - Over 95% of hip fractures are caused by falls.15 Each year, there are over 258,000 hip fractures, and the rate for women is almost twice the rate for men.17
>   - One out of five hip fractures individuals (16.9%) dies within a year of injury.

Involve All Hospital Personnel on Every Shift in the Fall Prevention Program

R: Approximately 14% of all falls in hospitals are accidental, another 8% are unanticipated physiologic falls, and 78% are anticipated physiologic falls.

- Always glance into the room of a high-risk person when passing his or her room.
- Alert other departments of high-risk individuals when off unit for tests, procedures.
- Address fall prevention and risks with every hand-off and transfer.
- Seek to identify reversible risk factors in all individuals. Be aware of changing individual conditions and a change in risk status.

- Identify in a private conference room the number of falls on the unit monthly (e.g., poster).

  R: Intradisciplinary approach to fall prevention is effective when falls are viewed not as inevitable accidents but as preventable events.

Identify the Individual's Risk for Falls

- Refer to Index for Fall Risk Assessment.
- Assess the person's ability to Timed Up and Go (TUG) (*Podsiadlo & Richardson, 1991). Refer to TUG in index for instructions.

  R: Numerous researchers have reported that the TUG test is reliable (87% sensitivity and specificity) for community-dwelling older adults (Beling & Roller, 2009). Loss of strength in legs and ankles is a common cause of falls in older persons; however, it is not an outcome of aging, but one of a sedentary lifestyle. It is not inevitable; it is preventable.

Identify High-Risk Individuals, and Initiate the Institution's Standard and Protocol to Prevent Falls

- One example is:

  Both Carondelet St. Joseph's Hospital (Tucson, AZ) and Providence Health Center used the Ruby Slippers Program as part of their fall prevention programs. Patients at high risk of falling were provided with a pair of bright red double treaded slipper socks. Staff throughout both organizations were oriented to the fact that patients wearing these socks were at high risk of falling. Staff not involved in direct patient care (for example, housekeepers) knew to summon help if they observed these patients trying to get out of bed or if they saw them unattended. At St. Joseph's, a picture of a ruby slipper on the door to patient rooms also alerted staff that the patient was at high risk of falling, whereas Providence used a red falling star on the doors and charts to identify these patients for staff. (Lancaster et al., 2007, p. 372)

R: Standard interventions to prevent any individual from falling are instituted on admission. In addition, high-risk individuals are identified using the institution's protocol (e.g., red slippers, colored bracelet.) Ensure that tables and chairs with side arms are stable. Persons with lower extremity weakness will benefit from sturdy chairs.

Reduce or Eliminate the Following Contributing Factors for Falls

Related to Unfamiliar Environment

- Orient to his or her environment (e.g., location of bathroom, bed controls, call bell). Leave a light on in the bathroom at night. Ensure that path to bathroom is clear.

  R: Orientation helps provide familiarity; a light at night helps the individual find the way safely.

- Teach him or her to keep the bed in the low position with side rails up at night.

  R: The low position makes it easier for the individual to get in and out of bed.

- Make sure that the telephone, eyeglasses, urinal, and frequently used personal belongings are within easy reach.

  R: Keeping objects at hand helps prevent falls due to overreaching and overextending.

- Instruct to request assistance whenever needed.

  R: Getting needed help with ambulation and other activities reduces an individual's risk of injury.

- For individuals with difficulty accessing toilet:
  - If urgency exists, evaluate for a urinary tract infection.

    R: New-onset urinary urgency can be a sign of an infection.

  - Provide an opportunity to use bathroom/urinal/bedpan every 2 hours while awake, at bedtime, and upon awakening.

    *R: Thirty percent of falls are related to attempting to access the bathroom and can be prevented by timed toileting schedule (*Alcee, 2000).*

- Frequently scan floor for wet areas, objects on floor.
  - Implement an elimination protocol (e.g., Toileting rounds every hour to offer bathroom assistance).

    R: Providing regular times for elimination can reduce getting OOB to toilet or incontinence.

Related to Gait Instability/Balance Problems

- Explain that gait and balance problems are due to underuse and deconditioning, *not aging*.
- Alert individuals that they may not be able to prevent a fall if they trip.

  R: Weak leg muscles and decreased range of motion (ROM) in ankles prevent a safe recovery from a slip or trip.

- Refer to Getting Started for strategies and exercises to improve gait and balance on thePoint.
- Instruct to wear slippers with nonskid soles and to avoid shoes with thick, soft soles.

  R: These precautions can help prevent falls from slipping. Thick soles require adequate lifting of feet as one walks, or the soles will catch and trip the person.

- Ensure that mobility aids are available and reachable. Wheelchairs should always be locked. Remind that IV poles are on wheels and are not sturdy.

  R: Falls occur when an individual is reaching for a mobility aid or for a wheelchair not in the locked position.

- Ensure that call bell, TV controls, and telephone are within reach.

  R: Stretching and reaching can contribute to rolling out of bed.

Related to Tethering Devices (IVs, Foley, Telemetry, Compression Devices)

- Evaluate whether tethering devices can be discontinued at night.
- Can the IV be converted to a saline port?
- If the individual is competent, teach him or her how to ambulate safely with devices to bathroom or advise to call for assistance.

  R: Individuals can become entangled in lines and tubes and fall.

Related to Medication Side Effects

- Review the person's medication reconciliation completed on admission.
  - Question regarding alcohol use.

    R: Alcohol can potentiate side effects of sombulence/dizziness.

  - Question whether the person has side effects when taking certain meds.
  - Question whether, in the person's opinion, he or she is taking a medication for pain that is not working.

    R: Some medications might need to be discontinued because of side effects or ineffective therapeutic response.

- Review with pharmacist/physicians/nurse practitioner the present medications, and evaluate those that can contribute to dizziness and whether they should be discontinued, have dose reduced, or replaced with an alternative (Kaufmann & Kaplan, 2015; *Riefkohl, Heather, Bieber, Burlingame, & Lowenthal, 2003).
  - Antidepressants (e.g., SSRIs)
  - Antipsychotics
  - Benzodiazepines
  - Antihistamines (e.g., Benadryl, hydroxyzine)
  - Anticonvulsants
  - Nonsteroidal anti-inflammatory drugs
  - Muscle relaxants
  - Narcotic analgesics
  - Antiarrhythmics (type 1A)
  - Digoxin

    *R: The use of medications is one of the many different factors that can contribute to balance problems and the risk of falls. Published research suggests an association between the use of these drugs or drug class and an increased risk of falling (*Riefkohl et al., 2003).*

Related to Confused/Uncooperative/Impaired Cognition

- Consider use of electronic devices in bed, chair, video surveillance.
- Follow institutional policy for side rails.
- Consider use of sitter.
- Move person to a more observable room.
- Plan to complete shift documentation in room of high-risk person.

R: In some cases, extra measures are necessary to ensure an individual's safety and prevent injury to him or her and others. The cost of extra surveillance will be less than the cost of injury and human suffering related to a fall.

- Explain that deficiencies in vitamin D interfere with one's postural balance, propulsion, and navigation and that vitamin B_{12} deficiencies cause weakness, tiredness, or light-headedness. Seek to include vitamin D, vitamin B_{12} levels in next laboratory tests. Explain that the normal range is 30 to 100 nmol/L.

  R: Vitamin D supplements improve gait performance and prevent falls by more than 22% in older adults (Annweiler et al., 2010). Researchers have reported that the level should be at least 60 nmol/L to effect a reduction of falls (Annweiler et al., 2010).

If a Person Falls or Reports a Fall

- Call out for help immediately, and continue to attend to the individual.
- Implement the following:
  - Do not move initially.
  - *If person hit head or if unknown, immobilize cervical spine.*
  - Assess whether loss of consciousness was experienced, or whether there are complaints of pain, or individual is confused.
  - Take baseline vital signs, blood glucose.
  - Determine baseline Glasgow Coma Scale.
  - Assess risk for intracranial bleed (anticoagulants, thrombocytopenia, coagulopathy).
  - Assess for lacerations, fractures, contusions, decreased ROM.
  - Clean and dress any wounds.
  - Implement neuro checks q 2 hours × 24 hours.
  - Contact the appropriate physician/nurse practitioner to discuss findings and implications.

    R: Immediate assessment with notification of medical staff is indicated in order to determine the extent of injuries and the need for diagnostic tests and or treatments.

SBAR *Situation:* Ask individual and witnesses what happened and at what time, and also get details about location and who witnessed it.

Background: Prior fall risk score? History of falls?

Assessment: Evaluate the following:

Side rails up/down	Fall risk alerts present (placards, wristband)	
Position of bed	Call light reachable	Sitter present
Nonskid footwear	Use of assistive devices	Visitors present
Presence of clutter	Bed alarm on	Presence of IV, Foley
Staffing ratios		

Recommendation: Communicate identified factors that caused or contributed to the fall.

- Engage in a postfall huddle within 1 hour of fall. Involve all staff. Avoid all discussions of blaming. Refer Institution's protocol for documentation guidelines of postfall huddles.

  R: Postfall huddles can identify falls amenable to prevention interventions as individual education, staff heightened awareness, and reduction of risk factors (*Gray-Miceli, Johnson, & Strumpf, 2005).

Teach Strategies to Decrease Risk of Falling at Home

- Ensure proper use of assistive devices. Consult with physical therapist.

  R: Expert instruction is needed to ensure proper equipment and use.

- Perform ankle-strengthening exercises daily (*Schoenfelder & Crowell, 1999*):
  - Stand behind a straight chair, with feet slightly apart.
  - Slowly raise both heels until body weight is on the balls of the feet; hold for a count of three (e.g., 1 Mississippi, 2 Mississippi, 3 Mississippi).
  - Do 5 to 10 repetitions; increase repetitions as strength increases.
- Walk at least two or three times a week.
  - Use ankle exercises as a warm-up before walking.
  - Begin walking with someone at side, if needed, for 10 minutes.
  - Increase time and speed according to capabilities.

> *R:Ankle strengthening and a walking program can improve balance, increase ankle strength, improve walking speed, decrease falls and fear of falling, and increase confidence in performing activities of daily living (*Schoenfelder & Crowell, 1999).*

- Go to thePoint and access Getting Started for take-home guidelines to prevent falls at home, and exercises to improve muscle strength and balance.

DEFICIENT FLUID VOLUME

NANDA-I Definition

Decreased intravascular, interstitial, and/or intracellular fluid. This refers to dehydration, water loss alone without change in sodium

Author's Note

Deficient Fluid Volume is frequently used to describe people who are NPO, in hypovolemic shock, or experiencing bleeding. This author recommends its use only when an individual can drink but has an insufficient intake for metabolic needs. If the individual cannot drink or needs intravenous therapy, refer to the collaborative problems in Section 2: *Risk for Complications of Hypovolemia* and *Risk for Complications of Electrolyte Imbalances.*

Defining Characteristics

Insufficient oral fluid intake	Dry skin*/mucous membranes*
Negative balance of intake and output	Weight loss
Increased serum sodium	Thirst*/nausea/anorexia
Concentrated urine or urinary frequency	Decreased urine output* or excessive urine output

Related Factors

Pathophysiologic

Related to excessive urinary output:

Uncontrolled diabetes
Diabetes insipidus

Related to increased capillary permeability and evaporative loss from burn wound (nonacute)
Related to losses secondary to:

Abnormal drainage	Excessive menses
Diarrhea	Fever or increased metabolic rate

Situational (Personal, Environmental)

Related to nausea/vomiting
Related to decreased motivation to drink liquids secondary to:

Depression
Fatigue

Related to high-solute tube feedings
Related to difficulty swallowing or feeding self secondary to:

Oral or throat pain   Fatigue

Related to excessive loss through (specify)
Related to excessive use of:

Laxatives or enemas
Diuretics, alcohol, or caffeine

Older Adult
Related to increased vulnerability secondary to decreased fluid reserve and decreased sensation of thirst

Goals

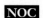 **NOC**
Electrolyte and Acid–
Base Balance, Fluid
Balance, Hydration

The individual will maintain urine-specific gravity within normal range as evidenced by the following indicators:

- Increase fluid intake to a specified amount according to age and metabolic needs.
- Identify risk factors for fluid deficit, and relate need for increased fluid intake as indicated.
- Demonstrate no signs and symptoms of dehydration.

Interventions

 NIC
Fluid/Electrolyte
Management, Fluid
Monitoring

Assess Causative Factors

Prevent Dehydration in High-Risk Individuals

- Monitor individual intake; ensure at least 2,000 mL of oral fluids every 24 hours unless contraindicated. Offer fluids that are desired hourly.
- Teach the individual to avoid coffee, tea, grapefruit juice, sugared drinks, and alcohol.

  R: Output may exceed intake, which may already be inadequate to compensate for insensible losses. Coffee, tea, grapefruit juice, sugared drinks, and alcohol have diuretic effects.

- Monitor output; ensure at least 0.5 mL/kg/hr.

  R: Monitoring of output will help to evaluate hydration status early.

- Monitor urine and serum electrolytes, blood urea nitrogen, osmolality, creatinine, hematocrit, and hemoglobin.

  R: These laboratory studies will reflect hydration status.

- Review the individual's medications. Do the medications contribute to dehydration (e.g., diuretics)? Do they require increased fluid intake (e.g., lithium)?

  R: Certain medications can contribute to dehydration.

Initiate Health Teaching as Indicated

- Give verbal and written directions for types of fluids and amounts needed at home.
- Include the individual/family in keeping a written record of fluid intake, output, and daily weights, if indicated.
- Explain the need to increase fluids during exercise, fever, infection, and hot weather.
- Teach the individual/family how to observe for dehydration (especially in infants, elderly) and to intervene by increasing fluid intake.

  R: Careful monitoring after transition will be needed for at-risk individuals.

 Clinical Alert Report
- Advise ancillary staff/student to report a decrease in usual urine output and oral intake.

EXCESS FLUID VOLUME

NANDA-I Definition

Increased isotonic fluid retention

Author's Note

Excess Fluid Volume is frequently used to describe pulmonary edema, ascites, or renal failure. These are all collaborative problems that should not be renamed as *Excess Fluid Volume*. Refer to Section 2 for collaborative problems such as *Risk for complications of renal/urinary dysfunction* or *pulmonary edema* or *hepatic dysfunction*. The interventions below focus on preventing or reducing peripheral edema. Nursing interventions center on teaching the individual or family how to minimize edema and protect tissue.

Defining Characteristics

Edema (peripheral, sacral)   Taut, shiny skin
Intake greater than output   Weight gain

Related Factors

Pathophysiologic

Related to portal hypertension, lower plasma colloidal osmotic pressure, and sodium retention secondary to:

Liver disease   Cirrhosis
Cancer   Ascites

Related to venous and arterial abnormalities secondary to:

Varicose veins   Phlebitis   Infection
Peripheral vascular disease   Immobility   Trauma
Thrombus   Lymphedema   Neoplasms

Treatment Related

Related to sodium and water retention secondary to corticosteroid therapy
Related to inadequate lymphatic drainage secondary to mastectomy

Situational (Personal, Environmental)

Related to excessive sodium intake/fluid intake
Related to a malnutrition
Related to dependent venous pooling/venostasis secondary to:

Standing or sitting for long periods   Tight cast or bandage
Immobility

Related to venous compression from pregnant uterus
Related to impaired venous return secondary to increased peripheral resistance and decreased efficiency of valves secondary to:

Aging   Obesity

Goals

NOC
Electrolyte Balance,
Fluid Balance, Hydration

The individual will relate:

• Causative factors.
• Methods of preventing edema.

Interventions

Identify Contributing and Causative Factors

NIC
Electrolyte
Management, Fluid
Management, Fluid
Monitoring, Skin
Surveillance, Nutritional
Counseling, Weight
Reduction Assistance

> **CLINICAL ALERT:**
> • Peripheral edema is caused by an alteration in capillary hemodynamics that favors the movement of fluid from the vascular space into the interstitium and/or the retention of dietary or intravenously administered sodium and water by the kidneys (Alguire & Scovell, 2015). Obesity is associated with sleep apnea and venous insufficiency.

• Explain the causes of chronic venous insufficiency, for example, family history of varicose veins, being overweight, being pregnant, not exercising enough, smoking, and standing or sitting for long periods of time (Alguire & Scovell, 2015).

R: Any problem that increases pressure in the veins in the legs can stretch the veins. This can damage the valves, leading to even higher pressures and worsened vein function, and can eventually lead to chronic venous disease (Alguire & Scovell, 2015).

Reduce or Eliminate Causative and Contributing Factors

High-Salt Diet (Dudek, 2014)

* Request a consult of nutritionist.
* Explain why salt intake contributes to leg edema.

  R: Excess dietary salt causes fluid retention, which increases capillary filtration pressure, which results in peripheral edema (Dudek, 2014).

* Assess dietary intake and habits that may contribute to fluid retention.
* Explain high-sodium foods, including salted snacks, bacon, cheese, olives, pickles, soy sauce, processed lunchmeats, monosodium glutamate (MSG), canned vegetables, ketchup, and mustard.
* Teach how to read labels for sodium content.
* Avoid canned vegetables; choose fresh or frozen.
* Cook without salt; use spices (e.g., lemon, basil, tarragon, mint) to add flavor.
* Use vinegar in place of salt to flavor soups, stews, etc. (e.g., 2 to 3 teaspoons of vinegar to 4 to 6 quarts, according to taste).
* Ascertain whether the individual may use salt substitute (caution that he or she must use the exact substitute prescribed).

  R: High-sodium intake leads to increased water retention. Drugs, such as antacids, are also high in sodium.

Dependent Venous Pooling

* Assess for evidence of dependent venous pooling or venous stasis.
* Encourage alternating periods of horizontal rest (legs elevated) with vertical activity (standing); this may be contraindicated in CHF.
  * Keep the edematous extremity elevated above the level of the heart whenever possible (unless contraindicated by heart failure).
  * Keep the edematous arms elevated on two pillows or with IV pole sling.
  * Elevate the legs whenever possible, using pillows under them (avoid pressure points, especially behind the knees).
  * Discourage leg and ankle crossing.

    R: These strategies reduce venous stasis by promoting lymphatic flow movement back into circulatory system.

* Reduce constriction of vessels.
* Assess clothing for proper fit and constrictive areas.
* Instruct the individual to avoid knee-highs and leg crossing and to practice elevating the legs when possible.
* Apply stockings while lying down (e.g., in the morning before arising).
* Check extremities frequently for adequate circulation and evidence of constrictive areas.

  R: Edema inhibits blood flow to the tissue, resulting in poor cellular nutrition and increased susceptibility to injury.

Overweight/Obesity

* Refer to *Obesity/Overweight* nursing diagnosis.

Sedentary Lifestyle

* Refer to thePoint, Getting Started to Moving More.

Protect Edematous Skin From Injury

* Inspect skin for redness and blanching.
* Reduce pressure on skin areas; pad chairs; use knee-high stockings and footstools.
* Prevent dry skin.
* Use soap sparingly.
* Rinse off soap completely.
* Use a lotion to moisten skin.

  R: Edema inhibits blood flow to the tissues, resulting in poor cellular nutrition, increased susceptibility to injury, and diminished healing ability.

Initiate Health Teaching and Referrals as Indicated

- Consider home care nurses referral to follow at home.
- Instruct to weigh self daily and record the weight.
- Instruct to call a primary care provider for a weight gain greater than 2 lb/day or increased shortness of breath at night or on exertion. Explain that these signs may indicate early heart problems and will require medication to prevent them from worsening.

R: Home management of edema will require specific instructions and monitoring. Readmission for heart failure often results from failure to take medications or from ignoring early signs of an exacerbation.

> ### *Clinical Alert Report*
> - Advise ancillary staff/student to report any signs/symptoms of edema, redness, tissue irritation/breakdown.

GRIEVING

NANDA-I Definition

A normal complex process that includes emotional, physical, spiritual, social, and intellectual responses and behaviors by which individuals, families, and communities, incorporate an actual, anticipated, or perceived loss into their daily lives.

Defining Characteristics

The individual reports an actual or perceived loss (person, pet, object, function, status, or relationship) with varied responses such as the following:

Denial	Disorganization
Suicidal thoughts	Feelings of worthlessness
Guilt	Numbness
Crying	Disbelief
Anger	Anxiety
Sorrow	Helplessness
Despair	

Related Factors

Many situations can contribute to feelings of loss. Some common situations follow.

Pathophysiologic

Related to loss of function or independence secondary to:

Loss of body part (planned, sudden)
Congenital anomaly
Sudden loss of function (e.g., amputation, ostomy)
Illness
Trauma
Visible scars

Treatment Related

Related to losses associated with:

Long-term dialysis
Surgery (e.g., mastectomy)

Situational (Personal, Environmental)

Related to losses associated with the death of someone's pet
Related to the losses associated with chronic pain and terminal illness
Related to losses in lifestyle associated with empty nest, divorce, and separation

Maturational

Related to losses/changes attributed to aging such as:

Friends
Function
Relocation (e.g., assisted living, living with adult children)
Occupation, retirement

Author's Note

Grieving, Anticipatory, and *Complicated Grieving (CG)* represent three types of responses of individuals or families experiencing a loss. *Grieving* describes normal grieving after a loss and participation in grief work. *Anticipatory Grieving* describes engaging in grief work before an expected loss. Refer to Palliative Care Plan for Interventions for Anticipated Grieving. *CG* represents a maladaptive process in which grief work is suppressed or absent or an individual exhibits prolonged exaggerated responses. The nurse should consult with a mental health nurse practitioner or physician.

In many clinical situations, the nurse expects a grief response (e.g., loss of body part, death of significant other). Other situations that evoke strong grief responses are sometimes ignored or minimized (e.g., abortion, newborn death, death of one twin or triplet, death of secret lover, suicide, loss of children to foster homes, or adoption).

Goals

NOC
Coping, Family Coping, Grief Resolution, Psychosocial Adjustment, Life Change

The individual will express his or her grief, as evidenced by the following indicators:

* Describe the meaning of the death or loss to him or her.
* Share his or her grief with significant others.

Interventions

Promote a Trust Relationship

Carp's Cues

NIC
Family Support, Grief Work Facilitation, Coping Enhancement, Anticipatory Guidance, Emotional Support

Too often, nurses believe that they must have the answers for individuals who are suffering. This belief creates a barrier, and the nurse is afraid she or he will say the wrong thing, so nothing is said. A nurse can gently touch a grieving person and say, "I am sorry for your loss," "I am so sorry you have cancer." This communication can create a flood of emotion and tears. This nurse should be proud that he or she is willing to enter this darkness because the true professional nurse is one who can sit in the cave of darkness and not talk about the light.

* Create a therapeutic milieu (convey that you care). "I am sorry." Provide a presence of simply "being" with the bereaved.
* Communicate clearly, simply, and to the point.
* Never try to lessen the loss (e.g., "She didn't suffer long"; or "You can have another baby").
* Offer support and reassurance.
* Establish a safe, secure, and private environment.
* Provide privacy, but be careful not to isolate the individual or family inadvertently.

R: Grief work cannot begin until the individual acknowledges the loss. Nurses can encourage this acknowledgment by engaging in open, honest dialogue, providing the family an opportunity to view the dead person, and recognizing and validating the grief (*Vanezis & McGee, 1999).

> **CLINICAL ALERT:** The following tasks of *Grieving* have been identified by Worden (*2002) and can assist the nurse in identifying the individual's current progression in the grief process:
> Task 1: To accept the reality of loss
> Task 2: To feel the pain of grief
> Task 3: To adjust to an environment in which the deceased is missing
> Task 4: To emotionally relocate the deceased and move on with life

Assess the Present Grief Response

• Ambivalence, Anger, Denial, Depression, Fear, Guilt

Explain the Normalcy of the Emotional and Physical Responses to a Significant Loss

• Emotional responses: Numbness, shock, anger, frustration, irritation, misdirected hostility, denial, sadness, fear, loneliness, relief, guilt, yearning, helplessness, a sense of being out of control, "Nothing seems real"
• Physical responses: Shakiness, edginess, insomnia, lack of energy, weakness
• Dry mouth, increased perspiration, stomach hollowness, "butterflies"
• Headache, chest or throat pain or tightness, breathlessness

> *R: Research findings have refuted the notion that grief is neat, orderly, linear, and completed at an arbitrary point (Wright & Hogan, 2008). Acknowledging that grief responses are expected and normal can support an anxious, grieving individual (*Hooyman & Kramer, 2006).*

> *R: Grief in older adults is often related to losses within the self, such as changes in roles or body image or decreased body function. These losses sometimes are less easily accepted than is the loss of a significant other (Miller, 2015).*

Demonstrate Respect for the Individual's Culture, Religion, and Values

> *R: Bereavement is a universal stressor, but the magnitude of stress and its meaning vary cross-culturally. The dominant US culture assumes that the death of a child is more stressful than that of an older relative. This belief can encourage nurses to ignore the profound grief experienced when one loses an older mother or father.*

Acknowledge the Difficulties and the Differences in Grief Related to HIV-Related Bereavement

• HIV-related bereavement is distinguished from other types of grief "with multiple losses and the overwhelming task of living in a situation where continual loss has become commonplace" (Kain, 2016).
• Disenfranchised grief occurs when social stigma is associated with a death or an illness (e.g., suicide, AIDS); the grieving person may be alone, emotionally isolated, or fearful of public expressions of grief (*Bateman, 1999; Lemming & Dickinson, 2010).
• Complex social issues of morality, sexuality, contagion, and shame associated with AIDS-related losses interfere with the process of bereavement and healing (*Cotton et al., 2006; *Mallinson, 1999).
• Gay men who have experienced multiple AIDS-related losses (e.g., loss of friends and community, disintegrating family structures and social networks) may receive little understanding from heterosexuals (*Cotton et al., 2006; *Mallinson, 1999).

Promote Family Cohesiveness

> *R: Understanding and strengthening families at the end of life and during bereavement are essential for health maintenance or restoration (O'Mallon, 2009).*

• Support the family at its level of functioning.

> *R: Each family member has his or her own perception of making sense of a loved one's death (O'Mallon, 2009).*

• Encourage self-exploration of feelings with family members.
• Explain the need to discuss behaviors that interfere with relationships.
• Recognize and reinforce the strengths of each family member.

> *R: Social supports, strong religious beliefs, and good prior mental health are resources that decrease psychosocial and physical dysfunction (*Hooyman & Kramer, 2006; Miller, 2015).*

Determine Signs/Symptoms of Complicated Grief (Shear, 2012)

R: "The difference between CG and normal grief is related to the heightened intensity and longer persistence of acute grief symptoms and to the presence of complicating processes" (Shear, 2012).

- Obsessed about the circumstances of the death
- Excessive worry about its consequences, or
- Excessive avoidance of reminders of the loss.
- Withdrawal from friends /family
- Difficulty in controlling strong emotions of sadness, guilt, envy, anger

R: About 7% of bereaved people do not cope effectively with bereavement (Kersting & Wagner, 2012).

Refer for Counseling Individuals/Families at High Risk for Complicated Grieving

R: CG can be reliably identified and responds best to specific treatment. Treatment targets resolving complications and facilitating healing, with addressing loss and restoration-related issues (Shear, 2012).
R: Research validates that professional interventions and professionally supported voluntary and self-help services are capable of reducing the risk of psychiatric and psychoanalytic disorders resulting from bereavement.

Provide Health Teaching and Referrals, as Indicated

Teach the Individual and Family Signs of Resolution

- Grieving person no longer lives in the past, but is future oriented and establishes new goals.
- Grieving person redefines relationship with the lost object/person.
- Grieving person begins to resocialize.

Identify Agencies that May be Helpful (e.g., Community Agencies, Religious Groups)

RISK FOR COMPROMISED HUMAN DIGNITY

NANDA-I Definition

At risk for perceived loss of respect and honor

Risk Factors

Treatment Related

Related to multiple factors associated with hospitalization, institutionalization, supervised group living environments, or any health care environment
Examples of factors are:

- Unfamiliar procedures
- Intrusions for clinical procedures
- Multiple, unfamiliar personnel
- Assistance needed for personal hygiene
- Painful procedures
- Unfamiliar terminology

Situational (Personal, Environmental)

Related to the nature of restrictions and environment of incarceration

Carp's Cues

Risk for Compromised Human Dignity was accepted by NANDA-I in 2006.

This nursing diagnosis presents a new application for nursing practice. All individuals are at risk for this diagnosis. Providing respect and honor to all individuals, families, and communities is a critical core element of professional nursing. Prevention of compromised human dignity must be a focus of all nursing interventions. It is the central concept of a caring profession.

This author recommends that this diagnosis be developed and integrated into a Standard Care of the Nursing Department for all individuals and families. The outcomes and interventions apply to all individuals, families, and groups. This Department of Nursing Standards of Practice could also include *Risk for Infection, Risk for Infection Transmission, Risk for Falls, and Risk for Compromised Family Coping.*

Goals

Refer to Generic Medical Care Plan.

Interventions

Refer to Generic Medical Care Plan.

BOWEL INCONTINENCE

NANDA-I Definition

Change in normal bowel habits characterized by involuntary passage of stool

Defining Characteristics*

Constant dribbling of soft stool
Fecal odor
Fecal staining of bedding
Fecal staining of clothing
Inability to delay defecation
Inability to recognize urge to defecate
Inattention to urge to defecate
Recognizes rectal fullness, but reports inability to expel formed stool
Red perianal skin
Self-report of inability to recognize rectal fullness
Urgency

Related Factors

Pathophysiologic (Robson & Lombo, 2015)

Related to rectal sphincter abnormality/Anal sphincter weakness secondary to:

Anal or rectal surgery   Peripheral neuropathy
Obstetric injuries   Anal or rectal injury

Related to overdistention of rectum secondary to chronic constipation
Related to overflow secondary to fecal retention and fecal impaction
Related to loss of rectal sphincter control secondary to:*

Cerebral vascular accident   Multiple sclerosis
Spinal cord compression   Progressive neuromuscular disorder
Spinal cord injury

Related to impaired reservoir capacity secondary to chronic rectal ischemia, inflammatory bowel disease*

Treatment Related

Related to impaired reservoir capacity secondary to colectomy, radiation proctitis, ulcerative proctitis, and proctectomy

Situational (Personal, Environmental)

Related to inability to recognize, interpret, or respond to rectal cues secondary to impaired cognition, depression neuropathy associated with diabetes mellitus, multiple sclerosis, dementia, meningomyelocele, and spinal cord injuries

Goals

NOC
Bowel Continence,
Tissue Integrity

The individual will evacuate a soft, formed stool every other day or every third day:

* Relate bowel elimination techniques.
* Describe fluid and dietary requirements.

> **CLINICAL ALERT:**
> * Fecal incontinence is one of the leading causes of institutionalization. It has a significant social and economic impact and significantly impairs quality of life (Robson & Lombo, 2015).
> * "Only 15% to 20% of individuals with urinary incontinence and 43% of those with fecal incontinence seek professional care for the problem" (Wilde, Bliss, Booth, Cheater, & Tannenbaum, 2014).

Interventions

NIC
Bowel Incontinence
Care, Bowel Training,
Bowel Management,
Skin Surveillance

Assess Contributing Factors

* Refer to Related Factors.

Assess the Individual's Ability to Participate in Bowel Continence

* Ability to reach toilet
* Control of rectal sphincter
* Intact anorectal sensation
* Orientation, motivation

> *R: To maintain bowel continence, an individual must have access to a toileting facility, be able to contract puborectals and external anal sphincter muscles, have intact anorectal sensation, be able to store feces consciously, and must be motivated and able to recognize bowel cues.*

Plan a Consistent, Appropriate Time for Elimination

* Institute a daily bowel program for 5 days or until a pattern develops, then move to an alternate-day program (morning or evening).
* Provide privacy and a nonstressful environment.
* Offer reassurance, and protect from embarrassment while establishing the bowel program.

> *R: Long-standing constipation or fecal impaction causes overdistention of the rectum by feces. This causes continuous reflex stimulation, which reduces sphincter tone. Incontinence will be either diarrhea leaking around the impaction or leaking of feces from a full rectum.*

* Implement prompted voiding program.

> *R: Research has shown prompted voiding results in an increase in bowel continence.*

* Assess perirectal tissue.

> *R: GI enzymes can erode tissue, cause discomfort, and increase the risk of infections.*

Consult With Physical Therapy for a Bowel Elimination Program

Explain Fluid and Dietary Requirements for Good Bowel Movements

* Ensure that individual drinks 8 to 10 glasses of water daily.
* Ensure diet high in bulk and fiber. Consider a bulking agent (e.g., methylcellulose 1 to 2 tablespoons/day).

R: Stool consistency and volume are important for continence. Large volumes of loose stool overwhelm the continence mechanism. Small, hard stools that do not distend or stimulate the rectum do not alert the individual of the need to defecate (*Bliss et al., 2001; Wilde et al., 2014).

Avoid Foods and Drinks That Cause Loose or Frequent Bowel Movements

- Examples include:
  - Dairy foods (for people who have trouble with dairy)
  - Spicy foods
  - Fatty or greasy foods
  - Drinks with caffeine, such as coffee
  - Diet foods or drinks
  - Sugar-free gum or candy
  - Alcohol

Advise to Eat Smaller Meals, More Often

- In some people, eating a large meal triggers the urge to have a bowel movement. It can also cause diarrhea. Eating smaller and more frequent meals can reduce the number of bowel movements you have.

Consult With Prescribing Professional for Antidiarrheal Agent

R: These medications reduce fecal incontinence. A systematic review of antidiarrheal therapy found a reduction in fecal urgency, episodes of incontinence, unformed stools, and use of pads (Omar & Alexander, 2013).

Initiate Health Teaching as Indicated

- Explain the hazards of using stool softeners, laxatives, suppositories, and enemas.
- Explain the signs and symptoms of fecal impaction and constipation.
- Ensure comprehension of a bowel program before discharge. If the individual is functionally able, encourage independence with the bowel program; if not, incorporate assistive devices or attendant care, as needed.
- Explain the effects of stool on the skin and ways to protect the skin (refer to *Diarrhea* for interventions).

  R: Laxatives cause unscheduled bowel movements, loss of colon tone, and inconsistent stool consistency. Enemas can overstretch the bowel and decrease tone. Stool softeners are not needed with adequate food or fluid intake.

- Emphasize self-management of condition
  - Advise to keep a change of underwear and toileting supplies in their car, handbag, briefcase, or backpack, and to wear darker clothing when away from home, if soiling should occur (Wilde et al., 2014).
  - Advise to use antidiarrheal medications on an as-needed, preemptory basis—such as before attending a public function (Wilde et al., 2014).

  R: Self-management behaviors use self-monitoring with individuals "becoming more knowledgeable about their needs and the management strategies that work best for them" (Wilde et al., 2014).

> ### *Clinical Alert Report*
> - Advise ancillary staff/student to report the number of bowel movements, character, and skin condition.

RISK FOR INFECTION

NANDA-I Definition

At risk for being invaded by pathogenic organisms

Risk Factors

See Related Factors.

Related Factors

Various health problems and situations can create favorable conditions that would encourage the development of infections.* Some common factors follow.

Pathophysiologic

Related to compromised host defenses secondary to:

Cancer	Renal failure	Alcoholism
Altered or insufficient leukocytes	Hematologic disorders	Immunosuppression*
Arthritis	Hepatic disorders	Immunodeficiency secondary to (specify)
Respiratory disorders	Diabetes mellitus*	
Periodontal disease	AIDS	

Related to compromised circulation secondary to:

Lymphedema	Obesity*	Peripheral vascular disease

Treatment Related

Related to a site for organism invasion secondary to:

Surgery	Dialysis	Total parenteral nutrition
Invasive lines	Intubation	Enteral feedings

Related to compromised host defenses secondary to:

Radiation therapy
Organ transplant
Medication therapy (specify) (e.g., chemotherapy, immunosuppressants)

Situational (Personal, Environmental)

Related to compromised host defenses secondary to:

History of infections	Prolonged immobility	Increased hospital stay
Malnutrition*	Stress	Smoking

Related to a site for organism invasion secondary to:

Trauma (accidental, intentional)	Bites (animal, insect, human)
Postpartum period	Thermal injuries
Warm, moist, dark environment (skinfolds, casts)	

Related to contact with contagious agents (nosocomial or community acquired)

Author's Note

All people are at risk for infection and increased wen in a health care facility. Thus *Risk for Infection* represents the activation of a standard of care to prevent infection, for example, handwashing, catheter-care protocols.

Secretion control, environmental control, and handwashing before and after contact can reduce the risk of transmission of organisms. Included in the population of those at risk for infection is a smaller group who are at high risk for infection. High *Risk for Infection* describes a person whose host defenses are compromised, thus increasing susceptibility to environmental pathogens or his or her own endogenous flora (e.g., a person with chronic liver dysfunction or with an invasive line). Nursing interventions for such a person focus on minimizing the introduction of organisms and increasing resistance to infection (e.g., improving nutritional status). For a person with an infection, the situation is best described by the collaborative problem *Risk for Complications of Sepsis/SIRS* (in Unit II Section 2).

Refer to Unit II Section I for *Risk for Infection* for infection prevention interventions.

RISK FOR INFECTION TRANSMISSION[2]

Definition

The state in which an individual is at risk for transferring an opportunistic or pathogenic agent to others

Risk Factors

Presence of risk factors (see Related Factors).

Related Factors

Pathophysiologic

Related to:

Colonization with highly antibiotic-resistant organism
Airborne transmission exposure (sneezing, coughing, spitting)
Contact transmission exposure (direct, indirect, contact droplet)
Vehicle transmission exposure (food, water, contaminated drugs or blood, contaminated sites [IV, catheter])
Vector-borne transmission exposure (animals, rodents, insects)

Treatment Related

Related to exposure to a contaminated wound
Related to devices with contaminated drainage (e.g., urinary, chest, endotracheal tubes, suction equipment)

Situational (Personal, Environmental)

Related to:

Unsanitary living conditions (sewage, personal hygiene)
Areas considered high risk for vector-borne diseases (malaria, rabies, bubonic plague)
Areas considered high risk for vehicle-borne diseases (hepatitis A, *Shigella*, *Salmonella*)
Exposures to sources of infection such as:
   Intravenous/intranasal/intradermal drug use (sharing of needles, drug paraphernalia [straws])
   Contaminated sex paraphernalia
   Multiple sex partners
   Natural disaster (e.g., flood, hurricane)
   Disaster with hazardous infectious material

Goals

NOC
Infection Status, Risk Control, Risk Detection

The individual will describe the mode of transmission of disease by the time of discharge as evidenced by the following indicators:

• Relate the need to be isolated until noninfectious (e.g., TB).
• Relate factors that contribute to the transmission of the infection.
• Relate methods to reduce or prevent infection transmission.
• Demonstrate meticulous handwashing.

Interventions

NIC
Teaching: Disease Process, Infection Control, Infection Protection

Identify People Who Are Susceptible for Infection and With a History of Exposure

Refer to *Risk for Infection* for Preventive Interventions in Health Care Settings

---

[2]This diagnosis is not currently on the NANDA-I list, but has been included for clarity or usefulness.

Teach the Mode of Transmission Based on Infecting Agent

- Airborne
- Contact:
    - Direct
    - Indirect
    - Contact droplet
- Vehicle-borne
- Vector-borne

  R: To prevent transmission of infection, the mode of transmission (i.e., airborne, contact, vehicle-borne, or vector-borne) must be known. For example, tuberculosis is spread airborne by coughing, sneezing, and spitting.

Related to Lack of Knowledge of Reducing the Risk of Transmitting HIV

Identify Susceptible Individuals

- Homosexual practices
- Bisexual practices
- Intravenous/intranasal/intradermal drug users
- Blood transfusions before 1985
- Multiple sexual partners with sexually transmitted infections
- Health care workers
- Tattoo by unlicensed persons
- First responders (e.g., police, rescue workers, ambulance, firefighters)

Counsel Susceptible Individuals to Be Tested for HIV

R: Testing can confirm whether the individual is HIV positive, which can then be treated.

Discuss the Mode of Transmission of the Virus

- Unprotected vaginal, anal, or oral sex with infected hosts or infected sex paraphernalia
- Unprotected sex with infected person
- Sharing intravenous needles and syringes; intranasal drug paraphernalia
- Contact of infected fluids with broken skin or mucous membrane
- Breastfeeding, perinatal transmission (when the pregnant woman and/or newborn are not treated)

  R: HIV is transmitted when infected body fluids/blood enters the vascular system of another.

Use Appropriate Universal Precautions for All Body Fluids

- Refer to *Risk for Infection* for specific precautions.
- Place used syringes immediately in a nearby impermeable container; do not recap or manipulate the needle in any way! Use retractable needle syringes when possible.

  R: Needlesticks can transmit infectious blood.

Teach How to Reduce the Risk of Transmission of HIV

- Explain low-risk sexual behaviors (e.g., mutual masturbation, intercourse with condom).

  R: The risk of developing sexually transmitted infections is prevented with abstinence. Activities that do not include penile, vaginal, anal, or oral contact carry low or no risk. Transmission is reduced by condom use and limiting partners.

- Explain other risks such as alcohol and drug use, sex aids, and having multiple partners.

  R: Use of alcohol and drugs reduces the individual's ability to make safe decisions regarding sexual activity. The risk of acquiring HIV increases as the number of partners increases.

- Teach individual to use condoms of latex rubber, not "natural membrane"; teach appropriate storage to preserve latex. Avoid spermicides with nonoxynol-9.
- Explain the need for water-based lubricants to reduce prophylactic breaks. Avoid petroleum-based lubricants, which dissolve latex.
- Explain that a condom with a spermicide may provide additional protection by decreasing the number of viable HIV particles.

  R: Nonoxynol-9 spermicides may increase the risk of HIV transmission. Natural membrane condoms do not prevent transfer of infected fluids.

Teach the Individual How to Disinfect at Home (e.g., Needles, Syringes, Drug Paraphernalia, Sex Aids)

- Wash under running water.
- Fill or wash with household bleach.
- Rinse well with water.

  R: Exposure to disinfecting agents rapidly inactivates HIV. Household bleach solution (dilute 1:10 with water) is an inexpensive choice.

Initiate Health Teaching and Referrals as Indicated

- Emphasize the need to be careful when choosing sex partners (past sexual partners, experimentation with drugs).
- Provide the community and schools with facts regarding AIDS transmission, and dispel myths.
- In a case of acute exposure to HIV (e.g., sexual assault, needlestick, break in barrier with HIV-infected person), immediately refer to health care facility for immediate initiation of postexposure prophylaxis of antiviral therapy.
- Refer to primary care provider to discuss the use of antiviral therapy to prevent HIV infection in HIV-negative persons.

  R: Protocols for exposure to body fluids possibly contaminated with HIV are available in all health care facilities. The FDA has approved the use of antiviral therapy in HIV-negative persons.

- Ensure that caregivers of HIV-positive individuals are knowledgeable regarding transmission and prevention.

  R: Misinformation can increase fears and unnecessarily isolate the individual and significant others.

LATEX ALLERGY RESPONSE

NANDA-I Definition

A hypersensitive reaction to natural latex rubber products

Defining Characteristics

Positive skin or serum test to natural rubber latex (NRL) extract
Allergic conjunctivitis
Urticaria
Rhinitis
Asthma

Carp's Cues

The prevalence of latex sensitization/allergy skyrocketed in the mid- to late-1990s owing to a significant increase in the use of latex gloves by clinicians and other health care employees (clinicians, nurses, dentists, laboratory workers, housekeepers, emergency medical technicians, patient transporters) (Hamilton, 2015). In response, there was widespread avoidance of powdered latex gloves in many hospitals, which resulted in a marked decrease in the number of new cases of latex allergy among health care workers and individuals receiving multiple surgeries in the US (Hamilton, 2015).

Frequent exposure to airborne latex has contributed to latex allergies. All individuals who do not have latex allergies should use nonpowder latex gloves to reduce inhalation (DeJong et al., 2011).

Related Factors

Biopathophysiologic

Related to hypersensitivity response to the protein component of NRL

Goals

NOC
Immune
Hypersensitivity
Control

The individual will report no exposure to latex as evidenced by the following indicators:

- Describe products of NRL.
- Describe strategies to avoid exposure.

Interventions

NIC
Allergy Management,
Latex Precautions,
Environmental Risk
Protection

Assess for the Presence of Food Allergies

- Food allergies that have high, moderate, or low prevalence with natural latex rubber allergies (American Latex Allergy Association, 2016)
  - High (Banana, Avocado, Chestnut, Kiwi)
  - Moderate (Apple, Carrot, Celery, Papaya, Potato, Tomato, Melons)
  - Low or undetermined (Pear, Mango, Sweet Pepper, Peach, Rye, Cayenne Pepper, Plum, Wheat, Shellfish, Cherry, Hazelnut, Sunflower Seed, Pineapple, Walnut, Citrus Fruits, Strawberry, Soybean, Coconut, Fig, Peanut, Chick Pea, Grape, Buckwheat, Castor Bean, Apricot, Dill, Lychee, Passion Fruit, Oregano, Zucchini, Nectarine, Sage, Persimmon)

  R: Individuals with certain food allergies may also have a coexisting latex allergy (American Latex Allergy Association, 2016).

- Collect personal history of any of the following:
  - Asthma
  - Urticaria
  - Contact dermatitis
  - Conjunctivitis
  - Eczema
  - Rhinitis
  - Anaphylactic reaction

  R: Frequently, individuals report they have a latex allergy. With further assessment, the latex allergy report may be able to be confirmed or ruled out.

- If there is a high clinical suspicion of latex allergy, consult with physician/nurse practitioner/allergy specialist for diagnostic testing for serum antilatex IgE.

  R: Skin testing or detection of Hevea-specific IgE in serum is used to confirm sensitization (Hamilton, 2015).

> **CLINICAL ALERT:**
> - If latex allergy or risk for latex allergy is confirmed or suspected, initiate the institution's protocol (e.g., armband, placards on beds and room entrances).

Teach Which Products are Commonly Made of Latex

- For a comprehensive listing, refer to American Latex Allergy Association (2016) accessed at http://latexallergyresources.org

Initiate Health Teaching as Indicated

- Explain the importance of completely avoiding direct contact with all NRL products.
- Advise that an individual with a history of a mild skin reaction to latex is at risk for anaphylaxis.
- Instruct the individual to wear a Medic-Alert bracelet stating "Latex Allergy" and to carry auto-injectable epinephrine.
- Evaluate whether the individual/family know what to do if an allergic reaction occurs (e.g., antihistamine, EpiPen, when to seek emergency treatment). Provide directions or access directions from physician/nurse practitioner or primary care provider.
- Advise to carry nonlatex gloves.

  R: Latex substitutes may not be available at all health care facilities or offices.

  R: The individual/family need to be aware of prevention strategies and actions to take if an allergic reaction occurs.

- Instruct the individual to warn all health care providers on each encounter (e.g., dental, provider/specialist appointments, surgical) of allergy.

  R: All personnel may not be aware of allergy even if it is documented.

> **Clinical Alert Report**
> - Advise ancillary staff/student to report immediately any signs of inflammation or c/o itchy eyes, runny nose, conjunctivitis, urticaria, and rhinitis.
> - Advise to report to nurse anyone who does not follow latex allergy protocol.

RISK FOR LATEX ALLERGY RESPONSE

NANDA-I Definition

Risk of hypersensitivity to natural latex rubber products that may compromise health

Risk Factors

Biopathophysiologic

Related to history of atopic eczema
Related to history of allergic rhinitis
*Related to history of asthma**

Treatment Related

*Related to multiple surgical procedures, especially beginning in infancy**
Related to frequent urinary catheterizations (e.g., spina bifida individuals)
Related to frequent rectal impaction removal
Related to frequent surgical procedures
Related to barium enema (before 1992)

Situational (Personal, Environmental)

*Related to history of allergies**

History of food allergy to banana, kiwi, avocado, chestnuts, tropical fruits (mango, papaya, passion fruit), poinsettia plants,* tomato, raw potato, peach
History of allergy to gloves, condoms, and so forth
Frequent occupational exposure to NRL,* such as:
   Workers making NRL products
   Food handlers
   Greenhouse workers
   Housekeepers
   Health care workers

General Considerations

Refer to *Latex Allergy Response.*

Focus Assessment Criteria

Refer to *Latex Allergy Response.*

Goals

NOC
Immune
Hypersensitivity Control

Refer to *Latex Allergy Response.*

Interventions

NIC
Allergy Management,
Latex Precautions,
Environmental Risk
Protection

Refer to *Latex Allergy Response.*

NAUSEA

NANDA-I Definition

A subjective phenomenon of an unpleasant feeling in the back of the throat and stomach that may or may not result in vomiting

Defining Characteristics*

Aversion toward food   Reports nausea
Increased swallowing   Increased salivation
Gagging sensation   Reports sour taste in mouth

Related Factors

Biopathophysiologic

Related to tissue trauma and reflex muscle spasms secondary to:

Gastrointestinal disorders   Drug overdose
Acute gastroenteritis   Pancreatitis
Peptic ulcer disease   Renal calculi
Infections (e.g., food poisoning)   Uterine cramps associated with menses
Irritable bowel syndrome   Motion sickness

Treatment Related

Related to effects of chemotherapy, theophylline, digitalis, antibiotics, iron supplements
Related to effects of anesthesia

Situational (Personal, Environmental)*

Anxiety   Pain
Noxious odors, taste   Psychological factors
Fear   Unpleasant visual stimulation

Goals

NOC
Comfort Level,
Nutrition Status,
Hydration

The individual will report decreased nausea as experienced by the following indicators:

- Name foods or beverages that do not increase nausea.
- Describe factors that increase nausea.

Interventions

NIC
Medication
Management, Nausea
Management,
Fluid/Electrolyte
Management, Nutrition
Management

- Aggressive management before, during, and after chemotherapy can prevent nausea (Yarbro, Wujcik, & Gobel, 2011).

    R: The objective of antiemetic therapy is the complete prevention of chemotherapy-induced nausea and vomiting (CINV), which is achievable in the majority of individuals receiving chemotherapy, even with highly emetic agents (Hesketh, 2015).

- Refer to Care Plan for individual receiving chemotherapy in Unit III Section 3.
- Determine the number of risk factors for postoperative nausea and vomiting (PONV) using the simplified risk score from Apfel.
- Consult with anesthesiologist/nurse anesthetist to prevent postoperative nausea and vomiting intraoperatively and postoperatively (Pasero & McCaffery, 2011).
- Use multimodal analgesics to reduce the dose of opioids to lowest possible.
- Use multimodal antiemetics preinduction and at the end of surgery.

    R: Postoperative nausea and vomiting can cause aspiration, tension on sutures, increased intracranial or intraocular pressure, and fluid and electrolyte imbalances (Pasero & McCaffery, 2011).

- Promote comfort during nausea and vomiting.
- Protect those at risk for aspiration (immobile, children).
- Address the cleanliness of the person and environment.
- Provide an opportunity for oral care after each episode.
- Apply a cool, damp cloth to the person's forehead, neck, and wrists.

    R: Comfort measures also reduce the stimuli for vomiting.

> **CLINICAL ALERT:**
> - Vomiting episodes should have an etiology.
> - Address reducing or preventing the stimulus or consult with physician/nurse practitioner for pharmacologic interventions.

Teach Acupressure at Pressure Points on His /Her Inner Wrist
(*Hickman, Bell, & Preston, 2005)

- Monitor for more specific instructions, if needed.
- Position your hand as shown.
- To find pressure point P-6, place the first three fingers of your opposite hand across your wrist. Then place your thumb on the point just below your index finger. You should be able to feel two large tendons under your thumb.
- Press on this point with your thumb or forefinger, and apply a circular motion for 2 to 3 minutes. The pressure should be firm but not cause discomfort.
- Repeat the process on your other wrist.
- Another option is wearing an acupressure band on wrist.

    *R: Acupressure has been proven to be effective for nausea after some surgeries, and discomforts related to cancer and treatments (Doran & Halm, 2010; *Hickman, Bell, & Preston 2005; *Streitberger et al., 2004).*

Reduce or Eliminate Noxious Stimuli

Pain
- Plan care to avoid unpleasant or painful procedures before meals.
- Medicate individuals for pain 30 minutes before meals according to physician/nurse practitioner's orders.
- Provide a pleasant, relaxed atmosphere for eating (no bedpans in sight; do not rush).
- Arrange the plan of care to decrease or eliminate nauseating odors or procedures near mealtimes.

Fatigue
- Advise to rest before meals.
- Teach the individual to spend minimal energy preparing food (cook large quantities, and freeze several meals at a time; request assistance from others).

Odor of Food

- Teach the individual to avoid cooking odors—frying food, brewing coffee—if possible (take a walk; select foods that can be eaten cold).
- Suggest using foods that require little cooking during periods of nausea.
- Suggest trying sour foods.

    R: Unpleasant sights or odors can stimulate the vomiting center.

Decrease Stimulation of the Vomiting Center

- Reduce unpleasant sights and odors.
- Teach individual to practice deep breathing and voluntary swallowing to suppress the vomiting reflex. Restrict activity.
- Explain ginger as a treatment for nausea/vomiting, for example, ginger ale (with real ginger), candied ginger.

    R: Meta-analysis supports benefits of ginger for seasickness, motion sickness, and postoperative nausea and vomiting, and pregnancy nausea/vomiting (Thomas, Corbin, & Leung, 2014).

- Restrict liquids with meals to avoid overdistending the stomach; also, avoid fluids 1 hour before and after meals.
- Encourage individual to sit in fresh air or use a fan to circulate air.

    R: The above strategies reduce gastric pressure and decrease stimuli that induce nausea and vomiting.

- Instruct the person to sit down after eating. Loosen clothing. Advise individual to avoid lying flat for at least 2 hours after eating.

    R: A person who must rest should sit or recline so the head is at least 4 inches higher than the feet to reduce gastro reflex.

- Suggest complementary approaches as music therapy and visual imagery.

    R: Music can serve as a diversional adjunct to antiemetic therapy (*Ezzone, Baker, Rosselet, & Terepka, 1998). Positive music therapy and visual imagery has positive effects on chemotherapy-induced anxiety, nausea and vomiting (Karagozoglu, Tekyasar, & Yilmaz, 2013).

- Offer muscle relaxation and distraction techniques to adult cancer patients.

    R: Both muscle relaxation and distraction techniques have been found to decrease nausea and vomiting in adults receiving chemotherapy (Cooke, 2015; *Miller & Kearney, 2004; Vasterling, *Jenkins, Tope, & Burish, 1993).

- Reinforce strategies utilized in hospital to prevent/reduce nausea.
- Advise individual to call primary care provider if nausea or vomiting continues or recurs.

> ### *Clinical Alert Report*
> - Advise ancillary staff/student to report increases in nausea, decrease in oral intake, and/or vomiting (description, amount, presence of blood).

UNILATERAL NEGLECT

NANDA-I Definition

Impairment in sensory and motor response, mental representation, and special attention of the body, and the corresponding environment characterized by inattention to one side and overattention to the opposite side. Left-side neglect is more severe and persistent than right-side neglect.

Defining Characteristics

Neglect of involved body parts and/or extrapersonal space (hemispatial neglect), and/or denial of the existence of the affected limb or side of body (anosognosia).

Positive Prevost's sign (with both eyes and the head fixed toward the right. This ipsilesional deviation of the head and eyes is specific to Unilateral Neglect (Becker & Karnath, 2010; *Berger et al., 2006).

Difficulty with spatial-perceptual tasks.

Hemiplegia (usually of the left side).

Related Factors

Pathophysiologic

Related to the impaired perceptual abilities secondary to:

Cerebrovascular accident (CVA)*
Brain injury/trauma
Cerebral aneurysms
Cerebral tumors
Infection (e.g., meningitis, encephalitis)
Refer to CVA for goals and interventions for *Unilateral Neglect*

IMBALANCED NUTRITION

NANDA-I Definition

Intake of nutrients insufficient to meet metabolic needs

Carp's Cues

Nurses are usually the primary diagnosticians and are usually the primary professionals for improving nutritional status. *Imbalanced Nutrition* is not a difficult diagnosis to validate. However, before interventions can be determined, it is necessary to identify the contributing factors, which are usually multiple and complex.

Nurses should not use this diagnosis to describe people who are NPO or cannot ingest food. For example, Imbalanced Nutrition related to parenteral therapy and NPO status.

This diagnosis represents a situation with which nurses are intricately involved (parenteral therapy). From a nutritional perspective, however, what interventions do nurses prescribe to improve the nutritional status of an NPO individual? Parenteral nutrition in an individual who is NPO influences several actual or potential responses that nurses treat, representing both nursing diagnoses, such as *Risk for Infection* and *Impaired Comfort*, and the collaborative problems *Risk for Complications of Hypovolemia* and *Risk for Complications of Negative Nitrogen Balance*.

Many factors influence food habits and nutritional status: personal, family, cultural, financial, functional ability, nutritional knowledge, disease and injury, and treatment regimens. Imbalanced Nutrition describes people who can ingest food but eat an inadequate or imbalanced quality or quantity. For instance, the diet may have insufficient protein or excessive fat. Quantity may be insufficient because of increased metabolic requirements (e.g., cancer, pregnancy, trauma, or interference with nutrient use [e.g., impaired storage of vitamins in cirrhosis]).

Defining Characteristics

The individual who is not NPO reports or is found to have food intake less than the recommended daily allowance (RDA) with or without weight loss
and/or
Actual or potential metabolic needs in excess of intake with weight loss
Weight 10% to 20% or more below ideal for height and frame
Triceps skinfold, midarm circumference, and midarm muscle circumference less than 60% standard measurement
Muscle weakness and tenderness
Mental irritability or confusion
Decreased serum prealbumin

Related Factors

Pathophysiologic

Related to increased caloric requirements and difficulty in ingesting sufficient calories secondary to:

Burns (postacute phase)	Chemical dependence
Cancer	GI complications/deformities
Infection	AIDS
Trauma	

Related to dysphasia secondary to:

CVA	Cerebral palsy
Muscular dystrophy	Neuromuscular disorders
Amyotrophic lateral sclerosis	Möbius syndrome
Parkinson's disease	Cleft lip/palate

Related to decreased absorption of nutrients secondary to:

Crohn's disease	Necrotizing enterocolitis
Lactose intolerance	Cystic fibrosis

Related to decreased desire to eat secondary to altered level of consciousness
Related to self-induced vomiting, physical exercise in excess of caloric intake, or refusal to eat secondary to anorexia nervosa
Related to reluctance to eat for fear of poisoning secondary to paranoid behavior
Related to anorexia, excessive physical agitation secondary to bipolar disorder
Related to anorexia and diarrhea secondary to protozoal infection
Related to vomiting, anorexia, and impaired digestion secondary to pancreatitis
Related to anorexia, impaired protein and fat metabolism, and impaired storage of vitamins secondary to cirrhosis
Related to anorexia, vomiting, and impaired digestion secondary to GI malformation or necrotizing enterocolitis
Related to anorexia secondary to gastroesophageal reflux
Related to anorexia secondary to indigestion, bloating, pain
Related secondary to gastric ulcer

Treatment Related

Related to protein and vitamin requirements for wound healing and decreased intake secondary to surgery, surgical reconstruction of mouth, radiation therapy, medications (chemotherapy), wired jaw
Related to inadequate absorption as a medication side effect of (specify) (Gröber & Kisters, 2007):

Colchicine	Antibiotics (clotrimazole, rifampicin)
Neomycin	Dexamethasone
Pyrimethamine	Antihypertensives (nifedipine, spironolactone)
para-Aminosalicylic acid	Antiretroviral drugs (ritononavir, saquinavir)
Antacid	Herbal medicines: Kava kava
Antiepileptics	St. John's wort (hyperforin)
Antineoplastic drugs	

Related to decreased oral intake, mouth discomfort, nausea, and vomiting secondary to:

Radiation therapy	Chemotherapy
Tonsillectomy	Oral trauma

Situational (Personal, Environmental)

Related to decreased desire to eat secondary to (specify):

Social isolation	Stress
Depression	Allergies
Nausea and vomiting	Excessive chronic alcohol intake

Related to increased metabolic rate with decreased intake secondary to the effects of substance abuse (e.g., cocaine, amphetamines)
Related to inability to procure food (physical limitation or financial or transportation problems)
Related to inability to chew (e.g., damaged or missing teeth, ill-fitting dentures)
Related to diarrhea secondary to (specify)*

Author's Note
Because of their 24-hour presence, nurses are usually the primary professionals responsible for improving nutritional status. Although *Imbalanced Nutrition* is not a difficult diagnosis to validate, interventions for it can challenge the nurse. Secondary screening for individuals determined to be at increased risk for nutritional deficits are performed by clinical nutritionists.

Many factors influence food habits and nutritional status: personal, family, cultural, financial, functional ability, nutritional knowledge, disease and injury, and treatment regimens. Imbalanced Nutrition: describes people who can ingest food but eat an inadequate or imbalanced quality or quantity. For instance, the diet may have insufficient protein or excessive fat. Quantity may be insufficient because of increased metabolic requirements (e.g., cancer, pregnancy, trauma, or interference with nutrient use [e.g., impaired storage of vitamins in cirrhosis]).

Nurses should not use this diagnosis to describe individuals who are NPO or cannot ingest food. They should use the collaborative problems *Risk for Complications of Fluid/ Electrolyte Imbalance* or *Risk for Complications of Negative Nitrogen Balance* to describe those situations.

Goals

NOC
Nutritional Status, Teaching: Nutrition, Symptom Control

The individual will ingest daily nutritional requirements in accordance with activity level and metabolic needs as evidenced by the following indicators:

* Relate importance of good nutrition for healing and preventing complications.
* Identify deficiencies in daily intake.
* Relate methods to increase appetite.

> **CLINICAL ALERT:**
> * In 2013, 85.7% of US households were food secure throughout the year. The remaining 14.3% (17.5 million households) were food insecure (Coleman-Jensen, Gregory, & Singh, 2013).
> * In 2013, 5.6% of US households (6.8 million households) had very low food security, essentially unchanged from 5.7% in 2011 and 2012 (Coleman-Jensen et al., 2013).

Interventions

NIC
Nutrition Management, Weight Gain Assistance, Nutritional Counseling

Ensure a Nutritional Screening Assessment Is Done on Admission According to Protocols

* Deficiencies identified in the screening assessment should be referred to a nutritionist.

   R: Nutritional Screening Assessments are required within 24 hours of admission to a hospital and within 14 days of admission to a long-term facility (The Joint Commission, 2015). One survey reported nurses were primarily responsible for nutrition screening, while dietitians had primary responsibility for assessment (Patel, Romano, & Corkins, 2014).

Evaluate the Appropriateness of Attempting to Increase Food/Fluid Intake in Individuals at the End of Life

* Refer to Unit III Section I Palliative Care Plan.

   R: Researchers report that "increased caloric intake may neither reverse weight loss nor improve survival" in individuals with end-stage disease (e.g., cancer, CHF, COPD, renal failure) (Cunningham & Hubmann, 2011).

Reinforce the Need for Adequate Consumption of Carbohydrates, Fats, Protein, Vitamins, Minerals, and Fluids

* Refer to Table II.1.

   R: Nutrients provide energy sources, build tissue, and regulate metabolic processes.

* When indicated, consult with a nutritionist to establish appropriate daily caloric and food-type requirements for the individual (Dudek, 2014; Hockenberry & Wilson, 2015).

   R: The body requires a minimum level of nutrients for health and growth. During the life span, nutritional needs vary.

* Assess whether there are cultural preferences in regard to food.
* Address the factors that are causing or contributing to decreased intake.
   * Related to decreased oral intake, mouth discomfort, nausea, and vomiting secondary to (e.g., depression, side effects of treatments).
   * Related to inability to chew.
   * Access a dental consult.

Table II.I Age-Related Daily Nutritional Requirements

Age	Daily Nutritional Requirements
Infants	
Newborn	100–120 kcal/kg/day for growth
2–3 months	12–18 oz formula or breast milk
4–5 months	20–30 oz formula or breast milk
6–7 months	25–35 oz formula or breast milk; strained vegetables and fruits; egg yolks
8–11 months	28–40 oz formula or breast milk; above solids, plus meat, finger foods
1–2 years	24 oz formula or breast milk; three regular meals, chopped table food
	24 oz formula or breast milk; 100 kcal/kg same as 8–11 months
Children	
Preschool (3–5 years)	90 kcal/kg; 76 g/kg protein
	Basic food groups
	Calcium 500–800 mg
School (6–12 years)	80 kcal/kg; 1.2 g/kg protein
	Basic food groups (as preschool)
	11 mg calcium
	400 units vitamin D
	1.5–3 L water
Adolescent (13–17 years)	2,200–2,400 kcal for girls
	3,000 kcal for boys
	Basic food groups (as preschool)
	50–60 g protein
	1,100 mg calcium (to age 25)
	400 units vitamin D
Adults	1,600–3,000 kcal range (based on physical activity, emotional state, body size, age, and individual metabolism)
	Basic food groups
	Men need increased protein, ascorbic acid, riboflavin, and vitamins E and B6
	Women need the above as well as increased iron, calcium, and vitamins A and B12
Pregnant women (second and third trimesters)	Daily calorie requirement
	11–15 years: 2,500
	16–22 years: 2,400
	23–50 years: 2,300
	Increase protein 10 g or 1 serving meat
	1.2–3.5 g calcium
	Increase vitamins A, B, and C
Lactating women	30–60 mg iron
	2,500–3,000 kcal (500 more than regular diet)
	Basic food groups
	4 servings protein
	5 servings dairy
	4+ servings grain
	5+ servings vegetables
	2+ servings vitamin C-rich
	1+ green leafy
	2+ others
	Fluids 2–3 qt (1 qt milk)
	Increase in vitamins A and C, niacin
Older than 65 years	Basic food groups (same as adult)
	Caloric requirements decrease with age (1,600–1,800 for women; 2,000–2,400 for men), but dependent on activity, climate, and metabolic needs
	Ensure intake of essential amino acids, fatty acids, vitamins, elements, fiber, and water
	60 mg ascorbic acid
	40–60 mg protein
	1,200 mg calcium (1,500 mg for women not taking estrogen)
	10 mg iron

Sources: Dudek, S. (2014). *Nutrition essentials for nursing practice.* Philadelphia, PA: Wolters Kluwer; Lutz, L., Mazur, E., & Litch, N. (2015). *Nutrition and diet therapy* (6th ed.). Philadelphia, PA: FA Davis.

- Related to decreased oral intake, mouth discomfort, nausea, and vomiting secondary to (e.g., radiation therapy, tonsillectomy, chemotherapy).
- Refer to specific care plans for radiation or chemotherapy. Refer to *Impaired Oral Mucous Membranes* in Unit II Section 1.

Assess for Factors That Contribute to Nutritional Deficiencies in Older Individuals (Lutz, Mazur, & Litch, 2015)

- Explain that their sense of smell and taste will diminish with aging, which may result in decreased intake due to bland taste and oversalting of foods (Miller, 2015).

  R: Seventy-five percent of individuals over 85 years old have decreased sense of smell. Smell is required for the sense of taste to function (Lutz et al., 2015).
- Explain the need to drink sufficient fluids even when not thirsty. Hydration can be evaluated by color of urine (e.g., goal is light yellow).

  R: The thirst sensation is diminished and can result in uncompensated dehydration.
- Explain that delayed gastric emptying can create bloating and decreased intake.

  R: Intestinal motility decreases with aging.
- Advise to reduce fluids with meals and to increase foods higher in protein (e.g., eggs, milk, cheese).
- Related to barriers of food procurement/preparation.

  R: Barriers affect functional ability, financial, transportation, and kitchen facilities.
- Refer to nutritionist/social services for an assessment and interventions.

Evaluate Whether Lactose Intolerance Is Present

R: The prevalence of primary lactose intolerance varies according to race. As many as 25% of the White population (prevalence in those from southern European roots) is estimated to have lactose intolerance, whereas among Black, Native American, and Asian American populations, the prevalence of lactose intolerance is estimated at 75% to 90% (Roy, 2011).

Identify Factors Such as Pain, Fatigue, Analgesic Use, and Immobility That Can Contribute to Anorexia

R: Identifying a possible cause enables interventions to eliminate or minimize it.

- When possible, attempt to have some socialization during mealtime (e.g., suggest to family that they eat with the individual, to bring permitted foods from home, if possible).

  *R: Evidence-based analysis demonstrates that nursing home residents who get up, get dressed, and get out of their rooms for meals are better nourished and better hydrated than their counterparts who eat in their rooms. In addition, those who do eat outside their rooms have increased mobility, greater socialization, and less depression than those who eat in-room (Shepherd, 2011; *Simmons & Levy-Storms, 2005).*
- Encourage and help the individual to maintain good oral hygiene.

  R: Poor oral hygiene leads to bad odor and taste, which can diminish appetite.

To Increase Intake, Teach the Individual to

- Arrange to serve the highest protein/calorie nutrients when the individual feels most like eating (e.g., if chemotherapy is in the early morning, serve food in the late afternoon).
- Eat dry foods (e.g., toast, crackers) on arising.
- Try salty foods, if permissible.
- Avoid overly sweet, rich, greasy, or fried foods.
- Try clear, cool beverages. Sip slowly through a straw.
- Try whatever the individual feels can be tolerated.
- Eat small portions low in fat. Eat more frequently.
- Review high-calorie versus low-calorie foods. Avoid empty-calorie foods (e.g., soda).
- Encourage significant others to bring in favorite home foods.

- Try commercial supplements available in many forms (e.g., liquids, powder, pudding); keep switching brands until some are found that are acceptable to the individual in taste and consistency.

  R: Varied techniques should be attempted to increase intake of nutritious foods and beverages. Attempts to vary the taste and texture can improve appetite and prevent food aversion.

Provide for Supplemental Dietary Needs Amplified by Acute Illness

R: Metabolic demands are increased by the catabolic processes that occur through stages of acute illness, usually increasing nutritional demand (Dudek, 2014).

Initiate Health Teaching and Referrals as Needed

- Refer to thePoint for a printable handout on "Getting Started to Better Nutrition."
- Refer to Dietary Guidelines for Americans at http://www.health.gov/dietaryguidelines/dga2010/dietaryguidelines2010.pdf

Initiate Health Teaching and Referrals, as Indicated

- Dietitian for meal planning
- Psychiatric therapy when indicated
- Community meal centers

  R: Resources in the community can assist the individual and family.

> ### *Clinical Alert Report*
> Before providing care, advise ancillary staff/student to report the following to the professional nurse assigned to the individual:
> - Significant decline in food and/or fluid intake
> - Urine darker than pale yellow

OBESITY

NANDA-I Definition

A condition in which an individual accumulates abnormal or excessive fat for age and gender that exceeds overweight.

Defining Characteristics

Adult: BMI of >30
Child <2 years: Term not applicable /not used with infants/children at this age
Child 2 to 18 years: BMI of >30 or >95th percentile for age and gender

Related Factors

Pathophysiologic

Genetic disorder
Heritability of interrelated factors (e.g., adipose tissue distribution, energy expenditure, lipoprotein lipase activity, lipid synthesis, lipolysis)

Situational (Personal, Environmental)

Average daily physical activity is less than recommended for gender and age
Consumption of sugar-sweetened beverages
Disordered eating behaviors
Disordered eating perceptions
Economically disadvantaged
Energy expenditure below energy intake based on standard assessment (e.g., WAVE assessment)
Excessive alcohol consumption
Fear regarding lack of food supply
Formula- or mixed-fed infants
Frequent snacking
High disinhibition and restraint eating behavior score
High frequency of restaurant or fried food
Low dietary calcium intake in children
Maternal diabetes mellitus
Maternal smoking
Parental obesity
Portion sizes larger than recommended
Sedentary behavior occurring for >2 hr/day
Shortened sleep time
Sleep disorder

Maturational

Maternal smoking
Overweight in infancy
Parental obesity
Portion sizes larger than recommended
Premature pubarche
Rapid weight gain during childhood
Rapid weight gain during infancy, including the first week, first 4 months, and first year
Sedentary behavior occurring for >2 hr/day
Shortened sleep time
Sleep disorder
Solid foods as major food source at <5 months of age

Author's Note

Given the public health problem of *Overweight* and *Obesity* across the life span, the above three diagnoses are excellent additions to NANDA-I Classification. The interventions for these diagnoses will focus on strategies to motivate and engage individuals/families to proceed to a healthy lifestyle.[3]

Obesity is a complex condition with sociocultural, psychological, and metabolic implications. When the focus is primarily on limiting food intake, as with many weight-loss programs, as bariatric as surgery, the chance of permanent weight loss is slim. To be successful, a weight-loss program in an individual needs to focus on behavior modification and lifestyle changes through exercise, decreased intake, and addressing their emotional component of overeating.

If someone is at a healthy weight, but routinely eats foods low in nutrients use *Risk-Prone Health Behavior* related to intake of insufficient nutrients that does not meet recommended dietary intake and/or inactivity in the presence of a healthy weight. For some people with dysfunctional eating, *Ineffective Coping* related to increased eating in response to stressors would be valid and require a referral after discharge.

---

[3]Imbalanced and Risk for Imbalance Nutrition has been deleted from the NANDA-I Classification.

Goals

NOC
Nutritional Status:
Nutrient Intake, Weight
Control, Exercise
Participation, Infant
Nutritional Status,
Weight Body Mass,
Adherence Behavior:
Healthy Diet, Weight
Loss Behavior

The individual will commit to a weight-loss program, as evidenced by the following indicators:

- Identify the patterns of eating associated with consumption/energy expenditure imbalance.
  - Can give examples of nutrient-dense foods versus those with "empty calories."
- Can identify three ways to increase his/her activity.
- Commit to increasing foods with high nutrient density and less with "empty calories."
- Commit to making 3 to 5 changes in food/fluid choices that are healthier.

Interventions

Carp's Cues

Individuals who are very ill are not ready for discussions about lifestyle changes.

NIC
Self-Efficacy
Enhancement,
Self-Responsibility
Enhancement,
Nutritional Counseling,
Weight Management,
Teaching: Nutrition (age
appropriate), Behavioral
Modification, Exercise
Promotion, Coping
Enhancement

Provide them with sources of help. Go to the Point and print Getting Started .... for example, smoking, to lose weight, move more; and provide it to the individual.

Refer to Appendix C Strategies to Increase Motivation and Engagement in Individuals /Families; For Specific Techniques to Improve Activation and Engagement

For Individuals Who Are Not Acutely Ill, Initiate Discussion: "How Can You Be Healthier?"

- Focus on the person's response (e.g., stop smoking, exercise more, eat healthier, and cut down on drinking).
- Refer to index for interventions for the targeted lifestyle change.

  R: The nurse should be cautioned against applying a nursing diagnosis for an overweight or obese person who does not want to participate in a weight-loss program. Motivation for weight loss must come from within.

Before a Person Can Change, He or She Must (Martin, Haskard, Zolnierek, & DiMatteo, 2010)

- Know what change is necessary (information) and why.
- Desire the change (motivation); and
- Have the tools to achieve and maintain the change (strategy).
- Trust the health care professional, who has a sympathetic presence (Pelzang, 2010).

  R: Empathic communication involving a thorough understanding of the individual's perspective improves adherence. Individuals who are informed and affectively motivated are also more likely to adhere to their treatment recommendations (*Martin, Williams, Haskard, & DiMatteo, 2005).

If Appropriate, Gently and Expertly Discuss the Hazards of Obesity, But Respect a Person's Right to Choose, the Right of Self-Determination

- Ask, "How do you think being overweight affects you?"

To Help to Activate Engagement in an Individual

- Ask one of the following questions. Pick the best question that applies to this person. Focus on only one or two effects of obesity on health. Use language they understand (e.g., blood tubes).
  - Do your legs swell during the day and go back to normal during the night?
    - Explain that fat tissue compresses tubes in the legs and prevents fluids from circulating well. Eventually, the swelling will be permanent, lasting the whole day, and will cause difficulty walking and wearing shoes.

- Do you have high blood pressure, or is it getting a little higher each year?
  - Explain that blood vessels are damaged when excess weight puts pressure on them and they stretch, become thinner, and lose their strength. Your heart now has to pump harder/causing high blood pressure. Over time, the heart enlarges and cannot pump well. This is heart failure.
- Are your cholesterol levels increasing each year?
  - Explain that the stretching of your blood vessels damages the inside of the blood tubes. Cholesterol sticks to the damaged tubes and slows the blood flow to your kidneys, eyes, brain, and legs. This can cause strokes, renal failure, vision problems, and blood clots in your legs.
- Although you may not feel that anything is wrong, high blood pressure can permanently damage your heart, brain, eyes, and kidneys before you feel anything. Even losing 10 lb can reduce your blood pressure.
  - Is your blood glucose test getting a little higher each year? Is there diabetes in your family?
  - Explain that the more fatty tissue you have, the more resistant your cells become to insulin.
  - Insulin carries sugar from the blood to the cells. When you are overweight, the cells are damaged and will not absorb the insulin. So your blood sugar goes up. High blood sugars damage blood vessels in the eyes, kidneys, and heart.
- Does your back and do your knees or other joints hurt?
  - Explain that extra weight puts pressure on your joints and bones. This pressure wears away the cartilage, the cushion at the ends of your bones. This causes the bone to rub against another bone, causing pain.
- Do you think people who are overweight have a problem healing from injuries or surgery?
  - Explain that fat tissue has less blood supply, which is needed for healing. The incision has more pressure against it when you are overweight, which can cause the wound to open up. If antibiotics are needed for infection, the medicine does not work well because of poor circulation to the wound.
- If the person does not identify any negative effects of excess weight felt, explain the effects of excess weight are slow and often not felt by the person until the effects threaten their health or cause pain (e.g., joint pain and swelling of legs).
- Advise not to focus on total weight loss goal. Focus on losing 5 lb. Use the example of how heavy 5 lb of sugar is, and imagine having 5 lb less weight on joints and how the heart will have less resistance.

  R: Losing 30 or 50 lb may seem impossible, but 5 lb at a time may be more manageable.

Eating Healthier

Review Usual Daily Intake to Identify Patterns That Contribute to Excess Weight

- Usual breakfast, usual lunch, usual dinner
- Snacks, nighttime eating
- Skipping meals

Explain Foods That Have "Empty Calories," Foods/Drinks That Are High in Calories But Have Little or No Nutritional Value such as Soda, Chips, French Fries

Carp's Cues

"Before you eat or drink something with "empty calories," ask yourself, "Is this worth it? If it is, *enjoy* it. There is no such thing as "bad foods," only bad amounts.

Promote Activation to Engage the Individual in Healthier Behavior. Focus on What the Person Wants to Change. Limit to Three Changes.

- Eat breakfast (e.g., cereal).
- Eliminate sugar drinks (e.g., soda, juice).
- Move more and park farther away from destination; walk down steps even when you cannot walk up steps; get off the bus a few blocks from your usual stop.

  R: "Activation refers to a person's ability and willingness to take on the role of managing their health and health care"(Hibbard & Cunningham 2008).

Address What Excesses or Deficiencies Exist, Using the Information He or She Gave, For Example

- What did you eat last night?
- I ate fried chicken wings last night for dinner.
- Anything else? No.
- How could you change what you ate to improve nutrients and decrease fat?
- Listen. If no response, suggest
  - One or two piece(s) of fried chicken instead of 12 wings.
  - One piece of fried chicken with no batter has 158 calories/thigh or 131 calories/breast.
  - One medium-fried chicken wing with no batter has 102 calories.
  - Ten (10) wings have 1,020 calories.
- What could you eat in addition to the fried chicken that is a vegetable (e.g., salad)?

  R: Chicken wings have more fat before frying than a chicken thigh or breast. White meat has fewer calories than dark meat.

Avoid Describing Foods as Bad or Good. Explain Nutrient Density of Foods (*Hunter & Cason, 2006)

R: The nutrient density of foods can be high, medium, low, or none. Foods with high nutrient density are low in calories and high in nutrients.

R: Nutrient-dense foods give the most nutrients for the fewest calories.

- Foods that are nutrient dense (low in calories):
  - Fruits and vegetables that are bright or deeply colored
  - Foods that are fortified
  - Lower-fat versions of meats, milk, dairy products, and eggs
- Foods that are less nutrient dense (high in calories, low or no nutrients)
  - Are lighter or whiter in color
  - Contain a lot of refined sugar
  - Contain refined products (white bread as compared with whole grains)
  - Contain high amounts of fat for the amount of nutrients compared with similar products (fat-free milk vs. ice cream). For example:
    - An apple is a better choice than a bag of pretzels with the same number of calories, but the apple provides fiber, vitamin C, and potassium.
    - An orange is better than orange juice because it has fiber.
    - Water is better than any sugar drink or even 100% fruit juice.

Keep a List of Positive Outcomes and Health Benefits (e.g., Sleep Better, Lower Blood Pressure)

R: Weight loss in the range of 2 to 4 kg is associated with systolic blood pressure declines in the range of 3 to 8 mm Hg, a clinically significant impact (Harsha & Bray, 2008).

Initiate Health Teaching and Referrals, as Indicated

- Refer to support groups (e.g., Weight Watchers, Overeaters Anonymous, TOPS).
- Suggest that the individual plan to walk or exercise with someone.

  R: Weight-loss strategies are lifelong and may require assistance from programs, support groups, and /or exercise partner.

OVERWEIGHT

NANDA-I Definition

A condition in which an individual accumulates abnormal or excessive fat for age and gender.

Defining Characteristics

Adult: BMI of >25 kg/m^2
Child <2 years: Weight-for-length >95th percentile
Child 2 to 18 years: BMI of > 85th but <95th percentile, or 25 kg/m^2 (whichever is smaller)

Related Factors

Physiologic

Genetic disorder
Heritability of interrelated factors (e.g., adipose tissue distribution, energy expenditure, lipoprotein
  lipase activity, lipid synthesis, lipolysis)

Treatment Related

Prolonged steroid therapy
  Diminished sense of taste/and/or smell (will diminish satiety)

Situational (Personal, Environment)

Economically disadvantaged
Fear regarding lack of food supply
Intake in excess of metabolic requirements
Reported undesirable eating patterns
  Frequent snacking
  High disinhibition and restraint eating behavior score
  High frequency of restaurant or fried food
  Portion sizes larger than recommended
  Consumption of sugar-sweetened beverages
  Disordered eating behaviors (e.g., binge eating, extreme weight control)
  Disordered eating perceptions
Energy expenditure below energy intake based on standard assessment (e.g., WAVE assessment)
  Sedentary activity patterns
  Sedentary behavior occurring for > 2 hr/day
  Average daily physical activity is less than recommended for gender and age
Sleep disorder, shortened sleep time
Excessive alcohol consumption
Low dietary calcium intake in children
Obesity in childhood
Parental obesity

Goals

NOC
Nutritional Status:
Nutrient Intake, Weight
Control, Exercise
Participation, Infant
Nutritional Status,
Weight Body Mass,
Adherence Behavior:
Healthy Diet, Weight
Loss Behavior

The individual will commit to a weight-loss program, as evidenced by the following indicators:

• Identify the patterns of eating associated with consumption/energy expenditure imbalance.
• Can give examples of nutrient-dense foods versus those with "empty calories."
• Can identify three ways to increase his/her activity.
• Commit to increasing foods with high nutrient density and avoiding those with "empty calories."
• Commit to making 3 to 5 changes in food/fluid choices that are healthier.

Interventions

Refer to *Risk for Overweight* for interventions for overweight individuals.

 NIC
Self-Efficacy
Enhancement,
Self-Responsibility
Enhancement,
Nutritional Counseling,
Weight Management,
Teaching: Nutrition (age
appropriate), Behavioral
Modification, Exercise
Promotion, Coping
Enhancement

RISK FOR OVERWEIGHT

NANDA-I Definition

Vulnerable to abnormal or excessive fat accumulation for age and gender, which may compromise health.

Risk Factors

Pathophysiologic

Genetic disorder
Heritability of interrelated factors (e.g., adipose tissue distribution, energy expenditure,
    lipoprotein lipase activity, lipid synthesis, lipolysis)

Situational (Personal, Environmental)

Average daily physical activity is less than recommended for gender and age
Consumption of sugar-sweetened beverages
Disordered eating behaviors
Disordered eating perceptions
Economically disadvantaged
Energy expenditure below energy intake based on standard assessment (e.g., WAVE assessment)
Excessive alcohol consumption
Fear regarding lack of food supply
Formula- or mixed-fed infants
Frequent snacking
High disinhibition and restraint eating behavior score
High frequency of restaurant or fried food
Low dietary calcium intake in children
Maternal diabetes mellitus
Maternal smoking
Parental obesity
Portion sizes larger than recommended
Sedentary behavior occurring for >2 hr/day
Shortened sleep time
Sleep disorder

Maturational

Maternal smoking
Overweight in infancy

Parental obesity

Portion sizes larger than recommended

Premature pubarche

Rapid weight gain during childhood

Rapid weight gain during infancy, including the first week, first 4 months, and first year

Sedentary behavior occurring for >2 hr/day

Shortened sleep time

Sleep disorder

Solid foods as major food source at <5 months of age

Adult: BMI approaching >25 kg/m^2

Average daily physical activity is less than recommended for gender and age

Child <2 years: Weight-for-length approaching 95th percentile

Child 2 to 18 years: BMI approaching 85th percentile, or 25 kg/m^2 (whichever is smaller)

Children who are crossing BMI percentiles upward

Children with high BMI percentiles

Consumption of sugar-sweetened beverages

Disordered eating behaviors (e.g., binge eating, extreme weight control)

Disordered eating perceptions

Eating in response to external cues (e.g., time of day, social situations)

Eating in response to internal cues other than hunger (e.g., anxiety)

Economically disadvantaged

Energy expenditure below energy intake based on standard assessment
   (e.g., WAVE assessment[3])

Excessive alcohol consumption

Fear regarding lack of food supply

Formula- or mixed-fed infants

Frequent snacking

Genetic disorder

Heritability of interrelated factors (e.g., adipose tissue distribution, energy expenditure,
   lipoprotein lipase activity, lipid synthesis, lipolysis)

High disinhibition and restraint eating behavior score

High frequency of restaurant or fried food

Higher baseline weight at beginning of each pregnancy

Low dietary calcium intake in children

Maternal diabetes mellitus

Maternal smoking

Obesity in childhood

Parental obesity

Portion sizes larger than recommended

Premature pubarche

Rapid weight gain during childhood

Rapid weight gain during infancy, including the first week, first 4 months, and first year

Sedentary behavior occurring for >2 hr/day

Shortened sleep time

Sleep disorder

Solid foods as major food source at <5 months of age

Goals

Nutritional Status,
Weight Control

The person will describe why he or she is at risk for weight gain as evidenced by the following indicators:

- Describe reasons for increased intake with taste or olfactory deficits.
- Discuss the nutritional needs during pregnancy.
- Discuss the effects of exercise on weight control.

Interventions

NIC
Self-Efficacy
Enhancement,
Self-Responsibility
Enhancement,
Nutritional Counseling,
Weight Management,
Teaching: Nutrition (age
appropriate), Behavioral
Modification, Exercise
Promotion, Coping
Enhancement

> **CLINICAL ALERT:**
> - Individuals can be malnourished even though they are obese or overweight because of intake of foods with high fat, high carbohydrates, which are low in nutrients per calorie intake. Individuals who are of healthy weight may also be nutritionally deficient by eating foods high in fat, high in carbohydrates. For individuals not overweight but who have poor nutrition > *refer to Imbalanced Nutrition.*

Refer to Appendix C, Strategies to Increase Motivation and Engagement in Individuals/Families; for Specific Techniques to Improve Activation and Engagement

Initiate Discussion: "How Can You Be Healthier?"

- Focus on the person's response (e.g., stop smoking, exercise more, eat healthier, and cut down on drinking).
- Refer to index for interventions for the targeted lifestyle change.

    R: The nurse should be cautioned against applying a nursing diagnosis for an overweight or obese person who does not want to participate in a weight-loss program. Motivation for weight loss must come from within.

Before a Person Can Change, They Must (Martin, Haskard, Zolnierek, & DiMatteo, 2010)

- Know what change is necessary (information) and why;
- Desire the change (motivation); and
- Have the tools to achieve and maintain the change (strategy).
- Trust the health care professional, who has a sympathetic presence (Pelzang, 2010).

    *R: Empathic communication involving a thorough understanding of the individual's perspective improves adherence. Individuals who are informed and affectively motivated are also more likely to adhere to their treatment recommendations (*Martin et al., 2005).*

If Appropriate, Gently and Expertly Teach the Hazards of Obesity, But Respect a Person's Right to Choose, the Right of Self-Determination

- Ask "How do you think being overweight affects you?"

Carp's Cues

If the person reports no complaints, explain that the effects of excess weight are insidious and often not felt by the person until they threaten their health or cause pain. Focus on what the person tells you (e.g., my sugar is high, my knees hurt). Do not overload him/her.

If the Person Does Not Identify any Negative Effects of Excess Weight Felt

- Ask one of the questions below. Pick the best question that applies to this person. Use language they understand (e.g., blood veins or that carry blood).
  - Do your legs swell during the day and go back to normal during the night?
    - Explain that fat tissue compresses tubes in your legs and prevents fluids from circulating well. Eventually, the swelling will be permanent, lasting the whole day, and cause difficulty walking and wearing shoes.
  - Do you have high blood pressure, or is it getting a little higher each year?
    - Explain that blood vessels are damaged when excess weight puts pressure on them and they stretch, become thinner, and lose their strength. Your heart now has to pump harder, causing high blood pressure. Over time, the heart enlarges and cannot pump well. This is heart failure.
  - Are your cholesterol levels increasing each year?
    - Explain that the stretching of your blood vessels damages the inside of the blood tubes. Cholesterol sticks to the damaged tubes and slows the blood flow to your kidneys, eyes, brain, and legs. This can cause strokes, renal failure, vision problems, and blood clots in your legs.

- Although you may not feel that anything is wrong, high blood pressure can permanently damage your heart, brain, eyes, and kidneys before you feel anything. Even losing 10 lb can reduce your blood pressure.
- Is your blood glucose test getting a little higher each year? Is there diabetes in your family?
  - Explain that the more fatty tissue you have, the more resistant your cells become to insulin.
  - Explain that insulin carries sugar from blood to the cells. When you are overweight, the cells are damaged and will not absorb the insulin. So your blood sugar goes up. High blood sugars damage blood vessels in the eyes, kidneys, and heart.
- Does your back or do your knees or other joints hurt?
  - Explain that extra weight puts pressure on your joints and bones. This pressure wears away the cartilage, the cushion at the ends of your bones. This causes the bone to rub against another bone, causing pain.
- Do you think people who are overweight have a problem healing from injuries or surgery?
  - Explain that fat tissue has less blood supply, which is needed for healing. The incision has more pressure acting against it when you are overweight, which can cause the wound to open up. If antibiotics are needed for infection, the medicine does not work well because of poor circulation to the wound.

Carp's Cues

It would be wise to mention that individuals who are thin or of normal weight can have hypertension, arthritis, high cholesterol, and diabetes, but not at the high rate experienced by people who are overweight.

Advise Them to Focus on a Goal of Losing 5 lb. Emphasize How Heavy 5 lb of Sugar Is and That Every 5 lb Lost Is Less Work for Their Heart and Less Strain on their Joints. A Reduction in Calories and Increase in Activity Can Cause a Weight Loss of About 2 lb a Week.

R: It can be discouraging to focus on losing 50 lb. 5 lb at a time is more realistic.

Refer Interested Individual to "Do You Know Some of the Health Risks of Being Overweight?" Accessed at http://www.niddk.nih.gov/health-information/health-topics/weight-control/health_risks_being_overweight/Pages/health-risks-being-overweight.aspx

Refer to *Obesity* nursing diagnosis under Eating Healthier.

IMPAIRED ORAL MUCOUS MEMBRANE

NANDA-I Definition

Disruption of the lips and/or soft tissue of the oral cavity

Defining Characteristics

Disrupted oral mucous membranes
Color changes—erythema, pallor, white patches, lesions, and ulcers
Moisture changes—increased or decreased saliva
Cleanliness changes—debris, malodor, discoloration of the teeth
Mucosal integrity changes—difficulty swallowing, decreased taste, difficulty weaning
Perception changes—difficulty swallowing, decreased taste, difficulty wearing dentures, burning, pain, and change in voice quality

Related Factors

Pathophysiologic

Related to inflammation secondary to:

Periodontal disease   Infection
Oral cancer

Treatment Related

Related to drying effects of:

NPO more than 24 hours
Radiation to head or neck
Prolonged use of steroids or other immunosuppressives and other medications including opioids, anti-
    depressants, phenothiazines, antihypertensives, antihistamines, diuretics, and sedatives
Use of antineoplastic drugs
Oxygen therapy
Mouth breathing
Blood and marrow stem cell transplant

Related to mechanical irritation secondary to:

Endotracheal tube   NG tube

Situational (Personal, Environmental)

Related to chemical irritants* secondary to:

Acidic foods   Drugs
Noxious agents   Alcohol
Tobacco   High sugar intake

Related to mechanical trauma secondary to

Broken or jagged teeth   Braces
Ill-fitting dentures

Related to malnutrition*
Related to inadequate oral hygiene

Goals

NOC
Oral Tissue Integrity, Oral Health Restoration, Chemotherapeutic Management, Oral Health Maintenance, Oral Health Promotion

The person will be free of oral mucosa irritation or exhibit signs of healing with decreased inflammation, as evidenced by the following indicators:

- Describe factors that cause oral injury.
- Demonstrate knowledge of optimal oral hygiene.
- Be free of oral discomfort during food and fluid intake.

Interventions

NIC
Oral Health Restoration, Chemotherapeutic Management, Oral Health Maintenance, Oral Health Promotion

Assess for Causative or Contributing Factors

- Assess with a valid and reliable tool as a first step toward preventing and treating oral mucositis (Eilers, Harris, Henry & Johnson, 2014).
- Refer to Related Factors.

Evaluate Person's Ability to Perform Oral Hygiene, Allow Person to Perform as Much Oral Care as Possible

> **CLINICAL ALERT:**
> • Too often, oral care and assessments are omitted in individual care.

• For high-risk individuals, inspect the oral cavity for lesions (e.g., white patches, broken teeth, signs of infection).

*R: Researchers have reported that for individuals with mechanical ventilation, only 32% had suctioning to manage oral secretions, 33% had their teeth brushed, 65% had swab cleansing, and 63% had a moisturizer applied to the oral mucosal tissues. In addition, nurses reported performing more oral care than actually completing (*Cutler & Davis, 2005; Fields, 2008; Goss, Coty, & Myers, 2011).*

Teach Preventive Oral Hygiene to Individuals at Risk for Development of Mucositis (e.g., Radiation)

R: Mucosal damage usually occurs 7 to 14 days after the start of radiation and 3 to 9 days after the start of chemotherapy.

• Instruct individual to:
  • Perform the regimen, including brushing, flossing, rinsing, and moisturizing, after meals and before sleep. If individual resists, have him or her rinse mouth with water after meals.
  • Avoid mouthwashes with alcohol content, lemon/glycerin swabs, or prolonged use of hydrogen peroxide.

  *R: These solutions can cause mucosal abnormalities, dryness, and discomfort (*Meurman et al., 1996; National Cancer Institute, 2014).*

Promote Healing and Reduce Progression of Mucositis

• Inspect oral cavity three times daily with tongue blade and light; if mucositis is severe, inspect mouth every 4 hours.
• Use normal saline solution as a mouthwash.
• Floss teeth only once in 24 hours.
• Omit flossing if bleeding is excessive.
• Ensure that oral hygiene regimen is done every 1 to 2 hours while awake and every 4 hours during the night.

R: Systematically applied protocols may significantly decrease the incidence, severity, and duration of oral problems (National Cancer Institute, 2014).

*R: Salt and soda rinses are effective and the least costly selection for the prevention of treatment of mucositis. Foam brushes are not equal to toothbrushes for removing plaque and bacteria for cavity prevention. The effectiveness of mouthwash preparations over normal saline has not been supported in the literature (*Dodd, Dibble, & Miaskowski, 2000; Oncology Nursing Society, 2007).*

R: Proper hydration must be maintained to liquefy secretions and prevent drying of oral mucosa.

Consult With Physician/Nurse Practitioner/Physician Assistant for an Oral Pain Relief Solution

• Xylocaine viscous 2% oral: swish and expectorate every 2 hours and before meals. (If throat is sore, the solution can be swallowed; if swallowed, Xylocaine produces local anesthesia and may affect the gag reflex.) The dose of the viscous Xylocaine is not to exceed 25 mm/day (National Comprehensive Cancer Network, 2008).
• A protective barrier may be applied and requires frequent applications because of limited duration (e.g. Episil, Gelclair, Mugard). Prophylaxis is not recommended (Eilers et al., 2014).
• Topical morphine provides a reduction in pain severity and duration of pain. If the morphine is in an alcohol-based formula, it may cause burning.

R: Proper hydration must be maintained to liquefy secretions and prevent drying of oral mucosa.

R: Dry oral mucosa causes discomfort and increases the risk of breakdown and infection.

Discuss the Importance of Daily Oral Hygiene and Periodic Dental Examinations

R: Plaque, microbial flora found in the mouth, is the primary cause of dental cavities and periodontal disease. Daily removal of plaque through brushing and flossing can help prevent dental decay and disease.

Perform Oral Hygiene on Individuals Who are Intubated and/or Mechanically Ventilated

- Gather equipment (same as for unconscious individual).
- Position head of bed higher than 30 degrees unless medically contraindicated.
- Follow protocol for oral care.

  R: Providing comprehensive oral care to decrease the bacterial load in the mouth and keeping the head of the bed elevated greater than 30 degrees helps decrease aspiration and may prevent pneumonia (Quinn et al., 2014).

Initiate Health Teaching and Referrals as Indicated

- Teach person and family the factors that contribute to stomatitis and its progression.
- Teach diet modifications to reduce oral pain and to maintain optimal nutrition.
- Have individual describe or demonstrate home care regimen.

  R: The frequency of oral health maintenance varies according to a person's health status and self-care ability, but minimum is in the morning and at bedtime. High-risk individuals (e.g., those with nasogastric tubes or suffering from cancer or who are poorly nourished) should have oral assessments daily.

- Explain that factors that contribute to oral disease are excessive use of alcohol and tobacco, microorganisms, inadequate nutrition (quantity, quality), inadequate hygiene, and trauma (ill-fitting dentures, sharp-edged teeth, sharp-edged prostheses, improper use of cleaning devices).
- Teach the factors that contribute to stomatitis and its progression.
- Teach diet modifications to reduce oral pain and to maintain optimal nutrition.
- Have individual describe or demonstrate home care regimen.
- Refer individuals with tooth and gum disorders to a dentist.

> ### Clinical Alert Report
> Advise ancillary staff/student to report any c/o mouth lesions, white patches, broken, sharp teeth.

RISK FOR IMPAIRED ORAL MUCOUS MEMBRANE

Definition[4]

At risk for disruption of the lips and soft tissue of the oral cavity

Risk Factors

Pathophysiologic

Related to inflammation secondary to:

Diabetes mellitus	Oral cancer
Periodontal disease	Infection

Treatment Related

Related to drying effects of:
NPO more than 24 hours
Radiation to head or neck
Prolonged use of steroids or other immunosuppressives and other medications, including opioids, antidepressants, phenothiazines, antihypertensives, antihistamines, diuretics, and sedatives
Use of antineoplastic drugs
Oxygen therapy
Mouth breathing
Blood and marrow stem cell transplant

---

[4] This diagnosis is not presently on the NANDA-I list, but has been added for clarity and usefulness.

Related to mechanical irritation secondary to:

Endotracheal tube
NG tube

Situational (Personal, Environmental)

Related to chemical irritants secondary to:

Acidic foods   Drugs
Noxious agents   Alcohol
Tobacco   High sugar intake

Related to mechanical trauma secondary to:

Broken or jagged teeth
Ill-fitting dentures
Braces

Related to malnutrition
Related to inadequate oral hygiene
Related to lack of knowledge of oral hygiene

Goals/Interventions

Refer to Generic Medical Care Plan.

ACUTE PAIN

NANDA-I Definition

Unpleasant sensory and emotional experience arising from actual or potential tissue damage or described in terms of such damage (International Association for the Study of Pain); sudden or slow onset of any intensity from mild to severe with anticipated or predictable end and a duration of <6 months

Defining Characteristics

Self-Report of Pain Quality and Intensity

(Attempt to use with all individuals.)

For Individuals Unable to Provide Self-Report (in Order of Preference)

Presence of pathological condition or procedure known to cause pain. Physical responses such as diaphoresis, changes in blood pressure or pulse, pupil dilation, change in respiratory rate, guarding, grimacing, moaning, crying, or restlessness.
Surrogate reporting (family members, caregivers).
Response to an analgesic trial.

Related Factors

Biopathophysiologic

Related to uterine contractions during labor
Related to trauma to perineum during labor and delivery
Related to tissue trauma and reflex muscle spasms secondary to (specify)
Related to inflammation of, or injury (specify)
Related to effects of cancer on (specify)
Related to abdominal cramps, diarrhea, and vomiting secondary to (specify)
Related to inflammation and smooth muscle spasms secondary to renal calculi

Treatment Related

Related to tissue trauma and reflex muscle spasms secondary to:

Surgery
Diagnostic tests (venipuncture, invasive scanning, biopsy)

 ## Carp's Cues

There is an ethical duty to relieve pain. Deandrea, Montanari, Moja, and Apolone. (2008) reported that 40% of individuals with cancer pain are undertreated. Nurses should be as aggressive in advocating for effective pain relief for their individuals as they would be if the individual were their child, mother, partner, or best friend. Those most in need of effective pain relief may be the poor, uneducated, substance abusers, and others who are voiceless in the health care system.

Goals

Comfort Level, Pain
Control

The person will report or exhibit a satisfactory relief measure as evidenced by (specify):

- Increased participation in activities of recovery
- Reduction in pain behaviors (specify)
- Improvement in mood, coping

Interventions

NIC
Pain Management, Medication Management, Emotional Support, Teaching: Individual, Hot/Cold Application, Simple Massage

Reduce or Eliminate Factors That Increase Pain

Disbelief From Others

- Establish a supportive accepting relationship.
- Acknowledge the pain.
- Listen attentively to individual's discussion of pain.
- Convey that you are assessing pain because you want to understand it better (not to determine whether it really exists).
- Assess the family for any misconceptions about pain or its treatment.

  R: Trying to convince health care providers that he or she is experiencing pain will cause the individual anxiety, which compounds the pain. Both are energy depleting.

Lack of Knowledge/Uncertainty

- Explain the cause of the pain, if known.
- Relate the severity of the pain and how long it will last, if known.
- Explain painful diagnostic tests and procedures in detail by relating the discomforts and sensations that the individual will feel; approximate the duration.
- Support individual in addressing specific questions regarding diagnosis, risks, benefits of treatment, and prognosis. Consult with the specialist or primary care provider.

  R: People who are prepared for painful procedures by explanations of the actual sensations experience less stress than those who receive vague explanations.

Fear

- Provide accurate information to reduce fear of addiction.
- Explore reasons for the fear.
- Explain the difference between drug tolerance and drug addiction.

  R: Addiction is a psychological syndrome characterized by compulsive drug-seeking behavior generally associated with a desire for drug administration to produce euphoria or other effects, not pain relief. There is no evidence that adequate administration of opioids for pain produces addiction (Pasero & McCaffery, 2011).

Fatigue

- Determine the cause of fatigue (sedatives, analgesics, sleep deprivation).
- Explain that pain contributes to stress, which increases fatigue.
- Assess present sleep pattern and the influence of pain on sleep.
- Provide opportunities to rest during the day and with periods of uninterrupted sleep at night.
- Consult with prescriber for an increased dose of pain medication at bedtime.
- Explain the options of nonpharmaceutical interventions and the rationale.

R: Relaxation and guided imagery effectively manage pain by increasing sense of control, reducing feelings of helplessness and hopelessness, providing a calming diversion, and disrupting the pain–anxiety–tension cycle.

Discuss the Use of Heat Applications, Their Therapeutic Effects, Indications, and Related Precautions

- Hot water bottle
- Warm tub
- Hot summer sun
- Electric heating pad
- Moist heat pack
- Thin plastic wrap over painful area to retain body heat (e.g., knee, elbow)

Discuss the Use of Cold Applications,* Their Therapeutic Effects, Indications, and Related Precautions

- Cold towels (wrung out)
- Ice bag
- Ice massage
- Cold water immersion for small body parts
- Cold gel pack

R: Nonpharmacologic interventions provide individuals with an increased sense of control, promote active involvement, reduce stress and anxiety, elevate mood, and raise the pain threshold (*McGuire, Sheidler, & Polomano, 2000).

Provide Optimal Pain Relief With Prescribed Analgesics

- Use oral route when feasible, intravenous or rectal routes if needed.

  R: Oral administration is preferred when possible. Liquid medications can be given to those who have difficulty swallowing. Avoid intramuscular routes. If frequent injections are necessary, the IV route is preferred because it is not painful and absorption is guaranteed. Intramuscular routes have erratic absorption and cause unnecessary pain. Side effects (decreased respirations and blood pressure), however, may be more profound (Pasero & McCaffery, 2011).

- When possible use patient-controlled analgesics (PCA).

  R: Undertreatment of pain in the elderly has been described by Denny and Guido (2012). Greco et al. (2014) reported that pain management of cancer has improved since last reported in 2008 but 1/3 of individuals "still do not receive pain medication proportional to their pain intensity."

- Use a preventive approach.
  - Medicate before an activity (e.g., ambulation) to increase participation, but evaluate the hazard of sedation.
  - Instruct individual to request p.r.n. pain medication before the pain is severe.
  - Collaborate with physician/nurse practitioner to order medications on a 24-hour schedule basis rather than p.r.n. unless the person is sedated.
  - Use the around the clock (ATC) approach, not p.r.n.

    R: Paice, Noskin, and Vanagunas (2005) reported the results of comparing the use of ATC scheduled opioid doses with p.r.n. opioid doses in medical inpatients and found that those who received ATC doses had lower pain intensity ratings. A significantly greater percentage of the prescribed opioid is administered when it was given ATC (70.8%) compared with p.r.n. (38%); however, there were no differences in adverse effects between the two groups (Pasero & McCafferty, 2011).

    R: The preventive approach may reduce the total 24-hour dose compared with the p.r.n. approach; it provides a constant blood level of the drug, reduces craving for the drug, and reduces the anxiety of having to ask and wait for p.r.n. relief.

Assess Individual's Response to the Pain-Relief Medication

- After administration, return in 30 minutes to assess effectiveness.
- Ask individual to rate severity of pain before the medication and amount of relief received.

- Ask person to indicate when the pain began to increase. How long since the last pain medication? After a certain activity (e.g., ambulation, dressing change)?
- Advise person to request pain medication earlier. Plan pain-relief measures before the activities.
- Consult with prescriber if a dosage or interval change is needed; the dose may be increased by 50% until effective.
- If pain management is ineffective, collaborate with the prescriber to consider multimodal analgesia.

    R: Multimodal analgesia is the use of a combination of acetaminophen and NSAIDS in combination with other analgesics (Pasero & McCaffery, 2011).

- If individual has a history of substance/alcohol abuse, refer also to care plan for substance abuse.

Reduce or Eliminate Common Side Effects of Opioids

- Sedation
    - Assess for signs of respiratory depression (decreased level of consciousness, respiratory rate below 8, decreased oxygen saturation).
- Identify individuals at risk for adverse effects of opioids (e.g., renal insufficiency, hepatic insufficiency).

    R: Clearance and excretion of opioids is delayed, and high concentrations of the drug can accumulate (Pasero & McCaffery, 2011).

- Respiratory disorders, obstructive sleep apnea syndrome

    R: Opioids decrease cough reflex, and dry secretions increase the risk of aspiration (Pasero & McCaffery, 2011).

- Constipation (Refer to *Constipation.*)
- Nausea and vomiting (Refer to *Nausea.*)
- Dry mouth
    - Explain that opioids decrease saliva production.
    - Instruct person to rinse mouth often, suck on sugarless sour candies, eat pineapple chunks or watermelon (if permissible), and drink liquids often.
    - Explain the necessity of good oral hygiene and dental care.

        R: Management of side effects can increase comfort level and use of medications.

\Minimize Procedural and Diagnostic Pain

- Anticipate pain, and premedicate the individual before painful procedures (e.g., sedation).
- Encourage the use of relaxation or guided imagery during procedures.

    R: Management of pain before a painful procedure can decrease the amount of analgesia needed and the effects of anxiety and fear, which will escalate the pain experience.

Initiate Health Teaching and Referrals as Indicated

- Review pain management strategies at home.
- Alert significant others on early signs of adverse effects and to call primary care provider.
- Instruct not to suddenly stop taking the pain medication.

    R: Tapering of opioids dose will prevent withdrawal symptoms. The longer the opioids have been taken, the longer it takes to wean off the medication (Pasero & McCaffery, 2011).

- Discuss the need to prevent constipation (e.g., optimal hydration [8 to 10 cups unless contraindicated], stool softener, laxatives).
- Explain the expected course of the pain (resolution) if known (e.g., fractured arm, surgical incision).

    R: Optimal pain management at home requires specific instructions to individual and significant others.

Clinical Alert Report

- Advise ancillary staff/student to report any changes in respiratory status and cognition and complaints of pain to the charge nurse.

LABOR PAIN

Definition

Sensory and emotional experience that varies from pleasant to unpleasant, associated with labor. (NANDA-I) Sensory and emotional experience that varies from cramping to severe pain and intense pressure which can be highly variable, associated with labor and childbirth (Personal Communication, T. Wilson).

Defining Characteristics

Altered muscle tension
Altered neuroendocrine function
Altered urinary function
Change in blood pressure
Change in heart rate
Change in respiratory rate
Diaphoresis
Distraction behavior
Expressive behavior
Facial mask
Increased appetite
Lack of appetite
Narrowed focus

Nausea
Noted evidence of contractions
Observed evidence of contractions
Perineum pressure sensation
Positioning to avoid pain
Protective gesture
Pupillary dilation
Reports pressure
Reports pain
Requests pain relief interventions[5]
Self-focused
Sleep pattern disturbance
Vomiting

Related Factors

Physiologic

Related to dilation period (uterine contractions, cervical stretching and dilation and distention of lower uterine segment)
Related to transition and expulsion period (uterine contractions and distension of pelvic floor, vagina and perineum, pressure on pelvic nerves)

Situational (Personal, Environmental)

Related to:

Fear
Anxiety
Emotional stress
Anticipation of pain
No prenatal education
Absent labor support
Fatigue
Anemia
Previous experience with pain
History of perinatal loss

History of neonatal death
History of neonatal health problems
Fetal position
Prior surgical procedures
Language barriers
Substance abuse (history, present)
History of abuse
History of sexual abuse/violence
History of trauma
Sexual orientation

Maturational

Adolescent
Developmental delay

Author's Note

This new NANDA-I nursing diagnosis contains the etiology of the pain in the diagnostic statement. What is problematic is identifying the related factors when a woman is experiencing normal labor pain. The experience of labor can be complicated when the mother is 14 years old or there is a history of perinatal loss. Labor pain is complicated by fear and anxiety; thus, these nursing diagnoses should be added with the related factors that reflect why this labor experience may be more difficult and necessitates additional nursing individuals.

---

[5]Added by T. Wilson, contributor.

Labor Pain may be more clinically useful as *Labor Syndrome*, which would include *Acute Pain, Impaired Comfort, Fear, Anxiety, Interrupted Family Processes*, etc.

Goals

Refer to *Acute pain*

The mother will report or exhibit satisfactory pain level as evidenced by

- Reduction in pain behaviors (specify)
- Increased relaxation between contractions
- Improved coping skills

Interventions

Refer to Acute Pain

Refer to nursing diagnosis *Acute Pain* for basic pain management interventions.

> **CLINICAL ALERT:**
> - The woman in labor experiences two types of pain: visceral and somatic.
>   - Visceral pain is related to contraction of the uterus and dilation and stretching of the cervix. Uterine pain during the first stage of labor results from ischemia caused by constriction and contraction of the arteries supplying the myometrium. Visceral pain is experienced primarily during the first stage of labor.
>   - Somatic pain is caused by pressure of the presenting part on the birth canal, vulva, and perineum. Somatic pain is experienced during transition and the second stage, and is more intense and localized.

Assess Progress in Labor

- Uterine contraction pattern
- Cervical dilation
- Fetal position and station

> *R: Location and intensity of pain vary with phase or stage of labor.*

Assess Support Person's Readiness to Participate

Determine effect of

- Age, developmental status
- Culture and religion on expectations

> *R: Perception and expression of pain are influenced by life experience, developmental stage, and cultural or religious norms.*

Provide Comfort Measures

- Gown and linen changes as needed
- Frequent pericare
- Cool damp cloth to forehead, neck, or upper back

Provide Labor Support

- Labor support, ideally, is continuous and provided by a variety of individuals.
- Labor support should begin in early labor and be continued through delivery.
- Assist the woman to cope with pain, build her self-confidence, and maintain a sense of mastery and well-being.
- Encourage verbalizations of feelings, pain, or pressure.
- Be supportive of individual's choices and wishes for her birth experience.
- Reassure, guide, and encourage the woman.
- Provide acceptance of her coping style.
- Reinforce positive coping mechanisms.
- Introduce and demonstrate new methods for coping with pain.

> *R: The element that best predicts a woman's experience of labor pain is her level of confidence in her ability to cope with labor (*Simkin & Bolding, 2004).*

R: Women who are provided continuously available support during labor have improved outcomes compared with women who do not have one-to-one continuously available support.

For women in labor, continuous support can result in the following:

- *Shorter labor*
- *Decreased use of analgesia/anesthesia*
- *Decreased operative vaginal births or cesarean births*
- *Decreased need for oxytocin/uterotonics*
- *Increase likelihood of breastfeeding*
- *Increased satisfaction with childbirth experience*

    R: Many of the mother's childbirth outcomes listed above also benefit the neonate (Association of Women's Health, Obstetric and Neonatal Nurses [AWHONN], 2011)

Encourage Adequate Intake of Oral Fluids by Monitoring Oral and IV Intake and by Offering

- Ice chips
- Popsicles
- Jell-O
- Suckers
- Wet washcloths

Encourage Woman to Void at Least Every 2 Hours if No Urinary Catheter

- Catheterize individual as indicated.

    R: Bladder distention can interfere with fetal descent and increase uterine contraction pain.

Guide and Support Woman and Her Support Person in Using Self-Comforting Techniques

Demonstrate and Encourage Support Person to Assist With Supportive Techniques as Needed

R: Qualitative research has demonstrated that one of the most significant aspects of the experience of labor for women is the presence of one or more support persons. Postpartum women report that one of the things contributing to a positive labor experience was the presence of a family member or friend in the room (Burke-Galloway, 2014).

Encourage Rest and Promote Relaxation Between Contractions

Encourage and Support Nonpharmacologic Pain Relief Measures

R: Achieving a state of relaxation is the basis of all nonpharmacologic interventions during labor. Relaxation enhances the effectiveness of nonpharmacologic and pharmacologic pain-management strategies (Burke-Galloway, 2014).

- Relaxation techniques
- Patterned breathing techniques

    R: Breathing techniques are used as a distraction during labor to decrease pain and promote relaxation (Burke-Galloway, 2014).

- Discourage supine position to prevent supine hypotension or vena cava syndrome.
- Patterned physical movement, frequent position changes, and ambulation
    - Leaning or leaning forward with support
    - Sitting
    - Standing
    - Side lying
    - Pillows to help with positioning
    - Squatting
    - Hands and knees
    - Rocking chair
    - Birthing ball

        R: Women naturally choose positions of comfort and are more likely to change positions in early labor (Burke-Galloway, 2014).

R: The birthing ball provides support for the woman's body as she assumes a variety of positions during labor. This may enhance maternal comfort. A birthing ball helps the woman use pelvic rocking, promotes mobility, and helps to provide support for the woman in the upright position (AWHONN, 2008).

- Biofeedback
- Hypnosis
- Attention focusing-focal point or imagery
- Music
- Aromatherapy
- Hydrotherapy
- Shower, pool, or tub

*R: With appropriate attention to water temperature, duration of the bath, and safety considerations, baths in labor are effective in reducing pain and suffering during labor (*Simkin & Bolding, 2004).*

- Touch
  - Massage, effleurage, and counterpressure
  - Application of heat or cold
  - Therapeutic touch and healing touch

    R: Various forms of touch can convey to the woman a sense of caring, reassurance, understanding, or nonverbal support (Simkin & Ancheta, 2011). Purposeful use of massage is employed during labor as a relaxation and stress-reduction technique that functions as a distraction, may stimulate cutaneous nerve fibers that block painful impulses, and stimulates the local release of endorphins (Burke-Galloway, 2014).

- Transcutaneous electrical nerve stimulation (TENS) decreases pain perception by providing alternate sensation

  R: TENS provides modest pain relief benefits and is a satisfying option for most women who use it (Simkin & Bolding, 2004).

- Acupuncture/Acupressure

  *R: Acupuncture provides an effective alternative to pharmacologic pain relief (*Simkin & Bolding, 2004).*

- Intradermal injections of sterile water

  *R: Intradermal injections of sterile water decrease lower back pain in most laboring women without any identified side effects on the fetus or mother (*Simkin & Bolding, 2004).*

Offer/Encourage Pharmacologic Pain Relief Measures Including (Burke-Galloway, 2014)

- Sedatives and hypnotics
  - Barbiturates—pentobarbital (Nembutal), secobarbital sodium (Seconal), zolipidem tartrate (Ambien)
  - H1-receptor antagonists— promethazine hydrochloride (Phenergan), hydroxyzine hydrochloride (Vistaril, Atarax)

    R: Barbiturates

    - *Provide sedation or sleep*
    - *Depress the central nervous system*
    - *Decrease anxiety*
    - *Rarely used in modern-day obstetrics because of long half-life*
    - *Historically, women experiencing prolonged latent labor were thought to benefit from the brief period of therapeutic rest or sleep following administration of barbiturates*

    R: H1-receptor antagonists may be administered with narcotics during labor to

    - *Decrease anxiety*
    - *Increase sedation*
    - *Decrease nausea and vomiting*
- Analgesics
  - Opioids—morphine and meperidine
  - Synthetic opioids—fentanyl (Sublimaze) and remifentanyl
  - Opioid agonist-antagonists—butorphanol (Stadol), nalbuphine (Nubain)

    R: Analgesics allow women to relax and rest between contractions by

    - *Blunting effect with increase in pain threshold*

- *Decreased perception of pain*
- *Somnolence*
- *Neuraxial analgesia*
- Epidural or spinal
- Combined spinal–epidural (CSE)
- Patient-controlled epidural analgesia (PCEA)

  R: Neuraxial analgesia in labor

  - *Provides superior pain relief*
  - *Goal is to provide sufficient analgesic effect with as little motor block as possible*
  - *Flexible and effective method of pain relief*
  - *Results in less central nervous system depression of mother and neonate than other pharmacologic methods*
- Regional anesthesia (rarely used in modern obstetrics)
  - Pudendal block—Provides vaginal, vulvar, and perineal anesthesia via injection of anesthetic agent through lateral walls into area of pudendal nerve
  - Paracervical block—injection of anesthetic agent around the cervix

Discuss the Maternal–Fetal–Neonatal Side Effects of Pharmacologic Pain Relief Measures (Burke-Galloway, 2014)

- Sedatives and hypnotics can
  - Potentiate respiratory depression in mother and neonate
- H1-receptor antagonists can cause
  - Drowsiness, sedation in mother and neonate
  - Anticholinergic effects
    - Dry mouth
    - Respiratory depression
- Opioids can cause
  - Nausea and vomiting
  - Respiratory depression in mother and neonate
  - Decreased fetal heart rate variability
  - Neonatal respiratory depression at birth
  - Neonate to exhibit decreased muscle tone and alertness
  - Inhibited neonatal suckling at the breast
- Maternal side effects of neuraxial analgesia
  - Hypotension
  - Inadequate, one-sided or failed block
  - Pruritis
  - Nausea/vomiting
  - Fever
  - Urinary retention
  - Back pain
  - Postdural headache
- Major complications of neuraxial analgesia
  - Intravascular injection of epinephrine and local anesthetic agent into an epidural vein
  - High spinal block due to inadvertent placement of epidural catheter and local anesthetic agent in the intrathecal space
  - Epidural hematoma due to bleeding within the spinal neuraxis
  - Respiratory depression
  - Neuraxial infection (meningitis)

    R: Intravascular injection of epinephrine and local anesthetic agent can result in
- *Systemic toxicity leading to*
  - *Immediate maternal heart rate*
  - *Palpitations*
  - *Elevated BP*

- *Numbness around the tongue or mouth*
- *Metallic taste*
- *Tinnitus*
- *Slurred speech*
- *Jitteriness or agitation*
- *Seizures*
- *Cardiac arrest*

> *R: High spinal block can result in*

- *Anesthetic agent ascending intrathecally into the brain stem leading to*
- *Respiratory paralysis*
- *Total autonomic blockage*
- *Loss of consciousness*

> *R: Epidural hematoma can result in*

- *Severe pain*
- *Progressive sensory or motor blockade*
- *Deteriorating function of the lower extremities and bowel and bladder*

> *R: Signs and symptoms of meningitis may occur within 12 hours to a few days following birth and include:*

- *Fever*
- *Severe unrelenting headache*
- *Neck stiffness*
- *Sensitivity to light*
- *Nausea and vomiting*
- *Drowsiness*
- *Confusion*
- *Seizures*

Monitor and Evaluate Effects of Pain Management Interventions on Mother and Fetus

- Assess comfort level before and after pain management interventions.
- Monitor FHR for nonreassuring characteristics. (Refer to *Nonreassuring Fetal Status in Risk for Complications of Reproductive Dysfunction.*)

> **CLINICAL ALERT:**
> - Notify the anesthesia provider if any of the following occurs:
>   - Hypotension
>   - High sensory level block
>   - Bradycardia
>   - Respiratory compromise
>   - Apnea
>   - Arm/hand numbness or paralysis
>   - Nausea
>   - Anxiety
>   - Decreasing level of consciousness

Initiate Health Teaching as Indicated

- Instruct mother and her family on labor process.
- Explain physiology of pain in labor.
- Provide information about analgesia/anesthesia measures, side effects, and potential complications.
- Provide information about procedures to the mother and her family.

CHRONIC PAIN

NANDA-I Definition

Unpleasant sensory and emotional experience arising from actual or potential tissue damage or described in terms of such damage (International Association for the Study of Pain); sudden or slow onset of any intensity from mild to severe with anticipated or predictable end and a duration of >3 months

Defining Characteristics

The individual reports that pain has existed for more than 6 months (may be the only assessment data present).

Discomfort

Anger, frustration, depression because of situation

Redness, swelling, heat

Color changes in affected area

Reflex abnormalities

Guarded movement

Muscle spasms

Facial mask of pain

Anorexia, weight loss

Insomnia

Related Factors

Related to tissue trauma and reflex muscle spasms secondary to:

Contractures

Arthritis

Fibromyalgia

Spinal cord disorders

Vasospasm

Occlusion

Vasodilatation (headache)

Related to inflammation of or injury of:

Nerve

Joint

Tendon

Muscle

Bursa

Pancreas, liver, GI tract, brain

Related to effects of cancer on (specify)

Related to tissue trauma and reflex muscle spasms secondary to (specify)

Carp's Cues

The American Society of Anesthesiologists (2010) defines "chronic pain as pain of any etiology not directly related to neoplastic involvement, extending in duration beyond the expected temporal boundary of tissue injury and normal healing and adversely affecting the function or well-being of the individual."

Chronic or persistent pain is common in 80% of older adults. One survey of 10,291 individuals revealed prevalence of 10.1% for back pain, 7.1% for leg and foot pain, 4.1% for hand and arm pain, and 3.5% for headache (Hardt, Jacobsen, Goldberg, Nickel, & Buchwald, 2008). Chronic pain is responsible for 1/2 million working days lost in the United States each year. Forty percent of the elderly report persistent pain with arthritis as the most frequent cause (Castillo-Bueno et al., 2010).

It is well known that chronic pain affects coping, sleep, sexual activity, socialization, family processes, nutrition, spirituality, and activity tolerance. Approximately 50% of individuals with persistent pain also suffer from depression or anxiety disorder (Weisburg & Boatwright, 2007).

Goals

NOC

Comfort Level, Pain: Disruptive Effects, Pain Control, Depression Control

The individual will relate:

• Increased understanding of his or her disease/disorder and resources/skills needed to cope.
• Will commit to practice at least one noninvasive pain-relief measure such as:
  • Music therapy
  • Stretching exercises, yoga, and/or walking
  • Massage
  • Guided imagery
  • Relaxation therapy
  • Heat/cold therapy

Interventions

NIC
Pain Management,
Medication
Management, Exercise
Promotion, Mood
Management, Coping
Enhancement

Establish a Supportive Accepting Relationship

- Acknowledge the pain. Listen attentively to individual's discussion of pain.
- Convey that you are assessing pain because you want to understand it better (not determine whether it really exists).

Assess the Family for Any Misconceptions About Pain or Its Treatment

R: Trying to convince health care providers that he or she is experiencing pain will cause the individual anxiety, which compounds the pain. Both are energy depleting.

Determine the Individual's Level of Understanding of His or Her Condition, and Causes of Pain and Pain-Relieving Techniques That He or She Uses

- Supplement the individual's information and correct misconceptions.

  R: The chronic pain self-management program (CPSMP) focuses on increasing an individual's understanding of his or her condition. This theory has validated that better knowledge of one's condition increases confidence and skill in managing a chronic condition (*Ledford, 1998).

Determine With Individual Factors That Decrease Pain Tolerance and/or Factors That Increase Pain

Determine With Individual and Family the Effects of Chronic Pain on the Individual's Life (Ferrell, 1995; Pasero & McCaffery, 2011)

- Physical well-being (fatigue, strength, appetite, sleep, function, constipation, nausea)
- Psychological well-being (anxiety, depression, coping, control, concentration, sense of usefulness, fear, enjoyment)
- Spiritual well-being (religiosity, uncertainty, positive changes, sense of purpose, hopefulness, suffering, meaning of pain, transcendence)
- Social well-being (family support, family distress, sexuality, affection, employment, isolation, financial burden, appearance, roles, relationships)

  R: Chronic pain is an intense experience for the individual and family members. Interventions focus on helping families understand pain's effects on roles and relationships.

Evaluate for the Presence of Depression

- Explain the relationship between chronic pain and mood disorders (e.g., anger, anxiety, depression).
- Refer to primary care provider or specialist for management of depression.

  R: The individual with chronic pain may respond with withdrawal, depression, anxiety, anger, frustration, and dependency, all of which can affect the family in the same way. Fifty percent of individuals with chronic pain have depression or anxiety disorders. Major depression is thought to be four times greater in people with chronic back pain than in the general population (*Sullivan, Reesor, Mikail, & Fisher, 1992). Currie and Wang (*2004) found that the greater the rate of major depression, the greater the pain severity.

Evaluate the Individual's Sleep Quality

- Refer to *Disturbed Sleep Pattern* for interventions.

  R: Depression and insomnia are the most common comorbid disorders experienced by chronic pain individuals (Wilson, Eriksson, D'Eon, Mikail, & Emery, 2002). Research suggests that interventions for insomnia and depression may yield improvements across a number of chronic pain-related variables, including pain intensity, affective/sensory pain ratings, and anxiety (Tang, Wright, & Salkovskis, 2007).

Provide Pain Relief With Prescribed Analgesics

* Determine preferred route of administration: oral, IM, IV, rectal.
* Assess individual's response to the medication. For those admitted to acute care settings:
* After administration, return in 30 minutes to assess effectiveness.
* Ask individual to rate severity of pain before the medication and amount of relief received.
* Consult with the physician/advanced practice nurse if a dosage or interval change is needed.

Monitor for Adverse Effects

* Carefully monitor individuals who are taking sedating medications and opioid analgesics for respiratory failure every hour for first 12 hours on opioids (Myers-Glower, 2013).
* Contact the prescribing professional if the individual is frequently drowsy, is arousable, but drifts off to sleep during conversation (Pasero & McCaffery, 2011).

    R: Monitoring of respiratory function usually includes respiratory rate and oxygen saturation (SaO$_2$). "Yet significant hypercapnia may arise before oxygen desaturation occurs. After a patient's pain has been relieved, he or she may fall asleep and slip into respiratory depression and apnea" (Myers-Glower, 2013).

Encourage the Use of Oral Medications as Soon as Possible

* Consult with physician/nurse practitioner for a schedule to change from IM to IV or oral.
* Explain to individual and family that oral medications can be as effective as IM.

Explain How the Transition Will Occur

* Begin oral medication at a larger dose than necessary (loading dose).
* Continue p.r.n. IV medication, but use as a backup for pain unrelieved by oral medication.
* Gradually reduce IM IV medication dose.
* Use the individual's account of pain to regulate oral doses.

Consult With Physician/Nurse Practitioner About Possibly Adding Aspirin or Acetaminophen to Medication Regimen

R: The oral route is preferred because it is convenient and cost effective. Intramuscular routes are painful and have unreliable absorption rates (Pasero & McCaffery, 2011).

If Using Long-Acting Opioids Such as Duragesic Patch, Evaluate Need for a Short-Acting Medication for Breakthrough Pain

R: "The routine treatment of breakthrough pain is considered, in general, to be conventional practice in populations for which opioid therapy is the mainstay for the long-term management of moderate to severe pain—specifically those with active cancer or other types of advanced medical illness" (Pasero, 2010, p. 38).

Discuss (Individual's/Family's) Fears of Addiction and Undertreatment of Pain

* Explain tolerance versus addiction.

    R: Control of pain effectively requires clarifying misconception about addiction and overdose. Opioid tolerance and physical dependence are expected with long-term opioid treatment. Addiction is different and not usual in individuals who use opioids for pain management (*APS, 2005; Pasero & McCaffery, 2011).

Teach and Demonstrate the Effectiveness of Distraction Techniques

* Watching a favorite movie
* Reading a book or listening to a book on tape
* Listening to only music (20 minutes to 1 hour daily)

    R: Distraction techniques focus one's attention away from negative or painful images to positive mental thoughts. Explain that the pain will return after the distraction is over.

Discuss the Use of Heat Applications (e.g., Hot Water Bottle, Warm Tub, Hot Summer Sun, Electric Heating Pad, Moist Heat Pack, Topical Analgesic Gels/Lotions, Single-Use Air-Activated Heating Pads, Thin Plastic Wrap over Painful Area to Retain Body Heat [e.g., Knee, Elbow]), Their Therapeutic Effects, Indications, and Related Precautions

- Refer to rationale to explain benefits.

   R: Heat causes an increase in blood flow to an area, and it brings along oxygen and nutrients that can help to speed healing. Heat relaxes muscles, which can decrease some types of pain sensations, and can increase flexibility and an overall feeling of comfort. The sensation of heat on the skin stimulates the sensory receptors in the skin, and therefore reduces the perception of pain by decreasing transmissions of pain signals to the brain. Heat therapy application facilitates stretching the soft tissues around the spine, including muscles, connective tissue, and adhesions, which increases flexibility (Pasero & McCaffery, 2011).

Discuss the Use of Cold Applications, Their Therapeutic Effects, Indications, and Related Precautions (e.g., Cold Towels [Wrung Out], Ice Bag, Cold Gel Pack)

- Refer to rationale to explain benefits to the individual.

   R: Cold therapy provides pain relief (analgesia) by decreasing muscle spasms and by inhibiting pain sensations by reducing the speed of impulses conducted by nerve fibers (Pasero & McCaffery, 2011).

Teach Relaxation Breathing

- Find a quiet, comfortable place to sit or lie down in a dark room.
- First, take a normal breath. Then try a deep breath: breathe in slowly through your nose, allowing your chest and lower belly to rise as you fill your lungs. Let your abdomen expand fully. Now breathe out slowly through your mouth (or your nose, if that feels more natural).
- Try to practice once or twice a day, always at the same time, in order to enhance the sense of ritual and establish a habit.
- Try to practice at least 10 to 20 minutes each day. Accessed from http://www.health.harvard.edu/fhg/updates/update1006a.shtml

   R: When the body's stress response is activated, breathing becomes shallow. Breathing slowly and deeply activates the relaxation response.

Initiate Health Teaching and Referrals as Indicated

- Discuss with individual and family the various treatment modalities available:
  - Family therapy
  - Group therapy
  - Behavior modification
  - Biofeedback
  - Hypnosis
  - Acupuncture
  - Exercise program
- Access a multitude of stress-relieving techniques at http://www.stress-relief-tools.com

RISK FOR PRESSURE ULCER

NANDA-I Definition

Vulnerable to localized injury to the skin and/or underlying tissue usually over a bony prominence as a result of pressure, or pressure in combination with shear (National Pressure Ulcer Advisory Panel [NPUAP], 2007).

Risk Factors

Pathophysiological

Adult: Braden Scale score of <18

Alteration in cognitive functioning

Alteration in sensation

American Society of Anesthesiologists (ASA) (2014) Physical Status classification score ≥2

Anemia

Cardiovascular disease

Child: Braden Q Scale of ≤16

Decrease in serum albumin level

Electrolyte imbalances, elevated urea, elevated creatinine above 1 mg/dL, lymphopenia, elevated C-reactive protein*

Decrease in tissue oxygenation

Decrease in tissue perfusion* (e.g., hypertension, hypotension, CVA, diabetes mellitus, renal disease, peripheral vascular disease)

Dehydration

Diabetes mellitus*

Edema

Elevated skin temperature by 1° C to 2° C

History of cerebral vascular accident

History of pressure ulcer

History of trauma

Hyperthermia

Impaired circulation

Low score on Risk Assessment Pressure Sore (RAPS) scale

Lymphopenia

New York Heart Association (NYHA) Functional Classification ≥2

Hip fracture

Nonblanchable erythema (Author's note: this is not a risk factor but instead represents Stage I pressure ulcer)

Treatment Related

Pharmaceutical agents (e.g., general anesthesia, vasopressors, antidepressant, norepinephrine)

Extended period of immobility on hard surface (e.g., surgical procedure ≥2 hours)

Shearing forces

Surface friction

Use of linen with insufficient moisture wicking property

Situational (Personal, Environmental)

Extremes of weight

Inadequate nutrition

Incontinence

Insufficient caregiver

Knowledge of pressure ulcer prevention

Physical immobilization

Pressure over bony prominence

Reduced triceps skin fold thickness

Scaly skin

Dry skin

Self-care deficit

Skin moisture

Smoking

Female gender

Decreased cognition[6]

Debilitated*

---

[6]Added by author source: NPUAP (2014)

Maturational

Extremes of age

> **CLINICAL ALERT:**
> • Pressure ulcers are among the most common conditions encountered in acutely hospitalized individuals (0% to 46%), in critical care (13.1% to 45.5%) or those requiring long-term institutional care (4.1% to 32.2%). An estimated 2.5 million pressure ulcers are treated each year in acute care facilities in the United States alone (Advisory Panel, European Pressure Ulcer Advisory Panel, 2014). The average hospital treatment cost associated with stage IV pressure ulcers and related complications was $129,248 for hospital-acquired ulcers during one admission and $124,327 for community-acquired ulcers over an average of 4 admissions (Brem et al., 2010). Studies have shown that the development of a pressure ulcer independently increases the length of an individual's hospital stay by 4 to 10 days. These prolonged hospital stays are also associated with an increased incidence of nosocomial infections and other complications. In the fourth quarter of 2011, on average, nursing homes had 6.9% of their long-stay high-risk residents with pressure ulcers (Berlowitz, 2014a; Ling & Mandl, 2013); the best nursing homes had a rate of 4%, and the worst had a rate of 12%. Of the facilities, 6.9% reported no pressure ulcers (Berlowitz, 2014a).

Goal

NOC

Immobility Consequences, Tissue Integrity: Skin and Mucous Membrane, Circulation Status, Nutrition Status, Risk Control, Urinary Continence

The individual will demonstrate skin integrity free of pressure ulcers (if able), as evidenced by the following indicators:

• Participate in risk assessment.
• Express willingness to participate in prevention of pressure ulcers.
• Describe etiology and prevention measures.

Interventions (NPUAP, 2014)

NIC

Pressure Management, Pressure Ulcer Care, Skin Surveillance, Positioning, Nutrition, Skin Surveillance Management, Perineal Care

• Determine the level of risk in the individual for pressure ulcers. Refer to back cover.
• Braden Scale for Predicting Pressure Sore Risk

Assess Dependent Skin Areas With Every Position Turn

• Use finger or transparent disk to assess whether skin is blanchable or nonblanchable.

    R: "Blanchable erythema is visible skin redness that become white when pressure is applied and reddens when pressure relieved" (NPUAP, 2014, p. 63). It may result from normal reactive hyperemia that should disappear within several hours or it may result from inflammatory erythema with intact capillary bed. Nonblanchable erythema is visible redness that persists with the application of pressure, which indicates structural damage to microcirculation. This represents Category/Stage I pressure ulcer (NPUAP, 2014, p. 63).

• Assess skin temperature, edema and change in tissue consistency as compared with surrounding tissue.

    R: Localized heat edema and change in tissue consistency as induration/hardness as compared with surrounding tissue are warning signs for pressure ulcer development (NPUAP, 2014).

• Observe the skin for pressure damage caused by medical devices (e.g., catheters and cervical collars).

> **CLINICAL ALERT:**
> • Do not wear gloves when assessing skin temperature and changes in tissue consistency. As indicated, cleanse skin before assessing and follow usual hand-washing procedures.

- Document all skin assessments, noting details of any pain possibly related to pressure damage.

    R: *The frequency of inspection may need to be increased in response to any deterioration in overall condition.*

- Ask the individual if they have any areas of discomfort or pain that could be attributed to pressure damage.

    R: *Studies reported that pain over the site was a precursor to tissue breakdown (NPUAP, 2014).*

Access the Wound Specialist, if There Are Changes in Skin Assessment (e.g., nonblanchable erythema)

R: *Researchers have reported that the failure to identify early stages of pressure damage results in greater numbers of people with darkly pigmented skin developing more severe forms of pressure damage (Baumgarten et al., 2004; NPUAP, 2014; Rosen et al., 2006). Early identification and initiation of corrective measure are critical for all types of skin tones.*

For Individuals With Darkly Pigmented Skin, Consider the Following (*Bennett 1995; Clark, 2010, p. 17)

- The color of intact dark pigmented skin may remain unchanged (does not blanch) when pressure is applied over a bony prominence.
- Local areas of intact skin that are subject to pressure may feel either warm or cool when touched. This assessment should be performed without gloves to make it easier to distinguish differences in temperature. Any body fluids should be cleansed before making this direct contact.
- Areas of skin subjected to pressure may be purplish/bluish/violet in color. This can be compared with the erythema seen in people with lighter skin tones.
- Complains of, or indications for, current or recent pain or discomfort at body sites where pressure has been applied should be considered.

    R: *Stage I pressure ulcers are underdetected in individuals with darkly pigmented skin. Visual cues for changes in skin appearance may be relatively easy to observe in Caucasian skin but with darker pigmentation it may be harder to spot visual signs of early changes due to pressure damage (Clark, 2010; NPUAP, 2014).*

Increase Frequency of the Turning Schedule if Any Nonblanchable Erythema Is Noted

- Consult with prescribing professional for the utilization of pressure-dispersing devices and microclimate manipulation devices in addition to repositioning.

    R: *Principles of pressure ulcer prevention include reducing or rotating pressure on soft tissue. If pressure on soft tissue exceeds intracapillary pressure (approximately 32 mm Hg), capillary occlusion and resulting hypoxia can cause tissue damage. The greater the duration of immobility, the greater the likelihood of the development of small vessel thrombosis and subsequent tissue necrosis (NPUAP, 2014).*

> **CLINICAL ALERT:**
> - Peterson, Gravenstein, Schwab, van Oostrom, and Caruso (2013) reported using pressure-mapping devices to measure pressure on skin/tissue, when high-risk individuals were positioned on their back, left side, and right side. "Bedridden individuals at risk for pressure ulcer formation exhibit high skin–bed interface pressures on specific skin areas that are likely always at risk (i.e., triple-jeopardy and always-at-risk areas) for the vast majority of the time they are in bed despite routine repositioning care. Triple jeopardy were skin areas that were consistently compressed in all three positions. Health-care providers are unaware of the actual tissue-relieving effectiveness (or lack thereof) of their repositioning interventions, which may partially explain why pressure ulcer mitigation strategies are not always successful. Relieving at-risk tissue is a necessary part of pressure ulcer prevention, but the repositioning practice itself needs improvement."

Place the Individual in Normal or Neutral Position With Body Weight Evenly Distributed

- Use 30 degrees laterally inclined position when possible. Avoid postures that increase pressure, such as the 90 degrees side-lying position, or the semirecumbent position.

    R: *Pressure is a compressing downward force on a given area. If pressure against soft tissue is greater than intracapillary blood pressure (approximately 32 mm Hg), the capillaries can be occluded and the tissue can be damaged as a result of hypoxia.*

Use Transfer Aids to Reduce Friction and Shear

* Lift—don't drag—the individual while repositioning.

  R: Shear is a parallel force in which one layer of tissue moves in one direction and another layer moves in the opposite direction. If the skin sticks to the bed linen and the weight of the body makes the skeleton slide down inside the skin (as with semi-Fowler's positioning), the subepidermal capillaries may become angulated and pinched, resulting in decreased perfusion of the tissue (Grossman & Porth, 2014).

  R: Friction is the physiologic wearing away of tissue. If the skin is rubbed against the bed linens, the epidermis can be denuded by abrasion.

* Avoid positioning the individual directly onto medical devices, such as tubes or drainage systems.
* Avoid positioning the individual on bony prominences with existing nonblanchable erythema.
* If sitting in bed is necessary, avoid head-of-bed elevation or a slouched position that places pressure and shear on the sacrum and coccyx.

  R: Reposition the individual in such a way that pressure is relieved or redistributed.

Promote Optimal Circulation When the Person Is Sitting

* Limit sitting time for those at high risk for ulcer development.
* Instruct to lift self using chair arms every 10 minutes, if possible, or assist in rising up off the chair at least every hour, depending on risk factors present.
* Do not elevate the legs unless calves are supported to reduce the pressure over the ischial tuberosities.
* Pad the chair with pressure-relieving cushion.
* Inspect areas at risk of developing ulcers with each position change.

  R: Pressure ulcer can result from soft tissue compression between a bony prominence and an external surface for a prolonged period of time (Berkowitz, 2014).

Use of Support Surfaces to Prevent Pressure Ulcers

R: Pressure ulcer can result from soft tissue compression between a bony prominence and an external surface for a prolonged period of time (Berkowitz, 2014).

* Use a pressure-redistributing seat cushion for individuals sitting in a chair whose mobility is reduced.
* Limit the time an individual spends seated in a chair without pressure relief.
* Use alternating-pressure active support overlays or mattress as indicated.

  R: A pressure-reducing surface must not be able to be fully compressed by the body. To be effective, a support surface must be capable of first being deformed and then redistributing the weight of the body across the surface. Comfort is not a valid criterion for determining adequate pressure reduction. A hand check should be performed to determine if the product is effectively reducing pressure. The palm is placed under the pressure-reducing mattress; if the individual can feel the hand or the caregiver can feel the individual, the pressure is not adequate.

Attempt to Modify Contributing Factors to Lessen the Possibility of a Pressure Ulcer Developing

Incontinence of Urine or Feces

* Determine the etiology of the incontinence.
* Maintain sufficient fluid intake for adequate hydration (approximately 2,500 mL daily, unless contraindicated); check oral mucous membranes for moisture and check urine specific gravity.
* Establish a schedule for emptying the bladder (begin with every 2 hours).
* If the individual is confused, determine what his or her incontinence pattern is and intervene before incontinence occurs.
* Explain problem to the individual; secure his or her cooperation for the plan.
* When incontinent, wash the perineum with a liquid soap.
* Apply a protective barrier to the perineal region (incontinence film barrier spray or wipes).
* Check the individual frequently for incontinence when indicated.
* For additional interventions, refer to *Impaired Urinary Elimination*.

  R: Maceration is a mechanism by which the tissue is softened by prolonged wetting or soaking. If the skin becomes waterlogged, the cells are weakened and the epidermis is easily eroded. Bowel incontinence is more damaging than urinary incontinence due to the additional digestive enzymes found in stool. Care must be taken to prevent excoriation (Wilkinson & Van Leuven, 2007).

Skin Care

- Whenever possible, do not turn the individual onto a body surface that is still reddened from a previous episode of pressure loading.
- Do not use massage for pressure ulcer prevention or do not vigorously rub skin that is at risk for pressure ulceration.

  R: Massage is contraindicated in the presence of acute inflammation and where there is the possibility of damaged blood vessels or fragile skin.

- Use skin emollients to hydrate dry skin in order to reduce risk of skin damage. Protect the skin from exposure to excessive moisture with a barrier product.

  R: Excessive moisture will contribute to maceration when tissues are softened by prolonged wetting, which breaks down the protective layer of epidermis/dermis.

- Avoid use of synthetic sheepskin pads; cutout, ring, or donut-type devices; and water-filled gloves.

  R: These products are irritating and create pressure, which compromises circulation.

- Monitor serum prealbumin levels.
  - Less than 5 mg/dL predicts a poor prognosis.
  - Less than 11 mg/dL predicts high risk and requires aggressive nutritional supplementation.
  - Less than 15 mg/dL predicts an increased risk of malnutrition (*Evans, 2005).

    R: Laboratory values, such as albumin, prealbumin, and transferrin, may not reflect the current nutritional state, especially in the critically ill individual. Other assessment factors such as weight loss, illness severity, co-morbid conditions, and gastrointestinal function should be considered for a nutrition plan of care (Doley, 2010).

Nutrition

- Ensure a nutritional assessment is completed by a registered dietician/nutritionist using the MNA, if possible.

  R: MNA is the only nutritional screening tool that has been specifically validated in individuals with pressure ulcers (NPUAP, 2014).

- Report to prescribing provider when food and/or fluid intake is decreased.

  R: Fortified foods and/or high-calorie, high-protein oral nutrition supplements between meals may be needed (NPUAP, 2014).

- Advise family/friends the importance of nutritionally dense foods/beverages versus calorie-dense foods/beverages.
  - Calorie-dense foods, also called energy-dense foods, contain high levels of calories per serving in fat and carbohydrates. Many processed foods are considered calorie-dense, such as cakes, cookies, snacks, doughnuts, and candies.
  - Nutrient-dense foods contain high levels of nutrients, such as protein, carbohydrates, fats, vitamins, and minerals, but with less calories. Some nutrient-dense foods are fresh fruits, vegetables, berries, melons, dark-green vegetables, sweet potatoes, tomatoes, and whole grains, including quinoa, barley, bulgur, and oats. Lean beef and pork are high in protein and contain high levels of zinc, iron, and B vitamins.

    R: Individuals with pressure ulcers need 30 to 35 kcal/kg body weight, 1.25 to 1.5 grams of protein/kg body weight daily, and vitamins and minerals (NPUAP, 2014). Calorie-dense foods do not provide the needed nutrients and can replace the needed nutrient-dense foods when the individual's appetite is poor.

- Refer to *Imbalance Nutrition* for interventions related to promoting optimal intake of required nutrients.

  R: Malnutrition is associated with impaired wound healing (NPUAP, 2014).

Initiate Health Teaching as Indicated

- Instruct the individual/family in specific techniques to use at home to prevent pressure ulcers.
- Teach how to use their finger to assess whether skin is blanchable or nonblanchable and when to notify primary care provider.
- Stress the importance of prevention and early identification of nonblanchable redness.

- Consider the use of long-term pressure-relieving devices for permanent disabilities.
  - Initiate a referral to a home health nurse for an in-home assessment.
    R: Pressure reduction is the one consistent intervention that must be continued at home.

IMPAIRED PHYSICAL MOBILITY

NANDA-I Definition

Limitation in independent, purposeful physical movement of the body or of one or more extremities

Defining Characteristics (*Levin, Krainovitch, Bahrenburg, & Mitchell, 1989)

Compromised ability to move purposefully within the environment (e.g., bed mobility, transfers, ambulation)
Range-of-motion (ROM) limitations
Imposed restriction of movement
Reluctance to move

Related Factors

Pathophysiologic

Related to decreased muscle strength* and endurance* secondary to:

Neuromuscular impairment
Autoimmune alterations (e.g., multiple sclerosis, arthritis)
Muscular dystrophy
Partial paralysis (spinal cord injury, stroke)
Nervous system diseases (e.g., Parkinson's disease, myasthenia gravis, tumors)
Trauma
Cancer
Musculoskeletal impairment
Fractures
Connective tissue disease (systemic lupus erythematosus)

Related to joint stiffness* or contraction* secondary to:

Inflammatory joint disease
Post–joint-replacement or spinal surgery
Degenerative joint disease
Degenerative disc disease

Related to peripheral edema

Treatment Related

Related to equipment (e.g., ventilators, enteral therapy, dialysis, total parenteral nutrition)
Related to external devices (casts or splints, braces, intravenous [IV] tubing)
Related to insufficient strength and endurance for ambulation with aids (e.g., prosthesis, crutches, walker) (specify)

Situational (Personal, Environmental)

Related to:

Fatigue	Deconditioning*
Depressive mood state*	Obesity
Decreased motivation	Dyspnea
Sedentary lifestyle*	Cognitive impairment*
Pain*	

Author's Note

Impaired Physical Mobility describes an individual with deconditioning from immobility resulting from a medical or surgical condition. The literature is full of the effects of immobility on body system function. Early progressive mobility programs or progressive mobility activity protocol (PMAP) are designed to prevent these complications. These programs are appropriate for individuals in intensive care units, other hospital units, and skilled nursing care facilities.

These programs necessitate continuous nursing attention. Several potential barriers for maintaining PMAP have been identified as lack of mobility education, safety concerns, and lack of interdisciplinary collaboration (King, 2012). Gillis , MacDonald, and MacIssac (2008) reported that time constraints due to increased acuity and staffing issues have lowered the priority and time available for basic mobility.

Acuity levels on units must address the workload associated with PMAP and factor this into staffing. Several studies have shown the cost-effectiveness of PMAP with decreased ICU stays, decreased ventilator use, and decreased hospital stays. In addition, complications of immobility as decreased deep-vein thrombosis ventilator–associated pneumonia and delirium.

Nursing interventions for *Impaired Physical Mobility* focus on early mobilization muscle strengthening and restoring function and preventing deterioration. *Impaired Physical Mobility* can also be utilized to describe someone with limited use of arm(s) or leg(s) or limited muscle strength.

Impaired Physical Mobility is one of the cluster of diagnoses in *Risk for Disuse Syndrome*. Limitation of physical movement of arms/legs also can be the etiology of other nursing diagnoses, such as *Self-Care Deficit* and *Risk for Injury*. If the individual can exercise but does not, refer to *Sedentary Lifestyle*. If the individual has no limitations in movement but is deconditioned and has reduced endurance, refer to *Activity Intolerance*.

Goals

NOC

Progressive Mobility Protocol[7]: Joint Mobility, Strength Training, Exercise Therapy: Positioning, Teaching: Prescribed Activity/ Exercise, Fall Prevention

The individual will report increased strength and endurance of limbs as evidenced by the following indicators:

- Demonstrate the use of adaptive devices to increase mobility.
- Use safety measures to minimize potential for injury.
- Describe rationale for interventions.
- Demonstrate measures to increase mobility.
- Evaluate pain and effectiveness of management.

Interventions

NIC

Progressive Mobility Protocol[7]: Joint Mobility, Strength Training, Exercise Therapy: Positioning, Teaching: Prescribed Activity/ Exercise, Fall Prevention

Assess for Barriers to Early Mobilization in the Health-Care Setting

- Refer to Box II.1

  R: Early mobility has been linked to decreased morbidity and mortality as inactivity has a profound adverse effect on the brain, skin, skeletal muscle, and pulmonary and cardiovascular systems.

Box II.1   BARRIERS AND FACILITATORS OF PROGRESSIVE MOBILITY ACTIVITY (Winkelman & Peereboom, 2010)

Faciltators

- The presence of a protocol in the institution, which guided decisions about readiness for increased activity
- Glasgow coma score greater than 10
- Beds that provided a chair position
- Prescriber's order
- Expert mentor (nurse, physical therapist)

Barriers

- Absence of the above facilitators
- Nurse's perception of the individual nonreadiness for increased activity
- Physical therapy not being consulted

---

[7]Added by Lynda Juall Carpenito.

> **CLINICAL ALERT:**
> • "Critically ill individuals who are older, with comorbid conditions such as diabetes and preexisting cardiac disease and/or the presence of vasoactive agents, will be at greater risk for not tolerating in-bed mobilization. It is critical that the nurse assess the risk factors and plan when activity will occur to allow sufficient physiological rest to meet the oxygen demand that positioning will place on the body" (Vollman, 2012, p. 174).

Consult With Physical Therapist for Evaluation and Development of a Mobility Plan

R: Physical therapists are professional experts on mobility.

Promote Optimal Mobility and Movement in All Health-Care Settings With Stable Individuals Regardless of the Ability to Walk

R: "As technology and medications have improved and increased, survival rates are also increasing in intensive care units (ICUs), so it is now important to focus on improving the individual outcomes and recovery. To do this, ICU individuals need to be assessed and started on an early mobility program, if stable" (Zomorodi, Topley, & McAnaw, 2012, p. 1).

Initiate an In-Bed Mobility Program Within Hours of Admission if Stable (Vollman, 2012)

- Maintain HOB 30 degrees, including individual on ventilators unless contraindicated

  R: This allows increased perfusion in all lung tissue.

- Initiate a turning schedule within hours of admission if stable.

  R: This can prevent prolonged gravitational equilibrium. Prolonged periods in a stationary position result in greater hemodynamic instability when the individual turned (Vollman, 2012).

- Assess tolerance to position change 5 to 10 minutes after apposition change.

  R: This time frame is needed to sufficiently assess response.

- Initially turn slowly to the right side.

  R: "The right lateral position should be used initially to prevent the hemodynamic challenges reported with use of the left lateral position" (Vollman, 2012, p. 174).

Initiate a Progressive Mobility Activity Protocol (PMAP) for Individuals in all Settings as Medical Stability Increases (e.g., Step-Down Unit, Medical, Surgical Units, Skilled Nursing Facilities)

R: The PMAP is a nursing and interdisciplinary team approach to increase movement through a series of progressive steps from passive range of motion to ambulating independently as their medical stability increases (Hopkins & Spuhler, 2009).

Explain to Individual and Family Why the Staff Are Frequently Moving the Individual

R: An explanation of what the moving is preventing (e.g., muscle wasting, blood clots, pneumonia) may improve cooperation.

Initiate Early Progressive Mobility Protocol. Consult With Physical Therapy and Prescribing Provider (American Association of Critical Care Nurses [AACN], 2012; American Hospital Association, 2014; Timmerman, 2007; Zomorodi et al., 2012)

Step 1: Safety Screening (AACN, 2012)
- M—Myocardial stability
  - No evidence of active myocardial ischemia × 24 hours.
  - No arrhythmia requiring new antidysrhythmic agent × 24 hours.
- O—Oxygenation adequate on:
  - $F_{IO_2} < 0.6$
  - PEEP < 10 cm H_2O
- V—Vasopressor(s) minimal
  - No increase of any vasopressor × 2 hours.

- E—Engages to voice
  - Individuals responds to verbal stimulation
- Reevaluate in 24 hours

Before Initiating Step 2, Level 1:

- Evaluate need for analgesics versus risk of increased sedation before activity.
- Progress each step to 30 to 60 minutes' duration depending on the individual's tolerance.
- Repeat each step until individual demonstrates hemodynamic and physical tolerance to the activity/position for 60 minutes, and then advance to next step at the next activity period.

Step 2: Progressive Mobility

- Follow protocol for progression from level 1 to level 4. If no protocol exists, consult with physical therapy for a written plan (American Critical Care Nurses Association, 2012)—Early Progressive Mobility Protocol, AACNPearl, http://www.aacn.org/wd/practice/docs/tool%20kits/early-progressive-mobility-protocol.pdf
- Encourage AAROM/AROM 3 times/day with RN, PCT, PT, OT, or family

Assess for Clinical Signs and Symptoms Indicating Terminating a Mobilization Session (Adler & Malone, 2012)

Heart Rate

- >70% age-predicted maximum heart rate
- >20% decrease in resting heart rate
- <40 beats/minute; >130 beats/min
- New onset arrhythmia
- New antiarrhythmia medication
- New myocardial infarction by ECG or cardiac enzymes

Pulse Oximetry/Saturation of Peripheral Oxygen (Spo$_2$)

- >4% decrease
- <88% to 90%

Blood Pressure

- Systolic BP >180 mm Hg
- >20% decrease in systolic/diastolic BP; orthostatic hypotension
- Mean arterial blood pressure <65 mm Hg; >110 mm Hg
- Presences of vasopressor medication; new vasopressor or escalating dose of vasopressor medication

Alertness/Agitation and Individual Symptoms

- Individual sedation or coma—Richmond Agitation Sedation Scale, ≤ –3
- Individual agitation requiring addition or escalation of sedative medication; Richmond Agitation Sedation Scale, >2
- Complaints of intolerable dyspnea on exertion

Promote Motivation and Adherence (*Addams & Clough, 1998; Halstead & Stoten, 2010)

- Explain the effects of immobility.
- Explain the purpose of progressive mobility, passive and active ROM exercises.
- Establish short-term goals.
- Ensure that initial exercises are easy and require minimal strength and coordination.
- Progress only if the individual is successful at the present exercise.
- Provide written instructions for prescribed exercises after demonstrating and observing return demonstration.
- Document and discuss improvement specifically (e.g., can lift leg 2 in higher).

    R: *Mobility is one of the most significant aspects of physiologic functioning because it greatly influences maintenance of independence (Miller, 2015). Motivation can be increased if short-term goals are accomplished.*

- Evaluate the level of motivation and depression. Refer to a specialist as needed.

    R: *Effective management of pain and depression is sometimes necessary. Inadequate pain relief may be a primary factor leading to depression in some people, but depression should not be discounted as a secondary feature of pain. Depression may require aggressive management, including drugs and other therapies.*

Increase Limb Mobility and Determine Type of ROM Appropriate for the Individual (Passive, Active Assistive, Active, Active Resistive)

- For passive ROM:
  - Begin exercises slowly, doing only a few movements at first.
  - Support the limb below the joint with one hand.
  - Move joint slowly and smoothly until you feel the stretch.
  - Move the joint to the point of resistance. Stop if the person complaints of discomfort or you observe a facial grimace.
  - Do the exercise 10 times and hold the position for a few seconds.
  - Do all exercises on one side and then repeat them on the opposite side if indicated.
  - If possible, teach the person or caregiver how to do the passive ROM.
  - Refer to http://alsworldwide.org/assets/misc/RANGE_OF_MOTION_EXERCISES_WITH_PHOTOS_copy.pdf for specific instructions and photos of passive ROM
- Perform active assistive ROM exercises (frequency determined by individual's condition):
  - If possible teach the individual/family to perform active ROM exercises on unaffected limbs at least four times a day, if possible.

    R: Active ROM increases muscle mass, tone, and strength and improves cardiac and respiratory functioning. Passive ROM improves joint mobility and circulation and decreases the likelihood of contractures.

Position in Alignment to Prevent Complications

- Use a footboard.

  R: This measure prevents foot drop.

- Avoid prolonged sitting or lying in the same position.

  R: This prevents hip flexion contractures.

- Change the position of the shoulder joints every 2 to 4 hours.

  R: This helps to prevent shoulder contractures.

- Use a small pillow or no pillow when in Fowler's position.

  R: This prevents flexion contracture of neck.

- Support the hand and wrist in natural alignment.

  R: This prevents dependent edema and flexion contractures of the hand.

- If supine or prone, place a rolled towel or small pillow under the lumbar curvature or under the end of the rib cage.

  R: This prevents flexion or hyperflexion of lumbar curvature.

- Place a trochanter roll alongside the hips and upper thighs.

  R: This presents external rotation of the femur and hips.

- If in the lateral position, place pillow(s) to support the leg from groin to foot, and use a pillow to flex the shoulder and elbow slightly. If needed, support the lower foot in dorsal flexion with a towel roll or special boot.

  R: These measures prevent internal rotation and adduction of the femur and shoulder and prevent foot drop.

RISK FOR INEFFECTIVE RESPIRATORY FUNCTION

NANDA-I Definition

At risk for experiencing a threat to the passage of air through the respiratory tract and/or to the exchange of gases (O_2–CO_2) between the lungs and the vascular system

Risk Factors

Presence of risk factors that can change respiratory function (see Related Factors).

Related Factors

Pathophysiologic

Related to excessive or thick secretions secondary to:

Infection	Cardiac or pulmonary disease
Inflammation	Smoking
Allergy	Exposure to noxious chemical

Related to immobility, stasis of secretions, and ineffective cough secondary to:

Diseases of the nervous system (e.g., Guillain–Barré syndrome, multiple sclerosis, myasthenia gravis)
Central nervous system (CNS) depression/head trauma
Cerebrovascular accident (stroke)
Quadriplegia

Treatment Related

Related to immobility secondary to:

Sedating or paralytic effects of medications, drugs, or chemicals (specify)
Anesthesia, general or spinal

Related to suppressed cough reflex secondary to (specify)
Related to effects of tracheostomy (altered secretions)

Situational (Personal, Environmental)

Related to immobility secondary to:

Surgery or trauma	Perception/cognitive impairment
Fatigue	Fear
Pain	Anxiety

Related to extremely high or low humidity

For infants, related to placement on stomach for sleep
Exposure to cold, laughing, crying, allergens, and smoke

 Carp's Cues

The author has added *Risk for Ineffective Respiratory Function* to describe a state that may affect the entire respiratory system, not just isolated areas, such as airway clearance or gas exchange. Allergy and immobility are examples of factors that affect the entire system; thus, it is incorrect to say *Impaired Gas Exchange Related to Immobility* because immobility also affects airway clearance and breathing patterns. The nurse can use the diagnoses *Ineffective Airway Clearance* and *Ineffective Breathing Patterns* when nurses can definitely alleviate the contributing factors influencing respiratory function (e.g., ineffective cough, stress).

The nurse is cautioned not to use this diagnosis to describe acute respiratory disorders, which are the primary responsibility of medicine and nursing together (i.e., collaborative problems). Such problems can be labeled *RC of Acute Hypoxia* or *RC of Pulmonary Edema*. When an individual's immobility is prolonged and threatens multiple systems—for example, integumentary, musculoskeletal, vascular, as well as respiratory—the nurse should use *Disuse Syndrome* to describe the entire situation.

REFER to Generic Care Plan for individual experiencing Surgery for prevention of respiratory complications in Unit III.

SELF-CARE DEFICIT SYNDROME

Definition

State in which an individual experiences an impaired motor function or cognitive function, causing a decreased ability in performing each of the five self-care activities

Defining Characteristics

Bathing Self-Care Deficit (Includes Washing Entire Body, Combing Hair, Brushing Teeth, Attending to Skin and Nail Care, and Applying Makeup)

Inability or unwilling to:

Access bathroom	Dry body
Get bath supplies	Obtain a water source
Wash body	Regulate bath water

Dressing Self-Care Deficits (Includes Donning Regular or Special Clothing, Not Nightclothes)

Inability or unwilling to:
- Choose clothing or put clothing on lower body
- Put clothing on upper body
- Put on necessary items of clothing
- Maintain appearance at a satisfactory level
- Pick up clothing
- Put on shoes/remove shoes
- Put on/remove socks
- Use assistive devices
- Use zippers
- Fasten, unfasten clothing
- Obtain clothing

Feeding Self-Care Deficit
Inability (or unwilling to):
- Bring food from a receptacle to the mouth
- Complete a meal
- Set food onto utensils
- Handle utensils
- Ingest food in a socially acceptable manner
- Open containers
- Pick up cup or glass
- Prepare food for ingestion
- Use assistive device

Instrumental Self-Care Deficits
Difficulty using telephone
Difficulty accessing transportation
Difficulty laundering, ironing
Difficulty managing money
Difficulty preparing meals
Difficulty with medication administration
Difficulty shopping

Toileting Self-Care Deficits
Unable or unwillingness to:
- Get to toilet or commode
- Carry out proper hygiene
- Manipulate clothing for toileting
- Rise from toilet or commode
- Sit on toilet or commode
- Flush toilet or empty commode

Instrumental ADLs
Difficulty to write checks and pay bills
Difficulty to handle cash transactions (simple, complex)

Difficulty with medication administration
Difficulty using telephone
Difficulty accessing transportation
Difficulty laundering, ironing
Difficulty managing money
Difficulty preparing meals
Difficulty shopping
Inadequate social supports:
   Support people
   Availability of help with transportation, shopping, money management, laundry, housekeeping, and
      food preparation
   Community resources

Related Factors

Pathophysiologic

Related to lack of coordination secondary to (specify)
Related to spasticity or flaccidity secondary to (specify)
Related to muscular weakness secondary to (specify)
Related to partial or total paralysis secondary to (specify)
Related to atrophy secondary to (specify)
Related to muscle contractures secondary to (specify)
Related to visual disorders secondary to (specify)
Related to nonfunctioning or missing limb(s)

Treatment Related

Related to external devices (specify) (e.g., casts, splints, braces, intravenous [IV] equipment)
Related to postoperative fatigue and pain

Situational (Personal, Environmental)

Related to cognitive deficits
Related to fatigue
Related to pain
Related to decreased motivation
Related to confusion
Related to disabling anxiety

Maturational

Older Adult
Related to decreased visual and motor ability, muscle weakness

Assess for Related Factors

Ability to remember
Judgment
Ability to follow directions
Ability to identify/express needs

Carp's Cues

Self-care encompasses the activities needed to meet daily needs, commonly known as activities of daily living (ADLs), which are learned over time and become lifelong habits. Self-care activities involve not only what is to be done (hygiene, bathing, dressing, toileting, feeding), but also how much, when, where, with whom, and how (Miller, 2015).

In every individual, the threat or reality of a self-care deficit evokes panic. Many people report that they fear loss of independence more than death. A self-care deficit affects the core of self-concept and self-determination. For this reason, the nursing focus for self-care deficit should be not on providing the care measure, but on identifying adaptive techniques to allow the individual the maximum degree of participation and independence possible.

Currently not on the NANDA-I list, the diagnosis *Self-Care Deficit Syndrome* has been added here to describe an individual with compromised ability in all five self-care activities. For this individual, the nurse assesses functioning in each area and identifies the level of participation of which the individual is capable. The goal is to maintain current functioning, to increase participation and independence, or both. The syndrome distinction clusters all five self-care deficits together to enable grouping of interventions when indicated, while also permitting specialized interventions for a specific deficit.

The danger of applying a Self-Care Deficit diagnosis lies in the possibility of prematurely labeling an individual as unable to participate at any level, eliminating a rehabilitation focus.

It is important to classify the individual's baseline functional level to evaluate changes in his or her ability to participate in self-care. Use the following scale to rate the individual's ability to perform:

0 = Is completely independent
1 = Requires use of assistive device
2 = Needs minimal help
3 = Needs assistance and/or some supervision
4 = Needs total supervision
5 = Needs total assistance or unable to assist

BATHING SELF-CARE DEFICIT

NANDA-I Definition

Impaired ability to perform or complete bathing activities for self

Defining Characteristics*

Inability (or unwilling) to:

Access bathroom	Dry body
Get bath supplies	Obtain a water source
Wash body	Regulate bath water

Goals/Interventions

Refer to Generic Medical Care Plan.

DRESSING SELF-CARE DEFICITS

NANDA-I Definition

Impaired ability to perform or complete dressing activities for self

Defining Characteristics

Inability or unwilling to:
Choose clothing
Put clothing on lower body
Put clothing on upper body

Put on necessary items of clothing
Maintain appearance at a satisfactory level
Pick up clothing
Put on shoes/remove shoes
Put on/remove socks
Use assistive devices
Use zippers
Fasten, unfasten clothing
Obtain clothing

Goals/Interventions

Refer to Generic Medical Care Plan.

FEEDING SELF-CARE DEFICIT

NANDA-I Definition

Impaired ability to perform or complete self-feeding activities

Defining Characteristics*

Inability (or unwilling to):
Bring food from a receptacle to the mouth
Complete a meal
Set food onto utensils
Handle utensils
Ingest food in a socially acceptable manner
Open containers
Pick up cup or glass
Prepare food for ingestion
Use assistive device

Goals/Interventions

Refer to Generic Medical Care Plan.

INSTRUMENTAL SELF-CARE DEFICITS

Definition

Impaired ability to perform certain activities or access certain services essential for managing a household

Defining Characteristics

Difficulty using telephone
Difficulty accessing transportation
Difficulty laundering, ironing

Difficulty managing money
Difficulty preparing meals
Difficulty with medication administration
Difficulty shopping

Goals/Interventions

- Initiate a home health assessment
- Consult with a home health nurse

R: For an accurate assessment and determination of assistance needed a home assessment is imperative.

TOILETING SELF-CARE DEFICIT

NANDA-I Definition

Impaired ability to perform or complete toileting activities for self

Defining Characteristics*

Unable (or unwilling) to:
Get to toilet or commode
Carry out proper hygiene
Manipulate clothing for toileting
Rise from toilet or commode
Sit on toilet or commode
Flush toilet or empty commode

Goals/Interventions

Refer to Generic Medical Care Plan.

DISTURBED SLEEP PATTERN

NANDA-I Definition

Time-limited interruptions of sleep amount and quality due to external factors

Defining Characteristics

Adults
Difficulty falling or remaining asleep
Fatigue on awakening or during the day
Agitation
Dozing during the day
Mood alterations

Related Factors

Many factors can contribute to disturbed sleep patterns. Some common factors follow.

Pathophysiologic

Related to frequent awakenings secondary to:

Impaired oxygen transport
    Angina
    Respiratory disorders
Impaired elimination; bowel or bladder
    Diarrhea
    Retention
    Constipation
Impaired metabolism
    Hyperthyroidism
    Hepatic disorders

Peripheral arteriosclerosis
Circulatory disorders

Dysuria
Incontinence
Frequency

Gastric ulcers

Treatment Related

Related to interruptions (e.g., for therapeutic monitoring, lab tests)*
Related to physical restraints*
Related to difficulty assuming usual position secondary to (specify)
Related to excessive daytime sleeping or hyperactivity secondary to (specify medication)

Tranquilizers
Sedatives
Amphetamines
Monoamine oxidase inhibitors
Hypnotics

Barbiturates
Antidepressants
Corticosteroids
Antihypertensives

Situational (Personal, Environmental)

Related to lack of sleep privacy/control*
Related to lighting, noise, noxious odors*
Related to sleep partner (e.g., snoring)*
Related to unfamiliar sleep furnishing*
Related to ambient temperature, humidity*
Related to caregiving responsibilities*
Related to change in daylight–darkness exposure*
Related to excessive hyperactivity secondary to:

Bipolar disorder
Attention-deficit disorder

Panic anxiety
Illicit drug use

Related to excessive daytime sleeping
Related to depression
Related to inadequate daytime activities
Related to pain
Related to anxiety response
Related to environmental changes (specify)

Hospitalization (noise, disturbing roommate, fear)

Author's Note

The following interventions can also be used for *Risk for Disturbed Sleep*.

Goals

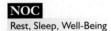

NOC
Rest, Sleep, Well-Being

The individual will report a satisfactory balance of rest and activity as evidenced by the following indicators:

- Complete at least four sleep cycles (100 minutes) undisturbed.
- State factors that increase or decrease the quality of sleep.

Interventions

NIC
Energy Management,
Sleep Enhancement,
Environmental
Management

Discuss the Reasons for Differing Individual Sleep Requirements, Including Age, Lifestyle, Activity Level, and Other Possible Factors

- Newborns (0 to 3 months): Sleep range narrowed to 14 to 17 hours each day (previously it was 12 to 18)
- Infants (4 to 11 months): Sleep range widened by 2 hours to 12 to 15 hours (previously it was 14 to 15)
- Toddlers (1 to 2 years): Sleep range widened by 1 hour to 11 to 14 hours (previously it was 12 to 14)
- Preschoolers (3 to 5): Sleep range widened by 1 hour to 10 to 13 hours (previously it was 11 to 13)
- School-age children (6 to 13): Sleep range widened by 1 hour to 9 to 11 hours (previously it was 10 to 11)
- Teenagers (14 to 17): Sleep range widened by 1 hour to 8 to 10 hours (previously it was 8.5 to 9.5)
- Younger adults (18 to 25): Sleep range is 7 to 9 hours (new age category)
- Adults (26 to 64): Sleep range did not change and remains 7 to 9 hours
- Older adults (65+): Sleep range is 7 to 8 hours (new age category)

   R: The above recommendations are from the National Sleep Foundation (2015)

Explain the Effects of Sleep Deprivation (e.g., Cognition, Stress Management)

R: Sleep deprivation results in impaired cognitive functioning (e.g., memory, concentration, judgment) and perception, reduced emotional control, increased suspicion, irritability, and disorientation (Colten & Altevogt, 2006). As sleep deprivation accumulates, individuals may experience reduced performance, increased risk for accidents and death, and detrimental effects on both psychological and physical health (Cirelli & Tononi, 2015).

> **CLINICAL ALERT:**
> - Sleep quality is determined by the number of arousals (or awakenings) from sleep during the night, as well as the percentage, duration, and type of sleep stages. It is possible for an individual to sleep eight or more hours and still be sleep deprived. In such cases, the sleep deprivation is usually due to disturbances in the quality of sleep.

Explain the Need for Sleep Cycle

R: Sleep cycle. An individual typically goes through four or five complete sleep cycles each night. Awakening during a cycle may cause him or her to feel poorly rested in the morning.

Assess With Individual and Family Their Usual Bedtime Routine—Time, hygiene Practices, Rituals Such as Reading—and Adhere to It as Closely as Possible

R: Sleep is difficult without relaxation, which the unfamiliar hospital environment can hinder.

Reduce or Eliminate Environmental Distractions and Sleep Interruptions

- Noise
  - Close the door to the room.
  - Pull the curtains.
  - Unplug the telephone.
  - Use "white noise" (e.g., fan; quiet music; recording of rain, waves).
  - Eliminate 24-hour lighting.
  - Provide night lights.
  - Decrease the amount and kind of incoming stimuli (e.g., staff conversations).
  - Cover blinking lights with tape.
  - Reduce the volume of alarms and televisions.
  - Place the individual with a compatible roommate, if possible.
- Interruptions

   R: Huang et al. (2015) found that "in simulated ICU noise and light, healthy subjects not only had greater anxiety and poorer subjective sleep quality, but also suffered from the disturbance of sleep structure, measured as shorter total sleep time, longer sleep-onset latency, longer REM latency, more light sleep, less REM sleep and more arousals and awakenings."

SBAR   *Situation:* Mr. Green has slept only 4 hours the last 24 hours.

Background: "He is not sleeping because...."

Assessment: He is complaints of more pain, wants a sleeping pill.

Recommendation: It would be useful to . . . (e.g., stop taking vital signs 10 p.m. to 6 a.m. unless needed, change the times for medications administration; provide treatments before 10 p.m. and after 6 a.m. when possible).

Discuss With Physician/Nurse Practitioner/Physician Assistant the Use of a "Sleep Protocol." This Will Allow the Nursing Staff/Student the Authority Not to Wake a Person for Blood Draws or Vital Signs if Appropriate (Bartick, 2009; Faraklas et al., 2013)

- Designate "quiet time" between 10 p.m. and 6 a.m.
- Play lullabies over public address system.
- Set a timer to turn off overhead hallway lights at 10 p.m.
- Mute phones close to patient rooms; avoid intercom use except in emergencies.
- Take vital signs at 10 p.m. and start again at 6 a.m., unless otherwise indicated.
- Order medications as b.i.d., t.i.d., q.i.d., but not "q" certain hours when possible.
- Do not administer a diuretic after 4 p.m.
- Avoid blood transfusions during "quiet time" due to frequent monitoring.

Provide Treatments Before 10 p.m. and After 6 a.m., When Possible

R: A small study reported that "sleep protocol" can reduce the number of individuals reporting disturbed sleep by 38% and reduce the number of individuals needing sedatives by 49% (Bartick, 2009). Results from another study of individuals, who received a sleep protocol in an intensive care unit reported to fall asleep more quickly and to experience fewer sleep disruptions (Faraklas et al., 2013).

Consider Using Ear Plug, Eye Masks, and, if Appropriate, Melatonin

R: Huang et al. (2015) reported in addition to earplugs and eye masks, melatonin 1 mg improves sleep quality and serum melatonin levels better in healthy subjects exposed to simulated ICU noise and light.

Encourage or Provide Evening Care Offer

- Use of bathroom or bedpan
- Personal hygiene (mouth care, bath, shower, partial bath)
- Clean linen and bedclothes (freshly made bed, sufficient blankets)

Cluster Procedures to Minimize the Times to Wake the Individual at Night. If Possible, Plan for at Least Four Periods of 90-Minute Uninterrupted Sleep

R: In order to feel rested, a person usually must complete an entire sleep cycle (70 to 90 minutes) four or five times a night.

Explain the Need to Avoid Sedative and Hypnotic Drugs

R: Sleep medications can increase awakenings and fewer total sleep hours. These medications begin to lose their effectiveness after a week of use, requiring increased dosages and leading to the risk of dependence (Arcangelo & Peterson, 2016).

Initiate Health Teaching as Indicated

- Refer to thePoint for a printable take-home guide: Getting Started to Sleep Better.

> **Clinical Alert Report**
>
> Advise ancillary staff/student to report the amount of time spent sleeping including naps and nighttime.

SPIRITUAL DISTRESS

NANDA-I Definition

A state of suffering related to impaired ability to experience meaning in life through connections with self, others, the world, or a superior being.

Defining Characteristics

Questions meaning of life, death, and suffering
Conveys meaning of life, death, and suffering
Reports no sense of meaning and purpose in life
Lacks enthusiasm for life, feelings of joy, inner peace, or love
Demonstrates discouragement or despair
Experiences alienation from spiritual or religious community
Expresses need to reconcile with self, others, God, or creator
Presents with sudden interest in spiritual matters (reading spiritual or religious books, watching spiritual or religious programs on television)
Displays sudden changes in spiritual practices (rejection, neglect, doubt, fanatical devotion)
Verbalizes that family, loved ones, peers, or health care providers opposed spiritual beliefs or practices
Questions credibility of religion or spiritual belief system
Requests assistance for a disturbance in spiritual beliefs or religious practice

Related Factors

Pathophysiologic

Related to challenge in spiritual health or separation from spiritual ties secondary to (e.g., hospitalization, pain, loss of body part or function, trauma, terminal illness, debilitating disease, miscarriage, stillbirth)

Treatment Related

Related to conflict between (specify prescribed regimen) and beliefs (e.g., isolation, surgery, termination, medical procedures, blood transfusion, dialysis, dietary restrictions, medications)

Situational (Personal, Environmental)

Related to death or illness of significant other*
Related to embarrassment of expressions of spirituality or religion, such as prayers, meditation, or other rituals
Related to barriers to practicing spiritual rituals

Restrictions of intensive care
Lack of privacy
Unavailability of special foods/diet or ritual objects
Confinement to bed or room

Related to spiritual or religious beliefs opposed by family, peers, health care providers
Related to divorce, separation from loved one, or other perceived loss

Author's Note

Weathers, McCarthy, and Coffey (2016) found the primary consequences that emerged from their concept analysis of spirituality in nursing care "were an alleviation of suffering, a sense of well-being, enhanced ability to adapt and cope with adversity, a sense of peace, and inner strength."

To promote positive spirituality, the nurse can assist people with spiritual concerns or distress by providing resources for spiritual help, by listening nonjudgmentally, and by providing opportunities to meet spiritual needs (O'Brien, 2010; *Wright, 2004).

Spirituality and religiousness are two different concepts. Burkhart and Solari-Twadell (*2001) define spirituality as the "ability to experience and integrate meaning and self, others, art, music, literature, nature, or a power greater than oneself" (p. 51). Religiousness is "the ability to exercise participation in the beliefs of a particular denomination of faith community and related rituals" (*Burkhart & Solari-Twadell, 2001, p. 51). Although the spiritual dimension of human wholeness is always present, it may or may not exist within the context of religious traditions or practices.

Goals

NOC
Hope, Spiritual
Well-Being

The individual will find meaning and purpose in life, including and during illness as evidenced by the following indicators:

- The individual expresses his or her feelings related to beliefs and spirituality.
- The individual describes his or her spiritual belief system as it relates to illness.
- The individual finds meaning and comfort in religious or spiritual practice.

Interventions

Carp's Cues

The nurse should consider the individual's spiritual nature as part of total care, along with the physical and psycho-social dimensions. Research indicates that most individuals feel religion is important in times of crisis (*Kendrick et al., 2000; Puchalski & Ferrell, 2010). The spiritual may include, but is not limited to, religion; spiritual needs include finding meaning, hope, relatedness, forgiveness or acceptance, or transcendence (*Mauk & Schmidt, 2004; *Kemp, 2006).

NIC
Spiritual Growth
Facilitation, Hope
Instillation, Active
Listening, Presence,
Emotional Support,
Spiritual Support

Create an Environment of Trust (Puchalski & Ferrell, 2010)

- Be open to listening to the individual's story, not just the medical facts.
- Listen for the content, emotion and manner, and spiritual meanings.
- Give "permission" to discuss spiritual matters with the nurse by bringing up the subject of spiritual welfare, if necessary.
- Be fully present.

    R: According to Hegarty (2007), "Caring presence disposition of the nurse is a state of being truly present alongside the patient for support and care, to stay there even when there are no easy solutions or answers to questions. "It becomes easy to incorporate into the day-to-day nursing practice an attentive and reflective approach to develop abilities and skills in that area."

    *R: The nurse should practice with a confidence to initiate spiritual dialogues and as an advocate in recognizing and respecting the individual's spiritual needs (*Mauk & Schmidt, 2004).*

    R: This spirit is named and experienced in various ways including as the human spirit, the spark of the divine, ground of being, higher self, and many names for aspects of the divine. Despite different names, it is a deep, inner resource on which people can draw.

Eliminate or Reduce Causative and Contributing Factors, if Possible

Feeling Threatened and Vulnerable Because of Symptoms or Possible Death
- Inform individuals and families about the importance of finding meaning in illness.
- Suggest using prayer, imagery, and meditation to reduce anxiety and provide hope and a sense of control.

Failure of Spiritual Beliefs to Provide Explanation or Comfort During Crisis of Illness/Suffering/ Impending Death
- Use questions about past beliefs and spiritual experiences to assist the individual in putting this life event into wider perspective.
- Offer to contact the usual or a new spiritual leader.

- Offer to pray/meditate/read with the individual if you are comfortable with this, or arrange for another member of the health care team if more appropriate.
- Provide uninterrupted quiet time for prayer/reading/meditation on spiritual concerns.

  *R: The nurse should practice with a confidence to initiate spiritual dialogues and as an advocate in recognizing and respecting the individual's spiritual needs (*Mauk & Schmidt, 2004).*

Conflict Between Religious or Spiritual Beliefs and Prescribed Health Regimen

- Lack of information about or understanding of spiritual restrictions
- Lack of information about or understanding of health regimen
- Informed, true conflict
- Parental conflict concerning treatment of their child
- Lack of time for deliberation before emergency treatment or surgery
- Practice as an advocate for the individual and family.

Doubting Quality of Own Faith to Deal With Current Illness/Suffering/Death

- Be available and willing to listen when individual expresses self-doubt, guilt, or other negative feelings.
- Silence, touch, or both may be useful in communicating the nurse's presence and support during times of doubt or despair.
- Offer to contact usual or new spiritual leader.

  R: Research shows that people with higher levels of spiritual well-being tend to experience lower levels of anxiety. For many people, spiritual activities provide a direct coping action and may improve adaptation to illness (Puchalski & Ferrell, 2010).

Anger Toward God/Supreme Deity or Spiritual Beliefs for Allowing or Causing Illness/Suffering/Death

- Express that anger toward God/Supreme Deity is a common reaction to illness/suffering/death.
- Help to recognize and discuss feelings of anger.

*R: The individual may view anger at God and a religious leader as "forbidden" and may be reluctant to initiate discussions of spiritual conflicts (*Kemp, 2006).*

- Allow to problem-solve to find ways to express and relieve anger.
- Offer to contact the usual spiritual leader or offer to contact another spiritual support person (e.g., pastoral care, hospital chaplain) if the individual cannot share feelings with the usual spiritual leader.

  R: The nurse should be the link between the family and other members of the health care team.

Lack of Information About Spiritual Restrictions

- Have the spiritual leader discuss restrictions and exemptions as they apply to those who are seriously ill or hospitalized.
- Provide reading materials on religious and spiritual restrictions and exemptions.
- Encourage the individual to seek information from and discuss restrictions with spiritual leader and/or others in the spiritual group.
- Chart the results of these discussions.

  R: Interventions focus on providing information about all alternatives and the consequences of each option.

Informed, True Conflict

- Encourage the individual and physician/nurse practitioner to consider alternative methods of therapy.
- Support the individual making an informed decision—even if the decision conflicts with nurses' own values.
- Encourage the involvement of their spiritual leader.

  R: Interventions focus on providing information about all alternatives and the consequences of each option.

RISK FOR SPIRITUAL DISTRESS

NANDA-I Definition

At risk for an impaired ability to experience and integrate meaning and purpose in life through connectedness with self, others, art, music, literature, nature, and/or a power greater than oneself.

Risk Factors

Refer to *Spiritual Distress*.

INEFFECTIVE TISSUE PERFUSION[8]

NANDA-I Definition

Decrease in oxygen resulting in failure to nourish tissues at capillary level

 Carp's Cues

The use of any *Ineffective Tissue Perfusion* diagnosis other than *Peripheral* merely provides new labels for medical diagnoses, for example, renal failure, congestive heart failure, and increased intracranial pressure labels that do not describe the nursing focus or accountability.

These situations required both medical and nursing intervention to maintain or restore physiologic stability. Instead of using *Ineffective Tissue Perfusion*, the nurse should focus on the nursing diagnoses and collaborative problems applicable because of altered renal, cardiac, cerebral, pulmonary, or gastrointestinal (GI) tissue perfusion, such as *Risk for Complications of GI Bleeding* or *Activity Intolerance related to insufficient oxygenation secondary to COPD*.

For each of the specific body Tissue Perfusion diagnoses listed above, refer to the discussion under its Carp's Cues.

INEFFECTIVE PERIPHERAL TISSUE PERFUSION

NANDA-I Definition

Decrease in blood circulation to the periphery that may compromise health

Defining Characteristics

Presence of one of the following types (see Key Concepts for definitions):

Claudication (arterial)*
Aching pain (arterial or venous)
Rest pain (arterial)
Diminished or absent arterial pulses* (arterial)
Skin color changes*
Pallor (arterial)
Reactive hyperemia (arterial)
Cyanosis (venous)
Skin temperature changes
Cooler (arterial)

Warmer (venous)
Decreased blood pressure (arterial)
Capillary refill longer than 3 seconds
    (arterial)*
Edema* (venous)
Change in sensory function (arterial)
Change in motor function (arterial)
Trophic tissue changes (arterial)
Hard, thick nails
Loss of hair
Nonhealing wound

---

[8]This diagnosis is not currently on the NANDA-I list, but has been included for clarity and usefulness.

Related Factors (Harris & Dryjski, 2015)

Pathophysiologic

Related to compromised blood flow secondary to:

Vascular disorders
  Arteriosclerosis
  Leriche's syndrome
  Venous hypertension
  Raynaud's disease/syndrome
  Aneurysm
Diabetes mellitus
Hypotension
Blood dyscrasias
Renal failure
Cancer/tumor

Varicosities
Alcoholism
Buerger's disease
Deep vein thrombosis
Sickle cell crisis

Collagen vascular disease
Cirrhosis
Rheumatoid arthritis

Treatment Related

Related to immobilization
Related to presence of invasive lines
Related to pressure sites/constriction (elastic compression bandages, stockings, restraints)
Related to blood vessel trauma or compression

Situational (Personal, Environmental)

Related to pressure of enlarging uterus on pelvic vessels
Related to pressure of enlarged abdomen on pelvic/peripheral vessels
Related to vasoconstricting effects of tobacco
Related to decreased circulating volume secondary to dehydration

Goals

NOC
Sensory Functions:
Cutaneous, Tissue
Integrity, Tissue
Perfusion: Peripheral

The individual will report a decrease in pain as evidenced by the following indicators:

- Define peripheral vascular problem in own words.
- Identify factors that improve peripheral circulation.
- Identify necessary lifestyle changes.
- Identify medical regimen, diet, medications, activities that promote vasodilation.
- Identify factors that inhibit peripheral circulation.
- State when to contact physician or health care professional.

> **CLINICAL ALERT:**
> - "Approximately 12% of the adult population has PAD, and the prevalence is equal in men and women. A strong association exists between advancing age and the prevalence of PAD. Almost 20% of adults older than 70 years have PAD. In an elderly hypertensive population from the Systolic Hypertension in the Elderly Program, the prevalence of PAD was 38% in black men, 25% in white men, 41% in black women, and 23% in white women" (Olin & Sealove, 2010).

Interventions

NIC
Peripheral Sensation
Management,
Circulatory Care:
Venous Insufficiency,
Circulatory Care:
Arterial Insufficiency,
Positioning, Exercise
Promotion, Smoking
Cessation Assistance

Assess Causative and Contributing Factors

- Tobacco use
- Type 2 diabetes
- Hypertension
- Dyslipidemia
- Obesity
- Sedentary lifestyle

- Metabolic syndrome
- COPD
- Mobility problems (e.g., arthritis)

   R: Peripheral arterial disease is typically due to aggressive atherosclerosis resulting from untreated cardiovascular disease (CVD) risk factors (Harris & Dryjski, 2015).

Discuss Specifically With the Individual His or Her Symptoms Associated With Mobility and Are Relieved by Rest as Pain, Numbness, and/or Weakness in Hips, Buttocks, Thigh, or Calf

R: Only 30% to 50% of older adults report typical claudication symptoms (e.g., calf pain when walking relieved with rest). Older, male, diabetic individuals may be asymptomatic (Harris & Dryjski, 2015).

Explain the Effects of Impaired Peripheral Circulation on Causing Substantial Walking Impairment, Diminished Quality of Life, Limb Ischemia/Amputation, and Increased CVD Morbidity and Mortality (Harris & Dryjski, 2015)

R: An explanation of the probable course of impaired peripheral circulation can increase motivation to modify risk factors.

Promote Factors That Improve Arterial Blood Flow

- Keep extremity in a dependent position.

   R: Arterial blood flow is enhanced by a dependent position and inhibited by an elevated position (gravity pulls blood downward, away from the heart).

- Keep extremity warm (do not use heating pad or hot water bottle).

   R: Peripheral vascular disease will reduce sensitivity. The person will not be able to determine if the temperature is hot enough to damage tissue; the use of external heat may also increase the metabolic demands of the tissue beyond its capacity.

Promote Factors That Improve Venous Blood Flow

- Teach to:
  - Elevate extremity above the level of the heart (may be contraindicated if severe cardiac or respiratory disease is present).

     R: Venous blood flow is enhanced by an elevated position and inhibited by a dependent position. (Gravity pulls blood downward, away from the heart.)

  - Change positions at least every hour.
  - Avoid leg crossing.

     R: Tight garments and certain leg positions constrict leg vessels, further reducing circulation.

  - Avoid pillows behind the knees or Gatch bed, which is elevated at the knees.
  - Avoid leg crossing.
  - Change positions, move extremities, or wiggle fingers and toes every hour.
  - Avoid tight elastic stockings above the knees.
  - Reduce external pressure points (inspect shoes daily for rough lining).
  - Avoid sheepskin heel protectors (they increase heel pressure and pressure across dorsum of foot).
  - Encourage range-of-motion exercises.

     R: Cellular nutrition and function depend on adequate blood flow through the microcirculation.

Explain the Process of Increasing Walking Distance and the Benefits of Walking (McDermott et al., 2014; *Oka, 2006)

- Walk until moderate pain is felt.
- Rest (standing or sitting) until pain subsides.
- Resume walking and repeat the rest–walk cycle.
- Increase walking time by 5 minutes each day walked, with a goal of walking at least 30 minutes three to five times a week.

- Emphasize the functional benefits (increased walking speed, distance, duration, and decreased symptoms) will occur gradually and can be noticed as early as 4 to 8 weeks. Greater benefit is achieved when the individual continues walking 6 months or longer.

    R: Exercise programs reduce the symptoms of claudication, including increasing the distance and time that one can walk before developing symptoms. Individuals who respond to an exercise program can expect improvement within 2 months. Motivated individuals who are supervised achieve the best results. The benefits of exercise diminish when exercise training stops (Mohler, 2015).

Emphasize the Need to Prevent Infection With Careful Foot Care

- Wear shoes that fit properly. Gradually "break in" new shoes.
- Inspect the inside of shoes daily for rough lining.
- Examine feet daily yourself or by someone else.
- Keep dry skin lubricated (cracked skin eliminates the physical barrier to infection).
- Pay attention to any reddened areas, cuts, scrapes, or injuries.
- Call primary care provider to report any changes or injuries.

    R: Tissues heal slowly and are more likely to get infected when there is decreased circulation.

> **CLINICAL ALERT:**
> - Any disruption of the skin integrity must be promptly assessed and treated to prevent infection, cellulitis, and the need for hospitalization and surgery.
> - Initiate transitional teaching, as indicated.

Discuss What Risk Factors That He or She Is Interested in Modifying

- Help him or her select goals that are seen as possible. Some examples are:
    - Will walk 15 minutes 5 days a week.
    - Will substitute sugar drinks with water or diet beverages.
    - Will eat one-third less portion of starches (potatoes, pasta, rice, bread).
    - Will eat three servings of vegetables each day.
    - Will delay the urge to smoke for 1 hour.

> **CLINICAL ALERT:**
> - Individuals with peripheral vascular insufficiency usually have more than three modifiable risk factors. Allow individual to identify his or her goals because unrealistic expectations of the nurse will result in rejection and failure.

Plan a Daily Walking Program

- Refer to Getting Started to Increase Activity on thePoint.

Initiate a Dialogue Regarding Interest in Smoking Cessation

- Refer to Getting Started to Quit Smoking on thePoint.

Explain the Effects of Excess Weight on Body Functions (e.g., Circulation, Lipids, Diabetes Mellitus, Cardiac Function, Hypertension)

R: Obesity increases peripheral resistance and venous pooling, excess weight increases cardiac workload, causing hypertension (Grossman & Porth, 2014).

- Refer to Getting Started to Losing Weight on thePoint.

> ### *Clinical Alert Report*
> Advise onsite staff first to report increase in edema, redness, and signs of trauma.

RISK FOR DECREASED CARDIAC TISSUE PERFUSION

NANDA-I Definition

Risk for a decrease in cardiac (coronary) circulation

NANDA-I Risk Factors*

Birth control pills (medication side effect of combination pills)[9]
Cardiac surgery (treatment)
Cardiac tamponade (clinical emergency)
Coronary artery spasm (clinical emergency)
Diabetes mellitus (medical diagnosis with multiple complications with associated modifiable risk lifestyles)
Drug abuse (clinical situations with multiple complications)
Elevated C-reactive protein (positive laboratory test)
Family history of coronary artery disease (factor with associated modifiable risk lifestyles)
Hyperlipidemia (medical diagnosis with associated modifiable risk lifestyles)
Hypertension (medical diagnosis with multiple complications with associated modifiable risk lifestyles)
Hypoxemia (complication)
Hypovolemia (complication)
Hypoxia (complication)
Lack of knowledge of modifiable risk factors (e.g., smoking, sedentary lifestyle, obesity)

Carp's Cues

Risk for Decreased Cardiac Tissue Perfusion can be used to describe a variety of physiologic events or pathology that can cause it as arrhythmias, left ventricular hypertrophy, drug abuse, septic shock, cardiomyopathies, and acute coronary syndrome. It would be more clinically specific to use instead *Risk for Complications of Decreased Cardiac Output, Risk for Complications of Dysrhythmias,* and *Risk for Complications of Septic Shock/SIRS.* Refer to Section 2 for specific collaborative problems. Nursing diagnoses related to these conditions may be *Activity Intolerance, Anxiety,* and *Acute Pain.* Refer to Section 2 for specific nursing diagnoses.

Some of the related factors as lack of knowledge of modifiable risk factors (e.g., smoking, sedentary lifestyle, obesity) can be addressed more appropriately with nursing diagnoses such as *Risk-Prone Health Behavior Risk for Overweight.* Refer to Section 2 for specific nursing diagnoses.

RISK FOR INEFFECTIVE CEREBRAL TISSUE PERFUSION

NANDA-I Definition

At risk for a decrease in cerebral tissue circulation that may compromise health

NANDA-I Risk Factors*

Abnormal partial thromboplastin time
Abnormal prothrombin time
Akinetic left ventricular segment
Aortic atherosclerosis
Arterial dissection
Atrial fibrillation
Atrial myxoma
Brain tumor

---

[9]Text in parentheses has been added by author.

Carotid stenosis
Cerebral aneurysm
Coagulopathies (e.g., sickle cell anemia)
Dilated cardiomyopathy
Disseminated intravascular coagulation
Embolism
Head trauma
Hypercholesterolemia
Hypertension
Endocarditis
Left atrial appendage thrombosis
Mechanical prosthetic valve
Mitral stenosis
Neoplasm of the brain
Recent myocardial infarction
Sick sinus syndrome
Substance abuse
Thrombolytic therapy
Treatment-related side effects (cardiopulmonary bypass, pharmaceutical agents)

Carp's Cues

This nursing diagnosis represents a collection of risk factors that have very different clinical implications. Some are physiologic complications that are related to a medical diagnosis or treatment. These situations are more accurately described as collaborative problems as *Risk for Complications of Increased Intracranial Pressure, RC of Seizures,* or *RC of Alcohol Withdrawal.* Refer to Section 2 for specific collaborative problems under Risk for Complications of Neurologic/Sensory Dysfunction or to a care plan for individuals with neurologic conditions (e.g., seizures, CVA). Some nursing diagnoses related to neurologic impairments are *Self-Care Deficits* and *Risk for Falls.* Refer to Section 2 for more specific nursing diagnoses.

RISK FOR INEFFECTIVE GASTROINTESTINAL TISSUE PERFUSION

NANDA-I Definition

At risk for decrease in gastrointestinal circulation

Risk Factors

Abdominal aortic aneurysm
Abdominal compartment syndrome
Abnormal partial thromboplastin time
Abnormal prothrombin time
Acute gastrointestinal bleed
Acute gastrointestinal hemorrhage
Age greater than 60 years
Anemia
Coagulopathies (e.g., sickle cell anemia)
Diabetes mellitus
Disseminated intravascular coagulation
Female gender
Gastric paresis (e.g., diabetes mellitus)
Gastrointestinal disease (e.g., duodenal or gastric ulcer, ischemic colitis, ischemic pancreatitis)
Liver dysfunction
Poor left ventricular performance
Hemodynamic instability

Stroke
Myocardial infarction
Renal failure
Treatment-related side effects (e.g., cardiopulmonary bypass, medications, anesthesia, gastric surgery)
Vascular disease (e.g., peripheral vascular disease, aortoiliac occlusive disease)
Dysfunctional gastrointestinal motility

Author's Note

This NANDA-I diagnosis Risk for Dysfunctional Gastrointestinal Motility and Dysfunctional Gastrointestinal Motility is too broad for clinical use. If the focus is to monitor gastrointestinal function for complications that require medical and nursing interventions, use a collaborative problem as *Risk for Complications of* (specify) as *Risk for Complications of Gastrointestinal Dysfunction, Risk for Complications of GI Bleeding, Risk for Complications of Paralytic Ileus.* Refer to Unit II Section 2 for interventions for these collaborative problems.

Examine the risk factors in the individual and determine if the focus of nursing interventions is prevention; if yes, use *Risk for Infection, Risk for Diarrhea,* or *Risk for Constipation.* Refer to Unit II Section 1 for interventions for these nursing diagnoses.

IMPAIRED URINARY ELIMINATION

NANDA-I Definition

Dysfunction in urinary elimination

Defining Characteristics

Reports or experiences a urinary elimination problem, such as:

Urgency*	Hesitancy*	Large residual urine volumes
Bladder distention	Incontinence*	Enuresis
Nocturia*	Dysuria*	Retention*
Dribbling	Frequency*	

Related Factors

Pathophysiologic

Related to incompetent bladder outlet secondary to congenital urinary tract anomalies
Related to decreased bladder capacity or irritation to bladder secondary to infection, glucosuria, trauma, carcinoma, urethritis, and congestive heart failure*
Related to diminished bladder cues or impaired ability to recognize bladder cues secondary to:

Cord injury/tumor/infection	Diabetic neuropathy	Brain injury/tumor/infection
Alcoholic neuropathy	Cerebrovascular accident	Multiple sclerosis
Demyelinating diseases	Parkinsonism	

Treatment Related

Related to effects of surgery on bladder sphincter secondary to (e.g., postprostatectomy, extensive pelvic dissection)
Related to diagnostic instrumentation
Related to decreased bladder tone post-indwelling catheters
Related to decreased muscle tone secondary to:

General or spinal anesthesia
Drug therapy (iatrogenic)

Antihistamines	Anticholinergics
Immunosuppressant therapy	Tranquilizers
Epinephrine	Sedatives
Diuretics	Muscle relaxants

Situational (Personal, Environmental)

Related to weak pelvic floor muscles secondary to (e.g., obesity, childbirth, aging, recent substantial weight loss)
Related to inability to communicate needs
Related to bladder outlet obstruction secondary to fecal impaction/chronic constipation
Related to decreased bladder muscle tone secondary to dehydration
Related to decreased attention to bladder cues secondary to (e.g., depression, delirium, intentional suppression [self-induced deconditioning], confusion)
Related to environmental barriers to bathroom secondary to (e.g., distant toilets, poor lighting, unfamiliar surroundings)
Related to inability to access bathroom on time secondary to (e.g., diuretics, caffeine/alcohol use, impaired mobility)

 ### Carp's Cues

Impaired Urinary Elimination is too broad a diagnosis for effective clinical use; however, it is clinically useful until additional data can be collected. With more data, the nurse can use a more specific diagnosis, such as *Stress Urinary Incontinence*, whenever possible. When the etiologic or contributing factors for incontinence have not been identified, the nurse could write a temporary diagnosis of *Impaired Urinary Elimination* related to unknown etiology, as evidenced by incontinence.

It is the second leading reason for placement of older adults into institutionalized care, and it is the primary reason why many elderly persons are not accepted into assisted living facilities.

CONTINUOUS URINARY INCONTINENCE

Definition

State in which an individual experiences continuous, unpredictable loss of urine without distention or awareness of bladder fullness

Defining Characteristics

Constant flow of urine at unpredictable times without uninhibited bladder contractions/spasm or distention
Lack of bladder filling or perineal filling
Nocturia
Unawareness of incontinence
Incontinence refractory to other treatments

Related Factors

Refer to *Impaired Urinary Elimination*.

Goals

NOC
Refer to *Functional Urinary Incontinence*.

The person will be continent (specify during day, night, 24 hours) as evidenced by the following indicators:

- Identify the cause of incontinence and rationale for treatments.
- Identify daily goal for fluid intake.

Interventions

NIC
See also *Functional Incontinence*, Environmental Management, Urinary Catheterization, Teaching: Procedure/Treatment, Tube Care: Urinary, Urinary Bladder Training

Develop a Bladder Retraining or Reconditioning Program, Which Should Include Communication, Assessment of Voiding Pattern, Scheduled Fluid Intake, and Scheduled Voiding Times

Promote Communication Among All Staff Members and Among Individual, Family, and Staff

- Provide all staff with sufficient knowledge concerning the program planned.
- Assess staff's response to program.

    R: Education of caregivers increases preparedness, decreases burden, and reduces role strain, thereby reducing overall stress when caring for an incontinent individual or family member.

Assess the Person's Potential for Participation in a Bladder-Retraining Program

- Cognition
- Desire to change behavior
- Ability to cooperate
- Willingness to participate

    R: Continence training programs are either self-directed or caregiver directed. Self-directed programs of bladder training, retraining, and exercises are for motivated, cognitively intact individuals (Miller, 2015). Caregiver-directed programs of scheduled toileting or habit training are appropriate for motivated caregivers of individuals with cognitive impairment.

Provide Rationale for Plan and Acquire Individual's Informed Consent

Encourage Person to Continue Program by Providing Accurate Information Concerning Reasons for Success or Failure

Assess Voiding Pattern

- Monitor and record:
    - Intake and output
    - Time and amount of fluid intake
    - Type of fluid
    - Amount of incontinence; measure if possible or estimate amount as small, moderate, or large
    - Presence of sensation of need to void
    - Amount of retention (amount of urine left in the bladder after an unsuccessful attempt at manual triggering or voiding)
    - Amount of residual (amount of urine left in the bladder after either a voluntary or manual triggered voiding; also called a *postvoid residual*)
    - Amount of triggered urine (urine expelled after manual triggering [e.g., tapping, Credé's method])
- Identify certain activities that precede voiding (e.g., restlessness, yelling, exercise).
- Record in appropriate column.

Schedule Fluid Intake and Voiding Times

- Provide fluid intake of 2,000 mL each day unless contraindicated.
- Discourage fluids after 7 p.m.
- Provide caregiver education.
- Initially, bladder emptying is done at least every 2 hours and at least twice during the night; goal is 2- to 4-hour intervals.
- If the person is incontinent before scheduled voids, shorten the time between voids.
- If the person has a postvoid residual greater than 100 to 150 mL, schedule intermittent catheterization.

    R: The essential components of any continence training program (self-directed or caregiver directed) include motivation, assessment of voiding and incontinence patterns, a regular fluid intake of 2,000 to 3,000 mL/day, timed voiding of 2- to 4-hour intervals in an appropriate place, and ongoing assessment (Miller, 2015).

Reduce Incontinence-Related Irritant Dermatitis (Burakgazi, Alsowaity, Burakgazi, Unal, & Kelly, 2012)

- Protect skin integrity from urine.

    R: Urine contains ammonia. Ammonia increases the pH of the skin, causing irritation. Ammonia is also a source of nutrition for bacteria, contributing to the reproduction of more microorganisms.

- Use a no-rinse perineal cleanser.
- Avoid fragrances, alcohol, and alkaline agents (found in many commercial soaps).
- Apply moisturizer immediately after bathing, when pores are open.
- Use a moisture-barrier product (e.g., Curity Moisture Barrier Cream; No Sting Barrier Film).
- Do not try to remove all of the ointment with cleansing.
- Gently wash skin using very little soap. Dry skin very gently by patting, not rubbing.

    R: Vigorous washing can injure tissue.

- Keep perineal area dry.

    R: Warm, damp skin provides an opportune environment for fungal infections.

    R: Dehydration can cause incontinence by eliminating the sensation of a full bladder (the signal to urinate) and also by reducing the person's alertness to the sensation.

Schedule Intermittent Catheterization Program (ICP), if Indicated
(Newman & Wilson, 2011)

- Monitor intake and output.
- Fluid intake should be at least 2,000 mL/day.
- Use sterile catheterization technique in the hospital and clean technique at home.
- Desired catheter volumes are less than 500 mL.
- Increase or decrease the interval between catheterizations to obtain the desired catheter volumes.
- Usual catheterization times are every 4 to 6 hours.
- Urine volumes may increase at night; thus, it may be necessary to catheterize more frequently at night.
- Encourage the individual to attempt to void before scheduled catheterization time.
- Initially obtain postvoid residuals at least every 6 hours.
- Terminate ICP when the bladder is consistently emptied voluntarily or by triggering with less than 50 mL residual urine after each void.

    R: Intermittent catheterization, when performed in a health care facility, should follow aseptic technique because the organisms present in such a facility are more virulent and resistant to drugs than the organisms in the home environment (Newman & Wilson, 2011).

Initiate Health Teaching and Referrals as Indicated

- Teach intermittent catheterization to person and family for long-term management of bladder.
- Explain the reasons for the intermittent catheterization.

    R: Long-term use of intermittent catheterization has a lower risk of infection and other complications when compared with indwelling urinary catheter (Newman & Willson, 2011).

> **CLINICAL ALERT:**
> - A cognitively impaired person with continuous incontinence requires caregiver-directed treatment. In institutional settings, indwelling and external catheters or disposal or washable incontinence briefs or pads are beneficial to the caregivers, but detrimental to the incontinent person. Aids and equipment should be considered only after other means have been attempted. In the home setting, the caregiver's needs may take precedence over the cognitively impaired person's. Urinary incontinence is cited as the major reason for seeking institutional care for people living at home (Miller, 2015).

Explain the Relation of Fluid Intake, Frequency of Catheterization, and Risk for Infection

R: Inadequate fluid intake can produce low urine volumes (less than 1,200 mL of urine per day). Decreased urine production may lead to fewer catheterizations, stasis of urine, and infection.

- Ensure total daily fluid intake (from foods and all types of beverages) is approximately 2.7 L/day for women and 3.7 L/day for men. Excessive fluid intake will produce periodic or regular bladder overdistention (volumes greater than 500 mL), possible overflow urinary incontinence, and urinary stasis. Distended bladder walls are susceptible to bacteria that circulate in retained urine (Newman & Willson,

2011, p. 15). When the bladder becomes stretched from retained urine, the capillaries become occluded, preventing the delivery of metabolic and immune substrates to the bladder wall, which are needed to maintain a physical barrier against colonization or invasion by pathogens (Heard & Buhrer, 2005).

- Advise of the possible need to catheterize more than six times a day.
- Encourage regular fluid intake, small volumes spaced hourly between breakfast and the evening meal, and reducing to sips thereafter (Newman & Willson, 2011, p. 15).
- Ensure that there is adequate emptying at the time of catheterization. Teach a gentle Crede's maneuver as one removes the catheter.

   R: Residual volume left in the bladder after catheterization promotes an environment for bacteria proliferation (Newman & Willson, 2011, p. 16).

Teach Individual and/or Family Member Intermittent Catheterization. Observe Them Performing Intermittent Catheterization for (Newman & Willson, 2011, p. 16)

- Ability
- Hygiene (hand washing, maintenance of catheter sterility)
- Correct technique (lubricant, position, prevention of trauma)
- Instruct individual/family member to wash perineum each day and after sexual activity.

Review Signs/Symptoms of Urinary Tract Infection With Individual and Family

- Dysuria: pain or burning during urination, lower abdominal pain
- Frequency: more frequent urination (or waking up at night to urinate), often with only a small amount of urine
- Urgency: the sensation of having to urinate urgently
- Hesitancy: the sensation of not being able to urinate easily or completely (or feeling that you have to urinate but only a few drops of urine come out)
- Cloudy, bad-smelling, or new onset bloody urine

   R: Bloody urine may be normal when intermittent catheterization is initiated (Newman & Willson, 2011).

- Mild fever (less than 101° F), chills, and "just not feeling well" (malaise)
- Upper urinary tract infection (pyelonephritis) may develop rapidly and may or may not include the symptoms for a lower urinary tract infection.
- Fairly high fever (higher than 101° F); shaking, chills
- Nausea, vomiting
- Flank pain: pain in back or side, usually on only one side at about waist level

CLINICAL ALERT:
- Elderly people may not have the usual signs/symptoms of UTI, but instead may have hypothermia, poor appetite, lethargy, and sometimes only a change in mental status.

   R: Of concern because when urethral damage occurs, the mucosal barrier to infection is compromised (Newman & Willson, 2011). In addition, another measure that may reduce infection is the acidification of urine with cranberry juice or capsules, foods containing lactobacillus, and vitamin C capsules (Newman & Willson, 2011). Cranberries inhibit bacterial adherence to the uroepithelial wall and have been primarily studied with Escherichia coli (E. coli) (Jepson & Craig, 2008).

CLINICAL ALERT:
- Incontinence management is a complex process. The nurse is advised to seek expert assistance from a nurse specialist. An excellent online resource is Newman, D. K., & Willson, M. M. (2011). Review of intermittent catheterization and current best practices. *Urologic Nursing, 31*(1), 12. Retrieved from http://www.suna.org/education/2013/article3101229.pdf
- Refer to community nurses for assistance in incontinence management at home if indicated.

Clinical Alert Report

Instruct staff/student to report incontinent episodes or change in medical status.

FUNCTIONAL URINARY INCONTINENCE

NANDA-I Definition

State in which a usually continent client experiences incontinence because of a difficulty or inability to reach the toilet in time

Carp's Cues

Functional incontinence is the inability or unwillingness of the person with a normal bladder and sphincter to reach the toilet in time. Functional incontinence may be caused by conditions affecting physical and emotional ability to respond and/or manage the act of urination.

Defining Characteristics

Incontinence before or during an attempt to reach the toilet

Related Factors

Pathophysiologic

Related to diminished bladder cues and impaired ability to recognize bladder cues secondary to:

Brain injury/tumor/infection	Alcoholic neuropathy	Cerebrovascular accident
Parkinsonism	Demyelinating diseases	Progressive dementia
Multiple sclerosis		

Treatment Related

Related to treatment barriers to access to bathroom (e.g., tether lines, IVs, urinary catheter, NG tube)
Related to decreased bladder tone secondary to:

Antihistamines	Immunosuppressant therapy	Epinephrine
Diuretics	Anticholinergics	Tranquilizers
Sedatives	Muscle relaxants	

Situational (Personal, Environmental)

Related to impaired mobility
Related to decreased attention to bladder cues secondary to depression
Related to decreased attention to bladder cues secondary to confusion
Related to environmental barriers to bathroom (e.g., distant toilets, toilet seat, bed too high, poor lighting, unfamiliar surroundings)

Maturational

Older Adult
Related to motor and sensory losses

CLINICAL ALERT: The Centers for Medicare & Medicaid Services (*CMS, 2005) have this requirement for residents in health care facilities.

Each resident who is incontinent of urine is identified, assessed, and provided appropriate treatment and services to achieve or maintain as much normal urinary function as possible:

- An indwelling catheter is not used unless there is valid medical justification;
- An indwelling catheter for which continuing use is not medically justified is discontinued as soon as clinically warranted;
- Services are provided to restore or improve normal bladder function to the extent possible, after the removal of the catheter; and
- A resident, with or without a catheter, receives the appropriate care and services to prevent infections to the extent possible.

Carp's Cues

Urinary incontinence (UI) has a major impact in long-term care facilities. It is the second leading reason for placement of older adults into institutionalized care, and it is the primary reason why many elderly persons are not accepted into assisted living facilities. In long-term care facilities, it has been estimated that about 50% of the residents are urinary incontinent and that many who are continent at admission tend to become incontinent over time. In a study of 430 newly admitted nursing home residents, 22% of women who were continent at admission were incontinent after 1 year. The conversion rate in men was even higher (56%). The causes for this increase involve cognitive and mobility impairment and adjustment to the nursing home environment. In addition to staff, many nursing home residents believe UI is inevitable. Residents will use self-management strategies for urine leakage to protect social and psychological integrity, privacy, and dignity. Not only does UI have a substantial social effect on residents, but it also has associated morbidities, including urinary tract infections (UTI), pressure ulcers, and falls with subsequent injury. In addition, caring for residents with UI adds considerably to the burden. An indwelling catheter is not used unless there is valid medical justification and, if not medically justified, it is discontinued as soon as clinically warranted (Roe et al., 2011; Vasavada, 2013).

Goals

NOC

Tissue Integrity, Urinary Continence, Urinary Elimination

The person will report no or decreased episodes of incontinence as evidenced by the following indicators:

* Remove or minimize environmental barriers at home.
* Use proper adaptive equipment to assist with voiding, transfers, and dressing.
* Describe causative factors for incontinence.

Interventions

NIC

Perineal Care, Urinary Incontinence Care, Prompted Voiding, Urinary Habit Training, Urinary Elimination Management, Teaching: Procedure/Treatment

Assess Causative or Contributing Factors

Obstacles to Toilet

* Poor lighting, slippery floor, misplaced furniture and rugs, inadequate footwear, toilet too far, bed too high, and side rails up
* Inadequate toilet (too small for walkers, wheelchair, seat too low/high, no grab bars)
* Inadequate signal system for requesting help
* Lack of privacy

Sensory/Cognitive Deficits

* Visual deficits (blindness, field cuts, poor depth perception)
* Cognitive deficits as a result of aging, trauma, stroke, tumor, and infection
* Psychological deficits

Motor/Mobility Deficits

* Limited upper and/or lower extremity movement/strength (inability to remove clothing)
* Barriers to ambulation (e.g., vertigo, fatigue, altered gait, hypertension)

  R: Barriers can delay access to the toilet and cause incontinence if the individual cannot delay urination. A few seconds' delay in reaching the bathroom can make the difference between continence and incontinence.

Reduce or Eliminate Contributing Factors, if Possible

Environmental Barriers

* Assess path to bathroom for obstacles, lighting, and distance.
* Assess adequacy of toilet height and need for grab bars.
* Assess adequacy of room size.
* Assess if individual can remove clothing easily.
* Provide a commode between bathroom and bed, if necessary.

Sensory/Cognitive Deficits

* For a person with diminished vision:
  * Ensure adequate lighting.
  * Encourage person to wear prescribed corrective lens.
  * Provide clear, safe pathway to bathroom.
  * Keep call bell easily accessible.
  * If bedpan or urinal is used, make sure it is within easy reach in the same location at all times.

- Assess person for safety in bathroom.
- Assess person's ability to provide self-hygiene.
- For a person with cognitive deficits:
  - Offer toileting reminders every 2 hours, after meals, and before bedtime.
  - Establish appropriate means to communicate need to void.
  - Answer call bell immediately.
  - Encourage wearing of ordinary clothes.
  - Provide a normal environment for elimination (use bathroom, if possible).
  - Allow for privacy while maintaining safety.
  - Allow sufficient time for task.
  - Reorient individual to where he or she is and what task he or she is doing.
  - Be consistent in your approach to person.
  - Give simple step-by-step instructions; use verbal and nonverbal cues.
  - Give positive reinforcement for success.
  - Assess person for safety in bathroom.
  - Assess need for adaptive devices on clothing to make dressing and undressing easier.
  - Assess person's ability to provide self-hygiene.

  R: An individual with a cognitive deficit needs constant verbal cues and reminders to establish a routine and reduce incontinence.

Maintain Optimal Hydration

- Increase fluid intake to 2,000 to 3,000 mL/day, unless contraindicated.
- Teach older adults not to depend on thirst sensations but to drink liquids even when not thirsty.
- Space fluids every 2 hours.
- Decrease fluid intake after 7 p.m.; provide only minimal fluids during the night.

  R: Dehydration can prevent the sensation of a full bladder and can contribute to loss of bladder tone. Spacing fluids helps promote regular bladder filling and emptying.

  R: Dehydration irritates the bladder lining, making the urgency worse (Griebling, 2009).

Explain Foods/Fluids That Increase Bladder Irritation and/or Volume, Increasing Urgency (Davis et al., 2013; Derrer, 2014; Gleason et al., 2013; Lukacz, Segall, & Wexner, 2015)

R: Caffienated beverages /foods (e.g., coffee, tea, chocolate) alcohol, red wine, highly acidic foods, and foods high in potassium can irritate the bladder, causing urgency and frequency (Griebling, 2009).

Maintain Adequate Nutrition to Ensure Bowel Elimination at Least Once Every 3 Days

Promote Personal Integrity and Provide Motivation to Increase Bladder Control

- Encourage person to share feelings about incontinence and determine its effect on his or her social patterns.
- Convey that incontinence can be cured or at least controlled to maintain dignity.
- Use protective pads or garments only after conscientious reconditioning efforts have been completely unsuccessful after 6 weeks.
- Work to achieve daytime continence before expecting nighttime continence:
  - Encourage socialization.
  - Discourage the use of bedpans.
  - Encourage and assist person to groom self.
  - If hospitalized, provide opportunities to eat meals outside bedroom (day room, lounge).
  - If fear or embarrassment is preventing socialization, instruct person to use sanitary pads or briefs temporarily until control is established.
  - Change clothes as soon as possible when wet to avoid indirectly sanctioning wetness.
  - Advise the oral use of chlorophyll tablets to deodorize urine and feces.
  - See *Social Isolation* and *Ineffective Coping* for additional interventions, if indicated.

    R: Wearing normal clothing or nightwear helps simulate the home environment, where incontinence may not occur. A hospital gown may reinforce incontinence. Use of bathroom rather than bedpans simulates the home environment.

> **CLINICAL ALERT:**
> • "Normal skin pH is acidic at 4 to 6.5, which helps protect the skin against microorganism invasion. Frequent use of soap can alter skin pH to an alkaline state, leaving it more vulnerable to microorganism invasion. Exposure to urine or diarrhea damages the skin and increases the risk of pressure ulcers. Urine is absorbed by keratinocytes (outermost layer of skin), and when these cells are softened, they cannot provide protection from pressure injury. Urine contains urea, and ammonia can damage the skin. In an incontinent individual with a urinary tract infection, urine will also be alkaline and injurious to the skin" (Langemo & Black, 2010, p. 61).

Promote Skin Integrity

- Identify individuals at risk for development of pressure ulcers.
- Avoid harsh soaps and alcohol products.
- Keep moisture away from the skin.
- Refer to *Risk for Impaired Skin Integrity* for additional information.

  R: Ammonia from urine makes the skin more alkaline and more vulnerable to irritants (*Scardillo & Aronovitch, 1999).

Teach Prevention of Urinary Tract Infections

- Encourage regular, complete emptying of the bladder.
- Ensure adequate fluid intake.
- Keep urine acidic; avoid citrus juices, dark colas, coffee, tea, and alcohol, which act as irritants.
- Monitor urine pH.
- Teach individual to recognize abnormal changes in urine properties.
  - Increased mucus and sediment
  - Blood in urine (hematuria)
  - Change in color (from normal straw colored) or odor
- Teach individual to monitor for signs and symptoms of infection:
  - Elevated temperature, chills, and shaking
  - Changes in urine properties
  - Suprapubic pain
  - Painful urination
  - Urgency
  - Frequent small voids or frequent small incontinences
  - Increased spasticity in spinal cord–injured individuals
  - Increased urine pH
  - Nausea/vomiting
  - Lower back and/or flank pain

  R: Bacteria multiply rapidly in stagnant urine retained in the bladder. Moreover, overdistention hinders blood flow to the bladder wall, increasing the susceptibility to infection from bacterial growth. Regular, complete bladder emptying greatly reduces the risk of infection.

Geriatric Interventions

Explain Not to Restrict Fluid Intake Because of Fear of Incontinence

R: Dehydration can cause incontinence by eliminating the sensation of a full bladder (the signal to urinate) and by reducing the individual's alertness to the sensation.

R: Studies have shown that mild dehydration impairs cognitive abilities and contributes to increased anxiety and fatigue in adults (Ganio et al., 2011). This may be even more problematic for someone of advanced age.

Teach Older Adults Not to Depend on Thirst Sensations But to Drink Liquids Even When Not Thirsty Every 2 Hour Especially in Hot Weather or When Exercising

R: The hypothalamus regulates body temperature, sleep, and appetite, monitors the blood's concentration of sodium and other substances and receives inputs from sensors in the blood vessels that monitor blood volume and pressure (hydration). As one ages, the function of the hypothalamus diminishes (Grossman & Porth, 2014).

Explain Age-Related Effects on Bladder Function and That Urgency and Nocturia Do Not Necessarily Lead to Incontinence

Initiate Health Teaching Referral, When Indicated

- Refer to visiting nurse (occupational therapy department) for assessment of bathroom facilities at home.
- Emphasize that incontinence is not an inevitable age-related event.

  R: Explaining the cause can motivate the person to participate.

- Explain not to restrict fluid intake for fear of incontinence.

  R: Dehydration can cause incontinence by eliminating the sensation of a full bladder (the signal to urinate) and also by reducing the person's alertness to the sensation.

- Explain not to rely on thirst as a signal to drink fluids.

  R: The older adult has an age-related decrease in thirst (Miller, 2015).

- Teach the need to have easy access to bathroom at night. If needed, consider commode chair or urinal.

  R: This is to prevent falls.

> **Clinical Alert Report**
>
> Instruct staff/student to report incontinent episodes or changes in mental status.

OVERFLOW URINARY INCONTINENCE

NANDA-I Definition

Involuntary loss of urine associated with overdistention of the bladder

Defining Characteristics*

Bladder distention
High postvoid residual volume
Observed involuntary leakage of small volumes of urine
Reports involuntary leakage of small volumes of urine
Nocturia

Related Factors

Pathophysiologic

Related to sphincter blockage secondary to:

Strictures	Prostatic enlargement
Ureterocele	Perineal swelling
Bladder neck contractures	Severe pelvic prolapse

Related to impaired afferent pathways or inadequacy secondary to:

Cord injury/tumor/infection	Multiple sclerosis
Brain injury/tumor/infection	Diabetic neuropathy
Cerebrovascular accident	Alcoholic neuropathy
Demyelinating diseases	Tabes dorsalis

Treatment Related

Related to bladder outlet obstruction* or impaired afferent pathways secondary to drug therapy (iatrogenic)

Antihistamines   Decongestants*
Theophylline   Anticholinergics*
Epinephrine   Calcium channel blockers*
Isoproterenol

Situational (Personal, Environmental)

Related to bladder outlet obstruction secondary to:

Fecal impaction*

Related to detrusor hypocontractility* secondary to:

Deconditioned voiding
Association with stress or discomfort

Refer to *Impaired Urinary Elimination.*

Goals

Refer to Neurogenic Bladder

Interventions

Refer to Neurogenic Bladder.

STRESS URINARY INCONTINENCE

NANDA-I Definition

Sudden leakage of urine with activities that increase the intra-abdominal pressure

Defining Characteristics*

Observed or reported involuntary leakage of small amounts of urine:
In the absence of detrusor contraction
In the absence of an overactive bladder
On exertion
With coughing, laughing, sneezing, or all of these

Related Factors

Pathophysiologic

Related to incompetent bladder outlet secondary to congenital urinary tract anomalies
Related to degenerative changes in pelvic muscles* and structural supports secondary to estrogen deficiency
Related to intrinsic urethral sphincter*

Situational (Personal, Environmental)

Related to high intra-abdominal pressure* and weak pelvic muscles* secondary to:

Obesity   Poor personal hygiene
Sex   Smoking
Pregnancy

Related to weak pelvic muscles and structural supports secondary to:

Recent substantial weight loss
Childbirth

Maturational

Older Adult
Related to loss of muscle tone

Goals

NOC
Refer to *Functional Urinary Incontinence.*

The person will report a reduction or elimination of stress incontinence as evidenced by the following indicator:

- Be able to explain the cause of incontinence and rationale for treatments.

Interventions

NIC
See also *Functional Incontinence, Pelvic Muscle Exercise, Weight Management*

Routinely Assess Women of All Ages For Their Knowledge of Pelvic Floor Health and Stress Incontinence. Specifically Ask if They Experience Leaking of Urine

R: Nygaard, Thompson, Svengalis, and Albright (*1994) reported a "study of elite nulliparous college athletes that 32% of the athletes leaked urine during their sports, 13% beginning in junior high." "Gymnastic athletes had the highest incidence of urinary leakage at 67%, with basketball close behind at 66%, and tennis at 50%" (*Nygaard et al. 1994; *Smith, McCrery, & Appell, 2006).

Determine Contributing Factors That Can Be Reduced as (*Smith et al., 2006)

- Obesity (refer also to Obesity/Overweight nursing diagnoses)
- Lack of knowledge of pelvic muscle structures and effects of weakness caused by, for example, obesity, vaginal childbirth, sports, loss of estrogen (perimenopause, menopause)
- With aging, a stretching or sagging of the pelvic floor may result in hernia-like positions of the bladder, the uterus, or the rectum
- Chronic constipation—frequent straining and bearing down to have a bowel movement stretches the pelvic muscles
- Hysterectomy—the removal of the uterus removes one of the support structures for the other pelvic organ
- Situational—prolonged standing, lifting, or carrying weight for a job or exercise
- Smoking and chronic coughing add extra stress to the pelvic floor muscles and ligaments

    R: The above situations are important times to keep the pelvic muscles exercised, increasing the blood supply to the muscles and providing strength and tone of the fibers for support. Pelvic floor weakness with incontinence or pelvic organ prolapse can interfere with social, recreational, and career activities (*Smith et al., 2006).

> **CLINICAL ALERT:**
> - The following myths held by health care professional and women are barriers to discussions and successful management of stress incontinence (*Smith et al., 2006):
>   - Underappreciation and the lack of knowledge of the complex nature of the pelvic floor and its function
>   - That it is difficult to isolate pelvic muscles
>   - That pelvic floor weakness is a natural result of aging
>   - That women are not comfortable discussing pelvic floor

Explain the Effect of Incompetent Floor Muscles on Continence

R: Urinary continence is maintained by the junction of the bladder and the urethra, support from the perineal floor, and the muscle around the urethra. Stress incontinence is the leakage of small amounts of urine when the urethral outlet cannot control passage of urine in the presence of increased intra-abdominal pressure (Grossman & Porth, 2014).

> **CLINICAL ALERT:**
> - "Effective and consistent pelvic muscle exercises can provide many benefits across the lifespan of women. Beginning in young healthy women, strengthening the pelvic floor muscles provides support for the bladder and urethra against the forces of increased intra-abdominal pressures from activity or exertion, provides increased sensation and control during sexual activity, and prepares the pelvic floor for pregnancy and childbirth" (*Smith et al., 2006).

Teach Pelvic Muscle Exercises (*Dougherty, 1998)

* Explain it will take 4 to 6 months before results can be noted (*Smith et al., 2006).

    *R: Like other muscles in the body, the muscles in the pelvic floor are subject to fatigue and injury. They can also be actively exercised to increase their tone and size to prevent fatigue and injury (*Smith et al., 2006).*

Teach How to Self-Assess Whether Exercises Are Being Done Correctly

* Stand with one foot elevated on a stool, insert finger in vagina, and feel the strength of the contraction. Evaluate the strength of the contraction on a scale of 0 to 5 (*Sampselle et al., 1998):
    * 0 = No palpable contraction
    * 1 = Very weak, barely felt
    * 2 = Weak but clearly felt
    * 3 = Good but not maintained when moderate finger pressure is applied
    * 4 = Good but not maintained when intense finger pressure is applied
    * 5 = Maximum strength with strong resistance
* Consult an incontinence specialist for use of vaginal weights for pelvic floor strengthening if indicated.

Provide Instructions for Pelvic Muscle Exercises (Kegel Exercises) and Explain

*R: Pelvic floor muscle rehabilitation is an important treatment for strengthening perineal muscles and is an effective exercise to prevent stress and urgency incontinence (Dumoulin, Hay-Smith, & Mac Habee-Segui, 2014). Pelvic floor muscle training should be encouraged and taught to all young women and older and for all incontinence episodes mixed, urge, or stress (*Wilson et al., 2005).*

* To learn which muscles to exercise and tightening muscles as you are urinating to stop urination; this includes tightening the rectal muscles (Wilkinson & Van Leuven, 2007).

    R: This will indicate if you are tightening the correct muscles.

* Empty your bladder before doing Kegel exercises

> **CLINICAL ALERT:**
> * Don't make a habit of using Kegel exercises to start and stop your urine stream. Doing Kegel exercises while emptying your bladder can actually weaken the muscles, as well as lead to incomplete emptying of the bladder—which increases the risk of a urinary tract infection.

* Hold the contractions for 5 to 10 seconds and release. Relax between contractions, taking care to keep contraction and relaxation times equal. Gradually increase the time of contracting from 2 to 10 seconds. If you contract for 10 seconds, relax for 10 seconds before next contraction (Wilkinson & Van Leuven, 2007).
* Perform 40 to 60 contractions divided in 2 to 4 sessions each time. These should be spread out through the day and incorporate different positions (sitting, standing, and lying; Wilkinson & Van Leuven, 2007).
* "For best results, focus on tightening only your pelvic floor muscles. Be careful not to flex the muscles in your abdomen, thighs, or buttocks. Avoid holding your breath. Instead, breathe freely during the exercises" (Mayo Clinic, 2012).
* A good way to help to remember to do exercises is to incorporate them into daily routine, such as stopping at a traffic light or washing dishes (Wilkinson & Van Leuven, 2007). Refer individuals to "How to do Kegel Exercises," accessed at http://www.mayoclinic.org/healthy-lifestyle/womens-health/in-depth/kegel-exercises/art-20045283?pg=1

⊗ HEALTH PROMOTION DIAGNOSES

DECISIONAL CONFLICT

NANDA-I Definition

Uncertainty about course of action to be taken when choice among competing actions involves risk, loss, or challenge to values and beliefs

Defining Characteristics*

Verbalized uncertainty about choices
Verbalizes undesired consequences of alternatives being considered
Vacillation among alternative choices
Delayed decision making
Self-focusing
Verbalizes feeling of distress while attempting a decision
Physical signs of distress or tension (e.g., increased heart rate, increased muscle tension, restlessness)
Questioning of personal values and/or beliefs while attempting to make a decision
Questioning moral values while attempting a decision
Questioning moral rules while attempting a decision
Questioning moral principles while attempting a decision

Related Factors

Many situations can contribute to decisional conflict, particularly those that involve complex medical interventions of great risk. Any decisional situation can precipitate conflict for an individual; thus, the examples listed below are not exhaustive, but reflective of situations that may be problematic and possess factors that increase the difficulty.

Treatment Related

Related to lack of relevant information
Related to risks versus the benefits of (specify test, treatment):

Surgery
   Tumor removal   Orchiectomy   Mastectomy
   Cosmetic surgery   Prostatectomy   Joint replacement
   Amputation   Hysterectomy   Cataract removal
   Transplant   Laminectomy   Cesarean section
Diagnostics
   Amniocentesis   X-rays   Ultrasound
Chemotherapy
Radiation
Dialysis
Mechanical ventilation
Enteral feedings
Intravenous hydration
   Use of preterm labor medications   Participation in treatment study trials   HIV antiviral therapy

Situational (Personal, Environmental)

Related to perceived threat to value system
Related to:

Institutionalization (child, parent)
Foster home placement

Related to:

Lack of relevant information*
Confusing information

Related to:

Disagreement within support systems
Inexperience with decision making
Unclear personal values/beliefs*
Conflict with personal values/beliefs
Ethical or moral dilemmas (e.g., "do not resuscitate" orders, quality of life, termination of pregnancy, selective termination with multiple-gestation pregnancies, organ transplant, cessation of life-support systems)

Maturational

Related to risks versus benefits of:

Alcohol/drug use
Sexual activity
High-risk sexual activity
Illegal/dangerous situations

Carp's Cues

The nurse has an important role in assisting individuals and families with making decisions. Because nurses usually do not benefit financially from decisions made regarding treatments and transfers, they are in an ideal position to assist with decisions. Although, according to Davis (1989), "Nursing or medical expertise does not enable health care professionals to know the values of patients or what patients think is best for themselves," nursing expertise does enable nurses to facilitate systematic decision making that considers all possible alternatives and possible outcomes, as well as individual beliefs and values. The focus is on assisting with logical decision making, not on promoting a certain decision. "Nurses' judgments and decisions have the potential to help healthcare systems allocate resources efficiently, promote health gain and patient benefit and prevent harm" (Thompson et al., 2013, p. 1721).

Goals

NOC
Decision Making, Information Processing, Participation: Health Care Decisions

The individual/group will make an informed choice as evidenced by the following indicators:

* Relate the advantages and disadvantages of choices.
* Share fears and concerns regarding choices and responses of others.
* Define what would be most helpful to support the decision-making process.

Interventions

> **CLINICAL ALERT:**
> • Andrew Lansley wrote, "No decision about me without me" (Department of Health, 2010), which emphasizes that shared decision making (SDM) must be the norm rather than the exception (Lilly, Robinson, Holtzman, & Bottorff, 2012).

Reduce or Eliminate Causative or Contributing Factors

R: A National Health Survey (NHS) patient survey found 48% of inpatients and 30% of outpatients want to be more involved in decisions about their care (Department of Health, 2010).

NIC

Decision-Making
Support, Mutual Goal
Setting, Learning
Facilitation, Health
System Guidance,
Anticipatory Guidance,
Client Right Protection,
Values Clarification,
Anxiety Reduction

Lack of Experience With or Ineffective Decision Making

- Facilitate logical decision making:
  - Assist the individual in recognizing the problem and clearly identifying the needed decision.
  - Generate a list of all possible alternatives or options.
  - Help identify the probable outcomes of the various alternatives.
  - Aid in evaluating the alternatives on the basis of actual or potential threats to beliefs/values.
  - Encourage the individual to make a decision.
- Suggest that the individual use significant others as a sounding board when considering alternatives.
- Respect and support the role that the individual desires in the decision, whether it is active, collaborative, or passive.

  R: The role of nurses in situations of interpersonal/intrapersonal conflict reflects a culture broker framework incorporating advocacy, negotiation, mediation, and sensitivity to individuals' and families' needs. Decisional conflict is greater when none of the alternatives is good. Assist the individual in exploring personal values and relationships that may affect the decision. Explore obtaining a referral with the individual's spiritual leader (Lilly et al., 2012).

- Encourage the individual to base the decision on the most important values.
- Support the decision—even if the decision conflicts with your own values.

  R: Difficult decisions create stress and conflict because values and actions are not congruent. Conflict may lead to fear and anxiety that negatively affect decision making. External resources become very important for the individual in decisional conflict with a low level of self-confidence in making autonomous decisions.

Fear of Outcome/Response of Others

- Provide clarification regarding potential outcomes and correct misconceptions.
- Explore with the individual what the risks of not deciding would be.
- Encourage the individual to face fears and to share fears with significant others.
- Actively reassure the individual that the decision is his or hers to make and that he or she has the right to do so.
- Assist the individual in recognizing that it is his or her life; if he or she is comfortable with the decision, others will respect the conviction.

  R: The roles of individual values greatly influence the resolution of ethical decision-making dilemmas. Decisional conflict becomes more intense when it involves a threat to status, self-esteem, or family harmony.

Insufficient or Inconsistent Information

- Provide information comprehensively and sensitively. Correct misinformation.
- Ensure that the individual clearly understands what is involved in the decision and the various alternatives (i.e., informed choice).
- Encourage the individual to seek second professional opinions regarding health.
- Collaborate with other health care members/significant others to determine appropriate timing for truthfulness.

  R: Information that is valid, relevant, and understandable is required for informed decisions (Oxman, Lavis, Lewin, & Fretheim, 2009). Mastering content for effective decision making requires time. Time allows an individual to choose the option that provides the most benefit with the least risk.

Controversy With Support System as Indicated

- Reassure the individual that he or she does not have to give in to pressure from others, whether family, friends, or health professionals.
- Advocate for the individual's wishes if others attempt to undermine his or her ability to make the decision personally.
- Advocate for the individual if the family/significant others are excluding him or her from decision making.
- Recognize that the individual may become ambivalent about "choosing" when putting the needs of the support system above his or her own.

  R: "The role of nurses in situations of interpersonal/intrapersonal conflict reflects a culture broker framework incorporating advocacy, negotiation, mediation, and sensitivity to clients' and families' needs" (Thompson et al., 2013, p. 1721).

Conflicts Related to Cancer Treatment Options (Lilly et al., 2012)

* Establish a pretreatment quality of life using a tested instrument. Refer to Halyard and Ferrans (2008).
* Quality-of-life assessment for routine clinical practice. Refer to *Journal of Supportive Oncology* on reference list.

    R: *"Client ratings of quality of life before treatment have seen to be predictive of length of survival"* (Yarbro, Wujek, & Gobel, 2011, p. 202).

* Explore how cancer treatment decisions will affect quality of life with individual (Yarbro et al., 2011, p. 203).
* Consult with others for needed data. Avoid relinquishing your responsibility to the individual/family or others.
    * What are the long-term negative effects when survival is long?
    * Is supportive care only better than therapeutic regimen, when survival time is short (6- to 12-month median survival)?
    * Is a new therapy preferable?
    * What are the side effects of all the proposed therapies?

        R: *"Client ratings of quality of life before treatment have been to be predictive of length of survival"* (Yarbro et al., 2011, p. 202). *Discussions of the effects of treatment alternatives on quality of life can help individuals/ families make better informed decisions (p. 202). Nurses have no investments (ego, financial) in the decisions individual make and thus are in a position to provide unbiased information.*

Explore End-of-Life Decisions

* Refer to Palliative Care Plan in Unit III.

Initiate Health Teaching and Referrals as Indicated

* Refer families to the appropriate person for assistance with decisions regarding care of a family member (e.g., nurse ombudsman, religious leader, advanced practice nurse).

COMPROMISED ENGAGEMENT[10]

Definition

Insuffient participation of individual/family to a proposed health-promoting and/or therapeutic plan to achieve desired, optimal health care outcomes

Defining Characteristics

Reports Insufficient Involvement in Their Own Care

Reluctance to engage in health care discussions/decisions
Verbalization of confusion about therapy (e.g., medications, diet, treatments, follow-up care, referrals)
Persistence or exacerbation of symptoms or progression of condition
Verbalization or evidence of not:
    Making or keeping follow-up appointments
    Scheduling/completing diagnostic tests, specialist appointments, therapies (physical therapy, speech)
    Taking medications as prescribed
    Performing treatments as prescribed
    Reducing or eliminating high-risk behaviors (substance abuse, significant daily dietary indiscretions, e.g., diabetic with high carbohydrate intake, reckless behavior)

---

[10]Compromised Engagement and Risk for Compromised Engagement have been developed by this author to replace the nursing diagnosis Noncompliance. Refer to the Author's Notes for rationale for this change.

Related Factors

Pathophysiologic

Related to the complexity of managing the condition
Related to impaired ability to manage his or her condition secondary to:

Multiple other responsibilities
Impaired memory
Motor deficits/disabilities
Inadequate or no available support

Treatment Related

Related to:

Side effects of therapy
Financial cost of therapy
Past unsuccessful experiences with advised regimen
Complex, unsupervised, prolonged therapy

Situational (Personal, Environmental)

Health Care Setting/Insurance
Related to varying/inconsistent health care providers
Related to reported unsatisfactory relationship with health care provider
Reports unsatisfactory and/or unpleasant experiences in health care settings
Related to financial barriers of multiple copays, limited insurance coverage, or no health insurance
Related to unsatisfactory health care setting (e.g. impersonal, rushed visit, long waiting times, punitive, unresponsive)
Related to the barriers or complexity of accessing (e.g., referrals, telephone) contact after office hours, medical advice, refilling medications, treatment supplies, professional agencies, facilities that take personal insurance
Related to complexity of paperwork associated with health care
Related to inadequate accommodation for hearing, vision, and mobility deficits
Related to inadequate accommodation for non-English-speaking individuals/family
Related to inadequate accommodation for low health literacy

Personal
Related to the complexity of the mastering/maintaining treatment/monitoring devices (e.g., glucose monitor)
Related to cultural values incongruent with proposed plan
Related to health beliefs or expectations incongruent with plan
Related to insufficient social support
Related to insufficient knowledge about regimen
Related to insufficient skills to perform regimen
Related to low confidence about their ability to manage their health
Related to barriers to access of care secondary to:

Mobility problems   Transportation problems
Inclement weather   Lack of child care
Financial/insurance issues

Related to concurrent illness of a family member
Related to barriers to care secondary to homelessness
Related to barriers to comprehension secondary to:

Cognitive deficits   Hearing deficits
Anxiety   Decreased attention span
Visual deficits   Poor memory
Fatigue   Motivation

Author's Note

The nursing diagnosis *Noncompliance* was last revised in 1998. The label *Noncompliance* has never reflected a proactive approach to an individual/family, who was not participating in recommended treatments or lifestyle changes. *Noncompliance* is viewed by health care professional as an individual/family that decides to ignore directives from a health care provider.

Criticism of the term noncompliant surfaced in the literature a decade ago. Recently health care literature is full of alternative strategies directed for health care professional to improve health outcomes with individual/families.

This author has chosen to retire this nursing diagnosis and replace it with *Compromised Engagement* and *Risk for Compromised Engagement*.

Gruman (2011) wrote, "Saying 'engagement' when meaning 'compliance' supports the belief that we are the only ones who must change our behavior. Doing so misrepresents the magnitude of shifts in attitude, expectations and effort that are required for all health care stakeholders to ensure that we have adequate knowledge and support to make well-informed decisions. And it fails to recognize that our behaviors are powerfully shaped by many contingencies money, culture, time, illness status, and personal preference. Being engaged in our health and care does not mean following our clinicians instructions to the letter. Rather, it means being able to accurately weigh the benefits and risks of a new medication, of stopping smoking or getting a PSA test in the context of the many other demands and opportunities that influence our pursuit of lives that are free of suffering for ourselves and those we love."

Note: We = individuals, families

Goals

NOC

Adherence Behavior, Acceptance Behavior, Health Beliefs: Perceived Control, Health Beliefs: Perceived Ability to Perform, Health Beliefs: Perceived Resources, Health Beliefs: Perceived Threat, Risk Control: (specify), for example, tobacco, use, alcohol use, lipid disorder, Symptom Control, Treatment Behavior: Illness/Injury

The individual will report a desire to initiate change as evidenced by the following indicators:

- Describe the reasons for the suggested treatment/lifestyle change.
- Identify barriers that he or she may encounter with the suggested regimen.
- Relate the possible consequences of not engaging in the recommended treatment/lifestyle change.

Interventions

NIC

Mutual-Goal Setting, Self-Efficacy Enhancement, Health System Guidance, Truth Telling, Health Education, Decision-Making Support, Transition Planning, Support System Enhancement, Self-Responsibility Facilitation, Caregiver Support

 Carp's Cues

Ask yourself, how many times have you not complied with the advice or instructions from a health care professional? Why? How would you like that professional to interact with you? Like a parent to a disobedient child or a concerned person who understands that instructions are not always clear and that perhaps you did not agree with the recommendation or prescription. "Seeing the world from the shoes of the individual/family in your care" (Sofaer & Schumann, 2013, p. 15) may improve your tolerance of nonadherance and prompt you to find out why.

- Refer to Appendix C *Strategies to Promote Engagement of Individual/families for Healthier Outcomes* for specific one-to-one strategies to increase activation to participate and to reduce barriers (e.g., health illiteracy, complexity).

Initially, Literacy and Health Literacy Must Be Accessed

- Refer to Appendix C for a focus assessment and strategies to engage individuals/families with heath literacy.

  R: Health care literacy and language-appropriate interactions are essential for individuals, family, and clinicians to understand the components of individual engagement. Providers must maintain awareness of the language needs and health care literacy level of the individual and family and respond accordingly (Sofaer & Schumann, 2013).

Determine if Individual/Family Can, Read, Understand, and Write in English and/or Their Native Language

R: Health care literacy and linguistically appropriate interactions are essential for individual, family, and clinicians to understand the components of engagement (Sofaer & Schumann, 2013).

Before a Person Can Change, They Must (Martin Haskard-Zolnierek & DiMatteo, 2010)

* Know what change is necessary (information and why).
* Desire the change (motivation).
* Have the tools to achieve and maintain the change (strategy).
* Trust the health care professional, who has a sympathetic presence (Pelzang, 2010).

> *R: Empathic communication involving a thorough understanding of the individual's perspective improves adherence. Individuals who are informed and affectively motivated are also more likely to adhere to their treatment recommendations (*Martin, Williams, Haskard, & DiMatteo, 2005).*

Explain the Recommendation (e.g., Medication, Life-Style Change, Treatment, Referral). Offer Options if Possible. Determine if Individual Intents to Implement the Recommendation(s)

R: Although asking questions, discussing preferences, or disagreeing with a recommendation are communication skills used in everyday life, for many individuals these may be novel in the context of a medical consultation (Entwistle et al., 2010; Sofaer & Schumann, 2013).

* Ask the person to relate to you what you discussed.
* Do they have any concerns about the recommendation?
* Do they see this as possible?
* If not, why?

> *R: Martin et al. (2010) reported, "Individual intentions to adhere to recommended treatments are significantly correlated with having choices regarding medical treatments; having the opportunity to discuss their care with their physicians; having their preferences taken into account; and having a doctor who communicates well, who they trust."*

Encourage a Discussion That Prompts the Person/Family to Tell Why the Suggested Plan Is Problematic for Them (e.g., So What Do You Think About . . .)

R: "Overall, participants' comments strongly suggest that speaking up is easier when healthcare staff give the impression of caring, having time and welcoming and supporting them as legitimate contributors to their care" (Entwistle et al., 2010, p. 6).

Carp's Cues

In conclusion, Dirk writes on July 18, 2011:

> Truly the closer such exchanges between providers and patients can be to a conversation, versus a lecture, the better for all involved. And as the impacts of medical treatments, falls mainly on the patient there should be no doubt about who has the final word/authority on what treatments will be undertaken. But as long as we largely put providers in the position of having to treat patients regardless of their level of cooperation (not compliance) there will be an unnecessary level of tension/resentment involved. On the legislative side we must err on the side of treatment for all but we also need to develop a culture/ethos of mutual engagement that recognizes/values the human investments on all sides. (Accessed at http://www.cfah.org/blog/2011 /engagement-does-not-mean-compliance)

RISK FOR COMPROMISED ENGAGEMENT

Definition

Vulnerable to insufficient participation of individual/family to a proposed health-promoting and/or therapeutic plan, which may compromise health

Risk Factors

Refer to Related Factors under *Compromised Engagement*.

Author's Note

The strategies for improving engagement under the diagnosis *Compromised Engagement* are relevant to *Risk for Compromised Engagement* as prevention strategies.

RISK-PRONE HEALTH BEHAVIOR

Definition

Impaired ability to modify lifestyle/behaviors in a manner that improves health status (NANDA-I)
    State in which a person has an inability to modify lifestyle/behavior in a manner consistent with a change in health status[11]

Defining Characteristics*

Demonstrates nonacceptance of health status change
Failure to achieve optimal sense of control
Minimizes health status change
Failure to take action that prevents health problems

Related Factors

Situational (Personal, Environmental)

Related to unhealthy lifestyle choices (e.g., tobacco use, excessive alcohol use, overweight) secondary to:

Insufficient knowledge
Low self-efficacy*
Negative attitude toward health care*
Multiple stressors

Inadequate social support*
Inadequate resources, finances
Multiple responsibilities

Related to impaired ability to understand secondary to:

Low literacy
Language barriers

Author's Note

Risk-Prone Health Behavior describes a person with an unhealthy lifestyle, who is not participating in management of the health problem because of lack of knowledge, motivation, comprehension, or other personal barriers.

    Individuals hospitalized with unhealthy lifestyles have immediate medical or surgical priorities. An appropriate focus in the hospital for these individuals is to explore with this person how their unhealthy choices are contributing to their health problems, supplement their knowledge with facts, and provide them with resources to use after discharge. Resources to change unhealthy lifestyles can be found on thePoint (e.g., Getting Started to Quit Smoking).

---

[11]This additional definition has been included for clarity and usefulness.

Goals

NOC

Adherence Behavior,
Symptom Control,
Health Beliefs,
Treatment Behavior,
Illness/Injury

The person will verbalize intent to modify one behavior to manage health problem as evidenced by the following indicators:

* Describe the relationship of present lifestyle to his or her health problems.
* Identify two resources to access after discharge.
* Set a date to initiate change.

Interventions

NIC

Heath Education,
Mutual Goal Setting,
Self-Responsibility,
Teaching: Disease
Process, Decision-
Making Process

Carp's Cues

Behavior change depends on various factors, including motivation, perception of vulnerability, and beliefs about controlling or preventing illness, environment, quality of health instruction, and ability to access resources (cost, accessibility). "An important aspect of adherence is recognizing the patient's right to choose whether or not to follow treatment recommendations" (Robinson, Callister, Berry, & Dearing, 2008).

Engage in Collaborative Negotiation

* Ask individual, "How can you be healthier?" Focus on the area he or she chooses.
* Do not provide unsolicited advice.
* Accept that only the individual can make the change.
* Accept resistance.
* For example:
  * Diabetes
  * Exercise
  * Healthy eating
  * Medication
  * Blood glucose monitoring
  * Individual-defined choice

  > *R: Motivational interviewing involves helping the person identify the discrepancy between present behaviors and future health goals. Asking someone to identify an unhealthy lifestyle versus telling him or her that he or she needs to lose weight, stop smoking, exercise, eat better, and so forth, starts a mutual conversation versus a one-direction dictum.*

Assess for Barriers

* What do you think is causing your BP (blood sugar or weight) to remain high?
* What could you do to decrease your BP (weight, blood sugar)?
* Would you like to stop smoking (or drinking alcohol)?
* What is preventing you?

If Low Literacy Is Suspected

* Refer to Appendix C for practical ways to identify and help individuals with low literacy.

Determine How Confident the Person Is to Make the Change

* For example:
  * How confident are you that you can get more exercise? Rate from 0 to 10.
  * If the importance level is 7 or above, assess confidence level. If the importance level is low, provide more information regarding the risks of not changing behavior.
  * If the level of confidence is 4 or less, ask the person why it is not a 1.
  * Ask person what is needed to change the low score to an 8.

> *R: If the importance and/or the confidence is low, an action plan with specific behavior changes would not reflect true collaboration.*

Collaboratively, Set a Realistic Goal and Action Plan (e.g., How Often Each Week Could You Walk Around the Block Two Times?)

R: The person's level of confidence will increase with success. Advice that is not easily achievable sets the person up for failure (*Bodenheimer, MacGregor, & Sharifi, 2005).

Initiate Health Teaching if Indicated

- Refer to thePoint for printed material Getting Started to provide the person with strategies to improve health, for example, smoking cessation, exercise, eating better.

RISK FOR INEFFECTIVE HEALTH MANAGEMENT

NANDA-I Definition

Pattern in which a person is at risk to experience a pattern of regulating and integrating into daily living a therapeutic regimen for the treatment of illness and its sequelae that is unsatisfactory for meeting specific health goals

Risk Factors

Treatment Related

Related to:

Complexity of therapeutic regimen*

Financial cost of regimen

Complexity of health care system*

Side effects of therapy*

Situational (Personal, Environmental)

Related to:

Previous unsuccessful experiences

Deficient knowledge*

Family patterns of health care*

Family conflict*

Mistrust of health care personnel

Powerlessness*

Perceived barriers*

Mistrust of regimen

Health belief conflicts

Insufficient confidence

Perceived susceptibility

Economic difficulties*

Questions seriousness of problem

Questions benefits of regimen

Excessive demands (individual, family)*

Decisional conflicts*

Related to insufficient or unavailable family support
Related to barriers to comprehension secondary to:

Cognitive deficits

Motivation

Fatigue

Anxiety

Hearing impairments

Memory problems

Carp's Cues

Ineffective Health Management is a very useful diagnosis for nurses in most settings. Individuals and families experiencing various health problems, acute or chronic, usually face treatment programs that require changes in previous functioning or lifestyle. These changes or adaptations can be instrumental in influencing positive outcomes.

Ineffective Health Management focuses on assisting the person and family to identify barriers in management of the condition and to prevent complications at home. Risk-Prone Health Behavior, approved in 2006, is different. This diagnosis focuses on habits or lifestyles that are unhealthy and can aggravate an existing condition or contribute to developing a disorder.

Refer to Unit II to medical or surgical care plan for specific interventions indicated to assist your assigned individual/family manage as they transition to home.

⊗ INDIVIDUAL COPING DIAGNOSES

ANXIETY

NANDA-I Definition

Vague, uneasy feeling of discomfort or dread accompanied by an autonomic response (the source often unspecific or unknown to the individual); a feeling of apprehension caused by anticipation of danger. It is an alerting signal that warns of impending danger and enables the individual to take measures to deal with threat.

Defining Characteristics

Manifested by symptoms from any category—physiologic, emotional, and cognitive; symptoms vary according to level of anxiety.

Physiologic

Increased pulse*	Urinary frequency, hesitancy, urgency*
Elevated blood pressure*	Fatigue*
Increased respiratory*	Insomnia*
Dilated pupils*	Dry mouth*
Diaphoresis*	Facial flushing* or pallor
Trembling, twitching*	Restlessness*
Voice quivering*	Body aches and pains (especially chest, back, neck)
Nausea*	Faintness*/dizziness
Palpitations	Paresthesias
Diarrhea*	Anorexia*

Emotional
Individual states feelings of:

Apprehension*	Loss of control
Persistent increased helplessness*	Tension or being "keyed up"
Jittery*	Anticipation of misfortune
Vigilance*	

Individual exhibits:

Irritability*/impatience	Criticism of self and others
Angry outbursts	Withdrawal
Crying	Lack of initiative
Tendency to blame others*	Self-deprecation
Startle reaction	Poor eye contact*

Cognitive

Inability to concentrate	Blocking of thoughts (inability to remember)
Lack of awareness of surroundings	Hyperattentiveness
Rumination*	Preoccupation*
Orientation to past	Diminished ability to learn*

Related Factors

Pathophysiologic

Related to any factor that interferes with physiologic stability (examples):

Respiratory distress
Mind-altering drugs

Chest pain
Cancer diagnosis

Treatment Related

Related to impending surgery, invasive procedure, therapy

Situational (Personal, Environmental)

Related to loss of significant others secondary to:

Death
Divorce
Cultural pressures

Moving
Temporary or permanent separation

Related to threat to biologic integrity secondary to (e.g., terminal illness, chronic disease)
Related to change in unfamiliar hospital environment
Related to change in socioeconomic status secondary to (e.g., unemployment, displacement, foreclosure, retirement)

Maturational

Child/Adolescent
Related to:

Inconsistent methods of discipline
Poor social skills
Peer rejection

Parental rejection
Fear of failure

Young Adult
Related to inadequate psychological resources to adapt to:

Career choices
Parenthood
Marriage

Leaving home
Educational demands

Middle Adult
Related to inadequate psychological resources to adapt to:

Physical signs of aging
Social status needs
Problems with relatives

Child-rearing problems
Career pressures
Aging parents

Older Adult
Related to inadequate resources (psychological, social support. financial, instrumental) to adapt to:

Daily Stressors
Physical changes
Retirement

Changes in residence
Changes in financial status

Author's Note

Margaret O's son Nicholas age 26 diagnosed with schizophrenia died on a psychiatric unit of mixed drug toxicity. Margaret wrote to students in mental health, "To care for people with mental illness in times of crisis with insight and compassion. . . .these are my hopes for you" (Procter, Hamer, McGarry, Wilson, & Froggatt, 2014, p. vii).

World Health Organization (WHO, 2014) defines mental health "as a state of well-being in which every individual realizes his or her own potential, can cope with the normal stresses of life, can work productively and fruitfully, and is able to make a contribution to her or his community." In addition, WHO describes mental health and illness as follows:

- Mental health is an integral part of health; indeed, there is no health without mental health.
- Mental health is more than the absence of mental disorders. Stigma and discrimination against individuals and families prevent people from seeking mental health care.

Goals

NOC
Anxiety Level, Coping, Impulse Self-Control

The individual will relate increased psychological and physiologic comfort evidenced by the following indicators:

- Describe own anxiety and coping patterns.
- Identifies two strategies to reduce anxiety.

Interventions

NIC
Anxiety Reduction, Impulse Control Training, Anticipatory Guidance

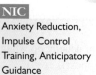

Carp's Cues

Procter et al. (2014) wrote, "When we listen to understand, we are present and available and are only listening to what the person is saying, not thinking about other things" (p. 93). It requires self-disciple rather than launching into our own agenda (Procter et al., 2014).

Nursing interventions for *Anxiety* can apply to any individual with anxiety regardless of etiologic and contributing factors.

Assist the Individual to Reduce Present Level of Anxiety

R: Lyon (*2002) has identified five factors that contribute to stressful lifestyles as idealistic expectations of self, unrealistic goals, toxic thoughts, negative self-talk, and procrastination.

- Assess level of anxiety: mild, moderate, severe, or panic
  - Provide reassurance and comfort.
  - Stay with the individual.
  - Support present coping mechanisms (e.g., allow the individual to talk, cry); do not confront or argue with defenses or rationalizations.
  - Speak slowly and calmly.
  - Be aware of your own concern and avoid reciprocal anxiety.
  - Convey empathic understanding (e.g., quiet presence, touch, allowing crying, talking).
  - Provide reassurance that a solution can be found.
  - Remind the individual that feelings are not harmful.
  - Respect personal space.
- If anxiety is at severe or panic level:
  - Ensure someone stays with the person with severe or panic levels of anxiety.
  - Do not make demands or ask the person to make decision.
  - Provide a quiet, nonstimulating environment with soft lighting.
  - Use short, simple sentences; speak slowly and calmly.
  - Focus on the present.
  - Remove excess stimulation (e.g., take the individual to a quieter room); limit contact with others who are also anxious (e.g., other individuals, family).
  - Avoid suggesting that the individual "relax." Do not leave the individual alone.
  - Provide assistance with all tasks during acute episodes of dyspnea.
  - During an acute episode, do not discuss preventive measures.
  - During nonacute episodes, teach relaxation techniques (e.g., tapes, guided imagery).
  - Consult a physician/nurse practitioner/physician assistant for possible pharmacologic therapy, if indicated.
- If the individual is hyperventilating or experiencing dyspnea:
  - Demonstrate breathing techniques; ask the individual to practice the technique with you.
  - Acknowledge the individual's fear and give positive reinforcement for efforts.
  - Acknowledge feelings of helplessness.

- Avoid suggesting that the individual "relax." Do not leave the individual alone.
- Provide assistance with all tasks during acute episodes of dyspnea.
- During an acute episode, do not discuss preventive measures.
- During nonacute episodes, teach relaxation techniques (e.g., tapes, guided imagery).

R: The severely anxious person tends to overgeneralize, assume, and anticipate catastrophe. Resulting cognitive problems include difficulty with attention and concentration, loss of objectivity, and vigilance. Providing emotional support and relaxation techniques and encouraging sharing may help an individual clarify and verbalize fears, allowing the nurse to give realistic feedback and reassurance. Exercise helps to dispel some anxiety (Halter, 2014).

If the Individual Is Hyperventilating or Experiencing Dyspnea, Ask the Person to Breathe With You (e.g., Slow Abdominal Breathing Rhythm)

R: This technique focuses on a slow rhythmic breathing, which with practice can distract and provide relaxation.

When Anxiety Diminishes, Assist in Recognizing Anxiety and Causes

- Help to see that mild anxiety can be a positive catalyst for change and does not need to be avoided.
- Request validation of your assessment of anxiety (e.g., "Are you uncomfortable now?").
- If the individual says yes, continue with the learning process; if the person cannot acknowledge anxiety, continue supportive measures until he or she can.
- When the individual can learn, determine usual coping mechanisms: "What do you usually do when you get upset?" (e.g., read, discuss problems, distance, use substances, seek social support).
- Assess for unmet needs or expectations; encourage recall and description of what the individual experienced immediately before feeling anxious.
- Assist in reevaluation of perceived threat by discussing the following:
  - Were expectations realistic? Too idealistic?
  - Was it possible to meet expectations?
  - Where in the sequence of events was change possible?
- "Keep focused on manageable problems; define them simply and concretely" (Varcarolis, 2011).
- Teach anxiety interrupters to use when the individual cannot avoid stressful situations:
  - Look up. Lower shoulders.
  - Control breathing.
  - Slow thoughts. Alter voice.
  - Give self-directions (out loud, if possible).
  - Exercise.
  - "Scruff your face"—changes facial expression.
  - Change perspective: imagine watching a situation from a distance (Grainger, 1990).

Reduce or Eliminate Problematic Coping Mechanisms

- Refer to *Ineffective Coping*.

Initiate Health Teaching and Referrals as Indicated

- Refer people identified as having chronic anxiety and maladaptive coping mechanisms for ongoing mental health counseling and treatment.
- Instruct in nontechnical, understandable terms regarding illness and associated treatments.

R: Simple and repeating explanations are needed because anxiety may interfere with learning.

> ### *Clinical Alert Report*
> - Advise ancillary staff/student to report an increase in anxiety and/or anger.

DEATH ANXIETY

NANDA-I Definition

Vague, uneasy feeling of discomfort or dread generated by perceptions of a real or imagined threat to one's existence

Defining Characteristics*

Reports:
Worry about the impact of one's own death on significant others
Feeling powerless over dying
Fear of loss of mental abilities when dying
Fear of pain related to dying
Fear of suffering related to dying
Deep sadness
Fear of the process of dying
Concerns of overworking the caregiver
Negative thoughts related to death and dying
Fear of prolonged dying
Fear of premature death
Fear of developing a terminal illness

Related Factors

A diagnosis of a potentially terminal condition or impending death can cause this diagnosis. Additional factors can contribute to death anxiety.

Situational (Personal, Environmental)

*Related to discussions on topic of death**
*Related to near-death experience**
*Related to perceived proximity of death**
*Related to uncertainty of prognosis**
*Related to anticipating suffering**
*Related to confronting reality of terminal disease**
*Related to observations related to death**
*Related to anticipating pain**
*Related to nonacceptance of own mortality**
*Related to uncertainty about life after death**
*Related to uncertainty about an encounter with a higher power**
*Related to uncertainty about the existence of a higher power**
*Related to experiencing the dying process**
*Related to anticipating impact of death on others**
*Related to anticipating adverse consequences of general anesthesia**
Related to personal conflict with palliative versus curative care
Related to conflict with family regarding palliative versus curative care
Related to fear of being a burden
Related to fear of unmanageable pain
Related to fear of abandonment
Related to unresolved conflict (family, friends)
Related to fear that one's life lacked meaning
Related to social disengagement

Goals/Interventions

 Carp's Cues

The detrimental impact of untreated, persistent anxiety was demonstrated in one multicenter study of over 600 individuals with advanced cancer that evaluated associations between anxiety disorders and multiple endpoints, including physician–individual relationships. Individuals with anxiety disorders had less trust in their clinicians compared with those without anxiety (Alici & Levin 2010; Irwin et al., 2011). Yun et al. (2010) reported a majority of individuals (58.0%) and caregivers (83.4%) were aware of the individual's terminal status. However, only 30% of individuals and 50% of caregivers were told directly by a physician. "For approximately 28% of patients and 23% of caregivers reported that they guessed it from the patient's worsening condition. The patient group was more likely than the caregiver group (78.6% v 69.6%) to prefer that patients be informed of their terminal status" (Yun et al., 2010).

Refer to Palliative Care Plan.

INEFFECTIVE COPING

NANDA-I Definition

Inability to form a valid appraisal of the stressors, inadequate choices of practiced responses, and/or inability to use available resources

Defining Characteristics

Verbalization of inability to cope or ask for help*
Inappropriate use of defense mechanisms
Inability to meet role expectations*
Chronic worry, anxiety
Sleep disturbance*
Fatigue*
High illness rate*
Reported difficulty with life stressors
Poor concentration*
Difficulty organizing information*
Decreased use of social support*
Inadequate problem solving*
Impaired social participation
Use of forms of coping that impede adaptive behavior*
Risk-taking*
Lack of goal-directed behavior*
Destructive behavior toward self or others*
Change in usual communication patterns*
High incidence of accidents
Substance abuse*

Related Factors

Pathophysiologic

Related to biochemical changes in brain secondary to (e.g., bipolar disorder, personality disorder, chemical dependency, attention-deficient disorders, schizophrenia)
Related to neurologic changes in brain secondary to (e.g., stroke, multiple sclerosis Alzheimer's disease, end-stage diseases)
Related to changes in body integrity secondary to (e.g., loss of body part, disfigurement secondary to trauma)

Treatment Related

Related to separation from family and home (e.g., hospitalization, nursing home)
Related to altered appearance from drugs, radiation, or other treatment

Situational (Personal, Environmental)

Related to poor impulse control and frustration tolerance
Related to disturbed relationship with parent/caregiver
Related to disorganized family system
Related to ineffective problem-solving skills
Related to increased food consumption in response to stressors
Related to the negative impact of (e.g., poverty, inadequate finances, relocation, foreclosure, homelessness, natural disaster)
Related to disruption of emotional bonds secondary to:

Death	Separation or divorce
Institutionalization	Foster care
Relocation	Imprisonment
Desertion	Educational institution

Related to unsatisfactory support system
Related to inadequate psychological resources secondary to:

Poor self-esteem	Lack of motivation to respond
Helplessness	Negative role modeling
Excessive negative beliefs about self	

Maturational

Child/Adolescent

Related to Inconsistent methods of discipline
Related to inadequate psychological resources to adapt to:

Physical and emotional changes	Educational demands
Sexual awareness	Sexual relationships
Independence from family	Career choices

Young Adult

Related to inadequate psychological resources to adapt to:

Career choices	Parenthood
Marriage	Leaving home
Educational demands	

Middle Adult

Related to inadequate psychological resources to adapt to:

Physical signs of aging	Social status needs
Problems with relatives	Child-rearing problems
Career pressures	Aging parents

Older Adult

Related to inadequate psychological resources to adapt to:

Physical changes	Response of others
Retirement	Changes in residence
Changes in financial status	

Carp's Cues

World Health Organization (WHO, 2014) defines mental health "as a state of well-being in which every individual realizes his or her own potential, can cope with the normal stresses of life, can work productively and fruitfully, and is able to make a contribution to her or his community." WHO (2014) reports:

- Mental disorders increase the risk of getting ill from other diseases such as HIV, cardiovascular disease, diabetes, and vice-versa. Human rights violations of people with mental and psychosocial disability are routinely reported in most countries.

Goals

NOC

Coping, Stress Level, Self-Esteem, Social Interaction Skills, Abusive Behavior, Self-Restraint, Social Support, Sleep, Decision-Making, Behavior Modification

The person will make decisions and follow through with appropriate actions to change provocative situations in the personal environment as evidenced by the following indicators:

- Verbalize feelings related to emotional state.
- Focus on the present.
- Identify response patterns and the consequences of resulting behavior.
- Identify personal strengths and accept support through the nursing relationship.

Interventions

NIC

Coping Enhancement, Counseling, Emotional Support, Active Listening, Assertiveness Training, Behavior Modification, Anger Control, Crisis Intervention, Self-responsibility Facilitation, Support System Enhancement

> **CLINICAL ALERT:**
> - Stigma and discrimination against individuals and families prevent people from seeking mental health care. One survey of adults reported that 57% believed that people are caring and sympathetic to persons with mental illness, while only 25% of individuals with mental illnesses reported that people are caring and sympathetic to persons with mental illness (CDC, 2013b).
> - Negative attitudes about mental illness often underlie stigma, which can cause affected persons to deny symptoms; delay treatment; be excluded from employment, housing, or relationships; and interfere with recovery (Procter et al., 2014).

Establish Rapport

- Spend time with the individual. Provide supportive companionship.
- Avoid being overly cheerful and clichés such as, "Things will get better."
- Offer support. Encourage expression of feelings. Let the individual know you understand his or her feelings. Do not argue with expressions of worthlessness by saying things such as, "How can you say that? Look at all you accomplished in life."
- Allow extra time for the person to respond.

  *R: The person with a chronic mental illness "must be helped to give up the role of being sick for that of being different" (*Finkelman, 2000).*

Assess Present Coping Status

- Determine the risk of the individual's inflicting self-harm; intervene appropriately.
- Assess for signs of potential suicide.
  - History of previous attempts or threats (overt and covert)
  - Changes in personality, behavior, sex life, appetite, and sleep habits
  - Preparations for death (putting things in order, making a will, giving away personal possessions, acquiring a weapon)
  - Sudden elevation in mood
- See *Risk for Suicide* for additional information on suicide prevention.

Assess Level of Depression

- Refer depressed people to specialists.

  R: Severely depressed or suicidal people need environmental controls, usually hospitalization.

Assist the Individual in Developing Appropriate Problem-Solving Strategies

- Ask the individual to describe previous encounters with conflict and how he or she resolved them.
- Evaluate whether his or her stress response is "fight or flight" or "tend and befriend."
- Encourage the individual to evaluate his or her behavior. "Did that work for you?" "How did it help?" "What did you learn from that experience?"
- Discuss possible alternatives (i.e., talk over the problem with those involved, try to change the situation, or do nothing and accept the consequences).
- Assist the individual in identifying problems that he or she cannot control directly; help the individual to practice stress-reducing activities for control (e.g., exercise, yoga).

    *R: Cognitive interventions help the person regain control over his or her life. They include identifying automatic thoughts and replacing them with positive thoughts (*Finkelman, 2000).*

Explore Outlets That Foster Feelings of Personal Achievement and Self-Esteem (e.g., Increase Activity)

- Identify activities that were previously gratifying but have been neglected: personal grooming or dress habits, shopping, hobbies, exercise, and arts and crafts.
- Encourage to include these activities in the daily routine for a set time span, for example,
    - I will walk 20 minutes every day.
    - I will plant a small garden.
    - I will walk down steps rather than using an elevator.
    - I will park my car farther from my destination and walk.
    - I will volunteer (e.g., literacy program, reading to children).
    - I will play the piano for 30 minutes every afternoon.

        R: Depression is immobilizing and immobilization increases depression. The person needs to make a conscious effort to fight inactivity to improve.

Facilitate Emotional Support From Others

- Identify persons, who understand your situation.
- Decide who can best act as a support system (do not expect empathy from people who themselves are overwhelmed with their own problems).
- Maintain a sense of humor.

    R: Coping effectively requires successful maintenance of many tasks: self-concept, satisfying relationships with others, emotional balance, and stress.

Address Coping With Caregiving Responsibilities

- Encourage sharing with "This situation must be very difficult, how is this for you?"

    R: Caregivers reiterated their need for someone to confide in, but felt that support was not easily found or was coupled with a fear of occupational repercussions. Ineffective coping often led to the accumulation of stressors, with a considerable impact on the caregiver and their working abilities. This highlighted the importance of coping, and the necessity to support caregivers and to put measures in place to prevent burnout and stress (Uren & Graham, 2013).

Refer to *Risk for Caregiver Role Strain* for Specific Interventions for Accessing Assistance

For Any Aged Individuals, Who Are Isolated, Compromised

Evaluate Coping Resources Available (Miller, 2015)
- Social supports, especially religious support
- Instrumental support (meals, transportation, personal care)
- Emotional support that he or she is valued, loved, and respected

- Information support regarding resources available

  R: Researchers have reported that stressful life events as predisposing factors and social connectedness as a buffer that serves to promote successful coping and reduce suicide risk in older adults (Conwell, Van Orden, & Caine, 2011).

Specifically Address Daily Stressors (Food Preparation, Medication Schedule, Self-Care, and Housekeeping)

Review Possible Options to Reduce Daily Stress (e.g., Weekly Pill Boxes, Frozen Complete Meals)

R: Adults who experience daily stressors more frequently reported their memory to be significantly worse and affects overall psychological functioning (Stawski, Mogle, & Sliwinski, 2013).

Clinical Alert Report
- Advise ancillary staff/student to report any changes in mood, angry outbursts, and/or references to not wanting to live.

Initiate Health Teaching and Referrals as Indicated

- Prepare for problems that may occur after discharge:
  - Medications—schedule, cost, misuse, and side effects
  - Increased anxiety
  - Sleep problems
  - Eating problems—access, decreased appetite
  - Inability to structure time
  - Family/significant other conflicts
  - Follow-up—forgetting, access, difficulty organizing time

    R: For depression-related problems beyond the scope of nurse generalists, therapist, psychologist, and psychiatrist will be needed.

- Instruct the individual in relaxation techniques; emphasize the importance of setting 15 to 20 minutes aside each day to practice relaxation.
  - Refer to Getting Started to Manage Stress on thePoint.

INEFFECTIVE DENIAL

NANDA-I Definition

Conscious or unconscious attempt to disavow the knowledge or meaning of an event to reduce anxiety and/or fear, leading to the detriment of health

Defining Characteristics (*Lynch & Phillips, 1989)

Delays seeking or refuses health care attention
Does not perceive personal relevance of symptoms or danger
Uses home remedies (self-treatment) to relieve symptoms
Does not admit fear of death or invalidism*
Minimizes symptoms*

Displaces the source of symptoms to other areas of the body
Cannot admit the effects of the disease on life pattern
Cannot admit the effects of substance abuse on life pattern
Makes dismissive gestures when speaking of distressing events*
Displaces the fear of effects of the condition
Displays inappropriate affect*

Related Factors

Pathophysiologic

Related to inability to tolerate consciously the consequences of (any chronic or terminal illness) secondary to (e.g., HIV infection, AIDS, cancer, progressive debilitating disorders [e.g., multiple sclerosis, myasthenia gravis])

Treatment Related

Related to preferences to continue treatment with no positive results (e.g., chemotherapy, radiation)

Situational/Psychological

Related to negative consequences of (e.g., financial crisis, inability to maintain employment obesity, domestic abuse, child neglect/abuse)
Related to inability to tolerate consciously physical and/or emotional dependence on (Halter, 2014):

Alcohol	Cannabis
Cocaine, crack	Barbituates/sedatives
Stimulants	Hallucinogens
Opiates	Tobacco use

Related to long-term self-destructive patterns of behavior and lifestyle (Varcarolis, 2011)
Related to genetic origins of alcoholism

Carp's Cues

Denial can be a constructive defense mechanism when reality is too painful as sudden death of loved one or a life-threatening diagnosis. When action is essential to change a threatening or damaging situation, denial is maladaptive; however, when no action is needed or when the outcome cannot be changed, denial can be positive and can help reduce stress (*Lazarus, 1985).

Ineffective Denial is not beneficial or constructive. When the person will not participate in regimens to improve health or the situation (e.g., denies substance abuse), his or her denial is a barrier. The focus for this diagnosis is the help the hospitalized individual acknowledge how his or her alcohol, drug, or tobacco abuse has negatively affected his or her health, relationships, and livelihood (e.g., employment) and to provide him or her resources to use after discharge.

Goals

NOC
Anxiety Self-Control, Coping, Social Support, Substance Addiction Consequences, Knowledge: Substance Use Control, Knowledge: Disease Process

The person will acknowledge an addiction problem and responsibility for own behavior:

* Identify three areas of one's life that drugs have negatively affected
* Acknowledge when using denial rationalization and projection in relation to their addiction
* Identify resources available in the community
* Express a sense of hope

Interventions

Teaching: Disease
Process, Anxiety
Reduction, Counseling,
Active Listening

Initiate a Therapeutic Relationship

- Assess effectiveness of denial.
- Avoid confronting the individual that he or she is using denial.
- Approach the individual directly, matter-of-factly, and nonjudgmentally.

  R: *Denial may be valuable in the early stages of coping, when resources are not sufficient to manage more problem-focused approaches (*Lazarus, 1985).*

Explore With the Individual How His or Her Addiction (Substance Abuse/Dependency, Pathological Gambling, Kleptomania, Pyromania, Compulsive Buying, Compulsive Sexual Behavior) Has Affected His or Her Life and Health (Present, Future)

Work/School Problems

- Absenteeism, frequent unexplained brief absences, loss of job, elaborate excuses, and failed assignments

Social Problems

- Daytime fatigue, mood swings, isolation (avoidance of others), arguments with partner/friends/family

Legal

- Traffic accidents/citations
- Violence while intoxicated
- Crimes (theft, fraud, assaults)

Physical Effects of Alcohol Abuse

- Blackout, liver dysfunction, pancreatitis, gastritis/gastric ulcers, cardiomyopathy, lower extremity paresthesias, brain atrophy, memory impairment, seizures, withdrawal symptoms (e.g., tremors, nausea, vomiting, increased blood pressure and pulse, sleep disturbances, disorientation, hallucinations, agitation, seizures)

Physical Effects of Opioid Abuse

- Blackout, liver dysfunction, pancreatitis, gastritis/gastric ulcers, chronic constipation, malnutrition, respiratory depression, increased risk for HIV, hepatitis C, cellulitis (sharing snorting equipment, needles)

Physical Effects of Amphetamine and Cocaine Abuse

- Hyperactivity, paranoia, decreased appetite/weight loss, cerebrovascular accident, cardiac arrhythmias, left ventricular hypertrophy, hallucinations, seizures, respiratory depression, hepatitis, HIV (sharing snorting equipment, needles)

Physical Effects of Tobacco Use (Smoked, Snuff)

- Cancers: lung, bronchial, laryngeal, oral cavity, pharyngeal, esophageal, stomach, pancreatic, kidney, urinary bladder, uterus, cervical, and acute myelogenous leukemia
- It also causes abdominal aortic aneurysms, peripheral vascular disease, strokes, and chronic obstructive lung disease and contributes to osteoporosis (CDC, 2014b).
- Exposure to secondhand smoke—sometimes called environmental tobacco smoke—causes nearly 50,000 deaths each year among adults in the United States. Secondhand smoke causes 3,400 annual deaths from lung cancer and causes 46,000 annual deaths from heart disease (CDC, 2014b).

Assist the Individual to Understand Addictions

- Be nonjudgmental. Explain addiction is a disorder with choices.
- Explain that addiction "does not cure itself" and that it requires abstinence and treatment of the underlying issues (Halter, 2014; Varcarolis, 2011).
- Have the individual identify triggers for his or her addiction. Discuss how to avoid.

  R: *Historically, individuals with addictions have been viewed as immoral and degenerate. Acknowledgment of their addiction as a disorder can increase the individual's sense of trust (Varcarolis, 2011).*

Openly Discuss the Reality of Relapse; Emphasize That Relapse Does Not Mean Failure

- Emphasize a "one day at a time" philosophy.

  R: Relapse must be addressed to increase motivation and to reduce abandoning all attempts to change behavior.

Initiate Health Teaching and Referrals as Indicated

- Advise the individual to consult with primary care provider regarding pharmaceutical treatment if indicated. For example, opioid antagonists (naltrexone, nalmefene), selective serotonin reuptake inhibitors (SSRIs).

  R: Opioid antagonists, such as naltrexone and nalmefene, which decrease dopamine release in the brain, have been found to reduce reward sensitivity and therefore may be effective in battling the urges that pathologic gamblers experience. Neurotransmitter glutamate has also been effective in reducing gambling behavior in pathologic gamblers. Selective serotonin reuptake inhibitors (SSRIs), most commonly referred to antidepressants, have shown mixed results in impulse control disorders.

- Refer to AA, Alanon, AlaTeen, or Gambling Anonymous.
- Refer for therapy and/or treatment facility.

  R: In controlled studies, several therapist-driven techniques, such as cognitive-behavioral therapy, motivational interviewing and relapse prevention have demonstrated efficacy with substance and behavioral addictions (Grant, 2011).

COMPROMISED FAMILY COPING

NANDA-I Definition

A usually supportive primary person (family member, significant other, or close friend) provides insufficient, ineffective, or compromised support, comfort, assistance, or encouragement that may be needed by the client to manage or master adaptive tasks related to his or her health challenge

Defining Characteristics*

Subjective

Individual reports a concern about significant person's response to health problem.

Significant person reports preoccupation with personal reaction (e.g., fear, anticipatory grief, guilt, anxiety) to individual's need.

Significant person reports inadequate understanding, which interferes with effective supportive behaviors.

Objective

Significant person attempts assistive or supportive behaviors with unsatisfactory results.

Significant person enters into limited personal communication with the individual.

Significant person displays protective behavior disproportionate to individual's need for autonomy.

Related Factors

Refer to *Interrupted Family Processes*.

Author's Note

Compromised Family Coping describes a family that reports usual constructive function but is experiencing an alteration from a current stress-related challenge. The family is viewed as a system, with interdependence among members. Thus, life challenges for individual members also challenge the family system. Certain situations may negatively influence family functioning; examples include illness, an older relative moving in, relocation, separation, and divorce. *Risk for Interrupted Family Processes* can represent such a situation.

Goals

NOC
Family Coping, Family
Environment: Internal,
Family Normalization,
Parenting

The family will maintain functional system of mutual support for one another, as evidenced by the following indicators:

- Frequently verbalize feelings to professional nurse and one another.
- Identify appropriate external resources available.

Interventions

NIC
Family Involvement
Promotion, Coping
Enhancement, Family
Integrity Promotion,
Family Therapy,
Counseling, Referral

Assess Causative and Contributing Factors

Illness-Related Factors
- Sudden, unexpected nature of illness
- Burdensome, chronic problems
- Potentially disabling nature of illness
- Symptoms creating disfiguring change in physical appearance
- Social stigma associated with illness
- Financial burden

Factors Related to Behavior of Ill Family Member
- Refuses to cooperate with necessary interventions
- Engages in socially deviant behavior associated with illness (e.g., suicide attempts, violence, substance abuse)
- Isolates self from family
- Acts out or is verbally abusive to health professionals and family members

Factors Related to Overall Family Functioning
- Unresolved guilt, blame, hostility, jealousy
- Inability to solve problems
- Ineffective communication patterns among members
- Changes in role expectations and resulting tension
- Unclear role boundaries

Factors Related to Illness in Family (See Also *Caregiver Role Strain*)
Factors Related to the Community
- Lack of support from spiritual resources (philosophical, religious, or both)
- Lack of relevant health education resources
- Lack of supportive friends
- Lack of adequate community health care resources (e.g., long-term follow-up, hospice, respite)

   R: Common sources of family stress are as follows (*Carson & Smith-DiJulio, 2006; Halter, 2014):

- External sources of stress (e.g., job or school related) one member is experiencing
- External sources of stress (e.g., finances, relocation) influencing the family unit
- Developmental stressors (e.g., childbearing, new baby, childrearing, adolescence, arrival of older grandparent, marriage of single parents, loss of spouse)
- Situational stressors (e.g., illness, hospitalization, separation, caregiving responsibilities)

Promote Cohesiveness
- Approach the family with warmth, respect, and support.
- Keep family members abreast of changes in ill family member's condition when appropriate.
- Avoid discussing what caused the problem or blaming.
- Encourage verbalization of guilt, anger, blame, and hostility and subsequent recognition of own feelings in family members.

   R: No family is 100% functional; however, healthy families are concerned with each other's needs and encourage expression of feelings (Halter 2014; *Varcarolis, Carson, & Shoemaker, 2006).

- Explain the importance of functional communications, which uses verbal and nonverbal communication to teach behavior, share feelings and values, and evolve decisions about family health practices (Kaakinen, Coelho, Steele, Tabacco, & Hanson, 2015).

   R: Effective communication is necessary in families to adapt to stressors and develop cohesiveness (Kaakinen et al., 2015).

Assist Family to Appraise the Situation

* What is at stake? Encourage family to have a realistic perspective by providing accurate information and answers to questions. Ensure all family members have input.
* What are the choices? Assist family to reorganize roles at home and set priorities to maintain family integrity and reduce stress.
* Initiate discussions regarding stressors of home care (physical, emotional, environmental, and financial).
* "Family-oriented approaches that include helping a family gain insight and make behavioral changes are most successful" (*Varcarolis et al., 2006).

Promote Clear Boundaries Between Individuals in Family

* Ensure that all family members share their concerns.
* Elicit the responsibilities of each member.
* Acknowledge the differences.

  R: An individual's emotional, social, and physical functioning is directly related to how clear his or her role is differentiated in the family (Halter, 2014).

Initiate Health Teaching and Referrals, as Necessary

* Assist family members to identify reliable friends (e.g., clergy, significant others); encourage seeking help (emotional, technical) when appropriate.
* Enlist help of other professionals (social work, therapist, psychiatrist, school nurse).

  R: Families in stress will need extra encouragement to participate in self-help or other community agencies (Hockenberry & Wilson, 2015).

RISK FOR SUICIDE

NANDA-I Definition

At risk for self-inflicted, life-threatening injury

Risk Factors

Suicidal behavior (ideation, talk, plan, available means) (Varcarolis, 2011)
Persons high risk for suicide
Poor support system*
Family history of suicide*
Hopelessness/helplessness*
History of prior suicidal attempts*
Alcohol and substance abuse*
Legal or disciplinary problems*
Grief/bereavement (loss of person, job, home)
Suicidal cues (Varcarolis, 2011)
Overt ("No one will miss me," "I am better off dead," "I have nothing to live for.")
Covert (making out a will, giving valuables away, writing forlorn love notes, acquiring life insurance)

Carp's Cues

This diagnosis focuses on the individual, who is at *Risk for Suicide* while hospitalized for a medical or surgical condition.

Goals

NOC
Impulse-Self Control,
Suicide Self-Restraint

The individual will identify suicidal thoughts if they occur as evidenced by the following indicators:

Short term (Varcarolis, 2011)

* Remain safe while in the hospital.
* Stay with a friend or family if person has a potential for suicide if discharged home.
* Report an intent to participate with family in family counseling.

Interventions

NIC

Active Listening, Coping Enhancement, Suicide Prevention, Impulse Control Training, Behavior Management: Self-Harm, Hope Instillation, Contracting, Surveillance: Safety

> **CLINICAL ALERT:**
> • In 2013, the highest suicide rate (19.1) was among people 45 to 64 years old. The second highest rate (18.6) occurred in those 85 years and older. The third highest rate (15%) is among persons 65 to 83 years old .Younger groups have had consistently lower suicide rates than middle-aged and older adults. In 2013, adolescents and young adults aged 15 to 24 had a suicide rate of 10.9. Of those who died by suicide in 2013, 77.9% were male and 22.1% were female. In 2013, firearms were the most common method of death by suicide, accounting for a little more than half (51.4%) of all suicide deaths (American Foundation for Suicide Prevention, 2015).

Access a Psychiatric Evaluation to Determine the Level of Risk for Suicide: High, Moderate, Low

Provide a Safe Environment Based on Level of Risk; Notify All Staff That the Individual Is at Risk for Self-Harm and the Level of Risk; Use Both Written and Oral Communication (Varcarolis, 2011)

- Initiate suicide precaution per institution's protocol for immediate management for the high-risk individual.
  - When the individual is being constantly observed, he or she is not to be allowed out of sight, even though privacy is lost. Arm's length is the most appropriate space for a high-risk individual.
- Initiate suicide observation for risk persons with visual check of mood, behaviors, and verbatim statements per protocol.

  R: The level of protection of the individual will be determined by his or her risk for suicide. Caregivers can become immobilized or drained by the acutely suicidal individual. Feelings of hopelessness are often communicated to the caregiver.

Ensure the Following

- Restrict glass, nail files, scissors, nail polish remover, mirrors, needles, razors, soda cans, plastic bags, lighters, electric equipment, belts, hangers, knives, tweezers, alcohol, and guns.
- Provide meals in a closely supervised area, usually on the unit or in individual's room.
  - Ensure adequate food and fluid intake.
  - Use paper/plastic plates and utensils.
  - Check to be sure all items are returned on the tray.
- When administering oral medications, check to ensure that all medications are swallowed.
- Designate a staff member to provide checks on the individual as designated by the institution's policy. Provide relief for the staff member.
- Restrict the individual to the unit unless specifically ordered by physician. When the individual is off unit, provide a staff member to accompany him or her.
- Instruct visitors on restricted items (e.g., ensure they do not give the individual food in a plastic bag).
- The individual may use restricted items in the presence of staff, depending on level of risk. For acutely suicidal persons, provide a hospital gown to deter the individual from leaving the facility.
- Conduct room searches periodically according to institution policy.
- Use seclusion and restraint if necessary (refer to *Risk for Violence* for discussion).
- Notify the police if the individual leaves the facility and is at risk for suicide.
- Keep accurate and thorough records of the individual's behaviors and all nursing assessments and interventions.

  R: High-risk suicidal persons should be admitted to a closely supervised environment and should not be allowed access to certain items. Although it is impossible to create a completely safe environment, removal of dangerous objects and close observation convey a nonverbal message of concern.

Emphasize the Following (Varcarolis, 2011)

- The crisis is temporary.
- Unbearable pain can be survived.

- Help is available.
- You are not alone.

  R: "These statements give perspective to the person and may help to offer hope for the future" (Varcarolis, 2011).

- Observe for a sudden change in emotions from sad and depressed to elated, happy, or peaceful.

  R: A sudden change in emotions can indicate the risk of suicide is very high as the individual seeks a way to lose the emotional pain.

Consider the Risks for Suicide for Older Adults, Particularly Men (Miller, 2015)

R: White men older than 65 years have twice the rate of suicide of all other age groups. They constitute 18.5% of the population but commit 23% of all suicides (Miller, 2015).

- Retirement
- Loss of vigor
- Loss of a meaningful role

  R: Older adults tend to complete suicide when they attempt it. The ratio of attempts to completion is 4:1, whereas for younger people it is approximately 25:1 (Miller, 2015).

Pediatric Interventions

> **CLINICAL ALERT:**
> - Suicide in children (5 to 14 years of age) tends to be more impulsive than in other age groups. Hyperactivity also seems to contribute to the impulsive nature. Suicide is the third leading cause of death among adolescents. A frequent factor is lack of or loss of a meaningful relationship (Hockenberry & Wilson, 2015).

With Older Children/Adolescents, Explore the Following (Hockenberry & Wilson, 2015):

- Chronic mental disorders (e.g., conduct disorders, autistic spectrum disorders, depression)
- Physical, emotional, and/or sexual abuse
- Family problems
- Strength of support systems
- Disruption of friendship or romantic relationship
- Presence of performance failure (e.g., examination, course)
- Recent or upcoming change (change of school, relocation)
- Sexual orientation (LGBT)

Convey Empathy Regarding Problems and/or Losses

- Do not minimize the loss; instead focus on their disappointment.

  R: Certain stressors are especially significant for adolescents, who are developmentally preoccupied with status, peers, and appearances (Varcarolis, 2011).

Monitor for Depression (Saewyc et al., 2007)

R: Recognition of depression in adolescents is often difficult because they mask their feelings with bored and angry behavior. Some symptoms include being sad or blue, withdrawal from social activities, trouble concentrating, somatic complaints, changes in sleep or eating patterns, and feelings of guilt or inadequacy.

Explore the Difficulties Encountered by Gay, Lesbian/Bisexual, Transgender Youth

R: Suicide is the leading cause of death among gay, lesbian/bisexual, transgender youth nationally. Thirty (30%) of gay youth attempt suicide near the age of 15 (CDC, 2011). Supportive friends, family, and relatives can be protective factors to prevent suicide (Saewyc et al., 2007).

Take All Suicide Threats Seriously. Listen Carefully

R: All threats or gestures to hurt oneself must be taken seriously regardless of the child's developmental age. Suicide attempts or threats may not represent a true desire to die, but they definitely represent a cry for help.

Determine Whether the Child Understands the Finality of Death (e.g., "What Does It Mean to Die?")

- "Have you ever seen a dead animal on the road? Can it get up and run?"
- Explore feelings and reason for suicidal feelings.

    R: Suicidal threats and ideation signal a crisis that requires specific care.

Consult With a Psychiatric Expert Regarding the Most Appropriate Environment for Treatment

R: Treatment strategies depend on the child's living situation, psychiatric history, and support system available.

Participate in Programs in School to Teach About the Symptoms of Depression and Signs of Suicidal Behavior

R: The preteen and early adolescent years are often when self-harm begins to manifest itself. Adults must be in tune with changes in behavior and changes in apparel and be highly suspicious of multiple "accidents" (Saewyc et al., 2007).

Initiate Health Teaching and Referrals as Indicated

- Refer for peer or group therapy.
- Refer for family therapy, especially when a child or adolescent is involved.
- Instruct significant others in how to recognize an increase in risk: change in behavior, verbal or nonverbal communication, withdrawal, or signs of depression.
- Supply the phone number of 24-hour emergency hotline.

    R: Interventions are based on the type of risk the individual presents. Long-term treatment is often more difficult to institute than emergency care in some communities.

> ### Clinical Alert Report
>
> Advise ancillary staff/student to report any changes in mood, angry outbursts, and/or references to not wanting to live. Remind staff/student to be diligent regarding activities and certain articles that can inflict self-injury with individual and visitors.

RISK FOR OTHER-DIRECTED VIOLENCE

Definition

Vulnerable for behaviors in which an individual demonstrates that he or she can be physically, emotionally, and/or sexually harmful to others (NANDA-I)

State in which an individual has been, or is at risk to be, assaultive toward others or the environment[12]

Risk Factors

Presence of risk factors (see Related Factors).

Related Factors

Pathophysiologic

Related to history of aggressive acts (e.g., kicking, hitting, spitting, throwing objects, breaking objects, inappropriate urinating/defecating (on floor, on others) and perception of environment) as threatening secondary to:
or
Related to history of aggressive acts and delusional thinking secondary to:

---

[12]This additional diagnosis has been included for clarity and usefulness.

or

Related to history of aggressive acts and manic excitement secondary to:

or

Related to history of aggressive acts and inability to verbalize feelings secondary to:

or

Related to history of aggressive acts and psychic overload secondary to:

Temporal lobe epilepsy

Head injury

Progressive CNS deterioration (brain tumor)

Hormonal imbalance

Viral encephalopathy

Mental retardation

Minimal brain dysfunction

Related to toxic response to alcohol or drugs

Related to organic brain syndrome

Treatment Related

Related to toxic reaction to medication

Situational (Personal, Environmental)

Related to history of overt aggressive acts

Related to increase in stressors within a short period

Related to acute agitation

Related to suspiciousness

Related to persecutory delusions

Related to verbal threats of physical assault

Related to low frustration tolerance

Related to poor impulse control

Related to fear of the unknown

Related to response to catastrophic event

Related to response to dysfunctional family throughout developmental stages

Related to dysfunctional communication patterns

Related to drug or alcohol abuse

Carp's Cues

"Health-care workers are hit, kicked, scratched, bitten, spat on, threatened and harassed by patients with surprising regularity. In a 2014 survey, almost 80 percent of nurses reported being attacked on the job within the past year" (Jacobson, 2014).

The diagnosis *Risk for Other-Directed Violence* describes an individual who has been assaultive or, because of certain factors (e.g., toxic response to alcohol or drugs, hallucinations or delusions, brain dysfunction), is at high risk for assaulting others. In such a situation, the nursing focus is on decreasing violent episodes and protecting the individual and others.

Goals

NOC

Abuse Cessation, Abusive Behavior Self-Restraint, Aggression Self-Control, Impulse Self-Control

The individual will have no or minimal aggressive responses as evidenced by the following indicators (Varcarolis, 2011):

- Refrains from threatening, loud language toward others
- Responds to external controls when at high risk for loss of control
- Explain rationales for interventions.

Interventions

> **CLINICAL ALERT:**
> - In 2011, 467,321 persons were injured or killed by firearm violence. Bats, hammers, and knives injure and kill more people than guns (National Institute of Justice, 2014).
> - Homicide is the 15th cause of death in the United States Homicide is the 4th cause of death in children ages 5 to 9 years; ages 10 to 14 3rd cause; 15 to 24 years 2nd cause (CDC, 2016K)

NIC

Anger Control
Assistance,
Environmental
Management: Violence
Prevention, Impulse
Control Training, Crisis
Intervention, Seclusion,
Physical Restraint

The nursing interventions for *Risk for Other-Directed Violence* apply to any individual who is potentially violent, regardless of related factors.

Establish an Environment That Reduces Agitation (Halter, 2014)

- Offer food, drink and a place to sit
- Decrease noise level.
- Give short, concise explanations.
- Control the number of persons present at one time.
- Provide a single or semiprivate room.
- Allow the individual to arrange personal possessions.
- Be aware that darkness can increase disorientation and enhance suspiciousness.
- Decrease situations in which the individual is frustrated.
- Provide music if the individual is receptive.

> *R: The individual is in an agitated/mentally compromised state. Environmental stimuli unnecessarily increase this state and can increase aggression.*

Use Verbal De-Escalation as a First-Line Intervention When Exposed to Violent and Aggressive Behaviour to (*National Institute of Clinical Excellence [NICE], 2005; *Royal College of Psychiatrists, 1998)

*R: De-escalation is defined as a "gradual resolution of a potentially violent and/or aggressive situation through the use of verbal and physical expressions of empathy, alliance and non-confrontational limit setting that is based on respect" (*Cowin et al., 2003, p. 65)*

Promote Interactions That Increase the Individual's Sense of Trust and to Ensure Safety of all (Kynoch & Wu, Chang, 2011; Stubb & Dickens, 2008)

*R: De-escalation enables the health care professional to develop rapport with the individual (*Cowin et al., 2003). This can promote trust.*

- Be genuine, calm, and empathetic.
- Acknowledge the individual's feelings (e.g., "You are having a rough time").
- Tell the individual that you will help him or her to control behavior and not do anything destructive.
- Be direct and frank ("I can see you are angry").
- Approach slowly with caution.
- Use open-ended questions.
- Use clear, simple language.
- Do not turn your back to the individual.
- Avoid challenges or promises.
- Do not threaten.
- Set limits when the individual poses a risk to others.

> *R: Setting limits clarifies rules, guidelines, and standards of acceptable behavior and establishes the consequences of violating the rules (Halter, 2014; Kynoch et al., 2011).*

Attend a Yearly Class on Protecting Yourself From a Physical Attack. Request These Sessions if They Are Presently Not Available

R: All staff must have training on techniques to de-escalate with role-playing, how to ward off a physical assault, and/or break away techniques if grab (Kynoch et al., 2011; Stubb & Dickens, 2008).

Be Aware of Your Own Feelings and Reactions

- Do not take verbal abuse personally.
- Remain calm if you are becoming upset; leave the situation to others, if possible.

- After a threatening situation, discuss your feelings with other staff.

  R: Staff activities may be counterproductive to managing aggressive behavior. Recognition and replacement of attitudes such as "I must be calm and relaxed at all times" with "No matter how anxious I feel, I will keep thinking and decide on the best approach" often prevent escalation of aggression.

Initiate Immediate Management of the High-Risk Behavior

Follow Protocol and Activate a Psychiatric Code Early in Order to Diffuse the Crisis in Its Early Stages (Halter, 2014)

- Always place staff safety first. The presence of three or four staff members reassures the individual that you will not let him or her lose control. The focus is respect, concern, and safety.
- Allow the individual with acute agitation space that is five times greater than that for an individual who is in control. Do not touch the individual.
- Avoid physical entrapment of individual or staff.
- Do not approach a violent individual alone. Often, the presence of three or four staff members is enough to reassure the individual that you will not let him or her lose control. Use a positive tone; do not demand or cajole.
- Maintain the same physical level (e.g., both people either sitting or standing prevents feelings of intimidation). The least aggressive stance is at a 45 degrees angle to the person, rather than face to face.
- Call the individual by name in a calm, quiet, and respectful manner.
- Avoid threats; refer to yourself, not policies, rules, or supervisors.
- Allow appropriate verbal expressions of anger. Give positive feedback.

  *R: Assaultive behavior tends to occur when conditions are crowded, are without structure, and involve activity "demanded" by staff (*Farrell et al., 1998).*

Assist the Individual to Maintain Control Over His or Her Behavior

- Establish the expectation that he or she can control behavior, and continue to reinforce the expectation. Explain exactly which behavior is inappropriate and why.
- Reassure the individual that you will provide control if he or she cannot ("I am concerned about you. I will get [more staff, medications] to keep you from doing anything impulsive").
- Set firm, clear limits when an individual presents a danger to self or others ("Put the chair down").
- Set limits on verbal abuse. Do not take insults personally. Support others (individuals, staff) who may be targets of abuse.
- Do not give attention to the individual who is being verbally abusive. Tell the individual what you are doing and why.

  R: Crisis management techniques can help prevent escalation of aggression and help the individual achieve self-control. The least restrictive safe and effective measure should be used (Halter, 2014).

Follow Protocol for Use of Seclusion and/or Restraint, if Indicated

- Remove individual from situation if environment is contributing to aggressive behavior, using the least amount of control needed (e.g., ask others to leave and take individual to quiet room).
- Reinforce that you are going to help the individual control himself or herself.
- When interpersonal and pharmacologic interventions fail to control the angry, aggressive individual, always follow hospital protocols or physical and chemical restraints (Halter, 2014).

  R: Hospital protocols should be clear regarding how, when, and for what time period an individual can be restrained or secluded and the associated nursing care needed (Halter, 2014).

  *R: Seclusion and restraint are options for an individual exhibiting serious, persistent aggression. The nurse must protect the individual's safety at all times. Use of the least restrictive measures allows the individual the most opportunity to regain self-control (*Farrell et al., 1998; Halter, 2014).*

Convene a Postcrisis Discussion After a Violent Episode With Involved Personnel

R: After a violent act, leading a postcrisis discussion of the event, outcome, and feelings can decrease anxiety, increase understanding of violence, and address preventable problems that occurred.

R: Postcrisis discussions can help to foster new and more effective approaches to management of aggressive persons (Halter, 2014).

> ### *Clinical Alert Report*
> • Advise ancillary staff/student to report an increase in anxiety, anger, or any displays of aggression.

Initiate Health Teaching and Referrals as Indicated

• Refer to appropriate program (e.g., counseling, family therapy).

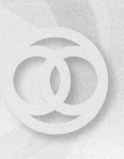

Section 2
Individual Collaborative Problems

RISK FOR COMPLICATIONS OF CARDIAC/VASCULAR DYSFUNCTION

Risk for Complications of Arrhythmias
Risk for Complications of Bleeding
Risk for Complications of Compartment Syndrome
Risk for Complications of Decreased Cardiac Output
Risk for Complications of Deep Vein Thrombosis/Pulmonary Embolism
Risk for Complications of Hypovolemia
Risk for Complications of Intra-Abdominal Hypertension/Abdominal Compartmental Pressure
Risk for Complications of Pulmonary Edema

Definition

Describes a person experiencing or at high risk to experience various cardiac and/or vascular dysfunctions

Carp's Cues

The nurse can use this generic collaborative problem to describe a person at risk for several types of cardiovascular problems. For example, for an individual in a critical care unit vulnerable to cardiovascular dysfunction, using *Risk for Complications of Cardiac/Vascular Dysfunction* would direct nurses to monitor cardiovascular status for various problems on the basis of focus assessment findings. Nursing interventions for this individual would focus on detecting and diagnosing abnormal functioning.

For an individual with a specific cardiovascular complication, the nurse would add the applicable collaborative problem to the individual's problem list, along with specific nursing interventions for that problem. For example, a standard of care for an individual after myocardial infarction could contain the collaborative problem *Risk for Complications of Cardiac/Vascular Dysfunction*, directing nurses to monitor cardiovascular status. If this individual later experienced an arrhythmia, the nurse would add *Risk for Complications of Arrhythmia* to the problem list, along with specific nursing management information (e.g., *Risk for Complications of Arrhythmia related to myocardial infarction*). When the risk factors or etiology is not directly related to the primary medical diagnosis, the nurse still should add them, if known (e.g., *Risk for Complications of Hypo/Hyperglycemia related to diabetes mellitus* in an individual who has sustained myocardial infarction).

For information on Focus Assessment Criteria, visit thePoint.

Significant Laboratory/Diagnostic Assessment Criteria

* Cardiac enzymes and proteins (Currently, the gross total values of CK, LDH, SGOT, and/or SGPT in the evaluation of cardiac injury are relatively low. Isoenzymes or bands as well as troponins are the only ones usually used. Elevated with cardiac tissue damage [e.g., in myocardial infarction].)
* Creatinine kinase (CK)
* Creatinine phosphokinase, isoenzymes (e.g., CK-MB, CK-BB, CK-MM)
* Creatinine kinase isoforms (CK-MB, CK-MM subforms)
* Lactic dehydrogenase (LDH), isoenzymes
* Myoglobin (troponin)

- Brain-type natriuretic peptide (BNP) (hormones released as a peripheral response to cardiac impairment) (e.g., heart failure)
- C-reactive protein, P-selectin (markers of inflammation and necrosis)
- Serum potassium (fluctuates with diuretic therapy, parenteral fluid replacement)
- Serum calcium, magnesium, phosphate
- White blood cell count (elevated with inflammation)
- Erythrocyte sedimentation rate (elevated with inflammation, tissue injury)
- Arterial blood gas (ABG) values (lowered Sao_2 indicates hypoxemia; elevated pH, alkalosis; lowered pH, acidosis)
- Coagulation studies (elevated with anticoagulant and/or thrombolytic therapy or coagulopathies)
- Hemoglobin and hematocrit (elevated with polycythemia, lowered with anemia)
- Invasive/noninvasive diagnostic tests (e.g., electrocardiograph [ECG] with or without stress test, Doppler ultrasonic flow meter, cardiac catheterization, echocardiography with or without stress test)

Clinical Alert Report

Advise ancillary staff/student to report:
- Signs and symptoms of arrhythmia/EKG changes
- Signs and symptoms of chest pain or abdominal discomfort
- Signs and symptoms of the individual being diaphoretic
- Signs and symptoms of acute pulmonary edema
- Signs of increased fluid retention
- Signs and symptoms of anxiety
- Any new change or deterioration in behavior (e.g., agitation, cognition)
- Change in systolic blood pressure >210 mm Hg or <90 mm Hg and/or diastolic >90 mm Hg
- Resting pulse >120 or <55 beats/min
- Change in rate of respirations >28 or <10/min
- Changes or new onset of dyspnea/palpitations
- Changes in EKG rhythms

RISK FOR COMPLICATIONS OF ARRHYTHMIAS

Definition

Describes a person experiencing or at high risk to experience a disorder of the heart's conduction system that results in an abnormal heart rate, abnormal rhythm, or a combination of both.

High-Risk Populations

A-type coronary artery disease (CAD):

- Angina
- Myocardial infarction (acute coronary syndrome [ACS])
- Congestive heart failure
- Significant hypoglycemia (Chou, 2016)
- Accidental hypothermia
    - Mild hypothermia > tachycardia
    - Moderate hypothermia > atrial fibrillation, junctional bradycardia
    - Severe hypothermia > bradycardia, ventricular arrhythmias (including ventricular fibrillation), and asystole (Mechem & Zafren, 2014)
- Sepsis
- Increased intracranial pressure
- Electrolyte imbalance (calcium, potassium, magnesium, phosphorus)
- Atherosclerotic heart disease

- COPD
- Cardiomyopathy, valvular heart disease
- Anemia
- Postoperative cardiac surgery
- Postoperative, after any major anesthesia
- Trauma
- Sleep apnea
- Hypoxia
  - Medication side effects (e.g., aminophylline; dopamine; stimulants; digoxin; beta blockers; calcium-channel blockers; dobutamine; lidocaine; procainamide; quinidine; diuretics; class 1C antiarrhythmic drugs; anticonvulsants such as phenytoin, tricyclic antidepressants, and some agents used to treat neuropathic pain; immunomodulators) (Heist & Ruskin, 2010)

Collaborative Outcomes

The individual will be monitored for early signs and symptoms of *Decreased Cardiac Output* and will receive collaborative interventions if indicated to restore physiologic stability.

Indicators of Physiologic Stability

Refer to *Decreased Cardiac Output* indicators.

Interventions and Rationales

Monitor for Signs and Symptoms of Arrhythmias

- Abnormal rate, rhythm
- Palpitations, chest pain, syncope, fatigue
- Decreased Sao_2
- ECG changes
- Hypotension
- Change in level of consciousness

  R: Ischemic tissue is electrically unstable, causing arrhythmias. Certain congenital cardiac conditions, electrolyte imbalances, and medications also can cause disturbances in cardiac conduction.

Monitor ECG Patterns and Changes as

- Acute coronary syndrome (ST-elevation, prolongation of Q wave, inversion of T wave)

  R: This is termed ST-elevation ACS (STE-ACS) and generally reflects an acute total coronary occlusion. Most of these individuals will ultimately develop an ST-elevation MI (STEMI). The therapeutic objective is to achieve rapid, complete, and sustained reperfusion by primary angioplasty or fibrinolytic therapy (Chou, 2016).

  R: ECG changes of infarction include ST elevation (indicating injury), Q waves (indicating necrosis), and T-wave inversion (indicating ischemia and evolution of the infarction). These signs of ischemia can be isolated to ECG leads overlying the involved myocardium and indicating localized ischemia. If they are present in many ECG leads, more widespread ischemia is suspected (Chou, 2016; Grossman & Porth, 2014).

> **CLINICAL ALERT:**
> - If the initial ECG is normal or inconclusive, additional recordings should be obtained if the individual develops symptoms. These should be compared with recordings obtained in an asymptomatic state (Chou, 2016).

Notify Physician, Physician Assistant, or Nurse Practitioner of ST Elevation and of Other Serious EKG Changes

Initiate Appropriate Protocols Depending on the Type of Arrhythmia

- Administer supplemental oxygen.

    R: It increases circulating oxygen levels and decreases cardiac workload.

- Monitor oxygen saturation (Sao₂) with pulse oximetry and ABGs as necessary.
- Monitor serum electrolyte levels (e.g., sodium, potassium, calcium, magnesium).

    R: High or low electrolyte levels may exacerbate an arrhythmia.

> ### Clinical Alert Report
>
> Advise ancillary staff/student to report:
> - Changes or new onset of dyspnea, palpitations, chest pain, syncope, fatigue
> - Signs of increased fluid retention
> - Decrease in urine output less than 0.5 mL/kg/hr

RISK FOR COMPLICATIONS OF BLEEDING

Definition

Describes a person experiencing or at high risk to experience a decrease in blood volume

High-Risk Populations

- Intraoperative status
- Postoperative status
- Postprocedural cannulation of any arterial vessel but particularly those at risk for retro-peritoneal bleed due to cannulation of femoral vessel.
- Anaphylactic shock
- Trauma
- A history of bleeding disease or dysfunction
- Anticoagulant use, including over-the-counter use of aspirin or nonsteroidal anti-inflammatory drugs (NSAIDs)
- Chronic steroid use
- Acetaminophen use with associated liver dysfunction
- Anemia
- Liver disease
- Disseminated intravascular coagulation (DIC)
- Rupture of esophageal varices
- Cirrhosis
- Dissecting aneurysms
- Trauma in pregnancy
- Pregnancy-related complications (placenta previa, molar pregnancy, abruption placenta)

Collaborative Outcomes

The individual will be monitored for early signs and symptoms of bleeding and will receive collaborative interventions, if indicated, to restore physiologic stability.

Indicators of Physiologic Stability

- Alert, oriented, calm
- Urine output >0.5 mL/kg/hr
- Neutrophils 60% to 70%
- Red blood cells
    - Male: 4.6 to 5.9 million/mm³
    - Female: 4.2 to 5.4 million/mm³

- Platelets 150,000 to 400,000/mm^3
- No petechiae or purpura
- No gum or nasal bleeding
- Regular menses
- No headache
- Clear vision
- Intact coordination, facial symmetry, and muscle strength
- No splenomegaly
- Identify risk factors that can be reduced
- Relate early signs and symptoms of infection
  - Oxygen saturation >95%
  - Normal sinus rhythm
  - No chest pain
  - No life-threatening arrhythmias
  - Skin warm and dry, usual skin color (appropriate for race)
  - Pulse: regular rhythm, rate 60 to 100 beats/min
  - Respirations 16 to 20 breaths/min
  - Blood pressure >90/60, <140/90 mm Hg, MAP >70, or CVP >11
  - Urine output >0.5 mL/kg/hr
  - Serum pH.7.35 to 7.45
  - Serum RCO$_2$ 35 to 45 mm Hg
  - Spo$_2$ goals >95% for those without history of lung disease
  - Breath sounds without evidence of new, abnormal sounds (rales)
  - No presence of distended neck veins (jugular vein distention [JVD])

Interventions and Rationales

Increase Monitoring of Urine Output to Hourly

R: Decreased blood volume reduces blood to kidneys, which decreases the glomerular filtration rate (GFR) causing a decrease urine output. When blood flow to the kidneys is less than 20% to 25% of normal, ischemic damage occurs (Grossman & Porth, 2014). Decreased urine output is an early sign of bleeding/hypovolemia.

Monitor the Surgical Site for Bleeding, Dehiscence, and Evisceration

R: Careful monitoring allows early detection of complications.

Teach Individual to Splint the Surgical Wound With a Pillow When Coughing, Sneezing, or Vomiting

R: Splinting reduces stress on suture line by equalizing pressure across the wound.

Monitor for Bleeding From Esophageal Varices

R: Varices are deflated tortuous veins in the lower esophagus. Portal hypertension caused by obstruction of the portal venous system from cirrhosis results in increased pressure on the vessels in the esophagus, making them fragile and at risk to bleed (Grossman & Porth, 2014).

- Hematemesis (vomiting blood)
- Melena (black, sticky stools)
- Dark or black streaks in stool

  R: If there is only a small amount of bleeding, this may be the only symptom (Garcia-Tsao, 2011).

- Black, tarry stools
- Bloody stools
- Light-headedness
- Paleness
- Symptoms of chronic liver disease
- Vomiting
- Vomiting blood

  R: If larger amounts of bleeding occur, the above signs/symptoms may be present (Garcia-Tsao, 2011).

> **CLINICAL ALERT:**
> • Contact physician/advanced practice nurse/physician assistant with a new onset of any of the above signs/symptoms assessment data that may indicate bleeding.
>   *R: An immediate endoscopic evaluation is indicated (Garcia-Tsao, 2011).*

If using the toilet, ask individual not to flush. Observe for streaks and darkening of color. Test stools daily for occult blood

R: Signs of gastrointestinal bleeding may be detected early (Garcia-Tsao, 2011).

R: The compensatory response to decreased circulatory volume aims to increase oxygen delivery through increased heart and respiratory rates and decreased peripheral circulation (manifested by diminished peripheral pulses and cool skin). Decreased oxygen to the brain alters mentation. Decreased circulation to the kidneys leads to decreased urine output. Hemoglobin and hematocrit values decline if bleeding is significant (Grossman & Porth, 2014).

Contact physician, advanced practice nurse, or physician assistant with assessment data that may indicate bleeding and to replace fluid losses at a rate sufficient to maintain urine output >0.5 mL/kg/hr. Follow protocols

If shock occurs, place individual in the supine position unless contraindicated (e.g., head injury)

R: This position increases blood return (preload) to the heart.

Insert an IV line; use a large-bore catheter if blood replacement is anticipated. Initiate appropriate protocols for shock (e.g., vasopressor therapy). Refer also to *Risk for Complications of Acidosis* or *Risk for Complications of Alkalosis*, if indicated, for more information

R: Protocols aim to increase peripheral resistance and elevate blood pressure.

Administer oxygen as ordered

R: Diminished blood volume causes decreased circulating oxygen levels.

Clinical Alert Report

Advise ancillary staff/student to report:
- Output hourly for individuals at high risk.
- Any sudden onset of a change in usual condition as:
  - Urine output <0.5 mL/kg/hr
  - Restlessness, agitation, decreased mentation
  - B/P >200 mm Hg (systolic), >115 mm Hg (diastolic), <90 mm Hg systolic
  - Respirations >10/min over baseline, <10/min under baseline, labored
  - Pulse >100 resting
  - Temperature (oral) over 100.5° F
  - Pulse oximetry <90%
  - Diminished peripheral pulses
  - Cool, pale, moist, or cyanotic skin
- Signs and symptoms of acute renal failure
- Signs and symptoms of anxiety
- Increased pulse rate with normal or slightly decreased blood pressure, narrowing pulse pressure, decrease in mean or mean arterial pressure (MAP)
- Increased respiratory rate, thirst
- Decreased oxygenation saturation (Sao_2, Svo_2), pulmonary artery pressures
- Decreased hemoglobin/hematocrit, cardiac output/index

RISK FOR COMPLICATIONS OF COMPARTMENT SYNDROME

Definition

Describes a person experiencing increased pressure in a limited space, such as a fascial envelope, which compromises circulation and function, usually in the forearm or leg. Compartment syndrome can also occur in the abdomen, when there is a sustained or repeated elevation of 12 mm Hg or greater. Refer to *Risk for Complications of Intra-Abdominal Hypertension*

High-Risk Populations

Internal Factors

- Fractures
- Musculoskeletal surgery
- Injuries (crush, electrical, vascular)
- Allergic response (snake, insect bites)
- Excessive edema
- Thermal injuries
- Vascular obstruction
- Intramuscular bleeding

External Factors

- Extravasation of IV fluids
- Drug abuse (arterial injection; Stracciolini & Hammerberg, 2014)
- Procedural cannulation of vessel for diagnostic or interventional reasons
  - Casts
  - Prolonged use of tourniquet
  - Tight dressings
  - Tight closure of fascial detects
  - Positioning during surgery (lithotomy)
  - Lying on limb for extended periods

Collaborative Outcomes

The individual will be monitored for early signs and symptoms of compartment syndrome and will receive collaborative interventions if indicated to restore physiologic stability.

Indicators of Physiologic Stability

- Pedal pulses 2+, equal
- Capillary refill <3 seconds
- Warm extremities
- No complaints of paresthesia (numbness), tingling
- Minimal swelling
- Ability to move toes or fingers

Interventions and Rationales

Assess for Specific Signs of Compartment Syndrome (Shadgan et al., 2010; Stracciolini & Hammerberg, 2014)

- Complaints of tingling or burning sensations > numbness

  R: Sensory deficits typically precede motor deficits and manifest distal to the involved compartment.

- Pain is out of proportion to the injury, unrelieved by narcotics.
- Pain with passive stretch of muscles in the affected compartment or hyperextension of digits (toes or fingers) (early finding)

R: Passive stretching of muscles decreases muscle compartment, thus increasing pain. Pain in response to passive stretching of muscles within the affected compartment is widely described as a sensitive early sign of ACS (Stracciolini & Hammerberg, 2014).

- A new and persistent deep ache in an arm or leg
- Electricity-like pain in the limb

R: Pain and paresthesia indicate compression of nerves and increasing pressure within muscle compartment.

- Increases with the elevation of the extremity

R: This increases the pressure in the compartment.

- Involved compartment or limb will feel tense and warm on palpation.
- Skin is tight and shiny.
- Late signs/symptoms
  - Diminished or absent pulse
  - Pallor, cool skin
  - Pale, grayish, or whitish tone to skin

  R: Arterial occlusion produces these late signs.

- Prolonged capillary refill (>3 seconds)

R: Delayed capillary refill or pale, mottled, or cyanotic skin indicates obstructed capillary blood flow.

- Complaints of weakness when moving affected limb
- Progresses to inability to move joint or fingers/toes
- Pulselessness

R: Decreased arterial perfusion results in pulselessness.

Examine Laboratory Findings of Compartment Syndrome

- Elevated white blood cell (WBC) count and erythrocyte sedimentation rate (ESR)

  R: These elevations are a result of the severe inflammatory response.

- Lowered serum pH

  R: This reflects tissue damage with acidosis.

- Elevated temperature

  R: This is due to necrosis of tissue.

- Elevated serum potassium

  R: Cellular damage releases potassium.

Assess Neurovascular Function at Least Every Hour for First 24 Hours

R: A delay in diagnosis is the most important determinant of a poor patient outcome.

Instruct to Report Unusual, New, or Different Sensations (e.g., Tingling, Numbness, and/or Decreased Ability to Move Toes or Fingers)

R: Early detection of compromise can prevent serious outcomes.

When the Individual Is Unconscious or Heavily Sedated and Unable to Complain or Report Sensations, Intensive Assessment Is Required

R: Permanent nerve injury can occur 12 to 24 hours of nerve compression.

If Pain Medications Become Ineffective, Consider Compartmental Syndrome

R: Opioids are ineffective for neurovascular pain (Pasero & McCaffery, 2011).

If Signs of Compartment Syndrome Occur

- Discontinue excessive elevation and ice applications.
- Keep the body part below the level of the heart.

  R: This will improve blood flow into the compartment.

- Remove restrictive dressings, splints.

   R: Elevation and external devices will impede perfusion.

Initiate Nasal Oxygen

R: This will improve oxygenation to compromised tissue.

> **CLINICAL ALERT:**
> - Immediately, advise physician, physician assistant/nurse practitioner of the need for the evaluation of the neurovascular changes assessed or reported by the individual. Immediate medical assessment will determine what specific interventions are needed (e.g., measurement of compartment pressures, emergency surgery [fasciotomy], removal of cast, splints) (Stracciolini & Hammerberg, 2014).

Monitor and Document Compartment Pressures According to Protocol; Report Elevated Pressures Promptly

R: "The normal pressure of a tissue compartment falls between 0 and 8 mmHg. Clinical findings associated with ACS generally correlate with the degree to which tissue pressure within the affected compartment approaches systemic blood pressures. Capillary blood flow becomes compromised when tissue pressure increases to within 25 to 30 mmHg of mean arterial pressure" (Stracciolini & Hammerberg, 2014).

> **CLINICAL ALERT:**
> - "Many surgeons involved in trauma care use a threshold based upon the difference between systemic blood pressures and compartment pressures to confirm the presence of ACS. These authors concur with this approach and suggest that a difference between the diastolic blood pressure and the compartment pressure (delta pressure) of 30 mmHg or less be used as the threshold for diagnosing ACS. The delta pressure is found by subtracting the compartment pressure from the diastolic pressure. Many clinicians use the delta pressure of 30 mmHg to determine the need for fasciotomy, while others use a difference of 20 mmHg." (Stracciolini & Hammerberg, 2014).

Carefully Maintain Hydration With at Least 0.5 mL/kg/hr of Urine Output

R: Muscle necrosis or rhabdomyolysis may lead to the accumulation of myoglobin in the kidneys, causing acute renal failure in up to 50% of individuals with rhabdomyolysis (Mabvuure, Malahias, Hindocha, Khan, & Juma, 2012).

Continue to Monitor Cardiovascular and Renal Status: Pulse, Respiration, Blood Pressure, and Urine Output

R: Eight liters of fluid can extravasate into a limb, causing hypovolemia, decreased renal function, and shock.

RISK FOR COMPLICATIONS OF DECREASED CARDIAC OUTPUT

Definition

Describes a person experiencing or at high risk to experience inadequate blood supply for tissue and organ needs because of insufficient blood pumping by the heart.

Deceased cardiac output is a phenomenon that is not restricted to individuals or environments that specifically focus on cardiovascular care. It is prevalent not only in cardiovascular care units, but also in postanaesthesia units and noncardiac care units among individuals with noncardiogenic disorders. A significant decrease in cardiac output is a life-threatening situation, demonstrating the need for developing a risk nursing diagnosis for early intervention (Pereira de Melo et al., 2011).

High-Risk Populations

- Acute coronary syndrome (ACS)
- Congestive heart failure
- Cardiogenic shock
- Hypertension
- Valvular heart disease
- Cardiomyopathy
- Cardiac tamponade
- Hypothermia
- Anaphylaxis
- Dilated cardiomyopathy
- Streptococcal toxic shock syndrome
- Severe diarrhea
- Systemic inflammatory response syndrome (SIRS)
- Coarctation of the aorta
- Chronic obstructive pulmonary disease (COPD)
- Pheochromocytoma
- Chronic renal failure
- Adult respiratory distress syndrome
- Hypotension/hypovolemia (e.g., postsurgery, severe bleeding or burns)
- Bradycardia
- Tachycardia

Collaborative Outcomes

The individual will be monitored for early signs and symptoms of *Decreased Cardiac Output* and will receive collaborative interventions if indicated to restore physiologic stability.

Indicators of Physiologic Stability

- Calm, alert, oriented
- Oxygen saturation >95%
- Normal sinus rhythm
- No chest pain
- No life-threatening arrhythmias
- Skin warm and dry
- Usual skin color (appropriate for race)
- Pulse: regular rhythm, rate 60 to 100 beats/min
- Respirations 16 to 20 breaths/min
- Blood pressure >90/60 and <140/90 mm Hg, MAP >70, or CVP >11
- Urine output >0.5 mL/kg/hr
- Breath sounds without evidence of new, abnormal sounds (rales)
- No presence of distended neck veins (jugular vein distention [JVD])

R: Low cardiac output can cause cardiac ischemia—perhaps more so for the heart than other organs because of the heart's already high rate of oxygen extraction. A vicious cycle ensues. Cardiac ischemia forces a shift towards anaerobic metabolism (2 ATP) from the much more efficient aerobic metabolism (36 ATP). With less energy available and increased intercellular acidity, the force of contraction weakens, causing a further reduction in stroke volume and cardiac output. The bottom line is that cardiac output is intimately coupled with energy production. For the heart, low cardiac output may in turn cause ischemia. Cardiac ischemia weakens contractility, further impacting cardiac output. When caring for individuals with cardiac ischemia, assess for signs and symptoms of poor cardiac output (shock).

Interventions and Rationales

Closely Monitor Urine Output Hourly

R: Decreased blood volume reduces blood to kidneys, which decreases the glomerular filtration rate (GFR) causing a decrease in urine output. When blood flow to the kidneys is less than 20% to 25% of normal, ischemic damage occurs (Grossman & Porth, 2014). Decreased urine output is an early sign of bleeding/hypovolemia.

Monitor for Signs and Symptoms of Decreased Cardiac Output/Index

- Increased, decreased, and/or irregular pulse rate
- Increased respiratory rate
- Decreased blood pressure, increased blood pressure
- Abnormal heart sounds
- Abnormal lung sounds (crackles, rales)
- Decreased urine output (<0.5 mL/kg/hr)
- Changes in mentation
- Cool, moist, cyanotic, mottled skin
- Delayed capillary refill time
- Neck vein distention

> *R: Decreased cardiac output/index leads to insufficient oxygenated blood to meet the metabolic needs of tissues. Decreased circulating volume can result in hypoperfusion of the kidneys and decreased tissue perfusion with a compensatory response of decreased circulation to extremities and increased pulse and respiratory rates. Changes in mentation may result from cerebral hypoperfusion. Vasoconstriction and venous congestion in dependent areas (e.g., limbs) produce changes in skin and pulses (Grossman & Porth, 2014).*

Initiate Appropriate Protocols or Standing Orders, Depending on the Underlying Etiology of the Problem Affecting Ventricular Function

> *R: Nursing management differs on the basis of etiology (e.g., measures to help increase preload for hypovolemia and to decrease preload for impaired ventricular contractility).*

Position the Individual With the Legs Elevated, Unless Contraindicated When Ventricular Function Is Impaired as With Congestive Heart Failure

> *R: This position can help increase preload and enhance cardiac output.*

Clinical Alert Report

Advise ancillary staff/student to report:
- Urine output <0.5 mL/kg/hr
- Any new change or deterioration in behavior (e.g., agitation, cognition, anxiety)
- Changes or new onset of dyspnea/palpitations
- B/P >200 mm Hg (systolic), >115 mm Hg (diastolic), <90 mm Hg systolic
- Respirations >10/min over baseline, <10/min under baseline, labored
- Pulse >100 resting
- Temperature (oral) over 100.5° F
- Pulse oximetry <90%
- Diminished peripheral pulses
- Cool, pale, moist, or cyanotic skin

RISK FOR COMPLICATIONS OF DEEP VEIN THROMBOSIS/PULMONARY EMBOLISM/FAT EMBOLISM

Definition

Describes a person experiencing venous clot formation because of blood stasis, vessel wall injury, or altered coagulation and/or experiencing or at high risk to experience obstruction of one or more pulmonary arteries from a blood clot, air, or fat embolus

High-Risk Populations (Barbar et al., 2010; Lip & Hull, 2016a)

- Active cancer (③)
- History of deep vein thrombosis (DVT) or pulmonary embolism (③)

- Reduced mobility >72 hours (③)
- Known thrombophilic condition (③) (e.g., polycythemia, blood dyscrasias)
- High levels of factor VIII in white people (Payne, Miller, Hooper, Lally, & Austin, 2014)
- High levels of factor VIII and von Willebrand factor in black people (Payne et al., 2014)
- Recent trauma/surgery (②)
- Over 70 years old (①)
- Obesity >30 BMI (①)
- Acute coronary or ischemic stroke (①)
- Acute infection and/or rheumatologic disorder (①)
- Ongoing hormonal therapy (①)
- Heart/respiratory failure (①)
- Age (risk rises steadily from age 40)
- Fractures (especially hip, pelvis, and leg)
- Chemical irritation of vein
- All major surgeries that involve general anesthesia and immobility (over 30 minutes) in the operative course (preop, periop, and postop combined), especially surgeries involving abdomen, pelvis, and lower extremities
- Orthopedic (hips/knees), urologic, or gynecologic surgery
- History of venous insufficiency
- Varicose veins
- Inflammatory bowel disease
- Pregnancy
- Surgery greater than 30 minutes (②)
- Over 40 years of age
- Valve malfunction
- Systemic lupus erythematosus
- Central venous catheters
- Nephrotic syndrome

Those risk factors with a score in parentheses have been identified in the Padua Prediction risk assessment for venous thrombolytic events. A score of ≥4 represents a high-risk individual (Barbar, 2010).

Air Embolism

- Central line insertion or removal, sheath central line tubing changes, manipulation, or disconnection

Fat Embolism (Eriksson, Quinlan, & Eikelboom, 2011)

- Fractures—closed fractures produce more emboli than open fractures. Long bones, pelvis, and ribs cause more emboli. Sternum and clavicle furnish less. Multiple fractures produce more emboli.
- Orthopaedic procedures—most commonly, intramedullary nailing of the long bones, hip, or knee replacements
- Massive soft tissue injury
- CPR is associated with a high incidence of PFE regardless of cause of death (Eriksson et al., 2011).
- Severe burns
- Bone marrow biopsy
- Nontraumatic conditions occasionally lead to fat embolism. These include conditions associated with:
  - Liposuction
  - Fatty liver
  - Prolonged corticosteroid therapy
  - Acute pancreatitis
  - Osteomyelitis
  - Conditions causing bone infarcts, especially sickle cell disease

Carp's Cues

In more than 90% of cases of PE, the thrombosis originates in the deep veins of the legs. Deep vein thrombosis (DVT) is a distressing but often avoidable condition that leads to long-term complications such as the postphlebitic syndrome and chronic leg ulcers in a large proportion of individuals who have proximal vein thrombosis. Pulmonary embolism remains the most common preventable cause of death in hospital (Lip & Hull, 2016a).

The incidence of FES varies from 1% to 29%. Fat emboli occur in all individuals with long-bone fractures, but only few patients develop systemic dysfunction, particularly the triad of skin, brain, and lung dysfunction known as the fat embolism syndrome (FES) (Eriksson et al., 2011).

Collaborative Outcomes

The individual will be monitored for early signs and symptoms of (a) deep vein thrombosis and (b) pulmonary embolism, and the individual will receive collaborative interventions if indicated to restore physiologic stability.

Indicators of Physiologic Stability

* No leg pain (a)
* No leg edema (a)
* No change in skin temperature or color (a, b)
* No acute dyspnea, restlessness, decreased mental status, or anxiety (b)
* No acute, sharp chest pain (b)
* Pulse: regular rhythm, rate 60 to 100 beats/min (b)
* Respirations 16 to 20 breaths/min (b)
* Blood pressure >90/60 and <140/90 mm Hg, MAP >70, or CVP >11
* Breath sounds without evidence of new, abnormal sounds (rales, crackles) (b)
* Absence of distended neck veins (jugular vein distention [JVD]) (b)

Interventions and Rationales

Identify Individuals Who Are High Risk for Bleeding if on Anticoagulant Therapy (Score ≥4) Using the Padua Prediction Score (Refer to List Under High-Risk Population)

R: Individuals at moderate or high risk by the Padua Prediction Score who are not bleeding or at high risk for bleeding should be given anticoagulant thromboprophylaxis with either low-molecular-weight heparin (enoxaparin/ Lovenox or others), unfractionated heparin (either b.i.d. or t.i.d.), or fondaparinux (Grade 1B; 1 = recommendation; B = moderate-quality evidence). This recommendation includes all critically ill individuals, as long as they are not at high bleeding risk (ACCP, 2012).

Consult With Physician/Nurse Practitioner/Physician Assistant to Evaluate the Need for Thromboprophylaxis

> **CLINICAL ALERT:**
> * If the individual is high risk for DVT and not high risk for bleeding and thromboprophylax is not prescribed, use SBAR to communicate the seriousness of the situation.

SBAR   *Situation:* I am concerned about Mr. Nedia and his risk for VTE (venous thrombolytic event).

Background: He is immobile, 72, obese, and has COPD and a Padua score of 6.

Assessment: Presently, he is resistant to getting out of bed and refuses to walk except to the chair.

Recommendation: Is there a reason why he is not on thromboprophylaxis?

R: This communication provides the physician/nurse practitioner/physician assistant with an opportunity to review the situation and to share his or her rationale why no thromboprophylaxis has been initiated.

Monitor for Onset or Status of Venous Thrombosis, Noting

- Diminished or absent peripheral pulses

  R: Insufficient circulation causes pain and diminished peripheral pulses.

- Unusual warmth and redness or coolness and cyanosis, increased leg swelling

  R: Unusual warmth and redness point to inflammation; coolness and cyanosis indicate vascular obstruction.

- Increasing leg pain

  R: Leg pain results from tissue hypoxia.

- A rapid heart rate and/or a feeling of passing out
- New chest pain with difficulty breathing

  R: These findings may indicate mobilization of thrombi to the lungs (pulmonary embolism)

> **CLINICAL ALERT:**
> - Stay will person and call for Rapid Response Team.

Monitor for the Most Common Symptoms of Pulmonary Embolism (Stein et al., 2007)

- Dyspnea at rest or with exertion (73%)
- Pleuritic pain (44%)
- Cough (37%)
- Orthopnea (28%)
- Calf or thigh pain and/or swelling (44%)
- Wheezing (21%)

  R: The most common symptoms in individuals with PE were identified in the Prospective Investigation of Pulmonary Embolism Diagnosis II (PIOPED II) study (Stein et al., 2007; Thompson & Hales, 2015).

Monitor for Other Signs and Symptoms (Stein et al., 2007; Thompson & Hales, 2015)

- Tachypnea (54%)
- Calf or thigh swelling, erythema, edema, tenderness, palpable cords (47%)
- Tachycardia (24%)
- Rales (18%)
- Decreased breath sounds (17%)
- An accentuated pulmonic component of the second heart sound (15%)
- Jugular venous distension (14%)
- Fever, mimicking pneumonia (3%)

  R: The most common symptoms in individuals with PE were identified in the Prospective Investigation of Pulmonary Embolism Diagnosis II (PIOPED II) study. Occlusion of pulmonary arteries impedes blood flow to the distal lung, producing a hypoxic state. Circulatory collapse is uncommon (8%) (Stein et al., 2007; Thompson & Hales, 2015). Among such individuals, either dyspnea or tachypnea is present in 91%. Massive PE may be accompanied by acute right ventricular failure, manifested by increased jugular venous pressure, a right-sided third heart sound, a parasternal lift, cyanosis, and obstructive shock (Thompson & Hales, 2015).

If These Manifestations Occur, Call Rapid Response Team and Promptly Initiate Protocols for Shock

- Establish an IV line (for medication and fluid administration).
- Administer fluid replacement therapy according to protocol.
- Insert indwelling urinary (Foley) catheter (to monitor circulatory volume through urine output).
- Initiate electrocardiograph (ECG) monitoring and invasive hemodynamic monitoring (to detect arrhythmias and guide therapy).

- Initiate unit protocols.
- Refer to *Risk for Complications of Hypovolemic Shock* for additional interventions.

   R: Because death from massive pulmonary embolism commonly occurs in the first 2 hours after onset, prompt intervention is crucial.

Initiate Oxygen Therapy; Monitor Oxygen Saturation

R: This measure rapidly increases circulating oxygen levels.

Monitor Serum Electrolyte Levels, ABG Values, Blood Urea Nitrogen, and Complete Blood Count Results

R: These laboratory tests help determine perfusion and volume status. Monitor D-Dimer & chest X-ray aids in diagnosis (Shaughnessy, 2007).

Provide Measures to Prevent Thrombosis

- Evaluate hydration status on the basis of urine specific gravity, intake/output, weights, and serum os-molality. Take steps to ensure adequate hydration.

   R: Increased blood viscosity and coagulability and decreased cardiac output may contribute to thrombus formation.

- Encourage to perform isotonic leg exercises, flexing knees and ankles hourly.

   R: They promote venous return.

- Ambulate as soon as possible with at least 5 minutes of walking each waking hour. Avoid prolonged chair sitting with legs dependent.

   R: Walking contracts leg muscles, stimulates the venous pump, and reduces stasis (Institute for Clinical Systems Improvement, 2008).

- Elevate the affected extremity above the level of the heart.

   R: This positioning can help reduce interstitial swelling by promoting venous return.

- Discourage smoking.

   R: Nicotine can cause vasospasms.

- Adhere to protocols for vascular access catchers (Burns, 2014; *Gorski, 2002; Luettel, Beaumont, & Healey, 2007).

 ## Carp's Cues

In 2002, the National Quality Forum created and endorsed a list of Serious Reportable Events (SREs), which was updated in 2006. There are 28 events that have been labeled as Serious Reportable Events, also called never events. "The 28 events on the list are largely preventable, grave errors and events that are of concern to the public and healthcare providers and that warrant careful investigation and should be targeted for mandatory public reporting" (*National Quality Forum, 2006). One of the 28 events is patient death or serious disability associated with intravascular air embolism that occurs while being cared for in a health care facility.

For Prevention of Air Embolism

- Refer to Box II.2 for the risks of catheter-related venous air embolism.

Box II.2 CATHETER-RELATED RISK FACTORS FOR VENOUS AIR EMBOLISM

The risk of catheter-related venous air embolism appears to be increased by the following factors:

- Fracture or detachment of catheter connections (which accounts for 60% to 90% of episodes)
- Failure to occlude the needle hub and/or catheter during insertion or removal
- Dysfunction of self-sealing valves in plastic introducer sheaths
- Presence of a persistent catheter tract following the removal of a central venous catheter
- Deep inspiration during insertion or removal, which increases the magnitude of negative pressure within the thorax
- Hypovolemia, which reduces central venous pressure
- Upright positioning of the patient, which reduces central venous pressure to below atmospheric pressure and places the patient at particular risk for entraining air very rapidly into the venous circulation.

Source: O'Dowd, L. C., & Kelley, M. A. (2015). Air embolism. In *UpToDate*. Retrieved from http://www.uptodate.com/contents /air-embolism?source=search_result&search=air+embolism&selectedTitle=1~114

R: A literature review reports that venous air embolism is a serious and underrecognized complication associated with the insertion of central venous catheters, hemodialysis catheters, and pulmonary artery catheters and with intravenous injections, particularly contrast injection. Arterial embolism can occur with the insertion of arterial catheters, angioplasty catheters, or other arterial interventions (e.g., intra-aortic balloon pump) (O'Dowd & Kelley, 2015).

- Before maintenance or removal of venous access device, explain to the individual what was going to happen and why it is important to follow the specific instructions.

  R: Cooperation with instructions and positioning during central line removal is a critical intervention to prevent air embolism.

- Maintain a sterile environment and maximal barrier precautions (Young, 2015).
  - Follow protocols, for example, wear a mask, sterile gown, and sterile gloves.
  - Perform hand hygiene and put on clean gloves. Remove the dressing carefully and discard it with your gloves.
  - Repeat hand hygiene and put on sterile gloves.
  - Assess the catheter insertion site for evidence of complications such as redness, swelling, or drainage. Notify the physician if you see any of these signs; she may order a culture. Clean the site according to facility policy, preferably with chlorhexidine. Never use scissors near the venous access device, as this could result in accidental severing of the catheter.
  - Remove the catheter-securing device.

- Before central line catheter insertion and tubing changes, place the person in supine or Trendelenburg's position and instruct him or her to perform Valsalva maneuver during the procedure. Instruct to take a deep breath and bear down simulating applying downward pressure as if having a bowel movement. Have person demonstrate it. Remove the catheter as the person bears down.

- If the individual is unable to cooperate with procedure, perform during positive pressure portion of respiratory cycle (Burns, 2014; Luettel, 2011).
  - Spontaneous breathing—during exhalation
  - Mechanical ventilation—during inhalation

  R: These measures increase intrathoracic pressure and help prevent air from entering the catheter.

- Follow protocol to remove central line catheter (Burns, 2014; O'Dowd & Kelley, 2015).
  - After you've removed the catheter, tell the person to breathe normally. Apply pressure with the sterile gauze until bleeding stops.
  - Apply a sterile air-occlusive dressing over the insertion site to prevent a delayed air embolism.
  - Assess the length and integrity of the catheter and visually inspect the tip for smoothness. Remove your gloves and perform hand hygiene.
  - Instruct individual to remain supine for 30 minutes after removal (O'Dowd & Kelley, 2015).
  - Document the date and time of CVC removal, noting the CVC's length and integrity, the site assessment, patient response, and nursing interventions.
  - Do not pull harder if resistance is met while removing a CVC.
  - Do not remove it when the person is inhaling.
  - Do not apply any dressing that is not air-occlusive; this would increase the risk of a delayed air embolism (O'Dowd & Kelley, 2015).

  R: These measures help prevent air entry and infection at insertion site (Burns, 2014; O'Dowd & Kelley, 2015).

- Monitor for signs and symptoms of air embolism during dressing and IV tubing changes and after any accidental separation of IV connections:
  - Sucking sound on insertion
  - Dyspnea
  - Tachypnea
  - Wheezing
  - Substernal chest pain
  - Anxiety

  R: Air embolism can occur with IV tubing changes, with accidental tubing separation, and during catheter insertion, removal, and disconnection (e.g., an individual can aspirate as much as 200 mL of air from a deep breath during subclavian line disconnection). Entry of air into the pulmonary arterial system can obstruct blood flow, causing bronchoconstriction of the affected lung area. Use luer lock connections to help prevent accidental disconnection.

- If air embolism is suspected, call the Rapid response team. Do not leave the person (von Jürgensonn, 2010).
  - Administer 100% oxygen.

    R: This promotes diffusion of nitrogen, which compresses an air embolism in about 80% of cases.

- Place person flat or in Trendelenburg position and turn on to left side.

    R: This position displaces air away from pulmonary valve and traps it in the ventricle for radiological aspiration.

RISK FOR COMPLICATIONS OF HYPOVOLEMIA

Definition

Describes a person experiencing or at high risk to experience inadequate cellular oxygenation and inability to excrete waste products of metabolism secondary to decreased fluid volume (e.g., from bleeding, plasma loss, prolonged vomiting, or diarrhea)

High-Risk Populations

- Intraoperative status
- Postoperative status
- Postprocedural cannulation of any arterial vessel but particularly those at risk for retro-peritoneal bleed due to cannulation of femoral vessel
- Anaphylactic shock
- Trauma
- Bleeding
- Diabetic ketoacidosis (DKA) or hyperosmolar hyperglycemic state (HHS) (Kitabchi, Hirsch, & Emmett, 2015)
- Prolonged vomiting or diarrhea
- Infants, children, older persons
- Acute pancreatitis
- Major burns
- Disseminated intravascular coagulation (DIC)
- Diabetes insipidus
- Ascites
- Peritonitis
- Intestinal obstruction
- Systemic inflammatory response syndrome (SIRS)/sepsis

Collaborative Outcomes

The individual will be monitored for early signs and symptoms of hypovolemia and will receive collaborative interventions if indicated to restore physiologic stability.

Indicators of Physiologic Stability

Refer to *Risk for Complications of Decreased Cardiac Output* for indicators.

Interventions and Rationales

For individual at risk for bleeding, refer to *Risk for Complications of Bleeding.*

Monitor Fluid Status; Evaluate

- Intake (parenteral and oral)
- Output and other losses (urine, drainage, and vomiting), nasogastric tube

R: Decreased blood volume reduces blood to kidneys, which decreases the glomerular filtration rate (GFR), causing a decrease in urine output. When blood flow to the kidneys is less than 20% to 25% of normal, ischemic damage occurs. Decreased urine output is an early sign of hypovolemia (Grossman & Porth, 2014).

Monitor for Signs and Symptoms of Shock

- Increased pulse rate with normal or slightly decreased blood pressure, narrowing pulse pressure, decrease in mean or mean arterial pressure (MAP)
- Urine output <0.5 mL/kg/hr
- Restlessness, agitation, decreased mentation
- Increased respiratory rate, thirst
- Diminished peripheral pulses
- Cool, pale, moist, or cyanotic skin

R: The compensatory response to decreased circulatory volume aims to increase oxygen delivery through increased heart and respiratory rates and decreased peripheral circulation (manifested by diminished peripheral pulses and cool skin). Decreased oxygen to the brain alters mentation. Decreased circulation to the kidneys leads to decreased urine output. Hemoglobin and hematocrit values decline if bleeding is significant (Grossman & Porth, 2014).

If Shock Occurs, Place Individual in the Supine Position Unless Contraindicated (e.g., Head Injury)

R: This position increases blood return (preload) to the heart.

Call a Code or for the Rapid Response Team. Follow Protocols (e.g., Insert Large-Bore IV Catheter)

R: Protocols aim to rapidly replace fluid volumes, increase peripheral resistance, and elevate blood pressure.

Administer Oxygen as Ordered

R: This will increase the circulating oxygen available for tissue use.

> ### *Clinical Alert Report*
>
> Advise ancillary staff/student to report:
> - Urine output <0.5 mL/kg/hr
> - Sudden restlessness, agitation, decreased mentation
> - Increased respiratory rate
> - Decreasing BP
> - Diminished peripheral pulses
> - Cool, pale, moist, or cyanotic skin

RISK FOR COMPLICATIONS OF INTRA-ABDOMINAL HYPERTENSION/ ABDOMINAL COMPARTMENTAL PRESSURE

Definition

Intra-abdominal hypertension (IAH) describes a person experiencing or at high risk to experience sustained or repeated pathologic elevation of intra-abdominal pressure (IAP) of 12 mm Hg or greater (The World Society of the Abdominal Compartment Syndrome [WSACS], 2013). Abdominal compartmental pressure is a sustained IAP greater than 20 mm Hg with new organ dysfunction or failure (WSACS, 2013).

High-Risk Populations (Gestring, 2015; Lee, 2012a, b; Lee et al., 2007)

- Causes of primary (i.e., acute) IAH include the following:
  - Penetrating trauma
  - Intraperitoneal hemorrhage
  - Pancreatitis
  - External compressing forces, such as debris from a motor vehicle collision or after a large structure explosion
  - Pelvic fracture
  - Rupture of abdominal aortic aneurysm
  - Perforated peptic ulcer
  - Liver transplant

> **CLINICAL ALERT:**
> - IAH caused by primary conditions when intra-abdominal pressure is ≥20 mm Hg may need surgical (e.g., decompression of the abdominal cavity) or interventional radiological treatment (e.g., paracentesis) (Lee, 2012a, b).

- Secondary IAH may occur in individuals without an intra-abdominal injury, when fluid accumulates in volumes sufficient to cause IAH. Causes include the following:
  - Large-volume resuscitation: The literature shows significantly increased risk with infusions greater than 3 L.
  - Large areas of full-thickness burns: Hobson et al. demonstrated abdominal compartment syndrome within 24 hours in individuals with burns who had received an average of 237 mL/kg over a 12-hour period.
  - Penetrating or blunt trauma without identifiable injury
  - Postoperative
  - Packing and primary fascial closure, which increases incidence
  - Sepsis
- Causes of chronic intra-abdominal hypertension include the following:
  - Peritoneal dialysis
  - Morbid obesity
  - Cirrhosis
  - Chronic alcohol abuse
  - Pancreatitis
  - Meigs's syndrome
  - Intra-abdominal mass

> **CLINICAL ALERT:**
> - IAP is also increased in persons who are morbidly obese, have chronic ascites, or are pregnant. In these chronic forms, the increase develops slowly and the body adjusts to the change (Lee, 2012a, b, p. 20).

Collaborative Outcomes

The individual will be monitored for early signs and symptoms of IAH and will receive collaborative interventions if indicated to restore physiologic stability.

Indicators of Physiologic Stability

- Intra-abdominal pressure 0 to 5 mm Hg
- No increase in abdominal girth
- Urine output >0.5 mL/kg/hr
- No melena

Interventions and Rationales

Monitor for IAH

R: Organ dysfunction with IAH is a product of the effects of IAH on multiple organ systems.

* Increase in abdominal girth

  R: The effect of IAH on the GI system leads to diminished perfusion, which results in ischemia, acidosis, capillary leak, intestinal edema, and release of GI flora into the lymph and vascular systems (Lee, 2012a, b; Lee et al., 2007).

* Wheezes, rales, increased respiratory rate, cyanosis
* Limited respiratory excursion

  R: As the abdomen distends, the diaphragm is pushed upward, preventing the lungs from full expansion and increasing intrathoracic pressure (Lee, 2012a, b; Lee et al., 2007).

* Decreased urine output

  R: Increasing abdominal distention compresses renal parenchyma and decreased renal perfusion (Lee, 2012a, b; Lee et al., 2007).

* Wan appearance, syncope, headache, confusion

  R: Increasing intrathoracic pressure causes back pressure on the jugular veins and impedes drainage of cerebrospinal fluid, producing increased intracranial pressure (Lee, 2012a, b; Lee et al., 2007).

> **CLINICAL ALERT:**
> IAH that increases to 20 mm Hg or greater and is associated with new organ dysfunction or failure is abdominal compartmental syndrome. Abdominal compartmental syndrome has a mortality rate of over 50%. Medical treatment focuses on attempting to reduce IAP with mechanical drainage and diuretics. If these methods are not effective, a decompressive laparotomy must be performed (Lee, 2012a, b).

To Manage Individual With IAH Appropriately, Nurses Must Perform IAP Measurements

The Gold Standard of Indirect Measurement Is Measurement via a Urinary Bladder Catheter

* Follow protocols for measuring intra-abdominal pressure.

  R: Hands-on assessments of the abdomen and serial measurements of abdominal girth are not sensitive as direct and indirect measurements of IAP (Lee, 2012a, b).

Monitor IAP in High-Risk Individuals Who (Gestring, 2015; Lee, 2012a, b)

R: Individuals who are difficult to ventilate may have high IAP.

* Are intubated with high peak and plateau pressures
* Have GI bleeding or pancreatitis, who are nonresponsive to intravenous (IV) fluids, blood products, and pressors
* Have severe burns or sepsis, who are not responding to IV fluids and pressors
* Have contradictory Swann-Ganz readings, when compared with clinical condition
* Therapeutic hypothermia
* Goal-directed fluid therapy in sepsis protocol
* Large blood transfusions (>10 units of packed red blood cells in 24 hours)
* Institute interventions to prevent or reduce abdominal distention
* Prevent constipation and fecal impactions

  R: These conditions will increase abdominal distention.

Maintain Patency of Nasogastric Tube and Monitor for Increased Residuals With Enteral Feedings

R: Increased residual feedings or retained GI fluids will further increase distention.

Ensure That Individuals Are Eating; Avoid All Gas-Producing Food

R: These gases can further aggravate abdominal distention.

Avoid the Prone Position and Elevating the Head of Bed More Than 20 Degrees

R: To improve abdominal wall compliance and reduce IAP, avoid the prone position and elevate the head of bed more than 20 degrees (Lee, 2012a, b).

Remove Heavy Blankets, Constrictive Abdominal Dressings

R: Any external pressure on the abdomen will increase pressure (must be avoided to prevent).

Aggressively Manage Fluid Balance to Aim for a Goal of an Equal or Negative Fluid Balance by Day 3 (Lee, 2012a, b)

R: Excess fluid replacement is a known risk factor for IAH, especially if a patient has capillary leak.

> ### *Clinical Alert Report*
> Advise ancillary staff/student to report:
> - Drinking more fluids than prescribed
> - All bowel movements
> - Any new change or deterioration in behavior (e.g., agitation, cognition, anxiety)
> - Changes or new onset of dyspnea/palpitations
> - BP >200 mm Hg (systolic), >115 mm Hg (diastolic), <90 mm Hg (systolic)
> - Respirations >10/min over baseline, <10/min under baseline, labored
> - Pulse >100 resting
> - Temperature (oral) over 100.5° F
> - Pulse oximetry <90%

RISK FOR COMPLICATIONS OF PULMONARY EDEMA

Definition

Cardiogenic pulmonary edema (CPE) is defined as pulmonary edema due to increased capillary hydrostatic pressure secondary to elevated pulmonary venous pressure. CPE reflects the accumulation of fluid with a low protein content in the lung interstitium and alveoli. Impaired LV contractility, resulting in reduced cardiac output, is the most common predisposing condition leading to cardiogenic pulmonary edema (Pinto & Kociol, 2015).

Pulmonary edema that is not caused by increased pressures in the heart is called noncardiogenic pulmonary edema (Givertz, 2015). One example of noncardiogenic pulmonary edema is high-altitude pulmonary edema.

High-altitude pulmonary edema seems to develop as a result of increased pressure from constriction of the pulmonary capillaries, although the exact cause is not completely understood.

A type of pulmonary edema called neurogenic pulmonary edema can occur after some nervous system conditions or procedures—such as after a head injury, seizure, or subarachnoid hemorrhage—or after brain surgery.

High-Risk Populations

Pulmonary edema can be caused by cardiac-related or noncardiac-related causes.

Cardiac Causes

This condition usually occurs when the diseased, compromised, or overworked left ventricle or heart valves are not able to pump out enough of the blood it receives through the pulmonary artery. The increased pressure extends into the left atrium and then to the pulmonary veins, causing fluid to accumulate in the lungs (Givertz, 2015).

- Hypertension (untreated or uncontrolled)
- arrhythmias
- Myocardial infarction
  - Acute cardiac syndrome (ACS)
  - Angina
- Congestive heart failure
- Cardiomyopathy
- Failed pacemaker, lead wires, and/or generator
- Coronary artery disease
- Aortic or mitral cardiac valve disease
- Congenital heart defects

Noncardiac Causes

In this condition, fluid may leak from the capillaries in the lungs' air sacs because the capillaries themselves become more permeable or leaky, even without the buildup of back pressure from the heart. The integrity of the alveoli become compromised as a result of underlying inflammatory response, and this leads to leaky alveoli that can fill up with fluid from the blood vessels (Givertz, 2015).

- Acute respiratory distress syndrome (ARDS)
- Diabetes mellitus (episodic severe hyperglycemia, underlying cause of CAD)
- Inhalation of toxins (ammonia and chlorine)
- Drug overdose (pathophysiology unknown) (e.g., heroin, cocaine, methadone, aspirin; Givertz, 2015)
- Smoke inhalation
- Neurologic trauma/surgery
- Volume overload (in the presence of compromised cardiac function)
- Renal failure (inability to excrete fluid from the body can cause fluid buildup in the blood vessels)
- Pulmonary embolism (PE can cause pulmonary edema by injuring the pulmonary and adjacent pleural systemic circulations, elevating hydrostatic pressures in pulmonary and/or systemic veins, and perhaps by lowering pleural pressure due to atelectasis [Givertz, 2015])
- Pneumothorax (pulmonary edema can occur with rapid expansion of the lung post collapse)
- Viral infections (rapidly progressive noncardiogenic pulmonary edema associated with profound hypotension and a high case fatality rate with, e.g., hantavirus infection, dengue, hemorrhagic fever, coronavirus infection, H1N1 influenza A; Givertz, 2015)
- Near-drowning
- High altitudes (an abnormally pronounced degree of hypoxic pulmonary vasoconstriction at a given altitude appears to underlie the pathogenesis of this disorder [Givertz, 2015])
- Hypothermia (when core temperatures reaches 32° C, metabolism, ventilation, and cardiac output begin to decline causing decreased cardiac output, which can lead to pulmonary edema, oliguria, areflexia, coma, hypotension, bradycardia, ventricular arrhythmias [including ventricular fibrillation], and asystole [Mechem & Zafren, 2014]).
- Circulating toxins (e.g., snake venom, alpha-naphthyl thiourea [rat poison inhaled])
- Systemic inflammatory response syndrome (SIRS)/sepsis (causes low cardiac output, low peripheral vascular pressure, and high pulmonary vascular resistance due to vasoconstriction, causing increased pulmonary congestion)

Collaborative Outcomes

The individual will be monitored for early signs and symptoms of pulmonary edema and will receive collaborative interventions if indicated to restore physiologic stability.

Indicators of Physiologic Stability

- Alert, calm, oriented
- Symmetrical, easy, rhythmic respirations

- Warm, dry skin
- Full breath sounds in all lobes
- No crackles and wheezing
- Usual color (for race)
- Refer to *Risk for Complications of Decreased Cardiac Output* for additional indicators.

Interventions and Rationales

Address the Overwhelming Terrifying Experience of Sudden, Critical Breathlessness

R: Individuals report breathlessness in terms of the feelings associated with bad episodes of breathlessness as distress, anxiety, panic, and fear of dying (Gysels & Higginson, 2011; Schneidman, Reinke, Donesky, & Carrieri-Kohlman, 2014).

- Validate how frighten he or she must be.
- Reassure the person and do not leave them alone.

   R: These strategies attempt to reduce anxiety/fear.

Elevate the Head of the Bed or Use Extra Pillows Under the Head and Shoulders

R: This position will decrease resistance to inspiration.

If Possible, Increase Air Flow Around Person (e.g., Fan, Open Window)

R: Increasing circulating cooler air can decrease breathlessness.

Monitor for Signs and Symptoms of Pulmonary Edema

- Dry, hacking cough, especially when lying down
- Confusion, sleepiness, and disorientation may occur in older people
- Dizziness, fainting, fatigue, or weakness
- Fluid buildup, especially in the legs, ankles, and feet
- Increased urination at night (Peripheral edema during the day returns to circulation when legs are elevated, resulting in nocturia.)
- Nausea, abdominal swelling, tenderness, or pain (may result from the buildup of fluid in the body and the backup of blood in the liver)
- Weight gain (Fluid accumulation increases weight.)
- Weight loss (Nausea causes a loss of appetite.)
- Rapid breathing, bluish skin, and feelings of restlessness, anxiety, and suffocation
- Shortness of breath and lung congestion
- Tiring easily
- Wheezing and spasms of the airways similar to asthma
- Jugular vein distention (JVD)
  - Persistent cough
  - Productive cough with frothy sputum
  - Cyanosis
  - Diaphoresis

   R: Impaired pumping of left ventricle accompanied by decreased cardiac output and increased pulmonary artery pressure produce pulmonary edema. Circulatory overload can result from the reduced size of the pulmonary vascular bed. Hypoxia causes increased capillary permeability that, in turn, causes fluid to enter pulmonary tissue. Venous pressure and pulmonary lungs become so congested with fluid that it affects the exchange of oxygen, which is considered pulmonary edema (Grossman & Porth, 2014). Some symptoms are caused by congestion in lungs from fluid accumulation.

Weigh Individual Daily

- Ensure accuracy by weighing at the same time every day on the same scale and with the individual wearing the same amount of clothing.

R: Daily weights and strict input and output (I&O) are vital in determining the effects of treatment and for early detections of fluid retention or worsening of condition.

Closely Monitor Urine Output Hourly

R: Decreased blood volume reduces blood to kidneys, which decreases the glomerular filtration rate (GFR) causing a decrease urine output. When blood flow to the kidneys is less than 20% to 25% of normal, ischemic damage occurs (Grossman & Porth, 2014). Decreased urine output is an early sign of bleeding or hypovolemia.

Monitor With Pulse Oximetry

R: This will provide for continuous monitoring of oxygen saturation.

Take Steps to Maintain Adequate Hydration While Avoiding Overhydration

R: Adequate hydration helps liquefy pulmonary secretions; overhydration can increase preload and worsen pulmonary edema.

Cautiously Administer Intravenous (IV) Fluids

• Consult with the physician/nurse practitioner if the ordered rate plus the PO intake exceeds 2 to 2.5 L/24 hr. Be sure to include additional IV fluids (e.g., antibiotics) when calculating the hourly allocation. Oral fluid intake must also be monitored and, if indicated, possibly restricted.

  R: Failure to regulate IV and oral fluids carefully can cause circulatory overload with worsening of the condition.

If Indicated, Administer Oxygen as Prescribed

R: Hypoxia produces increased capillary pressure, causing fluid to enter pulmonary tissue and triggering signs and symptoms of pulmonary edema.

Initiate Appropriate Treatments According to Protocol, Which May Include

• Diuretics

  R: To decrease preload

• Vasodilators

  R: To decrease preload and afterload

• Positive inotropics (e.g., digitalis)

  R: To enhance ventricular contractions

• Morphine

  R: To decrease anxiety, preload and afterload, and metabolic demands

Clinical Alert Report

Advise ancillary staff/student to report:
  • Any sudden onset of a change in usual condition as:
    • Increased peripheral edema
    • Increase in daily weight
    • Urine output <0.5 mL/kg/hr
  • Persistent cough or productive cough with frothy, pink-tinged sputum
  • Restlessness, agitation, decreased mentation
  • BP >200 mm Hg (systolic), >115 mm Hg (diastolic), <90 mm Hg (systolic)
  • Respirations >10/min over baseline, <10/min under baseline, labored
  • Pulse >100 resting
  • Temperature (oral) over 100.5° F
  • Pulse oximetry <90%
  • Diminished peripheral pulses
  • Cool, pale, moist, or cyanotic skin

RISK FOR COMPLICATIONS OF RESPIRATORY DYSFUNCTION

Risk for Complications of Atelectasis, Pneumonia
Risk for Complications of Hypoxemia

Definition

Describes a person experiencing or at high risk to experience various respiratory problems

Carp's Cues

The nurse uses the generic collaborative problem *Risk for Complications of Respiratory Dysfunction* to describe a person at risk for several types of respiratory problems and to identify the nursing focus—monitoring respiratory status for detection and diagnosis of abnormal functioning. Nursing management of a specific respiratory complication is then described under the appropriate collaborative problem for that complication. For example, a nurse using *Risk for Complications of Respiratory Dysfunction* for an individual in whom hypoxemia later develops would then add *Risk for Complications of Hypoxemia* to the individual's problem list. If the risk factors or etiology were not related directly to the primary medical diagnosis, the nurse would add this information to the diagnostic statement (e.g., *Risk for Complications of Hypoxemia* related to COPD in an individual with chronic obstructive pulmonary disease [COPD] who experiences respiratory problems after gastric surgery).

For a person vulnerable to respiratory problems because of immobility or excessive tenacious secretions, the nurse should apply the nursing diagnosis *Risk for Ineffective Respiratory Function* related to immobility rather than *Risk for Complications of Respiratory Dysfunction*.

For information on Focus Assessment Criteria, visit the**Point**.

Significant Laboratory/Diagnostic Assessment Criteria

- Blood pH (elevated in alkalosis, lowered in acidosis)
- Arterial blood gas (ABG) values:
  - pH (elevated in alkalemia, lowered in acidemia) (more commonly referred to as alkalosis and/or acidosis)
  - Pco_2 (elevated in pulmonary disease, lowered in hyperventilation)
  - Po_2 (lowered in pulmonary disease)
  - Co_2 content (elevated in COPD, lowered in hyperventilation)
- Sputum stain and culture
- Chest X-ray
- Pulmonary angiography
- Bronchoscopy
  - Thoracentesis
- Pulmonary function tests
- Ventilation/perfusion scanning
- Pulse oximetry
- End-tidal carbon monitoring ($ETCO_2$)

RISK FOR COMPLICATIONS OF ATELECTASIS, PNEUMONIA

Definition

Describes a person experiencing impaired respiratory functioning because of a complete or partial collapse of a lung or lobe of a lung, which can result in pneumonia[1]

---

[1]The nurse should use the nursing diagnosis *Risk for Ineffective Respiratory Function* for people at high risk for atelectasis and pneumonia, to focus on prevention. The collaborative problem *Risk for Complications of Atelectasis, Pneumonia* is applicable only if the condition occurs.

High-Risk Populations

- Mechanical ventilation
- Pulmonary edema
- Impaired swallowing (increased risk for aspiration)
- Shallow breathing (due to abdominal pain or rib fracture)
- Postoperative status (especially abdominal or thoracic surgery)
- Immobilization
- Decreased level of consciousness
- Nasogastric feedings
- Chronic lung disease (COPD, bronchiectasis, cystic fibrosis)
- Chronic heart, liver, or renal disease
- Diabetes mellitus
- Alcoholism
- Cancer
- Asplenia
- Immunosuppressed conditions or on immunosuppressing medications (within previous 3 months)
- Debilitation
- Decreased surfactant production
- Compression of lung tissue (e.g., from cancer, abdominal distention, obesity, pneumothorax)
- Airway obstruction
- Impaired ability to cough (e.g., poor cough reflex, too weak or in pain from recent surgery or an accident) or to cough vigorously

 ### Carp's Cues

Pneumonia can be classified as community acquired or hospital acquired. The following scoring helps to determine which individuals should be treated at home or admitted to the hospital.

CURB-65 uses five prognostic variables (Lim et al., 2003):
- Confusion (based on a specific mental test or disorientation to person, place, or time)
  - Urea (blood urea nitrogen in the United States) >7 mmol/L (20 mg/dL)
  - Respiratory rate ≥30 breaths/min
  - Blood pressure (systolic <90 mm Hg or diastolic ≤60 mm Hg)
  - Age ≥65 years
- "The authors (*Lim et al., 2003) of the original CURB-65 report suggested that patients with a CURB-65 score of 0 to 1, who comprised 45 percent of the original cohort and 61 percent of the later cohort, were at low risk and could probably be treated as outpatients. Those with a score of 2 should be admitted to the hospital, and those with a score of 3 or more should be assessed for care in the intensive care unit (ICU), particularly if the score was 4 or 5" (Bartlett, 2014).

Collaborative Outcomes

The individual will be monitored for early signs and symptoms of atelectasis and/or pneumonia, and the individual will receive collaborative interventions if indicated to restore physiologic stability.

Indicators of Physiologic Stability

- Alert, calm, oriented (baseline for individual)
- Respiratory rate 16 to 20 breaths/min
- Respirations easy, rhythmic
- Temperature 98° F to 99.5° F
- No change in usual skin color
- Pulse oximetry >95%

Interventions and Rationales

Evaluate the Individual's Risk for Mortality Using the CURB-65 Scale
(Bartlett, 2014; *Lim et al., 2003)

- One point is given for the presence of each of the following (Lim et al., 2003):
  - **C**onfusion—altered mental status
  - **U**remia—blood urea nitrogen (BUN) level >20 mg/dL
  - **R**espiratory rate—30 breaths or more per minute
  - **B**lood pressure—systolic pressure <90 mm Hg or diastolic pressure <60 mm Hg
  - Age older than 65 years

> **CLINICAL ALERT:**
> - Current guidelines suggest that individuals may be treated in an outpatient setting or may require hospitalization according to their CURB-65 score, as follows:
>   - Score of 0 to 1—Outpatient treatment
>   - Score of 2—Admission to medical unit
>   - Score of 3 or higher—Admission to intensive care unit (ICU)

Ensure Blood Culture Is Done Prior to the Start of Any Antibiotic

- Culture any suspected infection sites (urine, sputum, invasive lines).

  R: Poor outcomes are associated with inadequate or inappropriate antimicrobial therapy (i.e., treatment with antibiotics to which the pathogen was later shown to be resistant in vitro. They are also associated with delays in initiating antimicrobial therapy, even short delays (e.g., an hour) (Schmidt & Mandel, 2012).

> **CLINICAL ALERT:**
> - Blood culture obtained after antibiotic therapy has been initiated can be inaccurate. Research of individuals with septic shock demonstrated that the time to initiation of appropriate antimicrobial therapy was the strongest predictor of mortality (Schmidt & Mandel, 2012).

Monitor for Signs and Symptoms of Pneumonia, Atelectasis

- Increased respiratory rate >24 breaths/min (tachypnea) 45% to 70% frequency
- Fever (80% frequency) and chills (50%) (sudden or insidious)
- Productive cough with mucopurulent sputum
- Diminished or absent breath sounds
- Rales or crackles (30% frequency)
- Pleuritic chest pain (30% frequency)
- Marked dyspnea

  R: Bacteria can act as a pyrogen by raising the hypothalamic thermostat through the production of endogenous pyrogens, which may mediate through prostaglandins. Chills can occur when the temperature set point of the hypothalamus changes rapidly. High fever increases metabolic needs and oxygen consumption. The impaired respiratory system cannot compensate and tissue hypoxia results (Grosssman & Porth, 2014). In older adults, tachypnea >26 respirations/min is one of the earliest signs of pneumonia and often occurs 3 to 4 days before a confirmed diagnosis.

- Lethargy, change in mental status

  R: Delirium or mental status changes are often seen early in pneumonia in older individuals. Decreased blood flow to brain, heart, and kidneys triggers baroreceptors, and release of catecholamines increases heart rate/cardiac output, further increasing vasoconstriction (Grossman & Porth, 2014).

Monitor Laboratory and Other Diagnostic Tests

- White blood cells

  R: "The major blood test abnormality is leukocytosis (typically between 15,000 and 30,000 per mm³) with a leftward shift. Leukopenia can occur and generally connotes a poor prognosis" (Bartlett, 2014).

- Chest X-ray

    R: "The presence of an infiltrate on plain chest radiograph is considered the gold standard for diagnosing pneumonia when clinical and microbiologic features are supportive" (Bartlett, 2014).

Closely Monitor Individuals Over 65 Years of Age

R: Tracheobronchial inflammation, impaired alveolar capillary membrane function, edema, fever, and increased sputum production disrupt respiratory function and compromise the blood's oxygen-carrying capacity. Reduced chest wall compliance in older adults affects the quality of respiratory effort. In older adults, tachypnea (>26 respirations/min) is an early sign of pneumonia, often occurring 3 to 4 days before a confirmed diagnosis. Delirium or mental status changes are often seen early in pneumonia in older adults (Grossman & Porth, 2014).

Evaluate the Effectiveness of Cough Suppressants and Expectorants

R: A dry, hacking cough interferes with sleep and affects energy. Cough suppressants should be used judiciously, however, because complete depression of the cough reflex can lead to atelectasis by hindering movement of tracheobronchial secretions.

Monitor for Signs and Symptoms of Sepsis

R: Bacterial infections are the most common cause of sepsis. The infection can begin anywhere bacteria or other infectious agents can enter the body. Sepsis can be caused by skin laceration, appendicitis, pneumonia, or a urinary tract infection (Grossman & Porth, 2014).

- Altered body temperature (>38° C or <36° C)
- Hypotension (140/90, >90/60 mm Hg (MAP [mean arterial pressure] >70) (CVP >11)
- Decreased level of consciousness
- Weak, rapid pulse
- Rapid, shallow respirations or CO_2 <32

    R: Diminishing oxygen saturation as seen by pulse oximetry

- Cold, clammy skin
- Oliguria (urine output <0.5 mL/kg/hr)

    R: Sepsis is a systemic inflammatory response syndrome (SIRS) associated with infection because of microorganisms resulting in hypotension and perfusion abnormalities despite fluid resuscitation or vasopressors (Grossman & Porth, 2014).

> **CLINICAL ALERT:**
> - Immediate action is needed; call Rapid Response Team.

- Refer to *Risk for Complications of Systemic Inflammatory Response Syndrome (SIRS)/Sepsis*

RISK FOR COMPLICATIONS OF HYPOXEMIA

Definition

Describes a person experiencing or at high risk to experience insufficient plasma oxygen saturation (Po_2 less than normal for age) because of alveolar hypoventilation, pulmonary shunting, or ventilation–perfusion inequality

High-Risk Populations

- Heart failure
- COPD
- Asthma
- Acute lung injury
- Sepsis
- Pneumothorax
- Pleural effusion

- Pneumonia
- Atelectasis
- Pulmonary edema
- Adult respiratory distress syndrome
- Central nervous system depression
- Medulla or spinal cord disorders
- Guillain–Barré syndrome
- Myasthenia gravis
- Muscular dystrophy
- Obesity
- Compromised chest wall movement (e.g., trauma)
- Drug overdose
- Head injury
- Near-drowning
- Multiple trauma
- Anemia and/or hypovolemia
- Pulmonary embolism

Collaborative Outcomes

The individual will be monitored for early signs and symptoms of hypoxemia, and the individual will receive collaborative interventions if indicated to restore physiologic stability.

Indicators of Physiologic Stability

- Serum pH 7.35 to 7.45
- $Paco_2$ 35 to 45
- Pao_2 80 to 100
- Pulse: regular rhythm, rate 60 to 100 beats/min
- Respirations 16 to 20 breaths/min
- Blood pressure >90/60 mm Hg and <140/90 (MAP [mean arterial pressure] >70) (CVP >11)
- Urine output >30 mL/hr (use of a standardized volume that is weight based, e.g., >0.5 mL/kg/hr)

Interventions and Rationales

Identify High-Risk Individuals for Heart Failure (Boriaug, 2015)

- Systolic hypertension both with and without left ventricular hypertrophy (LVH)
- Aging
- Coronary heart disease
- Diabetes mellitus
- Sleep-disordered breathing
- Obesity
- Kidney disease

> *R: Classic heart failure with preserved ejection fraction (HFpEF) is typically associated with one or more of the above conditions (Boriaug, 2015).*

Monitor for Signs of Right-Sided Heart Failure

- Elevated diastolic pressure
- Distended neck veins
- Edema
- Elevated central venous pressure

> *R: The causes of right-sided heart failure are conditions that impede blood flow into the lungs. The heart must work harder to pump oxygen-rich blood throughout the body. The combination of arterial hypoxemia and respiratory acidosis acts locally as a strong vasoconstrictor of pulmonary vessels. This leads to pulmonary arterial hypertension, increased right ventricular systolic pressure, and, eventually, right ventricular hypertrophy and failure (Grossman & Porth 2014).*

Monitor for Signs of Acid–Base Imbalance

- ABG analysis: pH <7.35, $Paco_2$ >48 mm Hg

  R: ABG analysis helps evaluate gas exchange in the lungs. In mild to moderate COPD, the individual may have a normal $PaCO_2$ level as chemoreceptors in the medulla respond to increased $PaCO_2$ by increasing ventilation. In severe COPD, however, the individual cannot sustain this increased ventilation, and the $PaCO_2$ value gradually increases (Grossman & Porth, 2014).

- Increased and irregular pulse, and increased respiratory rate initially, followed by decreased rate

  R: Respiratory acidosis develops as a result of excessive CO_2 retention. An individual with respiratory acidosis from chronic disease at first experiences increased heart rate and respirations in an attempt to compensate for decreased oxygenation. After a while, he or she breathes more slowly and with prolonged expiration. Eventually, the respiratory center may stop responding to the higher CO_2 levels, and breathing may stop abruptly (Grossman & Porth, 2014).

- Changes in mentation (somnolence, confusion, irritability, anxiety)

  R: Changes in mentation result from cerebral tissue hypoxia.

- Decreased urine output (<0.5 mL/hr); cool, pale, or cyanotic skin

  R: The compensatory response to decreased circulatory oxygen aims to increase blood oxygen by increasing heart and respiratory rates and to decrease circulation to the kidneys and extremities (marked by decreased pulses and skin changes) (Grossman & Porth, 2014).

Administer Low-Flow (2 L/min) Oxygen as Needed Through Nasal Cannula; If Indicated, Titrate Up to Keep Pulse Oximetry Between 90% and 92%

R: Oxygen therapy increases circulating oxygen levels. Using a cannula rather than a mask may help reduce the individual's fears of suffocation.

Limit O_2 Flow to 1 to 2 L/min in Individuals With COPD

R: High concentrations of oxygen decrease the respiratory drive causing hypoventilation with increase in carbon dioxide ($PaCO_2$).

Evaluate the Effects of Positioning on Oxygenation, Using ABG Values as a Guide

- Change individual's position every 2 hours, avoiding positions that compromise oxygenation.

  R: This measure promotes optimal ventilation.

Ensure Adequate Hydration

- Teach individual to avoid dehydrating beverages (e.g., caffeinated drinks, grapefruit juice).

  R: Optimal hydration helps liquefy secretions. Avoid milk-based products.

Ensure Adequate Nutrition

- Advise to eat small, frequent meals.

  R: Small, frequent meals will be more comfortable and allow greater dietary intake. Individuals are often short of breath and fatigue while eating (Burns, 2014).

Refer to the Nursing Diagnosis *Activity Intolerance* in Unit II Section 1 for Specific Adaptive Techniques to Teach an Individual With Chronic Pulmonary Insufficiency

RISK FOR COMPLICATIONS OF METABOLIC/IMMUNE/ HEMATOPOIETIC DYSFUNCTION

Risk for Complications of Allergic Reaction
Risk for Complications of Electrolyte Imbalances
Risk for Complications of Hypo/Hyperglycemia
Risk for Complications of Systemic Inflammatory Response Syndrome (SIRS)/Sepsis

Definition

Describes a person experiencing or at high risk to experience various endocrine, immune, or metabolic dysfunctions

 ## Carp's Cues

The nurse can use this generic collaborative problem to describe a person at risk for several types of metabolic and immune system problems. For example, an individual with pituitary dysfunction who is at risk for various metabolic problems, using *Risk for Complications of Metabolic Dysfunction* directs nurses to monitor endocrine system function for specific problems, based on focus assessment findings. Under this collaborative problem, nursing interventions would focus on monitoring metabolic status to detect and diagnose abnormal functioning. If the individual developed a specific complication, the nurse would add the appropriate specific collaborative problem, along with nursing management information, to the individual's problem list. For an individual with diabetes mellitus, the nurse would add the diagnostic statement *Risk for Complications of Hypo/Hyperglycemia*. For an individual receiving chemotherapy, the nurse would use *Risk for Complications of Immunodeficiency*, a collaborative problem that encompasses leukopenia, thrombocytopenia, and erythrocytopenia. If thrombocytopenia were an isolated problem, it would warrant a separate diagnostic statement (i.e., *Risk for Complications of Thrombocytopenia*).

For an individual with a condition or undergoing a treatment that produces immunosuppression (e.g., acquired immunodeficiency syndrome [AIDS], graft-versus-host disease, immunosuppressant therapy), the collaborative problem *Risk for Complications of Immunosuppression* would be appropriate. When conditions have or possibly could have affected coagulation (e.g., chronic renal failure, alcohol abuse, anticoagulant therapy), a collaborative problem such as *Risk for Complications of Hemolysis* or *Risk for Complications of Erythrocytopenia* would be indicated. If the risk factors or etiology were not directly related to the primary medical diagnosis, they could be added (e.g., *Risk for Complications of Immunosuppression related to chronic corticosteroid therapy* in an individual who has sustained a myocardial infarction).

For information on Focus Assessment Criteria, visit thePoint

Significant Laboratory/Diagnostic Assessment Criteria

- Serum amylase (elevated in acute pancreatitis, lowered in chronic pancreatitis)
- Serum albumin (lowered in malnutrition)
- Lymphocyte count (lowered in malnutrition)
- Serum calcium (elevated in hyperparathyroidism, certain cancers, and acute pancreatitis, lowered in hypoparathyroidism)
- Blood pH (elevated in alkalosis, lowered in acidosis)
- Serum glucose (elevated in diabetes mellitus and pancreatic insufficiency, lowered in pancreatic islet cell tumors)
- Serum antidiuretic hormone (ADH) (elevated levels indicate syndrome of inappropriate antidiuretic hormone excretion [SIADH]), reduced levels indicate central diabetes insipidus)
- Urine specific gravity (reflects the kidneys' ability to concentrate and dilute urine)
- Serum osmolarity (represents concentration of particles in blood)
- Urine osmolarity (measures urine concentration—increased in Addison's disease, SIADH, dehydration renal disease; decreased in diabetes insipidus, psychogenic water drinking)
- Serum glycosylated hemoglobin (Hgb A1c) (reflects mean glucose levels for preceding 2 to 3 months)
- Urine acetone, urine glucose (present in diabetes mellitus)
- Urine ketone bodies (present in uncontrolled diabetes)
- Platelets (elevated in polycythemia and chronic granulocytic leukemia, lowered in anemia and acute leukemia)
- Immunoglobulins (elevated in autoimmune disease)
- Coagulation tests (elevated in thrombocytopenia, purpura, and hemophilia)
- Prothrombin time (elevated in anticoagulant therapy, cirrhosis, and hepatitis)
- Red blood cell (RBC) count (lowered in anemia, leukemia, and renal failure)
- Computed tomography (CT), magnetic resonance imaging (MRI) of targeted organ
- Bone marrow aspirate with diagnostic pathology
- Spinal tap with appropriate analysis, culture, and sensitivity

RISK FOR COMPLICATIONS OF ALLERGIC REACTION

Definition

Describes a person experiencing or at high risk to experience hypersensitivity and release of mediators to specific substances (antigens) and anaphylaxis. Type I hypersensitivities are Ig-E-mediated that develop upon exposure to the antigen. Common allergens are pollen proteins, house dust mites, animal dander, foods, household chemicals, and pharmaceutical agents. Depending on the site of entry, type I reactions may be localized as contact dermatitis or systemic as asthma and life-threatening anaphylaxis (Grossman & Porth, 2014).

High-Risk Populations

- History of allergies
- Asthma
- Immunotherapy
- Idiopathic anaphylaxis is more common (65%) in women (Greenberger, 2007)
- Individuals exposed to high-risk antigens:
  - Insect stings (e.g., bee, wasp, hornet, ant)
  - Animal bites/stings (e.g., stingray, snake, jellyfish)
  - Radiologic iodinated contrast media (e.g., used in arteriography, intravenous pyelography)
- Transfusion of blood and blood products
- High-risk individuals exposed to:
  - High-risk medications (e.g., aspirin, antibiotics, opiates, local anesthetics, animal insulin, chymopapain)
  - High-risk foods (e.g., peanuts, chocolate, eggs, seafood, shellfish, strawberries, milk)
  - Chemicals (e.g., floor waxes, paint, soaps, perfume, new carpets)

Collaborative Outcomes

The individual will be monitored for early signs and symptoms of allergic response and will receive collaborative interventions if indicated to restore physiologic stability.

Indicators of Physiologic Stability

- Calm, alert, oriented
- No complaints of urticaria or pruritus
- No complaints of tightness in throat
- No complaints of shortness of breath or wheezing

Interventions and Rationales

Review Allergy Profile Prior to Administrating Any Medications

Carefully Assess for History of Allergic Responses (e.g., Rashes, Difficulty Breathing)

R: Identifying a high-risk individual allows precautions to prevent anaphylaxis.

Screen Individual/Family for Hereditary Angioedema (HAE)

R: "Hereditary angioedema (HAE) is a rare disorder characterized by recurrent episodes of well-demarcated angioedema without urticaria, which most often affect the skin or mucosal tissues of the upper respiratory and gastrointestinal tracts. Although swelling resolves spontaneously in two to four days in the absence of treatment, laryngeal edema may cause fatal asphyxiation, and the pain of gastrointestinal attacks may be incapacitating" *(Atkinson, Cicardi, & Zuraw, 2014).*

> **CLINICAL ALERT:**
> - Determining that an allergic reaction is HAE is critical since the treatment needed targets specifically HAE. Plasma-derived C1INH is the best studied first-line therapy for acute episodes of angioedema in patients with HAE (Atkinson et al., 2014)

Assess for Sensitivities/Allergies to

- Foods, for example, most common food allergens are milk, eggs, peanuts, tree nuts, fish, shellfish, soy, and wheat, which account for over 90% of all food allergies. Foods commonly mistaken for IA include mustard and other spices (Burks, 2015).

    R: Food allergies are the commonest cause of anaphylaxis and occur in 1% to 2% of the population. Symptoms can start in minutes after ingestion, occasionally after 1 to 2 hours, but rarely any longer. Consider an alternative diagnosis if symptoms began many hours after ingestion or if the individual has since eaten the suspected food without any reaction (Auckland Allergy Clinic, 2012; Burks, 2015)

- Medications/drugs are another common cause of anaphylaxis.

    R: It is important to focus on drugs/supplements/herbal preparation (bee pollen, echinacea) and other over-the-counter formulations (especially aspirin and NSAIDs) in the history taking.

If the Individual has a History of Allergic Response, Consult With Physician/ Nurse Practitioner, or Physician Assistant Nurse Regarding Skin Tests, If Indicated

R: Skin testing can confirm hypersensitivity.

Monitor for Signs and Symptoms of Localized Allergic Reaction

- Wheals, flares (due to histamine release)
- Itching
- Nontraumatic edema (perioral, periorbital)

    R: The antigen–antibody reaction causes vasodilatation with pooling of blood (edema), histamine release (wheals, itching), and diminished perfusion to tissues followed by vascular and circulatory vasoconstriction (Burks, 2015).

At the First Sign of Hypersensitivity

- Consult with physician/nurse practitioner/physician assistant for pharmacologic intervention, such as epinephrine, corticosteroids, venous access. Follow protocol

    R: Establishing venous access prior to vasoconstriction is optimal for rapid medication administration. Epinephrine produces peripheral vasoconstriction, which raises blood pressure and acts as a β agonist to promote bronchial smooth muscle relaxation, and to enhance inotropic and chronotropic cardiac activity (Garzon, Kempker, & Piel, 2011).

Monitor for Signs and Symptoms of Systemic Allergic Reaction and Anaphylaxis (Simons, 2015)

- Anaphylaxis can cause symptoms throughout the body:
    - Skin—(occurs in 80% to 90% of reactions) itching, flushing, hives (urticaria), swelling (angioedema)
    - Eyes—itching, tearing, redness, swelling of the skin around the eyes
    - Nose and mouth—sneezing, runny nose, nasal congestion, swelling of the tongue, metallic taste
    - Lungs and throat—(occur in 70% of reactions) difficulty getting air in or out, repeated coughing, chest tightness, wheezing or other sounds of labored breathing, increased mucus production, throat swelling or itching, hoarseness, change in voice, sensation of choking
    - Heart and circulation—(occurs in 70% of reactions) dizziness, weakness, fainting, rapid, slow, or irregular heart rate, low blood pressure
    - Digestive system—nausea, vomiting, abdominal cramps, diarrhea
    - Nervous system—anxiety, confusion, sense of impending doom
- Light-headedness, skin flushing, angioedema, and slight hypotension result from histamine-induced vasodilation
- Throat or throat or palate tightness, wheezing, hoarseness, dyspnea, and chest tightness result from smooth muscle contraction from prostaglandin release
- Irregular increased pulse and decreased blood pressure result from leukotriene release, which constricts airways and coronary vessels
- Decreased level of consciousness, respiratory distress, and shock resulting from severe hypotension, respiratory insufficiency, and tissue hypoxia (Simons, 2015)

Promptly Initiate Emergency Protocol for Anaphylaxis and Access the Rapid Response Team Stat

> **CLINICAL ALERT:**
> - Progression from hives and itching to life-threatening symptoms of wheeze, loss of consciousness, and laryngeal edema may occur in 10 minutes to hours after onset (Grossman & Porth, 2014).
>   - "Anaphylaxis is an unpredictable condition. Many people who experience it have known allergies and some have *had* one or more allergic reactions previously. Others, who are not even aware that they have an allergy, can suddenly experience severe anaphylaxis. Even the first episode of anaphylaxis can be fatal" (Simons, 2015).

- Administer oxygen; establish a patent airway if indicated. Have suction available. Oropharyngeal intubation may be required.

  R: Laryngeal edema interferes with breathing.

Frequently Evaluate Response to Therapy

- Assess:
  - Vital signs
  - Level of consciousness
  - Lung sounds, peak flows
  - Cardiac function
  - Intake and output
  - ABG values

    R: Careful monitoring is necessary to detect complications of shock and identify the need for additional interventions (Garzon et al., 2011).

After Recovery, Discuss With the Individual and Family Preventive Measures for Anaphylaxis and the Need to Carry an Anaphylaxis Kit, Which Contains Injectable Epinephrine and Oral Antihistamines for Use in Self-Treating Allergic Reaction

- Stress the need to carry an anaphylaxis kit, which contains injectable epinephrine and oral antihistamines for use in self-treating allergic reaction and to seek emergency treatment.
- Have individual and family member practice with a nonactive demo autoinjector.
- Advise that serious reaction may require two injections.

  R: Demonstration of demo auto injectors explains the force needed to activate the auto injector and for the loud sound occurring with needle ejection is particularly helpful as many patients do not realize the force required to activate an auto injector, and are usually unaware and startled by the loud sound made as the needle ejects (Garzon et al., 2011).

Refer Individual/Family to Guidelines for the Diagnosis and Management of Food Allergy in the United States. More Information About Allergies, Accessed at https://www.niaid.nih.gov/topics/foodAllergy/clinical/Documents /FAguidelinesPatient.pdf

RISK FOR COMPLICATIONS OF ELECTROLYTE IMBALANCES

Risk for Complications of Hypokalemia
Risk for Complications of Hyperkalemia
Risk for Complications of Hyponatremia
Risk for Complications of Hypernatremia
Risk for Complications of Hypocalcemia
Risk for Complications of Hypercalcemia

Definition

Describes a person experiencing or at risk to experience a deficit or excess of one or more electrolytes

 Carp's Cues

For a person experiencing or at high risk to experience a deficit or excess in a single electrolyte, the diagnostic statement should specify the problem (e.g., Risk for Complications of Hypokalemia related to diuretic therapy). Usually collaborative problems do not need related factors unless they will add clarity.

High-Risk Populations

For Hypokalemia

- Crash dieting
- Diabetic ketoacidosis
- Metabolic or respiratory alkalosis
- Excessive intake of licorice
- Diuretic therapy
- Loss of gastrointestinal (GI) fluids (through excessive nasogastric suctioning, nausea, vomiting, or diarrhea)
- Steroid use
- Estrogen use
- Hyperaldosteronism
- Severe burns
- Decreased potassium intake
- Liver disease with ascites
- Renal tubular acidosis
- Malabsorption
- Severe catabolism
- Salt depletion
- Hemolysis
- Hypoaldosteronism
- Rhabdomyolysis
- Laxative abuse
- Villous adenoma
- Hyperglycemia
- Severe magnesium depletion

For Hyperkalemia

- Renal failure
- Excessive potassium intake (oral or IV)
- Cell damage (e.g., from burns, trauma, surgery)
- Crushing injuries
- Potassium-sparing diuretic use
- Adrenal insufficiency
- Lupus
- Sickle cell disease
- Post-transplant
- Chemotherapy
- Metabolic acidosis
- Transfusion of old blood
- Internal hemorrhage
- Hypoaldosteronism
- Acidosis
- Rhabdomyolysis

For Hyponatremia

- Water intoxication (oral or IV)
- Renal failure

- Gastric suctioning
- Vomiting, diarrhea
- Burns
- Potent diuretic use
- Excessive diaphoresis
- Excessive wound drainage
- Congestive heart failure
- Hyperglycemia
- Malabsorption syndrome
- Cystic fibrosis
- Addison's disease
- Psychogenic polydipsia
- Oxytocin administration
- Syndrome of inappropriate antidiuretic hormone (SIADH) (resulting from central nervous system [CNS] disorders, major trauma, malignancies, or endocrine disorders)
- Adrenal gland insufficiency
- Chronic illness (e.g., cirrhosis)
- Hypothyroidism (moderate, severe)

For Hypernatremia

- Older persons, infants
- Inadequate fluid intake
- Heat stroke
- Diarrhea
- Severe insensible fluid loss (e.g., through hyperventilation or sweating)
- Diabetes insipidus
- Excessive sodium intake (oral, IV, medications)
- Hypertonic tube feeding
- Coma
- High protein feeding with inadequate H_2O intake

For Hypocalcemia

- Renal failure (increased phosphorus)
- Protein malnutrition (e.g., due to malabsorption)
- Inadequate calcium intake
- Diarrhea
- Burns
- Malignancy
- Hypoparathyroidism
- Vitamin D deficiency
- Osteoblastic tumors

For Hypercalcemia

- Chronic renal failure
- Sarcoidosis and granulomatous disease
- Excessive vitamin D intake
- Hyperparathyroidism
- Decreased hypophosphatemia
- Bone tumors
- Cancers (Hodgkin's disease, myeloma, leukemia, neoplastic bone disease)
- Prolonged use of thiazide diuretics
- Paget's disease
- Parathyroid hormone-secreting tumors (e.g., lung, kidney)
- Hemodialysis
- Multiple fractures

- Prolonged immobilization
- Excessive calcium-containing antacids

Collaborative Outcomes

The individual will be monitored for early signs and symptoms of hypokalemia, hyponatremia, hyponatremia, hypercalcemia, or hypercalcemia and will receive collaborative interventions if indicated to restore physiologic stability.

Indicators of Physiologic Stability With Critical Value Alerts[2]
(Mayo, 2014; Stanford Medicine, 2009; Williamson & Snyder, 2014)

- Serum or plasma sodium: 135 to 145 mmol/L; alert levels: less than 120 ≥160 mmol/L
- Serum potassium: 3.6 to 5.4 mmol/L (plasma, 3.6 to 5.0 mmol/L); alert levels: less than 3.0 ≥6.0 mmol/L
- Serum or plasma chloride: 98 to 108 mmol/L
- Serum or plasma bicarbonate: 18 to 24 mmol/L (as total carbon dioxide, 22 to 26 mmol/L); alert levels: less than 10 and ≥40 mmol/L
- Serum calcium: 8.5 to 10.5 mg/dL (2.0 to 2.5 mmol/L); alert levels: less than 6.5 mg/dL and ≥13.0 mg/dL
- Ionized calcium: 1.0 to 1.3 mmol/L
- Serum phosphates 125 to 300 mg/dL
- Serum magnesium: 1.8 to 3.0 mg/dL (1.2 to 2.0 mEq/L or 0.5 to 1.0 mmol/L) alert level ≤1.0 and ≥9.0
- Osmolality (calculated) 280 to 300 mOsm/kg; alert levels: ≤190 mOsm/kg and ≥39

Interventions and Rationales

Identify the Electrolyte Imbalance(s) for Which the Individual is Vulnerable, and Intervene as Follows

- Refer to *High-Risk Populations* under the specific imbalance.

Risk for Complications of Hypo/Hyperkalemia

Monitor for Signs and Symptoms of Hyperkalemia

- Weakness to flaccid paralysis
- Muscle irritability
- Paresthesias
- Nausea, abdominal cramping, or diarrhea
- Oliguria
- Electrocardiograph (ECG) changes: tall, tented T waves, ST segment depression, prolonged PR interval (>0.2 seconds), first-degree heart block, bradycardia, broadening of the QRS complex, eventual ventricular fibrillation, and cardiac standstill (Grossman & Porth, 2014)

  R: Hyperkalemia can result from the kidneys' decreased ability to excrete potassium or from excessive potassium intake. Acidosis increases the release of potassium from cells. Fluctuations in potassium level affect neuromuscular transmission, producing cardiac arrhythmias, and reducing action of GI smooth muscle. There is an increase in cardiac irritability, and cardiac monitoring may show early changes as premature ventricular beats.

Monitor for Signs and Symptoms of Hypokalemia

- Weakness or flaccid paralysis
- Decreased or absent deep tendon reflexes
- Hypoventilation, change in consciousness
- Polyuria
- Hypotension
- Paralytic ileus
- ECG changes: Visible U wave, ST depression and flattening of the T wave, inverted T waves (DeJong, Patiwael, de Groot, Burdorf, & van Wijk, 2014)

[2]Critical values are defined as values that are outside the normal range to a degree that may constitute an immediate health risk to the individual or require immediate action (Stanford Medicine, 2009).

- Nausea, vomiting, anorexia

  R: Hypokalemia results from losses associated with vomiting, diarrhea, or diuretic therapy, or from insufficient potassium intake. Hypokalemia impairs neuromuscular transmission and reduces the efficiency of respiratory muscles. Kidneys are less sensitive to antidiuretic hormone and thus excrete large quantities of dilute urine. GI smooth muscle action also is reduced. Abnormally low potassium levels also impair electrical conduction of the heart (Grossman & Porth, 2014).

Risk for Complications of Hypo/Hypernatremia

Monitor for Signs and Symptoms of Hyponatremia

- CNS effects ranging from lethargy to coma, headache
- Weakness
- Abdominal pain
- Muscle twitching or convulsions
- Nausea, vomiting, diarrhea
- Apprehension

  R: Hyponatremia results from sodium loss through vomiting, diarrhea, or diuretic therapy; excessive fluid intake; or insufficient dietary sodium intake. Cellular edema, caused by osmosis, produces cerebral edema, weakness, and muscle cramps.

Monitor for Signs and Symptoms of Hypernatremia with Fluid Overload

- Thirst, decreased urine output
- CNS effects ranging from agitation to convulsions
- Elevated serum osmolality
- Weight gain, edema
- Elevated blood pressure
- Tachycardia

  R: Hypernatremia results from excessive sodium intake or increased aldosterone output. Water is pulled from the cells, causing cellular dehydration and producing CNS symptoms. Thirst is a compensatory response to dilute sodium.

Risk for Complications of Hypo/Hypercalcemia

Monitor for Signs and Symptoms of Hypocalcemia

- Altered mental status
- Numbness or tingling in fingers and toes
- Muscle cramps
- Seizures
- ECG changes: prolonged QT interval, prolonged ST segment, and arrhythmias
- Chvostek's or Trousseau's sign
- Tetany

  R: Hypocalcemia can result from the kidneys' inability to metabolize vitamin D (needed for calcium absorption). Retention of phosphorus causes a reciprocal drop in serum calcium level. A low serum calcium level produces increased neural excitability, resulting in muscle spasms (cardiac, facial, extremities) and CNS irritability (seizures). It also causes cardiac muscle hyperactivity, as evidenced by ECG changes.

- Assess for hyperphosphatemia or hypomagnesemia.

  R: Hyperphosphatemia inhibits calcium absorption; in hypomagnesemia, the kidneys excrete calcium to retain magnesium (Grossman & Porth, 2014).

Monitor for Signs and Symptoms of Hypercalcemia

- Altered mental status
- Anorexia, nausea, vomiting, constipation
- Numbness or tingling in fingers and toes

- Muscle cramps, hypotoxicity
- Deep bone pain
- AV blocks (ECG)

   R: Insufficient calcium level reduces neuromuscular excitability, resulting in decreased muscle tone, numbness, anorexia, and mental lethargy (Burns, 2014)

RISK FOR COMPLICATIONS OF HYPO/HYPERGLYCEMIA

Definition

Describes a person experiencing or at high risk to experience a blood glucose level that is too low (less than 50 mg/dL) (*Field, 1989) or too high (over 200 mg/dL) for metabolic function. A person with a consistent range between 100 and 126 mg/dL is considered hyperglycemic.

Carp's Cues

In 2006, NANDA approved the nursing diagnosis *Risk for Unstable Blood Sugar.* This author defines this condition as a collaborative problem. The nurse can choose which terminology is preferred. The student should consult with the instructor for direction. *If the person is not at risk for both, the diagnosis should specify the problem (e.g., Risk for Complications of Hyperglycemia related to corticosteroid therapy).*

High-Risk Populations

- Diabetes mellitus
- Parenteral nutrition
- Systemic inflammatory response syndrome (SIRS)/sepsis
- Enteral feedings
- Medications
- Hyperglycemia > corticosteroid therapy, acute response to stimulants as amphetamine, some psychotropic medications such as Zyprexa (olanzapine) and Cymbalta (duloxetine).
- Hypoglycemia > chronic use of stimulants
- Hypoglycemia
  - Excess alcohol intake
  - Pancreatic tumor > insulinoma
  - Lack (deficiency) of a hormone, such as cortisol or thyroid hormone
  - Severe heart, kidney, or liver failure or a body-wide infection
  - Some types of weight-loss surgery
- Pancreatitis (hyperglycemia), cancer of pancreas
- Addison's disease (hypoglycemia)
- Adrenal gland hyperfunction
- Liver disease (hypoglycemia)

Collaborative Outcomes

The individual will be monitored for early signs and symptoms of hyperglycemia and/or hypoglycemia and will receive collaborative interventions if indicated to restore physiologic stability.

Indicators of Physiologic Stability

- pH 7.35 to 7.45 and HCO_3 18 to 22 mmol/L
- Fasting blood glucose 70 to 130 mg/dL; No ketones in urine
- Serum sodium 135 to 145 mmol/L
- Serum osmolality >295 mOsm/kg
- Blood pressure <130/80 clear, oriented

- Pulse 60 to 100 beats/min
- Respiration 16 to 20 breaths/min
- Peripheral pulses, equal and full, capillary refill <3 seconds
- Warm, dry skin
- No vision changes
- Bowel sounds, present
- White blood cells 4,000 to 10,800 mm
- Urine, protein-negative
- Creatinine 0.8 to 1.3 mg/dL
- Blood urea nitrogen 5 to 25 mg/dL

Interventions and Rationales

Carp' Cues

Many labs and institutions require a repeat of or a second method of validation for treatment of "Critical Lab Values." The organizations define them and require them even for Point of Care (POC) testing for blood glucose values.

DKA is characterized by ketoacidosis and hyperglycemia, while hyperosmolar hyperglycemic state (HHS) usually has more severe hyperglycemia but no ketoacidosis. Each represents an extreme in the spectrum of hyperglycemia (Kitabchi, Hirsch, & Emmett, 2015)

Identify Individual at High Risk for Diabetic Ketoacidosis (DKA)

- Inadequate insulin treatment or noncompliance
- New onset diabetes (20% to 25%)
- Acute illness: Infection, frequently urinary, pneumonia (30% to 40%). Cerebral vascular accident. Myocardial infarction. Acute pancreatitis
- Drugs: Clozapine or olanzapine, cocaine, lithium, terbutaline

    R: A precipitating event can usually be identified in individuals with DKA or hyperosmolar HHS.

Identify Individuals at High Risk for HHS

- Previously undiagnosed diabetes
- Inadequate insulin treatment or noncompliance (21% to 41%)
- Acute illness: cardiac, endocrine, pulmonary, gastrointestinal infection (32% to 60%)
- Hypothermia
- Heat stroke
- Medications (e.g., β-adrenergic blockers, calcium-channel blockers, chlorpromazine, cimetidine, phenytoin)
- Propranolol
- Steroids
- Thiazide diuretics
- Total parenteral nutrition

Monitor for Signs and Symptoms of DKA With Type 1 Diabetes

- Recent illness/infection
- Blood glucose >300 mg/dL
- Malaise and generalized weakness
- Moderate/large ketones
- Dehydration
- Anorexia, nausea, vomiting, abdominal pain
- Kussmaul's respirations (shallow, rapid)
- Fruity acetone odor of the breath
- pH <7.30 and HCO_3 <15 mEq

- Decreased sodium, potassium, phosphates

    R: When insulin is not available, blood glucose (BG) levels rise and the body metabolizes fat for energy; the byproduct of this fat metabolism is ketones. Excessive ketone bodies results in ketoacidosis and a drop in pH and bicarbonate serum levels. This acidosis causes headaches, nausea, vomiting, and abdominal pain. Increased respiratory rate helps CO_2 excretion in effort to reduce acidosis. Elevated glucose levels inhibit water reabsorption in the renal glomerulus, leading to osmotic diuresis with loss of water, sodium, potassium, and phosphates, leading to severe dehydration and electrolyte imbalance (Vasudevan, Baheti, Naber, & Fredericson, 2012).

Monitor for Signs and Symptoms of HHS

- Blood glucose >600 mg/dL
- pH >7.30 and HCO_3 >15 mEq/L
- Severe dehydration
- Serum osmolality >320 mOsm/kg
- Hypotension, tachycardia
- Altered sensorium, lethargy
- Nausea, vomiting
- Urine ketones negative or <2+

    R: Hyperosmolar hyperglycemic state is marked by profound dehydration and hyperglycemia without ketoacidosis. Decreased renal clearance and utilization of glucose result in an osmotic dieresis and osmotic shift of fluid to the intravascular space, resulting in intracellular dehydration and loss of electrolytes. Cerebral impairment is due to this intracellular dehydration (Hemphill, 2012).

Monitor for Signs and Symptoms of Hypoglycemia

- Blood glucose <70 mg/dL
- Pale, moist, cool skin
- Tachycardia, diaphoresis
- Jitteriness, irritability
- Confusion
- Drowsiness
- Hypoglycemia unawareness

    R: Hypoglycemia unawareness is a defect in the body's defense system that impairs the ability to experience the warning symptoms usually associated with hypoglycemia. The individual may rapidly progress from being alert to unconsciousness.

> **CLINICAL ALERT:**
> - Hypoglycemia is defined as any BG <70 mg/dL and may be caused by too much insulin, too little food, or too much physical activity. Hypoglycemia symptoms are related to sympathetic system stimulation and brain dysfunction related to decreased levels of glucose. Sympathoadrenal activation and release of adrenaline causes diaphoresis, cool skin, tachycardia, anxiety, and jitteriness. Reduction in cerebral glucose will result in confusion, difficulty with concentration, focal impairments, and if severe, can cause seizures and eventually coma and death (Hamdy, 2012).

Institute "Rule of 15" With a Goal to Achieve BG >100 mg/dL

- If the individual is alert and cooperative: give 15 g of carbohydrate orally and monitor for 15 minutes; repeat BG—if above 100 mg/dL may give light snack if not time for a meal. If not above 70 mg/dL, repeat treatment with 15 g of carbohydrate—monitor and recheck BG in 15 minutes and may repeat until at goal.
- Nonalert individual: Call for Help—if IV access, give 24 g dextrose (1 amp D50); if none, give 1 mg glucagon IM, monitor for 15 minutes, and repeat BG; may repeat treatment q15 to 30 minutes depending on response.
- If hypoglycemia is severe (BG <40), recurrent, or caused by sulfonylurea or long-acting insulin, follow D50 treatment with D5 or D10 drip.

Continued Follow-Up is Mandatory Until Individual is Stable. Cause of the Hypoglycemia Should Always be Investigated (Inzucchi, 2012)

R: It is important to raise blood sugar with a goal of >100 mg/dL without causing hyperglycemia. Nonalert individual requires a rapid response.

Continue to Monitor Hydration Status Every 30 Minutes

- Assess skin moisture and turgor, urine output and specific gravity, and fluid intake.

  R: Accurate assessments are needed during the acute stage (first 10 to 12 hours) to prevent overhydration or underhydration.

Continue to Monitor Blood Glucose Levels According to Protocol

R: Careful monitoring enables early detection of medication-induced hypoglycemia or continued hyperglycemia.

Monitor Serum Potassium, Sodium, and Phosphate Levels

R: Acidosis causes hyperkalemia and hyponatremia. Insulin therapy promotes potassium and phosphate return to the cells, causing serum hypokalemia and hypophosphatemia.

Monitor Neurologic Status Every Hour

R: Fluctuating glucose levels, acidosis, and fluid shifts can affect neurologic functioning.

Carefully Protect Individual's Skin From Microorganism Invasion, injury, and Shearing Force; Reposition Every 1 to 2 Hours

R: Dehydration and tissue hypoxia increase the skin's vulnerability to injury.

Do Not Allow a Recovering Individual to Drink Large Quantities of Water

- Give a conscious individual ice chips to quench thirst.

  R: Excessive fluid intake can cause abdominal distension and vomiting.

Monitor Cardiac Function and Circulatory Status

- Evaluate:
  - Rate, rhythm (cardiac, respiratory)
  - Skin color
  - Capillary refill time, central venous pressure
  - Peripheral pulses
  - Serum potassium

    R: Severe dehydration can cause reduced cardiac output and compensatory vasoconstriction. Cardiac arrhythmias can result from potassium imbalances.

Follow Protocols for Ketoacidosis, as Indicated

Investigate for Causes of Ketoacidosis or Hypoglycemia, and Teach Prevention and Early Management

- Refer to Care Plan for Diabetes Mellitus in Unit III for teaching content.

RISK FOR COMPLICATIONS OF SYSTEMIC INFLAMMATORY RESPONSE SYNDROME (SIRS)/SEPSIS

Definition of Risk for Complications of Systemic Inflammatory Response Syndrome (SIRS)

Describes a person experiencing or at high risk to experience a life-threatening condition related to dysregulated systemic inflammation, organ dysfunction, and organ failure in response to both infectious processes (sepsis) and noninfectious insults, such as an autoimmune disorder, pancreatitis, vasculitis, and thromboembolism. The microorganisms may or may not be present in the bloodstream. SIRS has replaced the terminology *septic syndrome*. Sepsis is one contributing factor to SIRS (Neviere, 2016).

Definition of Risk for Complications of Sepsis

Describes a person experiencing or at risk for experiencing a loss of circulatory volume (hypovolemia) and impaired perfusion caused by an infectious agent (bacterial, viral) resulting in compromised tissue perfusion and cellular dysfunction (Neviere, 2016).

High-Risk Populations

- Bacterial infection (urinary, respiratory, wound)
- Viral infection
- Complication of surgery (GI, thoracic)
- Drug overdose
    - Burns, multiple trauma
    - Immunosuppression, AIDS
- Invasive lines (urinary, arterial, endotracheal, or central venous catheter)
- Pressure ulcers
    - Extensive slow-healing wounds
    - Immunocompromised (transplants, cancer, chemotherapy, AIDS, cirrhosis, pancreatitis)
- Diabetes mellitus
- Extreme age (<1 year and >65 years)

Collaborative Outcomes

The individual will be monitored for early signs and symptoms of septic shock and will receive collaborative interventions if indicated to restore physiologic stability.

Indicators of Physiologic Stability (Neviere, 2016)

- Alert
- No edema
- Temperature 98° F to 99.5° F
- Pulse 60 to 100 beats/min
- Capillary refill <2 seconds
- Urine output >0.5mL/kg/hr
- Urine specific gravity 1.005 to 1.030
- White blood count greater than 4,000 cells/mm^3 or less than 12,000 cells/mm^3
- Less than 10% immature neutrophils (band forms)
- Activated protein C (APC) 65 to 135 International Units/dL
- Platelets 150 to 400
- Prothrombin time 11 to 13.5 seconds
- INR 1.5 to 2.5

- Partial thromboplastin time (PTT) 30 to 45 seconds
- Serum potassium 3.5 to 5.0 mEq/L
- Serum sodium 135 to 145 mEq/L
- Blood glucose (fasting) <100 mg/dL
- Serum lactate levels 1.0 to 2.5 mmol/L
- Plasma C-reactive protein <0.8 mg/L
- Plasma procalcitonin >the normal value

Interventions and Rationales

Monitor for Septic Shock and SIRS (Halloran, 2009; Neviere, 2016)

- Urine output <0.5 mL/kg/hr

  R: Urine output is decreased when sodium shifts into the cells, which pulls water into cells. Decreased circulation to kidneys reduces their ability to detoxify the toxins that result from anaerobic metabolism (Grossman & Porth, 2014).

- Body temperature greater than 38° C or less than 36° C
- Heart rate greater than 90/min

  R: High heart rate decreases blood flow to brain, heart, and kidneys.

- Triggers baroreceptors and release of catecholamines, increasing heart rate/cardiac output and further increasing vasoconstriction
- Hyperkalemia

  R: Potassium moves into the cell with the sodium, impairing nervous, cardiovascular, and muscle cell function.

- Decreasing blood pressure

  R: Movement of water into the cell causes hypovolemia.

- Respiratory rate greater than 20/min

  R: Anaerobic metabolism decreases circulating oxygen. The body attempts to/increase oxgenation by increasing respiratory rate.

- Hyperglycemia

  R: The liver and kidneys produce more glucose in response to the release of epinephrine, norepinephrine, cortisol, and glucagon. Anaerobic metabolism reduces the effects of insulin. Insulin resistance contributes to multiple organ failure, nosocomial infection, and renal injury (Ball, deBeer, Gomm, Hickman, & Collins, 2007).

- White blood cell count greater than 12,000/µL or less than 4,000/µL or presence of 10% immature neutrophils

  R: Increased white cells indicate an infectious process.

- Plasma C-reactive protein more than two standard deviations above the normal value
- Plasma procalcitonin more than two standard deviations above the normal value

  R: CRP is increased by inflammatory disease as well as infection and is therefore not a good indicator of infection in patients with severe SIRS. PCT level is useful for diagnosis of sepsis and as an indicator of severity of organ failure in patients with SIRS (Kibel, Adams, & Barlow, 2011)

Ensure That Blood Culture is Done Prior to the Start of any Antibiotic

- Culture any suspected infection sites (e.g., urine, sputum, invasive lines).

  R: "Poor outcomes are associated with inadequate or inappropriate antimicrobial therapy (i.e., treatment with antibiotics to which the pathogen was later shown to be resistant in vitro. They are also associated with delays in initiating antimicrobial therapy, even short delays (e.g., an hour)" (Schmidt & Mandel, 2012)

> **CLINICAL ALERT:**
> - Blood culture obtained after antibiotic therapy has been initiated can be inaccurate. Research of individuals with septic shock demonstrated that the time to initiation of appropriate antimicrobial therapy was the strongest predictor of mortality (Schmidt & Mandel, 2012).

Assess Fluid Status

- Monitor CVP and follow protocol for fluid replacement.
- Early goal directed therapy (EGDT) with fluid replacement improves cardiac output, tissue perfusion, and oxygen delivery, improving mortality and morbidity.

  R: Sepsis causes vasodilation and capillary leak, resulting in hypovolemia.

Monitor Blood Pressure

- Administer replacement fluids and vasopressors (especially norepinephrine) to maintain mean arterial pressure (MAP) >65.

  *R: In EGDT, maintaining MAP >65 improves tissue perfusion and outcomes (*Picard, Donoghue, Young-Kershaw, & Russell, 2006).*

Assess for Evidence of Adequate Tissue Perfusion

- Heart rate
- Respirations
- Urine output
- Mentation
- $Scvo_2/Svo_2$

Monitor Older Adults for Changes in Mentation

- Weakness
- Malaise
- Normothermia or hypothermia
- Anorexia

  R: These individuals do not exhibit the typical signs of infection. Usual presenting findings—fever, chills, tachypnea, tachycardia, and leukocytosis—frequently are absent in older adults with significant infection (Neviere, 2016)

RISK FOR COMPLICATIONS OF RENAL/URINARY DYSFUNCTION

Risk for Complications of Acute Urinary Retention
Risk for Complications of Renal Calculi
Risk for Complications of Renal Insufficiency

Definition

Describes a person experiencing or at high risk to experience various renal or urinary tract dysfunctions

Carp's Cues

The nurse can use this generic collaborative problem to describe a person at risk for several types of renal or urinary problems. For such an individual (e.g., an individual in a critical care unit, who is vulnerable to various renal/urinary problems), using *Risk for Complications of Renal/Urinary Dysfunction* directs nurses to monitor renal and urinary status, based on the focus assessment, to detect and diagnose abnormal functioning. Nursing management of a specific renal or urinary complication would be addressed under the collaborative problem applying to the specific complication. For example, a standard of care for an individual recovering from coronary bypass surgery could contain the collaborative problem *Risk for Complications of Renal /Urinary Dysfunction*, directing the nurse to monitor renal and urinary status. If urinary retention developed in this individual, the nurse would add *Risk for Complications of Urinary Retention* to the problem list, along with specific nursing interventions to manage this problem. If the risk factors or etiology were not directly related to the primary medical diagnosis, the nurse still would specify them in the diagnostic statement (e.g., *Risk for Complications of Renal Insufficiency* related to chronic renal failure in an individual who has sustained a myocardial infarction).

Keep in mind that the nurse must differentiate those problems in bladder function that nurses can treat primarily as nursing diagnoses (e.g., incontinence, chronic urinary retention) from those that nurses manage using both nurse-prescribed and physician-prescribed interventions (e.g., acute urinary retention).

Significant Laboratory/Diagnostic Assessment Criteria
(MacGregor & Methven, 2011)

- Serum chemistries
- Albumin, prealbumin, and serum (lowered in renal disease)
- Amylase (elevated with renal insufficiency)
- Blood urea nitrogen (BUN) (elevated in acute or chronic renal failure)
- Calcium (lowered in uremic acidosis)
- Chloride (elevated with renal tubular acidosis)
- Creatinine (elevated with kidney disease)
- Magnesium (lowered in chronic nephritis)
- pH, base excess, bicarbonate (lowered in metabolic acidosis, elevated in metabolic alkalosis)
- Phosphorus (elevated with chronic glomerular disease, lowered with renal tubular acidosis)
- Potassium (elevated in renal failure, lowered with chronic diuretic therapy, renal tubular acidosis)
- Proteins (total, albumin, globulin) (lowered in nephritic syndrome)
- Sodium (elevated with nephritis, lowered with chronic renal insufficiency)
- Uric acid (elevated with chronic renal failure)
- Complete blood count
- Hemoglobin (lowered in chronic renal disorders)
- MCHC—normal or lowered with accompanying iron deficiency anemia
- MCV—normal or lowered with accompanying iron deficiency anemia
- White blood cell (WBC) count (elevated with acute infection)
- Urine
- Blood
  - Acute—present with hemorrhagic cystitis, renal calculi, renal, bladder tumors
  - Chronic—glomerular damage
- White blood cell (WBC) count (elevated with infection, obstruction). Obtain clean catch sample.
- Creatinine (elevated in acute/chronic glomerulonephritis, nephritis, lowered in advanced degeneration of kidneys)
- pH (decreased with metabolic acidosis, increased with metabolic alkalosis)
- Specific gravity (elevated with dehydration, lowered with overhydration, renal tubular disease)
- Protein to creatinine ratio (>200 mg/g is positive) or albumin to creatinine ratio (>30 mg/g is positive). Obtain random urine sample.
- Urine sodium and osmolarity (level depends on type—acute/chronic and site of kidney injury—prerenal or intrarenal)
- Culture and sensitivity—positive in infection
- 24-hour urine creatinine clearance—used in unstable clinical situations or to confirm clearance
- Imaging studies
- Helical non-contrast computerized tomography (CT) or ultrasonography
- Renal ultrasound—normal renal size 9 to 10 cm
- Magnetic resonance imaging for evaluating mass or cyst
- Kidneys, ureters, bladder x-ray—evaluating for overall size and obstructions
- Renal biopsy—diagnose specific kidney disease to determine treatment options
- Renal angiography—evaluate for stenosis

RISK FOR COMPLICATIONS OF ACUTE URINARY RETENTION

Definition

Describes a person experiencing or at high risk to experience an acute abnormal accumulation of urine in the bladder and the inability to void due to a temporary situation (e.g., postoperative status) or to a condition reversible with surgery (e.g., prostatectomy) or medication

High-Risk Populations (Barrisford & Steele, 2015; Selius & Subedi, 2008)

Acute urinary retention is most often secondary to obstruction, but may also be related to trauma, medication, neurologic disease, infection, and occasionally psychological issues

- Postoperative status (e.g., surgery of the perineal area, lower abdomen)
- Postpartum status
- Benign masses (e.g., fibroids)
- Malignant tumors of the pelvis, urethra, or vagina
- Postpartum vulvar edema
- Anxiety
- Prostate enlargement, prostatitis, prostate cancer
- Medication side effects (e.g., atropine, antidepressants, antihistamines)
- Postarteriography status
  - Bladder outlet obstruction (infection, tumor, calculi/stone, constipation, urethral stricture, perianal abscess)
  - Impaired detrusor contractility(spinal cord injuries, progressive neurologic diseases, diabetic neuropathy, cerebrovascular accidents)
  - Malignancy—bladder neoplasm, other tumors causing spinal cord compression
  - Other infections—genital herpes, varicella zoster, infected foreign bodies

Collaborative Outcomes

The individual will be monitored for early signs and symptoms of acute urinary retention and receive collaborative intervention to restore physiologic stability.

Indicators of Physiologic Stability

- Urinary output >1,500 mL/24 hr
- Can verbalize bladder fullness
- No complaints of lower abdominal pressure

Interventions and Rationales

Monitor a Postoperative Individual for Urinary Retention

R: Trauma to the detrusor muscle and injury to the pelvic nerves during surgery can inhibit bladder function. Anxiety and pain can cause spasms of the reflex sphincters. Bladder neck edema can cause retention. Sedatives and narcotics can affect the CNS and effectiveness of smooth muscles (Grossman & Porth, 2014; Urinary Retention, 2012).

Monitor for Urinary Retention by Palpating and Percussing the Suprapubic Area for Signs of Bladder Distention (Overdistention, etc.)

- Instruct individual to report bladder discomfort or inability to void.

  R: These problems may be early signs of urinary retention.

If Individual Does Not Void Within 8 to 10 Hours After Surgery or Complains of Bladder Discomfort, Take the Following Steps

- Warm the bedpan.
- Encourage individual to get out of bed to use the bathroom, if possible.
- Instruct a man to stand when urinating, if possible. If unable to stand, even sitting at the side of the bed helps.
- Run water in the sink as individual attempts to void.
- Pour warm water over individual's perineum.

  R: These measures help promote relaxation of the urinary sphincter and facilitate voiding.

After the First Voiding Postsurgery, Continue to Monitor and to Encourage Individual to Void Again in 1 Hour or So

R: The first voiding usually does not empty the bladder completely.

If the Individual Still Cannot Void After 10 hours, Follow Protocols for Straight Catheterization, as Ordered by Physician/Nurse Practitioner/Physician Assistant

* Consider bladder scanning to determine if the amount of urine in the bladder necessitates catheterization.

  R: Straight catheterization is preferable to indwelling catheterization because it carries less risk of urinary tract infection from ascending pathogens. Bladder scanning is not a risk for infection.

> **CLINICAL ALERT:**
> * If person is voiding small amounts, use straight catheterization; if postvoid residual is >200 mL, leave catheter indwelling. Notify physician/nurse practitioner/physician assistant.

> ***Clinical Alert Report***
>
> Prior to providing care, advice ancillary staff/student to report the following to the professional nurse assigned to the individual:
> * Inability to void
> * Voiding small quantities

RISK FOR COMPLICATIONS OF RENAL CALCULI

Definition

Describes a person with or at high risk for development of a solid concentration of mineral salts in the urinary tract

High-Risk Populations (Curhan, Aronson, & Preminger, 2015)

* History of renal calculi
* Family history of renal calculi
* Urinary infection
* Urinary stasis, obstruction
* Immobility
* Hypercalcemia (dietary)
* Enhanced enteric oxalate absorption (e.g., gastric bypass procedures, bariatric surgery, short bowel syndrome).
* Medications that may crystallize in the urine such as indinavir, acyclovir, sulfadiazine, and triamterene
* Low fluid intake is associated with increased stone risk
* A persistently acidic urine promotes uric acid precipitation (e.g., chronic diarrheal states, volume depletion leading to a concentrated acid urine, or with other metabolic defects, including gout, diabetes, insulin resistance, and obesity.
* Struvite stones form with an upper urinary tract infection due to a urease-producing organism such as Proteus or Klebsiella
* Conditions that cause hypercalcemia
  * Hyperparathyroidism
  * Renal tubular acidosis (decreased serum bicarbonate)
  * Myeloproliferative disease (leukemia, polycythemia vera, multiple myeloma)
  * Excessive excretion of uric acid
  * Inflammatory bowel disease
  * Gout
  * Dehydration

Collaborative Outcomes

The individual will be monitored for early signs and symptoms of renal calculi and the individual will receive collaborative interventions as indicated to restore physiologic stability.

Indicators of Physiologic Stability

- Temperature 98° F to 99.5° F
- Urine output >1,500 mL/24 hr
- Urine specific gravity 1.005 to 1.030
- Blood urea nitrogen 5 to 25 mg/dL
- Clear urine
- No flank pain

Interventions and Rationales

Monitor for Signs and Symptoms of Calculi

- Increased or decreased urine output
- Sediment in urine
- Flank or loin pain
- Hematuria(with symptomatic nephrolithiasis and also often present in asymptomatic individuals)
- Abdominal pain, distention, nausea, vomiting, diarrhea
- Flank pain or tenderness, ipsilateral testicle or labium.
- Dysuria, and urgency (when the stone is located in the distal ureter)

   R: Upper ureteral or renal pelvic obstruction lead to flank pain or tenderness, whereas lower ureteral obstruction causes pain that may radiate to the ipsilateral (same side as calcili) testicle or labium. Calculi-stimulating renointestinal reflexes can cause GI symptoms (Curhan et al., 2015)

Strain Urine to Obtain a Stone Sample; Send Samples to the Laboratory for Analysis

R: Acquiring a stone sample confirms stone formation and enables analysis of stone constituents.

If the Individual Complains of Pain

- Consult with the physician or advanced practice nurse for aggressive therapy (e.g., narcotics, antispasmodics).

   R: Calculi can produce severe pain from spasms and proximity of the nerve plexus.

Track the Pain by Documenting Location, any Radiation, Duration, and Intensity (Using a Rating Scale of 0 to 10)

R: This measure helps evaluate movement of calculi.

Instruct the Individual to Increase Fluid Intake, If not Contraindicated

R: Increased fluid intake promotes increased urination, which can help facilitate stone passage and flush bacteria and blood from the urinary tract.

Monitor for Signs and Symptoms of Pyelonephritis

- Fever, chills
- Costovertebral angle pain (a dull, constant backache below the 12th rib)
- Leukocytosis
- Bacteria, blood, and pus in urine
- Dysuria, frequency

   R: Urinary stasis or irritation of tissue by calculi can cause urinary tract infections. Signs and symptoms reflect various mechanisms. Bacteria can act as pyrogens by raising the hypothalamic thermostat through the production of endogenous pyrogen, which may be mediated through prostaglandins. Chills can occur when the temperature set-point of the hypothalamus changes rapidly. Costovertebral angle pain results from distention of the renal capsule. Leukocytosis reflects increased leukocytes to fight infection through phagocytosis. Bacteria and pus in urine indicate a urinary tract infection. Bacteria can irritate bladder tissue, causing spasms and frequency (Grossman & Porth, 2014).

Monitor for Early Signs and Symptoms of Renal Insufficiency

* Refer to *Risk for Complications of Renal Insufficiency.*

Explain Importance of Following Instructions for Current Care and Prevention or Minimization of Risk for Future Stone Formation

* Provide educational materials (e.g., Kidney Stones: Individual Fact Sheet http://www.suna.org/members /kidney_stones.pdf).

> ### *Clinical Alert Report*
>
> Prior to providing care, advice ancillary staff/student to report the following to the professional nurse assigned to the individual:
> * Complaints of sudden flank pain
> * Hematuria

RISK FOR COMPLICATIONS OF ACUTE RENAL INSUFFICIENCY/ CHRONIC KIDNEY DISEASE

Definition

Describes a person experiencing or at high risk to experience a decrease in glomerular filtration rate that results in changes in urine output, laboratory abnormalities, and hormonal alterations. Chronic kidney disease (CKD) is defined as the presence of kidney damage (usually detected as urinary albumin excretion of ≥30 mg/day, or equivalent) *or* decreased kidney function (defined as estimated glomerular filtration rate [eGFR] <60 mL/min/1.73 m^2) for 3 or more months, irrespective of the cause (Rosenberg, 2015).

High-Risk Populations
(Grossman & Porth, 2014; Kovesdy, Kopple, & Kalantar-Zadeh, 2015)

* Older persons
* High-risk individuals
* Gender
* Family history
* Race or ethnicity
* Genetic factors
* Smoking
* Obesity
* Postsurgical
* Major trauma
* Underlying chronic kidney disease
* Renal tubular necrosis from ischemic causes
    * Excessive diuretic use
    * Pulmonary embolism
    * Burns

- Intrarenal thrombosis
- Rhabdomyolysis
- Renal infections
- Renal artery stenosis/thrombosis
- Peritonitis
- Sepsis
- Hypovolemia
- Hypotension
- Congestive heart failure
- Myocardial infarction
- Aneurysm
- Aneurysm repair
- Renal tubular necrosis from toxicity
- Nonsteroidal anti-inflammatory drugs
- Gout (hyperuricemia)
- Hypercalcemia
- Certain street drugs (e.g., PCP)
- Gram-negative infection
- Radiocontrast media
- Aminoglycoside antibiotics
- Antineoplastic agents
- Methanol, carbon tetrachloride
- Snake venom, poison mushroom
- Phenacetin-type analgesics
- Heavy metals
- Insecticides, fungicides
- Diabetes mellitus
- Malignant hypertension
- Hemolysis (e.g., from transfusion reaction)

Collaborative Outcomes

The individual will be monitored for early signs and symptoms of renal insufficiency with a goal of preventing or minimizing chronic damage. The individual will receive collaborative interventions as indicated to restore and/or maintain physiologic stability.

Indicators of Physiologic Stability

- Blood pressure <120 (systolic) and <80 (diastolic)
- Urine specific gravity 1.005 to 1.030
- Urine output >0.5 mL/hr
- Urine sodium 40 to 220 mEq/L/24 hr (varies by dietary intake, medications)
- Blood urea nitrogen 10 to 20 mg/dL
- Serum potassium 3.8 to 5 mEq/L
- Serum sodium 135 to 145 mEq/L
- Serum phosphorus 2.5 to 4.5 mg/dL
- Serum creatinine clearance 100 to 150 mL/min (varies by age, gender, and race)
- Glomerular filtration rate over 90

Interventions and Rationales

Monitor for Hematauria and Proteinuria (Lewington & Kanagasundaram, 2013)

- Visible (macroscopic) haematuria (usually referred immediately to urology or to nephrology if acute renal pathology is suspected)
- Invisible (microscopic) haematuria without proteinuria, GFR >60 mL/min/1.73m^2
  - Age >40, usually refer to Urology (recommended age may vary locally)
  - Age <40, or >40 with negative urological investigations, refer to nephology

- Microscopic haematuria with prot/creat ratio >50 mg/mmol
  - Refer to nephrology if urological investigations negative
  - Refer nephrology

> **CLINICAL ALERT:**
> - Glomerular filtration rate, usually based on serum creatinine level, age, sex, and race. For Afro Caribbean black individuals, eGFR was 21% higher for any given creatinine. Most laboratory reports indicate a normal range for white and black individual (Lewington & Kanagasundaram, 2013).

Monitor for Early Signs and Symptoms of Renal Insufficiency

- Sustained elevated urine specific gravity, elevated urine sodium levels
- Sustained insufficient urine output (<30 mL/hr), elevated blood pressure
- Elevated BUN, serum creatinine, potassium, phosphorus, and decreased bicarbonate (CO_2); decreased creatinine clearance
- Dependent edema (periorbital, pedal, pretibial, sacral)
- Nocturia
- Lethargy
- Itching
- Nausea/vomiting

> *R: Hypovolemia and hypotension activate the renin–angiotensin system, which causes peripheral vasoconstriction and decreases glomerular filtration rate (blood flow.) The result is increased sodium and water reabsorption with decreased urine output. BUN is also reabsorbed. If this adaptive mechanism is inadequate, acute kidney injury from ischemia develops. Urine output remains low or diminishes and blood pressure is elevated (Fazia, Lin, & Staros, 2012). Decreased excretion of urea and creatinine in the urine elevates BUN and creatinine levels. Dependent edema results from increased plasma hydrostatic pressure, salt, and water retention, and/or decreased colloid osmotic pressure from plasma protein losses (Grosssman & Porth, 2014).*

> **CLINICAL ALERT:**
> - Notify physician/nurse practitioner/physician assistant of changes in condition or laboratory results, which reflect increasing renal insufficiency.

Weigh the Individual Daily at a Minimum

- Ensure accurate findings by weighing at the same time each day, on the same scale, and with the individual wearing the same amount of clothing.

> *R: Daily weights and intake and output records help evaluate fluid balance and guide fluid intake recommendations.*

Maintain Strict Intake and Output Records

Explain Prescribed Fluid Management Goals to Individual/Family

R: Individual and family understanding may enhance cooperation.

Refer to Unit III Section 1 for the Care Plan on Chronic Kidney Disease

> ### Clinical Alert Report
> Prior to providing care, advice ancillary staff/student to report the following to the professional nurse assigned to the individual:
> - Urine output <0.5 mL/hr
> - Nonadherance to fluid restrictions
> - Complaints of shortness (SOB) of breath or increased SOB
> - Behavioral changes

RISK FOR COMPLICATIONS OF NEUROLOGIC/SENSORY DYSFUNCTION

Risk for Complications of Alcohol Withdrawal
Risk for Complications of Increased Intracranial Pressure
Risk for Complications of Seizures

Definition

Describes a person experiencing or at high risk to experience various neurologic or sensory dysfunctions

Carp's Cues

The nurse can use this generic collaborative problem to describe a person at risk for several types of neurologic or sensory problems (e.g., an individual recovering from cranial surgery or who has sustained multiple traumas). For such a person, using *Risk for Complications of Neurologic/Sensory Dysfunction* directs nurses to monitor neurologic and sensory function on the basis of focus assessment findings. Should a complication occur, the nurse would add the applicable specific collaborative problem (e.g., *Risk for Complications of Seizure*) to the problem list to describe nursing management of the complication. If the risk factors or etiology were not related directly to the primary medical diagnosis or treatment, the nurse could add this information to the diagnostic statement. For example, for an individual with a seizure disorder admitted for abdominal surgery, the nurse would add *Risk for Complications of Seizures related to epilepsy* to the problem list.

In addition to the collaborative problem, the nurse should assess for other actual or potential responses that can compromise functioning. Some of these responses may represent nursing diagnoses (e.g., *Risk for Injury related to poor awareness of environmental hazards secondary to decreased sensorium*).

For information on Focus Assessment Criteria, visit the Point.

Significant Laboratory/Diagnostic Assessment Criteria

Cerebrospinal Fluid

Cloudy Presentation (Indicative of an Infection)
- Protein (increased in meningitis)
- White blood cell (WBC) count (increased in meningitis)
- Albumin (elevated with brain tumors)
- Glucose (decreased with bacterial meningitis)

Blood
- WBC count (elevated with bacterial infection, decreased in viral infection)
- Alcohol level
- Glucose calcium
- Mercury, lead levels if indicated

Radiologic/Imaging
- Skull, spine X-rays
- Computed tomography (CT)
- Magnetic resonance imaging (MRI)
- Cerebral angiography
- Position emission tomography (PET) (measures physiologic and biochemical process in the nervous system; can detect tumors, vascular diseases, and behavioral disturbances such as dementia or schizophrenia)
- Myelography

Other
- Doppler
- Lumbar puncture
- Electroencephalography (EEG)
- Continuous bedside cerebral blood flow monitoring

RISK FOR COMPLICATIONS OF ALCOHOL WITHDRAWAL

Definition

Describes a person experiencing or at high risk to experience the complications of alcohol withdrawal (e.g., delirium tremens, autonomic hyperactivity, seizures, alcohol hallucinosis, and hypertension)

 Carp's Cues

There are an estimated 8 million alcohol-dependent people in the United States. Approximately 500,000 episodes of withdrawal severe enough to require pharmacologic treatment occur each year (Hoffman & Weinhouse, 2015).

DT is associated with a mortality rate of up to 5%. Death usually is due to arrhythmia, complicating illnesses, such as pneumonia, or failure to identify an underlying problem that led to the cessation of alcohol use, such as pancreatitis, hepatitis, or central nervous system injury or infection. Older age, preexisting pulmonary disease, core body temperature greater than 40° C (104° F), and coexisting liver disease are associated with a greater risk of mortality (Hoffman & Weinhouse, 2015).

High-Risk Populations (Hoffman & Weinhouse, 2015),

"It is not entirely clear why some individuals suffer from more severe withdrawal symptoms than others, but genetic predisposition may play a role. Experiments in 1955 demonstrated that alcohol-naive volunteers given continual alcohol for longer periods developed more severe withdrawal than those who drank for shorter period. These results imply that most people are vulnerable to the effects of the abrupt cessation of prolonged, sustained ethanol intake" (Hoffman & Weinhouse, 2015).

- A history of sustained drinking
- A history of previous DT
- Age greater than 30
- The presence of a concurrent illness
- The presence of significant alcohol withdrawal in the presence of an elevated ethanol level
- A longer period (more than 2 days) between the last drink and the onset of withdrawal

Collaborative Outcomes

The individual will be monitored for early signs and symptoms of alcohol withdrawal and will receive collaborative interventions if indicated to restore physiologic stability.

Indicators of Physiologic Stability

- No seizure activity
- Calm, oriented
- Temperature 98° F to 99.5° F
- Pulse 60 to 100 beats/min
- Blood pressure >90/60 mm Hg and <140/90 mm Hg
- No reports of hallucinations
- No tremors

Interventions and Rationales

Carefully Attempt to Determine if the Individual Abuses Alcohol

- Consult with the family regarding their perception of alcohol consumption. Explain why accurate information is necessary.

    R: Data indicates that one in four medical-surgical patients admitted to a hospital has an alcohol use disorder (Elliott, Geyer, Lionetti, & Doty, 2012). It is critical to identify high-risk people so potentially fatal withdrawal symptoms can be prevented.

Obtain a Complete History of Prescription and Nonprescription Drugs Taken

R: Benzodiazepine or barbiturate withdrawal may mimic alcohol withdrawal and complicate the picture (Hoffman & Weinhouse, 2015).

If Alcohol Abuse Is Confirmed, Obtain History of Previous Withdrawals

- Delirium tremens
- Seizures

Maintain the Individual's IV Running Continuously

R: This may be necessary for fluid replacement and dextrose, thiamine bolus, benzodiazepine, and magnesium sulfate administration. Chlordiazepoxide and diazepam should not be given IM because of unpredictable absorption.

Monitor Vital Signs at Least Every 2 Hours

R: Individuals in withdrawal have elevated heart rate, respirations, and fever. Individuals experiencing delirium tremens can be expected to have a low-grade fever. Rectal temperature greater than 37.7° C (99.9° F) is a clue to possible infection.

Observe for Minor Withdrawal Symptoms
(Elliott et al., 2012; Hoffman & Weinhouse, 2015)

- Irritability
- Chills
- Insomnia
- Tremulousness
- Mild anxiety
- Gastrointestinal upset
- Anorexia
- Headache
- Diaphoresis
- Palpitations

R: Minor withdrawal symptoms are due to central nervous system hyperactivity. Withdrawal occurs 6 to 96 hours after drinking ends. Withdrawal can occur in people who are considered "social drinkers" (6 oz of alcohol daily for a period of 3 to 4 weeks). Withdrawal patterns may resemble those of previous episodes. Seizure patterns unlike previous episodes may indicate another underlying pathology.

> **CLINICAL ALERT:**
> - When alcohol abuse is suspected and/or minor withdrawal symptoms are assessed, notify the physician/nurse practitioner/physician assistant for initiation of benzodiazepine therapy, with dosage determined by assessment findings.
>
>   *R: Benzodiazepine requirements in alcohol withdrawal are highly variable and patient specific. Fixed schedules may oversedate or undersedate.*

Observe for the Desired Effects of Benzodiazepine Therapy

- Relief from withdrawal symptoms
- Peaceful sleep but rousable

R: Benzodiazepines are the drugs of choice in controlling withdrawal symptoms except with hepatic dysfunction. With hepatic dysfunction, the shorter half-life of lorazepam and the absence of active metabolites with oxazepam may prevent prolonged effects if oversedation occurs.

Monitor for Withdrawal Seizures

- Refer also to *Risk for Complications of Seizures.*

  R: Withdrawal seizures can occur 6 to 96 hours after drinking ends. They are usually nonfocal and grand mal, last minutes or less, and occur singularly or in clusters of two to six.

> **CLINICAL ALERT:**
> - Monitor for and intervene promptly in cases of status epilepticus. Follow institution's emergency protocol.
>
>   *R: Status epilepticus is life threatening if not controlled immediately with IV diazepam. For interventions of status epilepticus, refer to Care Plan for Seizure Disorder.*

Monitor and Determine Onset of Alcohol Hallucinosis

* Hallucinations are usually visual, although auditory and tactile phenomena may also occur. The person senses that the hallucinations are not real and is aware of surroundings.

    R: Alcoholic hallucinosis is not the same as delirium tremens. "Alcoholic hallucinosis refers to hallucinations that develop within 12–24 hours of abstinence and resolve within 24–48 hours (which is the earliest point at which delirium tremens typically develops). In contrast to delirium tremens, alcoholic hallucinosis is not associated with global clouding of the sensorium, but with specific hallucinations, and vital signs are usually normal" (Hoffman & Weinhouse, 2015).

> **CLINICAL ALERT:**
> * "Delirium tremens (DT) is a syndrome characterized by agitation, disorientation, hallucinations, and autonomic instability (tachycardia, hypertension, hyperthermia, and diaphoresis) in the setting of acute reduction or abstinence from alcohol. DT is associated with a mortality rate of up to 5 percent, but the rate can be substantially higher if the condition goes untreated. Alcoholic hallucinosis and DT are distinct clinical entities" (Hoffman & Weinhouse, 2015).

Monitor for Delirium Tremens

* Delirium component (vivid hallucinations, confusion, extreme disorientation, and fluctuating levels of awareness)
* Extreme hyperadrenergic stimulation (tachycardia, hypertension or hypotension, extreme tremor, agitation, diaphoresis, and fever)

    *R: Delirium tremens appears on days 3 to 5 after cessation of drinking and can persist for up to 7 days (*Bhardwaj, Mirskis, & Ulatowski, 2004; Hoffman & Weinhouse, 2015).*

Monitor Fluid and Electrolyte Status

R: Severe alcohol withdrawal can severely impact fluid and electrolyte status (Hoffman & Weinhouse, 2015).

If Indicated Refer to the Nursing Care Plan for Alcohol Withdrawal for Additional Interventions Such as Health Teaching and Referrals for Drug and Alcohol Counseling

> ***Clinical Alert Report***
>
> Before providing care, advise ancillary staff/student to report the following to the professional nurse assigned to the individual:
> * Change orientation
> * Complaints of new or worsening of headaches
> * Slowed responses (speech, movements)
> * Vomiting

RISK FOR COMPLICATIONS OF INCREASED INTRACRANIAL PRESSURE

Definition

Describes a person experiencing or at high risk to experience increased cranial pressure (>20 mm Hg) exerted by cerebrospinal fluid (CSF) within the brain's ventricles or the subarachnoid space

High-Risk Populations

(Rangel-Castillo, Gopinath, & Robertson, 2008; Smith & Amin-Hanjani, 2013)

Intracranial (Primary)

* Brain tumor
* Cerebral edema (such as in acute hypoxic ischemic encephalopathy, large cerebral infarction, severe traumatic brain injury)

- Nontraumatic intracerebral hemorrhage (aneurysm rupture and subarachnoid hemorrhage, hypertensive brain hemorrhage, intraventricular hemorrhage)
- Ischemic stroke
- Hydrocephalus
- Idiopathic or benign intracranial hypertension
- Idiopathic intracranial hypertension (pseudotumor cerebri)
- Other (e.g., pneumoencephalus, abscesses, cysts)
- Meningitis, encephalitis
- Status epilepticus

Extracranial (Secondary)

- Airway obstruction
- Hypoxia or hypercarbia (hypoventilation)
- Hypertension (pain/cough) or hypotension (hypovolemia/sedation)
- Posture (head rotation)
- Obstruction of venous outflow (e.g., venous sinus thrombosis, jugular vein compression, neck surgery)
- Hyperpyrexia
- Seizures
- Drug and metabolic (e.g., tetracycline, rofecoxib, divalproex sodium, lead intoxication)
- High altitude
- Hepatic failure (mass lesion [hematoma] edema)
- Increased cerebral blood volume (vasodilation)
- Decreased CSF absorption (e.g., arachnoid granulation adhesions after bacterial meningitis)
- Increased CSF production (e.g., choroid plexus papilloma)

Collaborative Outcomes

The individual will be monitored for early signs and symptoms of increased intracranial pressure (ICP) and will receive collaborative interventions if indicated to restore physiologic stability.

Indicators of Physiologic Stability

- Adult ICP 5 to 15 mm Hg (7.5 to 20 cm H_2O)
- ICP monitoring device (e.g., ventriculostomy)
- Pupils equal; reactive to light and accommodation
- Intact extraocular movements
- Pulse 60 to 100 beats/min
- Respirations 16 to 20 breaths/min
- Blood pressure >90/60 mm Hg and <140/90 mm Hg
- Stable pulse pressure (difference between diastolic and systolic readings)
- No nausea/vomiting

If Conscious:
- Alert, oriented, calm, or no change in usual cognitive status
- Appropriate speech
- Mild to no headache

Interventions and Rationales

Maintain ICP Monitoring

- If using an ICP monitoring device (e.g., ventriculostomy), refer to the procedure manual for guidelines.

  R: Ventriculostomy is utilized to monitor ICP and as an access to drain CSF to reduce ICP.

Monitor the System for Proper Functioning at Least Every 2 to 4 Hours, and Any Time There Is a Change in the ICP, Neurologic Examination, and CSF Output

R: The functioning of the monitoring system should be evaluated when malfunctioning is suspected.

CLINICAL ALERT:
- Report immediately an increase in ICP. "ICP values greater than 20 to 25 mm Hg require treatment in most circumstances. Sustained ICP values of greater than 40 mm Hg indicate severe, life-threatening intracranial hypertension" (Rangel-Castillo et al., 2008).

Differentiate Between Cerebral Perfusion Pressure (CPP) and ICP

R: Impaired cerebral perfusion results in decreased cerebral blood flow and a rise in ICP pressure. CPP can be impaired by an increase in ICP, a decrease in blood pressure, or a combination of both factors. With normal autoregulation, the brain is able to maintain a normal cerebral blood flow (CBF). After injury, the ability of the brain to pressure autoregulate may be absent or diminished (Rangel-Castillo et al., 2008).

Maintain Oxygenation and Ventilation to Keep PaO_2 >100, $PaCO_2$ 30 to 35.

R: This will increase the oxygenation of cerebral tissue.

Monitor for Signs and Symptoms of Increased ICP

- Asses the following (Glasgow Coma Scale [GCS]) (Hickey, 2014):
  - Best eye-opening response: spontaneously, to auditory stimuli, to painful stimuli, or no response
  - Best motor response: obeys verbal commands, localizes pain, flexion–withdrawal, flexion–decorticate, extension–decerebrate, or no response
  - Best verbal response: oriented to person, place, and time; confused conversation; inappropriate speech; incomprehensible sounds; or no response

    R: Deficiencies of cerebral blood supply resulting from hemorrhage, hematoma, cerebral edema, thrombus, or emboli compromise cerebral tissue. These responses evaluate the individual's ability to integrate commands with conscious and involuntary movement. The nurse can assess cortical function by evaluating eye opening and motor response. No response may indicate damage to the midbrain.

Assess for Changes in Vital Signs

- Pulse changes: slowing rate to 60 beats/min or lower or increasing rate to 100 beats/min or higher

  R: Bradycardia is a late sign of brain stem ischemia. Tachycardia may indicate hypothalamic ischemia and sympathetic discharge.

- Respiratory irregularities: slowing rate with lengthening apneic periods

  R: Respiratory patterns vary depending on the site of impairment. Cheyne-Stokes breathing (a gradual increase followed by a gradual decrease, then a period of apnea) points to damage in both cerebral hemispheres, midbrain, and upper pons. Central neurogenic hyperventilation occurs with midbrain and upper pontine lesions. Ataxic breathing (irregular with random sequence of deep and shallow breaths) indicates pontine dysfunction. Hypoventilation and apnea occur with medullary lesions (Hickey, 2014).

- Rising blood pressure and/or widening pulse pressure
- Bradycardia, increased systolic blood pressure, and increased pulse pressure

  R: These are late signs (known as Cushing response) of brain stem ischemia leading to cerebral herniation (Hickey, 2014).

Assess Pupillary Responses/Eye Movement

R: Changes indicate pressure on oculomotor or optic nerves.

- Inspect the pupils with a bright pinpoint light to evaluate size, configuration, and reaction to light. Compare both eyes for similarities and differences.

  R: The oculomotor nerve (cranial nerve III) in the brain stem regulates pupil reactions.

- Evaluate gaze to determine whether it is conjugate (paired, working together) or if eye movements are abnormal.

  R: Conjugate eye movements are regulated from parts of the cortex and brain stem.

- Evaluate the ability of the eyes to adduct and abduct.

  R: Cranial nerve VI, or the abducens nerve, regulates abduction and adduction of the eyes. Cranial nerve IV, or the trochlear nerve, also regulates eye movement.

Note Any Other Signs and Symptoms

- Vomiting

    R: Vomiting results from pressure on the medulla, which stimulates the brain's vomiting center.

- Headache: constant, increasing in intensity, or aggravated by movement
- Straining

    R: Compression of neural tissue increases ICP and causes pain.

- Subtle changes (e.g., lethargy, restlessness, forced breathing, purposeless movements, changes in mentation)

    R: These signs may be the earliest indicators of cranial pressure changes.

Elevate the Head of the Bed 20 to 30 Degrees Unless Contraindicated (e.g., Hypovolemia)

R: Slight elevation of the head of the bed to 30 degrees improves jugular venous outflow, reduces cerebrovascular congestion, and lowers ICP. In individuals who are hypovolemic, this may be associated with a fall in blood pressure and an overall fall in CPP. Care must therefore initially be taken to exclude hypovolemia. Positioning is very dependent on the type of surgery done and the approach used and should always be clarified before repositioning (Hickey, 2014).

Maintain Negative Fluid Balance

- Carefully monitor hydration status; evaluate fluid intake and output, serum osmolality, urine specific gravity, and osmolality.

    R: Significant departures from the normal intravascular volume can adversely affect ICP and/or cerebral perfusion. Increased intravascular volume will increase cranial pressure; decreased intravascular volume will decrease cardiac output and cerebral tissue perfusion (Hickey, 2014).

Monitor Intravenous (IV) Fluid Therapy (Hypertonic Saline, Mannitol); Carefully Administer IV Fluids With an Infusion Pump

R: Careful IV fluid administration is necessary to prevent overhydration, which increases ICP, and dehydration, which decreases cerebral tissue perfusion.

Monitor for Diabetes Insipidus (Hickey, 2014)

- More than 200 mL/hr of urine output for two consecutive hours

    R: Cerebral edema can damage the pituitary gland or hypothalamus where antidiuretic hormone (ADH) is produced. This results in decreased ADH and the development of central diabetes insipidus in individuals with traumatic brain injury (Hickey, 2014).

> **CLINICAL ALERT:**
> - Dehydration can occur rapidly and further compromise cerebral vascular perfusion. Immediate action is required.

Monitor Temperature

- As indicated, initiate antipyretics and cooling blankets per orders/institutional protocols.

    R: A fever increases metabolic rate by 10% to 13% per degree Celsius and is a potent vasodilator. Fever-induced dilation of cerebral vessels can increase cerebral blood flow and may increase ICP. Being an independent predictor of poor outcome after severe head injury, fever should be avoided as it increases ICP (Rangel-Castillo et al., 2008).

For Individuals With Posttraumatic Brain Injury

- Consult with physician/nurse practitioner/physician assistant for seizure prophylaxis (phenytoin).

    R: The risk of seizures after trauma is related to the severity of the brain injury; seizures occur in 15% to 20% of individuals with severe head injury. Seizures increase cerebral metabolic rate and ICP. Seizure prophylaxis is recommended for the first 7 days after severe brain injury (Rangel-Castillo et al., 2008).

Avoid the Following Situations or Maneuvers, Which Can Increase ICP
(Hickey, 2014; Smith & Amin-Hanjani, 2013)

* Carotid massage

  R: This slows the heart rate and reduces systemic circulation, which is followed by a sudden increase in circulation.

* Neck flexion or extreme rotation; if intubated, do not use securing device with circumferential wrapping.

  R: This inhibits jugular venous drainage, which increases cerebrovascular congestion and ICP.

* Digital anal stimulation, breath-holding, straining

  R: These can initiate the Valsalva maneuver, which impairs venous return by constricting the jugular veins, thus increasing ICP.

* Extreme flexion of the hips and knees

  R: Flexion increases intrathoracic pressure, which inhibits jugular venous drainage, increasing cerebrovascular congestion and, thus, ICP.

* Rapid position changes

Teach to Exhale During Position Changes

R: This helps prevent the Valsalva maneuver.

Consult with the Physician or Nurse Practitioner for Stool Softeners, if Needed

R: Stool softeners prevent constipation and straining during defecation, which can trigger the Valsalva maneuver.

Maintain a Quiet, Calm, Softly Lit Environment. Schedule Several Lengthy Periods of Uninterrupted Rest Daily. Minimize Interruptions

R: These measures promote rest and decrease stimulation, both of which can help decrease ICP.

> **CLINICAL ALERT:**
> * Avoid sequential performance of activities that increase ICP (e.g., coughing, suctioning, repositioning, bathing).
>
>   *R: Research has validated that such sequential activities can cause a cumulative increase in ICP (Hickey, 2014).*

Limit Suctioning Time to 10 Seconds at a Time; Hyperoxygenate Individual Both Before and After Suctioning

R: These measures help prevent hypercapnia, which can increase cerebral vasodilation and raise ICP, and prevent hypoxia, which may increase cerebral ischemia.

Consult With Physician/Nurse Practitioner/Physician Assistant About Administering Prophylactic Lidocaine Before Suctioning

R: This measure may help prevent acute intracranial hypertension.

Clinical Alert Report
Before providing care, advise ancillary staff/student to report the following to the professional nurse assigned to the individual:
* Increase in signs/symptoms (e.g., agitation, insomnia)
* Observed tremors
* Mild anxiety
* GI upset; decreased appetite
* Headache
* Diaphoresis

RISK FOR COMPLICATIONS OF SEIZURES

Definition

Describes a person experiencing or at high risk to experience paroxysmal episodes of involuntary muscular contraction (tonus) and relaxation (clonus)

 Carp's Cues

Alcohol abuse is one of the most common causes of adolescent- and adult-onset seizures. Seizures, nearly always generalized tonic-clonic, occur in about 10% of adults during withdrawal. Multiple seizures happen in about 60% of these individuals. The first seizure occurs 7 hours to 2 days after the last drink, and the time between the first and last seizure is usually 6 hours or less (Hoffman & Weinhouse, 2015). Less than one-half of epilepsy cases have an identifiable cause (Schachter, 2015).

High-Risk Populations

- Family history of seizure disorder
- Cerebral cortex lesions
- Head injury
- Infectious disorder (e.g., meningitis)
- Cerebral circulatory disturbance (e.g., cerebral palsy, stroke)
- Brain tumor
- Alcohol overdose or withdrawal, refer to *Risk for Complications of Alcohol Withdrawal*
- Drug overdose (e.g., cocaine)
- Poststroke
- Sudden withdrawal from certain antianxiety or antidepressant drugs such as benzodiazepines, barbiturates, and tricyclic antidepressants
- Medications (overdose, abrupt withdrawal) such as theophylline, meperidine, tricyclic antidepressants, phenothiazines, lidocaine, quinolones, penicillins, selective serotonin reuptake inhibitors, isoniazid, antihistamines, cyclosporine, interferons, lithium
- Electrolyte imbalances (e.g., hypocalcemia, pyridoxine deficiency)
- Hypoglycemia as a complication of diabetes mellitus
- High fever
- Eclampsia
- Metabolic abnormalities (e.g., renal, hepatic, electrolyte)
- Alzheimer's or other degenerative brain diseases in older persons
- Poisoning (e.g., mercury, lead, carbon monoxide)

Refer to Unit III Section 1 *Seizure Disorder* Care Plan.

RISK FOR COMPLICATIONS OF GASTROINTESTINAL/ HEPATIC/BILIARY DYSFUNCTION

Risk for Complications of GI Bleeding
Risk for Complications of Hepatic Dysfunction
Risk for Complications of Paralytic Ileus

Definition

Describes a person experiencing or at high risk to experience compromised function in the gastrointestinal (GI), hepatic, or biliary systems. (*Note:* These three systems are grouped together for classification purposes. In a clinical situation, the nurse would use either *Risk for Complications of Gastrointestinal Dysfunctional*, *Risk for Complications of Hepatic Dysfunction*, *Risk for Complications of GI Bleeding*, or *Risk for Complications of Biliary Dysfunction* to specify the applicable system.)

Carp's Cues

The nurse can use these generic collaborative problems to describe a person at risk for various problems affecting the GI, hepatic, or biliary system. Doing so focuses nursing interventions on monitoring GI, hepatic, or biliary status to detect and diagnose abnormal functioning. Should a complication develop, the nurse would add the applicable specific collaborative problem (e.g., *Risk for Complications of GI Bleeding*, *Risk for Complications of Hepatic Dysfunction*) to the problem list, specifying appropriate nursing management.

In most cases, along with these collaborative problems, the nurse treats other associated responses, using nursing diagnoses (e.g., *Impaired Comfort related to accumulation of bilirubin pigment and bile salts*).

Significant Laboratory/Diagnostic Assessment Criteria

- Urinalysis (to detect low amylase levels, which indicate pancreatic insufficiency)
- Serum *Helicobacter pylori (H. pylori)* (positive as a risk factor for peptic ulcer disease)
- Serum albumin (lowered in chronic liver disease)
- Serum amylase (elevated in biliary tract disease)
- Serum lipase (elevated in pancreatitis)
- Serum calcium (high total calcium levels in cancer of liver, pancreas, and other organs)
- Stool specimen (can be analyzed for blood, parasites, fat)
- Bilirubin (elevated in hepatic disease, newborn hyperbilirubinemia)
- Potassium (lowered in liver disease with ascites, vomiting, diarrhea)
- Blood urea nitrogen (BUN; increased in hepatic failure)
- Prothrombin time (PT) (elevated in cirrhosis, hepatitis)
- Hemoglobin, hematocrit (decreased with bleeding)
- Sodium (decreased with dehydration)
- Platelets (decreased with liver disease or bleeding)
- Serum ammonia level elevated in liver dysfunction
- Hepatitis panel for primary differential diagnosis of diseases of the liver
- Abdominal X-ray
- Ultrasound (to detect masses, obstruction, gallstones)
- CT scan, MRI (to evaluate soft tissue for abscesses, tumors, sources of bleeding)
- Colonoscopy, barium enema, sigmoidoscopy
- Endoscopy, upper GI series, endoscopic retrograde cholangiopancreatography (ERCP) (visual examination of the inside of the stomach and duodenum, with the injection of radiographic contrast into the ducts in the biliary tree and pancreas for visualization on X-rays)
- Balloon-assistive enteroscopy (visual examination of the small bowel using an instrument called an endoscope with a balloon, which allows the scope to pass further into the small bowel)
- Esophagogastroduodenoscopy (EGD) (to examine the lining of the esophagus, stomach, and first part of the small intestine)

RISK FOR COMPLICATIONS OF GI BLEEDING

Definition

Describes a person experiencing or at high risk to experience GI bleeding

Carp's Cues

The three nonsurgical modalities used to diagnose lower gastrointestinal bleeding (LGIB) are colonoscopy, radionuclide scans, and angiography. Apart from colonoscopy, endoscopic procedures such as esophagogastroduodenoscopy (EGD), wireless capsule endoscopy (WCE), push enteroscopy, and double-balloon enteroscopy are used depending on the clinical circumstance. The sequence of using various modalities depends on such factors as rate of bleeding, hemodynamic status of the individual, and inability to localize bleeding with the initial modality.

High-Risk Populations

Upper GI Bleeding

- Miscellaneous causes
  - Older persons
  - Daily use of aspirin or nonsteroidal anti-inflammatory drugs (NSAIDs)
  - Antiplatelet therapy and PPI cotherapy
  - Selective serotonin reuptake inhibitors or serotonin-specific reuptake inhibitor (SSRIs)
  - Prolonged mechanical ventilation >48 hours
  - Recent stress (e.g., trauma, sepsis)
  - Platelet deficiency
  - Coagulopathy
  - Shock, hypotension
  - Major surgery (>3 hours)
  - Head injury
  - Severe vascular disease
  - Disorders of GI, hepatic, and biliary systems
  - Transfusion of 5 units (or more) of blood
  - Burns (>35% of body)
  - Hematobilia, or bleeding from the biliary tree
  - Hemosuccus pancreaticus, or bleeding from the pancreatic duct
  - Severe superior mesenteric artery syndrome
- Esophageal causes
  - Esophageal varices
  - Esophagitis
  - Esophageal cancer
  - Esophageal ulcers
  - Mallory–Weiss tear
- Gastric causes
  - Gastric ulcer
  - Gastric cancer
  - Gastritis
  - Gastric varices
  - Gastric antral vascular ectasia
  - Dieulafoy's lesions
- Duodenal causes
  - Duodenal ulcer
  - Vascular malformation
  - Antithrombolytic therapy

LGIB in Adults With Causation Frequency (Strate, 2015a)

- Diverticular disease (most frequent cause)
  - Diverticulosis/diverticulitis of small intestine
  - Diverticulosis/diverticulitis of colon
- Inflammatory bowel disease (second frequent cause)
  - Crohn disease of small bowel, colon, or both
  - Ulcerative colitis
  - Noninfectious gastroenteritis and colitis
- Benign anorectal diseases (third most frequent cause)
  - Hemorrhoids
  - Anal fissure
  - Fistula-in-ano
- Neoplasia
  - Malignant neoplasia of small intestine
  - Malignant neoplasia of colon, rectum, and anus

- Coagulopathy
- Arteriovenous malformations (AVMs)
- Unknown causes (6% to 23%)

Collaborative Outcomes

The individual will be monitored for early signs and symptoms of GI bleeding and will receive collaborative interventions if indicated to restore physiologic stability.

Indicators of Physiologic Stability

- Negative stool occult blood
- Calm, oriented
- Hemodynamic stability (blood pressure, pulse, urine output)
- Refer to *Risk for Complications of Hypovolemia*

Interventions and Rationales

Initiate Prophylaxis Stress Ulcers Protocol for Persons on Mechanical Ventilation (e.g., oral Proton Pump Inhibitor [PPI] or Intravenous Histamine-2 Receptor Antagonist [H2 Blocker] or Intravenous PPI) (Weinhouse, 2016)

R: Researchers have reported an incidence of 46.7% of GI bleeding in individuals on mechanical ventilation (Chu et al., 2010, p. 34). Critically ill individuals experience a decrease in the protective mucous layer in the stomach, hyper secretion of acid due to excessive gastrin stimulation and inadequate perfusion to stomach secondary to shock, infection, or trauma (Weinhouse, 2016).

> **CLINICAL ALERT:**
> - Acute respiratory failure requiring mechanical ventilation (MV) for >48 hours has been shown to be one of the two strongest independent risk factors for clinically important GI bleeding in the ICU (Chu et al., 2010).

Monitor for Complications Associated With MV, Such as Stress Ulcer and GI Hypomotility

R: Positive pressure ventilation for greater than 48 hours is a risk factor for clinically important GI bleeding due to stress ulceration. Positive airway pressure (especially PEEP) is also associated with decreased splanchnic perfusion. The mechanism underlying this association is unknown, but may be related to decreased cardiac output (Hyzy, 2015).

- Diarrhea
- Decreased bowel sounds
- High gastric residuals
- Constipation
- Ileus

Monitor for Signs and Symptoms of Acute Upper GI Bleeding

- Hematemesis (vomiting blood)
- Melena (dark stool)
- Dysphasia, dyspepsia
- Epigastric pain
- Heartburn
- Diffuse abdominal pain
- Weight loss
- Presyncope, syncope

R: Clinical manifestations depend on the amount and duration of upper GI bleeding. Early detection enables prompt intervention to minimize complications.

Monitor for Lower GI Bleeding

- Maroon-colored stools
- Bright red blood

    R: LGIB ranges from trivial hematochezia (blood in stool) to massive hemorrhage with shock and accounts for up to 24% of all cases of GI bleeding. This condition is associated with significant morbidity and mortality (10% to 20%). LGIB is one of the most common gastrointestinal indications for hospital admission, particularly in older persons. Diverticulitis accounts for up to 50% of cases, followed by ischemic colitis and anorectal lesions.

Monitor for Occult Blood in Gastric Aspirates and Bowel Movements

R: An individual can lose 100 mL of blood in stool and may have normal-appearing stools. Testing stool for occult blood is more accurate.

- Test nasogastric aspirate with Gastroccult.

    R: The Hemoccult test's sensitivity is reduced by the acidic environment, and the Gastroccult test is the most accurate.

- Test stool for occult blood with FOBT.

    R: The Gastroccult test is not recommended for use with fecal samples.

> **CLINICAL ALERT:**
> - Massive LGIB is a life-threatening condition; although this condition manifests as maroon stools or bright red blood from the rectum, individuals with massive upper gastrointestinal bleeding (UGIB) may also present with similar findings. Regardless of the level of the bleeding, one of the most important elements of the management of individuals with massive UGIB or LGIB is restoring hemodynamic stability (Strate, 2015b).

Institute Protocols for Volume Replacement (e.g., Two Large-Bore Intravenous [IV] Catheters and Isotonic Crystalloid Infusions)

R: Orthostatic hypotension (i.e., a blood pressure fall of >10 mm Hg) is usually indicative of blood loss of more than 1,000 mL.

Prepare for Transfusion per Physician/Physician Assistant/Advanced Practice Nurse Orders and Protocol

R: The goal is to increase blood volume and treat or prevent hypovolemic shock.

Monitor Hemoglobin, Hematocrit, Red Blood Cell Count, Platelets, PT, Partial Thromboplastin Time (PTT), Type Blood and Cross Match, and Blood Urea Nitrogen (BUN) Values

R: These values reflect the effectiveness of therapy.

If Hypovolemia Occurs, Refer to *Risk for Complications of Hypovolemia* for More Information and Specific Interventions

Educate Individuals/Family of the Risks of Daily Aspirin/NSAID Use and the Increased Risk With Long-Acting NSAIDS

- Long-term NSAID use is associated with a 20% to 25% incidence in the development of mucosal ulceration (Massó González, Patrignani, Tacconelli, & García Rodríguez, 2010).
- Drugs that have a long half-life or slow-release formulation and/or are associated with profound and coincident inhibition of both COX isozymes are associated with a greater risk of upper GI bleeding/perforation (Massó González et al., 2010).

Clinical Alert Report

Before providing care, advise ancillary staff/student to report the following to the professional nurse assigned to the individual:

- Occult testing results
- Streaks of blood in stool
- Hematemesis (vomiting blood)
- Melena (dark stool)
- Dysphasia, dyspepsia
- Epigastric pain
- Diffuse abdominal pain
- Presyncope, syncope

RISK FOR COMPLICATIONS OF HEPATIC DYSFUNCTION

Definition

Describes a person experiencing or at high risk to experience progressive liver dysfunction

High-Risk Populations

- Infections
  - Hepatitis A, B, C, D, E, non-A, non-B, non-C
  - Herpes simplex virus (types 1 and 2)
  - Epstein–Barr virus
  - Varicella zoster
  - Dengue fever virus
  - Rift Valley fever virus
- Drugs/toxins
  - Industrial substances (vinyl chloride, chlorinated hydrocarbons, phosphorus, carbon tetrachloride)
  - *Amanita phalloides* (mushrooms)
  - Aflatoxin (herb)
  - Medications (isoniazid, rifampin, halothane, methyldopa, tetracycline, valproic acid, monoamine oxidase inhibitors, phenytoin, nicotinic acid, tricyclic antidepressants, isoflurane, ketoconazole, cotrimethoprim, sulfasalazine, pyrimethamine, octreotide, antivirals)
  - Acetaminophen toxicity
  - Cocaine
  - Alcohol
- Hypoperfusion (shock liver)
  - Venous obstructions
  - Budd-Chiari syndrome
  - Veno-occlusive disease
  - Ischemia
- Metabolic disorders
  - Hyperbilirubinemia
  - Hereditary (Wilson's disease, hemochromatosis)
  - Tyrosinemia
  - Heat stroke
  - Galactosemia
  - Nutritional deficiencies
- Surgery
  - Traumatized liver
  - Jejunoileal bypass

- • Partial hepatectomy
  - • Liver transplant failure
- • Other
  - • Reye's syndrome
  - • Acute fatty liver of pregnancy
  - • Massive malignant infiltration
  - • Autoimmune hepatitis
  - • Rh incompatibility
  - • Ingestion of raw contaminated fish
  - • Thalassemia

Collaborative Outcomes

The individual will be monitored for early signs and symptoms of hepatic dysfunction and will receive collaborative interventions, if indicated, to restore physiologic stability.

Indicators of Physiologic Stability

- • PT 9.5 to 13.8 seconds
- • PTT 25 to 35 seconds
- • Aspartate aminotransferase (AST) male 8 to 48 units/L, female 6 to 18 units/L
- • Alanine aminotransferase (ALT) 7 to 55 units/L
- • Alkaline phosphatase 45 to 115 units/L
- • Serum barbiturates 2 to 21 μmol/L
- • Serum electrolytes within normal range

Interventions and Rationales

Monitor for Signs and Symptoms of Hepatic Dysfunction

- • Anorexia, indigestion

  R: GI effects result from circulating toxins.

- • Jaundice

  R: Yellowed skin and sclera result from excessive bilirubin production.

- • Petechiae, ecchymoses

  R: These skin changes reflect impaired synthesis of clotting factors.

- • Clay-colored stools

  R: This can result from decreased bile in stools.

- • Elevated liver function tests (e.g., serum bilirubin, serum transaminase)

  R: Elevated values indicate extensive liver damage.

- • Bleeding, prolonged PT

  R: This reflects reduced production of clotting factors.

- • Edema, ascites

  R: Decreased synthesis of protein results in hypoalbuminemia and fluid shifts into extravascular space.

With Hepatic Dysfunction, Monitor for Hemorrhage

R: The liver has a central role in hemostasis. Decreased platelet count results from impaired production of new platelets from the bone marrow. Decreased clearance of old platelets by the reticuloendothelial system also results. In addition, synthesis of coagulation factors (II, V, VII, IX, and X) is impaired, resulting in bleeding. The most frequent site is the upper GI tract. Other sites include the nasopharynx, lungs, retroperitoneum, kidneys, and intracranial and skin puncture sites (Grossman & Porth, 2014).

Teach Individual to Report Any Unusual Bleeding (e.g., in the Mouth After Brushing Teeth)

R: Mucous membranes are prone to injury because of their high surface vascularity.

Monitor for Hepatic Encephalopathy by Assessing Orientation, Cognition, Speech Patterns (Goldberg & Chopra, 2015)

- Grade I: Changes in behavior, mild confusion, slurred speech, disordered sleep
- Grade II: Lethargy, moderate confusion
- Grade III: Marked confusion (stupor), incoherent speech, sleep but awakening with stimulation
- Grade IV: Coma, unresponsive to pain

    R: Profound liver failure results in accumulation of ammonia and other toxic metabolites in the blood. The blood–brain barrier permeability increases, and both toxins and plasma proteins leak from capillaries to the extracellular space, causing cerebral edema (Goldberg & Chopra, 2015).

Create a Quiet Environment

- Explain to family the reason.
- Post a sign to remind staff (e.g., a sign suggesting maintaining a quiet environment)
- Decrease audible stimuli (e.g., alarms, loud voices)
- Reduce harsh lights

    R: Stimulation can contribute to increased intracranial pressure and should be minimized (Goldberg & Chopra, 2015).

Monitor for Signs and Symptoms of (Refer to the Index Under Each Electrolyte for Specific Signs and Symptoms)

- Hypoglycemia

    R: Hypoglycemia is caused by loss of glycogen stores in the liver from damaged cells and decreased serum concentrations of glucose, insulin, and growth hormones.

- Hypokalemia

    R: Potassium losses occur from vomiting, NG suctioning, diuretics, or excessive renal losses.

- Hypophosphatemia

    R: The loss of potassium ions causes the proportional loss of magnesium ions. Increased phosphate loss, transcellular shifts, and decreased phosphate intake contribute to hypophosphatemia.

- Acid–base disturbances

    R: Hepatocellular necrosis can result in accumulation of organic anions, resulting in metabolic acidosis. People with ascites often have metabolic alkalosis from increased bicarbonate levels resulting from increased sodium/hydrogen exchange in the distal tubule.

Assess for Side Effects of Medications

- Avoid administering narcotics, sedatives, and tranquilizers and exposing the individual to ammonia products.

    R: Liver dysfunction results in decreased metabolism of certain medications (e.g., opiates, sedatives, tranquilizers), increasing the risk of toxicity from high drug blood levels. Ammonia products should be avoided because of the individual's already high serum ammonia level.

Monitor for Signs and Symptoms of Renal Failure

- Refer to *Risk for Complications of Renal Failure* for more information.

    R: Obstructed hepatic blood flow results in decreased blood to the kidneys, impairing glomerular filtration and leading to fluid retention and decreased urinary output.

Teach Individual and Family to Report Signs and Symptoms of Complications, Such as

- Increased abdominal girth

    R: Increased abdominal girth may indicate worsening portal hypertension.

- Rapid weight loss or gain

  R: Weight loss points to negative nitrogen balance; weight gain points to fluid retention.

- Bleeding

  R: Unusual bleeding indicates decreased PT and clotting factors.

- Tremors

  R: Tremors can result from impaired neurotransmission because of failure of the liver to detoxify enzymes that act as false neurotransmitters.

- Increasing confusion and/or sombulence

  R: Cognitive impairments will worsen as cerebral hypoxia increases caused by continuing increases in serum ammonia levels resulting from the liver's impaired ability to convert ammonia to urea.

The Stages of Hepatic Failure Will Impact the Functioning of the Individual and Family. When Indicated Refer to Individual Nursing Diagnoses in Section 2 Part 1 as *Fatigue, Risk for Injury, Confusion, Risk for Pressure Ulcers, Compromised Family Coping*

RISK FOR COMPLICATIONS OF PARALYTIC ILEUS

Definition

Describes a person experiencing or at high risk to experience neurogenic or functional bowel obstruction

High-Risk Populations

- Bacteria or viruses that cause intestinal infections (gastroenteritis)
- Thrombosis or embolus to mesenteric vessels
- Any major surgery with use of general anesthesia and subsequent limitation of mobility, as well as minor surgery of the abdomen
- Postoperative status (bowel, retroperitoneal, or spinal cord surgery)
- Perioperative complications (e.g., postoperative pneumonia, intra-abdominal abscess)
- Kidney or lung disease
- Use of certain medications, especially narcotics
- Decreased blood supply to the intestines (mesenteric ischemia)
- Postshock status
- Hypovolemia
- Infections inside the abdomen, such as appendicitis
- Chemical, electrolyte, mineral imbalances (e.g., hypokalemia)
- Posttrauma (e.g., spinal cord injury)
- Uremia
- Spinal cord lesion
- Mechanical causes of intestinal obstruction may include (Townsend et al., 2012):
  - Adhesions or scar tissue that forms after surgery
  - Foreign bodies that block the intestines
  - Gallstones (rare)
  - Hernias
  - Impacted stool
  - Intussusception (telescoping of one segment of bowel into another)
  - Tumors blocking the intestines
  - Volvulus (twisted intestine)

Collaborative Outcomes

The individual will be monitored for early signs and symptoms of paralytic ileus and will receive collaborative interventions, if indicated, to restore physiologic stability.

Indicators of Physiologic Stability

- Bowel sounds present
- No nausea and vomiting
- No abdominal distention
- No change in bowel function
- Evidence of flatus

Interventions and Rationales

Auscultate Each of the Four Abdominal Quadrants to Evaluate the Specific Function of Large (Colon) and Small Intestines as

- The right upper quadrant contains lower margin of the liver, the gallbladder, part of the large intestine, and a few loops of the small intestine.
- The right lower quadrant contains the appendix, the connection between the large and small intestines, and loops of bowel.
- The left upper quadrant contains the lower margin of the spleen, part of the pancreas, and some of the stomach and duodenum.
- The left lower quadrant contains bowel loops and the descending colon.

  R: Knowing the structures under the stethoscope will help to determine the nature of the bowel sounds. Large intestine (colon) function can be auscultated at the outer (distal) aspects of each quadrant. Small intestine function can be auscultated in the inner aspect of each quadrant.

- Refer to Figure II.1.

In a Postoperative Individual, Monitor Bowel Function, Looking For

- Bowel sounds in small intestines can return within 24 to 48 hours of surgery.
- Bowel sounds in large intestines can return within 3 to 5 days of surgery.
- Flatus and defecation resuming by the second or third postoperative day.

  R: Resolution of normal bowel function starts in the proximal or right colon and progresses to the distal or left colon. Normally the small bowel regains function within hours whereas it may take 3 to 5 days for the colon to regain function. Bowel sounds should be auscultated to help differentiate paralytic ileus from a mechanical ileus. Continued absence of bowel sounds suggests paralytic ileus whereas hyperactive bowel sounds may indicate a mechanical ileus (McCutcheon, 2013).

Restrict Fluids Until Bowel Sounds Are Present. When Indicated, Begin With Small Amounts of Clear Liquids Only

- Monitor individual's response to resumption of fluid and food intake, and note the nature and amount of any emesis or stools.

  R: The individual will not tolerate fluids until bowel sounds resume.

Monitor for Signs and Symptoms of Paralytic Ileus: For One or More of the Following Symptoms or Signs That Persist for More Than 3 to 5 days (Depending on the Nature of the Surgery and What Is Considered "Typical") (Kalf, Wehner, & Litkoubi, 2015)

- Abdominal distention, bloating, and "gassiness"
- Diffuse, persistent abdominal pain
- Nausea and/or vomiting
- Delayed passage of or inability to pass flatus

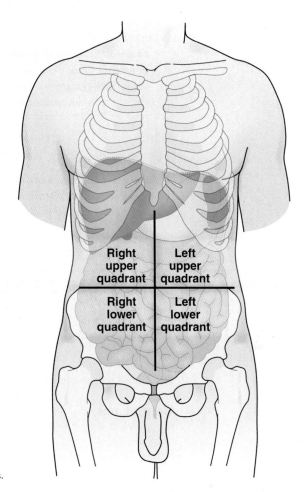

FIGURE II.I Diagram of the location of small and large intestines in quadrants for auscultation. From Weber J., & Kelley, J. (2014). *Health assessment in nursing* (5th ed.). Philadelphia, PA: Wolters Kluwer Health | Lippincott Williams & Wilkins.

- Inability to tolerate an oral diet

  R: Intraoperative manipulation of abdominal organs and the depressive effects of narcotics and anesthetics on peristalsis reduces bowel motility. The physiologic postoperative ileus that usually follows surgery has a benign and self-limited course. However, when ileus is prolonged, it leads to increasing discomfort and must be differentiated from other potential complications (e.g., bowel obstruction, intra-abdominal abscess) (McCutcheon, 2013).

Differentiated Between Paralytic Ileus and Mechanical Bowel Obstruction

> **CLINICAL ALERT:**
> - "It is useful to note that nearly all individuals with early postoperative bowel obstruction have an initial return of bowel function and oral intake, which is then followed by nausea, vomiting, abdominal pain, and distention, whereas patients with ileus generally do not experience return of bowel function" (Kalf et al., 2015).

- Abdominal distention, vomiting, obstipation: may be present with both
- Bowel sounds: paralytic ileus—usually quiet or absent
  - Bowel obstruction: may be high pitched, may be absent
- Pain: paralytic ileus—mild and diffuse
  - Bowel obstruction: moderate to severe, colicky
- Fever, tachycardia: paralytic ileus—absent
  - Bowel obstruction: should raise suspicion

  R: Localized tenderness, fever, tachycardia, and peritoneal signs suggest bowel ischemia or perforation, which indicate the need for emergent surgical intervention.

CLINICAL ALERT:
- Notify physician/nurse practitioner/physician assistant with new onset or increasing signs and symptoms of paralytic ileus. If the obstruction blocks the blood supply to the intestine, it may cause infection and tissue death (gangrene). The longer duration of the blockage and its cause are risk factors for tissue death. Hernias, volvulus, and intussusception carry a higher gangrene risk (Townsend et al., 2012).

When Bowel Obstruction Is Suspected, a Plain Abdominal X-Ray or Computed Tomographic (CT) Scan With Contrast Is Indicated

R: Small bowel obstruction can be diagnosed on X-ray if the more proximal small bowel is dilated and the more distal small bowel is not dilated. The stomach may also be dilated. However, if there remains any suspicion for small bowel obstruction or another diagnosis, we suggest computed tomography (CT) of the abdomen (Kalf et al., 2015).

RISK FOR COMPLICATIONS OF MUSCULAR/SKELETAL DISORDERS

Risk for Complications of Pathologic Fractures

Definition

Describes a person experiencing or at high risk to experience various musculoskeletal problems

Carp's Cues

The nurse can use this generic collaborative problem to describe people at risk for several types of musculoskeletal problems (e.g., all individuals who have sustained multiple trauma). This collaborative problem focuses nursing management on assessing musculoskeletal status to detect and to diagnose abnormalities.

For an individual exhibiting a specific musculoskeletal problem, the nurse would add the applicable collaborative problem (e.g., *Risk for Complications of Pathologic Fractures*) to the problem list. If the risk factors or etiology were not related directly to the primary medical diagnoses, the nurse would add this information to the diagnostic statement (e.g., *Risk for Complications of Pathologic Fractures related to osteoporosis*).

Because musculoskeletal problems typically affect daily functioning, the nurse must assess the individual's functional patterns for evidence of impairment. Findings may have significant implications—for instance, a casted leg that prevents a woman from assuming her favorite sleeping position and impairs her ability to perform housework. After identifying any such problems, the nurse should use nursing diagnoses to address specific responses of actual or potential altered functioning.

Significant Laboratory/Diagnostic Assessment Criteria

- Laboratory
  - Serum calcium (decreased in osteoporosis)
  - Serum phosphorus (decreased in osteoporosis)
  - Sedimentation rate (increased in inflammatory disorders)
- Diagnostic
  - X-ray
  - Bone scan (uses a radioactive material to evaluate bone tissue, such as fractures, tumors, areas of inflammation [arthritis])
  - Bone density test—Dexa Scan, DXA (measures and calculates the relative density of that bone, primarily to diagnose osteopenia or osteoporosis)
  - Computed tomography (CT) scan (exams bone for bone detail and cortical destruction)
  - Magnetic resonance imaging (MRI)
  - Arthrography (multiple X-rays of a joint using a fluoroscope to examine ligaments, cartilage, tendons, or the joint capsule, e.g., hip, shoulder)
  - Discography (uses injection of contrast medium into one or more spinal discs to determine source of back pain)

RISK FOR COMPLICATIONS OF PATHOLOGIC FRACTURES

Definition

A pathologic fracture occurs when a bone breaks without adequate trauma in an area that is weakened by another disease process. Causes of weakened bone include tumors (metastatic cancer), infection, and certain inherited bone disorders (osteoporosis, Paget's disease)

Carp's Cues

Pathologic fractures can be caused by any type of bone tumor, but the overwhelming majority of pathologic fractures in older persons are secondary to metastatic carcinomas. Multiple myeloma is also common in older persons and has a high incidence of pathologic fractures.

High-Risk Populations

- Tumors
  - Primary
  - Benign (fibroxanthoma)
  - Secondary (metastatic) (most common) (e.g., fibrous dysplasia, osteosarcoma, Ewing's, malignant fibrous histiocytoma, fibrosarcoma)
- Metabolic
  - Osteoporosis (most common)
  - Paget's disease
  - Hyperparathyroidism (Brown tumors)
  - Renal failure
  - Cushing's syndrome
  - Malnutrition
  - Long-term corticosteroid therapy
  - Osteogenesis imperfecta
  - Prolonged immobility
  - Radiation osteonecrosis (Ewing's, Lyme's disease)
  - Rickets
  - Osteomalacia
  - Multiple myeloma
  - Lymphatic leukemia
  - Unicameral bone cyst
  - Infection

Collaborative Outcomes

The individual will be monitored for early signs and symptoms of pathologic fractures and will receive collaborative interventions, if indicated, to restore physiologic stability.

Indicators of Physiologic Stability

- No new onset of pain
- No changes in range of motion

Interventions and Rationales

In Individuals With Cancer, Identify Those at High Risk for Pathologic Fractures. Primary Site With % of Frequency of Metastasis to Bone (Balach & Peabody, 2011)

- Breast 50 to 85
- Kidneys 30 to 50
- Thyroid 40

- Lung 30 to 50
- Melanoma 30 to 40
- Prostate 50 to 70
- Bladder 12 to 25
- Hodgkin's 50 to 70

R: The majority of bone metastases originate from cancers of the breast, lung, and prostate, followed by the thyroid and kidney. The most common sites of spread in the skeleton include the spine, pelvis, ribs, skull, upper arm, and leg long bones. These sites correspond to areas of bone marrow that demonstrate high levels of red blood cell production, the cells responsible for carrying oxygen to tissues in the body (Balach & Peabody, 2011; Damron, Bogart, & Bilsky, 2015; Monczewski, 2013).

> **CLINICAL ALERT:**
> - "A pathologic fracture should always be considered when patients with known bone metastases or a history of cancer develop the sudden onset of pain even in the absence of deformity or inability to ambulate" (Damron et al., 2015). This is particularly true in the upper extremity and spine, where pain may be the only manifestation. In many cases, pain or discomfort precedes the actual fracture itself, and this is another clue to the presence of a true pathologic fracture.

Monitor for Signs and Symptoms of Pathologic Fractures

- Hip pain (61% of all pathologic fractures occur in the femur)
- Thoracic or lumbar spine pain typically present with sitting or standing
- Localized pain that is continuous and unrelenting (back, neck, pelvic, or extremities)
- Visible bone deformity
- Crepitation on movement
- Loss of movement or use
- Localized soft tissue edema
- Skin discoloration/bruising

R: Detection of pathologic fractures enables prompt intervention to prevent or minimize further complications.

If a Fracture Is Suspected, Maintain Proper Alignment and Immobilize the Site Using Pillows or a Splint; Notify the Physician or Advanced Practice Nurse Promptly

R: Timely, appropriate intervention can prevent or minimize soft tissue damage.

For Some Individuals With Pathological Fractures, Surgical Fixation Is Indicated

R: In individuals with tumors destroying >50% of the diameter of bone or with lesions >2.5 cm, prophylactic internal fixation will be needed because of the increased risk to fracture.

For Postoperative Radiation Therapy Following Surgery, Individual Will Be Referred to Radiation Oncology to (O'Donnell, 2012)

- Decrease pain
- Slow progression
- Treat remaining tumor burden not removed at surgery

In Individuals With Fracture, Radiation Therapy May Be Indicated

R: Radiation alone can provide complete pain relief in 50% of individuals and partial pain relief in 35% (O'Donnell, 2012).

In an Individual With Osteoporosis, Teach Him or Her the Signs and Symptoms of Vertebral, Hip, and Wrist Fractures, Such as

- Pain in the lower back, neck, or wrist
- Localized tenderness

- Pain radiating to abdomen and flank
- Spasm of paravertebral muscles

    R: Progressive osteoporosis more readily affects bones with high amounts of trabecular tissue (e.g., hip, vertebrae, wrist).

RISK FOR COMPLICATIONS OF MEDICATION THERAPY ADVERSE EFFECTS

Risk for Complications of Anticoagulant Therapy Adverse Effects

Definition

Describes an individual experiencing or at high risk to experience potentially serious effects or reactions related to medication therapy

Carp's Cues

The nurse can use these collaborative problems to describe an individual who has experienced or who is at risk for adverse effects of medication therapy. In contrast to side effects, which are troublesome and annoying but rarely serious, adverse effects are unusual, unexpected, and potentially serious reactions. Adverse drug reactions are drug-induced toxic reactions. Examples of adverse effects include arrhythmias, gastric ulcers, blood dyscrasias, and anaphylactic reactions; examples of side effects include drowsiness, dry mouth, nausea, and weakness. Side effects usually can be managed by changing the dose, form, route of administration, or diet, or by using preventive measures with continuation of the medication. Adverse effects usually require discontinuation of the medication. A care plan will not contain a collaborative problem for every medication that the individual is taking. Nurses routinely teach individuals about side effects of medications and monitor for side effects as part of the standard of care for every individual. These collaborative problems are indicated for individuals who are at high risk for adverse effects or reactions because of the duration of the therapy, high predictability of their occurrence, the potential seriousness if they occur, and previous history of an adverse response. Students may add these collaborative problems to care plans. Practicing nurses could have access to electronic sources for *adverse effects* for major medications.

High-Risk Populations

- Prolonged medication therapy
- History of hypersensitivity
- History of adverse reactions
- High single or daily doses
- Changes in daily doses
- Multiple medication therapy
- Mental instability
- Hepatic insufficiency
- Renal insufficiency
- Disease or condition that increases the risk of a specific adverse response (e.g., history of gastric ulcer)

RISK FOR COMPLICATIONS OF ANTICOAGULANT THERAPY ADVERSE EFFECTS

High-Risk Populations

- Diabetes mellitus
- Hypothyroidism
- Gastrointestinal (GI) bleeding

- Bleeding tendency, comply with
- Hyperlipidemia
- Elderly women
- Compromised cognitive function
- History of noncompliance (e.g., missed appointments, failure to comply with lab test monitoring)
- Vitamin K deficiency
- Debilitation
- Congestive heart failure
- Children
- Mild hepatic or renal dysfunction
- Tuberculosis
- Pregnancy
- Immediately postpartum

Collaborative Outcomes

The individual will be monitored for early signs and symptoms of adverse effects of anticoagulant therapy and will receive collaborative interventions if indicated to restore physiologic stability.

Indicators of Physiologic Stability

Identify signs and symptoms that need immediate reporting (e.g., bleeding gums, skin bruises, dark stools, hematuria, epistaxis).

Interventions and Rationales

Refer Also to a Pharmacology Text for Specific Information on the Individual Drug

Assess for Contraindications to Anticoagulant Therapy

- History of hypersensitivity
- Wounds
- Presence of active bleeding
- Blood dyscrasias
- Anticipated or recent surgery
- GI ulcers
- Subacute bacterial endocarditis
- Pericarditis
- Severe hypertension
- Impaired renal function
- Impaired hepatic function
- Hemorrhagic cerebrovascular accident
- Use of drugs that affect platelet formation (e.g., salicylates, dipyridamole, nonsteroidal anti-inflammatory drugs [NSAIDs])
- Presence of drainage tubes
- Eclampsia
- Hemorrhagic tendencies
- Threatened abortion
- Ascorbic acid deficiency
- Spinal puncture
- Regional anesthesia
- Pregnancy (Coumadin)
- Inadequate lab facilities
- Compliance risk
- Spinal puncture

Explain Possible Adverse Effects

- Systemic
  - *Hypersensitivity* (fever, chills, runny nose, headache, nausea, vomiting, rash, itching, tearing)
    - Bleeding, hemorrhage
      - Fatigue/malaise/lethargy
      - Alopecia
      - Rash
      - Fever
      - Cold intolerance
      - Anemia
- Gastrointestinal
  - Vomiting
  - Diarrhea
  - Dark, tarry colored stools
  - Abdominal cramps
  - Hepatitis
  - Flatulence/bloating
- Cardiovascular
  - Hypertension
  - Chest pain
  - Edema
  - Vasculitis
- Renal
  - Impaired renal function
- Neurologic
  - Dizziness
  - Paresthesias

Monitor for and Reduce the Severity of Adverse Effects

- For warfarin (Coumadin), monitor laboratory results of activated partial thromboplastin time (APTT) for heparin therapy and prothrombin time (PT) and international normalized ratio (INR) for oral therapy. Report values over target for therapeutic range.

  R: The therapeutic range for PT is 1.3 to 1.5× control or INR of 2.0 to 3.0.

- For Dabigatran (Paradoxa), no PT/INR monitoring is needed.
- Monitor for signs of bleeding (e.g., bleeding gums, skin bruises, dark stools, hematuria, epistaxis).
- For an individual receiving heparin therapy, have protamine sulfate available during administration. For warfarin, the antidote is vitamin K.

  R: Protamine sulfate is the antidote to reverse the effects of heparin.

- Carefully monitor older adult patients.

  R: They are more sensitive to the effects of anticoagulants.

- Consult with the pharmacist about medications that can potentiate (e.g., antibiotics, cimetidine, salicylates, phenytoin, acetaminophen, antifungals, NSAIDs, bismuth) or inhibit (e.g., barbiturates, dicloxacillin, carbamazepine, nafcillin, bile acid binding agents, griseofulvins) anticoagulant action.
- Monitor for signs and symptoms of heparin-induced thrombocytopenia (fever, weakness, difficulty speaking, seizures, yellowing of skin/eyes, dark or bloody urine, petechiae).

  R: Antibodies directed against platelet membrane are produced in the presence of heparin, causing increased platelet consumption.

- Reduce hematomas and bleeding at injection sites.
- Use small-gauge needles.
- Do not massage sites.
- Rotate sites.
- Use subcutaneous route.

- Apply steady pressure for 1 to 2 minutes.

  R: These techniques reduce the trauma to tissues and avoid highly vascular areas (e.g., muscles).

- Instruct individual to avoid use of razors or to use electric razors.
- Instruct individual to avoid pregnancy while on therapy.

  R: Warfarin is toxic to fetuses.

Teach Individual and Family How to Prevent or Reduce the Severity of Adverse Effects

- Instruct them to monitor for and report signs of bleeding.
- Tell them to inform physicians, dentists, and other health care providers of anticoagulant therapy before invasive procedures.

  R: Precautions may be needed to prevent bleeding.

- Instruct them to contact physician or advanced practice nurse immediately after the onset of a fever or rash.

  R: These can indicate an infection or allergic response.

- Tell them that it takes 2 to 10 days for PT levels to return to normal after warfarin (Coumadin) is stopped.
- Explain that certain medications can inhibit or potentiate anticoagulant effect, and advise them to consult with a pharmacist before taking any prescribed or over-the-counter drug (e.g., aspirin, antibiotics, ibuprofen, diuretics).
- Teach persons on Coumadin to avoid or learn how to incorporate foods high in vitamin K if desired; such foods include turnip greens, asparagus, broccoli, watercress, cabbage, beef liver, lettuce, and green tea.

  R: Vitamin K decreases anticoagulant action. If desired, plan to consume foods high in potassium in portions that are consistent daily. Keeping the portion consistent daily will establish their Coumadin dose to maintain an INR within range for effective anticoagulation. Explain to persons on Paradoxa that there are no dietary restrictions.

- Advise individual to avoid alcohol, which potentates the effects of the anticoagulant if hepatic disease is also present.
- Instruct individual to wear Medic-Alert identification.
- Stress the importance of regular follow-up care and regular monitoring of blood levels.
- Instruct the individual and family to report the following:
  - Bleeding
  - Dark stools
  - Fever
  - Chills
  - Sore throat, difficulty speaking
  - Itching
  - Dark urine
  - Yellowing of skin or eyes
  - Mouth sores
  - Severe headache
  - New rash
  - Major illness
  - Persistent abdominal pain
  - Episode of fainting

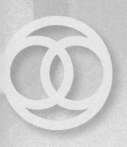

Unit III

Individual and Family-Centered Care Plans

Unit III

Unit III comprises care plans for clinical situations. These care plans represent the nursing diagnoses and collaborative problems known to occur frequently in these clinical situations and to be of major importance. Data collected about an individual must confirm the diagnosis.

Components of Each Care Plan

Definition

Each care plan begins with a description of the clinical situation. This information summarizes the current science on the condition, focusing on risk populations, diagnosis, treatment, and complications.

Time Frame

An individual's response to certain situations or conditions can vary depending if this is a new diagnosis, an exacerbation of a chronic disorder. For example, an individual with newly diagnosed diabetes mellitus will have additional educational needs from an individual with an exacerbation of the same disease. The focus of the care plans in this book is the initial diagnosis. The nurse can also use the care plan if an individual is readmitted for the same condition; however, the nurse may delete some of the care if not indicated.

Diagnostic Cluster

A diagnostic cluster represents a set of collaborative problems and nursing diagnoses anticipated and of key significance in a selected clinical situation of course, can experience many collaborative problems and nursing diagnoses. The diagnostic cluster represents those with high predictability, as the result of a validation study described beginning on page xii. Individuals will usually have additional nursing diagnoses and/ or collaborative problems beyond those identified for their condition. The limited hospital stays mandate that the nurse only address priority problems. Refer to Priority Identification Chapter 5 for guidelines in determining priorities.

Unit II

Section 1 contains Individual Nursing Diagnoses and Section 2 contains Individual Collaborative Problems. These two sections target an individual nursing diagnosis or collaborative problem to increase the reader's understanding. It prevents the repetition of these nursing diagnoses/collaborative problems throughout the care plans on specific conditions in Unit III.

For example, interventions associated with the treatment of the nursing diagnosis *Acute Pain* is found in Unit II Section 1. The nursing diagnosis of *Acute Pain* is in the diagnostic cluster in the Pancreatitis Care Plan. The reader will receive an explanation of the causes of acute pain in an individual with pancreatitis and then will be referred to Unit II Section 1 for the complete assessment and management of *Acute Pain*.

The collaborative problem *Risk for Complications of Deep Vein Thrombosis* (DVT) is described in Unit II Section 2. When DVT is a risk under a specific condition or situation such as postorthopedic surgery, the reader will receive an explanation of why and then be referred to Unit II Section 2 for a complete discussion of monitoring and interventions indicated.

In addition, the single file of collaborative problems can be used if an individual is admitted for a surgical procedure and also has diabetes mellitus. The nurse will select the appropriate surgical procedure care plan in Unit II Section 2. In addition, the collaborative problem > Risk for Complications of Hypo/Hyperglycemia will be added because the individual also has diabetes mellitus.

Transition to Home/Community Agencies

The old concept of discharge as a single event has been transformed into a process that begins on admission. Certain risk factors increase the vulnerability of the individual to experience an adverse event or complication. Occurrence of an adverse event or complication can increase the individual's morbidity and may cause death. This can increase suffering, extend hospitalization, and increase utilization of resources. Failure to address these risk factors can cause unsuccessful management at home and increase the likelihood of re-admission. This is emphasized with the Transition to Home/Community Facilities utilizing four elements:

1. **Transition Criteria:** These criteria are the individual or family behaviors desired to maintain or to achieve maximum functioning after transition. The transition needs of individuals and families can necessitate two types of nursing actions: teaching the individual and family to manage the situation at home, and referring the individual and family to agencies for assistance with continuing care management at home or transfer to a facility in the community. The transition criteria cited in each care plan represent those that a staff nurse can usually achieve with an individual or family during a typical length of stay.

2. **Transitional Risk Assessment Plan (TRAP):** Certain factors in individual increase their risk for complications as falls, infections, and pressure ulcers. When these complications occur, they increase morbidity and suffering and extend hospitalization with increased costs. These complications are often preventable. Each care plan in Unit III begins with the following:

> ### Transitional Risk Assessment Plan (TRAP)
>
> Begin this plan on admission.
> Implement the Transitional Risk Assessment Plan (TRAP):
> * Refer to inside back cover for an assessment tools to validate Risk for Surgical Site Infection, Risk for Falls, and Risk for Pressure Ulcers.
> * Add each validated high-risk problem to individual's problem list with the risk code in ().
> * Refer to Unit II for the individual high-risk nursing diagnoses/collaborative problems for outcomes and interventions.
>
> > *R:* "*Close coordination of care in the post-acute period, early discharge follow-up care, enhanced patient education and self-management training, proactive end-of-life counseling, and extending the resources and clinical expertise over time via multidisciplinary team management*" *can lower readmission rates and improve health outcomes (Boutwell & Hwu, 2009, p. 14). Interventions are utilized to activate the individual and family to select changes in their everyday lifestyle choices to improve their health (Hibbard & Greene, 2013).*

3. **Transition to Home/Community Care:** This feature addresses the assessment of risk factors that increase the likelihood that transition will be delayed or that problems may occur at home that can complicate recovery or cause readmission to the acute care agency. Preparing family members/support persons for home care is addressed in each care plan in Unit III. If a support system is not present, nonexistent, or incapable to providing home care, a referral to the appropriate resource in the institution as early as possible (e.g., social service, home care).

4. **Risk for Ineffective Health Management:** Every care plan ends with this nursing diagnosis. This diagnosis refers to the teaching needed for individual/family for management at home and referrals as indicated. Teaching the individual/family the early signs/symptoms that need immediate attention are emphasized.

Collaborative Problems

Collaborative problems have collaborative outcomes such as:

The individual will be monitored for early signs and symptoms of bleeding and will receive collaborative interventions if indicated to restore physiologic stability. Collaborative goals are followed with indicators that represent physiologic stability. Assessment of changes in these indicators warrants notifying the appropriate physician, nurse practitioner, or physician assistant. The nurse-prescribed interventions consist of monitoring for the onset of the complication or for worsening of a complication. Other nurse-prescribed interventions may include positioning, activity restrictions, prevention of pressure ulcer, anxiety reducing strategies, and the like. Keep in mind that collaborative problems are not physiologic nursing diagnoses. Physiologic nursing diagnoses that nurses use to prescribe treatment for or prevent are listed in the care plan as nursing diagnoses (e.g., *Risk for Pressure Ulcer, Risk for Fluid Volume Deficit, Imbalanced Nutrition*).

Nursing Diagnoses

Each care plan has at least two problem or risk nursing diagnoses. Keep in mind that the nurse should have validation for the diagnosis before initiating the care plan. Appropriate major signs and symptoms validate problem nursing diagnoses. Appropriate risk factors validate risk nursing diagnoses. Some of the nursing diagnoses are cross-referenced to Unit II Section 1 as Acute Pain.

Goals

The goals outlined for each nursing diagnosis consist of measurable behaviors of the individual or family that represent a favorable status. In addition, goals are from the Nursing Outcomes Classification (NOC), and interventions from the Nursing Interventions Classification (NIC) developed at the University of Iowa have been included for use in electronic systems.

Rationales

A supporting rationale is presented for each nursing intervention for both collaborative problems and nursing diagnoses. The rationale explains why the intervention is appropriate and why it will produce the desired response. Rationales may be scientific principles derived from the natural, physical, and behavioral sciences, or they may be drawn from the nursing, medical, and other health professionals (physical therapy, occupational therapy, nutritional therapy, sociology, psychology), research, and literature. Medical literature is used extensively for collaborative problems, since they represent medical complications. Some topics in nursing and medicine are well studied, whereas others have had little or no research. When a reference that is 10 or more years old is used, it is usually treated as a classic or continues to represent the most recent source on the subject, and such references will be indicated with an asterisk (*).

Documentation

Electronic health records represent the method of documentation for clinical nurses. Recommended elements to document are listed. Electronic flow records are utilized to document assessment data. Free texting is utilized to document unusual events or significant discussions/observations.

Addendum Diagnoses

Frequently the nurse will identify and validate the presence of a risk or actual diagnosis that is not included in the given care plan for the situation or diagnostic cluster. The nurse can refer to Unit II Section 1 and 2 for specific nursing diagnoses and collaborative problems. For example, Mr. Jamie has had an acute coronary syndrome; the nurse initiates the care plan for an individual experiencing an acute coronary syndrome. In addition, Mr. Jamie has just experienced the sudden death of his brother. The nurse can find *Grieving* in Unit II Section 1 and retrieve information about that diagnosis. Then, the diagnosis can be added as an additional or addendum diagnosis.

Features

STAR

STAR (stop, think, act, review) is an evidence-based model to help the nurse assess a situation prior to intervening and to evaluate the response after acting. The nurse/student nurse is encouraged to utilize this decision-making tool whenever a situation occurs that is problematic. The following is an example of using STAR to evaluate an individual's/family's ability to safely transition to home.

STAR **Stop**

Think Is this person at high risk for injury, falls, medical complications, and/or inability to care for self (activities of daily living)?

Is a support person available?

Is the person competent to manage self-administration of medications, treatment procedures? Are additional resources needed?

Can the person explain how to monitor the condition (e.g., blood glucose, signs/symptoms of complications, dietary/mobility restrictions, and when to call his or her primary provider or specialist)?

Act Contact or provide the appropriate resource (e.g., contacting a support person, home health assessment, additional teaching, printed materials).

Review Has the problem been addressed? If not, use SBAR to communicate to the appropriate person.

SBAR Nurses are taught to use detailed, narrative form in reports in contrast to physicians, who are taught to communicate using only the key information. SBAR serves to bridge the communication gap.

SBAR (situation, background, assessment, recommendation) is a framework for clearly and consistently, and communicating pertinent information among health care professionals. SBAR quickly organize the briefing information in your mind or on paper.

This format is useful in handoffs (shift report) when an urgent response is needed and in conflict situations (Leonard, Graham, & Bonacum, 2004). SBAR examples are found throughout the plans. For additional information on SBAR. Refer to Chapter 2.

Unit III Contents

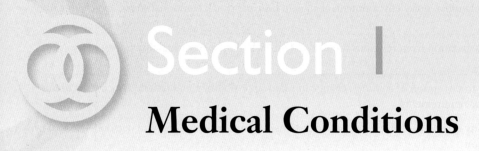

Section I

Medical Conditions

GENERIC MEDICAL CARE PLAN FOR THE HOSPITALIZED ADULT INDIVIDUAL

> **Carp's Cues**
>
> This care plan presents nursing diagnoses and collaborative problems that commonly apply to individuals (and their significant others) undergoing hospitalization for any medical disorder. It represents a basic standard of care. For beginning students, it can represent the care that they are prepared to provide. As the student progresses in the curriculum, the care plans for specific medical conditions such as pneumonia, diabetes mellitus, and congestive heart failure, and those focusing on the care of individuals undergoing surgery or therapies such as chemotherapy or anticoagulant therapy will be their focus of care.

◼◼◼◼◼ DIAGNOSTIC CLUSTER**

Collaborative Problems

Risk for Complications of Cardiovascular Dysfunction

Risk for Complications of Respiratory Insufficiency

Nursing Diagnoses

Anxiety related to unfamiliar environment, routines, diagnostic tests, treatments, and loss of control

Risk for Injury related to unfamiliar environment and physical and mental limitations secondary to condition, medications, therapies, and diagnostic tests

Risk for Infection related to increased microorganisms in environment, risk of person-to-person transmission, and invasive tests and therapies

(Specify) Self-Care Deficit related to sensory, cognitive, mobility, endurance, or motivation problems

Risk for Imbalanced Nutrition related to decreased appetite secondary to treatments, fatigue, environment, and changes in usual diet, and to increased protein and vitamin requirements for healing

Risk for Constipation related to change in fluid and food intake, routine, and activity level; effects of medications; and emotional stress

Risk for Pressure Ulcer related to prolonged pressure on tissues associated with decreased mobility, increased fragility of the skin associated with dependent edema, decreased tissue perfusion, malnutrition, and urinary/fecal incontinence

Disturbed Sleep Pattern related to unfamiliar, noisy environment, change in bedtime ritual, emotional stress, and change in circadian rhythm

Risk for Spiritual Distress related to separation from religious support system, lack of privacy, or inability to practice spiritual rituals

Interrupted Family Processes related to disruption of routines, change in role responsibilities, and fatigue associated with increased workload and visiting hour requirements

Risk for Compromised Human Dignity related to multiple factors (intrusions, unfamiliar procedures and personnel, loss of privacy) associated with hospitalization

Risk for Ineffective Health Management related to complexity and cost of therapeutic regimen, complexity of health care system, shortened length of stay, insufficient knowledge of treatment, and barriers to comprehension secondary to language barriers, cognitive deficits, hearing and/or visual impairment, anxiety, and lack of motivation

**This medical condition was not included in the validation study.

Transition Criteria

Specific discharge criteria vary depending on the individual's condition. Generally, all diagnoses in the above diagnostic cluster should be resolved before discharge.

Collaborative Problems

Risk for Complications of Cardiovascular Dysfunction

Risk for Complications of Respiratory Insufficiency

Collaborative Outcomes

The individual will be monitored for early signs and symptoms of (a) cardiovascular dysfunction, and (b) respiratory insufficiency and will receive collaborative interventions if indicated to restore physiologic stability.

Indicators of Physiologic Stability

- Calm, alert, oriented (a, b)
- Respiration 16 to 20 breaths/min, relaxed and rhythmic (b)
- Breath sounds present all lobes, no rales or wheezing (b)
- Pulse 60 to 100 beats/min (a, b)
- BP >90/60, <140/90 mm Hg (a, b)
- Capillary refill <3 seconds; skin warm and dry (a, b)
- Peripheral pulses full, equal (a)
- Temperature 98.5° F to 99° F (a, b)

Transitional Risk Assessment Plan (TRAP)

Begin this plan on admission.
Implement the Transitional Risk Assessment Plan (TRAP):
- Refer to inside back cover.
- Add each validated high-risk diagnosis to individual's problem list with the risk code in ( ).
- Refer to Unit II to the individual high-risk nursing diagnoses/collaborative problems for outcomes and interventions.

  R: "Close coordination of care in the post-acute period, early discharge follow-up care, enhanced patient education and self-management training, proactive end-of-life counseling, and extending the resources and clinical expertise over time via multidisciplinary team management" can lower readmission rates and improve health outcomes (Boutwell & Hwu, 2009, p. 14). Interventions are utilized to activate the individual and family to select changes in their everyday lifestyle choices to improve their health (Hibbard & Greene, 2013).

Interventions	*Rationales*
1. Monitor cardiovascular status:	1. Physiologic mechanisms governing cardiovascular function are very sensitive to any change in body function, making changes in cardiovascular status important clinical indicators.
a. Radial pulse (rate and rhythm)	a. Pulse monitoring provides data to detect cardiac arrhythmia, blood volume changes, and circulatory impairment.
b. Apical pulse (rate and rhythm)	b. Apical pulse monitoring is indicated if the individual's peripheral pulses are irregular, weak, or extremely rapid.
c. Blood pressure	c. Blood pressure represents the force that the blood exerts against the arterial walls. Hypertension (systolic pressure >140 mm Hg, diastolic pressure >85 mm Hg) may indicate increased peripheral resistance, cardiac output, blood volume, or blood viscosity. Hypotension can result from significant blood or fluid loss, decreased cardiac output, and certain medications.
d. Skin (color, temperature, moisture) and temperature	d. Skin assessment provides information evaluating circulation, body temperature, and hydration status.
e. Pulse oximetry	e. Pulse oximetry is a noninvasive method (probe sensor on fingertip) for continuous monitoring of oxygen saturation of hemoglobin.
2. Monitor respiratory status: rate, rhythm, breath sounds	2. Respiratory assessment provides essential data for evaluating the effectiveness of breathing and detecting adventitious or abnormal sounds, which may indicate airway moisture, narrowing, or obstruction.
3. Monitor for changes in mentation (increased drowsiness, confusion, irritability, anxiety).	3. Changes in mentation result from cerebral tissue hypoxia.
4. Monitor for decreased urine output (<0.5 mL/hr); cool, pale, or cyanotic skin.	4. The compensatory response to decreased circulatory oxygen aims to increase blood oxygen by increasing heart and respiratory rates and to decrease circulation to the kidneys and extremities (marked by decreased pulses and skin changes).
5. Administer low-flow (2 L/min) oxygen as prescribed through nasal cannula, titrate up per protocol to keep pulse oximetry between 90% and 92%.	5. Oxygen therapy increases circulating oxygen levels. Using a cannula rather than a mask may help reduce the individual's fears of suffocation.

Clinical Alert Report

Before providing care, advise ancillary staff/student to report the following to the professional nurse assigned to the individual:
- Change in cognitive status
- Oral temperature >100.5° F
- Systolic BP <90 mm Hg
- Resting pulse >100, <50 beats/min
- Respiratory rate >28, <10/min
- Oxygen saturation <90%

Documentation

Pulse rate and rhythm
Blood pressure
Respiratory assessment
Abnormal findings

Nursing Diagnoses

Anxiety Related to Unfamiliar Environment, Routines, Diagnostic Tests, Treatments, and Loss of Control

NOC
Anxiety Control, Coping, Impulse Control

Goal

The individual will communicate feelings regarding the condition and hospitalization.

NIC
Anxiety Reduction, Impulse Control Training, Anticipatory Guidance

Indicators

- Verbalize, if asked, what to expect regarding routines and procedures.
- Explain restrictions.

Interventions	Rationales

1. Explain hospital policies and routines:
  a. Visiting hours, mealtimes, and availability of snacks
  b. Vital-sign monitoring
  c. Television rental and operation
  d. Storage of valuables
  e. Telephone use
  f. No Smoking policy
2. Determine their knowledge of his or her condition, its prognosis, and treatment measures. Reinforce and supplement their understanding as necessary.
	1, 2. Providing accurate information can help decrease the individual's anxiety associated with the unknown and unfamiliar.

3. Explain any scheduled diagnostic tests, covering the following: description, purpose, pretest routines, expected sensations, posttest routines, timing of results 4. Explain any prescribed diet: purpose, duration, allowed, and restricted foods/fluids.	3–4. Teaching the individual about tests and treatment measures can help decrease his or her fear and anxiety associated with the unknown, and improve his or her sense of control over the situation.
5. Provide the individual with opportunities to make decisions about his or her care whenever possible.	5. Participating in decision making can help give an individual a sense of control, which enhances his or her coping ability. Perception of loss of control can result in a sense of powerlessness, then hopelessness.
6. Provide reassurance and comfort. Encourage him or her to share feelings and concerns, listen attentively, and convey empathy and understanding.	6. Providing emotional support and encouraging sharing may help an individual clarify and verbalize his or her fears, allowing the nurse to get realistic feedback and reassurance.
7. Encourage the support people to share their fears and concerns, and encourage them in providing meaningful and productive support.	7. Supporting the individual's support, people can enhance their ability to help the individual.

Documentation

Unusual responses or situations
Individual's knowledge/information provided related to diagnosis, treatment, and hospital routine

Risk for Falls[1] Related to Unfamiliar Environment and Physical or Mental Limitations Secondary to the Condition, Medications, Therapies, and Diagnostic Tests

NOC

Risk Control, Safety
Status: Falls Occurrence

Goal

The individual will not injure him- or herself during hospital stay.

NIC

Fall Prevention,
Environmental
Management: Safety,
Health Education,
Surveillance: Safety, Risk
Identification

Indicators

* Identify factors that increase risk of injury.
* Describe appropriate safety measures.

Interventions	Rationales
1. Involve all hospital personnel on every shift in the Fall Prevention Program. a. Always glance into the room of a high-risk person when passing his or her room. b. Alert other departments of high-risk individuals when off unit for tests, procedures. c. Address fall prevention and risks with every handoff and transfer. d. Seek to identify reversible risk factors in all individuals. Be aware of changing individual. e. Conditions and a change in risk status. f. Identify in a private conference room number of falls on the unit monthly (e.g., poster).	1. Approximately 14% of all falls in hospitals are accidental, another 8% are unanticipated physiologic falls, and 78% are anticipated physiologic falls (*Morse, 2002). Ancillary staffs are in an optimal position to witness high-risk situations, which can be addressed to prevent injury. e. Interdisciplinary approach to fall prevention is effective when falls are not viewed as inevitable accidents but preventable events.

2. Reduce or eliminate contributing factors for falls:
 a. Related to Unfamiliar Environment
 • Orient the individual to his or her environment (e.g., location of bathroom, bed controls, call bell). Leave a light on in the bathroom at night. Ensure path to bathroom is clear.
 • Teach him or her to keep the bed in the low position with side rails up at night.
 • Make sure that the telephone, eyeglasses, urinal, and frequently used personal belongings are within easy reach.
 • Instruct the individual to request assistance whenever needed.
 • For individuals with difficulty accessing toilet:
  • If urgency exists, evaluate for a urinary tract infection.
  • Provide an opportunity to use bathroom/urinal/bedpan every 2 hours while awake, at bedtime, and upon awakening.
  • Frequently scan floor for wet areas, objects on floor.
	• Orientation helps provide familiarity; a light at night helps the individual find his or her way safely.
	
	 • The low position makes it easier for the individual to get in and out of bed.
	 • Keeping objects at hand helps prevent falls from overreaching and overextending.
	
	 • Getting needed help with ambulation and other activities reduces an individual's risk of injury.
	  • New onset urinary urgency can be a sign of an infection.
	  • Thirty percent of falls are related to attempting to access the bathroom and can be prevented by timed toileting schedule (Tzeng, 2010).

(continued)

---

[1]Using the Risk Assessment tool for Falls on the inside back cover, calculate the score and record it in the ( ).

Interventions	*Rationales*

b. Related to Gait Instability/Balance Problems
  • Refer to Unit II Section 1 to Risk for Falls for interventions and rationale
c. Related to Medication Side Effects
  • Review the person's medication reconciliation completed on admission.
    • Question regarding alcohol use.
    • Question if the individual has side effects when taking certain meds.

  • Review present medications with pharmacist/ physician/nurse practitioner and evaluate those that can contribute to dizziness and if they should be discontinued, have dose reduction, or replaced with an alternative (*Riefkohl, Heather, Bieber, Burlingame, & Lowenthal, 2003).
    • Antidepressants (e.g., SSRIs)
    • Antipsychotics
    • Benzodiazepines
    • Antihistamines, Benadryl, hydroxyzine
    • Anticonvulsants
    • Nonsteroidal anti-inflammatory drugs
    • Muscle relaxants
    • Narcotic analgesics
    • Antiarrhythmics (type IA)
    • Digoxin
d. Related to Confused/Uncooperative/Impaired Cognition
  • Consider use of electronic devices in bed, chair, video surveillance.
  • Follow institutional policy for side rails.
  • Consider use of sitter.
  • Move person to a more observable room.
  • Plan to complete shift documentation in room of high-risk person.
e. Related to Tethering Devices (IVs, Foley, telemetry, compression devises)
  • Evaluate if tethering devices can be discontinued at night.
  • Can the IV be converted to saline port?
  • If individual is able, teach him or her how to safely ambulate with devices to bathroom or advise to call for assistance.
f. Related to Orthostatic Hypotension
  • Refer to Risk for Falls in Unit II Section 1.

Rationales (right column):

• Alcohol can potentiate side effects of sombulence/ dizziness.
• Some medications might need to be discontinued because of side effects or ineffective therapeutic response.
• The use of medications is one of the many different factors that can contribute to balance problems and the risk of falls. Published research suggests an association between the use of these drugs or drug classes and an increased risk of falling (*Riefkohl et al., 2003).

• Individuals can become entangled in lines and tubes and fall.

3. If individual falls, refer to Risk for Falls for interventions and documentation guidelines.

Clinical Alert Report

Advise ancillary staff/student to report:
  • Any incident of an almost fall or accident.
  • Attempts of a vulnerable individual to get out of bed without assistance.
  • Other risk situations (e.g., attempts of visitors who are not capable, to assist an individual).

Documentation

Individual/family teaching
Post fall documentation
  Document circumstances, assessment, interventions in health record
  Complete incident report

Risk for Infection[2] Related to Increased Microorganisms in the Environment, Risk of Person-to-Person Transmission, and Invasive Tests or Therapies

NOC
Infection Status, Wound Healing: Primary Intention, Immune Status

Goal

The individual will describe or demonstrate appropriate precautions to prevent infection.

NIC
Infection Control, Wound Care, Incision Site Care, Health Education

Interventions	Rationales
1. Use appropriate universal precautions for every individual. a. Hand hygiene b. Antiseptic hand hygiene ([quoted from Diaz & Newman, 2015]; Centers for Disease Control and Prevention [CDC], 2016b) • Wash with antiseptic soap and water for at least 15 seconds followed by alcohol-based hand rub. • If hands were not in contact with anyone or thing in the room, use an alcohol-based hand rub and rub till dry (CDC, 2016b). • Plain soap is good at reducing bacterial counts but antimicrobial soap is better, and alcohol-based handrubs are the best (CDC, 2016b). • Before putting on gloves and after taking them off • Before and after touching an individual, before handling an invasive device (foley catheter, peripheral vascular catheter) regardless of whether or not gloves are used • After contact with body fluids or excretions, mucous membranes, nonintact skin, or wound dressings • If moving from a contaminated body site to another body site during the care of the same individual • After contact with inanimate surfaces and objects (including medical equipment) in the immediate vicinity of the individual; • After removing sterile or nonsterile gloves • Before handling medications or preparing food c. Personal protective equipment (PPE) (CDC, 2013a) • Wear PPE when the individual interaction indicates that contact with blood/body fluids may occur.	1. Assume everyone is potentially infected or colonized with an organism that could be transmitted in the health care setting (CDC, 2016b). a,b. Numerous studies have proved that health care workers' hands transmit microorganisms to patients. Evidence proves that effective hand washing is the cornerstone for preventing health care–associated infections. It is also important in preventing specific site infections such as catheter-related bloodstream infections, catheter-related urinary tract infections, ventilator-associated pneumonia, and surgical site infections (SSIs) studies continue to demonstrate that hand hygiene practices among health care workers is at an abysmally low rate (Diaz, & Newman, 2015).

(continued)

[2]Using the Risk Assessment tool for Infection on the inside back cover, calculate the score and record it in the ( ).

Interventions	*Rationales*
d. Gloves • Wears gloves when providing direct individual care. • Wear gloves for potential contact with nonintact skin, mucous membranes blood, and body fluids. Handle the blood of all individuals as potentially infectious. • Remove gloves properly to prevent hand contamination. Deposit gloves in the proper container in the room. • After removing gloves, wash hands with soap and water. • Do not substitute alcohol-based hand rubs when the physical action of washing and rinsing hands with antimicrobial or no antimicrobial soap and water when any contact with individuals or any object in the room. Alcohol, chlorhexidine, and other antiseptic agents alone have poor activity against some organisms (e.g., spores *C. difficile*) (CDC, 2016b). e. Masks • Use PPE (masks, goggles, face shields) to protect the mucous membranes of your eyes, mouth, nose during procedures and individual care activities that may generate splashes or sprays of blood, body fluids, secretions, and excretions. f. Gowns • Wear a gown for direct contact with uncontained secretions or excretions. • Remove gown and perform hand hygiene before leaving the individual's room/cubicle. • Do not reuse gowns even with the same individual. When suctioning oral secretion. Wear gloves and mask/goggles or a face shield—sometimes gown (CDC, 2013a).	d. Gloves provide a barrier from contact with infectious secretions and excretions. These precautions prevent the transmission of pathogens to the caregiver and then to others (e.g., other individuals, visitors, other staff/student. f. Gowns are needed to prevent soiling or contamination of clothing during procedures and individual care activities. • This will prevent contamination of clothing and skin during the process of care. • Before leaving room, remove and discard all PPE in the room or cubicle. • These precautions prevent the transmission of pathogens to the caregiver and then to others (e.g., other individuals, visitors, other staff).
2. Educate all staff/student, visitors, and individuals on the importance preventing droplet and infectious organisms' transmission from themselves to others (CDC, 2015a). a. Offer a surgical mask to persons who are coughing to decrease contamination of the surrounding environment. b. Cover the mouth and nose during coughing and sneezing. c. Use tissues to contain respiratory secretions with prompt disposal into a no-touch receptacle. Wash hands with soap and water. d. Turn the head away from others and maintaining spatial distance, ideally >3 feet, when coughing.	2. These measures are targeted to all individuals with symptoms of respiratory infection and their accompanying family members or friends beginning at the point of initial encounter with a health care setting (e.g., reception/triage in emergency departments, ambulatory clinics, health care provider offices) (CDC, 2015a).

> **CLINICAL ALERT:**
> • If an individual or visitors refuse to comply with infection prevention requirements, report situation to manager or infection control officer.

Interventions	*Rationales*

3. Determine the individual placement based on:
  a. Route of transmission of known or suspected infectious agent
  b. Risk factors for transmission in the infected individual
  c. Risk factors for adverse outcomes resulting from an hospital-acquired infection (HAI) in other individuals in the area or room.
  d. Availability of single-individual rooms.
  e. Client options for room-sharing (e.g., placing individuals with the same infection in the same room).	

4. Immediately report any situation that increases the risk of infection transmission to individuals, visitors, or staff/students.	

5. Before confirmation of infectious agent, initiate specific precautions for the suspected agent:
  a. Meningitis: droplet, airborne precautions
  b. Maculopapular rash with cough, fever
  c. Rubella > airborne precautions
  d. Abscess > MRSA > contact, droplet precautions
  e. Cough/fever/pulmonary infiltrate in HIV infected or someone at high risk of HIV infection
  f. Tuberculosis > airborne/contact (respirators)
	5. Prevention strategies are indicated when high-risk infections are suspected but not yet confirmed.

6. Reduce entry of organisms into individuals:
  a. Urinary tract (catheter-associated urinary tract infection [CAUTI])
    • Refer to Unit II Section 1 Risk for Infection for interventions to prevent urinary tract (CAUTI)
  b. Invasive access sites
	6a. Every attempt to minimize urinary catheter use and duration of use in all individuals must be instituted, especially with those at higher risk for CAUTI or mortality from catheterization such as women, older persons, and individuals with impaired immunity.
	  b. Invasive lines provide a site for organism entry. Interventions focus on prevention and identification of early signs of infection.
	      Transparent, semi-permeable polyurethane dressings permit continuous visual inspection of the catheter site. Transparent dressings can be safely left on peripheral venous catheters for the duration of catheter insertion without increasing the risk for thrombophlebitis (O'Grady et al., 2011).
	      The CDC (2016c) reported a 46% decrease in central line-associated bloodstream infection (CLABSI) was reported between 2008 and 2013, which is attributed to adhering to protocols.

CLINICAL ALERT:
- O'Grady et al. (2011) summarized research which "reports spanning the past four decades have consistently demonstrated that risk for infection declines following standardization of aseptic care, and that insertion and maintenance of intravascular catheters by *inexperienced* staff might increase the risk for catheter colonization and CRBSI. Specialized "IV teams" have shown unequivocal effectiveness in reducing the incidence of CRBSI, associated complications, and costs additionally, infection risk increases with nursing staff reductions below a critical level.

(continued)

Interventions	Rationales

- Follow protocol for invasive access sites for insertion and maintenance. Some general interventions are (O'Grady et al., 2011):
  - Evaluate the catheter insertion site daily by palpation through the dressing to discern tenderness and by inspection if a transparent dressing is in use. If the individual is diaphoretic or if the site is bleeding or oozing, use gauze dressing until this is resolved.
  - Gauze and opaque dressings should not be removed if the individual has no clinical signs of infection.
  - If the individual has local tenderness or other signs of possible CRBSI, an opaque dressing should be removed and the site inspected visually (O'Grady et al., 2011).
  - Encourage the individual to report any changes in their catheter site or any new discomfort to their nurse.
  - Monitor temperature at least every 24 hours or more often as indicated; notify proscribing physician, nurse practitioner/physical assistant if greater than 100.8° F.
  - Remove peripheral venous catheters if the individual develops signs of phlebitis (warmth, tenderness, erythema or palpable venous cord), infection, or a malfunctioning catheter
  - Maintain aseptic technique for all invasive devices, changing sites, dressings, tubing, and solutions per policy schedule.
  - Use maximal sterile barrier precautions, including the use of a cap, mask, sterile gown, sterile gloves, and a sterile full body drape, for the insertion of CVCs, PICCs, or guidewire exchange.
  - Use a 2% chlorhexidine wash instead of soap and water for daily skin cleansing
  - Daily cleansing of ICU individuals with a 2% chlorhexidine-impregnated washcloth may be a simple, effective strategy to decrease the rate of primary blood stream infections (O'Grady et al., 2011).
  - Evaluate all abnormal laboratory findings, especially cultures/sensitivities and CBC.

c. Respiratory tract infections
  - Prevent and monitor for respiratory infections
    - Monitor temperature at least every 8 hours and notify physician if greater than 100.8° F.
    - Evaluate sputum characteristics for frequency, purulence, blood, and odor.
    - Evaluate sputum and blood cultures, if done, for significant findings.
    - Assess lung sounds every 8 hours or p.r.n.
    - If individual has abdominal/thoracic surgery, instruct before surgery on importance of coughing, turning, and deep breathing.
    - Prompt to cough and deep breathe hourly.
    - If individual has had anesthesia, monitor for appropriate clearing of secretions in lung fields.
    - Evaluate need for suctioning if individual cannot clear secretions adequately.
    - Assess for risk of aspiration, keeping head of bed elevated 30 degrees unless otherwise contraindicated.
    - Ensure optimal pain management.

c. Individuals with pain, postanesthesia, compromised ability to move, and those with ineffective cough are at risk for infection due to pooling of respiratory secretions.

Interventions	Rationales

d. Surgical site infection
Refer to Generic Care Plan for an individual
pre-/postsurgery.

Documentation

Catheter and insertion site care
Abnormal findings

(Specify) Self-Care Deficit Related to Sensory, Cognitive, Mobility, Endurance, or Motivational Problems

NOC

See Self-Care: Bathing, Self-Care: Hygiene, Self-Care: Eating, Self-Care: Dressing, Self-Care: Toileting, and/or Self-Care: Instrumental Activities of Daily Living

Goal

The individual will perform self-care activities (feeding, toileting, dressing, grooming, bathing), with assistance as needed.

NIC

See Feeding, Bathing, Dressing, and/or Instrumental Self-Care Deficit

Indicators

- Demonstrate optimal hygiene after care is provided.
- Describe restrictions or precautions as needed.

Interventions	Rationales

1. Consult with a physical therapist to assess present level of participation and for a plan.
  a. Determine areas for potentially increased participation in each self-care activity.
  b. Explore the individual's goals and determine what the learner perceives as his or her own needs.
  c. Compare what the nurse believes are the learner's needs and goals, and then work to establish mutually acceptable goals.
  d. Allow ample time to complete activities without help. Promote independence, but assist when the individual cannot perform an activity.
	1. Offering choices and including the individual in planning care reduces feelings of powerlessness; promotes feelings of freedom, control, and self-worth; and increases the individual's willingness to comply with therapeutic regimens. Optimal education promotes self-care.

2. Evaluate the individual's ability to participate in each self-care activity (feeding, dressing, bathing, and toileting).	2. Enhancing an individual's self-care abilities can increase his or her sense of control and independence, promoting overall well-being.
3. Use the following scale to rate the individual's ability to perform 0 = Is completely independent 1 = Requires use of assistive device 2 = Needs minimal help 3 = Needs assistance and/or some supervision 4 = Needs total supervision 5 = Needs total assistance or unable to assist Reassess ability frequently and revise code as appropriate.	3. This coding allows for establishing a baseline from which to evaluate progress.

(continued)

Interventions	Rationales

4. Refer to interventions under each diagnosis—feeding, bathing, dressing, toileting, and instrumental self-care deficit as indicated.
   a. Provide common nursing interventions for feeding.
   b. Ascertain from the individual or family members what foods the individual likes or dislikes.
   c. Ensure that the individual eats meals in the same setting with pleasant surroundings that are not too distracting.
   d. Maintain correct food temperatures (hot foods hot, cold foods cold).
   e. Provide pain relief because pain can affect appetite and ability to feed self.
   f. Provide good oral hygiene before and after meals.
   g. Encourage the individual to wear dentures and eyeglasses.
   h. Assist the individual to the most normal eating position suited to his or her physical disability (best is sitting in a chair at a table).
   i. Encourage an individual who has trouble handling utensils to eat "finger foods" (e.g., bread, sandwiches, fruit, nuts).
   j. Provide needed adaptive devices for eating, such as a plate guard, suction device under the plate or bowl, padded-handle utensils, wrist or hand splints with clamp, and special drinking cup.
   k. Provide social contact during eating.
   l. If individual is not eating or drinking enough, consult with nutritionist.

4a. These strategies attempt to normalize mealtime to increase participation and intake.

5. Provide general nursing interventions for inability to bathe.
   a. Bathing time and routine should be consistent to encourage optimal independence.
   b. Encourage the individual to wear prescribed corrective lenses or hearing aid.
   c. Keep the bathroom temperature warm; ascertain the individual's preferred water temperature.
   d. Provide for privacy during bathing routine.
   e. Elicit from the individual his or her usual bathing routine.
   f. Keep the environment simple and uncluttered.
   g. Observe skin condition during bathing.
   h. Provide all bathing equipment within easy reach.
   i. Provide for safety in the bathroom (nonslip mats, grab bars).
   j. When the individual is physically able, encourage the use of either a tub or shower stall, depending on which he or she uses at home.
   k. Provide for adaptive equipment as needed:
      • Chair or stool in bathtub or shower
      • Long-handled sponge to reach back or lower extremities
      • Grab bars on bathroom walls where needed to assist in mobility
      • Bath board for transferring to tub chair or stool
      • Safety treads or nonskid mat on floor of bathroom, tub, and shower
      • Washing mitts with pocket for soap
      • Adapted toothbrushes
      • Shaver holders
      • Handheld shower spray

5j. The individual should practice in the hospital in preparation for going home.

Interventions	*Rationales*
l. Provide for relief of pain that may affect the individual's ability to bathe self.	l. Offering choices and including the individual in planning care reduces feelings of powerlessness; promotes feelings of freedom, control, and self-worth; and increases the individual's willingness to comply with therapeutic regimens. Assistive devices can improve self-care abilities.
m. Consider use of nondetergent, no-rinse, prepackaged bathing products.	m. Individual aggression may be precipitated by baths or showers. Soap, towels in a warm environment have been found to reduce aggression.
n. For confused individuals, preserve dignity and decrease agitation: • Provide verbal warning before doing anything (e.g., touching, spraying with water). • Apply firm pressure to the skin when bathing; it is less likely to be misinterpreted than a gentle touch. • Use a warm shower or bath to help a confused or agitated individual to relax. • Add lavender oil to bath water. • Determine the best method to bathe person (e.g., bed bath, shower, tub bath).	
6. Provide general nursing interventions for self-dressing. a. Obtain clothing that is larger-sized and easier to put on, including clothing with elastic waistbands, wide sleeves and pant legs, dresses that open down the back for women in wheelchairs, and Velcro fasteners or larger buttons.	6. Inability to care for oneself produces feelings of dependency and poor self-concept. With increased ability for self-care, self-esteem increases. Optimal personal grooming promotes psychological well-being.
b. Encourage the individual to wear prescribed corrective lenses or hearing aid.	
c. Promote independence in dressing through continual and unaided practice.	
d. Allow sufficient time for dressing and undressing because the task may be tiring, painful, or difficult.	
e. Plan for the individual to learn and demonstrate one part of an activity before progressing further.	
f. Lay clothes out in the order in which the individual will need them to dress.	
g. Provide dressing aids as necessary.	g. Some commonly used aids include dressing stick, Swedish reacher, zipper pull, buttonhook, long-handled shoehorn, and shoe fasteners adapted with elastic laces.
h. If needed, increase participation in dressing by medicating for pain 30 minutes before it is time to dress or undress, if indicated.	
i. Provide for privacy during dressing routine.	
j. Provide for safety by ensuring easy access to all clothing and by ascertaining the individual's performance level.	

Documentation

Assistance needed for self-care

Risk for Imbalanced Nutrition Related to Decreased Appetite Secondary to Treatments, Fatigue, Environment, and Changes in Usual Diet, and to Increased Protein and Vitamin Requirements for Healing

NOC
Nutritional Status,
Teaching: Nutrition

Goal

The individual will ingest daily nutritional requirements in accordance with activity level, metabolic needs, and restrictions.

NIC
Nutrition Management,
Nutritional Monitoring

Indicators

- Relate the importance of good nutrition.
- Relate restrictions, if any.

Interventions	Rationales
1. Ensure that a nutritional assessment is done on admission according to protocols.	1. Nutritional assessments are required within 24 hours of admission to a hospital and within 14 days of admission to a long-term facility (The Joint Commission, 2010).

> **CLINICAL ALERT:**
> - In 2013, 85.7% of US households were food secure throughout the year. The remaining 14.3% (17.5 million households) were food insecure (Coleman-Jensen, Gregory, & Singh, 2013).

Interventions	Rationales
2. Explain the need for adequate consumption of carbohydrates, fats, protein, vitamins, minerals, and fluids.	2. Nutrients provide energy sources, build tissue, and regulate metabolic processes.
3. When indicated, consult with a nutritionist to establish appropriate daily caloric and food type requirements for the individual.	3. The body requires a minimum level of nutrients for health and growth. During the life span, nutritional needs vary (Lutz, Mazur, & Litch, 2015).
4. Assess if there are cultural preferences in regard to food.	

5. Address the factors that are causing or contributing to decrease intake (Dudek, 2014)
a. Related to decreased oral intake, mouth discomfort, nausea, and vomiting secondary to
  • Alcohol abuse
  • Drug use
  • Depression
  • Inability to chew
b. Related to decreased oral intake, mouth discomfort, nausea, and vomiting secondary to (e.g., radiation therapy, tonsillectomy, chemotherapy, oral trauma)
c. Related to factors associated with aging	

6. Assess for factors that contribute to nutritional deficiencies in older individuals.	6. In general, older adults need the same kind of balanced diet as any other group, but fewer calories. Diets of older individuals, however, tend to be insufficient in iron, calcium, and vitamins. The combination of long-established eating patterns, income, transportation, housing, social interaction, and the effects of chronic or acute disease influence nutritional intake and health (Miller, 2015).
7. When possible, attempt to reduce barriers of food procurement/preparation (e.g., functional ability, financial, transportation, kitchen facilities)	7. Factors such as pain, fatigue, analgesic use, and immobility can contribute to anorexia. Identifying a possible cause enables interventions to eliminate or minimize it.
8. Refer to nutritionist/social services for an assessment and interventions.	
9. Determine if individual has lactose intolerance. Refer to dietician if present.	9. Estimates vary, but generally it is believed that as much as 80% of the black population is affected, 53% of the Mexican-American population, and about 15% of the white population. In Europe, it varies widely from about 2% in Scandinavia to about 70% in Sicily. The prevalence is almost 100% in some Asian countries. Most people are born with the ability to digest lactose, but for many, that ability lessens significantly after about age 2 (Webb, 2015).

Interventions	Rationales
10. Provide the following generic interventions for individuals with decreased appetite regardless of etiology:	
a. When possible, attempt to have some socialization during mealtime (e.g., suggest to family that they eat with individual if appropriate).	10a. In nursing home settings, residents' nutritional status is significantly better in those who eat in the general dining room, rather than isolated in their own rooms (*Simmons & Levy-Storms, 2005).
b. Offer frequent, small meals instead of a few large ones; offer foods served cold.	b. Even distribution of total daily caloric intake helps prevent gastric distention, possibly increasing appetite.
c. With decreased appetite, restrict liquids with meals and avoid fluids 1 hour before and after meals.	c. Restricting fluids with meals helps prevent gastric distention.
d. Encourage and help the individual to maintain good oral hygiene.	d. Poor oral hygiene leads to bad odor and taste, which can diminish appetite.
e. Arrange to have high-calorie and high-protein foods served at the times that the individual usually feels most like eating.	e. Presenting high-calorie and high-protein food when the individual is most likely to eat increases the likelihood that he or she will consume adequate calories and protein.
f. Decrease amounts of food on tray, if it is anticipated that the person will eat only some.	f. Unrealistic amounts of food can discourage the individual before he or she starts.

Interventions	Rationales
11. Take steps to promote appetite:	11. Diet planning focuses on avoiding nutritional excesses. Reducing fats, salt, and sugar can reduce the risk of heart disease, diabetes, certain cancers, and hypertension.
a. Determine the individual's food preferences and arrange to have them provided, as appropriate.	
b. Eliminate any offensive odors and sights from the eating area.	
c. Control any pain and nausea before meals.	
d. Encourage the individual's support people to bring permitted foods from home, if possible.	
e. Provide a relaxed atmosphere and some socialization during meals.	
f. When anorexia is present, stress the importance of consuming foods higher in nutrition. Avoid describing foods as bad or good. Explain nutrient density of foods (*Hunter & Cason, 2006)	f. Nutrient dense foods give the most nutrients for the fewest amounts of calories.

  • Foods that are nutrient dense:
    • Fruits and vegetables that are bright or deeply colored
    • Foods that are fortified
    • Lower fat versions of meats, milk, dairy products, and eggs
  • Foods that are less nutrient dense:
    • Be lighter or whiter in color
    • Contain a lot of refined sugar
    • Be refined products (white bread as compared to whole grains)
    • Contain high amounts of fat for the amount of nutrients compared to similar products (fat-free milk vs. ice cream)
      • For example:
        • Apple is a better choice than a bag of pretzels with the same number of calories, but the apple provides fiber, vitamin C, and potassium.
        • An orange is better than orange juice because it has fiber

12. Give the individual printed materials outlining a nutritious diet. Refer to Getting Started to Better Nutrition on thePoint.

Clinical Alert Report

Before providing care, advise ancillary staff/student to report the following to the professional nurse assigned to the individual with marginal fluid or nutritional status:
- The amount/types of food ingested
- The amount/types of fluids

Documentation

Dietary intake
Daily weight
Diet instruction
Use of assistive devices

Risk for Constipation Related to Change in Fluid or Food Intake, Routine, or Activity Level; Effects of Medications; and Emotional Stress

NOC
Bowel Elimination, Hydration, Symptom Control

Goal

The individual will maintain prehospitalization bowel patterns.

NIC
Bowel Management, Fluid Management, Constipation/Impaction Management

Indicators

- State the importance of fluids, fiber, and activity.
- Report difficulty promptly.

Interventions	Rationales
1. Auscultate bowel sounds. **CLINICAL ALERT:** • Constipation is often viewed as expected and benign. • Constipation can be responsible for undiagnosed pain and exacerbating confusion in individuals who cannot communicate. • Almost all episodes of constipation can be prevented.	1. Bowel sounds indicate the nature of peristaltic activity.

2. Explain the risks of constipation when hospitalized
  a. Reduced activity
  b. Insufficient fluid intake
  c. Inadequate food intake with low fiber
  d. Opioids, diuretics, anticholinergics, antiemetics
Consult with physician/nurse practitioner/physician assistant for stool-softener medication.
	2. Factors that decrease peristalsis are some medications, for example, opioids, antiemetics, anticholinergics, and reduced activity. Insufficient fluid intake and diuretics reduce produce hard feces (Dudek, 2014).
	
	Stool softeners draw water into the intestines to help prevent dry, hard stools (Arcangelo & Peterson, 2016).

3. If severe constipation is present; consult with physician/nurse practitioner for an evaluation.	

4. Promote corrective measures.
  a. Regular time for elimination
    • Review daily routine.
    • Provide a stimulus to defecation (e.g., coffee, prune juice).
    • Advise the individual to attempt to defecate about 1 hour or so after meals and that remaining in the bathroom for a suitable length of time may be necessary.
	4a. The gastrocolic and duodenocolic reflexes stimulate mass peristalsis two or three times a day, most often after meals.

Interventions

Rationales

b. Adequate exercise
  • Provide frequent ambulation of hospitalized when tolerable.
  • Perform range-of-motion exercises for the individual who is bedridden.

c. Balanced diet
  • Avoid food low in fiber (e.g., starches, white bread, pasta, white rice, dairy products, processed foods).
  • Review list of foods high in fiber (e.g., fresh fruits, fruit juices, and vegetables with skins).
  • Beans (navy, kidney, lima), nuts and seeds, whole-grain breads, cereal, and bran
  • Include approximately 800 g of fruits and vegetables (about four pieces of fresh fruit and large salad) for normal daily bowel movement. Avoid cooked fruits.
  • Suggest moderate use of bran at first (may irritate gastrointestinal tract, produce flatulence, cause diarrhea, or blockage). Explain the need for fluid intake with bran.

d. Adequate fluid intake
  • Encourage intake of at least 2 L (8 to 10 glasses) unless contraindicated.
  • Discuss fluid preferences. Set up regular schedule for fluid intake.
  • Advise avoiding grapefruit juice, apple juice, coffee, tea, cola, and chocolate drinks as daily fluid intake.

b. Regular physical activity promotes muscle tonicity needed for fecal expulsion. It also increases circulation to the digestive system, which promotes peristalsis and easier feces evacuation.

  • Low-fiber foods pass slowly in the large intestines and thus become dry, hard, and difficult to defecate. Diets low in fiber and high in concentrated refined foods produce small, hard stools that increase the colon's susceptibility to disease.
  • Diets high in unrefined fibrous food produce large, soft stools that decrease the colon's susceptibility to disease. An increase in fiber without an optimal hydration will worsen constipation.

  • Sufficient fluid intake, at least 2 L daily, is necessary to maintain bowel patterns and to promote proper stool consistency.

  • These beverages have a diuretic effect.

Clinical Alert Report

Advise ancillary staff/student to report:
  • Any changes in bowel function (e.g., diarrhea, hard stools).
  • If no bowel movement occurs during shift.

Documentation

Bowel movements
Bowel sounds
Individual/family teaching

Risk for Pressure Ulcers[3] Related to Prolonged Pressure on Tissues Associated with Decreased Mobility, Increased Fragility of the Skin Associated with Dependent Edema, Decreased Tissue Perfusion, Malnutrition, Urinary/Fecal Incontinence

NOC

Tissue Integrity: Skin and Mucous Membranes

Goal

The individual will maintain present intact skin/tissue.

NIC

Pressure Management, Pressure Ulcer Care, Skin Surveillance, Positioning

Indicators

  • No redness (erythema)
  • Relate risk factors to skin/tissue trauma.

[3]Using the risk assessment tool for pressure ulcers on the inside back cover, calculate the score and record it in the ( ).

Interventions	Rationales
1. Using the Risk Assessment Score on the inside back cover, identify individuals as High Risk for Pressure Ulcers (PUs). Refer to Risk for Pressure Ulcers in Unit II Section 1 for intrinsic and extrinsic factors for PUs.	1. The risk assessment score using the Braden Scale should be completed if not already completed on admission using the criteria.
2. Upon admission, all skin surfaces, bony prominences, and skin folds will be inspected for evidence of redness or skin breakdown. a. Inspect the skin from head-to-toe to assess skin integrity and detect existing PUs. b. Look closely at all bony prominences and body surfaces subject to pressure or pressure in combination with shear. c. Examine the skin/soft tissue under and around tubing and other medical devices. d. Palpate suspect skin to assess temperature, moisture, and consistency. e. Document the skin condition with location, description, and measurement of lesions. Take photos with permission.	2a. A physical assessment must be completed within 24 hours of hospital admission in accordance with The Joint Commission regulations. This physical assessment should include a skin assessment and a PU risk assessment. Individual health care agencies can require this assessment to be completed earlier (e.g. 2 to 4 hours., 6 to 8 hours).
3. Perform a skin assessment at least every 8 hours or more often depending on risks factors. High-risk areas for PUs are: a. The backs of the heels b. The back of the head (occipital) c. Knees d. Elbows e. Buttocks and tailbone (coccyx, sacrum) f. Hipbone when lying on side (greater trochanter). g. Any area of the body with cast, boot, restraint, tubing, cervical collar, etc.	
4. For individuals, with increased risk for PUs, refer to Unit II, Section 2, Risk for Pressure Ulcers a. Ensure high-risk individuals have pressure-relieving devices. If needed utilize SBAR: **SBAR** *Situation:* I just assessed Mr. Jones. I am concerned because he had several risk factors for PU. *Background:* Mr. Jones is underweight, not eating well, and not moving on his own in bed. He is resistant to getting out of bed His heels and sacral area are reddened even with repositioning every hour. *Assessment:* Not applicable *Recommendation:* I would like an order for a pressure-relieving device. I would also like a nutritional consult to increase his protein intake.	4. Prevention strategies are indicated (e.g., pressure-relieving devices).

Clinical Alert Report

Advise ancillary staff/student to report:
- Skin condition of vulnerable areas (back, heels, and elbows)
- New onset of incontinence

Documentation

Turning and repositioning
Skin assessment

Disturbed Sleep Pattern Related to an Unfamiliar, Noisy Environment, a Change in Bedtime

NOC
Rest, Sleep, Well-Being

Goal

The individual will report a satisfactory balance of rest and activity.

NIC
Energy Management,
Sleep Enhancement,
Environmental
Management

Indicators

- Complete at least four sleep cycles (100 minutes) undisturbed.
- State factors that increase or decrease the quality of sleep.

Interventions	Rationales
1. Explain the effects of sleep deprivation on cognitive changes and risk of falls/injury. **SBAR** *Situation:* Mr. Green has slept only 4 hours in the last 24 hours. *Background:* "He is not sleeping because...." *Assessment:* He complaints of more pain, wants a sleeping pill. *Recommendation:* It would be useful to ... (e.g., stop taking vital signs 10 p.m. to 6 a.m. unless needed, change the times for med. administration; provide treatments before 10 p.m. and after 6 a.m. when possible).	1. Sleep deprivation results in impaired cognitive functioning (e.g., memory, concentration, and judgment) and perception, reduced emotional control, increased suspicion, irritability, and disorientation. It also lowers the pain threshold and decreases production of catecholamines, corticosteroids, and hormones (Arthritis Foundation, 2008). Sleep disturbance is the leading cause of hospital complications, such as falls, delirium (Institute of Medicine, 2009).
2. Discuss with physician/nurse practitioner/physical assistant the use of a "sleep protocol." This will allow the nursing staff/student the authority not to wake a person for blood draws or vital signs if appropriate, and (Bartick, 2009; Faraklas et al., 2013): a. Designate "quiet time" between 10 p.m. and 6 a.m. b. Play lullabies over public address system. c. Set a timer to turn off overhead hallway lights at 10 p.m. d. Mute phones close to patient rooms; avoid intercom use except in emergencies. e. Take vital signs at 10 p.m., and start again at 6 a.m. unless otherwise indicated. f. Order medications as b.i.d., t.i.d., q.i.d., but not "q" certain hours when possible. g. Do not administer a diuretic after 4 p.m. h. Avoid blood transfusions during "quiet time" due to frequent monitoring.	2. A small study reported that "sleep protocol" can reduce the number of individuals reporting disturbed sleep by 38% and reduce the number of individuals needing sedatives by 49% (Bartick, 2009).

(continued)

Interventions	Rationales

3. Encourage or provide evening care, offer:
  a. Use of bathroom or bedpan
  b. Personal hygiene (mouth care, bath, shower, partial bath)
  c. Clean linen and bedclothes (freshly made bed, sufficient blankets)	

4. Reduce or eliminate environmental distractions and sleep interruptions.
  a. Noise
  b. Close the door to the room.
  c. Pull the curtains.
  d. Unplug the telephone.
  e. Use "white noise" (e.g., fan; quiet music; tape of rain, waves).
  f. Eliminate 24-hour lighting.
  g. Provide night lights.
  h. Decrease the amount and kind of incoming stimuli (e.g., staff conversations).
  i. Cover blinking lights with tape.
  j. Reduce the volume of alarms and televisions.
  k. Place the individual with a compatible roommate, if possible.
  l. Interruptions
  m. Cluster procedures to minimize the times to wake the individual at night. If possible, plan for at least four periods of 90-minute uninterrupted sleep.
	4. Sleep is difficult without relaxation, which the unfamiliar hospital environment can hinder. Ensure that the individual has at least four or five periods of at least 90 minutes each of uninterrupted sleep every 24 hours. Researchers have reported that the chief deterrents to sleep in critical care individuals were activity, noise, pain, physical condition, nursing procedures, lights, and hypothermia.
	
	  m. In order to feel rested, a person usually must complete an entire sleep cycle (70 to 90 minutes) four or five times a night.

5. Document the amount of the individual's uninterrupted sleep each shift.	5. To feel rested, an individual usually must complete an entire sleep cycle (70 to 100 minutes) four or five times a night.
6. Provide health teaching and referrals, as indicated.	
7. Refer to Getting Started to Sleeping Better on thePoint. Print and give to individual.	

> ### *Clinical Alert Report*
>
> Before providing care, advise ancillary staff/student to report the following to the professional nurse assigned to the individual:
> - The actual time (minutes) of uninterrupted sleep/including naps taken during their shift.

STAR

Stop		
Think	Determine how many 90-minute cycles of undisturbed sleep the person has had in the last 24 hours.	
Act	If not sufficient, identify causes and address them.	
Review	Evaluate if sleep has improved, if not return to Act and reevaluate Clinical Alert Report. Before providing care, advise ancillary staff/student to report the following to the professional nurse assigned to the individual the actual time (minutes) of uninterrupted sleep/naps taken during the nurse's shift.	

Documentation

Amount (hours) of sleep, nap times
Reports of unsatisfactory sleep

Risk for Spiritual Distress Related to Separation from Religious Support System, Lack of Privacy, or Inability to Practice Spiritual Rituals

NOC
Hope, Spiritual
Well-Being

NIC
Spiritual Growth
Facilitation, Hope
Instillation, Active
Listening, Presence,
Emotional Support,
Spiritual Support

Goal

The individual will maintain usual spiritual practices not detrimental to health.

Indicators

* Ask for assistance as needed.
* Relate support from staff as needed.

Interventions	Rationales
1. Explore whether the individual desires to engage in an allowable religious or spiritual practice or ritual. If so, provide opportunities for him or her to do so.	1. For an individual who places a high value on prayer or other spiritual practices, these practices can provide meaning and purpose and can be a source of comfort and strength.
2. Provide privacy and quiet for spiritual rituals, as the desires and as practicable.	2. Privacy and quiet provide an environment that enables reflection and contemplation.
3. Offer to contact a religious leader or hospital clergy to arrange for a visit. Explain available services (e.g., hospital chapel, Bible).	3. These measures can help the individual maintain spiritual ties and practice important rituals.
4. Advise individual/family to share if any usual hospital practices conflict with their beliefs (e.g., diet, hygiene, treatments). If so, try to accommodate the individual's beliefs to the extent that policy and safety allow.	4. Many religions prohibit certain behaviors; complying with restrictions may be an important part of the individual's worship.
5. Discuss religious conflicts with the appropriate persons (e.g., spiritual leader, physician/nurse practitioner, nurse manager).	

Documentation

Spiritual concerns

Risk for Compromised Family Functioning Related to Disruption of Routines, Changes in Role Responsibilities, and Fatigue Associated With Increased Workload, and Visiting Hour Requirements

NOC
Family Coping, Family
Normalization, Family
Environment: Internal,
Parenting

NIC
Family Involvement
Promotion, Coping
Enhancement, Family
Integrity Promotion,
Family Therapy,
Counseling, Referral

Goal

The individual and family members will verbalize feelings regarding the diagnosis and hospitalization.

Indicators

* Identify signs of family dysfunction.
* Identify appropriate resources to seek when needed.

Interventions	Rationales
1. Explain the importance of functional communications, which uses verbal and nonverbal communication to teach behavior, share feelings and values, and evolve decisions about family health practices (Kaakinen, Gedaly-Duff, & Hanson, 2010). a. Assist family to appraise the situation • What is at stake? Encourage family to have a realistic perspective by providing accurate information and answers to questions. Ensure all family members have input. • What are the choices? Assist family to reorganize roles at home and set priorities to maintain family integrity and reduce stress. • Initiate discussions regarding stressors of home care (physical, emotional, environmental, and financial).	1. Effective communication is necessary in families to adapt to stressors and develop cohesiveness (Kaakinen et al., 2010). An individual's emotional, social, and physical functioning is directly related to how clear his or her role is differentiated in the family (Halter, 2014). "Family-oriented approaches that include helping a family gain insight and make behavioral changes are most successful" (Halter, 2014).
2. Explore the family members' perceptions of the situation. Realistic? Denial?	2. Evaluating family members' understanding can help identify which interventions would be indicated.
3. Provide accurate information using simple terms. If needed, consult with physician, nurse practitioner, or physical assistant to provide the family with concrete information.	3. Moderate or high anxiety impairs the ability to process information. Simple explanations impart useful information most effectively (Halter, 2014).
4. Involve family members in caring for the individual to the extent that they want to.	4. These measures may help maintain an existing family structure, allowing it to function as a supportive unit.
5. Adjust visiting hours to accommodate family schedules.	5. This measure may help promote regular visitation, which can help maintain family integrity.

Documentation

Interactions with family
Assessment of family functioning
End-of-life decisions, if known
Advance directive in chart

Risk for Compromised Human Dignity Related to Multiple Factors (Intrusions, Unfamiliar Environment and Personnel, Loss of Privacy) Associated With Hospitalization

NOC
Abuse Protection,
Comfort Level,
Knowledge: Illness
Care, Self-Esteem,
Dignified Dying,
Spiritual Well-Being,
Information Processing

Goal

The individual will report respectful and considerate care.

NIC
Patient Rights
Protection, Anticipatory
Guidance, Counseling,
Emotional Support,
Preparatory Sensory
Information, Family
Support, Humor,
Mutual Goal Setting,
Teaching: Procedure/
Treatment, Touch

Indicators

• Respect for privacy
• Consideration of emotions
• Asked for permission
• Given options
• Minimization of body part exposure

Carp's Cues

"Dignity is the ability to feel important and valuable in relation to others, in contexts which are perceived as threatening. Dignity is a dynamitic subjective belief but also has a shared meaning among humanity. Dignity is striven for and its maintenance depends on one's ability to keep intact the boundary containing beliefs about oneself and the extent of the threat. Context and possession of dignity within oneself affects one's ability to maintain or promote the dignity of another" (*Haddock, 1996).

Interventions	Rationales
1. Determine if the agency/hospital has a policy for prevention of compromised human dignity (Note: This type of policy or standard may be titled differently [e.g., Mission Statement]).	1. Agency policies can assist the nurse when problematic situations occur. However, the moral obligation to protect and defend the dignity of individuals and their families does not depend on the existence (or lack) of a policy.
2. Ensure that there are clear guidelines regarding the number of personnel (e.g., students, nurses, physicians [residents, interns]) that can be present when confidential and/or stressful information is discussed, or when procedures that leave an individual exposed need to be done.	2. This type of policy can project the philosophy and culture of moral and respectful care of the institution among its personnel. "Practice expecting that honoring and protecting the dignity of individual/groups is not a value but a way of being" (*Söderberg, Gilje, & Norberg, 1998).
3. Role-model and advocate to maintain the dignity when living and after death.	3. Role-modeling considerate and respectful care can assist others to a heightened awareness and encourage them to perform this care themselves.
4. When appropriate, request the individual or family members to provide the following information: a. Person to contact in the event of emergency b. Person whom the individual trusts with personal decisions, power of attorney c. Signed living will/desire to sign a living will d. Decision on organ donation e. Funeral arrangements; burial, cremation	4. Individuals and families should be encouraged to discuss their directions to be used to guide future clinical decisions, and their decisions should be documented. One copy should be given to the person designated as the decision maker in the event the individual becomes incapacitated or incompetent, with another copy retained in a safe deposit box and one copy on the chart.
5. Make a priority to provide the individual with choices and control in their care and in accordance with their ability.	5. Choice and control are key defining aspects of dignity. Withdrawal of respect inhibits choice and control (European Commission, 2010). Individuals have reported that in unavoidable, embarrassing situations (e.g., bowel or bladder accident), a nurse who was matter-of-fact and who made them feel at ease with small talk or humor made the situation better (*Walsh & Kowanko, 2002).
6a. Engage in dialogue with the individual and family regarding their understanding of the individual's condition, prognosis, and present plan of care, and decisions that may need to be explained. If experienced consult an experienced nurse. • How do you think you are doing? How do you think he/she is doing? • What have you been told about your condition? Your _____ condition? • To family, how well do you think your _____ will be in 1 month? • If the person is terminally ill, what are his or her end-of-life decisions? • Does the family agree with the decision? • Explain the present situation (e.g., renal function, metastasis, congestive heart failure)	6. Providing directions in questions may help to uncover misunderstandings, denial, secrets and the need for clarifications and/or other interventions.

(continued)

Interventions	*Rationales*

b. Contact the physician, nurse practitioner, or physical assistant, who is primarily responsible for the care of the need to clarify misunderstandings and/or deliberate isolation of the individual from prognosis information.

> **CLINICAL ALERT:**
> * It is imperative for the individuals and families that they are provided with current, accurate information about the person's condition, prognosis, and treatment options. The expected sequela or the after effects of the disease, condition, or injury should be explained. Treatment options are outlined addressing purpose (cure, palliative hospice), risks, and advantages. If the person is terminally ill, what are their end-of-life decisions?
> * Decisions that protect an individual from unnecessary pain and suffering and protect dignity come from informed individuals and/or families. This information should be provided by the physician, nurse practitioner, or physical assistant, who is primarily responsible for the care. The nurse's responsibility is to assess understanding, to encourage dialogue, questioning and to ensure truth-telling.

7. Gently explore the individual/family end-of-life decisions

a. Explain the options (e.g., "If you or your loved one dies . . .")
   * Give medications, oxygen
   * Cardio defibrillation (shock)
   * Cardiopulmonary resuscitation
   * Intubation and use of respirator

b. Advise the individual/family that they can choose all, some, or none of the above. The family, however, needs to support the individual's decisions.
   * If family members disagree, the individual can be advised to name the family member that supports their decisions as their legal delegate/power of attorney.

c. Differentiate between prolonging life versus prolonging dying.

d. Document the discussion and decisions according to institute on policy.

7. Protecting dignity is the acknowledgment of humanity in people, alive or dead, rather than treating them as inanimate objects (*Haddock, 1996). When people are helpless or unconscious, preserving their dignity is of the utmost priority (*Mairis, 1994). Protecting dignity and privacy always applies to unconscious or deceased individuals (*Mairis, 1994).

a. When someone is dying avoid using terms like "If you or your loved one stops breathing or their heart stops. . .." This may imply to the individual or family that the event is unexpected and therefore CPR should be initiated. Successful resuscitation will be painful and temporary and unfortunately the person will die gain from the same cause.

b. Direct but gentle inquiries and discussions can assist the individual/family to examine the situation clearly and the implications of treatment options and decisions.

Interventions	*Rationales*

> **CLINICAL ALERT:**
> • "The choices and values of the competent patient should always be given highest priority, even when these wishes conflict with those of the health care team and family. An exception to this is when one or more physicians determine that CPR attempts would be medically ineffective or if the decision of the patient/surrogate is in conflict with the informed opinion of the agency/provider as to what constitutes beneficent care of the patient. In this situation, requests from a patient or surrogate will not be honored" (American Nurses Association, 2012; *Ditillo, 2002).

8. If indicated, explain "no code" status and explain the focus of palliative care that replaces aggressive and futile care (e.g., pain management, symptom management, less or no intrusive/painful procedures).	8. Often, families think that "no code" status means no care. Palliative care focuses on comfort during the dying process.
9. When extreme measures that are futile are planned or are being provided for an individual, discuss the situation with the physician/nurse practitioner/physical assistant.	9. "Extreme measures, when futile, are an infringement of the basic respect for the dignity innate in being a person" (*Walsh & Kowanko, 2002, p. 146).

> **CLINICAL ALERT:**
> • "Use the chain of command to share and discuss issues that have escalated beyond the problem-solving ability and/or scope of those immediately involved" (LaSala & Bjarnason, 2010, p. 6).
> • The urgency of the situation requires immediate attention.

SBAR   *Situation:* (To physician/nurse practitioner/physical assistant) I have just assessed Mr. Black. Pulse ox is 90, with labored breathing.

Background: As you know, he is in end-stage congestive heart failure. He is lethargic and not eating or drinking. The family are questioning if he should have a feeding tube.

Assessment: I cared for him yesterday. His condition is deteriorating.

Recommendation: I would like a consult for the palliative care specialist to speak to the family regarding his changing condition and comfort measures that can be implemented to prevent prolonging his suffering with enteral nutritional therapy.

Refer to Palliative Care Plan if indicated.

(continued)

Interventions	*Rationales*

10. Discuss with involved personnel any incident that was disrespectful to the individual or his or her family. Professionals have a responsibility to practice ethical and moral care and to address situations and personnel that compromise human dignity.

STAR

Stop Did you witness or have reported to you an unsatisfactory treatment of individual and/or family?

Think Can I discuss this with the involved personnel or is it serious enough to report it to nurse manager?

Act If desired, discuss the situation with a trusted colleague. Report the incident to nurse manager. Complete an incident report. Do not document the incident in the individual's record, unless instructed to by manager.

Review Are you satisfied with the actions taken in response to your report? If not, discuss your options with a trusted colleague.

> **CLINICAL ALERT:**
> • A zero tolerance for abuse or neglect should be the institution's model. Report repetitive incidents or any egregious incident that is a violation of individual's dignity to the appropriate personnel.

11. If you decide to speak to the involved coworker, use SBAR.

SBAR

Situation: I overheard you talking to Mr. White's family. You told them to "stop ringing the call bell" and that they were being too demanding.

Background: Mr. White is critically ill with a poor prognosis.

Assessment: Do you know how much his family knows about his condition? Do they understand the concept of palliative care?

Recommendation: I would suggest you assess for their understanding of the situation. Ask them "How do you think your father is doing?" Engage in dialogue with individual and family regarding their thoughts on the present plan of care and decisions that may need explanation. If more information is needed, contact the appropriate person (e.g., physician/nurse practitioner, nurse manager).

Interventions	Rationales

> **CLINICAL ALERT:**
> • If you are dissatisfied with the response of the nurse to your discussion, discuss this with the nurse manager.

>> **Carp's Cues**
> Please refer the web site for access to all of the ANA's position statements under *The Nurse's Role in Ethics and Human Rights: Protecting and Promoting Individual Worth, Dignity, and Human Rights in Practice Settings*, Nursing Care and do not Resuscitate (DNR) and Allow Natural Death (AND) Decisions, accessed at http://www.nursingworld.org /MainMenuCategories/EthicsStandards /Ethics-Position-Statements

Documentation

Care plan
  Specify preferences

> **TRANSITION TO HOME/COMMUNITY CARE**
> If indicated, review the high-risk diagnoses identified for this individual on admission:
> • Is the person still at high risk?
> • Can the family reduce the risks?
> • Is the person at higher risk at home?
> • Is a home health nurse assessment needed?
> • Refer to discharge planner/case manager/social service
> • When is this person scheduled for follow-up with primary provider? Specialists? Record dates of appointments.
> • Complete a medication reconciliation before discharge. Refer to front/back cover.

STAR

Stop

Think   Is this person at high risk for injury, falls, medical complications, and/or inability to care for self (activities of daily living)?
    Is there a support person available?
    Is the person competent to manage self-administration of medications, treatment procedures? Are additional resources needed?
    Can the person explain how to monitor the condition (e.g., blood glucose, signs/symptoms of complications, dietary/mobility restrictions, and when to call his or her primary provider or specialist)?

Act   Contact or provide the appropriate resource (e.g., a support person, home health assessment, additional teaching, printed materials).

Review   Has the problem been addressed? If not, use SBAR to communicate to the appropriate person.

Risk for Ineffective Health Management Related to Complexity and Cost of Therapeutic Regimen, Complexity of Health Care System, Insufficient Knowledge of Treatment, and Barriers to Comprehension Secondary to Language Barriers, Cognitive Deficits, Hearing and/or Visual Impairment, Anxiety, and Lack of Motivation

NOC

Compliance Behavior, Knowledge: Treatment Regimen, Participation in Health Care Decisions, Treatment Behavior: Illness or Injury

Goal

The individual or primary caregiver will describe disease process, causes, and factors contributing to symptoms, and the regimen for disease or symptom control.

NIC

Anticipatory Guidance, Learning Facilitation, Risk Identification, Health Education, Teaching: Procedure/ Treatment, Health System Guidance

Indicators

- Relate the intent to practice health behaviors needed or desired for recovery from illness/symptom management and prevention of recurrence or complications.
- Describe signs and symptoms that need reporting.

Interventions	*Rationales*
1. Determine the individual's knowledge of his or her condition, prognosis, and treatment measures. Reinforce and supplement the physician's explanations as necessary.	1. Assessing the individual's level of knowledge will assist in the development of an individualized learning program. Providing accurate information can decrease the individual's anxiety associated with the unknown and unfamiliar.
2. Identify factors that influence learning.	2. The individual's ability to learn will be affected by a number of variables that need to be considered. Denial of illness, lack of financial resources, and depression may affect the individual's ability and motivation to learn. Cognitive changes associated with this might influence the individual's ability to learn new information.
3. Explain and discuss with individual and family/caregiver (when possible): a. Disease process b. Treatment regimen (medications, diet, procedures, exercises, equipment use) c. Rationale for regimen d. Side effects of regimen e. Signs or symptoms of complications f. Lifestyle changes needed. Refer to the Getting Started documents on thePoint. g. Follow-up care needed h. Resources and support available	3. Depending on individual's physical and cognitive limitations, it may be necessary to provide the family/caregiver with the necessary information for managing the treatment regimen. In order to assist the individual with postdischarge care, the individual needs information about the disease process, treatment regimen, symptoms of complications, etc., as well as resources available for assistance.
4. Identify referrals or community services needed for follow-up. Direct the family to community agencies and other sources of emotional and financial assistance, as needed.	4. Additional resources may be needed to help with management at home.

Documentation

Specific discharge needs and plans
Referrals made
Individual/family teaching about disease

CARDIOVASCULAR AND PERIPHERAL VASCULAR DISORDERS

Heart Failure

Heart failure (HF) is a syndrome that occurs when there is a structural or functional impairment in the ability of the heart to fill with or eject blood. HF can present in a myriad of ways, from minimal symptoms to those that are totally debilitating. These symptoms include fatigue, exercise intolerance, shortness of breath, breathing difficulty, retention, pulmonary congestion, peripheral edema, rapid weight gain, dizziness, and/or confusion. HF can cause cardiogenic pulmonary edema (CPE).

CPE is defined as pulmonary edema due to increased capillary hydrostatic pressure secondary to elevated pulmonary venous pressure. CPE reflects the accumulation of fluid with a low protein content in the lung interstitium and alveoli. Impaired left ventricular (LV) contractility, resulting in reduced cardiac output, is the most common predisposing condition leading to CPE (Pinto & Kociol, 2015).

Individuals are usually graded by their functional capacity and quality of life. The measurements are often assessed with the New York Heart Association (NYHA) function classification assessment as (*The Criteria Committee of the New York Heart Association, 1994):

- Class I—Individuals with heart disease without resulting limitation of physical activity. Ordinary physical activity does not cause HF symptoms such as fatigue or dyspnea.
- Class II—Individuals with heart disease resulting in slight limitation of physical activity. Symptoms of HF develop with ordinary activity but there are no symptoms at rest.
- Class III—Individuals with heart disease resulting in marked limitation of physical activity. Symptoms of HF develop with less than ordinary physical activity but there are no symptoms at rest.
- Class IV—Individuals with heart disease resulting in inability to carry on any physical activity without discomfort. Symptoms of HF may occur even at rest.

HF is the most non-Medicare diagnosis-related group (i.e., hospital transition diagnosis. At least 20% hospital admissions among persons older than 65 are due to HF). More Medicare dollars are spent for the diagnosis and treatment of HF than for any other diagnosis. The total estimated direct and indirect costs for HF in 2009 were approximately $37.2 billion (Lloyd-Jones et al., 2010).

 Time Frame
Initial diagnosis (nonintensive care unit)
Exacerbation of chronic condition

DIAGNOSTIC CLUSTER

Collaborative Problems

▲ Risk for Complications of Pulmonary Edema

▲ Risk for Complications of Hypoxia

▲ Risk for Complications of Deep Vein Thrombosis (refer to Unit II)

▲ Risk for Complications of Cardiogenic Shock (refer to Acute Coronary Syndrome)

▲ Risk for Complications of Arrhythmias (refer to Unit II)

▲ Risk for Complications of Renal Insufficiency

△ Risk for Complications of Hepatic Insufficiency (refer to Unit II)

Nursing Diagnoses

▲ Activity Intolerance related to insufficient oxygen for activities of daily living (refer to Chronic Obstructive Pulmonary Disease)

▲ Anxiety related to breathlessness (refer to Chronic Obstructive Pulmonary Disease)

Imbalanced Nutrition related to nausea; anorexia secondary to venous congestion of gastrointestinal tract, and fatigue (refer to Unit II)

Disturbed Sleep Pattern related to nocturnal dyspnea and inability to assume usual sleep position secondary to the extra fluid in the lungs (refer to Unit II)

Powerlessness related to progressive nature of condition (refer to Unit II)

▲ Risk for Ineffective Self-Health Management related to lack of knowledge of low-salt diet, drug therapy (diuretic, digitalis, and vasodilators), activity program, signs and symptoms of

Transition Criteria

The staff/student will:

1. Explain the causes of the symptoms.
2. Describe the signs and symptoms that must be reported to a health care professional.
3. Relate the importance of adhering to dietary restrictions and understand amount of fluid intake ordered.
4. Explain the importance of daily weights.
5. Explain who they need to report to if the individual gains 3 lb in 1 day or 5 lb in a week.
6. Explain the importance of adherence to prescribed medications.

Transitional Risk Assessment Plan (TRAP)

Begin this plan on admission.
Implement the Transitional Risk Assessment Plan (TRAP):

- Refer to inside back cover.
- Add each validated risk diagnosis to individual's problem list with the risk code in ( ).
- Refer to Unit II to the individual nursing diagnoses/collaborative problems for outcomes and interventions.

R: *"Close coordination of care in the postacute period, early transition follow-up care, enhanced client education and self-management training, proactive end-of-life counseling, and extending the resources and clinical expertise over time via multidisciplinary team management" can lower readmission rates and improve health outcomes (Boutwell & Hwu, 2009, p. 14). Interventions are utilized to activate the individual and family to select changes in their everyday lifestyle choices to improve their health (Hibbard & Greene, 2013).*

Collaborative Problems

Risk for Complications of Cardiogenic Pulmonary Edema

Risk for Complications of Hypoxia

Risk for Complications of Renal Insufficiency

Collaborative Outcomes

The individual will monitor for early signs and symptoms of multiple organ failure (a) early signs of pulmonary edema, (b) hypoxia, (c) early signs of acute kidney failure, (d) metabolic acidosis, (e) electrolyte imbalances, and (f) hypotension and will receive collaborative interventions if indicated to restore physiologic stability.

Indicators of Physiologic Stability

- Alert, calm, oriented (a, b, c, e)
- Blood pressure (BP) >90/160 mm Hg (a, b, f)
- Respiration relaxed and rhythmic (a, b)
- Pulse 60 to 100 beats/min (a, b, c, f)
- Full breath sounds in all lobes (a, b)
- No crackles and/or wheezing (a, b)
- Flat neck veins
- No edema (pedal, sacral, periorbital)
- No muscle cramps
- Serum sodium 135 to 145 mEq/L
- Serum potassium 3.8 to 5 mEq/L

Interventions	Rationales
1. Address the overwhelming terrifying experience of sudden, critical breathlessness. a. Validate how frightened he or she must be. b. Reassure the person and do not leave them alone. c. Elevate the head of the bed or use extra pillows under the head and shoulders. d. If possible, increase air flow around person (e.g., fan, open window).	1. These strategies attempt to reduce anxiety/fear. Individuals report breathlessness in terms of the feelings associated with bad episodes of breathlessness as distress, anxiety, panic and fear of dying (Gysels & Higginson, 2011; Schneidman, Reinke, Donesky, & Carrieri-Kohlman, 2014). c. This position will decrease resistance to inspiration. d. Increasing circulating cooler air can decrease breathlessness
2. Weigh individual daily. Ensure accuracy by weighing at the same time every day on the same scale and with the individual wearing the same amount of clothing.	2. Daily weights and strict input and output (I&O) are vital in determining the effects of treatment and for early detections of fluid retention.

3. Monitor for signs and symptoms of acute pulmonary edema:
 a. Dyspnea, cyanosis
  • Tachypnea, labored breathing
  • Adventitious breath sounds, crackles
  • Persistent cough or productive cough with frothy, pink-tinged sputum
  • Abnormal arterial blood gases (ABGs)
  • Decreased O$_2$ saturation by pulse oximetry
  • Decreased cardiac output/cardiac index
  • Elevated pulmonary artery pressure
  • Tachycardia
  • Abnormal heart sounds (S$_3$)
 b. Jugular vein distention (JVD)
  • Persistent cough
  • Productive cough with frothy sputum
  • Cyanosis
  • Diaphoresis
	3b. Impaired pumping of left ventricle accompanied by decreased cardiac output and increased pulmonary artery pressure produce pulmonary edema. Hypoxia produces increased capillary congestion, causing fluid to enter pulmonary tissue and triggering signs and symptoms. (Venous pressure and pulmonary lungs become so congested with fluid that it affects the exchange of oxygen, which is considered pulmonary edema.) Diuretics help the body to rid itself of excess fluids and sodium through urination. Helps to relieve the heart's workload (Pinto et al., 2016).

(continued)

Interventions	*Rationales*
	Decreased cardiac output leads to insufficient oxygenated blood to meet the tissues' metabolic needs. Decreased circulating volume/cardiac output can cause hypoperfusion of the kidneys and decreased tissue perfusion with a compensatory response of decreased circulation to the extremities and increased pulse and respiratory rates. Changes in mentation may result from cerebral hypoperfusion. Vasoconstriction and venous congestion in dependent areas (e.g., limbs) produce changes in skin and pulses.

4. Monitor with pulse oximetry
  a. Monitor for signs and symptoms of acute pulmonary edema:
    • Severe dyspnea with use of accessory muscles
    • Tachycardia
    • Adventitious breath sounds
	4. The pulse oximeter is an accurate, noninvasive monitor of oxygen concentrations.

5. Cautiously administer intravenous (IV) fluids. Consult with the physician/nurse practitioner/physical assistant if the ordered rate plus the PO intake exceeds 2 to 2.5 L/24 hr. Be sure to include additional IV fluids (e.g., antibiotics) when calculating the hourly allocation.	5. Failure to regulate IV fluids carefully can cause circulatory overload.

6. Initiate appropriate treatments according to protocol, which may include (National Institute for Health and Clinical Excellence [NICE], 2016):
  a. Diuretics
  b. Vasodilators
  c. β-Blockers
 	
  d. Angiotensin-converting enzyme inhibitors (ACE inhibitors) or
 	
  e. Angiotensin-II receptor blockers (ARBs)
 	
  f. Digitalid
 	
  g. Sedatives
	6a. Diuretics decrease preload.
	  b. Vasodilators decrease preload and afterload.
	  c. β-Blockers when combined with diuretics and ACE inhibitors, β-blockers improve symptoms, lower morbidity, and reduce hospital admissions
	  d. Angiotensin-converting enzyme inhibitors (ACE inhibitors) block the renin–angiotensin–aldosterone system, which helps to reduce the effects of one of the maladaptive compensatory mechanisms.
	  e. ARBs are an alternative to ACE inhibitors for individuals with HF due to left ventricular systolic dysfunction who have intolerable side effects with ACE inhibitors.
	  f. Digoxin is often used in individuals with systolic dysfunction who remain symptomatic despite optimal therapy.
	  g. Sedatives decrease anxiety, preload and afterload, and metabolic demands.
	Additional medications may be indicated.

7. Assist the individual with measures to conserve strength, such as resting before and after activities (e.g., meals).	7. Adequate rest reduces oxygen consumption and decreases the risk of hypoxia.
8. Monitor individuals for signs for renal insufficiency. Refer to Unit II Section 2 Risk for Complications of Renal Insufficiency for interventions.	8. Hypoxemia will compromise renal function and decreased urine output can be the first sign.

Clinical Alert Report

Advise ancillary staff/student to report:

- Any new change or deterioration in behavior (e.g., agitation, cognition)
- Any change in systolic BP >210 mm Hg, <90 mm Hg and/or diastolic >90 mm Hg
- Resting pulse >120 or <55 beats/min
- Change in rate of respirations and/or >28 or <10/min
- Changes or new onset of dyspnea/palpitations
- Decrease in urine output less than 0.5 mL/kg/hr

Documentation

Vital signs
Intake and output
Assessment data
Daily weight
Pulse oximeter
Change in physiologic status
Interventions
Individual response to interventions

TRANSITION TO HOME/COMMUNITY CARE

If indicated, review the risk diagnoses identified for this individual on admission:

- Is the person still at risk?
- Can the family reduce the risks?
- Is the person at higher risk at home?
- Is a home health nurse assessment needed?
- Refer to transition planner/case manager/social service.
- When is this person scheduled for follow-up with primary provider? Specialists? Record dates of appointments.
- Complete a medication reconciliation prior to transition. Refer to index.

STAR

Begin this plan on admission.
Education on HF needs to begin as soon as there is a diagnosis.
Education on daily weights, with a log and individual teach-back is very important.
The individual needs to start discussing what signs and symptoms may occur.
Education on what level of risk the signs and symptoms may be at and when they need to call their primary care provider (PCP).

Stop

Think Is this person at risk for fluid overload, acute renal fluid, increased shortness of breath, and/or inability to care for self (ADLs)?

Is the person competent to manage self-administration of medications, perform daily weights, prepare foods with low sodium, and understand the plan of care if weight gain occurs? Are additional resources needed?

Can the person explain how to monitor daily weights, sign/symptoms of complications, dietary restrictions, and when to call his or her primary provider or specialist?

Act Contact or provide the appropriate resource (e.g., contacting a support person, home health assessment, additional teaching, and printed materials).

Review Has the problem been addressed? If not, use SBAR to communicate to the appropriate person.

SBAR   *Situation:* Mr. Smith will be scheduled to be transitioned to his home.

Background: Mr. Smith lives alone. He (state his disabilities, self-care needs, treatments)

Action: A more thorough reevaluation of where he can be transitioned is needed.

Recommendation: Referral to social service/transition planner/case manager

Nursing Diagnoses

Risk for Ineffective Health Management Related to Insufficient Knowledge of Low-Salt Diet, Activity Program, Drug Therapy (Diuretics, Digitalis, Vasodilators), and Signs and Symptoms of Complications

NOC

Compliance/ Engagement Behavior, Knowledge: Treatment Regimen, Participation in Health Care Decisions, Treatment Behavior: Illness or Injury

NIC

Anticipatory Guidance, Risk Identification, Health Education, Self-Modification Assistance, Learning Facilitation

Goal

The goals for this diagnosis represent those associated with transition planning. Refer to the transition criteria.

Interventions	Rationales
1. Teach individual and family about HF and its causes.	1. Teaching reinforces the need to comply with prescribed treatments (diet, activity, and medications).
2. Explain the need to adhere to a low-sodium (<2 mg/day) and fluid-restricted (2 L/day) diet, as prescribed. Ensure a consult with a nutritionist.	2. Excess sodium intake increases fluid retention, which in turn increases vascular volume and cardiac workload.
3. Explain the actions of prescribed medications, particularly digitalis preparations, vasodilators, and diuretics.	3. Such explanations can help increase individual understanding and reduce errors in self-administration.
4. Teach the individual how to measure his or her pulse rate.	4. Pulse-taking can detect an irregular rhythm or a high (<120) or low (>60) rate, which may indicate a drug side effect or disease complication.
5. Acknowledge the complaints of fatigue and dyspnea. Explain the need to increase activity gradually, and to rest if dyspnea and fatigue occur. Acknowledge the complaints of fatigue and dyspnea. Explain the need to increase activity gradually, and to rest if dyspnea and fatigue occur. Ensure a referral to an outpatient cardiac rehabilitation.	5. Individuals with heart failure (HF) often have limited exercise capacity because of dyspnea and fatigue. Symptoms of exercise-induced dyspnea resemble those of deconditioning-related dyspnea and these symptoms make individuals fearful of being active and may interpret deconditioning as worsening of their disease. Research has demonstrated the benefits of exercise therapy, including improved walking tolerance, modified inflammatory/hemostatic markers, enhanced vasoresponsiveness, adaptations within the limb (angiogenesis, arteriogenesis, and mitochondrial synthesis) that enhance oxygen delivery and metabolic responses, potentially delayed progression of the disease, enhanced quality-of-life indices, and extended longevity (Haas et al., 2013; Pinto et al., 2016).

Interventions	Rationales
6. Explain the effects of smoking, exposure to secondhand smoke and obesity on cardiac function. Refer to the index for specific strategies to activate an individual to lose weight and stop smoking.	6. Nicotine is a powerful vasoconstrictor. Obesity causes compression of vessels, leading to peripheral resistance, which increases cardiac workload.
7. Instruct individual to seek help—Call 911 if the following occur (Colucci, 2016): a. Severe shortness of breath b. Chest discomfort or pain that lasts more than 15 minutes and does not get better with rest or nitroglycerin. c. Fainting or passing out. d. Call your doctor or nurse if you develop any of the following, which can be signs of worsening heart failure: e. Increasing or new shortness of breath. f. New or worsened cough, especially if you are coughing up frothy or bloody material. g. Worsened swelling in your legs or ankles. h. Weight gain of 2 lb (1 kg) or 4 lb in 1 week	7. Early detection and prompt intervention can reduce the risk of severe drug side effects or worsening HF. h. Gaining weight suddenly is one sign that you may be retaining more fluid than you should be.
8. Provide information about or initiate referrals to community resources (e.g., American Heart Association, community nursing agency).	8. They may provide the individual and family with needed assistance in home management and self-care.

Documentation

Individual/family teaching
Outcome achievement or status
Referrals, if indicated

Deep Vein Thrombosis

Describes a person experiencing venous clot formation because of blood stasis, vessel wall injury, or altered coagulation and/or experiencing or at high risk to experience obstruction of one or more pulmonary arteries from a blood clot, air, or fat embolus. In more than 90% of cases of pulmonary embolism (PE), the thrombosis originates in the deep veins of the legs. A major theory delineating the pathogenesis of venous thromboembolism (VTE), often called Virchow's triad, proposes that VTE occurs as a result of (Bauer & Lip, 2015):

- Alterations in blood flow (i.e., stasis)
- Vascular endothelial injury
- Alterations in the constituents of the blood (i.e., inherited or acquired hypercoagulable state).

The most serious complication of a deep vein thrombosis (DVT) is when a piece of the clot breaks off and travels through the bloodstream into the lungs, causing a blockage called a PE. In more than 90% of cases of PE, the thrombosis originates in the deep veins of the legs. DVT is a distressing but often avoidable condition that leads to long-term complications such as the postphlebitic syndrome and chronic leg ulcers in a large proportion of individuals who have proximal vein thrombosis. PE remains the most common preventable cause of death in hospital (Lip & Hull, 2016a). Refer also to Pulmonary Embolism.

High-Risk Populations (Barbar et al., 2010; Lip & Hull, 2016a)

- Active cancer (3)
- History of DVT or PE (3)
- Reduced mobility >72 hours (3)
  - Known thrombophilic condition (3) (e.g., polycythemia, blood dyscrasias)
  - High levels of factor VIII in white people (Payne, Miller, Hooper, Lally, & Austin, 2014)

- High levels of factor VIII and von Willebrand factor in black people (Payne et al., 2014).
- Recent trauma/surgery (2)
- Over 70 years old (1)
- Obesity >30 BMI (1)
- Acute coronary or ischemic stroke (1)
- Acute infection and/or rheumatologic disorder (1)
- Ongoing hormonal therapy (1)
- Heart/respiratory failure (1)
- Age (risk rises steadily from age 40)
- Fractures (especially hip, pelvis, and leg)
- Chemical irritation of vein
- All major surgeries that involve general anesthesia and immobility (over 30 minutes) in the operative course (pre-op, peri-op, and post-op combined), especially surgeries involving abdomen, pelvis, and lower extremities
- Orthopedic (hips/knees), urologic, or gynecologic surgery
- History of venous insufficiency
- Varicose veins
- Inflammatory bowel disease
- Pregnancy
- Surgery greater than 30 minutes (2)
- Over 40 years of age
- Valve malfunction
- Systemic lupus erythematosus
- Central venous catheters
- Nephrotic syndrome

These risk factors have been identified in the Padua Prediction risk assessment for venous thrombolytic events. A score of ≥4 denotes a high-risk individual (Barbar et al., 2010).

Time Frame

Initial diagnosis

Recurrent acute episodes

▪▪■■ DIAGNOSTIC CLUSTER

Collaborative Problems

▲ Risk for Complications of Pulmonary Embolism (refer to Risk for Complications of Pulmonary Embolism in Unit II.)

> **CLINICAL ALERT:**
> - Approximately half of the individuals with DVT who develop PE have no symptoms of deep venous disease. This causes a delay in the administration of appropriate prophylactic and therapeutic measures (Davies et al., 2010).

Nursing Diagnoses

▲ Acute pain related to impaired circulation (refer to Acute Pain)

△ Risk for Ineffective Health Management related to lack of knowledge of prevention of recurrence of deep vein thrombosis and signs and symptoms of complications

▲ This diagnosis was reported to be monitored for or managed frequently (75% to 100%).
△ This diagnosis was reported to be monitored for or managed often (50% to 74%).

Transition Criteria

The staff/student will:

1. Explain the risk factors and management of DVT.
2. Describe the signs and symptoms that must be reported to a health care professional.
3. Review risk assessment and the various management strategies of the risk, to reduce mortality and aid secondary prevention.
4. Review their understanding on the need to be assessed regularly.
5. Review diagnosis and laboratory tests.
6. Explain the importance of adherence to prescribed medications for secondary prevention.

Before transition, the individual or family will:

1. Identify factors that contribute to occurrence or recurrence of thrombosis.
2. Relate the signs and symptoms that must be reported to a health care professional.
3. Verbalize intent to implement lifestyle changes.

Transitional Risk Assessment Plan (TRAP)

Begin this plan on admission.

Implement the Transitional Risk Assessment Plan (TRAP):

- Refer to inside back cover.
- Add each validated risk diagnosis to individual's problem list with the risk code.
- Refer to Unit II to the individual risk nursing diagnoses/collaborative problems for outcomes and interventions.

  R: "Close coordination of care in the postacute period, early discharge follow-up care, enhanced client education and self-management training, proactive end-of-life counseling, and extending the resources and clinical expertise over time via multidisciplinary team management" can lower readmission rates and improve health outcomes (Boutwell & Hwu, 2009, p. 14). Interventions are utilized to activate the individual and family to select changes in their everyday lifestyle choices to improve their health (Hibbard & Greene, 2013).

Documentation

Position in bed and activity restrictions
Leg measurements and changes in measurement, color, or pain
Individual/family teaching

TRANSITION TO HOME/COMMUNITY CARE

If indicated, review the risk diagnoses identified for this individual on admission:

- Is the person still at risk?
- Can the family reduce the risks?
- Is the person at higher risk at home?
- Is a home health nurse assessment needed?
- Refer to transition planner/case manager/social service.
- When is this person scheduled for follow-up with primary provider? Specialists? Record dates of appointments.
- Complete a medication reconciliation prior to transition. Refer to index.

STAR   **Stop**

Think   Is this person at risk for injury, falls, medical complications, and/or inability to care for self (ADLs)?

Is the person competent to manage self-administration of medications, treatment procedures? Are additional resources needed?

Can the person explain how to monitor condition (e.g., blood glucose, sign/symptoms of complications, dietary/mobility restrictions, and when to call his or her primary provider or specialist)?

Act   Use SBAR to notify the appropriate professional.SBAR

SBAR   *Situation:* Mr. Smith will be scheduled to be transitioned to his home.

Background: Mr. Smith lives alone. He (state his disabilities, self-care needs, treatments)

Action: A more thorough reevaluation of where he can be transitioned is needed.

Recommendation: Referral to social service/transition planner/case manager

Review   Is the response/solution the right option for the individual? If not, discuss the situation with the appropriate person, department, and/or agency (using SBAR).

Nursing Diagnoses

Risk for Ineffective Health Management Related to Lack of Knowledge of Prevention of Recurrence of Deep Vein Thrombosis and Signs and Symptoms of Complications

NOC

Compliance/
Engagement Behavior,
Knowledge: Treatment
Regimen, Participation in
Health Care Decisions,
Treatment Behavior:
Illness or Injury

NIC

Anticipatory Guidance,
Risk Identification,
Health Education,
Learning Facilitation

Goal

The goals for this diagnosis represent those associated with transition planning. Refer to the transition criteria.

> **CLINICAL ALERT:**
> • Individuals should be followed up for 3 years to ensure that there is no recurrent thromboembolic event (Lip & Hull, 2016a).

Interventions	Rationales

1. Explain relevant venous anatomy and physiology, including:
  a. Leg vein anatomy
  b. Function of venous valves
  c. Importance of muscle pumping action
2. Teach the pathophysiology of DVT, including:
  a. Effect of thrombosis on valves
	1,2. This teaching helps reinforce the need to comply with instructions (restrictions, exercises).
	
	a,b,c. Venous valvular incompetence occurs after DVT. This is supported by natural history studies that have demonstrated a correlation between segment thrombosis and subsequent valvular incompetence (Davies et al., 2010). Education on what to watch out for is important.

b. Hydrostatic pressure in venous system	b. Venous stasis is the most important feature predisposing to venous thrombosis. The venous sinuses of the veins are especially vulnerable to stasis and thrombosis. Propagation of the thrombus may then follow upstream or the process may spread retrograde (Davies et al., 2010).

Interventions	Rationales
c. Pressure transmitted to capillary system d. Pressure in subcutaneous tissue	c, d. Deep venous thrombi can propagate into the superficial system (Davies et al., 2010).

> **CLINICAL ALERT:**
> • Indefinite anticoagulation may be appropriate for individuals with a first, unprovoked episode of proximal DVT and/or unprovoked symptomatic PE as well those with recurrent unprovoked venous thromboembolism (VTE). It can also be indicated for individuals with recurrent provoked VT and those with provoked VTE with persistent, irreversible, or multiple major risk factors (e.g., active cancer, antiphospholipid syndrome) (Lip & Hull, 2016b).

Interventions	Rationales
3. Explain postthrombotic syndrome (PTS)	3. Up to half of individuals with proximal DVT will develop post-thrombotic syndrome. Importantly, 50% of legs at 3 years still demonstrate some residual thrombus causing partial obstruction.
4. Explain the importance of ambulation as prescribed	4. Despite prior concerns regarding the potential for embolization, early ambulation is safe in individuals with acute DVT (Lin & Hull, 2016a).

5. Explain signs and symptoms
  a. Aching, heaviness, swelling, cramps, or itching of the affected limb.
  b. Symptoms can be episodic or persistent, are often aggravated by ambulation, and improve with leg elevation and rest
  c. May experience venous claudication, with bursting leg pain during mobilization.
	5. The inflammatory response to acute thrombosis and the process of recanalization directly damages venous valves, resulting in valvular reflux, venous obstruction, and calf muscle dysfunction. The size of residual thrombus also contributes to PTS.

> **CLINICAL ALERT:**
> • Adequate anticoagulation and use of elastic compression stockings (ECS) following DVT can reduce the incidence of PTS. Catheter-directed thrombolysis and mechanical thrombectomy of acute DVT may preserve valvular function.

Interventions	Rationales

6. Teach preventive measures:
  a. Initiate a regular exercise program (e.g., walking or swimming). Consult with physical therapy to determine, what type of exercise, frequency and duration of exercise session.
 	
  b. Avoid immobility.
    • Encourage the individual to move around as soon as possible after having been confined to bed, such as after surgery, illness, or injury (Lip & Hull, 2016b)
  c. Elevate the legs whenever possible.
 	
  d. Avoid over-the-counter elastic support stockings.
	6a. These measures can help to prevent subsequent episodes of DVT. DVT is preventable and treatable if discovered early (Lip & Hull, 2016b). Exercise increases muscle tone and promotes the pumping effect in the veins.
	  b. Immobility increases venous stasis.
	
	  c. Elevation reduces venous pooling and promotes venous return
	  d. The use of over-the-counter support stockings is discouraged; improperly fitted stockings may produce a tourniquet effect.

(continued)

Interventions	*Rationales*

7. If gradual compression stockings (GCS) for the prevention of PTSn are prescribed, advise to use daily as directed.
   a. Compression stockings may be useful for symptomatic relief and the promotion of ambulation.
	7. Small randomized trials of individuals with acute DVT (first or recurrent) suggested that GCS that apply an ankle pressure of 30 to 40 mm Hg started within 2 weeks and continued for 2 years to reduce the occurrence of PTS by 50% without increasing the frequency of recurrent VTE (*Brandjes et al., 1997; Lip, & Hull, 2016a; *Prandoni et al., 2004)
	
	   Individuals most likely to benefit included those with a proximal DVT, prior DVT, and those with symptoms (Lip, & Hull, 2016a).

8. Explain to individuals the rationale for anticoagulant and the importance of taking the medications as prescribed.	8. Several large randomized studies have demonstrated that longer term anticoagulation is associated with a reduced risk of recurrent VTE

9. Explain the need to do the following:
   a. Maintain a fluid intake of 2,500 mL/day, unless contraindicated.
   b. Stop smoking. Refer to Getting Started to Quit Smoking on thePoint.
   c. Achieve or Maintain ideal weight. Refer to Unit II Section 1 nursing diagnoses under Obesity or Overweight.
   d. Avoid tight constricting clothes as slimming body shapers and over-the-counter (OTC) knee-high stockings.
	9. These practices help to decrease risk of recurrence.
	   a. Adequate hydration prevents increased blood viscosity.
	   b. Nicotine is a potent vasoconstrictor.
	
	   c. Obesity increases compression of vessels and causes hypercoagulability.
	   d. Slimming body shapers and knee-high stockings constrict vessels, causing venous pooling.

10. Teach to watch for and promptly report these symptoms to PCP (or call 911):
   a. Diminished sensation in legs or feet
   b. Coldness or bluish color in legs or feet
   c. Increased swelling or pain in legs or feet
   d. In case of sudden chest pain or dyspnea, call 911.
	10. Early detection enables prompt intervention to prevent serious complications.
	   a, b, c. These changes in the legs and feet may point to an extension of the clot with resulting compromised circulation and inflammation.
	   d. Sudden chest pain or dyspnea may indicate a PE.

11. Instruct the individual and family to advise health care providers of the history of DVT (e.g., before surgery).	11. Individuals with previous DVT are at four times greater risk for developing new DVT (Grossman & Porth, 2014).
12. Explain the importance of wearing a bracelet, necklace, or similar alert tag at all times.	12. If medical treatment is required and the person is too ill to explain his or her condition, the tag will alert responders about the individual's use of anticoagulants and risk of excessive bleeding.

13. Advise on the risk of prolonged travel. Instruct to (Pai & Douketis, 2015):
   a. Flex and extend the ankles and knees periodically, avoid crossing the legs, and change positions frequently while seated. Every half hour or so, bend and straighten your legs, feet and toes when you are seated.
   b. Press the balls of your feet down hard against the floor or foot rest every so often. This helps to increase the blood flow in your legs.
   c. Take a walk up and down the airplane aisle in the plane every hour or so, when the aircraft crew say it is safe to do so.
   d. Make sure you have as much space as possible in front of you for your legs to move. So avoid having bags under the seat in front of you, and recline your seat where possible.
	13. Long-distance travel, either by air or land, confers a two- to fourfold increased risk of symptomatic venous thromboembolism (VTE), although the overall incidence is small. The rates are highest in those who spend longer periods of time traveling (e.g., more than 6 hours). The peak rate occurs within the first 2 weeks after travel (Pai & Douketis, 2015).

Interventions	*Rationales*
e. Take all opportunities to get up to stretch your legs, when there are stops in your journey. f. Avoid medications (e.g., sedatives, sleeping pills) or alcohol, which could impair your ability to get up and move around. g. Wear loose-fitting, comfortable clothing	
14. Consult with PCP to advise if additional measure are needed, if prolonged travel is planned, for example, anticoagulant therapy, graduated compression stockings (GCS) are indicated. Advise NOT to purchase compression stocking over the counter.	14. Anticoagulant therapy may be indicted for individuals at risk for travel-associated venous thromboembolism (VTE) (e.g., travel more than 6 hours in individuals with risk factors for VTE). GCS require care measurement to assure proper fit and avoidance of constriction that can actually contribute to DVT occurrence.

Clinical Alert Report

Advise ancillary staff/student to report:

- Any new change or deterioration diastolic in behavior (e.g., agitation, cognition, anxiety)
- Any swelling on extremities
- Individual complaint of pain and/or tenderness on extremities
- Redness of the skin
- Difficulty breathing
- Faster than normal or irregular heartbeat
- Chest pain or discomfort, which usually worsens with a deep breath or coughing
- Coughing up blood
- Very low BP, lightheadedness, or fainting

Documentation

Individual/family teaching
Outcome achievement or status

Hypertension

The following chart reflects BP categories defined by the American Heart Association (2012).
BP for adults 18 years of age and older:

Normal	Systolic:	Less than 120 mm Hg	Diastolic: Less than 80 mm Hg
PREHYPERTENSION			
Borderline	Systolic:	120 to 139 mm Hg	Diastolic: 80–89 mm Hg
HYPERTENSION	≥140/90 mm Hg		
Stage 1:	Systolic:	140 to 159 mm Hg	Diastolic: 90–99 mm Hg
Stage 2:	Systolic:	≥160 mm Hg	Diastolic: ≥100 mm Hg
HYPERTENSIVE CRISIS			
	Systolic:	≥180 mm Hg	Diastolic: ≥110 mm Hg

Hypertension is the major cause of coronary heart disease (CHD), cerebrovascular accident, and renal failure, which are the leading causes of death in the United States (CDC, 2012). Sustained hypertension and accompanying increased peripheral resistance cause a disruption in the vascular endothelium, forcing plasma and lipoproteins into the vessel's intimal and subintimal layers and causing plaque formation (atherosclerosis). Increased pressure also causes hyperplasia of smooth muscle, which scars the intima and results in thickened vessels with narrowed lumina. Elevated systemic BP increases the work of the left ventricle, leading to hypertrophy and increased myocardial oxygen demand.

The National Health and Nutrition Examination Survey (NHANES) conducted from 2005 through 2008 contained data, that approximately 76.4 million Americans over the age of 20 years have hypertension (Wright, Hughes, Ostchega, Yoon, & Nwankwo, 2011). Among adults with hypertension, nearly 83% were aware, nearly 76% were taking medication to lower their BP, and nearly 52% were controlled. There was no change in awareness, treatment, and control from 2009–2010 to 2011–2012 (Carson et al., 2011). Hypertension tends to be more common, be more severe, occur earlier in life, progress faster and be associated with greater target-organ damage in blacks. The causative factors are not well understood (Basile & Bloch, 2016).

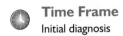

Time Frame
Initial diagnosis

■■■■■ DIAGNOSTIC CLUSTER**

Collaborative Problems

Risk for Complications of Vascular Insufficiency

Nursing Diagnoses

Risk for Compromised Engagement[4] related to negative side effects of prescribed therapy versus the belief that treatment is not needed without the presence of symptoms

Risk for Ineffective Health Management related to lack of knowledge of condition, diet restrictions, medications, risk factors, and follow-up care

**This medical condition was not included in the validation study.

Transition Criteria

The staff/student will:

1. Explain the risk factors and management of hypertension risk factors.
2. Describe the signs and symptoms that must be reported to a health care professional.
3. Review risk assessment and the various management strategies of the risk, to reduce mortality and aid secondary prevention.
4. Review the individual's understanding on the need to be assessed regularly.
5. Review diagnosis and laboratory tests.
6. Explain the importance of adherence to prescribed medications. Drug therapy for secondary prevention.

Before transition the individual will:

1. Demonstrate BP self-measurement.
2. Identify risk factors for hypertension.
3. Explain the action, dosage, side effects, and precautions for all prescribed medications.
4. Verbalize dietary factors associated with hypertension.
5. Relate an intent to comply with lifestyle changes and prescriptions post transition.
6. Describe the signs and symptoms that must be reported to a health care professional.
7. Articulate commonly identified goals for BP.

---

[4]The nursing diagnosis has been developed by Lynda Juall Carpenito.

Transitional Risk Assessment Plan (TRAP)

Begin this plan on admission.

Implement the Transitional Risk Assessment Plan (TRAP):

* Refer to inside back cover.
* Add each validated risk diagnosis to individual's problem list with the risk code in ( ).
* Refer to Unit II to the individual risk nursing diagnoses/collaborative problems for outcomes and interventions.

> *R: "Close coordination of care in the postacute period, early transition follow-up care, enhanced client education and self-management training, proactive end-of-life counseling, and extending the resources and clinical expertise over time via multidisciplinary team management" can lower readmission rates and improve health outcomes (Boutwell & Hwu, 2009, p. 14). Interventions are utilized to activate the individual and family to select changes in their everyday lifestyle choices to improve their health (Hibbard & Greene, 2013).*

Collaborative Problems

Risk for Complications of Vascular Insufficiency

Collaborative Outcomes

The individual will be monitored for early signs and symptoms of vascular insufficiency and will receive collaborative interventions if indicated to restore physiologic stability.

Indicators of Physiologic Stability

* No new visual defects
* Oriented
* Equal-strength upper/lower extremities

CLINICAL ALERT:
* In most individuals ≥60 years, the goal is to initiate pharmacologic treatment to lower BP at systolic blood pressure (SBP) ≥150 mm Hg or diastolic blood pressure (DBP) ≥90 mm Hg and treat to a goal SBP <150 mm Hg and goal DBP <90 mm Hg (James et al., 2014).

Interventions	Rationales
1. Monitor for evidence of tissue ischemia.	1. Hypertension adversely affects the entire cardiovascular system. Chronic increases in perfusion pressure result in hypertrophy of vascular smooth muscle and increased collagen concentration. These changes reduce the lumen size of the blood vessels, change the vessels' shape, and give rise to cyclospasm of the vessel cells. The results are plaque formation from increased adherence of monocytes to the endothelium. The increase in the wall-to-lumen ratio in the arteries causes greater vessel resistance and a reduced ability to dilate in response to increased metabolic need for oxygen (Grossman & Porth, 2014).
a. Visual defects including blurring, spots, and loss of visual acuity	a. Evidence of blood vessel damage in the retina indicates similar damage elsewhere in the vascular system.

(continued)

Interventions	Rationales

b. Cerebrovascular deficits
  • Orientation or memory deficits
  • Weakness
  • Paralysis
  • Mobility, speech, or sensory deficits
	b. In the brain, sustained hypertension causes progressive cerebral arteriosclerosis and ischemia. Interruption of cerebral blood supply caused by cerebral artery occlusion or rupture results in sensory and motor deficits.

c. In addition to extreme readings, a person in hypertensive crisis may experience:
  • Severe headaches (brain swelling and dysfunction)
  • Severe anxiety (brain swelling and dysfunction)
  • Lightheadedness, vertigo, (brain swelling and dysfunction)
  • Nosebleeds (rupture of a blood vessel within the richly perfused nasal mucosa)
	c. Severely elevated BP (equal to or greater than a systolic 180 or diastolic of 110—sometimes termed *malignant* or *accelerated hypertension*) is referred to as a "hypertensive crisis," as BPs above these levels are known to confer a risk of complications (e.g., left ventricular failure, acute renal injury).

d. Renal insufficiency
  • Decreased serum protein level
  • Sustained elevated urine specific gravity
  • Elevated urine sodium levels
  • Increased blood urea nitrogen (BUN), serum potassium, creatinine, potassium, phosphorus, and ammonia levels; decreased creatinine clearance.
  • Sustained insufficient urine output (<0.5 mL/kg/hr)
	d. With decreased blood supply to the nephrons, the kidney loses some ability to concentrate and form normal urine (Grossman & Porth, 2014).
	  • Further structural abnormalities may cause the vessels to become more permeable and allow leakage of protein into the renal tubules.
	  • Decreased ability of the renal tubules to reabsorb electrolytes causes increased urine sodium levels and increased urine specific gravity.
	  • Decreased renal function impairs the excretion of urea and creatinine in the urine, thus elevating BUN and creatinine levels.
	  • Decreased glomerular filtration rate eventually causes insufficient urine output and stimulates renin production, which results in increased BP in an attempt to increase blood flow to the kidneys.

e. Explain that:
  • Hypertension is both a cause and complication of chronic kidney disease.
  • BP control is the key to slowing the progression of chronic kidney disease (CKD) (Basile & Bloch, 2016; Grossman & Porth, 2014).	

f. Cardiac insufficiency	f. Microvascular coronary atherosclerotic plaques or vasospasm reduce the caliber of vessel and its ability to oxygenate tissue (Grossman & Porth, 2014).

Clinical Alert Report

Advise ancillary staff/student to report:
- Blood spots in the eyes or subconjunctival hemorrhage
- Facial flushing
- Individual complaint of chest pain or discomfort
- Dizziness
- Any change in systolic BP >180 mm Hg or <90 mm Hg, and/or diastolic BP >90 mm Hg
- Resting pulse >120 or <55 beats/min

Documentation

        Vital signs
        Intake and output
        Laboratory values
        Status of individual
        Unusual events
        Changes in behavior

Nursing Diagnoses

Risk for Compromised Engagement[5] Related to Negative Side Effects of Prescribed Therapy versus the Belief that Treatment Is Not Needed Without the Presence of Symptoms

NOC

Engagement Behavior, Symptom Control, Treatment Behavior: Illness or Injury

NIC

Health Education, Self-Modification Assistance, Self-Responsibility Facilitation, Coping Enhancement, Decision-Making Support, Health System Guidance, Mutual Goal Setting, Teaching: Disease Process

Goal

The individual will
- Verbalize feelings related to following the prescribed regimen.
- Identify sources of support for assisting with compliance.
- Verbalize the potential complications of noncompliance.
- Eat a better diet, which may include reducing salt.
- Enjoy regular physical activity.
- Maintain a healthy weight.
- Manage stress.
- Avoid tobacco smoke.

Interventions	Rationales

1. Identify any factors that may predict failure to engage in recommended treatments, lifestyle changes, such as:
  a. Lack of knowledge, cost
  b. Low literacy
  c. Failure to perceive the seriousness or chronicity of hypertension
  d. Belief that the condition will go away
  e. Belief that the condition is hopeless
	1. Motivation improves when individuals have positive experiences with and trust in their clinicians. Empathy builds trust and is a potent motivator (*Barrier, Li, & Jensen, 2003). "Clients need to recognize the importance of BP control and that in most cases they will need a combined approach of lifestyle changes and medication for effective treatment." This emphasis may encourage the individual to comply with treatment by pointing out the seriousness of hypertension.

2. Point out that BP elevation typically produces no symptoms.	2. Absence of symptoms often encourages noncompliance.
3. Discuss the likely effects of a future stroke, renal failure, or coronary disease on significant others (spouse, children, grandchildren).	3. This discussion may encourage compliance by emphasizing the potential impact of the individual's hypertension on his or her significant others.
4. Include the individual's significant others in teaching sessions whenever possible.	4. Significant others also should understand the possible consequences of noncompliance; this encourages them to assist the individual to comply with treatment.
5. Emphasize to the individual that, ultimately, it is his or her choice whether or not to comply with the treatment plan.	5. Helping the individual to understand that he or she is responsible for compliance may enhance the individual's sense of control and self-determination, which may help to improve compliance.
6. Refer to Appendix C for Strategies to Promote Engagement of Individual/Families for Healthier Outcomes	

(continued)

[5]Risk for Compromised Engagement has been developed by Lynda Juall Carpenito and can be found in Unit II Section 1.

Interventions	*Rationales*
8. Instruct the individual to check or have someone else check his or her BP at least once a week and to keep an accurate record of readings.	8. Weekly BP readings are needed to evaluate the individual's response to treatments and lifestyle changes.
9. Explain the possible side effects of antihypertensive medications (e.g., impotence, decreased libido, vertigo); instruct the individual to consult the physician/nurse practitioner for alternative medications should these side effects occur.	9. An individual who experiences these side effects may be tempted to discontinue medication therapy on his or her own.
10. If the cost of antihypertensive medications is a burden, consult with social services.	10. Financial assistance may be needed to prevent medication access due to financial reasons.

Documentation

Individual/family teaching
Response to interventions

> **TRANSITION TO HOME/COMMUNITY CARE**
> If indicated, review the risk diagnoses identified for this individual on admission:
> - Is the person still at risk?
> - Can the family reduce the risks?
> - Is the person at higher risk at home?
> - Is a home health nurse assessment needed?
> - Refer to transition planner/case manager/social service.
> - When is this person scheduled for follow-up with primary provider? Specialists? Record dates of appointments.
> - Complete a medication reconciliation prior to transition. Refer to index.

STAR **Stop**

Think Is this person at risk for injury, falls, medical complications, and/or inability to care for self (ADLs)?
Is the person competent to manage self-administration of medications, treatment procedures? Are additional resources needed?
Can the person explain how to monitor the condition (e.g., blood glucose, sign/symptoms of complications, dietary/mobility restrictions, and when to call his or her primary provider or specialist)?

Act Contact or provide the appropriate resource (e.g., contacting a support person, home health assessment, additional teaching, printed materials).

Review Has the problem been addressed? If not, use SBAR to communicate to the appropriate person.

Risk for Ineffective Management Related to Lack of Knowledge of Condition, Diet Restrictions, Medications, Risk Factors, and Follow-up Care

NOC

Compliance Behavior, Knowledge: Treatment Regimen, Participation in Health Care Decisions, Treatment Behavior: Illness or Injury

Goal

The goals for this diagnosis represent those associated with transition planning. Refer to the transition criteria.

NIC

Anticipatory Guidance, Risk Identification, Health Education, Learning Facilitation

Interventions	Rationales

1. Discuss BP concepts using terminology the individual and significant other(s) can understand:
  a. Normal values (target/goals). The clinician and the individual must agree upon BP goals. An individual-centered strategy to achieve the goal and an estimation of the time needed to reach that goal are important (*Boulware, Daumit, & Frick, 2001).
  b. Effects of sustained high BP on the brain, heart, kidneys, and eyes
  c. Control versus cure
	1. Risk of stroke rises directly with a person's BP (both systolic and diastolic). The reported decline in strokes coincides with the aggressive treatment and effective control of hypertension during the past several years (American Heart Association, 2012).

2. Teach the individual BP self-measurement, or teach significant other(s) how to measure the individual's BP.	2. Self-monitoring is more convenient and may improve compliance.

3. Discuss lifestyle modification (e.g., smoking cessation, weight control, exercising) that can reduce hypertension. Refer to the index for strategies for life style changes. Emphasize:
 	
  a. Eating a heart-healthy diet is important for managing your BP and reducing your risk of heart attack, heart disease, stroke, and other diseases.
 	
  b. The D.A.S.H. plan is proven effective for lowering BP.
 	
  c. Combinations of two (or more) lifestyle modifications can achieve even better results.
 	
  d. Achieve weight loss to within 10% of ideal weight.
 	
  e. Limit alcohol intake daily (2 oz liquor, 8 oz wine, or 24 oz beer).
  f. Engage in regular exercise (30 to 45 minutes) three to five times a week.
  g. Reduce sodium intake to 4.6 g of sodium chloride.
  h. Reduce saturated fat and cholesterol to <30% of dietary intake.
  i. Ensure the daily allowance of calcium, potassium, and magnesium in diet.
Refer also to Unit II Section 1 to Overweight, Sedentary Lifestyle nursing diagnoses if indicated (Basile & Bloch, 2016). If indicated refer to index to smoking cessation.
	3. Adoption of healthy lifestyles by all persons is critical for the prevention of high BP and is an indispensable part of the management of those with hypertension. Major lifestyle modifications shown to lower BP include weight reduction in those individuals who are overweight or obese.
	  a. Obesity-related hypertension has become an epidemic health problem and a major risk factor for the development of cardiovascular disease (CVD) (Purkayastha, Zhang, & Cai, 2011). Metabolic syndrome is the presence of three or more of the following conditions: abdominal obesity (waist circumference >40 inches in men or >35 inches in women), glucose intolerance (fasting glucose >100 mg/dL), BP >130/85 mm Hg, high triglycerides (>150 mg/dL), or low HDL (<40 mg/dL in men or <50 mg/dL in women).
	  b. Alcohol is a vasodilator causing rebound vasoconstriction that has been associated with increased BP.
	  c. The decline in arterial function with aging is considered to be part of a physiologic process reflecting elevated BP. However, the extent and rate of this decline can be manipulated. Various types of exercise programs are recommended for improving and/or maintaining the arterial function in middle-aged to older individuals (Miura, 2012).
	  d. Sodium controls water distribution throughout the body. An increase in sodium causes an increase in water, thus increasing circulating volume and raising BP.
	  e. A high-fat diet contributes to plaque formation and narrowing vessels.
	  f. These elements maintain the cardiovascular and muscular systems.

(continued)

Interventions	*Rationales*

4. Provide with medication guidelines for all prescribed medications. Explain the following:
  a. Dosage
  b. Action
  c. Side effects
  d. Precautions
	4. This teaching conveys which side effects should be reported and precautions that should be taken.

5. Instruct to call 911 (Basile & Bloch, 2016)
  a. Blurry vision or other vision changes
  b. Headache
  c. Nausea or vomiting
  d. Confusion
  e. Passing out or seizures—seizures are waves of abnormal electrical activity in the brain that can make people move or behave strangely.
  f. Weakness or numbness on one side of the body, or in one arm or leg
  g. Difficulty talking
  h. Trouble breathing
  i. Chest pain
  j. Pain in the upper back or between the shoulders
  k. Urine that is brown or bloody
  l. Pain when urinating
  m. Pain in the lower back or on the side of the body
  n. Women may experience (Gulati, Shaw, & Merz, 2012; *Pepine et al., 2004)
    • Neck or jaw pain
    • Shoulder or arm pain
    • A fast heartbeat
    • Shortness of breath when you are physically active
    • Nausea and vomiting
    • Sweating
    • Fatigue
	5. These signs and symptoms may indicate elevated BP or other cardiovascular complications that require immediate care.
	   Women appear to have different symptom presentations than men. The higher prevalence of nonobstructive coronary artery disease (CAD) among the CASS women compared with the CASS men suggested symptoms were less diagnostic in women (Gulati, Shaw, & Merz, 2012).

6. Stress the importance of follow-up care by PCP, cardiologist.	6. Follow-up care is important to determine if the person if normotensive, has any new complaints and if they are participating in lifestyle changes that are indicated.

Documentation

Status of goal attainment
Status at transition
Transition instructions
Referrals

Acute Coronary Syndrome

Acute coronary syndrome (ACS) is the umbrella term that encompasses myocardial ischemia, unstable angina, and all types of myocardial infarction: Q-wave, non–Q-wave, ST segment elevation myocardial infarction, and those without ST wave elevations, non-ST segment elevation myocardial infarction. Myocardial infarction (MI) is the death of myocardial tissue resulting from impaired myocardial coronary blood flow. The cause of inadequate blood flow most commonly is the narrowing or occlusion of the coronary artery resulting from atherosclerosis, or decreased coronary blood flow from shock or hemorrhage. Diminished ability to bind oxygen to the hemoglobin can also result in an MI. Heart disease (HD) is caused by atherosclerosis, which involves a gradual buildup of plaque in the lumen of the coronary arteries. The development of atherosclerosis is influenced by risk factors such as smoking, hypertension, hyperlipidaemia, and diabetes. ACS occurs as a result of disruption of an atherosclerotic coronary artery plaque, either through rupture or erosion. This causes thrombosis and possibly vasoconstriction, leading to a sudden and significant reduction in blood flow and myocardial oxygen supply (Bassand et al., 2007). The diagnosis of acute coronary ischemia depends upon the characteristics of the chest pain, specific associated symptoms, abnormalities on electrocardiogram (ECG), and levels of serum markers of cardiac injury (Reede &, Awtry, 2016).

 Time Frame
Initial diagnosis
Post–intensive care
Recurrent episodes

■■■DIAGNOSTIC CLUSTER

Collaborative Problems

▲ Risk for Complications of arrhythmias

▲ Risk for Complications of Cardiogenic Shock

▲ Risk for Complications of Heart Failure

▲ Risk for Complications of Thromboembolism

▲ Risk for Complications of Recurrent Acute Coronary Syndrome

* Risk for Complications of Pericarditis

* Risk for Complications of Pericardial Tamponade/Rupture

* Risk for Complications of Structural Defects

* Risk for Complications of Extension of Infarct

Nursing Diagnoses

▲ Anxiety/Fear (individual, family) related to unfamiliar situation status, unpredictable nature of condition, negative effect on lifestyle, fear of death, possible sexual dysfunction

▲ Pain related to cardiac tissue ischemia or inflammation

▲ Activity Intolerance related to insufficient oxygenation for ADLs secondary to cardiac tissue ischemia, prolonged immobility, narcotics, or medications (refer to Unit II)

△ Grieving related to actual or perceived losses secondary to cardiac condition (refer to Unit II)

△ Risk for Ineffective Health Management related to lack of knowledge of hospital routines, procedures, equipment, treatments, conditions, medications, diet, activity progression, signs and symptoms of complications, reduction of risks, follow-up care, community resources

▲This diagnosis was reported to be monitored for or managed frequently (75% to 100%).
△This diagnosis was reported to be monitored for or managed often (50% to 74%).
* This diagnosis was not included in the validation study.
* This medical condition was not included in the validation study.

Transition Criteria

The staff/student will:

1. Explain the risk factors and management of cardiovascular risk factors.
2. Describe the signs and symptoms that must be reported to a health care professional.
3. Review risk assessment and the various management strategies of the risk, to reduce mortality and aid secondary prevention.
4. Review the individuals' understanding on the need to be assessed regularly.
5. Review diagnosis and laboratory test.
6. Explain the importance of adherence to prescribed medications. Drug therapy for secondary prevention.
7. Review the importance of cardiac rehab.

Transitional Risk Assessment Plan (TRAP)

Begin this plan on admission.

Implement the Transitional Risk Assessment Plan (TRAP):

* Refer to inside back cover.
* Add each validated risk diagnosis to individual's problem list with the risk code in ( ).
* Refer to Unit II to the individual risk nursing diagnoses/collaborative problems for outcomes and interventions.

> *R: "Close coordination of care in the postacute period, early transition follow-up care, enhanced client education and self-management training, proactive end-of-life counseling, and extending the resources and clinical expertise over time via multidisciplinary team management" can lower readmission rates and improve health outcomes (Boutwell & Hwu, 2009, p. 14). Interventions are utilized to activate the individual and family to select changes in their everyday lifestyle choices to improve their health (Hibbard & Greene, 2013).*

* Add other rationale indicators.

Collaborative Problems

Risk for Complications of Arrhythmias

Risk for Complications of Cardiogenic Shock

Risk for Complications of Heart Failure

Risk for Complications of Thromboembolism

Risk for Complications of Recurrent Acute Coronary Syndrome

Risk for Complications of Pericarditis

Risk for Complications of Pericardial Tamponade/Rupture

Risk for Complications of Structural Defects

Risk for Complications of Extension of Infarct

Collaborative Outcomes

The individual will be monitored for early signs and symptoms of (a) cardiogenic shock, (b) heart failure, (c) thromboembolism, (d) recurrent ACS, (e) pericarditis, (f) pericardial tamponade/rupture, (g) structural defects, and will receive collaborative interventions if indicated to restore physiologic stability.

Indicators of Physiologic Stability

* Oxygen saturation >95% (pulse oximeter)
* Normal sinus rhythm
* No life-threatening arrhythmias
* No chest pain
* Pulse: regular rhythm, rate 60 to 100 beats/min
* Respiration 16 to 20 breaths/min
* BP: Systolic >120 mm Hg, Diastolic >85 mm Hg
* Urine output >0.5 mL/kg/hr

Interventions	Rationales
1. Per protocol, initiate pharmacologic reperfusion therapy (e.g., thrombolytics).	1. These agents restore full blood flow through the blocked artery.
2. Maintain continuous electrocardiography (EKG), BP, and pulse oximetry monitoring; report changes.	2. Continuous monitoring allows for early detection of complications.

Interventions	*Rationales*
3. Administer medications, as indicated, and continue to monitor for side effects. Consult pharmaceutical reference for specifics.	3. It is important to manage individuals effectively when they first present with acute chest pain to reduce the risk of further adverse events. Early administration of antiplatelet therapy, pain relief, and oxygen therapy, if required, will help to reduce this risk (Marshall, 2011).

4. Monitor for signs and symptoms of arrhythmias:
  a. Abnormal rate, rhythm
  b. Palpitations, syncope
  c. Hemodynamic compromise (e.g., hypotension)
  d. Cardiac emergencies (arrest, ventricular fibrillation)
 	
 CLINICAL ALERT:
  • Not all individuals present with typical chest pain.
  • Older individuals and those with diabetes are particularly prone to atypical presentation, such as fatigue, shortness of breath, presyncope, or syncope. Atypical symptoms may include pain in the epigastric region or back, rather than the centre of the chest (Marshall, 2011).
	4. Myocardial ischemia results from reduced oxygen to myocardial tissue. Ischemic tissue is electrically unstable, causing arrhythmias, such as premature ventricular contractions, that can lead to ventricular fibrillation and death. Arrsrhythmias can result from reperfusion of ischemic tissue secondary to thrombolytics.

5. Maintain oxygen therapy, as prescribed. Evaluate pulse oximeter readings.	5. Supplemental oxygen therapy increases the circulating oxygen available to myocardial tissue. Pulse oximeter readings should be >95%. Exceptions may be necessary for those with chronic obstructive pulmonary disease.

6. Monitor for signs and symptoms of cardiogenic shock:
  a. Tachycardia
  b. Urine output >30 mL/hr
  c. Restlessness, agitation, change in mentation
  d. Tachypnea
  e. Diminished peripheral pulses
  f. Cool, pale, or cyanotic skin
  g. Mean arterial pressure >60 mm Hg
  h. Cardiac index >2.0 L
  i. Increased systemic vascular resistance
	6. Cardiogenic shock results most often from loss of viable myocardium and impaired contractility. This manifests as decreased stroke volume and cardiac output. The compensatory response to decreased circulatory volume aims to increase blood oxygen levels by increasing heart and respiratory rates, and to decrease circulation to extremities (marked by decreased pulses and cool skin). Diminished oxygen to the brain causes changes in mentation.

7. Monitor for signs and symptoms of HF and decreased cardiac output:
  a. Gradual increase in heart rate
  b. Increased shortness of breath
  c. Adventitious breath sounds
  d. Decreased systolic BP
  e. Presence of or increase in S_3 or S_4 gallop
  f. Peripheral edema
  g. Distended neck veins
  h. Elevation in BNP (β-type natriuretic peptide)
	7. Myocardial ischemia causes HF. Ischemia reduces the ability of the left ventricle to eject blood, thus decreasing cardiac output and increasing pulmonary vascular congestion. Fluid enters pulmonary tissue, causing rales, productive cough, cyanosis, and possibly signs and symptoms of respiratory distress.

8. Monitor for signs and symptoms of thromboembolism:
 	
  a. Diminished or no peripheral pulses, decreased Ankle–Brachial index
  b. Leg pain localized to calf area
	8. Prolonged bed rest, increased blood viscosity and coagulability, and decreased cardiac output contribute to thrombus formation.
	  a. Insufficient circulation causes pain and diminished peripheral pulse.
	  b. Unusual warmth and redness point to inflammation; coolness and cyanos is indicate vascular obstruction. Leg pain results from tissue hypoxia.

(continued)

Interventions	*Rationales*
c. Sudden severe chest pain, increased dyspnea	c. Obstruction to pulmonary circulation causes sudden chest pain and dyspnea.
d. Claudication	d. Pain with walking is caused by insufficient circulation.

9. Monitor for signs and symptoms of pericarditis:
  a. Chest pain influenced by change in respiration or position
  b. Pericardial rub
  c. Temperature elevation >101° F
  d. Diffuse ST segment electrocardiogram (ECG) changes
	9. Pericarditis is inflammation of the pericardial sac. Damage to the epicardium causes it to become rough, which tends to irritate and inflame the pericardium.

10. Monitor for signs and symptoms of pericardial tamponade/cardiac rupture:
  a. Hypotension
  b. Distended neck veins
  c. Tachycardia
  d. Pulsus paradoxus
  e. Equalization of cardiac pressures
  f. Narrowed pulse pressure
  g. Muffled heart tones
  h. Electrical alternans
	10. Cardiac tamponade results from accumulation of fluid in the pericardial space, causing impaired cardiac function and decreased cardiac output. Cardiac rupture occurs most often from 3 to 10 days after MI, resulting from leukocyte scavenger cells removing necrotic debris, which thins the myocardial wall. The onset is sudden, with bleeding into the pericardial sac.

11. Monitor for signs and symptoms of structural defects:
  a. Severe chest pain
  b. Syncope
  c. Hypotension
  d. New loud holosystolic murmur
  e. CHF
  f. Left-to-right shunt
	11. Ventricular aneurysm, ventricular septal defect, and papillary muscle rupture all result from ischemia or necrosis to the structures.

12. Monitor for signs and symptoms of recurrent MI:
  a. Classic symptoms: Sudden, severe chest pain with nausea/vomiting and diaphoresis; pain may or may not radiate. ACS can occur without pain and without change in EKG.
  b. Increased dyspnea
  c. Increased ST elevation and abnormal Q waves on ECG
	12. These signs and symptoms indicate myocardial tissue deterioration with increasing hypoxia.
	
	Clinical Alert:
	 • Not all individuals present with typical chest pain.
	 • Older individuals and those with diabetes are particularly prone to atypical presentation, such as fatigue, shortness of breath, presyncope, or syncope. Atypical symptoms may include pain in the epigastric region or back, rather than the centre of the chest (Marshall, 2011).

13. Progressive activity after chest pain is controlled; involve individual in cardiac rehabilitation.	13. These measures actively promote venous return.

Clinical Alert Report

Advise ancillary staff/student to report:
- Any new change or deterioration diastolic in behavior (e.g., agitation, cognition)
- Any changes in the individual's rhythm/arrhythmias
- Individual complaint of chest pain or discomfort
- Individual diaphoretic
- Any change in systolic BP >210 mm Hg and <90 mm Hg, and/or diastolic >90 mm Hg
- Resting pulse >120 or >55 beats/min
- Change in rate of respirations >28 or <10/min
- Changes or new onset of dyspnea/palpitations
- Decrease in urine output <0.5 mL/kg/hr

Intravenous Therapy

IV access for medication administration, IV access for blood sampling, arterial access for ABGs and BP monitoring, sheath access for coronary interventions

Laboratory Studies

Arterial blood gas analysis, electrolytes, cholesterol, white blood count, triglycerides, sedimentation rate, coagulation studies, chemistry profile, creatinine kinase, MB isoenzyme, troponin I, troponin T, myoglobin, CK-MB isoforms

Diagnostic Studies

ECG, stress test, chest X-ray film, cardiac catheterization, echocardiogram, digital subtraction angiography, nuclear imaging studies, thallium scans, magnetic resonance imaging, thoracic electrical bioimpedance (IEB), Svo$_2$ monitoring, hemodynamic monitoring, stroke volume (SV) and stoke volume variations (SVV), cardiac output (CO) and cardiac index (CI), systemic vascular resistance (SVR), central venous pressure (CVP)

Therapies

Oxygen via cannula; (in selected cases) pacemakers, transcutaneous, transvenous, and permanent single or dual chamber; therapeutic diet (low salt, low saturated fats, low cholesterol); cardiac rehabilitation program; pulse oximetry

Interventional Therapies

Percutaneous transluminal coronary angioplasty, intracoronary stents, atherectomy, intra-aortic balloon pump

Documentation

Vital signs
Intake and output
Rhythm strips
Status of individual
Unusual events

Nursing Diagnoses

Anxiety/Fear (Individual, Family) Related to Unfamiliar Situation, Unpredictable Nature of Condition, Fear of Death, Negative Effects on Lifestyle, or Possible Sexual Dysfunctions

NOC
Anxiety Level, Coping, Impulse Control

Goal

The individual or family will relate increased psychological and physiologic comfort.

NIC
Anxiety Reduction, Impulse Control Training, Anticipatory Guidance

Indicators

- Verbalize fears related to the disorder.
- Share concerns about the disorder's effects on normal functioning, role responsibilities, and lifestyle.
- Use at least one relaxation technique.

Interventions	Rationales

1. Assist the individual to reduce anxiety:
  a. Provide reassurance and comfort.
  b. Convey understanding and empathy. Do not avoid questions.
  c. Encourage the individual to verbalize any fears and concerns regarding MI and its treatment.
  d. Identify and support effective coping mechanisms.
	1. An anxious individual has a narrowed perceptual field and a diminished ability to learn. He or she may experience symptoms caused by increased muscle tension and disrupted sleep patterns. Anxiety tends to feed on itself, trapping the individual in a spiral of increasing anxiety, tension, and emotional and physical pain.

CLINICAL ALERT:
- Depression and anxiety co-occur, appear to inhibit recovery, and have a negative impact on social functioning and capacity to perform ADLs in individuals who develop an ACS (Tisminetzky, Bray, Miozzo, Aupont, & McLaughlin, 2012).

(continued)

Interventions	*Rationales*
2. Assess the individual's anxiety level. Plan teaching when level is low or moderate.	2. Some fears are based on inaccuracies; accurate information can relieve them. An individual with severe or panic anxiety does not retain learning.
3. Encourage family and friends to verbalize fears and concerns.	3. Verbalization allows sharing and provides the nurse with an opportunity to correct misconceptions.
4. Provide the individual and family valid reassurance; reinforce positive coping behavior.	4. Praising effective coping can reinforce future positive coping responses.
5. Encourage the individual to use relaxation techniques, such as guided imagery and relaxation breathing.	5. These techniques enhance the individual's sense of control over her or his body's responses to stress.
6. Contact the physician/nurse practitioner immediately if the individual's anxiety is at severe or panic level. Sedate if necessary.	6. Severe anxiety interferes with learning and compliance and also increases heart rate.

> **CLINICAL ALERT:**
> • High levels of correlation among depression, anxiety, and impaired function in ACS individuals over time may cause important information to be missed that may be crucial to understanding how and when an intervention should be implemented and in which populations its implementation would be most effective (Tisminetzky et al., 2012).

7. Refer also to the nursing diagnosis Anxiety in the Generic Medical Care Plan, for general assessment and interventions.

Documentation

Present emotional status
Response to interventions
Teaching sheets

Pain Related to Cardiac Tissue Ischemia or Inflammation

NOC
Comfort Level, Pain Control

Goal

The individual will report satisfactory control of chest pain within an appropriate time frame.

NIC
Pain Management, Medication Management, Emotional Support, Teaching: Individual, Heat/Cold Application, Simple Massage

Indicators

• Report pain relief after pain-relief measures.
• Demonstrate a relaxed mode.

Interventions	*Rationales*
1. Instruct the individual to immediately report any pain episode.	1. Less pain medication generally is required if administered early. Acute intervention can prevent further ischemia or injury.

Interventions	Rationales
2. Administer nitrates and oxygen or analgesics, per physician/nurse practitioner order. Document administration and degree of relief the individual experiences.	2. Severe, persistent pain unrelieved by analgesics may indicate impending or extending infarction.
3. Instruct the individual to rest during a pain episode.	3. Activity increases oxygen demand, which can exacerbate cardiac pain.
4. Reduce environmental distractions as much as possible.	4. Environmental stimulation can increase heart rate and may exacerbate myocardial tissue hypoxia, which increases pain.
5. After acute pain passes, explain its cause and possible precipitating factors (physical and emotional).	5. Calm explanation may reduce the individual's stress associated with fear of the unknown.
6. Obtain and evaluate a 12-lead ECG and rhythm strip during pain episodes. If *immediately* available, do so before nitrates administration. Notify the physician/nurse practitioner.	7. Cardiac monitoring may help to differentiate variant angina from extension of the infarction.

> **CLINICAL ALERT**
> • Administrator nitrates with caution. Nitrates lower BP.

Interventions	Rationales

8. Explain and assist with alternative pain-relief measures:
  a. Positioning
  b. Distraction (activities, breathing exercises)
  c. Massage
  d. Relaxation exercises
	9. These measures can help to prevent painful stimuli from reaching higher brain centers by replacing the painful stimuli with another stimulus. Relaxation reduces muscle tension, decreases heart rate, may improve stroke volume, and enhances the individual's sense of control over the pain.

Documentation

Medication administration
Unsatisfactory pain relief
Status of pain

STAR

Stop

Think Is this person at risk for injury, falls, medical complications, and/or inability to care for self (ADLs)?
  Is the person competent to manage self-administration of medications, treatment procedures? Are additional resources needed?
  Can the person explain how to monitor condition (e.g., blood glucose, sign/symptoms of complications, dietary/mobility restrictions, and when to call his or her primary provider or specialist?)

Act Use SBAR to notify the appropriate professional

SBAR *Situation:* Mr. Smith will be scheduled to be transitioned to his home.
Background: Mr. Smith lives alone. He (state his disabilities, self-care needs, treatments)
Action: A more thorough reevaluation of where he can be transitioned is needed.
Recommendation: Referral to social service/transition planner/case manager

Review Is the response/solution the right option for the individual? If not, discuss the situation with the appropriate person, department, and/or agency (using SBAR).

Risk for Ineffective Health Management Related to Lack of Knowledge of Condition, Hospital Routines (Procedures, Equipment), Treatments, Medications, Diet, Activity Progression, Signs and Symptoms of Complications, Reduction of Risks, Follow-Up Care, and Community Resources

NOC

Compliance Behavior, Knowledge: Treatment Regimen, Participation in Health Care Decisions, Treatment Behavior: Illness or Injury

NIC

Anticipatory Guidance, Risk Identification, Health Education, Learning Facilitation

Goal

The goals for this diagnosis represent those associated with transition planning. Refer to the transition criteria.

Interventions	Rationales
1. Explain the pathophysiology of MI using teaching aids appropriate for individual's educational level (e.g., pictures, models, written materials).	1. Such explanations reinforce the need to comply with instructions on diet, exercise, and other aspects of the treatment regimen.
2. Explain risk factors for MI that can be eliminated or modified: a. Obesity Refer to Getting Started to Losing Weight on thePoint. Print and give to individual. b. Tobacco Refer to Getting Started to Quit Smoking on thePoint. Print and give to individual. c. Diet high in fat or sodium Refer to Getting Started to Better Nutrition on thePoint. Print and give to individual. d. Sedentary lifestyle Refer to Getting Started to Increase Activity on thePoint. Print and give to individual. e. Excessive alcohol intake f. Hypertension g. Oral contraceptives h. Diabetes	2. Focusing on controllable factors can reduce the individual's feelings of powerlessness. a. Obesity increases peripheral resistance and cardiac workload. Fifty percent of CAD in women is attributed to overweight (*American Heart Association, 2005). Refer to the Obesity Care Plan. b. Smoking unfavorably alters lipid levels. It impairs oxygen transport while increasing oxygen demand (Grossman & Porth, 2014). c. A high-fat diet contributes to plaque formation in the arteries; excessive sodium intake increases water retention. d. A sedentary lifestyle leads to poor collateral circulation and predisposes the individual to other risk factors. e. Alcohol is a potent vasodilator; subsequent vasoconstriction increases cardiac workload. f. Hypertension with increased peripheral resistance damages the arterial intima, which contributes to arteriosclerosis. g. Oral contraceptives alter blood coagulation, platelet function, and fibrinolytic activity, thereby affecting the integrity of the endothelium. h. Elevated glucose levels damage the arterial intima.
3. Teach the individual the importance of stress management through relaxation techniques and regular, appropriate exercise.	3. Although the exact effect of stress on CAD is unclear, release of catecholamines elevates systolic BP, increases cardiac workload, induces lipolysis, and promotes platelet clumping (Grossman & Porth, 2014).

Interventions	Rationales
4. Teach the individual how to assess radial pulse and instruct her or him to report any of the following: a. Dyspnea b. Chest pain unrelieved by nitroglycerin c. Unexplained weight gain or edema d. Unusual weakness, fatigue e. Irregular pulse or any unusual change	4. These signs and symptoms may indicate myocardial ischemia and vascular congestion (edema) secondary to decreased cardiac output.
5. Instruct the individual to report side effects of pre-scribed medications which may include diuretics, digitalis, β-adrenergic blocking agents, ACE inhibitors, or aspirin.	5. Recognizing and promptly reporting medication side effects can help to prevent serious complications (e.g., hypokalemia, hypotension).
6. Reinforce the physician's/nurse practitioner's explanation for the prescribed therapeutic diet. Consult with a dietitian, if indicated.	6. Repetitive explanations may help to improve com-pliance with the therapeutic diet as well as promote understanding.
7. Explain the need for activity restrictions and how activity should progress gradually. Instruct the individual to a. Increase activity gradually. b. Avoid isometric exercises and lifting objects weighing more than 30 lb. c. Avoid jogging, heavy exercise, and sports until the physician/nurse practitioner advises otherwise. d. Consult with the physician/nurse practitioner on when to resume work, driving, sexual activity, recreational activi-ties, and travel. e. Take frequent 15- to 20-minute rest periods, four to six times a day for 1 to 2 months. f. Perform activities at a moderate, comfortable pace; if fa-tigue occurs, stop and rest for 15 minutes, then continue.	7. Increasing activity gradually allows cardiac tissue to heal and accommodate increased demands. Overexertion increases oxygen consumption and cardiac workload.
8. Reinforce the necessity of follow-up care.	8. Proper follow-up is essential to evaluate if and when progression of activities is advisable.
9. Provide information on community resources such as the American Heart Association, self-help groups, counseling, and cardiac rehabilitation groups.	9. Such resources can provide additional support, informa-tion, and follow-up assistance that the individual and family may need post transition.

Documentation

Follow-up instructions
Status at transition (pain, activity, wound)
Achievement of goals (individual or family)

Peripheral Arterial Disease (Atherosclerosis)

Atherosclerosis is a systemic disease of the large and medium-sized arteries causing luminal narrowing (fo-cal or diffuse) as a result of the accumulation of lipid and fibrous material between the intimal and medial layers of the vessel. Atherosclerosis of the noncardiac vessels is defined as peripheral artery disease (PAD) (Harris & Dryjski, 2015). When atherosclerotic plaque and blood clots reduce blood flow to the legs or, less often, to the arms, the condition is called PAD. PAD makes walking painful and slows injury healing. It is characterized by specific changes in the arterial wall as well as the development of an intraluminal plaque. Atherosclerosis can lead to MI, renal hypertension, stroke, and amputation.

Approximately 8 million people in the United States have PAD, including 12% to 20% of individuals older than age 60 (CDC, 2016d). The known risk factors for atherosclerosis include hyperlipidemia, smok-ing history, hypertension, diabetes mellitus, and a family history of strokes or heart attacks, especially at an early age. Altering modifiable risk factors has been shown to reduce significantly the chances of progressing to the morbid consequences of this disease. Teaching the risk factors and modifying behaviors that reduce risk factors are important components of nursing interventions for atherosclerotic disease.

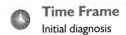

Time Frame

Initial diagnosis

■■■■■■ DIAGNOSTIC CLUSTER**

Collaborative Problems

Risk for Complications of Stroke

Risk for Complications of Ischemic Ulcers

Risk for Complications of Acute Arterial Thrombosis

Nursing Diagnoses

Activity Intolerance related to Claudication

Risk for Falls related to effects of orthostatic hypotension (refer to Unit II)

Risk for Ineffective Health Management related to lack of knowledge of condition, management of claudication, risk factors, foot care, and treatment plan

**This medical condition was not included in the validation study.

Transition Criteria

The staff/student will:

1. Explain the risk factors and management of PAD.
2. Review risk assessment and the various management strategies of the risk, to reduce mortality and aid secondary prevention.
3. State specific activities to manage claudication.
4. Describe the need for and steps of proper foot care.
5. Describe any lifestyle changes indicated (e.g., cessation of smoking, low-fat diet, regular exercise program).
6. State goal to reduce low-density lipoprotein (LDL) cholesterol to less than 100 optimal, 100 to 129 near optimal/above optimal (NCEP, 3rd Report ATP III).
7. Relate the signs and symptoms that must be reported to a health care professional.
8. Identify community resources available for assistance.

Transitional Risk Assessment Plan (TRAP)

Begin this plan on admission.

Implement the Transitional Risk Assessment Plan (TRAP):

- Refer to inside back cover.
- Add each validated risk diagnosis to individual's problem list with the risk code in ( ).
- Refer to Unit II to the individual risk nursing diagnoses/collaborative problems for outcomes and interventions.

R: "Close coordination of care in the postacute period, early transition follow-up care, enhanced client education and self-management training, proactive end-of-life counseling, and extending the resources and clinical expertise over time via multidisciplinary team management" can lower readmission rates and improve health outcomes (Boutwell & Hwu, 2009, p. 14). Interventions are utilized to activate the individual and family to select changes in their everyday lifestyle choices to improve their health (Hibbard & Greene, 2013).

Collaborative Problems

Risk for Complication of Stroke

Risk for Complication of Ischemic Ulcers

Risk for Complication of Acute Arterial Thrombosis

Risk for Complications of Hypertension

Collaborative Outcomes

The individual will be monitored for early signs and symptoms of (a) stroke, (b) ischemic ulcers, and (c) acute arterial thrombosis and will receive collaborative interventions if indicated to restore physiologic stability.

Indicators of Physiologic Stability

- BP >90/60, <140/90 mm Hg
- Oriented and alert
- Palpable peripheral pulses
- Warm, dry skin
- Intact motor/sensation of extremities
- Ankle–brachial index (difference between the BP of the arm to the ankle. If the ankle pressure is 50% or less than the arm, indicates impaired circulation.)
- Claudication, sudden onset or progressive deterioration

Interventions	Rationales

1. Teach the individual about the signs and symptoms of transient ischemic attack (TIA) and the importance of reporting to the physician/nurse practitioner if they occur (Grossman & Porth, 2014).
  a. Dizziness, loss of balance, or fainting
  b. Changes in sensation or motor control in arms or legs
  c. Numbness in face
  d. Speech changes
  e. Visual changes or loss of vision
  f. Temporary loss of memory
	1. The risk of stroke increases in individuals who have had a TIA. Disruption of cerebral circulation can result in motor or sensory deficits.

> **CLINICAL ALERT:**
> - Prevalences of cerebral infarction and carotid artery stenosis were markedly higher in individuals with peripheral arterial disease than in controls, indicating that peripheral arterial disease is a meaningful risk factor for cerebral infarction, lacunar infarction, and carotid artery stenosis. This suggests that screening for cerebral infarction and carotid artery stenosis is important for managements in peripheral arterial disease, as with screening for peripheral arterial disease in individuals with stroke (Filho, 2015).

Interventions	Rationales
2. Assess for ischemic ulcers in extremities. Report ulcers or darkened spots of skin to the physician/nurse practitioner/physical assistant.	2. Atherosclerosis causing arterial stenosis and subsequent decreased tissue perfusion interferes with and may prevent healing of skin ulcers. Darkened spots of skin distal to arterial stenosis may indicate tissue infarctions related to ischemia.

> **CLINICAL ALERT:**
> - The most severe stage of PAD is critical limb ischemia, in which blood flow is so reduced that sores do not heal and gangrene can develop.
> - Only 1% to 2% of individuals with PAD develop threatened limb (critical limb ischemia), but all of them will need surgery to restore blood flow, and for almost 30%, amputation will ultimately be required (Neschis & Golden, 2014).

(continued)

Interventions	Rationales
3. Reinforce teaching of foot care. (Refer to the nursing diagnosis Risk for Ineffective Management of Therapeutic Regimen in this plan for more information.)	3. Protection from skin loss may preserve tissue by preventing access to infective agents.
4. Monitor peripheral circulation (pulses, sensation, skin color, and temperature). Report any changes immediately.	4. In acute arterial thrombosis, loss of sensation distal to the thrombosis occurs first with accompanying ischemic pain. This may be followed by a decrease in motor function.

Clinical Alert Report

Advise ancillary staff/student to report:
- Any change in systolic BP >210 mm Hg, <90 mm Hg, and/or diastolic >90 mm Hg
- Any new change or deterioration diastolic in behavior (e.g., agitation, cognition)
- Nonpalpable or very weak peripheral pulses
- Cool, pale, and even numb
- Weak motor/sensation of extremities
- Pain with walking (claudication), sudden onset or progressive deterioration

Documentation

Assessment results
Changes in condition

Nursing Diagnoses

Activity Intolerance Related to Claudication

NOC
Activity Tolerance

Goal

The individual will progress activity to (specify level of activity desired).

NIC
Activity Tolerance,
Energy Management,
Exercise Promotion,
Sleep Enhancement,
Mutual Goal Setting

Indicators

- Identify activities that cause claudication.
- State why pain occurs with activity.
- Develop a plan to increase activity and decrease claudication.

Interventions	Rationales
1. Teach the individual about the physiology of blood supply, in relation to activity and the pathophysiology of claudication. And the benefits of exercise.	1. Research has demonstrated the benefits of exercise therapy, including improved walking tolerance, modified inflammatory/hemostatic markers, enhanced vasoresponsiveness, adaptations within the limb (angiogenesis, arteriogenesis, and mitochondrial synthesis) that enhance oxygen delivery and metabolic responses, potentially delayed progression of the disease, enhanced quality of life indices, and extended longevity (Haas et al., 2012). Understanding of the condition may promote compliance with restrictions and the exercise program.

Interventions	Rationales
2. Reassure the individual that activity does not harm the claudicating tissue.	2. The individual may be tempted to discontinue activity when pain occurs in an attempt to avoid further injury.
3. Plan activities to include a scheduled ambulation time, try to have a walking partner: a. Start slow 10 minutes and increase 15 minutes as indicated. b. Institute a daily walking regimen of at least 30 minutes. c. Teach individual to "walk into" the pain, to pause when claudication occurs, and then to continue as soon as discomfort disappears. d. Start slowly. e. Emphasize that the *action* of walking is important, not the speed or distance.	

Documentation

Individual/family teaching
Outcome achievement or status
Referrals

> **TRANSITION TO HOME/COMMUNITY CARE**
> If indicated, review the risk diagnoses identified for this individual on admission:
> * Is the person still at risk?
> * Can the family reduce the risks?
> * Is the person at higher risk at home?
> * Is a home health nurse assessment needed?
> * Refer to transition planner/case manager/social service.
> * When is this person scheduled for follow-up with primary provider? Specialists? Record dates of appointments.
> * Complete a medication reconciliation prior to transition. Refer to inside back cover.

STAR

Stop

Think   Is this person at risk for injury, falls, medical complications, and/or inability to care for self (ADLs)?

Is the person competent to manage self-administration of medications, treatment procedures? Are additional resources needed?

Can the person explain how to monitor condition, for example, blood glucose, sign/symptoms of complications, dietary/mobility restrictions, and when to call his or her primary provider or specialist?

Act   Use SBAR to notify the appropriate professional

SBAR   *Situation:* Mr. Smith will be scheduled to be transitioned to his home.

Background: Mr. Smith lives alone. He (state his disabilities, self-care needs, treatments).

Action: A more thorough reevaluation of where he can be transitioned is needed.

Recommendation: Referral to social service/transition planner/case manager.

Review   Is the response/solution the right option for the individual? If not, discuss the situation with the appropriate person, department, and/or agency (using SBAR).

Risk for Ineffective Health Management Related to Lack of Knowledge of Condition, Management of Claudication, Risk Factors, Foot Care, and Treatment Plan

NOC

Compliance Behavior, Knowledge: Treatment Regimen, Participation in Health Care Decisions, Treatment Behavior: Illness or Injury

NIC

Anticipatory Guidance, Risk Identification, Health Education, Learning Facilitation

Goal

The outcome criteria for this diagnosis represent those associated with transition planning. Refer to the transition criteria.

Interventions	Rationales
1. Explain atherosclerosis and its effects on cardiac, circulatory, renal, and neurologic functions.	1. Health education offers individuals some control over the direction of their disease.

2. Briefly explain the relationship of certain risk factors to the development of atherosclerosis:
a. Smoking
  • Vasoconstriction
  • Decreased blood oxygenation
  • Elevated BP
  • Increased lipidemia
  • Increased platelet aggregation
	2a. The effects of nicotine on the cardiovascular system contribute to CAD, stroke, hypertension, and peripheral vascular disease. Exposure to tobacco raises the risk of atherosclerosis by constricting arteries and promoting inflammation. A 2011 report from the Women's Health Study found that compared with nonsmokers, smokers whose lifetime exposure to cigarettes was 10 to 29 pack-years were six times more likely to develop PAD; those with a lifetime exposure of 30 or more pack-years had 11 times the risk.

b. Hypertension
  • Constant trauma of pressure causes vessel lining damage, which promotes plaque formation and narrowing.
c. Hyperlipidemia
  • Promotes atherosclerosis
d. Sedentary lifestyle
  • Decreases muscle tone and strength
  • Decreases circulation
e. Excess weight (>0% of ideal)
  • Fatty tissue increases peripheral resistance.
  • Fatty tissue is less vascular.
Refer to Getting Started to Healthy Eating on thePoint.
	b. Changes in arterial walls increase the incidence of stroke and CAD (Grossman & Porth, 2014).
	
	c. High-circulating lipids increase the risk of CHD, peripheral vascular disease, and stroke.
	d. Lack of exercise inhibits the pumping action of muscles that enhance circulation. With peripheral vascular disease, exercise promotes collateral circulation.
	e. Overweight increases cardiac work load, thus causing hypertension.

3. Encourage the individual to share feelings, concerns, and understanding of risk factors, disease process, and effects on life.	3. This dialogue will provide data to assist with goal setting.
4. Assist the individual to select lifestyle behaviors that he or she chooses to change (*Burch et al., 1991). a. Avoid multiple changes. b. Consider personal abilities, resources, and overall health. c. Be realistic and optimistic.	4. An older individual may have lifestyle patterns of inactivity, smoking, and high-fat diet.

Interventions	*Rationales*

5. Assist the individual to set goal(s) and the steps to achieve them (e.g., will walk 30 minutes daily.)
   a. Will walk 10 minutes daily.
   b. Will walk 10 minutes daily and 20 minutes three times a week.
   c. Will walk 20 minutes daily.
   d. Will walk 2 minutes daily and 30 minutes three times a week.
	5. Attaining short-term goals can foster motivation to continue the process.

6. Suggest a method to self-monitor progress (e.g., graph, checklist).	6. A structured monitoring system increases individual involvement beyond the goal-setting stage.
7. Provide specific information to achieve selected goals (e.g., self-help programs, referrals, techniques).	7. The educational program should not overload the individual.
8. Refer to Index for interventions for smoking cessation and weight reduction.	

9. Explain the risks that atherosclerotic disease poses to the feet:
   a. Diabetes-related peripheral neuropathy and microvascular disease
 	
   b. Pressure ulcers
	9. Understanding may encourage compliance with necessary lifestyle changes.
	   a. Diabetes accelerates the atherosclerotic process. Diabetic neuropathy prevents the individual from feeling ischemic or injured areas. One in three people who are over age 50 and have diabetes will develop PAD.
	   b. Healing of open lesions requires approximately 10 times the blood supply necessary to keep live tissue intact.

10. Teach foot care measures.
   a. Daily inspection
     • Use a mirror.
     • Look for corns, calluses, bunions, scratches, redness, and blisters.
     • If vision is poor, have a family member or other person inspect the feet.
   b. Daily washing
     • Use warm, not hot, water (check the water temperature with the hand or elbow before immersing feet).
     • Avoid prolonged soaking.
     • Dry well, especially between the toes.
   c. Proper foot hygiene
     • Clip nails straight across; use an emery board to smooth edges.
     • Avoid using any chemicals on corns or calluses.
     • Avoid using antiseptics, such as iodine.
     • If feet are dry, apply a thin coat of lotion. Avoid getting lotion between the toes.
	10a. Daily foot care can reduce tissue damage and helps to prevent or detect early further injury and infection.
	   • This will prevent burning in sensitive tissue.
	   • This can macerate tissue.
	   • They can cause an injury that will not heal.
	   • These can damage healthy tissue.

11. Teach the individual to
   a. Avoid hot water bottles and heating pads.
   b. Wear wool socks to warm the feet at night.
   c. Wear warm foot covering before going out in cold weather (wool socks and lined boots).
   d. Avoid walking barefoot.
	11. These precautions help to reduce the risk of injury.

(continued)

Interventions	Rationales
12. Instruct the individual to wear well-fitting leather shoes (may require shoes made with extra depth), to always wear socks with the shoes, to avoid sandals with straps between the toes, and to inspect the insides of the shoes daily for worn areas, protruding nails, or other objects.	12. Well-fitting shoes help to prevent injury to skin and underlying tissue.
13. Teach the individual to a. Wear socks that fit well. b. Avoid socks with elastic bands. c. Avoid sock garters. d. Avoid crossing the legs.	13. Tight garments and certain leg positions constrict the leg vessels, which further reduces circulation.
14. Emphasize the importance of visiting a podiatrist for nail/callus/corn care if the individual has poor vision or any difficulty with self-care.	14. The individual may require assistance with foot care to ensure adequate care and prevent self-inflicted injuries.
15. Explain that if the individual cannot inspect his or her feet, he or she should arrange for another person to inspect them regularly.	15. Daily inspection helps to ensure early detection of skin or tissue damage.

Documentation

Individual/family teaching
Outcome achievement or status
Referrals when indicated

RESPIRATORY DISORDERS

Asthma

Asthma is a chronic inflammatory disorder of the airway characterized by airway hyperresponsiveness, mucus hypersecretion, and reversible airflow limitation. Chronic inflammation associated with asthma thickens the airway walls or changes their structure, a process known as airway remodeling. In an acute episode, the individual also has airway edema and bronchoconstriction. It is characterized symptomatically by cough, chest tightness, shortness of breath, increased sputum production, and wheezing as a result of decreased airflow.

Asthma attacks can be mild, moderate, or serious and even life-threatening (CDC, 2016a). One in 12 Americans have asthma; 18.7 million adults, 6.8 million children (CDC, 2016a). According the World Health Organization (2013), it is estimated that 235 million have been diagnosed with asthma. Asthma is the most common chronic disease in children and occurs in all countries regardless of level of development. Over 80% of asthma deaths occur in low- and lower-middle-income countries (World Health Organization [WHO], 2013). Exposure to common aeroallergens (e.g., animal dander, tobacco smoke, dust, molds, and air pollution) can trigger an acute episode up to 24 hours after exposure (WHO, 2013). Additional triggers include emotional and hormonal changes, cold temperatures, certain exercise activities, medications, and viral or occupational exposures (Grossman & Porth, 2014). Urbanization has been associated with an increase in asthma. But the exact nature of this relationship is unclear (WHO, 2013).

Time Frame
Acute episode

■■■ DIAGNOSTIC CLUSTER

Collaborative Problems

▲ Risk for Complications of Hypoxemia

△ Risk for Complications of Acute Respiratory Failure (refer to Unit II)

△ Risk for Complications of Status Asthmaticus

Nursing Diagnoses

Anxiety related to breathlessness (refer to Anxiety)

Risk for Ineffective Health Management related to insufficient knowledge of signs/symptoms of exacerbation. Pharmacological therapy, preventions of or early treatment of infection, monitoring peak flows, and environmental hazards (tobacco smoke, environmental allergens [e.g., dust mites, weather such as high humidity])

▲ This diagnosis was reported to be monitored for or managed frequently (75% to 100%).
△ This diagnosis was reported to be monitored for or managed often (50% to 74%).

Transition Criteria

Before transition, the individual or family will:

1. Describe methods to reduce the risk of exacerbations.
2. Describe asthma action plan.
3. State signs and symptoms that must be reported to a health care professional.

Transitional Risk Assessment Plan (TRAP)

Begin this plan on admission.
Implement the Transitional Risk Assessment Plan (TRAP):
- Refer to inside back cover.
- Add each validated risk diagnosis to individual's problem list with the risk code in ( ).

- Refer to Unit II to the individual risk nursing diagnoses/collaborative problems for outcomes and interventions.

  R: "Close coordination of care in the post-acute period, early discharge follow-up care, enhanced patient education and self-management training, proactive end-of-life counseling, and extending the resources and clinical expertise over time via multidisciplinary team management" can lower readmission rates and improve health outcomes (Boutwell & Hwu, 2009, p. 14). Interventions are utilized to activate the individual and family to select changes in their everyday lifestyle choices to improve their health (Hibbard & Greene, 2013).

Collaborative Problems

Risk for Complications of Hypoxemia

Risk for Complications of Respiratory Failure

Risk for Complications of Status Asthmaticus

Collaborative Outcomes

The individual will be monitored for early signs and symptoms of hypoxemia, respiratory failure, and status asthmaticus, and will receive collaborative interventions if indicated to restore physiologic stability.

Indicators of Physiologic Stability

- Serum pH 7.35 to 7.45
- Serum Pco_2 35 to 45 mm Hg
- Pulse: regular rhythm, rate 60 to 100 beats/min
- Blood pressure (BP): >90/60, <140 to 90 mm Hg
- Urine output >0.5 mL/kg/hr
- Alert, oriented
- No abnormal breath sounds
- Oxygen saturation >95% (pulse oximetry)
- No confusion or agitation

Interventions	Rationales

1. Obtain a thorough history from either the individual or family (frequency of short-acting β_2 agonist use). Assess the origins of the exacerbation as
   a. What triggered the event?
   b. What methods have been used to alleviate the symptoms? Did they work?
   c. What medications are generally prescribed?
   d. How frequently is the using short-acting β_2 agonist inhaler (albuterol)?
   e. What stimulants exacerbate the asthma?
	1. History taking is an essential factor in the treatment of asthma and prevention of exacerbations

> **CLINICAL ALERT:**
> - Currently, the majority of medical visits for asthma are for urgent care. Effective asthma management, however, requires a proactive, preventive approach, similar to the treatment of hypertension, or diabetes (Fanta, 2014a).

    f. How long did the individual wait before seeking treatment?

    g. Was the asthma action plan used? If so, what zone was the individual in and for how long? How was the individual's peak flow?

    h. Was the individual within the target range?

Interventions	Rationales
2. Monitor for hypercapnia, increased intracranial pressure (ICP) (when appropriate), headache, confusion, combativeness, hallucinations, transient psychosis, stupor, coma, or any significant change in mental status.	2. Acid–base analysis helps to evaluate gas exchange in the lungs. Anxiety and air hunger will lead to an increase in the respiratory rate. In severe cases, a decreased Po_2 will lead to hypoxemia. Respiratory alkalosis will be exhibited. In status asthmaticus, the individual will tire and air trapping will worsen. Acid–base results will return to baseline, which is an ominous sign. The Pco_2 will then rise quickly. Respiratory acidosis and failure will result. Intubation will be required (Grossman & Porth, 2014).
a. Increased/decreased BP b. Monitor intake and output c. Cool, pale, cyanotic skin	a, b, c. First the individual will have an elevated BP resulting from anxiety and feelings of air hunger. As the individual's condition and air trapping worsen, pressure in the thoracic cavity will increase, which decreases venous return. Thus the individual will then exhibit a decrease in BP and the signs and symptoms of decreased cardiac output.
d. Tachypnea and dyspnea at rest. Respiratory rate >20 breaths/min	d. The individual experiences dyspnea because of narrowed passages and air trapping related to bronchospasms (Grossman & Porth, 2014).
e. Abnormal breath sounds	e. Auscultation of the chest is often misleading. Initially, wheezing may be heard throughout all lung fields during both phases of respiration. As airflow becomes restricted because of severe obstruction and mucus secretion, breath sounds become diminished or absent. This is a sign of impending respiratory failure.
f. Cough	f. For some with asthma, cough may be their only symptom. Spasmodic contractions of the bronchi produce the cough.
g. Changes in mental status	g. The individual is often anxious and restless. However, changes in mentation reflect changes in oxygenation. Confusion, agitation, and lethargy are signs of imminent respiratory failure.
3. Administer O_2 via nasal cannula.	3. Hypoxemia is common due to ventilation/perfusion disturbances. Air trapping and increased respiratory rate impede gas exchange. Po_2 <60 mm Hg requires supplemental oxygen. Administration of O_2 via nasal cannula is preferred to reduce the individual's feelings of suffocation. In severe cases, however, intubation and mechanical ventilation may be required.
4. Ensure optimal hydration. Consult with physician/nurse practitioner/physical assistant for intravenous fluids if indicated. (Excess mucus production is common.)	4. Adequate hydration prevents dehydration and enhances clearance of secretions. Daily fluid intake of 2 to 4 L is recommended.
5. Obtain sputum specimen (if possible).	5. Sputum, if present, is generally clear, mucoid, or white during exacerbation of asthma. Discoloration of sputum can be indicative of infection. Administration of antihistamines and decongestants is common to decrease mucus production.
6. Assess for gastrointestinal (GI) reflux symptoms. a. Heartburn b. Sour or bitter-tasting acid in throat or mouth c. Bloating, burping d. Sensation of food being stuck in your throat e. Persistent hiccups f. Nausea g. Wheezing, dry cough, hoarseness, or chronic sore throat	6. Gastroesophageal (GE) reflux is common in individuals with asthma and has been identified as a potential trigger for asthma GE reflux is thought to affect asthma through the activation of vagal reflexes and/or microaspiration. A systematic review of 28 studies of individuals with asthma found GE reflux symptoms in 59% (Havemann, Henderson, & El-Serag, 2007).

(continued)

Interventions	Rationales
7. Ask individual to breath with you, for example, breathe slowly and deeply in through nose and out through mouth.	7. Individuals are often anxious, which will intensify the situation. Relaxation techniques that include diaphragmatic breathing, breathing through the nose, and relaxation exercises to reduce anxiety have been shown to reduce asthma symptoms by one-third by assisting with anxiety and hyperventilation (Mayor, 2007).
8. Monitor for status asthmaticus: a. Labored breathing b. Prolonged exhalation c. Engorged neck veins d. Wheezing	8. Status asthmaticus does not respond to conventional therapy. As status asthmaticus worsens, the $Paco_2$ increases and pH falls. The extent of wheezing does not indicate the severity of the attack (Grossman & Porth, 2014).
9. Evaluate level of hypoxia with arterial blood gases and (Pco_2, Pao_2, pH, Sao_2) pulse oximetry.	9. During an acute episode, the Pao_2 and serum pH will decrease. Blood gases will show respiratory alkalosis in the early stages of an asthma attack and then move toward a neutral pH. As the episode intensifies in severity, blood gases will confirm respiratory acidosis, paralleling the rising $Paco_2$ (*Sims, 2006).
10. Call rapid response team if indicated. Ensure that someone stays with individual.	10. Intense monitoring is required to rapidly assess responses to medications (e.g., corticosteroids, albuterol) and need for emergency measures (e.g., intubation).

Clinical Alert Report

Prior to providing care, advise ancillary staff/student to report the following to the professional nurse assigned to the individual:

- Complaints of shortness of breath, wheezing
- New onset coughing
- Pco_2 <35 mm Hg or >45 mm Hg
- Pulse: >100 beats/min
- New onset of anxiousness
- Abnormal breath sounds
- Oxygen saturation <95% (pulse oximetry)

Nursing Diagnoses

STAR   **Stop**

Think   Is this person at risk for injury, falls, medical complications, and/or inability to care for self (activities of daily living)?

Is the person competent to manage self-administration of medications, treatment procedures? Are additional resources needed?

Can the person explain how to monitor condition (e.g., blood glucose, signs/symptoms of complications, dietary/mobility restrictions, and when to call his or her primary provider or specialist)?

Act   Contact or provide the appropriate resource (e.g., contacting a support person, home health assessment, additional teaching, printed materials).

Review   Has the problem been addressed? If not, use SBAR to communicate to the appropriate person.

Risk for Ineffective Health Management Related to Insufficient Knowledge of Signs/Symptoms of Exacerbation. Pharmacological Therapy, Preventions of or Early Treatment of Infection, Monitoring Peak Flows, and Environmental Hazards (Tobacco Smoke, Environmental Allergens [e.g., Dust Mites, Weather such as High Humidity])

NOC

Compliance Behavior, Knowledge: Treatment Regimen, Participation: Health Care Decisions, Treatment Behavior: Illness or Injury

NIC

Anticipatory Guidance, Risk Identification, Health Education, Learning Facilitation

Goal

The goals for this diagnosis represent those associated with transition planning. Refer to transition criteria.

Interventions	Rationales
1. Teach about the diagnosis and treatment regimen. **CLINICAL ALERT** • Many individuals/parents ignore the seriousness of this disease. Frequent hospitalizations result from disregarding the warning signs of impending asthma attacks and noncompliance with the therapeutic regimen. Status asthmaticus refers to a severe case of asthma that does not respond to conventional treatment. This life-threatening situation requires prompt action. According to the CDC (2016e), approximately nine people die from asthma each day, 3,630 yearly.	1. Understanding may help to encourage compliance and participation in self-care.
2. Explain the asthma action plan and the use of peak flow monitoring and what actions are indicated for each zone, with teach-back techniques for green, yellow, and red zones as Green: 80% to 100% of personal best, Yellow: 50% to 80% of personal best, Red: <50% of personal best. Refer to Figure III.1	2. Peak flow monitoring can assist in determining if asthma is getting worse and the actions to take before symptoms can be felt. This may prevent or reduce emergency room visits. Individuals are assisted to determine their personal best peak flows and then to monitor and manipulate their own therapy or to seek medical attention when the condition approaches the red zone. Additionally, measurements with a peak flow meter can help your health care provider make decisions about treatment and adjust medications as necessary (American Lung Association, 2013).
3. Teach sources of respiratory irritants. a. Smoke (cigarette, fireplace, ashes) b. Dust, pet dander c. Aerosol sprays, perfumes d. Cooking odors, musty odors, shower steam, traffic fumes, air pollution, desert dust, and workplace irritants	3. Exposure to these respiratory irritants can cause bronchospasm and increase mucus production. Smoking destroys the ciliary cleansing mechanism of the respiratory tract. Heat raises the body temperature and increases the body's oxygen requirements, possibly exacerbating the symptoms.

(continued)

My Asthma Action Plan

Patient Name: _____

Medical Record #: _____

Physician's Name: _____   DOB: _____

Physician's Phone #: _____   Completed by: _____   Date: _____

Long-Term-Control Medicines	How Much To Take	How Often	Other Instructions
		_____ times per day **EVERY DAY!**	
		_____ times per day **EVERY DAY!**	
		_____ times per day **EVERY DAY!**	
		_____ times per day **EVERY DAY!**	

Quick-Relief Medicines	How Much To Take	How Often	Other Instructions
		Take ONLY as needed	NOTE: If this medicine is needed frequently, call physician to consider increasing long-term-control medications.

Special instructions when I feel ⬤ *good,* ◯ *not good,* and ⬤ *awful.*

GREEN ZONE

I feel *good.*

(My peak flow is in the GREEN zone.)

My Personal Best Peak Flow

PREVENT asthma symptoms everyday:

☐ Take my long-term-control medicines (above) every day.

☐ Before exercise, take _____ puffs of _____

☐ Avoid things that make my asthma worse like:

YELLOW ZONE

I do *not* feel *good.*

(My peak flow is in the YELLOW zone.)

My symptoms may include one or more of the following:
- Wheeze
- Tight chest
- Cough
- Shortness of breath
- Waking up at night with asthma symptoms
- Decreased ability to do usual activities
- _____

80% Personal Best

CAUTION. I should continue taking my long-term-control asthma medicines every day AND:

☐ Take _____

If I still do not feel good, or my peak flow is not back in the *Green Zone* within 1 hour, then I should:

☐ Increase _____

☐ Add _____

☐ Call _____

RED ZONE

I feel *awful.*

(My peak flow is in the RED zone.)

Warning signs may include one or more of the following:
- It's getting harder and harder to breathe
- Unable to sleep or do usual activities because of trouble breathing

50% Personal Best

Liters/Min.

Peak Flow Meter

MEDICAL ALERT! *Get help!*

☐ Take _____ until I get help immediately.

☐ Take _____

☐ Call _____

Danger! Get help immediately!

Call 9–1–1 if you have trouble walking or talking due to shortness of breath or lips or fingernails are gray or blue.

FIGURE III.1 Components of an asthma action plan. (Source: National Heart, Lung, and Blood Institute; National Institutes of Health; U.S. Department of Health and Human Services.)

Interventions	*Rationales*

4. Explain how the reduce exposure to irritants
   a. Complete avoidance of the trigger (e.g., do not own pets if allergic to them, mop or wet wipe instead of sweeping or dusting).

Interventions	*Rationales*
b. Limit exposure to the trigger if it cannot be completely avoided (e.g., leave the room if someone starts smoking, move to another seat if someone with strong perfume sits near you, have someone else dust and clean the house if dust mite allergic).	
c. Take an extra dose of bronchodilator and an antihistamine before trigger exposure, for example, extremely cold or warm temperatures. Advise not to exceed the amount of normally prescribed medication.	4c. This approach should be implemented only if the first two options are not feasible. Individuals should consult with their clinician to be sure before instituting this approach.

5. Explain the exercise-induced asthma and weather effects on asthma:
   a. Hot, humid air
   b. Wet conditions and thunderstorms
	5. Exercise-triggered symptoms typically develop 5 to 15 minutes after a brief (e.g., 5 minutes) period of exertion or about 15 minutes into prolonged exercise and resolve with rest over approximately 30 to 60 minutes (Fanta, 2014b). Temperature and humidity may play a role in exercise-induced asthma. While the precise mechanism is not clear, the inhalation of cold and dry air appears to increase bronchoconstriction during or shortly after exercise (Bailey & Miller, 2016).
	
	   Hot sunny days that increase ozone-related asthma symptoms. Hot, humid air can cause bronchoconstriction. Studies of weather events have found increased levels of respiratory allergens present in the air, particularly pollen.

6. Teach and have the individual demonstrate breathing exercises:
 	
   a. Use incentive spirometer.
 	
   b. Assume a leaning-forward position.
 	
   c. Use pursed-lip breathing.
	6. Individuals experiencing asthma frequently become anxious and assume an ineffective breathing pattern. Decreasing labored breathing through positioning and effective breathing patterns may reduce asthmatic episodes and prevent hospitalization.
	   a. Incentive spirometry encourages deep, sustained inspiratory efforts.
	   b. Leaning forward enhances diaphragmatic excursions and diminishes the use of accessory muscles.
	   c. Pursed-lip breathing prolongs exhalation, which prevents air trapping and air gulping.

7. Explain the hazards of infection and ways to reduce the risk (Fanta, 2014c):
   a. Avoid contact with infected persons.
 	
   b. Teach importance of hand hygiene.
 	
   c. Receive immunization against influenza yearly and bacterial pneumonia (Pneumovax, Prevnar per guidelines).
 	
   d. Advise individual that if there is a need for increased use of rescue inhaler (albuterol) or home nebulizer to call primary care provider (PCP).
	7a. Colds, influenza, respiratory syncytial virus (RSV), bronchitis, ear infections, sinus infections, and pneumonia are very common asthma triggers because they can cause airway inflammation and increased mucus production. Asthma attacks that occur with a respiratory infection are frequently more severe than those occurring at other times (Bailey & Miller, 2016).
	   b. Hand hygiene is the most effective way to prevent illness. Encourage to ask friends and family to participate in hand hygiene.
	   c. Influenza vaccines will decrease the likelihood of contracting the flu, or decrease the severity of the occurrence. Individuals with asthma should receive the inactivated form only (Bailey, 2008). Pneumovax vaccine reduces the incidence of infections due to the bacteria *Streptococcus pneumoniae*.
	   d. When an individual, previously controlled, needs increased doses of albuterol, an evaluation is needed to rule out an upper respiratory infection early.

(continued)

Interventions	*Rationales*

8. Notify PCP if there is:
  a. Change in sputum characteristics or failure of sputum to return to usual color after 3 days of antibiotic therapy.
 	
  b. Elevated body temperature.
 	
  c. Increase in cough, weakness, or shortness of breath.
	8a. Sputum changes may indicate an infection or resistance of the infective organism to the prescribed antibiotic.
	  b. Circulating pathogens stimulate the hypothalamus to elevate body temperature.
	  c. Hypoxia is chronic; exacerbations must be detected early to prevent complications. In addition to infection, yellow or green sputum may also be due to eosinophil peroxidase, which enhances destruction of bacteria.

9. Instruct the individual to seek medical attention immediately if asthma is not relieved after using method outlined in their therapeutic regimen.	9. Unrelieved symptoms of asthma may lead to status asthmaticus. It is documented that individuals with asthma repeatedly ignore the warning signs and seek medical attention only when the condition becomes life-threatening.

10. During hospitalization, assess the individual using handheld inhaler and nebulizer if used. Observe if the individual
  a. For liquid inhalers:
    • Shake canister.
    • Blow out air.
    • Put inhaler to mouth, release medication, and breathe in deeply.
    • Hold breath for 10 seconds; then exhale slowly.
    • Wait for 1 minute, then repeat.
    • Rinse mouth if using a corticosteroid inhaler.
    • Add a spacer if needed.
  b. For dry powder inhaler:
    • Breathe out normally—but not into the inhaler.
    • Put your mouth on the mouthpiece.
    • Breathe in quickly and steadily, and as deeply as possible.
    • Remove your mouth from the mouthpiece and hold your breath for 5 to 10 seconds.
    • Let your breath out—but **not** into the inhaler.
  c. For nebulizer:
    • Assemble correctly.
    • Using mouthpiece or mask, slowly take deep breaths and exhale.
    • Stops treatment when mist is gone.
	10. Accurate instructions can help to prevent medication underdose or overdose. Improper use of inhalers has been identified as a cause of asthma exacerbation. Individuals tend to overuse inhalers, which leads to inhaler ineffectiveness.

11. Clarify which inhaler is needed every day and which is the rescue inhaler for p.r.n. use.	11. Improper use of inhalers can result in underdosing or overdosing.
12. Advise of the importance of an exercise routine.	12. Exercise increases stamina. Warn that improper exercise may also trigger asthma. Instruct that use of inhaler prior to exercise may be needed and will assist in exercise endurance. Instruct to avoid exercising in extremely hot or cold weather. Wearing a paper mask may reduce the sensitivity to stimulants. Emphasize the importance of a cool-down period. Suggest swimming and exercising indoors to avoid exposure to irritants.

Interventions	Rationales
13. Receive yearly immunization against influenza and vaccines against bacterial pneumonia (Pneumovax, Prevnar 13) as indicated.	13. Influenza vaccines will decrease the likelihood of contracting the flu, or decrease the severity of the occurrence. Individuals with asthma should receive the inactivated form only. Pneumovax is indicated for adults 65 years and older, people with certain medical conditions, and cigarette smokers. Prevnar 13 is approved for adults 50 years of age and older for the prevention of pneumococcal pneumonia and invasive disease caused by 13 Streptococcus pneumoniae strains. (CDC, 2016f).

Documentation

Individual/family teaching/returned demonstrations
Referrals if indicated

Chronic Obstructive Pulmonary Disease

Chronic obstructive pulmonary disease (COPD) is initiated by exposure to cigarette smoke and other noxious particles, which results in lung inflammation. Lung tissue is destroyed in response to increased presence of macrophages and CD-8 T lymphocytes. As part of the pathophysiologic cascade, protective antiproteinases are inactivated, which reduces lung-tissue repair and promotes alveolar-wall destruction. In chronic bronchitis, the airways thicken and the mucociliary elevator is inactivated while mucus production increases. As airway diameter narrows, airflow decreases.

- In emphysema, destruction of the alveolar septa reduces the surface area available for gas exchange. Elastic recoil (in which the lungs return to their original size after expanding during inspiration) decreases with loss of lung-tissue structure, resulting in air trapping and hyperinflation.

WHO defines an exacerbation of COPD as "an acute event characterized by a worsening of the patient's respiratory symptoms that is beyond normal day-to-day variations and leads to a change in medication" (Global strategy for the diagnosis, management, and prevention of COPD). Although death rates for COPD have declined among US men between 1999 (57.0/100,000) and 2010 (47.6/100,000) in the United States, there has been no significant change among death rates in women (35.3/100,000 in 1999 and 36.4/ in 2010) (CDC, 2014a).

COPD is the second leading cause of disability in the United States (Boardman, 2008).

The more familiar terms of *chronic bronchitis* and *emphysema* are no longer used; they are now included within the COPD diagnosis (CDC, 2014a). The most common symptoms of COPD are breathlessness, abnormal sputum, and a chronic cough.

COPD is preventable and the primary cause is tobacco smoke (including secondhand or passive exposure). COPD affects men and women almost equally due to tobacco use in high-income countries and the higher risk of exposure to indoor air pollution (CDC, 2014a). Effective education has been proven recently to have a profound role in the decrease in individual morbidity, due to the resultant behavior modification (Boardman, 2008).

 Time Frame
Acute episode (nonintensive care)

■■■■■ DIAGNOSTIC CLUSTER

Collaborative Problems

▲ Risk for Complications of Hypoxemia

▲ Risk for Complications of Right-Sided Heart Failure

Nursing Diagnoses

▲ Ineffective Airway Clearance related to excessive and tenacious secretions (refer to Unit II)

▲ Activity Intolerance related to fatigue and inadequate oxygenation for (refer to Unit II)

▲ Anxiety related to breathlessness and fear of suffocation

△ Disturbed Sleep Pattern related to cough, inability to assume recumbent position, environmental stimuli (refer to Unit II)

△ Risk for Imbalanced Nutrition related to anorexia secondary to dyspnea, halitosis, and fatigue (refer to Pressure Ulcers) (refer to Unit II)

▲ Risk for Ineffective Health Therapeutic Regimen Management related to lack of knowledge of condition, treatments, prevention of infection, breathing exercises, risk factors, signs and symptoms of complications

▲ This diagnosis was reported to be monitored for or managed frequently (75% to 100%).
△ This diagnosis was reported to be monitored for or managed often (50% to 74%).

Transition Criteria

Before transition, the individual or family will:

1. Identify long- and short-term goals to modify risk factors (e.g., diet, smoking, exercise).
2. Identify adjustments needed to maintain self-care.
3. State how to prevent further pulmonary deterioration.
4. State signs and symptoms that must be reported to a health care professional.
5. Identify community resources that can provide assistance with home management.

Transitional Risk Assessment Plan (TRAP)

Begin this plan on admission.
Implement the Transitional Risk Assessment Plan (TRAP):
• Refer to inside back cover.
• Add each validated risk diagnosis to individual's problem list with the risk code in ( ).
• Refer to Unit II to the individual risk nursing diagnoses/collaborative problems for outcomes and interventions.

> *R:* "Close coordination of care in the post-acute period, early discharge follow-up care, enhanced patient education and self-management training, proactive end-of-life counseling, and extending the resources and clinical expertise over time via multidisciplinary team management" can lower readmission rates and improve health outcomes (Boutwell & Hwu, 2009, p. 14). Interventions are utilized to activate the individual and family to select changes in their everyday lifestyle choices to improve their health (Hibbard & Greene, 2013).

Collaborative Problems

Risk for Complications of Hypoxemia

Risk for Complications of Right-Sided Heart Failure

Collaborative Outcomes

The individual will be monitored for early signs and symptoms of hypoxemia and right-sided heart failure and will receive collaborative interventions if indicated to restore physiologic stability.

Indicators of Physiologic Stability

- Serum pH 7.35 to 7.45
- Serum P_{CO_2} 35 to 45 mm Hg
- Pulse: regular rhythm and rate 60 to 100 beats/min
- Respiration 16 to 20 breaths/min
- BP <140/90, >90/60 mm Hg
- Urine output >0.5 mL/kg/hr

Interventions	Rationales
1. Monitor for hypercapnia (increased carbon dioxide) (Feller-Kopman & Schwartzstein, 2015)	1. It has been estimated that COPD, which increase dead space are responsible for the majority of cases of hypercapnic respiratory failure, while a smaller proportion are due to extrapulmonary conditions (e.g., sedatives, neuromuscular or thoracic cage disorders) (Feller-Kopman & Schwartzstein, 2015).
a. Increased ICP (when appropriate), headache, confusion, combativeness, hallucinations, transient psychosis, stupor, coma, or any significant change in mental status	a. Acute hypercapnia may produce a depressed level of consciousness carbon dioxide (CO_2) (narcosis) and increase in cerebral blood flow and ICP.
b. Arterial blood gas (ABG) analysis: pH <7.35 and P_{CO_2} >46 mm Hg	b. ABG analysis helps to evaluate gas exchange in the lungs. In mild to moderate COPD, the individual may have a normal Pa_{CO_2} level because of chemoreceptors in the medulla responding to increased Pa_{CO_2} by increasing ventilation. In severe COPD, the individual cannot sustain this increased ventilation and the Pa_{CO_2} value increases.
c. Increased and irregular pulse, increased respiratory rate, followed by decreased rate	c. Respiratory acidosis develops due to excessive CO_2 retention. The individual with respiratory acidosis from chronic disease at first increases heart rate and respiration in an attempt to compensate for decreased oxygenation. Eventually, the respiratory center may stop responding to the higher CO_2 levels, and breathing may stop abruptly.
d. Decreased urine output (<0.5 mL/hr) e. Cool, pale, or cyanotic skin	d, e. The compensatory response to decreased circulatory oxygen is to increase blood oxygen by increasing heart and respiratory rates and to decrease circulation to the kidneys and to the extremities (marked by decreased pulse and skin changes).
CLINICAL ALERT: • It is estimated that 14% of individuals admitted for an exacerbation of COPD will die within 3 months of admission (Feller-Kopman & Schwartzstein, 2015).	
2. Administer low-flow oxygen, as needed, through a cannula.	2. This measure increases circulating oxygen levels. Higher flow rates increase carbon dioxide retention. The use of a cannula rather than a mask reduces the fears of suffocation.
3. Obtain a sputum sample for culture and sensitivity.	3. Sputum culture and sensitivity determine if an infection is contributing to the exacerbation of symptoms.
4. Monitor electrocardiogram (ECG) for arrhythmias.	4. Arrhythmias can be caused by altered ABGs.
5. Initiate preventive measures for deep vein thrombosis (DVT) and pulmonary embolism (PE)	5. Hospitalization for exacerbations of COPD increases the risk for DVT and PE (Stoller, 2015).
6. Monitor for signs of right-sided heart failure: a. Elevated diastolic pressure b. Distended neck veins c. Peripheral edema	6. The combination of arterial hypoxemia and respiratory acidosis acts locally as a strong vasoconstrictor of pulmonary vessels. This leads to pulmonary arterial hypertension, increased right ventricular systolic pressure, and, eventually, right ventricular hypertrophy and failure.

(continued)

Interventions	Rationales

7. Refer to the Heart Failure Care Plan for additional interventions if right-sided failure occurs.

Clinical Alert Report

Prior to providing care, advise ancillary staff/student to report the following to the professional nurse assigned to the individual:
- Change in cognitive status
- Oral temperature > 100.5° F
- Systolic BP <90 mm Hg
- Resting pulse >100, <50 beats/min
- Respiratory rate >28, <10/min labored
- Sputum color
- Oxygen saturation <90%
- Urine output <0.5 mL/kg/hr

Documentation

Vital signs
Intake and output
Assessment data
Change in status
Interventions
Individual's response to interventions

Nursing Diagnoses

Anxiety Related to Breathlessness and Fear of Suffocation

NOC

Anxiety Self-Control, Coping, Impulse Self-Control

Goal

The individual will verbalize increased psychological and physiologic comfort.

NIC

Anxiety Reduction, Impulse Control Training, Anticipatory Guidance

Indicators

- Verbalize feelings of anxiety.
- Demonstrate breathing techniques to decrease dyspnea.

Interventions	Rationales
1. Provide a quiet, calm environment when the individual is experiencing breathlessness.	1. Reducing external stimuli promotes relaxation.
2. Do not leave the individual alone during periods of acute breathlessness.	2. Fear triggers dyspnea and dyspnea increases fear. Individuals report a nurse's acknowledgment of their fear assuaged their fear and alleviated their breathing difficulty.

Interventions	*Rationales*
3. Encourage the individual to use breathing techniques especially during times of increased anxiety. Coach the individual through the breathing exercises.	3. Concentrating on diaphragmatic or pursed-lip breathing slows the respiratory rate and gives the individual a sense of control.
4. During nonacute episodes, teach relaxation techniques (tapes, guided imagery).	4. Relaxation techniques have been shown to decrease anxiety, dyspnea, and airway obstruction.

Documentation

Acute anxiety episodes
Interventions
Individual's response to interventions

> **TRANSITION TO HOME/COMMUNITY CARE**
> If indicated, review the risk diagnoses identified for this individual on admission:
> * Is the person still at risk?
> * Can the family reduce the risks?
> * Is the person at higher risk at home?
> * Is a home health nurse assessment needed?
> * Refer to transition planner/case manager/social service.
> * When is this person scheduled for follow-up with primary provider? Specialists? Record dates of appointments.
> * Complete a medication reconciliation prior to transition. Refer to index.

STAR

Stop

Think   Is this person at risk for injury, falls, medical complications, and/or inability to care for self (activities of daily living)?

Is the person competent to manage self-administration of medications, treatment procedures? Are additional resources needed?

Can the person explain how to monitor the condition (e.g., blood glucose, sign/symptoms of complications, dietary/mobility restrictions, and when to call his or her primary provider or specialist)?

Act   Contact or provide the appropriate resource (e.g., contacting a support person, home health assessment, additional teaching, printed materials).

Review   Has the problem been addressed? If not, use SBAR to communicate to the appropriate person.

Risk for Ineffective Health Regimen Management Related to Lack of Knowledge of Condition, Treatments, Prevention of Infection, Breathing Exercises, Risk Factors, Signs and Symptoms of Complications

NOC

Compliance Behavior, Knowledge: Treatment Regimen, Participation: Health Care Decisions, Treatment Behavior: Illness or Injury

NIC

Anticipatory Guidance, Learning Facilitation, Risk Identification, Health Education, Teaching: Procedure/ Treatment, Health System Guidance

Goal

The goals for this diagnosis represent those associated with transition planning. Refer to the transition criteria.

Interventions	*Rationales*
1. Teach about the diagnosis and the treatment regimen. **CLINICAL ALERT:** • The management of COPD is particularly challenging, as individuals have complex health and social needs requiring life-long monitoring and treatment (Fletcher & Dahl, 2013).	1. Understanding may help to encourage compliance and participation in self-care.
2. Help to formulate and accept realistic short- and long-term goals. Ask, "What is one change in your life that could make you healthier?"	2. This may help the individual to realize that he or she has some control over his or her quality of life.

3. Teach the individual measures to help control dyspnea and infections:
  a. Eat a well-balanced diet.
 	
  b. Take sufficient rest periods. Gradually increase activity.
  c. Increase fluids, unless contraindicated.
 	
  d. Avoid exposure to:
    • Smoke, dust
    • Severe air pollution (rush hour traffic)
    • Extremely cold or warm temperatures
	3a. Weight loss and, specifically, malnutrition decrease the individual's ability to exercise, and increases fatigue, dyspnea, and the likelihood of respiratory infections (Grossman & Porth, 2014).
	  b. Activity improves optimism.
	  c. Hydration liquefies secretions, which will assist with effective coughing.
	  d. Exposure to these respiratory irritants can cause bronchospasm and increased mucus production. Smoking destroys the ciliary cleansing mechanism of the respiratory tract. Heat raises body temperature and increases the body's oxygen requirements, possibly exacerbating the symptoms.

4. Teach and have the individual demonstrate diaphragmatic breathing exercises.
 	
  a. Diaphragm exercise: Place fingers on the lower ribs; inhale, pushing out against light pressure of fingers.
	4. An individual with COPD typically breathes shallowly from the upper chest. Breathing exercises increase alveolar ventilation and reduce respiratory rate.
	  a. Expanding and contracting the diaphragm muscle can help to strengthen it. Counterpressure forces the individual to breathe harder, which strengthens muscles and aerates lung apexes.

5. Receive yearly immunization against influenza and vaccines against bacterial pneumonia (Pneumovax, Prevnar 13) as indicated.	5. Influenza vaccines will decrease the likelihood of contracting the flu, or decrease the severity of the occurrence. Individuals with asthma should receive the inactivated form only. Pneumovax is indicated for adults 65 years and older, people with certain medical conditions, and cigarette smokers. Prevnar 13 is approved for adults 50 years of age and older for the prevention of pneumococcal pneumonia and invasive disease caused by 13 Streptococcus pneumoniae strains (CDC, 2016f).
6. Teach importance of hand hygiene as the most effective way to prevent illness. Instruct friends and family to participate in hand hygiene. Request that ill visitors wear masks and avoid direct contact with ill individual.	6. An individual with COPD is prone to infection due to inadequate primary defenses (i.e., decreased ciliary action and stasis of secretions). Minor respiratory infections can cause serious problems in an individual with COPD. Chronic debilitation and retention of secretions (which provide a medium for microorganism growth) put the individual at risk for complications.

Interventions	Rationales

7. Instruct the individual/family to respond:
  a. When at home. Instruct the individual/family to report change in sputum characteristics or failure of sputum to return to usual color after 3 days of antibiotic therapy.
  b. Elevated temperature
  c. Increase in cough, weakness, or shortness of breath
  d. Increased or new onset confusion or drowsiness
	7. Early identification a viral upper respiratory tract infection—the most common cause of COPD exacerbations, may prevent hospitalization (Stoller, 2015).

8. During hospitalization, assess the individual use of handheld inhaler and nebulizer if used. Explain which inhalers are needed every day versus those are p.r.n. Observe the individual using:
  a. Spray inhalers:
    • Shake canister.
    • Blow out air.
    • Put inhaler to mouth, release medication, and breathe in deeply.
    • Hold breath for 10 seconds; then exhale slowly.
    • Wait for 1 minute, then repeat.
    • Rinse your mouth with water after using the inhaler. Do not swallow the rinse water.
  b. Powder inhalers
    • Breathe out fully, away from the inhaler. Never exhale into or on the inhaler. Add a spacer if needed.
    • Nebulizer: have the individual
    • Assemble correctly.
    • Using mouthpiece or mask, slowly take deep breaths and exhale.
    • Stop treatment when mist is gone.
	8. Accurate instructions can help to prevent medication underdose or overdose. Improper use of inhalers has been identified as a cause of asthma exacerbation.

9. Teach to conserve energy.
 	
 Carp's Cues
  Smokers know that smoking is harming their health. Everyone tells them to quit. This implies quitting is in fact easy. Addiction to tobacco is stronger than addiction to heroin. About 70% of smokers say they want to quit and about half try to quit each year, but only 4% to 7% succeed without help. This is because smokers not only become physically dependent on nicotine; but also have a strong psychological dependence (CDC, 2014b).
  Nicotine reaches the brain within seconds after taking a puff. Nicotine alters the balance of chemicals in your brain. It mainly affects chemicals called dopamine and noradrenaline. Nicotine induces pleasure and reduces stress and anxiety. Smokers use it to modulate levels of arousal and to control mood (CDC, 2014b).
  On average, women metabolize nicotine more quickly than men, which may contribute to their increased susceptibility to nicotine addiction and may help to explain why, among smokers, it is more difficult for women to quit (CDC, 2014b).
	9. Energy conservation helps prevent exhaustion and exacerbation of hypoxia. See the nursing diagnosis Fatigue in the Inflammatory Joint Disease Care Plan for more information.

10. During hospitalization, focus on the individual's readiness to quit, and clarify misinformation. Ask the individual:
  a. How smoking has affected their health?
  b. Have they ever tried to quit?
  c. How long did they stop?
  d. Do they want to quit?
	10. People who are in hospital because of a smoking-related illness are likely to be more receptive to help to give up smoking (Rigotti, Clair, Munafò, & Stead). Focusing the discussion on the person's experiences and perceptions may provide insight into assisting the person to quit.

(continued)

Interventions	*Rationales*
11. Explain that there is no such thing as "a few cigarettes a day." **Carp's Cues** More deaths are caused by cigarette smoking than by all deaths from HIV, illegal drug use, alcohol use, motor vehicle accidents, suicide, and murders combined (CDC, 2015b). Refer to Getting Started to Quit Smoking on the**Point**.	11. Smoking 1 to 4 cigarettes/day increases one's risk of death from ischemic heart disease and from all other causes. Studies also report there is a steady increase in consumption over 10 to 20 years.
12. Discuss with prescribing professional the addition of nicotine replacement therapy (NRT) (transdermal patch, gum, spray).	12. A Cochrane review reported that adding NRT to an intensive counseling intervention increased smoking cessation rates compared with intensive counseling alone (Rigotti et al., 2012).
13. Discuss various available methods to quit smoking. Explain that most individual take several attempts at quitting before success. a. Individual/group counseling b. Self-help materials (written, audio, video) c. NRT (transdermal patch, gum, spray)	13. Each of these modalities has varying degrees of effectiveness. Individuals should be encouraged to continue trying different therapies until they succeed. Practical smoking cessation guidelines are available at http://www.cdc.gov/tobacco/campaign/tips/quit-smoking/?gclid=CKSN26non8sCFYE9gQodwg0Leg; http://www.lung.org/stop-smoking/i-want-to-quit/how-to-quit-smoking.html?referrer=https://www.google.com/
14. Provide information about or initiate referrals to community resources such as the American Lung Association, self-help groups, Meals-on-Wheels, and home health agencies. As indicated.	14. These resources can provide with needed assistance with home management and self-care.

Documentation

Individual/family teaching
Referrals, if indicated

Pneumonia

In 2009, 1.1 million people in the United States were hospitalized with pneumonia and more than 50,000 people died from the disease (CDC, 2016g). Pneumonia is an infection of the lungs that is usually caused by bacteria or viruses. Globally, pneumonia causes more deaths than any other infectious disease. It can often be prevented and can usually be treated. Signs of pneumonia can include coughing, fever, fatigue, nausea, vomiting, rapid breathing or shortness of breath, chills, or chest pain. Certain people are more likely to become ill with pneumonia. This includes adults 65 years of age or older and children younger than 5 years of age. People up through 64 years of age who have underlying medical conditions (like diabetes or HIV/AIDS) and people 19 through 64 who smoke cigarettes or have asthma are also at increased risk.

Globally, pneumonia kills more than 1.5 million children younger than 5 years of age each year. This is greater than the number of deaths from any other infectious disease, such as AIDS, malaria, or tuberculosis (CDC, 2016g). Access to vaccines and treatment (like antibiotics and antivirals) can help prevent many pneumonia-related deaths. Pneumonia experts are also working to prevent pneumonia in developing countries by reducing indoor air pollution and encouraging good hygiene practices.

 Time Frame
Acute episode with hospitalization

▪▪■■ DIAGNOSTIC CLUSTER

Collaborative Problems

▲ Risk for Complications of Respiratory Insufficiency

▲ Risk for Complications of Septic Shock

▲ Risk for Complications of Paralytic Ileus

Nursing Diagnoses

▲ Activity Intolerance related to insufficient oxygenation for activities of daily living (ADLs) (refer to Unit II)

▲ Ineffective Airway Clearance related to pain, increased tracheobronchial secretions, and fatigue (refer to Unit II)

△ Risk for Impaired Oral Mucous Membrane related to mouth breathing, frequent expectorations, and decreased fluid intake secondary to malaise (refer to Unit II)

△ Risk for Imbalanced Nutrition related to anorexia, dyspnea, and abdominal distention secondary to air swallowing (refer to Unit II)

△ Risk for Ineffective Health Regimen Management related to lack of knowledge of condition, infection transmission, prevention of recurrence, diet, signs and symptoms of recurrence, and follow-up care

▲ This diagnosis was reported to be monitored for or managed frequently (75% to 100%).
△ This diagnosis was reported to be monitored for or managed often (50% to 74%).

Transitional Risk Assessment Plan (TRAP)

Begin this plan on admission.
Implement the Transitional Risk Assessment Plan (TRAP):

- Refer to inside back cover.
- Add each validated risk diagnosis to individual's problem list with the risk code in ( ).
- Refer to Unit II to the individual risk nursing diagnoses/collaborative problems for outcomes and interventions.

  R: "Close coordination of care in the post-acute period, early discharge follow-up care, enhanced patient education and self-management training, proactive end-of-life counseling, and extending the resources and clinical expertise over time via multidisciplinary team management" can lower readmission rates and improve health outcomes (Boutwell & Hwu, 2009, p. 14). Interventions are utilized to activate the individual and family to select changes in their everyday lifestyle choices to improve their health (Hibbard & Greene, 2013).

Transition Criteria

Before transition, the individual or family will:

1. Describe how to prevent infection transmission.
2. Describe rest and nutritional requirements.
3. Describe methods to reduce the risk of recurrence.
4. State signs and symptoms that must be reported to a health care professional.

Collaborative Problems

Risk for Complications of Respiratory Insufficiency

Risk for Complications of Septic Shock

Risk for Complications of Paralytic Ileus

Collaborative Outcomes

The individual will be monitored for early signs and symptoms of (a) hypoxia, (b) septic shock, and (c) paralytic ileus and will receive collaborative interventions if indicated to restore physiologic stability.

Indicators of Physiologic Stability

- Alert (a, b)
- Temperature 98° F to 99.5° F (a, b)
- Pulse regular rhythm rate 60 to 100 beats/min (a)
- Pulse oximetry >95 (a, b)
- BP >90/60, <140/90 mm Hg (a, b)
- Urine output >0.5 mL/kg/hr (a, b)
- Bowel sounds detected (c)
- No nausea and vomiting (c)
- No abdominal distention (c)
- No change in bowel function (c)
- Evidence of flatus (c)

Interventions	Rationales
1. Closely monitor risk individuals for hospital-acquired (nosocomial) pneumonia as: a. The elderly and very young b. Those with chronic or severe medical conditions, such as lung problems, heart disease, nervous system (neurologic) disorders, and immune compromised (AIDS, cancer). c. Those postsurgery as over age 80 post splenectomy, abdominal aortic aneurysm repair, or any factor that impairs coughing. d. Those in the intensive care unit (ICU), in prolonged prone positions, on mechanical ventilators e. Those sedated	1. Community acquitted pneumonia (CAP) is a common and potentially serious illness. It is associated with considerable morbidity and mortality, particularly in older adult individuals and those with significant comorbidities. The mortality rate ranged from 5.1% for combined ambulatory and hospitalized individuals (data were not reported for ambulatory individuals alone) to 13.6% in hospitalized individuals to 36.5% in individuals admitted to the ICU (Fil, 2015).
2. Evaluate the individual's risk for mortality using the CURB-65 scale (*Lim et al., 2003; Yealy & Fine, 2015) a. One point is given for the presence of each of the following (*Lim et al., 2003): • **C**onfusion—Altered mental status • **U**remia—Blood urea nitrogen (BUN) level greater than 20 mg/dL • **R**espiratory rate—30 breaths or more per minute • **B**P—Systolic pressure less than 90 mm Hg or diastolic pressure less than 60 mm Hg • Age older than **65** years b. Current guidelines suggest that individuals may be treated in an outpatient setting or may require hospitalization according to their CURB-65 score, as follows (Yealy & Fine, 2015): • Score of 0 to 1—Outpatient treatment • Score of 2—Admission to medical ward • Score of 3 or higher—Admission to ICU	2. CURB-65 is a scoring system developed from a multivariate analysis of 1,068 individuals that identified various factors that appeared to play a role in individual mortality (*Lim et al., 2003).

Interventions	Rationales

3. Monitor for signs and symptoms of hyperthermia:
  a. Fever of 103° F or above, chills
  b. Tachycardia
  c. Signs of shock: Restlessness or lethargy, confusion, decreased systolic BP
	3. Bacteria can act as a pyrogen by raising the hypothalamic thermostat through the production of endogenous pyrogens, which may mediate through prostaglandins. Chills can occur when the temperature setpoint of the hypothalamus changes rapidly. High fever increases metabolic needs and oxygen consumption. The impaired respiratory system cannot compensate, and tissue hypoxia results (Grossman & Porth, 2014).

4. Monitor respiratory status and assess for signs and symptoms of hypoxia:
  a. Increased respiratory rate (tachypnea), marked dyspnea, cyanosis
  b. Fever, chills (sudden or insidious)
  c. Productive (pink, rusty, purulent, green, yellow, or white sputum) or nonproductive cough
  d. Diminished or absent breath sounds
  e. Crackles, rhonchi, bronchial breath sounds, positive bronchophony, increased tactile fremitus, and/or dullness on percussion (Dillon, 2007)
  f. Pleuritic pain
  g. Tachycardia
	4. Tracheobronchial inflammation, impaired alveolar capillary membrane function, edema, fever, and increased sputum production disrupt respiratory function and alter the blood's oxygen-carrying capacity. Reduced chest wall compliance in older adults also affects the quality of respiratory effort. In older adults, tachypnea >26 respirations/min is one of the earliest signs of pneumonia and often occurs 3 to 4 days before a confirmed diagnosis. Delirium or mental status changes are often seen early in pneumonia in older individuals.

5. Monitor for Sepsis and Systemic Inflammatory Response Syndrome (SIRS). Use criteria in Institution to diagnosis sepsis.
 	
  a. New, simpler criteria to diagnosis sepsis are Glasgow Coma Scale (GCS) score of 13 or less, systolic BP of 100 mm Hg or less, and respiratory rate of 22/min or more (1 point each; score range, 0 to 3) (Seymour et al., 2016)
  b. SIRS criteria >2 of the four findings:
    • Temperature >38.3° C or <36° C
    • Heart rate >90 beats/min or more than two standard deviations above the normal value for age
    • Tachypnea, respiratory rate >20 breaths/min
  c. White blood cell count greater than 12,000/µL with greater than 10% bands
    • Sepsis criteria >SIRS +source of infection
    • Severe sepsis criteria (organ dysfunction, hypotension, or hypoperfusion)
    • Lactic acidosis, SBP <90 or SBP drop ≥ 40 mm Hg of normal
	5. The hypothalamus resets in sepsis, so that heat production and heat loss are balanced in favor of a higher temperature (Bartlett, 2015).
	  a. Decreased blood flow to brain, heart, and kidneys triggers baroreceptors and release of catecholamines increases heart rate/cardiac output and further increasing vasoconstriction (Bartlett, 2015).
	  b. Anaerobic metabolism decreases circulating oxygen. The body attempts to increase oxygenation by increasing respiratory rate (Bartlett, 2015).
	
	  c. Increased white cells indicate an infectious process. Biologic markers are sometimes used to try to distinguish between bacterial and nonbacterial causes of pneumonia.

6. Monitor
  a. C-reactive protein more than two standard deviations above the normal value
  b. Plasma procalcitonin more than two standard deviations above the normal value
	6. The two most promising are procalcitonin (PCT) and C-reactive protein (CRP), which are elevated in bacterial pneumonia (Bartlett, 2015).

7. Ensure blood culture is done prior to the start of any antibiotic. Culture any suspected infection sites (urine, sputum, invasive lines).	7. Blood cultures should be obtained (prior to initiation of antimicrobial therapy) for any individual in whom there is suspicion of bacteremia or fungemia, including hospitalized individuals and selected outpatients with fever and leukocytosis or leukopenia (Barlett, 2015).
8. Refer to Risk for Complications of Sepsis/SIRS in Unit II.	

Clinical Alert Report

Prior to providing care, advise ancillary staff/student to report the following to the professional nurse assigned to the individual:

- Change in cognition, increasing drowsiness
- Temperature >100
- Pulse irregular rhythm rate <60, >100 beats/min
- BP <90/60, >140/90 mm Hg
- Urine output <0.5 mL/kg/hr (a, b)
- Decreased or no bowel sounds
- Abdominal distention
- Nausea/vomiting

Documentation

Medication (type, dosage, routes)
    Vital signs
    Assessments
    Treatments

Nursing Diagnoses

TRANSITION TO HOME/COMMUNITY CARE

If indicated, review the risk diagnoses identified for this individual on admission:

- Is the person still at risk?
- Can the family reduce the risks?
- Is the person at higher risk at home?
- Is a home health nurse assessment needed?
- Refer to transition planner/case manager/social service.
- When is this person scheduled for follow-up with primary provider? Specialists? Record dates of appointments.
- Complete a medication reconciliation prior to transition. Refer to index.

STAR   **Stop**

    Think   Is this person at risk for injury, falls, medical complications, and/or inability to care for self (activities of daily living)?

        Is the person competent to manage self-administration of medications, treatment procedures? Are additional resources needed?

        Can the person explain how to monitor condition (e.g., blood glucose, sign/symptoms of complications, dietary/mobility restrictions, and when to call his or her primary provider or specialist)?

    Act   Contact or provide the appropriate resource (e.g., contacting a support person, home health assessment, additional teaching, printed materials).

    Review   Has the problem been addressed? If not, use SBAR to communicate to the appropriate person.

Risk for Ineffective Health Management Related to Lack of Knowledge of Condition, Infection Transmission, Prevention of Recurrence, Diet, Signs and Symptoms of Recurrence, and Follow-Up Care

NOC

Compliance Behavior, Knowledge: Treatment Regimen, Participation: Health Care Decisions, Treatment Behavior: Illness or Injury

NIC

Anticipatory Guidance, Risk Identification, Health Education, Learning Facilitation, Amputation Care

Goal

The goals for this diagnosis represent those associated with transition planning. Refer to the transition criteria.

Interventions	Rationales
1. Explain the pathophysiology and expected course of pneumonia using teaching aids (e.g., illustrations, models) appropriate for the individual's or family's educational level.	1. Understanding the disease process and its possible complications may encourage engagement with the therapeutic regimen.

2. Explain measures to prevent the spread of infection:
  a. Cover the nose and mouth when sneezing or coughing.
  b. Dispose of used tissues in a paper bag; when the bag is half full, close it securely and place it in a larger disposal unit.
  c. Explain the importance of hand hygiene.
	2. Although pneumococcal pneumonia is not highly communicable, the individual should refrain from visiting with persons predisposed to pneumonia during the acute phase (e.g., elderly or seriously ill persons, those with sickle cell disease, postsurgical individuals, or persons with chronic respiratory disease, compromised immune system).

3. Advise individual/family to call PCP if there is no improvement in 72 hours or symptoms are worse.

> **CLINICAL ALERT:**
> • If there is no response to treatment within 72 hours, a reevaluation should be initiated. Possibly there has been an inaccurate diagnosis, the causative organism is resistant to prescribed antibiotic, or dosage has to be adjusted. More invasive techniques for obtaining respiratory secretions for culture may be required. Because most individuals notice a decrease in symptoms after 72 hours of treatment, they sometimes do not recognize the importance of continuing the antibiotic as prescribed. The course of medication is usually 7 to 14 days, but may be as long as 21 days, depending on severity of illness, presence of underlying disease, and individual response. Antibiotics should be continued until completed and a follow-up X-ray film confirms that infection has subsided.

4. Keep scheduled follow-up medical appointments.

(*continued*)

Interventions	*Rationales*
5. Explain that a follow-up chest X-ray at 7 to 12 weeks is indicated in certain individuals. Provide individual with the prescription with the date to go written.	5. "Follow-up chest radiograph is particularly important for males and smokers, who are over age 50 years" (Filho, 2015). Little et al. (2014) found that in 32 of 618 individuals (5.2%), significant new pulmonary diagnoses were established during follow-up imaging of suspected pneumonia.
6. Advise to continue deep breathing exercises for 6 to 8 weeks during the convalescent period.	6. Deep breathing increases alveolar expansion and thus facilitates movement of secretions from the tracheobronchial tree with coughing. Routine planned deep breathing and coughing sessions increase vital capacity and pulmonary compliance. Sometimes dry cough occurs with chest wall pain related to myalgias of the intercostal muscles, so increased efforts must be made to encourage regular lung expansion. A pillow may be used to splint the chest wall while coughing.
7. Receive yearly immunization against influenza and vaccines against bacterial pneumonia (Pneumovax, Prevnar 13) as indicated.	7. Individuals with asthma should receive the inactivated form only. Pneumovax is indicated for adults 65 years and older, people with certain medical conditions, and cigarette smokers. Prevnar 13 is approved for adults 50 years of age and older for the prevention of pneumococcal pneumonia and invasive disease caused by 13 Streptococcus pneumoniae strains (CDC, 2016f).
8. Encourage adequate hydration with intake of 3,000 mL/day, if not contraindicated.	8. Insensible fluid losses from hyperthermia and productive cough predispose the individual to dehydration, particularly an elderly individual.
9. Encourage adequate, nutritious food intake and use of high-protein supplements, if necessary.	9. Increased metabolism raises the individual's calorie requirements; however, dyspnea and anorexia sometimes prevent adequate caloric intake. High-protein supplements provide increased calories and fluids if anorexia and fatigue from eating interfere with food intake.
10. If the individual smokes, explain how smoking contributes to infections. Refer to Getting Started to Quit Smoking on thePoint.	10. Chronic smoking destroys the tracheobronchial ciliary action, the lungs' first defense against infection. It also inhibits alveolar macrophage function and irritates the bronchial mucosa.

Documentation

Transition instructions
Follow-up instructions
Status at transition

METABOLIC AND ENDOCRINE DISORDERS

Cirrhosis

Cirrhosis is a disease in which the liver becomes permanently damaged and the normal structure of the liver is changed. Healthy liver cells are replaced by scarred tissue. The liver is not able to do its normal functions, such as detoxifying harmful substances, purifying blood, and making vital nutrients. In addition, scarring slows down the normal flow of blood through the liver, causing blood to find alternate pathways (e.g., ascites). Once decompensation occurs (e.g., the individual develops variceal bleeding, hepatic encephalopathy, or spontaneous bacterial peritonitis), mortality rates are high (Goldberg & Chopra, 2015a,b).

Cirrhosis is the end result of chronic liver damage caused by chronic liver diseases. Common causes of chronic liver disease in the United States include:

- Long-term alcohol abuse
- Chronic viral hepatitis (hepatitis B, C)
- Alcoholic liver disease
- Hemochromatosis
- Nonalcoholic fatty liver disease

Other causes of cirrhosis include:

- Autoimmune hepatitis
- Primary and secondary biliary cirrhosis
- Primary sclerosing cholangitis
- Medications (e.g., methotrexate, isoniazid)
- Wilson disease
- α-1 antitrypsin deficiency
- Celiac disease
- Idiopathic adulthood ductopenia
- Granulomatous liver disease
- Idiopathic portal fibrosis
- Polycystic liver disease
- Infection (e.g., brucellosis, syphilis, echinococcosis, schistosomiasis)
- Right-sided heart failure
- Hereditary hemorrhagic telangiectasia
- Veno-occlusive disease

Cirrhosis is the 7th leading cause of death in the United States. Every year, about 36,427 people in the United States die from cirrhosis, mainly due to alcoholic liver disease and chronic hepatitis C (Xu, Murphy, Kochanek, & Bastian, 2016). In individuals with hepatitis B or C, the five-year survival rate after a diagnosis of cirrhosis ranges between 71% and 85%. Alcohol abuse and viral hepatitis are the most common causes of cirrhosis, although nonalcoholic fatty liver disease is emerging as an increasingly important cause. Primary care physicians share responsibility with specialists in managing the most common complications of the disease, screening for hepatocellular carcinoma, and preparing individuals for referral to a transplant center. Individuals with cirrhosis should be screened for hepatocellular carcinoma with imaging studies every 6 to 12 months (Starr & Raines, 2011).

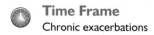

Time Frame
Chronic exacerbations

▪▪▪▪▪▪ DIAGNOSTIC CLUSTER

Collaborative Problems

▲ Risk for Complications of Ascites

* Risk for Complications of Spontaneous Bacterial Peritonitis

△ Risk for Complications of Hepatitis Encephalopathy

▲ Risk for Complications of Portal Hypertension/Variceal Bleeding

△ Risk for Complications of Metabolic Disorders

△ Risk for Complications of Hepatorenal Syndrome

* Risk for Complications of Medication Toxicity (opiates, short-acting barbiturates, major tranquilizers)

Nursing Diagnoses

▲ Imbalanced Nutrition related to anorexia, nausea impaired protein, fat, glucose metabolism, and impaired storage of vitamins (A, C, K, D, E)

▲ Impaired Comfort related to pruritus secondary to accumulation of bilirubin pigment and bile salts

▲ Excess Fluid Volume related to portal hypertension, lowered plasma colloidal osmotic pressure, and sodium retention

▲ Pain related to liver enlargement and ascites (pancreatitis)

▲ Diarrhea related to excessive secretion of fats in stool secondary to liver dysfunction (refer to Pancreatitis Care Plan)

▲ High Risk for Infection related to leukopenia secondary to enlarged, overactive spleen and hypoproteinemia (refer to Leukemia Care Plan)

▲ Risk for Ineffective Health Management related to lack of knowledge of pharmacologic contraindications, nutritional requirements, signs and symptoms of complications, and risks of alcohol ingestion

▲ This diagnosis was reported to be monitored for or managed frequently (75% to 100%).

△ This diagnosis was reported to be monitored for or managed often (50% to 74%).

* This medical condition was not included in the validation study.

Transition Criteria

Before transition, the individual or family will:

1. Describe the causes of cirrhosis.
2. Describe activity restrictions, nutritional requirements, and the need for alcohol abstinence.
3. State actions that reduce anorexia, edema, and pruritus at home.
4. Relate community resources available for drug and alcohol counseling.
5. State the signs and symptoms that must be reported to a health care professional.

Collaborative Problems

Risk for Complications of Ascites

Risk for Complications of Spontaneous Bacterial Peritonitis

Risk for Complications of Hepatitis Encephalopathy

Risk for Complications of Portal Hypertension

Risk for Complications of Variceal Bleeding

Risk for Complications of Metabolic Disorders

Risk for Complications of Hepatorenal Syndrome

Risk for Complications of Medication Toxicity (Opiates, Short-Acting Barbiturates, Major Tranquilizers)

Collaborative Outcomes

The individual will be monitored for early signs and symptoms of (a) ascites, (b) spontaneous bacterial peritonitis, (c) hepatic encephalopathy, (d) portal hypertension, (e) variceal bleeding, (f) metabolic disorders, (g) hepatorenal syndrome, and (h) medication toxicity and will receive collaborative interventions if indicated to restore physiologic stability.

Indicators of Physiologic Stability

- BP >90/60, <140/90 mm Hg
- Heart rate 60 to 100 beats/min
- Respiration 16 to 20 breaths/min
- Hemoglobin: Male 14 to 18 g/dL, female 12 to 16 g/dL
- Hematocrit:
  - Male 42% to 52%
  - Female 37% to 47%
- Stools negative occult blood (e)
- Prothrombin time 11 to 12.5 seconds (e)
- Electrolytes within normal range
- Serum pH 7.35 to 7.45
- Serum Pco_2 35 to 45 mm Hg
- Oxygen saturation >95% (pulse oximeter)
- Urine output >0.5 mL/kg/hr
- Urine specific gravity 1.005 to 1.030
- Sodium 135 to 145 mEq/L (f, g, h)
- Creatinine 0.7 to 1.4 mg/dL (f, g, h)
- Albumin 3.5 to 5.0 m/units/mL (f, g, h)
- Prealbumin 16 to 40 m/units/mL (f, g, h)
- Blood urea nitrogen 5 to 25 mg/dL
- Temperature greater than 37.8° C (100° F)
- No reports of new onset or increased abdominal pain and/or tenderness (b)
- No change in mental status (b, c)
- Ascitic fluid PMN count, <250 cells/mm^3 (b)
- Serum-to-ascites albumin gradient (SAAG) <1.1 g/dL (calculated to determine the presence of portal hypertension-related ascites)

Transitional Risk Assessment Plan (TRAP)

Begin this plan on admission.

Implement the Transitional Risk Assessment Plan (TRAP):

* Refer to inside back cover.
* Add each validated high-risk diagnosis to individual's problem list with the risk code in ( ).
* Refer to Unit II to the individual high-risk nursing diagnoses/collaborative problems for outcomes and interventions.

> *R: "Close coordination of care in the post-acute period, early discharge follow-up care, enhanced client education and self-management training, proactive end-of-life counseling, and extending the resources and clinical expertise over time via multidisciplinary team management" can lower readmission rates and improve health outcomes (Boutwell & Hwu, 2009, p. 14). Interventions are utilized to activate the individual and family to select changes in their everyday lifestyle choices to improve their health (Hibbard & Greene, 2013)*

Interventions	Rationales
1. If chronic alcoholism is suspected, refer also to Alcohol Withdrawal Syndrome Care Plan.	1. Undetected alcoholism can result in fatal withdrawal symptoms.

2. Monitor for ascites.
  a. Increased abdominal girth
  b. Rapid weight gain
	2. Obstruction of blood flow in the portal vein increases hydrostatic pressure in the peritoneal capillaries and decreased albumin decreases osmotic pressure; both of which cause the fluid shift into the peritoneal cavity (Grossman & Porth, 2014).

3. Explain ascites and treatments	3. Ascites is typically treated with a combination of diuretics and sodium restriction, though some individuals require repeated therapeutic paracenteses or TIPS placement (Goldberg & Chopra, 2015a, b).
4. Explain need for dietary salt restriction. Access a nutritionist.	4. Dietary salt should be restricted to a no-added-salt diet of <2,000 mg/day (Dudek, 2014).
5. Explain paracentesis if needed for comfort and/or diagnostic purposes. a. Cirrhotic individuals should undergo diagnostic paracentesis in cases of unexplained fever, abdominal pain, or encephalopathy or when admitted to the hospital for any cause.	5. Abdominal paracentesis should be performed and ascetic fluid should be obtained with clinically apparent new-onset ascites for analysis of cell count and total protein, serum-ascites albumin gradient (SAGG), and obtaining cultures only in symptomatic individuals if the fluid is cloudy (Such & Runyon, 2016).
6. Explain diuretic-resistant ascites and the need for serial therapeutic paracentesis.	6. "Serial large-volume paracenteses (LVPs) are mainstays in the treatment of diuretic-resistant ascites, both for those awaiting liver transplantation and for those who are not transplantation candidates. Individuals who are consuming 88 mEq (2,000 mg) of sodium per day and are excreting no sodium in the urine should require paracentesis of approximately 8 L every 2 weeks (Such & Runyon, 2016).

Interventions	Rationales
7. Monitor for hepatic encephalopathy. Continually assess for causes of hepatic encephalopathy include constipation, infection, gastrointestinal (GI) bleeding, certain medications, electrolyte imbalances, and noncompliance with medical therapy.	7. Hepatic encephalopathy describes a spectrum of potentially reversible neuropsychiatric abnormalities seen in individuals with liver dysfunction and/or portosystemic shunting. Overt hepatic encephalopathy develops in 30% to 45% of individuals with cirrhosis (Ferenci, 2013). Profound liver failure results in accumulation of ammonia and other identical toxic metabolites in the blood. The blood–brain barrier permeability increases, and both toxins and plasma proteins leak from capillaries to the extracellular space, causing cerebral edema (Grossman & Porth, 2014).
8. Closely monitor cognitive status.	8. Cognitive findings with hepatic encephalopathy vary from subtle deficits that are not apparent without specialized testing (minimal hepatic encephalopathy), to more overt findings, with impairments in attention, reaction time, and working memory (Ferenci, 2013).

9. Monitor for hepatorenal syndrome.
  a. A progressive rise in serum creatinine
  b. An often normal urine sediment
  c. No or minimal proteinuria (less than 500 mg/day)
  d. A very low rate of sodium excretion (i.e., urine sodium concentration less than 10 mEq/L)
  e. Oliguria
	9. The hepatorenal syndrome represents the end-stage of a sequence of reductions in renal perfusion induced by increasingly severe hepatic injury. The hepatorenal syndrome is a diagnosis of exclusion and is associated with a poor prognosis (Runyon, 2015).

10. Monitor for portal hypertension and bleeding.
  a. Bleeding from esophageal varices:
  b. Hematemesis (vomiting blood)
  c. Melena (black, sticky stools)
	10. Any of the complications of cirrhosis are the result of portal hypertension (increased pressure within the portal venous system). This can lead to the formation of venous collaterals (varices) as well as circulatory, vascular, functional, and biochemical abnormalities that contribute to the pathogenesis of ascites and other complications (Goldberg & Chopra, 2015a, b).

11. Teach the individual port unusual bleeding (e.g., in the mouth after brushing teeth) and ecchymotic areas.	11. Portal hypertension caused by obstruction of the portal venous system results in increased pressure on the vessels in the esophagus, making them fragile (Grossman & Porth, 2014). Mucous membranes are more prone to injury because of their great surface vascularity.
12. Monitor for signs and symptoms of hyponatremia (serum sodium concentration below 135 mEq/L)	12. Hyponatremia is a common problem in individuals with advanced cirrhosis. The pathogenesis of hyponatremia is directly related to the hemodynamic changes and secondary neurohumoral adaptations that occur in the setting of cirrhosis, resulting in an impaired ability to excrete ingested water. The severity of the hyponatremia is related to the severity of the cirrhosis.

13. Assess for adverse effects of medications in the presence of impaired liver function. Evaluate the medications that require:
  a. Reduced doses because they decrease metabolizing enzymes (cimetidine, rantidine, diazepam, lorazepam, morphine, meperidine, phenytoin, verapamil, ketoconzole, fluoxetine)
  b. Increased dosing because they increase metabolizing enzymes (e.g., rifampin, phenobarbital).
	13. Most medications are metabolized by enzymes in the liver. Impaired liver function can increase circulating drug levels.

(continued)

Interventions	Rationales
14. Ensure vitamin D levels are measured and monitored	14. Many studies have shown low serum levels of 25-hydroxyvitamin D due to impaired synthesis in individuals with chronic liver disease and levels fall with disease progression in cirrhosis (Nair, 2010)

15. If individual is in end-stage hepatic failure, consult physician/nurse practitioner regarding the need for palliative care. Refer to Palliative Care Plan.

Clinical Alert Report

Prior to providing care, advise ancillary staff/student to report the following to the professional nurse assigned to the individual:

- Temperature >37.8° C (100° F)
- Resting pulse >100, <50 beats/min
- New irregular pulse
- Systolic BP >200 mm Hg or <9 mm Hg
- Diastolic BP >90
- Oxygenation saturation <90%
- Weight gain
- Any change in mental status
- Complaints of abdominal pain/tenderness
- Observed tremors
- Urine output for shift or hourly if indicated
- Hemoptasis, streaks of blood in stools, dark stools
- Prolonged bleeding for venipuncture sites
- Reports of bleeding gums, excess menstrual bleeding

Documentation

Weight
Vital signs
Stools for occult blood
Urine specific gravity
Intake and output
Evidence of bleeding
Evidence of tremors or confusion

Nursing Diagnoses

Imbalanced Nutrition Related to Anorexia, Nausea Impaired Protein, Fat, and Glucose Metabolism, and Impaired Storage of Vitamins (A, C, K, D, E)

NOC
Nutritional Status, Knowledge: Diet

Goal

The individual will relate the importance of nutritional intake and complying with the prescribed dietary regimen.

NIC
Nutrition Management, Nutrition Monitoring

Indicators

- Describe the reasons for nutritional problems.
- Relate which foods are high in protein and calories.
- Gain weight (specify amount) without increased edema.
- Explain the rationale for sodium restrictions.

Interventions	*Rationales*
1. Discuss the causes of anorexia, dyspepsia, and nausea. Causes include poor oral nutritional intake, malabsorption, ongoing alcohol use, chronic nausea, and early satiety due to abdominal compression from ascites. Explain that obstructed hepatic blood flow causes GI vascular congestion (which results in gastritis and diarrhea or constipation), and that impaired liver function causes metabolic disturbances (fluid, electrolyte, glucose metabolism), resulting in anorexia and fatigue.	1. Helping the individual understand the condition can reduce anxiety and may help improve compliance.
CLINICAL ALERT: • Malnutrition represents a negative prognostic factor for cirrhosis and consists of muscle wasting, hypoalbuminemia, decreased resistance to infections, and variceal bleeding (Grattagliano, Ubaldi, Bonfrate, & Portinc, 2011).	
2. Explain the treatment consists of avoidance of alcohol, excess fat intake and having 4 to 6 small meals of carbohydrates and protein daily. Request a nutritional consult.	2. Careful balancing of protein intake is required. Protein is required, however ammonia is produced when digestive enzymes breakdown protein. Excessive ammonia causes hepatic encephalopathy (Lutz, Mazur, & Litch, 2015).
3. Teach and assist the individual to rest before meals.	3. Fatigue further decreases the desire to eat.
4. Offer frequent small feedings (six per day plus snacks).	4. Increased intra-abdominal pressure from ascites compresses the GI tract and reduces its capacity.
5. Restrict liquids with meals and avoid fluids 1 hour before and after meals.	5. Fluids can over distend the stomach, decreasing appetite and intake.
6. Arrange to have foods with the highest protein/calorie content served at the time the individual feels most like eating.	6. This increases the likelihood of the individual consuming adequate amounts of protein and calories.
7. Teach the individual measures to reduce nausea. Refer to Nausea nursing diagnosis in Unit II.	7. Venous congestion in the GI tract predisposes the individual to nausea.

Documentation

Weight
Intake (type, amount)
Abdominal girth

Impaired Comfort Related to Pruritus Secondary to Accumulation of Bilirubin Pigment and Bile Salts

NOC
Symptom Control

Goal

The individual will verbalize decreased pruritus.

NIC
Pruritus Management,
Fever Treatment,
Environmental
Management: Comfort

Indicators

• Describe factors that increase pruritus.
• Describe factors that improve pruritus.

Interventions	Rationales
1. Explain causes of pruritus. **CLINICAL ALERT:** • Fifty percent of individuals with primary biliary cirrhosis initially present with pruritus (100% report pruritus at some point). Pruritus is reported in 20% of individuals with Hepatitis C. Pruritus from Hepatitis C may be localized to a specific body part, such as hands and feet, or generalized, involving the entire body (Garcia-Albea & Limaye, 2012).	1. Etiology is related to the increased level of bile salts, elevated plasma and tissue levels of opioid peptides, and downregulation of opioid peptide receptors (James, Berger, & Elston, 2011).
2. Explain the itch–scratch cycle. Inflammation causes scratching > stimulates excitation of C-nerve fibers > causes itching > causes scratching, etc. Instruct to apply firm pressure to pruritic areas instead of scratching. Or apply cold cloth. Explain stress, fear, loss of sleep, and anxiety can make itch worse.	2. Successful treatment of itch requires interruption of this cycle.
3. Maintain hygiene without causing dry skin: a. Give frequent baths using cool water and mild soap (castile, lanolin) or a soap substitute. b. Blot skin dry; do not rub. c. Apply *Cooling agents* are over-the-counter preparations which usually contain menthol, camphor, or phenol. Apply immediately after bathing to promote hydration of the skin by preventing water loss thru evaporation (*Yosipovitch & Hundley, 2004).	3. Dryness or rubbing increases skin sensitivity by stimulating nerve endings. These substances stimulate nerve fibers which transmit the sensation of cold, thereby masking the itch sensation (*Yosipovitch & Hundley, 2004).
4. Prevent excessive warmth by maintaining cool room temperatures and with humidity at 30% to 40%, using light covers with a bed cradle, and avoiding overdressing.	4. Excessive warmth aggravates pruritus by increasing sensitivity through vasodilation.
5. Avoiding hot or spicy foods and alcoholic beverages, which induce histamine secretin (*Yosipovitch & Hundley, 2004).	5. These products increased histamines stimulate itching.
6. Consult with the physician/nurse practitioner/physical assistant for a pharmacologic treatment (e.g., antihistamines, antipruritic lotions), if necessary.	6. If pruritus is unrelieved or if the skin is excoriated from scratching, topical or systemic medications are indicated.

Documentation

Unrelieved pruritus
Excoriated skin

Excess Fluid Volume Related to Portal Hypertension, Lowered Plasma Colloidal Osmotic Pressure, and Sodium Retention

NOC
Electrolyte Balance,
Fluid Balance, Hydration

Goal

- The individual will relate actions that decrease fluid retention.
- The individual will list foods high in sodium.

NIC
Electrolyte
Management, Fluid
Management, Fluid
Monitoring, Skin
Surveillance

Interventions	Rationales
1. Assess their diet for inadequate protein or excessive sodium intake. 2. Encourage the individual to decrease salt intake. Refer to nutritional specialist.	1,2. Decreased renal flow results in increased aldosterone and antidiuretic hormone secretion, causing water and sodium retention and potassium excretion.
3. Take measures to protect edematous skin from injury:	3. Edematous skin is taut and easily injured. Dry skin is more vulnerable to breakdown and injury.
4. Inspect the skin for redness and blanching.	
5. Reduce pressure on skin (e.g., pad chairs and footstools).	
6. Prevent dry skin by using soap sparingly, rinsing off soap completely, and using a lotion to moisten skin.	

Documentation

Presence of edema

> **TRANSITION TO HOME/COMMUNITY CARE**
> If indicated, review the risk diagnoses identified for this individual on admission:
> * Is the person still at risk?
> * Can the family reduce the risks?
> * Is the person at higher risk at home?
> * Is a home health nurse assessment needed?
> * Refer to transition planner/case manager/social service.
> * When is this person scheduled for follow-up with primary provider? Specialists? Record dates of appointments.
> * Complete a medication reconciliation prior to transition. Refer to index.

STAR   **Stop**

Think   Is this person at risk for injury, falls, medical complications, and/or inability to care for self (activities of daily living)?

Is there a support person available?

Is the person competent to manage self-administration of medications, treatment procedures? Are additional resources needed?

Can the person explain how to monitor the condition (e.g., blood glucose, signs/symptoms of complications, dietary/mobility restrictions, and when to call his or her primary provider or specialist)?

Act   Contact or provide the appropriate resource (e.g., contacting a support person, home health assessment, additional teaching, printed materials).

Review   Has the problem been addressed? If not, use SBAR to communicate to the appropriate person.

Risk for Ineffective Health Management Related to Lack of Knowledge of Pharmacologic Contraindications, Nutritional Requirements, Signs and Symptoms of Complications, and Risks of Alcohol Ingestion

NOC

Compliance Behavior, Knowledge: Treatment Regimen, Participation in Health Care Decisions, Treatment Behavior: Illness or Injury

NIC

Anticipatory Guidance, Risk Identification, Health Education, Learning Facilitation

Goal

The goals for this diagnosis represent those associated with transition planning. Refer to the transition criteria.

Interventions	Rationales
1. Teach the individual or family about the condition and its causes and treatments.	1. This teaching reinforces the need to comply with the therapeutic regimen, including diet and activity restrictions.
2. Explain portal system encephalopathy to the family. Teach them to observe for and report any confusion, tremors, night wandering, or personality changes. a. The onset often is insidious and is characterized by subtle and sometimes intermittent changes in memory, personality, concentration, and reaction times. Hepatic encephalopathy is a diagnosis of exclusion; therefore, all other etiologies of altered mental status must be effectively ruled out (Starr & Raines, 2011).	2. Confusion and altered speech patterns result from cerebral hypoxia because of high serum ammonia levels caused by the liver's impaired ability to convert ammonia to urea. Family members typically first note the development of encephalopathy.
3. Explain the risk of osteoporosis. Advise to discuss the need for a dexa scan with primary care provider.	3. Some studies have shown increased bone resorption, in the presence of chronic liver disease, whereas most others have shown decreased bone formation (*Collier, Ninkovic, & Compston, 2002).
4. Advise of lifestyle choices that can prevent osteoporosis as adequate dietary calcium intake, (1 g/day) + vitamin D_3 (dose dependent on serum levels), regular weight-bearing exercise.	4. Many studies have shown low serum levels of 25-hydroxyvitamin D due to impaired synthesis in individuals with chronic liver disease and levels fall with disease progression in cirrhosis (Nair, 2010).
5. Explain the hazards of certain medications, including narcotics, sedatives, tranquilizers, and ammonia products.	5. Impaired liver function slows the metabolism of some drugs, causing levels to accumulate and increasing toxicity.

6. Teach to watch for and report signs and symptoms of complications:
 	
   a. Bleeding (gums, stools), prolonged, heavy period
 	
   b. Hypokalemia (muscle cramps, nausea, vomiting)
 	
   c. Rapid weight loss or gain
	6. Progressive liver failure affects hematopoietic function and electrolyte and fluid balance, causing potentially serious complications that require prompt intervention.
	   a. Bleeding indicates decreased platelets and clotting factors.
	   b. Hypokalemia results from overproduction of aldosterone, which causes sodium and water retention and potassium excretion.
	   c. Rapid weight loss points to negative nitrogen balance; weight gain, points to fluid retention.

Interventions	Rationales
7. Explain the need to avoid alcohol. Refer to D&A program if indicated.	7. Alcoholism is a complex physiologic, psychological, and social disorder.
8. Stress the importance of follow-up care and laboratory studies. Ensure appointments are made before leaving the facility. Ensure all needed prescriptions are provided	8. Timely follow-up enables evaluation of liver function and early detection of relapse or recurrence.

Documentation

Flow records
> Individual/family teaching
> Referrals when indicated
> Unachieved outcomes

Diabetes Mellitus

Diabetes mellitus is a chronic disease of abnormal glucose metabolism requiring lifelong management through nutrition, exercise, and often medication and increasing in adults and children every year. Of the 29.1 million Americans who have diabetes, 21.0 million were diagnosed, and 8.1 million were undiagnosed, and 86 million are prediabetes. Uncontrolled diabetes affects all body systems, causing serious complications such as retinopathy, nephropathy, neuropathy, and vascular disease. The diagnosis of diabetes is made based on: two fasting plasma glucose measurements greater than or equal to 126 mg/dL; a 2-hour plasma glucose >200 mg/dL after an oral glucose tolerance test; classic symptoms of diabetes—polyuria, polydipsia, unexplained weight loss—and a random plasma glucose of >200 mg/dL; or an A1C >6.5 (American Diabetes Association, 2016)

The classification of diabetes includes four clinical classes: type 1 diabetes, which results from beta cell destruction leading to absolute insulin deficiency; type 2 diabetes, which results from an insulin secretory defect coupled with insulin resistance; gestational diabetes (GDM) occurs during pregnancy; and other diabetes due to other causes such as genetic defects, chemical induced, diseases of exocrine pancreas (American Diabetes Association, 2016).

The causative factor of type 1 diabetes is an autoimmune destruction of the beta cell and accounts for less than 10% of all diabetes diagnoses. The cause of the more prevalent type 2 diabetes, accounting for over 90% of diabetes diagnoses, is multifactorial including genetic and environmental influences. Risk factors for type 2 diabetes include family history of the disease, age, obesity, and inactivity. Type 2 diabetes occurs more frequently in those with hyperlipidemia or hypertension, females with a history of GDM, and in those with certain ethnic background such as African American, American Indian, Hispanic/Latino, or Asian American (American Diabetes Association, 2016).

■■■■ DIAGNOSTIC CLUSTER

Collaborative Problems

▲ Risk for Complications of Diabetic Ketoacidosis (DKA)—type 1

▲ Risk for Complications of Hypoglycemia

▲ Risk for Complications of Hypoglycemia

▲ Risk for Complications of Infections

▲ Risk for Complications of Vascular Disease

▲ Risk for Complications of Neuropathy

▲ Risk for Complications of Retinopathy

▲ Risk for Complications of Nephropathy

(continued)

Nursing Diagnoses

▲ Overweight related to intake in excess of activity expenditures, lack of knowledge, or ineffective coping

Δ Risk for Ineffective Health Management related to insufficient knowledge of disease process, self-monitoring of blood glucose, medications, nutrition and meal planning, recognition and treatment of hypoglycemia, weight control, sick day care, exercise, foot care, signs and symptoms of complications, and the need for comprehensive diabetes outpatient education

▲ This diagnosis was reported to be monitored for or managed frequently (75% to 100%).
Δ This diagnosis was reported to be monitored for or managed often (50% to 74%).

Transition Criteria

Before transition, the individual or family will:

1. Define diabetes as a chronic disease requiring lifelong management through nutrition, exercise, and usually, medications for control.
2. Identify carbohydrates as foods that affect blood glucose, and create a meal using the plate method.
3. State the relationship of food and exercise to blood glucose.
4. State the effects of weight loss on BG control with type 2 diabetes.
5. State the value of monitoring BG and knowledge of normal blood glucose values.
6. Demonstrate the ability to perform self-blood-glucose monitoring and knowledge of obtaining testing supplies.
7. Explain the importance of foot care and regular assessments.
8. Describe self-care measures that may prevent or delay progression of chronic complications (microvascular, macrovascular, neuropathy).
9. Agree to attend comprehensive outpatient diabetes education programs.
10. Identification of the health care provider who will provide diabetes care after discharge.

For Individuals Requiring Medications

Oral Agents

1. State name, dose, action, potential side effects, and schedule to take diabetes medications.
2. State risk of hypoglycemia with delayed meals or increased activities.
3. State signs, symptoms, and treatment of hypoglycemia.
4. State intent to wear diabetes identification.
5. Describe self-care measures during illness.

Transitional Risk Assessment Plan (TRAP)

Begin this plan on admission.
Implement the Transitional Risk Assessment Plan (TRAP):
- Refer to inside back cover.
- Add each validated high-risk diagnosis to individual's problem list with the risk code in ( ).
- Refer to Unit II to the individual high-risk nursing diagnoses/collaborative problems for outcomes and interventions.

R: "Close coordination of care in the post-acute period, early discharge follow-up care, enhanced patient education and self-management training, proactive end-of-life counseling, and extending the resources and clinical expertise over time via multidisciplinary team management" can lower readmission rates and improve health outcomes (Boutwell & Hwu, 2009, p. 14). Interventions are utilized to activate the individual and family to select changes in their everyday lifestyle choices to improve their health (Hibbard & Greene, 2013).

Insulin

1. Demonstrate technique for insulin administration.
2. State brand, type, onset, peak, duration, and dose of insulin.
3. State recommendations for site rotation, storage of insulin, and disposal of syringes.
4. State signs, symptoms, and treatment of hypoglycemia.
5. State intent to wear diabetes identification.
6. Describe self-care measures during illness.

Collaborative Problems

Risk for Complications of Diabetic Ketoacidosis (DKA)

Risk for Complications of Hyperosmolar Hyperglycemic State

Risk for Complications of Hypoglycemia

Risk for Complications of Infections

Risk for Complications of Vascular Disease

Risk for Complications of Neuropathy

Risk for Complications of Retinopathy

Risk for Complications of Nephropathy

Collaborative Outcomes

The individual will be monitored for early signs and symptoms of (a) diabetic ketoacidosis, (b) hyperosmolar hyperglycemic state, (c) hypoglycemia, (d) infections, (e) vascular, (f) neurological, (g) retinal, and (h) renal complications, and will receive collaborative interventions if indicated to restore physiologic stability.

Indicators of Physiologic Stability

- pH 7.35 to 7.45 and HCO_3 18 to 22 mmol/L (a, b)
- Fasting blood glucose 70 to 130 mg/dL (a, b, c)
- No ketones in urine (a, b)
- Serum sodium 135 to 145 mmol/L (a, b, h)
- Serum osmolality, >295 mOsm/kg (a, b, h)
- BP <130/80 (e)
- Clear, oriented (a, b, e, f)
- Pulse 60 to 100 beats/min (e)
- Respiration 16 to 20 breaths/min (a, b, e)
- Peripheral pulses, equal and full, capillary refill <3 seconds (e)
- Warm, dry skin (a, b, e)
- No vision changes (f, g)
- Bowel sounds, present (f)
- White blood cells 4,000 to 10,800 mm (d)
- Urine, protein-negative (h)
- Creatinine 0.8 to 1.3 mg/dL (h)
- Blood urea nitrogen 5 to 25mg/dL (h)

Interventions	*Rationales*
1. Monitor for signs and symptoms of DKA with type 1 diabetes: a. Recent illness/infection b. Blood glucose >300 mg/dL c. Malaise and generalized weakness d. Moderate/large ketones e. Dehydration f. Anorexia, nausea, vomiting, abdominal pain g. Kussmaul's respirations (shallow, rapid) h. Fruity acetone odor of the breath i. pH <7.30 and HCO_3 <15 mEq j. Decreased sodium, potassium, phosphates	1. When insulin is not available, blood glucose levels rise and the body metabolizes fat for energy; the byproduct of this fat metabolism is ketones. Excessive ketone bodies results in ketoacidosis and a drop in pH and bicarbonate serum levels. This acidosis causes headaches, nausea, vomiting, and abdominal pain. Increased respiratory rate helps CO_2 excretion in effort to reduce acidosis. Elevated glucose levels inhibit water reabsorption in the renal glomerulus, leading to osmotic diuresis with loss of water, sodium, potassium, and phosphates, leading to severe dehydration and electrolyte imbalance (Kitabchi, Hirsch, & Emmett, 2015).
2. Monitor for signs and symptoms of hyperosmolar hyperglycemic state (HHS) type 2: a. Blood glucose >600 mg/dL b. pH >7.30 and HCO_3 >15 mEq/L c. Severe dehydration d. Serum osmolality >320 mOsm/kg e. Hypotension f. Altered sensorium	2. HHS is marked by profound dehydration and hyperglycemia without ketoacidosis. Decreased renal clearance and utilization of glucose result in an osmotic dieresis and osmotic shift of fluid to the intravascular space, resulting in intracellular dehydration and loss of electrolytes. Cerebral impairment is due to this intracellular dehydration (Kitabachi et al., 2015).

3. Monitor for signs and symptoms of hypoglycemia (Hamdy, 2016):
a. Blood glucose <70 mg/dL
b. Pale, moist, cool skin
c. Tachycardia, diaphoresis
d. Jitteriness, irritability
e. Confusion
f. Drowsiness
g. Hypoglycemia unawareness
  • Hypoglycemia is defined as any BG <70 mg/dL and may be caused by too much insulin, too little food, or too much physical activity. Hypoglycemia symptoms are related to sympathetic system stimulation and brain dysfunction related to decreased levels of glucose. Sympathoadrenal activation and release of adrenaline causes diaphoresis, cool skin, tachycardia, anxiety, and jitteriness. Reduction in cerebral glucose will result in confusion, difficulty with concentration, focal impairments, and if severe, can cause seizures and eventually coma and death (Hamdy, 2016).
  • Treatment of hypoglycemia is considered emergent.
	3. Hypoglycemia unawareness is a defect in the body's defense system that impairs the ability to experience the warning symptoms usually associated with hypoglycemia. The individual may rapidly progress from being alert to unconsciousness affecting about 25% of type 1 diabetics (Hamdy, 2016).

4. Institute "Rule of 15" with a goal to achieve BG >100 mg/dL: a. If individual is alert and cooperative: give 15 g of carbohydrate orally and monitor for 15 minutes; repeat BG—if above 100 mg/dL may give light snack if not time for a meal. If not above 70 mg/dL, repeat treatment with 15 g of carbohydrate—monitor and recheck BG in 15 minutes and may repeat until at goal. b. Nonalert individual: Call for Help—if IV access, give 24 g dextrose (1 amp D50); if none, give 1 mg glucagon IM, monitor for 15 minutes, and repeat BG; may repeat treatment q15–30 minutes depending on response.	

Interventions	Rationales
c. If hypoglycemia is severe (BG <40), recurrent, or caused by sulfonylurea or long-acting insulin, follow D50 treatment with D5 or D10 drip. d. Continued follow-up is mandatory until individual is stable. Cause of the hypoglycemia should always be investigated (Inzucchi, 2012).	
5. Monitor for signs and symptoms of infection. Refer to Risk for Infection in Unit II for preventive intervention. a. Upper respiratory tract infection b. Urinary tract infection c. Otitis media d. Red, painful, or warm skin e. Furunculosis, carbuncles	5. Infection is the primary cause of metabolic abnormalities in individuals with diabetes. Increased glucose in epidermis and urine promotes bacterial growth. The early diagnosis and prompt treatment of infection are essential to prevent issues that can lead to major complications (e.g., cellulitis spreading to the bone necessitating amputations) (Edelman & Henry, 2014).
6. Assess for risk factors and monitor for signs and symptoms of macrovascular complications: a. Family history of heart disease b. Male: over age 40 c. Cigarette smoker d. Hypertension e. Hyperlipidemia f. Obesity g. Uncontrolled diabetes	6. Diabetes is associated with severe degenerative vascular changes; heart disease is the number one cause of death for people with diabetes. Lesions of the blood vessels strike at an earlier age and tend to produce more severe pathologic changes. Early atherosclerotic changes are probably caused by high blood glucose and lipid levels characteristic of persistent hyperglycemia. Atherosclerosis leads to premature coronary artery disease (American Diabetes Association, 2016).
7. Monitor for signs and symptoms of retinopathy: a. Blurred vision b. Black spots c. "Cobwebs" d. Sudden loss of vision e. Floaters	7. Retinopathy does not cause visual symptoms until at a fairly advanced stage, usually when macular edema or proliferative retinopathy has occurred. The incidence and severity of retinopathy are thought to be related to the duration and the degree of control of blood glucose as well as blood pressure (Tarr, Kaul, Chopra, Kohner, & Chibber, 2013).
8. Monitor for signs and symptoms of peripheral neuropathy: a. Pain, burning sensation in feet, legs b. Decreased sensation, numbness in feet, fingers c. Decreased deep tendon response (Achilles and patella) d. Charcot's foot ulcer e. Decreased proprioception f. Paresthesia	8. Sensory symptoms usually predominate and include numbness, tingling, pain, or loss of sensation in feet. This nerve damage may lead to long-term chronic pain, ulcers, and eventually amputation. Current treatments include improved control of blood glucose and use of antidepressant drugs as well as aldose reductase inhibitors.
9. Monitor for signs and symptoms of autonomic neuropathy: a. Orthostatic hypotension b. Impotence c. Abnormal sweating d. Bladder paralysis e. Nocturnal diarrhea f. Gastroparesis	9. Autonomic nervous system modulates many body functions, both parasympathetic or sympathetic. The degree of autonomic dysfunction may be clinically irrelevant or symptoms may be disabling (Vinik, Erbas, & Casellini, 2013).

(continued)

Interventions	Rationales
10. Monitor for signs and symptoms of nephropathy: a. Proteinuria, casts in urine b. Abnormal blood urea nitrogen (BUN) and creatinine c. Urine for microalbumin, goal <30 mg d. Urine for proteinuria >300 mg albumin	10. In nephropathy, the capillary basement membrane thickens, due to chronic filtering of high glucose. The membrane becomes more permeable, causing increased loss of blood proteins in urine. Increased filtration requirements increase the pressure in renal blood vessels, contributing to sclerosis.
11. Consult with the physician to order a 24-hour urine test.	11. Clinical manifestations of nephropathy occur late in the disease. Proteinuria is the first sign of the disorder. If urine is positive for protein, then a 24-hour quantitative measure with a CrCl is important to obtain. When decreased kidney function is identified early, more aggressive therapy may be initiated to prevent or slow progression to overt kidney failure (Edelman & Henry, 2014).
12. Carefully monitor blood pressure.	12. Aggressive blood pressure control can reduce proteinuria and delay the progression of renal damage (American Diabetes Association, 2016).
13. Teach the individual about the risk factors that may contribute to renal damage: a. Uncontrolled blood glucose b. Hypertension c. Neurogenic bladder d. Urethral instrumentation e. Urinary tract infection f. Nephrotoxic drugs g. Making the individual aware of risk factors may help to reduce renal impairment.	

Clinical Alert Report

Prior to providing care, advise ancillary staff/student to report the following to the professional nurse assigned to the individual:

- Signs and symptoms of infection: elevated temperature, reddened skin, odor, or discharge from surgical sites or injuries
- Blood glucose >300 mg/dL or <70 mg/dL
- Nausea and vomiting
- Change in mental status/behavior
- Decrease in urine output

Diagnostic Studies

Fasting blood glucose, glucose tolerance test

Therapies

Self-monitoring blood glucose (SMBG), meal plan, exercise

Documentation

Vital signs
Blood glucose
HgbA$_{1c}$
BUN/creatinine
Lipid profile
    Date last eye exam
    Date last 24-hour urine test

Individual complications
Abnormal labs
Episodes of hypoglycemia
Changes in medications

> **TRANSITION TO HOME/COMMUNITY CARE**
>
> If indicated, review the risk diagnoses identified for this individual on admission:
> * Is the person still at risk?
> * Can the family reduce the risks?
> * Is the person at higher risk at home?
> * Is a home health nurse assessment needed?
> * Refer to transition planner/case manager/social service.
> * When is this person scheduled for follow-up with primary provider? Specialists? Record dates of appointments.
> * Complete a medication reconciliation prior to transition. Refer to index.

STAR

Stop

Think   Is this person at risk for injury, falls, medical complications, and/or inability to care for self (activities of daily living)?

Is there a support person available?

Is the person competent to manage self-administration of medications, treatment procedures? Are additional resources needed?

Can the person explain how to monitor condition (e.g., blood glucose, sign/symptoms of complications, dietary/mobility restrictions, and when to call his/her primary provider or specialist)?

Act   Contact or provide the appropriate resource (e.g., contacting a support person, home health assessment, additional teaching, printed materials).

Review   Has the problem been addressed? If not, use SBAR to communicate to the appropriate person.

Nursing Diagnoses

Risk for Ineffective Health Management Related to Insufficient Knowledge of Diabetes, Monitoring of BG, Medications, Meal Planning, Treatment of Hypoglycemia, Weight Control, Sick Day Management, Exercise Routine, Foot Care, Risks of Complications

NOC

Compliance/
Engagement Behavior,
Knowledge: Treatment
Regimen, Participation
in Health Care
Decisions, Treatment
Behavior: Illness or
Injury

NIC

Anticipatory Guidance,
Risk Identification,
Learning Facilitation,
Health Education,
Teaching: Procedure/
Treatment, Health
System Guidance

Goal

The goals for this diagnosis represent those associated with transition planning. Refer to the transition criteria.

Interventions	*Rationales*

1. Explore with the individual and significant others the actual or perceived effects of diabetes on:
  a. Finances
  b. Occupation (sick time)
  c. Lifestyle
  d. Energy level
  e. Relationships
	1. Common frustrations associated with diabetes stem from problems involving the disease itself, the treatment regimen, and the health care system. The American Diabetes Association recommends that all individuals with diabetes receive diabetes self-management education and support (DSME/S) with diagnosis and as needed throughout illness (Powers et al., 2015).

2. Instruct the individual and family on the components of diabetes treatment—meal planning, monitoring, exercise, and medications: effective self-management and quality of life are the key outcomes of an education program (American Diabetes Association, 2016).	

3. Increase awareness of the role of uncontrolled diabetes in the development of complications:
  a. Chronic:
    • Coronary artery disease
    • Peripheral vascular disease
    • Retinopathy
    • Neuropathy
    • Nephropathy
  b. Acute:
    • Hypoglycemia
    • Hyperglycemia
    • Diabetic ketoacidosis
    • Hyperosmolar hyperglycemia state
	3. When teaching the risks of complications, stress the importance personal self-management and the responsibility of each individual to follow-up with health care provider, including ophthalmologic and podiatric specialists (Powers et al., 2015).

4. Teach the individual the signs and symptoms of hyperglycemia:
  a. Blood glucose >200 mg/dL
  b. Polyuria
  c. Polydipsia
  d. Polyphagia
  e. Fatigue
  f. Blurred vision
  g. Weight loss
	4. Elevated BG causes dehydration from osmotic diuresis. Potassium is elevated because of hemoconcentration. Because carbohydrates are not metabolized, the individual loses weight (Grossman & Porth, 2014).

5. Teach the individual the causes of hyperglycemia:
  a. Increased food intake
  b. Omitting oral medications
  c. Decreased insulin dosing
  d. Decreased exercise
  e. Infection/illness
  f. Dehydration
	5. Increased food intake requires increased insulin or exercise; otherwise hyperglycemia will ensue. Infections, illnesses, or both increase insulin requirements (Grossman & Porth, 2014).

6. Discuss BG monitoring: its purpose, utilization of results, record keeping
  a. Advise the individual to obtain a third-party reimbursement for BG monitoring supplies. Medicare will pay for BG supplies for anyone who has diabetes.
 	
  b. Discuss with the individual his or her specific BG goal, the frequency of BG monitoring, and the value of recording the results.
	6. BG monitoring assists individuals to control diabetes by regulating food, exercise, and medications, and has become an essential component of diabetes management. BG monitoring has allowed flexible mealtimes, made strenuous exercise safe, and made successful pregnancy outcomes more likely.
	  b. BG records help the individual and health care provider evaluate patterns of food intake, insulin administration, and exercise.

Interventions	Rationales
c. Teach the individual the need for increased BG monitoring when meals are delayed, before exercise, and when sick, as these situations may change dietary or insulin requirements.	
d. Assist the individual in identifying the brand, type, dosage, action, and side effects of prescribed medications for controlling diabetes.	d. An individual needs to know the dose, action, and side effects to make appropriate decisions for adjusting food intake and exercise.
e. Advise the individual about prescription drugs and over-the-counter remedies, such as cough syrups and throat lozenges that affect BG levels.	e. Oral agents, insulin, glucagon, aspirin, and beta–adrenergic blockers decrease blood glucose; whereas corticosteroids, birth control pills, diuretics, and cold remedies containing decongestants increase BG.

7. Teach the individual insulin administration and storage, including
  a. Measuring an accurate dose
  b. Mixing insulins
  c. Injecting insulin
  d. Rotating injection sites
  e. Refer the individual and family to a community diabetes education program, the local American Diabetes Association and registered dietitian for medical nutrition therapy (MNT).
  f. Continued monitoring and teaching at home will be needed after transition.	

8. Discuss strategies to improve nutrition:
  a. Provide information regarding food groups: carbohydrates (CHO) which includes starches, starchy vegetables, milk, and fruit, protein group, and vegetables group. Instruct on use of the "plate method" as easy way of meal planning and maintaining healthy nutrition.
  b. Show the individual and family a paper plate that is divided into quarter sections:
  • Fill ½ of plate with nonstarchy vegetables (lettuce, tomato, broccoli).
  • Fill ¼ with protein (meat, beans, fish, eggs).
  • Fill ¼ with starches (rice, potatoes, pasta, bread).
  • Add one cup of skim milk.
  • Add one piece of fruit.
  c. Teach the individual to lower fat intake by:
  • Trimming fat off meat
  • Avoiding fried foods
  • Limiting salad dressings, selecting low fat
  d. Advise the individual to:
  • Drink water. Limit diet soda, coffee, and tea. Avoid all sugar drinks (juice, soda, power drinks).
  • Eat breakfast every day (high-fiber cereal, low-fat milk)
  • Do not skip meals.
  • Make effort to eat same amount at each meal.
  • Avoid seconds.
  • Watch portion sizes.
	8. Balanced nutrition helps to maintain normal blood glucose level. The American Diabetes Association recommends an individualized meal plan based on individual assessment. The "plate method," carbohydrate counting, and portion control are easy and acceptable methods of meal planning. Low-fat foods, water as a beverage, and portion controls of CHO and protein can reduce weight and lower BG.

9. Encourage the individual to access self-management information at American Diabetes Association (www.diabetes.org), National Diabetes Education Program (www.ndep.nih.gov/diabetes), American Dietetic Association (www.eatright.org).	9. Proficiency in self-management: The many daily decisions the person with diabetes needs to make regarding medications, food, and activity is crucial due to the complexity and burden of the disease (Powers et al., 2015).

(continued)

Interventions	*Rationales*

10. Teach recognition of the signs and symptoms of hypoglycemia to the individual and family.
  a. Sweaty
  b. Tingling in hands, lips, and tongue
  c. Cold, clammy, and pale skin.
  d. Fast heartbeat, shakiness
  e. Uncooperative, irritable, confused
  f. Light-headed, dizzy
  g. Slurred speech
  h. Lack of motor coordination
  i. Seizure or coma/convulsions
	10. Early detection of hypoglycemia enables prompt intervention and may prevent serious complications. Insulin reaction, insulin shock, and hypoglycemia are all synonymous with low blood glucose (<70 mg/dL). Hypoglycemia may result from too much insulin, too little food, or too vigorous activity. Low BG may occur just before meal times, during or after exercise, and/or when insulin is at its peak action (American Diabetes Association, 2016).

> **CLINICAL ALERT:**
> • Hypoglycemia is sudden and can progress to seizures and loss of consciousness if untreated.

11. Teach the individual and family appropriate treatment for hypoglycemia using the "Rule of 15" to achieve BG goal of >100 mg/dL (American Diabetes Association, 2015).
  a. Take 15 g of carbohydrates (½ cup of juice, ½ cup regular soda, 3 teaspoon jelly, 1 cup milk, 3 glucose tablets, 5 Lifesavers candy).
  b. Wait 15 minutes, test BG again. Take another 15 g of carbohydrates if BG is still not at goal.
  c. Glucose gel, honey, jelly on the inside of the cheek are treatments of choice for a semiconscious person or someone having difficulty in swallowing.
  d. If hypoglycemia is severe, loss of consciousness, having seizures, or the individual cannot swallow, administer 1 mg of glucagon IM. Turn person onto side as treatment often causes nausea. If the individual does not respond, seek emergency assistance.
  e. After BG >100 mg/dL, individual may have a snack if not scheduled mealtime.
  f. Do not overtreat hypoglycemia with excessive carbohydrates.
	11. Prescription glucagon is an injectable treatment for severe hypoglycemia. Glucagon should be prescribed for all individuals at significant risk of severe hypoglycemia. The stability of glucagon is short; therefore, it must be mixed just before use. Because glucagon must be administered by another person, the individual's family or friends must be taught how to prepare and administer it in case of an emergency (American Diabetes Association, 2016).

12. Teach the individual to prevent hypoglycemia:
  a. Routine BG monitoring
  b. Schedule medications with meal times
  c. Schedule meals, never skip meals
  d. BG monitoring before exercise or strenuous activity
  e. Awareness of changes in daily routines that may precipitate hypoglycemia
  f. Carry some form of glucose at all times
  g. Never drink alcohol on an empty stomach (drink in moderation)
  h. Need to wear diabetes identification	

13. Teach the individual the importance of achieving and maintaining normal weight. Refer to the Obesity Care Plan for specific strategies.	13. An obese individual has fewer available insulin receptors. Weight loss restores the number of insulin receptors, making insulin more effective. Weight loss may also reduce or eliminate the need for oral agents (Grossman & Porth, 2014).

Interventions	Rationales

14. Teach the individual about Sick Day Treatment:
   a. Never fail to take diabetic medicine.
 	
   b. Monitor blood glucose every 3 to 4 hours. Test urine for ketones when two BG levels are >250 mg/dL (type 1).
   c. Drink 6 to 8 ounces of water each hour.
   d. Immediate interventions are required to prevent dehydration and severe hyperglycemia.
	14. Anticipating the effects of illness on the BG level may alert the individual to take precautions. Extra fluids help to prevent dehydration.
	   b. Early detection of ketones in urine can enable prompt intervention to prevent ketoacidosis. Individuals with type 1 diabetes are susceptible to ketosis (Grossman & Porth, 2014).

15. Call health care provider or seek emergency room care if:
   a. Vomiting or diarrhea persists for more than 6 hours
   b. Ketone values are moderate or large
   c. Fevers over 100 for >24 to 48 hours
   d. Blood glucose levels are over 250 mg/dL consistently
   e. You do not know what to do	

16. Teach the individual to take insulin or oral medications and maintain carbohydrate (CHO) intake when ill by substituting liquids or easily digested solids for regular food. Examples of CHO for sick days:
   a. Bread exchange = 15 g CHO
     • 1 slice bread or toast
     • ½ English muffin or ½ bagel (2 oz)
     • ½ cup cooked cereal
     • 6 saltines or 6 pretzels
     • 20 oyster crackers
   b. Fruit exchange = 15 g CHO
     • 1 cup Gatorade
     • ½ twin bar popsicle
     • ½ cup fruit juice
     • ½ cup unsweetened applesauce
     • ½ cup ginger ale or cola (not diet)
   c. CHO content of other foods
     • ½ cup regular Jello = 24 g
     • 2 level tsp. sugar = 8 g
	16. Illness often causes loss of appetite. Liquids or semi-soft foods may be substituted for the individual's normal diet. An individual on insulin therapy needs to maintain a consistent CHO intake that will supply glucose. When there is a lack of CHO, fats are used for energy. Ketones form from the metabolism of fat.

17. Explain the effects of exercise on glucose metabolism:
   a. Explain the benefits of regular exercise:
     • Improved fitness
     • Psychological benefits (e.g., enhanced ability to relax, increased self-confidence, and improved self-image)
     • Reduction of body fat
     • Weight control
	17. Emphasizing the benefits of exercise may help the individual to succeed with the prescribed exercise regimen.

18. Explain that the goal is to engage in a total of 30 minutes of moderate-intensity physical activity every day. For example, walk 10,000 steps in a day (usual is 4,000 to 6,000 steps). Wear a pedometer to monitor and motivate. Refer to thePoint to print out "Getting Started to Move More" or refer individual to www.walkinginfo.org.
   a. Instruct the individual to seek the advice of a health care provider before beginning an exercise program.
   b. Exercise may be contraindicated with certain complications (e.g., severe nephropathy, proliferative retinopathy).
   c. Teach the individual to avoid injecting insulin into a body part that is about to be exercised.
	18c. Insulin absorption increases in a body part that is exercised, which alters the insulin's absorption.

(continued)

Interventions	Rationales
d. Encourage the individual to exercise with others or where other informed persons are nearby, always wear diabetes identification, always carry a fast-acting CHO. e. Explain how to reduce serious hypoglycemic episodes related to exercise: • Monitor BG before and after exercise. • Exercise when BG level tends to be higher, such as shortly after a meal. • Always carry a source of fast-acting sugar for emergency.	d. Exercising with others ensures that assistance is available should hypoglycemia occur. e. Proper timing of exercise, monitoring BG, and adjusting food or insulin decreases the risk of exercise-induced hypoglycemia. In the event of a severe reaction, a semiconscious or unconscious individual may require glucagon (American Diabetes Association, 2016).
19. Explain the importance of foot care and risks to the feet: a. Teach the importance of daily foot inspection: make foot care a daily routine, visually inspect the bottom of feet and between toes looking for injury, reddened areas. b. Teach the individual to prevent foot problems: good fitting shoes, protective socks, never walk barefoot, good nail care, use of cream to prevent dry skin. c. Teach good nail care: trim toenails straight across, never cut too short, seek professional care for ingrown or thickened toenails. d. Never cut corns or calluses, gently use pumice stone or seek professional care.	19. Foot lesions result from peripheral neuropathy, vascular disease, and superimposed infection. Feet that are deformed, insensitive, and ischemic are prime targets for lesions and susceptible to trauma (Grossman & Porth, 2014)
20. Provide smoking cessation support. Refer to Getting Started to Quit Smoking on thePoint (printable to give to individual).	20. Diabetes makes the feet more prone to injury from decreased circulation. Daily inspections are vital to detect problems early. Injury can be reduced with proper shoes; proper nail trimming; attention to calluses, corns, and thickened nails; and avoiding extreme temperatures. Removing shoes and socks with each visit to a health care provider will remind the provider to examine the feet. Tobacco use will increase vasoconstriction and decrease circulation to the feet.
21. Teach to contact a health care provider when any of these occur: a. Unexplained fluctuations in BG b. A foot injury that does not show signs of healing in 24 hours c. Changes in vision d. Vomiting/diarrhea for more than 24 hours e. Signs of infection	
22. Provide informational materials and/or referrals that may assist the individual to reach goals: a. Comprehensive outpatient diabetes education b. Medical nutrition therapy c. Support groups d. Magazines for persons with diabetes (e.g., *Diabetes Forecast*, *Diabetes Self-Management*) e. American Diabetes Association (www.diabetes.org) f. American Association of Diabetes Educators (www.diabeteseducator.org)	22. An individual who feels well-supported can cope more effectively. A chronically ill person with multiple stressors needs to identify an effective support system. Knowing a friend or neighbor with diabetes, participating in a walk-a-thon for the American Diabetes Association, and reading about people successfully coping with diabetes are some helpful examples (Powers et al., 2015).

Interventions	Rationales

23. Ensure that supplies/prescriptions are provided as (American Diabetes Association, 2015):
  a. Insulin (vials or pens), if needed
    • Syringes or pen needles, if needed
  b. Oral medications, if needed
  c. Blood glucose meter and strips
  d. Lancets and lancing devices
    • Urine ketone strips (type 1 diabetes)
  e. Glucagon emergency kit (insulin treated individuals)
  f. Medical alert application/charms
	23. Information on medication changes, pending tests and studies, and follow-up needs must be accurately and promptly communicated to the primary care provider as soon as possible after transition (American Diabetes Association, 2015).

24. Ensure appointments have been scheduled for primary care provider, specialists, home nursing assessment, diagnostic tests as indicated.	24. Appointment-keeping behavior is enhanced when the inpatient team schedules outpatient medical follow-up prior to discharge. Ideally, the inpatient care providers or case managers/transition planners will schedule follow-up visit(s) with the appropriate professionals, including primary care provider, endocrinologist, and diabetes educator (American Diabetes Association, 2015).

Documentation

Individual/family teaching
Status at transition
Referrals

Pancreatitis

Pancreatitis can be acute or chronic. Acute pancreatitis can be precipitated by mechanical and/or metabolic causes. Mechanical causes are those that obstruct or damage the pancreatic duct system, such as cancer, cholelithiasis, abdominal trauma, radiation therapy, parasitic diseases, and duodenal disease. Metabolic causes are those that alter the secretory processes of the acinar cells, such as alcoholism, certain medications (mesalazine, azathioprine, simvastatin, sulfonamides, NSAIDs, corticosteroid, tetracycline), genetic disorders, and diabetic ketoacidosis. The most common cause is gallstones (Vege, 2015). Alcohol is responsible for 30% of cases of acute pancreatitis in the United States (Vege, 2014a). Though the overall mortality in all hospitalized individuals with acute pancreatitis is approximately 10% (range 2% to 22%), the mortality in the subset with severe acute pancreatitis may be as high as 30% (Vege, 2015). Chronic pancreatitis is a chronic, continuing inflammatory process of the pancreas with irreversible morphologic changes. Chronic pancreatitis is caused by excessive alcohol consumption (60%), hereditary pancreatitis (1%), idiopathic (unknown etiology) (30%), drug-induced (0.1% to 2%), and from blunt trauma or accidents (obstructive) (Huffman, 2015; Pezzilli, Corinaldesi, & Morselli-Labate, 2010; Zagaria, 2011). The prognosis for chronic pancreatitis is associated with age at diagnosis, smoking, continued use of alcohol, and the presence of liver cirrhosis.

■ ■ ■ DIAGNOSTIC CLUSTER

Collaborative Problems

▲ Risk for Complications of Hypovolemia/Shock

*   Risk for Complications of Acute Respiratory Distress Syndrome

*   Risk for Complications of Systemic Inflammatory Response Syndrome (SIRS)

*   Risk for Complications of Metabolic Instability

*   Risk for Complications of Alcohol Withdrawal (refer to Alcohol Abuse Care Plan)

Nursing Diagnoses

▲ Acute Pain related to nasogastric suction, distention of pancreatic capsule, and local peritonitis

▲ Ineffective Denial related to acknowledgment of alcohol abuse or dependency (refer to Alcohol Abuse Care Plan)

▲ Risk for Ineffective Self Health Management to insufficient knowledge of home care needed, treatments, early signs/symptoms of complications, dietary management, and follow-up care.

▲ This diagnosis was reported to be monitored for or managed frequently (75% to 100%).
* This diagnosis was not included in the validation study.

Transition Criteria

The individual or family will:

1. Explain the causes of the symptoms.
2. Describe signs and symptoms that must be reported to a health care professional.
3. Relate the importance of adhering to dietary restrictions and avoiding alcohol.
4. If alcohol abuse is present, admit to the problem.
5. Relate community resources available for treatment of alcohol abuse.

Transitional Risk Assessment Plan (TRAP)

Begin this plan on admission.
Implement the Transitional Risk Assessment Plan (TRAP):
• Refer to inside back cover.
• Add each validated risk diagnosis to individual's problem list with the risk code in ( ).
• Refer to Unit II to the individual risk nursing diagnoses/collaborative problems for outcomes and interventions.

> *R: "Close coordination of care in the post-acute period, early transition follow-up care, enhanced client education and self-management training, proactive end-of-life counseling, and extending the resources and clinical expertise over time via multidisciplinary team management" can lower readmission rates and improve health outcomes (Boutwell & Hwu, 2009, p. 14). Interventions are utilized to activate the individual and family to select changes in their everyday lifestyle choices to improve their health (Hibbard & Greene, 2013).*

Collaborative Problems

Risk for Complications of Hypovolemia/Shock

Risk for Complications of Acute Respiratory Distress Syndrome

Risk for Complications of Systemic Inflammatory Response Syndrome (SIRS)

Risk for Complications of Metabolic Instability

Risk for Complications of Alcohol Withdrawal

Collaborative Outcomes

The individual will be monitored for early signs and symptoms of (a) hypovolemia/shock, (b) acute respiratory distress syndrome, (c) systemic inflammatory response syndrome (SIRS), (d) metabolic complications, (e) alcohol withdrawal, and (g) hematologic complications, and will receive collaborative interventions if indicated to restore physiologic stability.

Indicators of Physiologic Stability

- Calm, alert (all)
- Cardiac: rhythm regular, rate 60 to 100 beats/min (a, b)
- BP >90/60, <140/90 mm Hg (a, b)
- Respiratory rate 16 to 20 breaths/min (a, b)
- Oxygen saturation (pulse oximeter) >96% (a, b, e)
- Capillary refill <3 seconds (a, b, c, e, f)
- Temperature 98° F to 99.5° F (c, e)
- pH 7.35 to 7.45 (a, b, c, e)
- Urine output >0.5 mL/kg/hr (a, b, c, e, f)
- Urine specific gravity 1.005 to 1.030 (f)
- Dry skin (a, b)
- No nausea or vomiting (c, e)
- White blood cells 4,300 to 10,800 mm^3 56 to 190 IV/L (c, e)
- Serum amylase alkaline phosphatase 30 to 85 mU/mL (c)
- Fasting serum glucose 70 to 115 mg/dL (c)
- Aspartate aminotransferase (AST) (c)
  - Male: 7 to 21 units/L
  - Female: 6 to 18 units/L
- Alanine aminotransferase 5 to 35 units/L (c)
- Lactate dehydrogenase (LDH) 100 to 225 units/L (c)
- Hematocrit (a, b, g)
  - Male: 42% to 52%
  - Female: 37% to 47%
- Serum calcium 8.5 to 10.5 mg/dL (c, f)
- Stool occult blood negative (g)
- Serum potassium 3.8 to 5 mEq/L (a, c, e)
- Serum creatinine 0.6 to 1.2 mg/dL (f)

Interventions	Rationales

CLINICAL ALERT:
- Several studies have concluded that older age is a predictor of a worse prognosis (Vege, 2014a). Individuals older than 75 years had more than a 15-fold greater chance of dying within 2 weeks and a more than 22-fold greater chance of dying within 91 days compared with individuals aged 35 years or younger (Vege, 2014a). Obesity is a risk factor for severe acute pancreatitis.

1. Monitor for signs and symptoms of hypovolemia and shock:

   a. Increasing pulse rate, normal or slightly decreased blood pressure
   b. Increasing respiratory rate
   c. Urine output >0.5 mL/kg/hr

1. Autodigestion of the pancreas results in increased capillary permeability, causing a plasma shift from the circulatory system to the peritoneal cavity. Hypovolemic shock can result. The compensatory response to decreased circulatory volume is to (Grossman & Porth, 2014):

   a,b. Increase heart and respiratory rates in an attempt to increase blood oxygen levels.

   c. Hypovolemia and hypotension activate the renin-angiotensin system; this results in increased renal vasculature resistance, which decreases renal plasma flow and glomerular filtration rate. Hourly urine output monitoring is essential for early detection.

(continued)

Interventions	Rationales
d. Restlessness, agitation, change in mentation	d. Diminish oxygen to the brain causes changes in mentation.
e. Diminished peripheral pulses f. Cool, pale, or cyanotic skin	e,f. Decrease circulation to the extremities, causing decreased pulse and cool skin.

2. Monitor for respiratory complications:
  a. Hypoxemia
  b. Atelectasis
  c. Pleural effusion
  d. Acute respiratory distress syndrome (ARDS)
	2. Death within the first several days of acute pancreatitis is attributed to cardiovascular instability or respiratory failure.

3. Monitor for SIRS. Evaluate the SIRS score using
 	
  a. The following criteria
    • Body temperature $>38°$ C or $<36°$ C
    • Heart rate >90/min
    • Respiratory rate >20/min or $Paco_2$ <32 mm Hg
    • White blood cell count $>12,000$/µL equal to or presence of 10% immature neutrophils
    Or
  b. New, Simpler Criteria to diagnosis sepsis are Glasgow Coma Scale (GCS) score of 13 or less, systolic blood pressure of 100 mm Hg or less, and respiratory rate of 22/min or more (1 point each; score range, 0 to 3) (Seymour et al., 2016).
    • Sepsis criteria $>$ SIRS +source of infection
    • Severe sepsis criteria (organ dysfunction, hypotension, or hypoperfusion)
    • Lactic acidosis, SBP <90 or SBP
    • Drop ≥ 40 mm Hg of normal
	3. SIRS has replaced the terminology *septic syndrome*. Sepsis is one contributing factor to SIRS, which is a life-threatening condition related to systemic inflammation, organ dysfunction, and organ failure. The SIRS score is determined by assigning 1 point for each vital sign measure listed. This SIRS is probably mediated by activated pancreatic enzymes (phospholipase, elastase, trypsin, etc.) and cytokines (tumor necrosis factor, platelet activating factor) released into the circulation from the inflamed pancreas (Vege, 2014b).
	a,b. A SIRS score of 0 or 1 indicates absence of SIRS. A SIRS score of 2 (mild), 3 (moderate), or 4 (severe) indicates the occurrence of SIRS.

4. Monitor for metabolic complications
  a. Hypokalemia:
  b. Hiccups
    • Polyuria
    • Polydipsia
	4. Pancreatic enzymes are high in potassium; losses into the peritoneal cavity may result in a potassium deficiency.
	    Hiccups may be related to phrenic nerve irritation resulting from subdiaphragmatic collection of purulent debris.

5. Monitor for hematologic complications:
  a. Thrombosis
  b. Disseminated intravascular coagulation (DIC)
	5. Early intravascular consumption of coagulation factors secondary to circulating pancreatic enzymes and vascular injury contribute to DIC (*Munoz & Katerndahl, 2000).

6. Monitor:
  a. Coagulation profiles
  b. Hemoglobin/hematocrit
  c. For hypoalbuminemia
    • Stool, urine, and GI drainage for occult blood
    • For ecchymosis (blackened bruises)
	6. Early detection of signs of bleeding or DIC can reduce morbidity/mortality.

7. Explain the use of nasogastric tube and suctioning.	7. Nasogastric suctioning is used to remove gastric juices, which, if present, will stimulate the release of secretions in the duodenum. These secretions, in turn, stimulate the pancreas to secrete enzymes.

Interventions	Rationales
8. Evaluate whether or not the individual abuses alcohol. Discuss with individual his/her drinking patterns (e.g., binging, daily drinking, amounts). Separately, question the family regarding the individual's alcohol intake.	8. Alcohol stimulates pancreatic secretions and can trigger excess production of hydrochloric acid, which causes spasms partial obstruction of the ampulla of Vater. This contributes to inflammation and the destruction of pancreatic cells (Grossman & Porth, 2014).
9. Monitor for early signs and symptoms of alcohol withdrawal: a. Agitation b. Tremors c. Diaphoresis d. Anorexia, nausea, vomiting e. Increased heart rate and respiratory rate **CLINICAL ALERT:** • Denial is a common defense mechanism for individuals who abuse alcohol and for their families (Halter, 2014; Varcarolis, 2011). If one suspects alcohol abuse, even when denied, monitor individual closely.	9. Because chronic alcohol abuse can cause pancreatitis, the nurse must be alert for the signs even when the individual denies alcoholism. Denial is a major coping mechanism for individuals and families. Signs of alcohol withdrawal begin 24 hours after the last drink and can continue for 1 to 2 weeks. Refer to Alcohol Withdrawal Care Plan for specifics.
10. Alert the physician/nurse practitioner when alcohol withdrawal is suspected.	10. Alcohol withdrawal often requires large doses of sedatives to prevent seizures.
11. Refer to collaborative problem index under thrombosis and DIC for specific monitoring criteria.	
12. If enteral feeding is initiated, refer to Enteral Feeding Care Plan.	12. Enteral nutrition is preferred over total parenteral nutrition because of less septic complications, surgical interventions, total hospitalization time, and decreased costs because of less septic complications (Ioannidis, Lavrentieva, & Botsios, 2008). Oral intake should not be resumed until abdominal pain subsides and serum amylase levels are normal.
13. If total parenteral nutrition (TPN) is used, refer to TPN Care Plan.	13. TPN may be needed if the person cannot tolerate enteral nutrition such as paralytic ileus.

 Clinical Alert Report

Advise ancillary staff/student to report:
- Any new change or deterioration diastolic in behavior (e.g., agitation, cognition)
- Any change in systolic BP >210 mm Hg, <90 mm Hg, and/or diastolic >90 mm Hg
- Resting pulse >120 or <55 beats/min
- Change in rate of respirations >28 or <10/min
- Changes or new onset of dyspnea/palpitations
- Decrease in urine output less than 0.5 mL/kg/hr
- Temperature >101° F oral

Nursing Diagnoses

Acute Pain Related to Nasogastric Suction, Distention of Pancreatic Capsule, and Local Peritonitis

NOC

Comfort Level, Pain
Control

Goal

The individual will relate satisfactory relief after pain-relief interventions.

NIC

Pain Management,
Medication
Management, Emotional
Support, Teaching:
Individual, Heat/Cold
Application, Simple
Massage

Indicators

- Relate factors that increase pain.
- Relate effective interventions.
- Rate pain level lower after measures.

Interventions	Rationales
1. Collaborate with individual to determine what methods could be used to reduce the pain's intensity.	1. Pain related to pancreatitis produces extreme discomfort in addition to increasing metabolic activity, with a corresponding increase in pancreatic secretory activity.
2. Discuss with the physician the use of analgesics such as meperidine, barbiturates, and fentanyl. Avoid the p.r.n. approach and morphine. a. For interventions to manage acute pain, refer to Acute Pain in Unit II.	2. These analgesics do not cause spasm of the Sphincter of Oddi (*Munoz & Katerndahl, 2000). A regular time schedule maintains a steady drug blood level.
3. Provide nasogastric tube care, if indicated: a. Explain why nasogastric tube is needed. b. Apply a water-soluble lubricant around the nares to prevent irritation. c. Monitor the nares for pressure points and signs of necrosis. Retape or reposition the tube when it gets detached or soiled. d. Provide frequent oral care with gargling; avoid alcohol-based mouthwashes that dry mucosa.	3. Removal of stomach fluids may be needed to control vomiting and pain. These interventions can reduce some discomfort associated with nasogastric tube use.
4. Explain the need for bed rest.	4. Bed rest decreases metabolism, reduces gastric secretions, and allows available energy to be used for healing.
5. Position the individual sitting upright in bed with knees and spine flexed.	5. This position relieves tension on the abdominal muscles.
6. When the individual is NPO, avoid all exposure to food (e.g., sight and smell).	6. The sight and smell of food can cause pancreatic stimulation.
7. Nutritionally, the person may (Lutz et al., 2015) a. Have nothing by mouth (IV, enteral feedings) b. Clear fluids c. Soft to low-fat diet over 3 to 4 days as tolerated	7. This avoids stimulating the pancreas, which will reduce pain and inflammation. Can be initiated when pain has been controlled for 24 hours. The person's progress (e.g., pain, nausea) will be evaluated.

Ineffective Denial Related to Acknowledgment of Alcohol Abuse or Dependency

NOC

Anxiety Level, Coping, Social Support, Substance Addiction Consequences, Knowledge: Substance Abuse Control, Knowledge: Disease Process

Goal

The individual will acknowledge an alcohol/drug abuse problem.

NIC

Coping Enhancement, Anxiety Reduction, Counseling, Mutual Goal Setting, Substance Abuse Treatment, Support System Enhancement, Support Group

Indicators

- Explain the physiologic effects of alcohol or drug use.
- Elicit the negative effects of alcoholism on family unit, jobs, legal issues.
- Report an intent to participate in drug/alcohol treatment program. Abstain from alcohol/drug use.

Interventions	Rationales
1. Approach nonjudgmentally. Some causes of pancreatitis are not alcohol-related, about 30%. Be aware of your own feelings regarding alcoholism. Refer to Care Plan on Alcohol Abuse.	1. The probably has been reprimanded by many and is distrustful. The nurse's personal experiences with alcohol may increase or decrease empathy for the individual.

> **TRANSITION TO HOME/COMMUNITY CARE**
> If indicated, review the risk diagnoses identified for this individual on admission:
> - Is the person still at risk?
> - Can the family reduce the risks?
> - Is the person at higher risk at home?
> - Is a home health nurse assessment needed?
> - Refer to transition planner/case manager/social service.
> - When is this person scheduled for follow-up with primary provider? Specialists? Record dates of appointments.
> - Complete a medication reconciliation prior to transition. Refer to index.

STAR   **Stop**

Think   Is this person at risk for injury, falls, medical complications, and/or inability to care for self (activities of daily living)?
    Is there a support person available?
    Is the person competent to manage self-administration of medications, treatment procedures?
    Are additional resources needed?
    Can the person explain how to monitor condition (e.g., blood glucose, sign/symptoms of complications, dietary/mobility restrictions, and when to call his or her primary provider or specialist)?

Act   Use SBAR to notify the appropriate professional.

SBAR   *Situation:* Mr. Smith will be scheduled to be transitioned to his home.

Backgound: Mr. Smith lives alone. He (state his disabilities, self-care needs, treatments)

Action: A more thorough reevaluation of where he can be transitioned is needed.

Recommendation: Referral to social service/transition planner/case manager

Review   Is the response/solution the right option for the individual? If not, seek discuss the situation with the appropriate person, department, and/or agency (using SBAR).

Risk for Ineffective Health Management Related to Lack of Knowledge of Disease Process, Treatments, Contraindications, Dietary Management, and Follow-Up Care

NOC

Compliance Behavior, Knowledge: Treatment Regimen, Participation in Health Care Decisions, Treatment Behavior: Illness or Injury

NIC

Health Education, Health System Guidance, Learning Facilitation, Learning Readiness Enhancement, Risk Identification, Self-Modification Assistance

Goals

The goals for this diagnosis represent those associated with transition planning. Refer to the transition criteria.

Interventions	Rationales
1. Explain the causes of acute and chronic pancreatitis. **CLINICAL ALERT:** • "Cessation of alcohol consumption and tobacco smoking are important. In early stage alcohol-induced chronic pancreatitis, lasting pain relief can occur after abstinence from alcohol, but in advanced stages, abstinence does not always lead to symptomatic improvement. Patients continuing to abuse alcohol develop either marked physical impairment or have a death rate 3 times higher than do patients who abstain" (Huffman, 2015).	1. Inaccurate perceptions of health status usually involve misunderstanding the nature and seriousness of the illness, susceptibility to complications, and need to modify behaviors that may exacerbate the natural history of the disease
2. Explain the risks of alcohol use and tobacco use: a. Alcohol and its metabolites produce changes in the acinar cells, which may promote premature intracellular digestive enzyme activation thereby predisposing the gland to auto-digestive injury.	2. Current smokers with ≥20 pack-years of smoking had a fourfold higher risk than never-smokers. Elevated risk for non–gallstone-related pancreatitis in former smokers persisted 20 years after smoking cessation in those who drank ≥400 g monthly but only 10 years in those who drank less (Sadr-Azodi, Andrén-Sandberg, Orsini, & Wolk, 2012).
3. During hospitalization, focus on the individual's readiness to quit, and clarify misinformation. Ask the individual: a. How alcohol smoking has affected their health? b. Have they ever tried to quit? c. How long did they stop? d. Do they want to quit?	3. People who are in hospital because of a smoking-related illness are likely to be more receptive to help to give up smoking (Rigotti, Clair, Munafò, & Stead, 2012). Focusing the discussion on the person's experiences and perceptions may provide insight into assisting the person to quit tobacco and/or alcohol.

 Carp's Cues

More deaths are caused by cigarette smoking than by all deaths from HIV, illegal drug use, alcohol use, motor vehicle accidents, suicide, and murders combined (CDC, 2015b).

Interventions	Rationales
4. Discuss with prescribing professional the addition of nicotine replacement therapy (transdermal patch, gum, spray).	4. A Cochrane review reported that adding nicotine replacement therapy (NRT) to an intensive counseling intervention increased smoking cessation rates compared with intensive counseling alone (Rigotti et al., 2012).
5. Refer to Getting Started to Quit Smoking on thePoint.	
6. Teach report early these worsening of symptoms: a. Clay-colored stools b. Increase in pain in upper left side, mid-abdominal and/or radiating to back c. Persistent gastritis, nausea, or vomiting d. Weight loss e. Elevated temperature	6. These symptoms can indicate worsening of inflammation and increased malabsorption. An elevated temperature could indicate infection or abscess formation. Early reporting can ensure immediate attention and possibly prevention of readmission.
7. Explain the need to monitor BS at home. Teach use of glucometer. Advise to contact primary provider if BS are above 200 in a.m., p.m., or more than 2 hours after eating.	7. Pancreatitis can decrease insulin production, causing hyperglycemia.
8. Ensure a consult with nutrition specialist. Reinforce with printed dietary recommendations: low-fiber diet, high protein, moderate low fat (Dudek, 2014). a. Pureed vegetable soups, steamed vegetables; avoid raw vegetables b. Lean cuts of meat, preferably filets of chicken, turkey, rabbit and veal, only steaming or poaching, absolutely no frying or grilling c. Fish, especially cold-water varieties d. Eggs should supplement any diet for chronic pancreatitis. e. Organic dairy products (e.g., low-fat yogurt, cheese, kefir). These should be introduced slowly and after 2 to 3 weeks of a recent attack. f. A good breakfast, oatmeal has a smooth consistency and coats the stomach. g. Water and herbal teas are great sources of hydration and should be preferred over strong coffee, tea, carbonated, and alcoholic beverages. h. Oil from olive, grapeseed, and flax seed can be added into your salads, soups, or side dishes right before serving. i. Fruits initially baked or steamed. When recovered, slowly introduce raw fruits.	8. Intake of incorrect foods can exacerbate pancreatitis and cause exacerbation and the need for readmission. a. Antioxidants/vitamins/minerals that are easily absorbed are needed for healing. Raw vegetables require too many enzymes to process rough fiber and thus can cause pain. b. They are low in fat and high in proteins, iron, zinc, and essential amino acids to maintain good health. c. Refer to a, b. d. They are great sources of protein and amino acids and gentle on the digestive system. e. These contain high doses of active probiotic cultures that will help normalize your digestion. f. Oatmeal provides B vitamins and other nutrients. g. Great sources of hydration and nonirritating to the GI tract as coffee, tea, carbonated, and alcoholic beverages h. Omega 3 and Omega 6 fatty acids and make them easy to digest by your pancreas. i. High-fiber foods need to be introduced slowly to prevent GI irritation.
9. Initiate referrals as indicated; a. Substance abuse programs, Alcoholics Anonymous b. Practical smoking cessation guidelines are available at http://www.cdc.gov/tobacco/campaign/tips/quit-smoking/?gclid=CKSN26non8sCFYE9gQodwg0Leg; http://www.lung.org/stop-smoking/i-want-to-quit/how-to-quit-smoking.html?referrer=https://www.google.com/	

(continued)

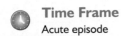

GASTROINTESTINAL DISORDERS

Gastroenterocolitis/Enterocolitis

Most cases of acute infectious gastroenteritis are viral, with norovirus being the most common cause of acute gastroenteritis and the second most common cause of hospitalization for acute gastroenteritis. Other common pathogens causing viral gastroenteritis are rotavirus, enteric adenovirus, and astrovirus. Consumption of contaminated food and water, noroviruses are efficiently spread person-to-person and are responsible for large outbreaks (Alexandraki & Smetana, 2015).

An infectious agent (bacterial or viral) can cause inflammation of the lining of the stomach, gastroenterocolitis small intestine, and large intestine (enterocolitis). Parasites can also cause a gastroenteritis attack. Enterocolitis causes cramps and diarrhea, whereas gastroenterocolitis produces nausea, vomiting, diarrhea, and cramps. Hospitalization is indicated with severe fluid and electrolyte imbalances or for risk individuals (older adults, individuals with diabetes, or with compromised immune systems).

Time Frame
Acute episode

■■■■■ DIAGNOSTIC CLUSTER**

Collaborative Problems

Risk for Complications of Fluid/Electrolyte Imbalance

Nursing Diagnoses

Risk for Deficient Fluid Volume related to losses secondary to vomiting and diarrhea (refer to Unit II nursing diagnosis Risk for Deficient Fluid Volume)

Acute Pain related to abdominal cramping, diarrhea, and vomiting secondary to vascular dilatation and hyperperistalsis (refer to Unit II nursing diagnosis Nausea)

Risk for Ineffective Health Management related to lack of knowledge of condition, dietary restrictions, and signs and symptoms of complications

**This medical condition was not included in the validation study.

Transition Criteria

Before transition, the individual or family will

1. Describe the causes of gastroenteritis and its transmission.
2. Identify dietary restrictions that promote comfort and healing.
3. State signs and symptoms of dehydration.
4. State signs and symptoms that must be reported to a health care professional.

> ### Transitional Risk Assessment Plan (TRAP)
>
> Begin this plan on admission.
> Implement the Transitional Risk Assessment Plan (TRAP):
> * Refer to inside back cover.
> * Add each validated risk diagnosis to individual's problem list with the risk code in ( ).
> * Refer to Unit II to the individual risk nursing diagnoses/collaborative problems for outcomes and interventions.
>
> *R: "Close coordination of care in the post-acute period, early transition follow-up care, enhanced client education and self-management training, proactive end-of-life counseling, and extending the resources and clinical expertise over time via multidisciplinary team management" can lower readmission rates and improve health outcomes (Boutwell & Hwu, 2009, p. 14). Interventions are utilized to activate the individual and family to select changes in their everyday lifestyle choices to improve their health (Hibbard & Greene, 2013).*

Collaborative Problems

Risk for Complications of Fluid/Electrolyte Imbalance

Collaborative Outcomes

The individual will be monitored for early signs and symptoms of fluid/electrolyte imbalance and will receive collaborative interventions if indicated to restore physiologic stability.

Indicators of Physiologic Stability

* Urine output >0.5 mL/kg/hr (a, b)
* Urine specific gravity 1.005 to 1.030 (a)
* Moist skin/mucous membranes (a)
* Serum sodium 135 to 145 mEq/L (b)
* Serum potassium 3.8 to 5 mEq/L (b)
* Serum chloride 95 to 105 mEq/L (b)

Interventions	Rationales

1. Monitor for signs and symptoms of dehydration:
  a. Dry skin and mucous membrane
  b. Elevated urine specific gravity
  c. Thirst
	1. Rapid propulsion of feces through the intestines decreases water absorption. Low circulatory volume causes dry mucous membranes and thirst. Concentrated urine has an elevated specific gravity (Alexandraki & Smetana, 2015).

2. Carefully monitor intake and output	2. Intake and output records help to detect early signs of fluid imbalance.
3. Monitor for electrolyte imbalances of sodium, chloride, potassium.	3. Rapid propulsion of feces through the intestines decreases electrolyte absorption. Vomiting also causes electrolyte loss.
4. Monitor for Bloody stool/rectal bleeding	4. Stool studies should be obtained in the following situations: Adults presenting with persistent fever, dehydration, blood or pus in the stool, or other alarm symptoms and signs, and when there is clinical suspicion of a nonviral, inflammatory etiology of acute gastroenteritis (Alexandraki & Smetana, 2015).

Clinical Alert Report

Prior to providing care, advise ancillary staff/student to report the following to the professional nurse assigned to the individual:

- Temperature >37.8° C (100° F)
- Resting pulse >100, <50 beats/min
- Systolic BP >200 mm Hg or <9 mm Hg
- Diastolic BP >90
- Complaints of abdominal pain/tenderness
- Urine output for shift or hourly if indicated

Documentation

Intake and output
Stools (amount, consistency)

TRANSITION TO HOME/COMMUNITY CARE

If indicated, review the risk diagnoses identified for this individual on admission:

- Is the person still at risk?
- Can the family reduce the risks?
- Is the person at higher risk at home?
- Is a home health nurse assessment needed?
- Refer to transition planner/case manager/social service.
- When is this person scheduled for follow-up with primary provider? Specialists? Record dates of appointments.
- Complete a medication reconciliation prior to transition. Refer to index.

STAR

Stop

Think Is this person at risk for injury, falls, medical complications, and/or inability to care for self (activities of daily living)?

Is there a support person available?

Is the person competent to manage self-administration of medications, treatment procedures?

Are additional resources needed?

Can the person explain how to monitor condition (e.g., blood glucose, sign/symptoms of complications, dietary/mobility restrictions) and when to call his or her primary provider or specialist?

Act Contact or provide the appropriate resource (e.g., contacting a support person, home health assessment, additional teaching, printed materials).

Review Has the problem been addressed? If not, use SBAR to communicate to the appropriate person.

Risk for Ineffective Health Regimen Management Related to Lack of Knowledge of Condition and transmission precautions, Dietary Restrictions, and Signs and Symptoms of Complications

NOC

Compliance Behavior, Knowledge: Treatment Regimen, Participation in Health Care Decisions, Treatment Behavior: Illness or Injury

NIC

Health Education, Health System Guidance, Learning Facilitation, Learning Readiness Enhancement, Risk Identification, Self-Modification Assistance

Goal

The goals for this diagnosis represent those associated with transition planning. Refer to the transition criteria.

Interventions	Rationales
1. Discuss the disease process in understandable terms; explain the following: a. Causative agents b. Reason for enteric precautions c. Prevention of transmission	1. The individual's understanding may increase compliance with dietary restrictions and hygiene practices.
2. Avoid anti-inflammatory drugs (e.g., NSAIDs). Advise to use acetaminophen for aches/pains if needed unless contraindicated.	2. NSAIDs can cause gastric irritation.
3. Provide fluids often and in small amounts so that the urge to urinate occurs every 2 hours: a. Broths, noncarbonated soft drinks, sports drinks, caffeine-free soft drinks b. Electrolyte-supplemented drink	3. Certain beverages replace sodium and potassium lost in diarrhea and vomiting without irritating the GI tract (Graves, 2013).
4. Explain dietary restrictions: a. High-fiber foods (e.g., bran, fresh fruit) b. High-fat foods (e.g., whole milk, fried foods) c. Very hot or cold fluids d. Caffeine e. High carbohydrate foods	4. These foods can stimulate or irritate the intestinal tract.
5. Instruct on dietary options: a. Rice b. Toast, crackers c. Bananas d. Tea e. Applesauce (not juice)	5. Foods with complex carbohydrates facilitate fluid absorption into the intestinal mucosa.
6. Encourage frequent intake of small amounts of cool clear liquids (e.g., dilute tea, flat ginger ale, Jell-O, water): 30 to 60 mL every ½ to 1 hour. a. Foods to avoid with all age groups include caffeine; fatty foods; spicy foods; sharp foods such as seeds, nuts, and chips; sugary foods and desserts; carbonated drinks; fruit juices; and alcohol (Graves, 2013).	6. Diet is a large portion of acute gastroenteritis treatment. The goal is to aid in individual comfort while maintaining hydration and nutrition (Graves, 2013). a. Small amounts of fluids do not distend the gastric area, and thus do not aggravate the symptoms.

Interventions	Rationales
7. Eliminate unpleasant sights and odors from the individual's environment.	7. Unpleasant sights or odors can stimulate the vomiting center.
8. Instruct the individual to avoid hot or cold liquids, foods containing fat or fiber (e.g., milk, fruits), caffeine.	8. Cold liquids can induce cramping; hot liquids can stimulate peristalsis. Fats also increase peristalsis, and caffeine increases intestinal motility.
9. Protect the perianal area from irritation with petroleum cream, barrier creams.	9. Frequent stools of increased acidity can irritate perianal skin.
10. Explain the benefits of rest and encourage adequate rest.	10. Inactivity reduces peristalsis and allows the GI tract to rest.
11. Explain preventive measures (Graves, 2013): a. Proper food storage/refrigeration b. Proper cleaning of kitchen utensils especially wooden cutting boards. • Disinfect surfaces at home with ½ cup of bleach to 1 gallon of water. Apply the solution to surfaces and let it dry for 5 minutes. Rinse thoroughly and allow it to air-dry. Clean eating utensils and thermometers with products that contain alcohol, or use dishwasher for eating utensils and dishes. c. Proper cleaning of bathroom d. Hand-washing before and after handling food	11a. The most common cause of gastroenteritis is ingestion of bacteria-contaminated food (Graves, 2013). The spread of bacteria and viruses can be controlled by disinfecting surface areas (bathrooms). Disinfectants with antibacterial properties are effective against some bacteria and viruses. d. The transmission of getting or spreading viral gastroenteritis can be reduced by washing hands thoroughly with soap and warm water for 20 seconds after using the bathroom or changing diapers and before eating or handling food.
12. Advise to call primary care provider if the following occurs: a. Severe volume depletion/dehydration • Dry mucous membranes (lips, gums) • Dark colored urine • Continued weight loss • Severe abdominal pain • Prolonged symptoms (more than 1 week)	12. Early detection and reporting of the signs of dehydration enable prompt interventions to prevent serious fluid or electrolyte imbalances. These signs/symptoms indicate the need for an immediate evaluation.

Documentation

Transition instructions
Status at transition

Inflammatory Bowel Syndrome

Irritable bowel syndrome (IBS) is a condition that affects the function and behavior of the intestines. Normally, the muscles lining the intestines intermittently contract and relax to move food along the digestive tract. In IBS, this pattern is disturbed, resulting in uncomfortable symptoms. More than 40 million people are affected by IBS. It is important to remember that individuals with inflammatory bowel diseases (IBD) can also have IBS.

IBD are a group of inflammatory conditions in which the body's own immune system attacks parts of the digestive system. The two most common inflammatory bowel diseases are Crohn's disease (CD) and ulcerative colitis (UC).

The pathogenesis of IBS appears to be multifactorial. There is evidence to show that the following factors play a central role in the pathogenesis of IBS: heritability and genetics, environment and social learning, dietary or intestinal microbiota, low-grade inflammation, and disturbances in the neuroendocrine system (NES) of the gut (El-Salhy et al., 2010; Peppercorn & Cheifetz, 2015).

IBS is a generic term comprising both Crohn's disease and ulcerative colitis. Both are inflammatory conditions of the gastrointestinal (GI) tract and have similar clinical presentations. IBS is a chronic, relapsing, and often life-long disorder. It is characterized by the presence of abdominal pain or discomfort, which may be associated with defecation and/or accompanied by a change in bowel habit. Symptoms may include disordered defecation (constipation or diarrhea or both) and abdominal distension, usually referred to as bloating. Symptoms sometimes overlap with other GI disorders such as nonnuclear dyspepsia or celiac disease.

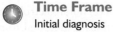 **Time Frame**
Initial diagnosis
Recurrent acute episodes

■■■■DIAGNOSTIC CLUSTER

Collaborative Problems

▲ Risk for Complications of Fluid/Electrolyte Imbalances

▲ Risk for Complications of GI Bleeding

▲ Chronic Pain related to intestinal inflammatory process (refer to Unit II nursing diagnosis Chronic Pain)

Nursing Diagnoses

▲ Chronic Pain related to intestinal inflammatory process (refer to Unit II nursing diagnosis Chronic Pain))

▲ Imbalanced Nutrition related to dietary restrictions, nausea, diarrhea, and abdominal cramping associated with eating or painful ulcers of the oral mucous membrane

▲ Diarrhea related to intestinal inflammatory process (refer to Unit II nursing diagnosis Diarrhea)

Δ Risk for Ineffective Coping related to chronicity of condition and lack of definitive treatment (refer to Unit II nursing diagnosis Ineffective Coping)

▲ Risk for Ineffective Health Management related to lack of knowledge of condition, diagnostic tests, prognosis, treatment, and signs and symptoms of complications

Related Care Plan

Corticosteroid Therapy

▲ This diagnosis was reported to be monitored for or managed frequently (75% to 100%).
Δ This diagnosis was reported to be monitored for or managed often (50% to 74%).

Transition Criteria

Before transition, the individual or family will:

1. Discuss management of activities of daily living.
2. State signs and symptoms that must be reported to a health care professional.
3. Verbalize an intent to share feelings and concerns related to IBS with significant others.
4. Identify available community resources or self-help groups.

Collaborative Problems

Risk for Complications of Fluid/Electrolyte Imbalances

Risk for Complications of GI Bleeding

Risk for Complications of Anemia

Collaborative Outcomes

The individual will be monitored for early signs and symptoms of (a) fluid/electrolyte imbalances, (b) GI bleeding, and (c) anemia, and will receive collaborative interventions if indicated to restore physiologic stability.

Indicators of Physiologic Stability

- Temperature 98° F to 99.5° F
- Respiratory rate 16 to 20 breaths/min (a, b)
- Normal breath sounds, no adventitious sounds (a, b)
- Pulse 60 to 100 beats/min (a)
- Blood pressure >90/60, <140/90 mm Hg
- No nausea or vomiting
- Urine output >0.5 mL/kg/hr (a)
- Urine specific gravity within range
- Red blood cells (c)
  - Male 4.6 to 5.9 million/mm^3
  - Female 4.2 to 5.4 million/mm^3
- Serum potassium 3.5 to 5.0 mEq/L (a)
- Creatinine clearance (a)
  - Male 95 to 135 mL/mm
  - Female 85 to 125 mL/mm
- Bowel sounds present in all quadrants
- Stool occult blood negative
- No abdominal pain
- Hemoglobin (b, c)
  - Males 13.18 g/dL
  - Females 12.16 g/dL
- No rectal pain

Carp's Cues

IBS is a GI disorder characterized by chronic abdominal pain and altered bowel habits in the absence of any organic cause. It is the most commonly diagnosed GI condition and accounts for approximately 30% of all referrals to gastroenterologists (Wald, 2014).

IBS is a common functional bowel disorder characterized by abdominal pain or discomfort and associated with such alterations in bowel patterns as diarrhea, constipation, or both. Other supportive signs and symptoms may include hard, lumpy, loose, or watery stools; bloating; passing mucus; straining to defecate; bowel urgency; and the feeling of incomplete bowel evacuation. The condition is nearly 50% more common among women than men.

Per the extensive, international work of the Rome Foundation, The Rome III Classification System of Functional Gastro-Intestinal Disorder, IBS can be diagnosed 6 months after symptom onset in individuals who, on at least 3 days/month for the past 3 months, have experienced recurrent abdominal pain or discomfort and at least two of the following (Anastasi, Capili, & Chang, 2013):

- Pain improvement with defecation
- Change in stool frequency at onset
- Change in stool form or appearance at onset

More recent studies have considered the role of inflammation, alterations in fecal flora, and bacterial overgrowth. Also being considered is the role of food sensitivity. Whether a genetic predisposition exists is also being investigated (Wald, 2014). "Because no single drug effectively relieves all IBS symptoms, management relies on dietary and lifestyle modifications, as well as pharmacologic and nonpharmacologic therapies" (Anastasi et al., 2013).

Interventions	*Rationales*

> **CLINICAL ALERT:**
> • There has been and currently is a belief by health care professionals that IBS is caused by psychological factors. The historical difficulty of explaining the pathophysiology of IBS has contributed to these misconceptions. "IBS client are offered non effective treatments, are treated with mistrust and neglect by health care professionals, feel that they are labeled as hypochondriacs and believe that they receive no support from society. It could be expected that IBS clients would be more anxious and depressed."

1. Clarify the following (*Drossman, 2006a, b; Wald, 2014): a. Epidemiologic studies show that IBS aggregates in families, suggesting a genetic component to the disorder. b. An international group of experts have formalized Diagnostic Criteria for Functional Gastrointestinal Disorders. c. These disorders have genetics, psychosocial, and physiologic contributing factors.	1. Researchers have reported that quality of life improved after participants anticipated in a health program of reassurance, diet management, probiotics, and regular exercise (El-Salhy et al., 2010).
2. Explain the effects of an impaired neuroendocrine system (NES) of the gut as disturbances in digestion, GI motility, and visceral hypersensitivity (Wald, 2014). a. Changes the motility of bowels (how fast food moves through the system) b. Affects how much fluid, such as mucus, is secreted in intestines c. Affects how sensitive the intestines are to sensations like pain and fullness	2. Low levels of serotonin appear to contribute to symptom development and may play a central role in the pathogenesis of IBS. Genetic differences have been found between IBS individuals and healthy subjects in genes controlling the serotonin signaling system and CCK.
3. Monitor laboratory values for electrolyte imbalances.	3. Chronic diarrhea and inadequate oral intake can deplete electrolytes. Small intestine inflammation impairs absorption of fluid and electrolytes (Grossman & Porth, 2014).
4. Monitor for signs and symptoms of dehydration: a. Tachycardia b. Dry skin/mucous membrane c. Elevated urine specific gravity d. Thirst	4. When circulating volume decreases, heart rate increases in an attempt to supply tissues with oxygen. Low circulatory volume causes dry mucous membranes and thirst. Concentrated urine has an elevated specific gravity (Grossman & Porth, 2014).
5. Monitor for signs and symptoms of GI bleeding: a. Decreased hemoglobin and hematocrit b. Fatigue c. Irritability d. Pallor e. Tachycardia f. Dyspnea g. Anorexia Refer to Unit II Collaborative Problems—Risk for Complications of GI Bleeding	5. Chronic inflammation can cause erosion of vessels and bleeding.

Interventions	*Rationales*

6. Monitor for signs of anemia:
  a. Decreased hemoglobin
  b. Decreased red blood cells
  c. B_{12} deficiency
  d. Folate deficiency
	6. Anemia may result from GI bleeding, bone marrow depression (associated with chronic inflammatory diseases), and inadequate intake or impaired absorption of vitamin B_{12}, folic acid, and iron. Sulfasalazine therapy can cause hemolysis, which contributes to anemia

Clinical Alert Report

Prior to providing care, advise ancillary staff/student to report the following to the professional nurse assigned to the individual:

- Immediately: severe abdominal pain, abdominal swelling, tenderness, nausea, vomiting, fever
- Change in cognitive status
- Oral temperature >100.5° F
- Systolic BP <90 mm Hg
- Resting pulse >100, <50 beats/min
- Respiratory rate >28, <10/min
- Oxygen saturation <90%
- Occult testing results
- Streaks of blood in stool

Documentation

Vital signs
Intake and output
Bowel sounds
Diarrhea episodes
Vomiting episodes
Drainage (wound, rectal, vaginal)
Urine specific gravity

Nursing Diagnoses

Imbalanced Nutrition Related to Dietary Restrictions, Nausea, Diarrhea, and Abdominal Cramping Associated with Eating or Painful Ulcers of the Oral Mucous Membrane

Carp's Cues

"Most clients with IBS believe diet plays a significant role in their symptoms and 63% were interested in knowing what food to avoid. It has been shown that the IBS clients have nonspecific diet intolerance. This lack of specificity causes considerable difficulty for IBS clients in choosing their diets" (El-Salhy et al., 2010).

NOC

Nutritional Status, Teaching: Nutrition

Goal

The individual will have positive nitrogen balance as evidenced by weight gain of 2 to 3 lb/week.

NIC

Nutrition Management, Nutritional Monitoring

Indicators

- Verbalize understanding of nutritional requirements
- List foods to avoid

Interventions	Rationales
1. Ensure a nutritional consult	1. Nutritional therapy is the cornerstone of treatment of IBS.
2. Discuss the importance of fiber intake on constipation-predominant IBS symptoms (Hsiu-Feng et al., 2011): a. Hastens oral-anal transit time, decreases the whole gut transition time, holds water to prevent excess dehydration of stool, and adds bulk to the stool that may relieve the GI symptom of constipation (Anderson et al., 2009). b. Decreases intracolonic pressure either by direct effect or by binding bile salts that can reduce visceral pain caused by colon wall tension. 3. Determine the individual's usual fiber intake.	2,3. In one study fiber intake found in the individuals with IBS was similar to the general population in the United States. The 2000 National Health Interview Survey found that the mean dietary fiber intake was 19.2 g/day for men and 14.4 g/day for women (*Thompson et al., 2005). Both IBS individuals as well as the general population, however, consume less than the recommended daily amount of fiber (25 to 30 g) (American Dietetic Association [ADA], 2008). Studies have confirmed that there is a beneficial effect in increasing fiber and fluid intake for constipation-predominant individuals with IBS (Hsiu-Feng et al., 2011).
4. Advise the individual to alert staff/student if there are beverages or food on tray that are irritating.	4. Individuals with IBS are the best resources for foods/beverages that need to be avoided.
5. Assist with progression to soft, bland, and low-residue solids and encourage small frequent feedings high in calories, protein, vitamins, and carbohydrates.	5. Gradual introduction of solid foods is needed to reduce pain and increase tolerance.
6. Ensure vitamin D levels are determined.	6. Vitamin D deficiency is highly prevalent in individuals with IBS and these results seem to have therapeutic implications. Vitamin D supplementation could play a therapeutic role in the control of IBS.

Documentation

Type and amount of food taken orally
Daily weight

Diarrhea Related to Intestinal Inflammatory Process

NOC
Bowel Elimination, Electrolyte & Acid/Base Balance, Fluid Balance, Hydration, Symptom Control

Goal

The individual will report less diarrhea.

NIC
Bowel Management, Diarrhea Management, Fluid/Electrolyte Management, Nutrition Management, Enteral Tube Feeding

Indicators

- Describe factors that cause diarrhea
- Explain the rationales for interventions
- Have fewer episodes of diarrhea
- Verbalize signs and symptoms of dehydration and electrolyte imbalances

Interventions	Rationales
1. Assess stools for frequency, consistency, characteristics, presence of pain, urgency.	1. Stool assessment helps to evaluate the effectiveness of antidiarrheal agents and their relationship to intake.
2. Ensure good perianal care.	2. Perianal irritation from frequent liquid stool should be prevented.
3. Decrease physical activity during acute episodes of diarrhea.	3. Decreased physical activity decreases bowel peristalsis.
4. Determine the relationship between diarrheal episodes and ingestion of specific foods.	4. Identification of irritating foods can reduce diarrheal episodes.
5. Observe for signs and symptoms of electrolyte imbalance: a. Decreased serum potassium b. Decreased serum sodium	5. In osmotic diarrhea, impaired fluid absorption by the intestines is caused by ingested solutes that cannot be digested or by a decrease in intestinal absorption. Water and electrolytes are drawn into the intestine in greater quantities than can be absorbed, and the diarrheal fluid is high in potassium (Grossman & Porth, 2014). Secretory diarrhea occurs when the gut wall is inflamed or engorged or when it is stimulated by bile salts. The resulting diarrheal stool is high in sodium.
6. Replace fluid and electrolytes with oral fluid containing appropriate electrolytes: a. Gatorade, a commercial preparation of glucose-electrolyte solution b. Apple juice, which is high in potassium but low in sodium c. Colas, root beer, and ginger ale that contain sodium but negligible potassium. De-fizz with a pinch of sugar or salt.	6. The type of fluid replacement depends on the electrolyte(s) needed.
7. Encourage the use of probiotics. Advise to consult with physician/nurse practitioner/physical assistant regarding the use of probiotics.	7. Probiotics alter colonic fermentation and stabilize the colonic microbiota. Several studies on probiotics have shown improvements in flatulence and abdominal distension (El-Salhy et al., 2010; Spiller & Garsed, 2009).

Documentation

Intake and output
Number of stools
Consistency of stools

Risk for Ineffective Coping Related to Chronicity of Condition and Lack of Definitive Treatment

NOC
Coping, Self-Esteem, Social Interaction Skills

Goal

The individual will make appropriate decisions to cope with condition.

NIC
Coping Enhancement, Counseling, Emotional Support, Active Listening, Assertiveness Training, Behavior Modification

Indicators

- Verbalize factors that contribute to anxiety and stress
- Verbalize methods to improve the ability to cope with the chronic condition

Interventions	*Rationales*

CLINICAL ALERT:
- Halpert and Godena (2011) conducted a qualitative study, which revealed that a major concern of individuals with IBS is related to being heard and receiving empathy. Some responses of participants were "I need more empathy and listening from my HCP about how much IBS affects my life" (27%), "Nothing my HCP does helps my IBS" (25%), "My HCP has been helpful and reassuring" (17%), and "My HCP thinks I'm crazy" (8%) (Halpert & Godena, 2011).

Interventions	*Rationales*
1. Elicit from individual the effects of IBS on daily activities and life.	1. Researchers have reported individuals with IBS "would give up 25% of their remaining life (average 15 years) and 14% would risk a 1/1,000 chance of death to receive a treatment that would make them symptom free" (El-Salhy et al., 2010).
2. Clear up misconceptions about IBS. Stress that psychological symptoms are a component of IBS.	2. A Cochrane Review found that psychological therapies, including cognitive behavioral therapy (CBT), psychotherapy, and hypnotherapy, and in combination with other therapies were found to be beneficial in reducing global symptoms of IBS (Zijdenbos et al., 2009).
3. Explain comprehensive self-management (CSM) strategies of diet adjustments (composition, trigger foods, meal size or timing, and eating behaviors), relaxation (specific relaxation strategies and lifestyle behaviors), and psychological therapies, including CBT, psychotherapy, and hypnotherapy, engaging in alternative thoughts (identifying thought distortions, challenging underlying beliefs, and other strategies) (Zia, Barney, Cain, Jarrett, & Heitkemper, 2016).	3. A CSM program that combines CBT with relaxation and dietary strategies included nine sessions (1 hour each) over 13 weeks were shown to reduce GI symptoms and increase quality of life (Zia et al., 2016).
4. Emphasize that after 13 weeks the strategies reported to be most frequently used were "specific relaxation strategies" (95%), "diet composition" (90%), and "identify thought distortions" (90%) (Zia et al., 2016).	4. Selecting these strategies affirms that self-help strategies did improve physiologic outcomes (Zia et al., 2016).
5. Discuss with family members or significant others their impressions of IBS. Clarify misconceptions.	5. Family members and others play a very important role in supporting individuals and helping them to cope with and accept their disease.
6. Refer to the Irritable Bowel Syndrome Association at http://www.ibsgroup.org/ibsassociation.	6. Discussing IBS with others with the same problem can reduce feelings of isolation and anxiety. Sharing experiences in a group led by professionals gives the individual the benefit of others' experiences with IBS and the interpretation of those experiences by health care professionals.

Documentation

Participation in self-care
Emotional status

TRANSITION TO HOME/COMMUNITY CARE

If indicated, review the risk diagnoses identified for this individual on admission:

* Is the person still at risk?
* Can the family reduce the risks?
* Is the person at higher risk at home?
* Is a home health nurse assessment needed?
* Refer to transition planner/case manager/social service.
* When is this person scheduled for follow-up with primary provider? Specialists? Record dates of appointments.
* Complete a medication reconciliation prior to transition. Refer to index.

STAR

Stop

Think Is this person at risk for injury, falls, medical complications, and/or inability to care for self (activities of daily living)?

Is there a support person available?

Is the person competent to manage self-administration of medications, treatment procedures?

Are additional resources needed?

Can the person explain how to monitor condition (e.g., blood glucose, sign/symptoms of complications, dietary/mobility restrictions) and when to call his or her primary provider or specialist?

Act Contact or provide the appropriate resource (e.g., contacting a support person, home health assessment, additional teaching, printed materials).

Review Has the problem been addressed? If not, use SBAR to communicate to the appropriate person.

Risk for Ineffective Health Management Related to Lack of Knowledge of Condition, Diagnostic Tests, Prognosis, Treatment, and Signs and Symptoms of Complications

NOC

Compliance Behavior, Knowledge: Treatment Regimen, Participation in Health Care Decisions, Treatment Behavior: Illness or Injury

Goal

The goals for this diagnosis represent those associated with transition planning. Refer to the transition criteria.

NIC

Health Education, Health System Guidance, Learning Facilitation, Learning Readiness Enhancement, Risk Identification, Self-Modification Assistance

Interventions	Rationales
1. Assure the individual that even though the pathology of IBS is not well understood. It is a credible disorder with international criteria for diagnosis. Acknowledge the reality of their symptoms. **CLINICAL ALERT:** • IBS symptoms frequently have a frightful impact on self-esteem, relationships work, social activities, quality of life, and health care resource utilization. Individuals with IBS consistently report increased absences from school and work, limitations in social activities, and the need to make lifestyle modifications.	1. Researchers have reported that quality of life improved after participants participated in a health program of reassurance, diet management, probiotics, and regular exercise (El-Salhy et al., 2010).
2. Explain the ROME	2. An individual with IBS may have been led to believe that anxiety or psychological problems caused the disorder. Dispelling this belief can help the individual to accept the disorder and encourage compliance with treatment.
3. Explain the familial aspects of IBS	3. Although the cause of IBS is unknown, 15% to 35% of individuals with IBS have a relative with the disorder; thus, it is considered a familial disorder (Saito, 2011; Turner, 2010).

4. Discuss the symptomatic treatment of IBS
  a. Medications
  b. Diet (refer to the nursing diagnosis Altered Nutrition in this care plan)	

5. Advise to:
  a. Eat smaller meals more frequently.
 	
  b. Stress the need to have optimal water intake daily. Advise to monitor hydration by urine color.
  c. Slowly increase fiber intake with fiber-rich foods or supplements.
 	
  d. Consider taking a supplement.
	5a. Avoiding three meals a day can help reduce the strength of contractions in your intestines.
	  b. The lighter the urine, the more hydrated. Adequate hydration is also needed to prevent constipation.
	  c. Fiber helps to keep stool soft but does not lower pain. Gradual introduction may help to reduce the risk of increased gas and bloating.
	  d. Supplemental fiber usually causes less gas than getting fiber through your diet. Consult with PCP if indicated and take your supplement with plenty of water.

6. Determine if the following cause symptoms and should be avoided:
  a. Caffeine in coffee, cola beverages, and tea; nicotine in tobacco
  b. Alcohol
	6. They are muscle stimulants that may have severe effects on hypersensitive bowel muscles.
	    Liquor and other alcoholic beverages are proven gastric irritants and often contribute to symptoms of IBS.

7. Instruct to keep a food diary in a small notebook:
  a. What you eat
  b. When you eat it
  c. How you are feeling when you eat it
  d. Occurrence of any symptoms and their intensity
	7. A food diary will help the person understand what types of food/fluids exacerbate symptoms.

Interventions	Rationales
8. Teach measures to preserve perianal skin integrity: a. Use soft toilet tissue. b. Cleanse area with mild soap after bowel movements. c. Apply a protective ointment (e.g., A&D, Desitin, Sween Cream).	8. These measures can help prevent skin erosion from diarrheal irritation.
9. Teach the individual to report the following signs and symptoms: a. Increasing abdominal pain or distention b. Persistent vomiting c. Unusual rectal or vaginal drainage or rectal pain d. Continued amber urine	9. Early reporting enables prompt intervention to reduce the severity of complications. a. Increasing abdominal pain or distention may indicate obstruction or peritonitis. b. Persistent vomiting may point to obstruction. c. Unusual drainage or rectal pain may indicate abscesses or fistulas. d. Amber urine indicates dehydration.
10. Provide information on available community resources (e.g., self-help groups, counseling) and individual education material on how to live with IBS.	10. Communicating with others with IBS may help the individual to cope better with the disorder's effect on his or her lifestyle.

Documentation

Individual/family teaching
Status at transition
Referrals, if indicated

Peptic Ulcer Disease

A peptic ulcer is a defect in the gastric or duodenal mucosa that extends through the muscularis mucosa (thin layer of muscle of the GI tract) into the deeper layers of the wall. Peptic ulcers may present with dyspeptic or other GI symptoms, or may be asymptomatic and present with complications such as hemorrhage or perforation (Vaki, 2015b). Approximately 80% of individuals, with endoscopically diagnosed ulcers, have epigastric pain (Barkun & Leontiadis, 2010). "The 'classic' pain of duodenal ulcers occurs two to five hours after a meal when acid is secreted in the absence of a food buffer and at night (between about 11 PM and 2 AM) when the circadian stimulation of acid secretion is maximal" (Vakil, 2015a).

It is now evident that the epidemiology of peptic ulcer disease largely reflects environmental factors, primarily *Helicobacter pylori* infection, nonsteroidal anti-inflammatory drug (NSAID) use, and smoking (Vakil, 2014).

Time Frame
Initial diagnosis
Recurrent acute episodes

▪▪▪▪▪DIAGNOSTIC CLUSTER

Collaborative Problems

▲ Risk for Complications of Stress-Related Mucosal Disease (SRMD)

▲ Risk for Complications of Hemorrhage

△ Risk for Complications of Perforation

Nursing Diagnoses

▲ Acute/Chronic Pain related to lesions secondary to increased gastric secretions (refer to Acute Pain)

Δ Risk for Ineffective Therapeutic Regimen Management related to lack of knowledge of disease process, contraindications, signs and symptoms of complications, and treatment regimen

▲ This diagnosis was reported to be monitored for or managed frequently (75% to 100%).
Δ This diagnosis was reported to be monitored for or managed often (50% to 74%).

Transition Criteria

Before transitions, the individual or family will:

1. Identify the causes of disease symptoms.
2. Identify lifestyle changes that are needed to prevent ulcers
3. Identify necessary adjustments to prevent ulcer formation.
4. State signs and symptoms that must be reported to a health care professional.
5. Relate community resources that can provide assistance with lifestyle modifications.

Transitional Risk Assessment Plan (TRAP)

Begin this plan on admission.
Implement the Transitional Risk Assessment Plan (TRAP):

* Refer to inside back cover.
* Add each validated risk diagnosis to individual's problem list with the risk code in ( ).
* Refer to Unit II to the individual risk nursing diagnoses/collaborative problems for outcomes and interventions.

  R: "Close coordination of care in the post-acute period, early transition follow-up care, enhanced client education and self-management training, proactive end-of-life counseling, and extending the resources and clinical expertise over time via multidisciplinary team management" can lower readmission rates and improve health outcomes (Boutwell & Hwu, 2009, p. 14). Interventions are utilized to activate the individual and family to select changes in their everyday lifestyle choices to improve their health (Hibbard & Greene, 2013).

Collaborative Problems

Risk for Complications of Stress-Related Mucosal Disease (SRMD)

Risk for Complications of Hemorrhage

Risk for Complications of Perforation

Collaborative Outcomes

The individual will be monitored for early signs and symptoms of hemorrhage perforation and stress-related mucosal disease and will receive collaborative interventions if indicated to restore physiologic stability.

Indicators of Physiologic Stability

* Heart rate 60 to 100 beats/min, rhythm regular
* Respiratory rate 16 to 20 breaths/min
* BP >90/60, <40/90 mm Hg
* Urinary output >0.5 mL/kg/hr
* No abdominal pain
* Alert, oriented, calm
* Capillary refill <3 seconds
* Gastric pH 3.5 to 5.0
* Gastric aspirates negative for occult blood

Interventions   *Rationales*

> **CLINICAL ALERT:**
> Vakil (2015a) reported:
>
> Approximately 70 percent of peptic ulcers are
> asymptomatic. Individuals with silent peptic
> ulcers may later present with ulcer-related
> complications. Between 43 and 87 percent of
> individuals with bleeding peptic ulcers present
> without antecedent dyspepsia or other heralding
> GI symptoms. Older adults and individuals on
> NSAIDs are more likely to be asymptomatic and
> later present with ulcer complications.

1. Identify individuals at risk for stress ulcers
   a. Critically ill
   b. Respiratory failure requiring mechanical ventilation for more than 48 hours[6]
   c. Coagulopathies (international normalized ratio >1.5 or platelet count <50,000 mm^3)[6]
   d. Acute renal insufficiency
   e. Acute hepatic failure
   f. Sepsis syndrome
   g. Hypotension
   h. Thermal injury involving more than 35% of the body surface area
   i. Severe head or spinal cord injury
   j. Anticoagulation
   k. History of GI bleeding
   l. Low intragastric pH
   m. Major surgery (lasting more than 4 hours)
   n. Administration of high-dose corticosteroids (250 mg/day of steroids or equivalent hydrocortisone)
   o. Enteral feedings

1a. Stress-related mucosal disease (SRMD) is the broad term used to describe the spectrum of pathology attributed to the acute, erosive, inflammatory insult to the upper GI tract associated with critical illness.

2. Monitor for occult bleeding in gastric aspirates and bowel movements.

2. Frequent and careful assessment can help diagnose clinically important bleeding before the individual's status is compromised.

3. Monitor for signs and symptoms of hemorrhage and report promptly:
   a. Hematemesis
   b. Dizziness
   c. Generalized weakness
   d. Melena
   e. Increasing pulse rate with normal or slightly decreased blood pressure
   f. Urine output <0.5 mL/hr
   g. Restlessness, agitation, change in mentation
   h. Increasing respiratory rate
   i. Diminished peripheral pulses
   j. Cool, pale, or cyanotic skin
   k. Thirst

3. Signs and symptoms of hemorrhage may present gradually, or may have a sudden onset. The mortality rate due to ulcer hemorrhage is approximately 5% over the last 20 years (Plummer, Blaser, & Deane, 2014)

---

[6]Independent risk factors for bleeding.

Interventions	Rationales
4. Monitor for gastric ulcer perforation (Vakil, 2015b) Sudden, severe, diffuse abdominal pain.	4. Perforations complicate 2% to 10% of individuals with peptic ulcer diseases. The pain typically becomes more intense, of longer duration, and is frequently referred to the lower thoracic or upper lumbar spine region. Penetrating posterior ulcers classically present with a shift from the typical vague visceral discomfort to a more localized and intense pain that is felt in the back and is not relieved by food or antacids. This change in symptom pattern may be gradual or sudden.

CLINICAL ALERT:
- Call Rapid Response Team if there is a sudden onset of the above symptoms.

Clinical Alert Report

Prior to providing care, advise ancillary staff/student to report the following to the professional nurse assigned to the individual:
- Report immediately: severe abdominal pain, abdominal swelling, tenderness, nausea, vomiting, fever
- Change in cognitive status
- Oral temperature >100.5° F
- Systolic BP <90 mm Hg
- Resting pulse >100, <50 beats/min
- Respiratory rate >28, <10/min
- Oxygen saturation <90%
- Occult testing results
- Streaks of blood in stool

Documentation

Vital signs
Intake and output
Weight
Gastric pH
Stool characteristics
Bowel sounds
Unusual events

Nursing Diagnoses

TRANSITION TO HOME/COMMUNITY CARE

If indicated, review the risk diagnoses identified for this individual on admission:
- Is the person still at risk?
- Can the family reduce the risks?
- Is the person at higher risk at home?
- Is a home health nurse assessment needed?
- Refer to transition planner/case manager/social service.
- When is this person scheduled for follow-up with primary provider? Specialists? Record dates of appointments.
- Complete a medication reconciliation prior to transition. Refer to index.

STAR   **Stop**

              Think   Is this person at risk for injury, falls, medical complications, and/or inability to care for self (activities of
                          daily living)?
                                  Is there a support person available?
                                  Is the person competent to manage self-administration of medications, treatment procedures?
                                  Are additional resources needed?
                                  Can the person explain how to monitor condition (e.g., blood glucose, sign/symptoms of complica-
                                  tions, dietary/mobility restrictions) and when to call his or her primary provider or specialist?

                Act   Contact or provide the appropriate resource (e.g., contacting a support person, home health assessment,
                          additional teaching, printed materials).

             Review   Has the problem been addressed? If not, use SBAR to communicate to the appropriate person.

Risk for Ineffective Health Management Related to Lack of Knowledge of Disease Process, Contraindications, Signs and Symptoms of Complications, and Treatment Regimen

NOC

Compliance Behavior,
Knowledge: Treatment
Regimen, Participation
in Health Care
Decisions, Treatment
Behavior: Illness

Goal

The goals for this diagnosis represent those associated with transition planning. Refer to transition criteria.

NIC

Health Education,
Health System
Guidance, Learning
Facilitation, Learning
Readiness Enhancement,
Risk Identification, Self-
Modification Assistance

Interventions	Rationales
1. Explain the pathophysiology of peptic ulcer disease, using terminology and media appropriate to the individual's and family's levels of understanding. a. Ask individual that foods/beverages increase their discomfort?	1. Understanding helps to reinforce the need for restrictions and may improve engagement.
2. Advise the individual to eat regularly and to avoid bedtime snacks.	2. Although frequently advised in the past, there is no evidence that dietary manipulations, such as a bland diet, enhance healing. During the day, regular amounts of food particles in the stomach help to neutralize the acidity of gastric secretions. Bedtime snacks stimulate nocturnal acid secretion.
3. Explain the risks of NSAIDs (e.g., ibuprofen [Motrin, Aleve, Relafen]) and low-dose aspirin. Discuss with primary care provider what agents can be used for pain (e.g., arthritis, headaches).	3. Peptic ulcer disease (PUD) is associated with two major factors: *Helicobacter pylori* infection; and the consumption of NSAIDs. The older the person the more risk for gastric ulcers with NSAIDs and aspirin use (Vakil, 2014).

Interventions	Rationales
4. Explain the effects of smoking on the GI tract by inhibiting factors that protect or heal the lining, including (Vakil, 2014): a. Blood flow to the lining b. Secretion of mucus, a clear liquid that protects the lining from acid c. Decrease in pancreatic secretion of bicarbonate; this increases duodenal acidity	4. Smoking does increase the production of other substances that may harm the lining, such as pepsin, an enzyme made in the stomach that breaks down proteins.
5. Avoid foods/beverages that increase discomfort.	5. There is no evidence that dietary intake, or moderate intake of caffeine or alcohol causes peptic ulcers (Lutz, Mazur, & Litch, 2015).
6. If the individual is being transitioned on antacid therapy, teach the following (Arcangelo & Peterson, 2016): a. Chew tablets well and follow with a glass of water to enhance absorption. b. Lie down for ½ hour after meals to delay gastric emptying. c. Take antacids 1 hour after meals to counteract the gastric acid stimulated by eating.	6. Proper self-administration of antacids can enhance their efficacy and minimize side effects.
7. If on therapy for *Helicobacter pylori*, explain triple therapy: PPI (e.g., *lansoprazole* 30 mg twice daily, *omeprazole* 20 mg twice daily, *pantoprazole* 40 mg twice daily, *rabeprazole* 20 mg twice daily, or *esomeprazole* 40 mg once daily); Amoxicillin, (1 g twice daily); *Clarithromycin* (500 mg twice daily) for 7 to 14 days. We suggest treatment for 10 days to 2 weeks. a. The need to be on therapy for prescribed number of days b. The need to take all three types of medication c. Possible side effects and the need to call primary care provider with concerns before discontinuing treatment prior to completion	7. Recommended treatment duration is 10 days to 2 weeks. Triple therapy for 2 weeks eradicates *H. pylori* at an 80% rate (Crowe, 2015).
8. Discuss the importance of continued treatment, even in the absence of overt symptoms.	8. Continued therapy is necessary to prevent recurrence or development of another ulcer.
9. Instruct to watch for and report these symptoms: a. Red or black stools b. Persistent epigastric pain c. Constipation (not resolved) d. Unexplained temperature elevation e. Persistent nausea f. Vomiting g. Unexplained weight loss h. Call 911 if the following occurs: • Develop sudden, sharp abdominal pain • Have a rigid, hard abdomen that is tender to touch • Have symptoms of shock such as fainting, excessive sweating, or confusion • Vomit blood or have blood in your stool (especially if it is maroon or dark, tarry black)	

(*continued*)

Interventions	Rationales

> **CLINICAL ALERT:**
> • Explain that these signs and symptoms may point to complications such as peritonitis, perforation. Early detection and emergency treatment is needed:
>   • Change in cognitive status
>   • Oral temperature >100.5° F
>   • Systolic BP <90 mm Hg
>   • Resting pulse >100, <50 beats/min
>   • Respiratory rate >28, <10/min
>   • Oxygen saturation <90%

10. Refer to community resources, if indicated (e.g., smoking cessation program, stress management class).

10. The individual may need assistance with lifestyle changes after transition.

Documentation

Individual/family teaching
Referrals

RENAL AND URINARY TRACT DISORDERS

Acute Kidney Injury

Acute kidney injury (AKI) is a syndrome characterized by an abrupt deterioration of renal function, resulting in the accumulation of metabolic wastes, fluids, and electrolytes, and usually accompanied by a marked decline in urinary output. AKI is one of the few types of total organ failure that may be reversible if the underlying cause is corrected. Although AKI has many causes, ischemia and toxicity are the most common. Depending on where the problem originates, ischemia and toxicity also determine if AKI is prerenal, intrarenal, or postrenal (Fallone & Cotton, 2015).

Prerenal AKI occurs when decreased blood flow to the kidneys causes ischemia of the nephrons. Blood loss, severe dehydration, septicemia, and cardiogenic shock are common underlying causes of prerenal AKI. *Intrarenal AKI* is associated with damage to the renal parenchyma. Prerenal AKI can trigger the problem, but a major cause of intrinsic AKI and AKI in general is acute tubular necrosis (damage to the renal tubules caused by ischemia or toxins). *Postrenal AKI* occurs as a result of conditions that block urine flow, causing it to back up into the kidneys. Prostatic hypertrophy, urethral obstruction (usually bilateral), and bladder outlet obstruction are common causes of postrenal AKI (Fallone & Cotton, 2015).

 Time Frame
Initial diagnosis (post intensive care)
Recurrent acute episodes

■■■ DIAGNOSTIC CLUSTER

Collaborative Problems

▲ Risk for Complications of Fluid Overload

▲ Risk for Complications of Metabolic Acidosis

▲ Risk for Complications of Electrolyte Imbalances

* Risk for Complications of Acute Albuminemia

* Risk for Complications of Hypertension

* Risk for Complications of Pulmonary Edema

* Risk for Complications of Arrhythmias

* Risk for Complications of Gastrointestinal Bleeding

Nursing Diagnoses

▲ Risk for Infection related to invasive procedure (refer to Unit II)

Δ Imbalanced Nutrition related to anorexia, nausea, vomiting, loss of taste, loss of smell, stomatitis, and unpalatable diet (refer to Chronic Kidney Disease Care Plan)

Related Care Plans

Hemodialysis or Peritoneal Dialysis

Chronic Kidney Disease

▲ This diagnosis was reported to be monitored for or managed frequently (75% to 100%).

Δ This diagnosis was reported to be monitored for or managed often (50% to 74%).

* This diagnosis was not included in the validation study.

Transition Criteria

The individual or family will:

1. Relate the intent to comply with agreed-on restrictions and follow-up
2. State signs and symptoms that must be reported to a health care professional
3. Identify how to reduce the risk of infection

Transitional Risk Assessment Plan (TRAP)

Begin this plan on admission.

Implement the Transitional Risk Assessment Plan (TRAP):

- Refer to inside back cover.
- Add each validated risk diagnosis to individual's problem list with the risk code in ( ).
- Refer to Unit II to the individual risk nursing diagnoses/collaborative problems for outcomes and interventions.

R: "Close coordination of care in the post-acute period, early transition follow-up care, enhanced client education and self-management training, proactive end-of-life counseling, and extending the resources and clinical expertise over time via multidisciplinary team management" can lower readmission rates and improve health outcomes (Boutwell & Hwu, 2009, p. 14). Interventions are utilized to activate the individual and family to select changes in their everyday lifestyle choices to improve their health (Hibbard & Greene, 2013).

Collaborative Problems

Risk for Complications of Fluid Overload

Risk for Complications of Metabolic Acidosis

Risk for Complications of Electrolyte Imbalances

Risk for Complications of Hypertension

Risk for Complications of Pulmonary Edema

Risk for Complications of Arrhythmias

Risk for Complications of Decreased Level of Consciousness (to Coma)

Risk for Complications of Gastrointestinal Bleeding

Collaborative Outcomes

The individual will be monitored for early signs and symptoms of (a) fluid overload, (b) metabolic acidosis, (c) electrolyte imbalances, (d) hypertension, (e) pulmonary edema, (f) arrhythmias, (g) decreased level of consciousness, and (h) gastrointestinal bleeding, and the individual will receive collaborative interventions if indicated to restore physiologic stability.

Indicators of Physiologic Stability

- Alert, calm, oriented (a, c, g)
- No seizure activity (b, c, g)
- BP >90/60, <140/90 mm Hg (a, d, e)
- Respirations relaxed and rhythmic (a, e); 16 to 20 breaths/min (a, e, f, g)
- Pulse 60 to 100 beats/min; regular rate and rhythm (a, e, f, g)
- EKG normal sinus rhythm (b, c, f)
- Flat neck veins, no edema (pedal, sacral, periorbital) (a)
- Usual or desired weight (a)
- Skin warm, dry, usual color (a, e, f, g, h)
- Bowel sounds all quadrants (c)
- Intact strength, no complaints of numbness/tingling in fingers or toes, no muscle cramps (b, c)
- Serum albumin 3.5 to 5 g/dL (b, c)
- Serum prealbumin 1 to 3 g/dL (b, c)
- Serum sodium 135 to 145 mEq/L (b, c)
- Serum potassium 3.8 to 5 mEq/L (b, c)
- Serum calcium 8.5 to 10.5 mg/dL (b, c)
- Serum phosphates 3 to 5 mg/dL (b, c)
- Blood urea nitrogen 10 to 20 mg/dL (b)
- Creatinine 0.5 to 1.2 mg/dL (men in the slightly higher range) (b)
- Alkaline phosphate 30 to 150 International Units/mL (b)
- Creatinine clearance 100 to 150 mL/min (a, b)
- Oxygen saturation (Sao_2) >94% (a, e, g)
- Carbon dioxide ($Paco_2$) 35 to 45 mm Hg (a)
- Urine output >0.5 mL/kg/hr (a, h)
- Urine specific gravity 1.005 to 1.030 (a)
- Normal stool formation, stool negative for hemoglobin (h)
- No vomitus positive for hemoglobin (h)

Interventions	Rationales

1. Monitor for signs of fluid overload:
  a. Weight gain (1 kg = 1 L)
  b. Increased blood pressure and pulse rate, neck vein distention
  c. Dependent edema (periorbital, pedal, pretibial, sacral)
  d. Adventitious breath sounds (e.g., wheezes, crackles)
  e. Urine specific gravity <1.010
	1. The oliguric phase of acute kidney failure usually lasts from 5 to 15 days and often is associated with excess fluid volume retention. Functionally, the changes result in decreased glomerular filtration, tubular transport of substances, urine formation, and renal clearance (Fallone & Cotton, 2015).

2. Weigh the individual daily. (Weigh more often, if indicated.) Ensure accuracy by weighing at the same time every day on the same scale and with the individual wearing the same amount of clothing.	2. Weighing the individual daily can help to determine fluid balance and appropriate fluid intake (Fallone & Cotton, 2015).
3. Maintain strict intake and output records. Include all fluid loss—urine, vomit, diarrhea, wound, and nasogastric drainage. Include all fluid intake—oral, intravenous, and nasogastric. Consider all sensible and insensible losses when calculating replacement fluids. Adjust the individual's fluid intake so it approximates fluid loss plus 300 to 500 mL/day. Compare with daily weight loss or gain for correlation of fluid balance.	3. A 1-kg weight gain should correlate with excess intake of 1 L (1 L of fluid weighs 1 kg, or 2.2 lb). Insensible losses include respirations and perspiration. Careful replacement can prevent fluid overload or deficit.

Interventions	*Rationales*
4. Manage fluids: a. Administer oral medications with meals whenever possible. If medications must be administered between meals, give with the smallest amount of fluid necessary. b. Avoid continuous IV fluid infusion whenever possible. Dilute all necessary IV drugs in the smallest amount of fluid safe for IV administration. c. Engage in discussions about fluid management goals and strategies. 　• Encourage their input, questions, and suggestions. 　• Provide ongoing clinical updates. 　• Allow time for the individual to express feelings. 　• Give her or him positive feedback. d. The individual's and family's understanding of the need for fluid management can help gain their cooperation and lessen feelings of uncertainty or frustration. e. Consult with dietitian regarding fluid plan and overall diet.	4a. This prevents the fluid allowance from being used up unnecessarily. b. A small IV bag or an infusion pump will avoid accidental infusion of a large volume of fluid. c. The individual's and family's understanding of the need for fluid management can help gain their cooperation and lessen feelings of uncertainty or frustration. d. Toxins can accumulate with decreased fluid and cause nausea and sensorium changes. It may be necessary to match fluid intake with loss every 8 hours or even every hour if the individual is critically imbalanced. e. Fluid content of nonliquid food, amount and type of liquids, liquid preferences, and sodium content are all important in fluid management. Nutritional needs will change as kidney function improves or declines. Dietitians assist in calculating caloric, protein, electrolyte, lipid, and micronutrient requirements (Fallone & Cotton, 2015).
5. Monitor for signs and symptoms of metabolic acidosis: a. Rapid, shallow respiration b. Headache c. Nausea and vomiting d. Low plasma bicarbonate e. Low arterial blood pH (<7.35) f. Behavior changes, drowsiness, and lethargy **CLINICAL ALERT:** • Metabolic acidosis with a blood pH less than 7.2 can result in life-threatening vasodilation, cardiac arrhythmias, and hyperkalemia. Emergent treatment with medications and possible dialysis needs to be initiated (Fallone & Cotton, 2015).	5. Acidosis results from the kidney's inability to excrete hydrogen ions, phosphates, sulfates, and ketone bodies. Bicarbonates are lost when the kidney reduces its reabsorption. Hyperkalemia, hyperphosphatemia, and decreased bicarbonate levels aggravate metabolic acidosis. Excessive ketone bodies cause headaches, nausea, vomiting, and abdominal pain. Increases in respiratory rate and depth enhance CO_2 excretion and reduce acidosis. Acidosis affects the central nervous system (CNS) and can increase neuromuscular irritability because of the cellular exchange of hydrogen and potassium (Fallone & Cotton, 2015).
6. Ensure sufficient caloric intake and nutritional balance by consulting a dietitian for appropriate diet of adequate carbohydrate, fat, and protein intake.	6. Fats provide 9 kcal/g and protein and carbohydrates provide 4 kcal/g. Renal insufficiency and uremia alter metabolism of these nutrients so adjustments will be needed based on cause and degree of AKI (Fallone & Cotton, 2015).
7. Assess for signs and symptoms of hypocalcemia, hypokalemia, and alkalosis as acidosis is corrected.	7. Rapid correction of acidosis may cause rapid excretion of calcium and potassium and rebound alkalosis.

Interventions	*Rationales*

8. Monitor for signs and symptoms of hypernatremia with fluid overload:
  a. Thirst
  b. CNS effects ranging from agitation to convulsions
  c. Edema, weight gain
  d. Hypertension
  e. Tachycardia
  f. Dyspnea
  g. Rales
	8. Hypernatremia results from excessive sodium intake or increased aldosterone output. Water is pulled from the cells, which causes cellular dehydration and produces CNS symptoms. Thirst is a compensatory response to dilute sodium (Axley, 2015).

9. Maintain sodium restriction	9. Hypernatremia must be corrected slowly to minimize CNS deterioration (Axley, 2015).

10. Monitor for signs and symptoms of hyponatremia:
  a. CNS effects ranging from lethargy to coma
  b. Weakness
  c. Abdominal pain
  d. Muscle twitching or convulsions
  e. Nausea, vomiting, and diarrhea
	10. Hyponatremia results from sodium loss through vomiting, diarrhea, or diuretic therapy; dilution from excessive fluid intake or excessive hypotonic IV fluid; or insufficient dietary sodium. Cellular edema, caused by osmosis, produces cerebral edema, weakness, and muscle cramps (Axley, 2015).

11. Monitor for signs and symptoms of hyperkalemia:
  a. Anxiety
  b. Weakness to paralysis
  c. Muscle irritability
  d. Paresthesias
  e. Nausea, abdominal cramping, or diarrhea
  f. Irregular pulse
  g. Electrocardiogram (ECG) changes: tall, tented T-waves, ST segment depression, prolonged PR interval (>0.2 second), first-degree heart block, bradycardia, broadening the ORS complex, eventual ventricular fibrillation, and cardiac standstill.
	11. Hyperkalemia results from the kidney's decreased ability to excrete potassium or from excess intake of potassium. Acidosis increases release of potassium from cells. Fluctuations in potassium affect neuromuscular transmission; this produces cardiac arrhythmias, reduces action of GI smooth muscle, and impairs electrical conduction (Axley, 2015; Fallone & Cotton, 2015).

12. Intervene for hyperkalemia:
  a. Restrict potassium-rich foods and fluids. Do not allow salt substitute that contains potassium as the cation (Hensley & McCarthy, 2015).
  b. Correction of acidosis will help alleviate hyperkalemia.
  c. Emergency medications as ordered with follow-up labs.
    • Insulin and glucose to push potassium back into cells
    • Calcium to temporarily stabilize cardiac electrical activity
    • Exchange resin (e.g., sodium polystyrene sulfonate) to pull potassium into bowel
  d. Hemodialysis on a low or potassium-free bath removes K+ rapidly and efficiently from the plasma.
  e. Administer blood transfusions during hemodialysis to remove excess K+.
	12. High potassium levels necessitate a reduced potassium intake. Intervention needs to begin when elevation is noted. This can be done with dietary changes, medication adjustments, and dialysis.

> **CLINICAL ALERT:**
> • Potassium levels greater than 6.5 mmol/L are an immediate emergency. Persons on chronic dialysis may be less likely to exhibit signs and symptoms than those experiencing acute kidney injury (Axley, 2015).

(continued)

Interventions	Rationales

13. Monitor for signs and symptoms and risks of hypokalemia:
  a. Weakness or paralysis
  b. Decreased or no deep-tendon reflexes
  c. Hypoventilation
  d. Polyuria
  e. Hypotension
  f. Constipation; paralytic ileus
  g. ECG changes: U wave, flat T-wave, arrhythmias, and prolonged Q-T interval
  h. Increased risk of digitalis toxicity
  i. Nausea, vomiting, and anorexia
	13. Hypokalemia results from losses associated with vomiting, diarrhea, diuresis occurring as the oliguric phase resolves, diuretic therapy, or from insufficient potassium intake. Hypokalemia impairs neuromuscular transmission and reduces the efficiency of respiratory muscles. Kidneys are less sensitive to antidiuretic hormone (ADH) and thus excrete large quantities of dilute urine. Gastrointestinal (GI) smooth muscle action is also reduced. Abnormally low potassium levels also impair electrical conduction of the heart (Axley, 2015; Fallone & Cotton, 2015).

14. Intervene for hypokalemia:
  a. Evaluation of lab values when hyperkalemia is being corrected
  b. Encourage increased intake of potassium-rich foods
  c. Dietary consult
  d. Intravenous potassium replacement as ordered
  e. Medication adjustment as ordered (e.g., change in diuretic to preserve potassium)
  f. Individual education regarding signs and symptoms of low potassium and rationale for dietary recommendations
	14. Correct or prevent potassium deficit to avoid potentially life-threatening consequences. Overcorrection of hyperkalemia can cause hypokalemia. Increased potassium intake helps to ensure potassium replacement (Axley, 2015; Fallone & Cotton, 2015).

15. Monitor for signs and symptoms of hypocalcemia:
  a. Altered mental status
  b. Numbness or tingling in fingers and toes and around the mouth
  c. Muscle cramps
  d. Seizures
  e. ECG changes: prolonged Q-T interval, prolonged ST segment, and arrhythmias
	15. Hypocalcemia results from the kidneys' inability to metabolize vitamin D (needed for calcium absorption); retention of phosphorus causes a reciprocal drop in serum calcium level. Low serum calcium level produces increased neural excitability resulting in muscle spasms (cardiac, facial, extremities) and CNS irritability (seizures). It also causes cardiac muscle hyperactivity as evidenced by ECG changes (Axley, 2015).

16. Intervene for hypocalcemia. Administer a high-calcium, low-phosphorus diet as prescribed. Acute decreases may require intravenous administration.	16. Elevated phosphate levels lower serum calcium level, necessitating dietary replacement.

17. Monitor for signs and symptoms of hypermagnesemia:
  a. Weakness
  b. Hypoventilation
  c. Hypotension
  d. Flushing
  e. Behavioral changes
	17. Hypermagnesemia results from the kidneys' decreased ability to excrete magnesium. Its effects include CNS depression, respiratory depression, and peripheral vasodilation (Axley, 2015).

18. Monitor for signs and symptoms of hyperphosphatemia:
  a. Tetany
  b. Numbness or tingling in fingers and toes
  c. GI disturbance—nausea, vomiting, anorexia
  d. Tachycardia
	18. Hyperphosphatemia results from the kidneys' decreased ability to excrete phosphorus and from the breakdown of lean muscle mass due to catabolism. Symptoms that occur from elevated phosphorus are usually a result of hypocalcemia (Fallone & Cotton, 2015).

Interventions	Rationales
19. For an individual with hyperphosphatemia, administer phosphorus-binding antacids, calcium supplements, or vitamin D, and restrict phosphorus-rich foods.	19. The individual needs supplements to overcome vitamin D deficiency or compensate for a calcium deficit through low diet intake, poor intestinal absorption, or calcium loss during diuretic phase of recovery. High phosphate decreases calcium, which increases parathyroid hormone (PTH) secretion. During AKI, PTH is less effective in removing phosphates and absorbing calcium from the gut. The result is calcium reabsorption from the bones and decreases tubular reabsorption of phosphate (Fallone & Cotton, 2015).
20. Monitor for signs and symptoms of hypertension: a. Headache b. Fatigue c. Dizziness d. Blurred vision	20. Hypertension is a common manifestation of renal failure. It is caused by systemic and central fluid volume excess and increased renin production. In the presence of renal ischemia the renin-angiotensin system is triggered, which results in increased blood pressure and increased renal blood flow (Dutka & Szromba, 2015).
21. Monitor for signs and symptoms of pulmonary edema: a. Cough with possible pink frothy sputum b. Dyspnea and tachypnea with use of accessory muscles for breathing c. Rales, decreased oxygen saturation d. Anxiety e. Excessive sweating and pale skin	21. Pulmonary edema is usually a result of cardiac failure but can also be caused by renal failure due to fluid volume excess and electrolyte imbalance (Axley, 2015; Fallone & Cotton, 2015; Williams, 2015).
22. Monitor for signs and symptoms of change in level of consciousness: a. Fatigue and lethargy b. Altered mental status c. Decreased range of movement	22. A decrease in mental functioning is a direct result of an accumulation of nitrogenous waste products from impaired renal excretion and metabolic acidosis (Axley, 2015; Fallone & Cotton, 2015).
23. Monitor for signs and symptoms of GI bleeding: a. Abdominal pain with or without vomiting of blood b. Black tarry stool c. Tachycardia d. Hypotension	23. Increasing levels of uremic toxins are the primary contributors to GI manifestations. As urea decomposes in the GI tract, it releases ammonia. Ammonia in the GI tract increases capillary fragility and GI mucosal irritation, small mucosal ulcerations may develop, causing GI bleeding (Axley, 2015; Fallone & Cotton, 2015).
24. Consult with the physician or advanced practice nurse, who may order renal replacement therapy (RRT) usually as intermittent hemodialysis (IHD) or continuous renal replacement therapy (CRRT) if medical management is not sufficient to control symptoms and complications of AKI.	24. CRRT offers advantages of greater hemodynamic stability with slower but continuous fluid removal and fluid/electrolyte balance. IHD provides more rapid fluid removal and electrolyte balance in a shorter time frame but has increased risk of hypotensive events (Williams, 2015).

Clinical Alert Report

Prior to providing care, advise ancillary staff/student to report the following to the professional nurse assigned to the individual:

- AKI can present with a rapidly changing clinical picture, which may require urgent intervention. Infections are the primary cause of morbidity and mortality in AKI. Therefore, advise ancillary staff/student to report.
- Any new changes or deteriorations in individual's behavior or symptoms (e.g., level of consciousness, agitation, confusion).
- Blood pressure or pulse outside of the range established for that individual (see Indicators for baseline).
- Difficulty breathing or respirations less than 10/min.
- Temperature (oral) 1° F to 2° F over baseline. Uremia suppresses temperature, so lower reading may still indicate fever and possible infection.
- Change in urine output from baseline. Fluid and medication management may need adjustment as kidney function changes.
- Any redness, warmth, drainage, or tenderness at IV or catheter sites.

Nursing Diagnoses

TRANSITION TO HOME/COMMUNITY CARE

If indicated, review the risk diagnoses identified for this individual on admission:

- Review risk diagnoses and interventions identified on admission.
- Use STAR (Stop, Think, Act, Review) to help assess current risk and SBAR (Situation, Background, Action, Recommendation) to develop feasible plan.
- Individual and family need to continue good infection control measures especially hand washing and avoidance of ill individuals.
- Do individual and family have resources to maintain adequate hygiene, obtain prescribed medications, return for scheduled follow-up appointments, and understand how to contact appropriate health care personnel for after transition questions or concerns?
- Consider referral to transition planner, case manager, and/or social service prior to transition if risk diagnoses are still present.
- Consider referral for home health for additional services if indicated.

STAR

Stop

Think What are the individual's risks upon transition?
Does the individual/family understand how to minimize risk of infection in home environment?

Act Does individual have support system? Use SBAR

SBAR *Situation:* Individual is being transitioned to his home.

Background: Individual lives alone and cares for several farm animals. Individual still feels weak.

Action: More thorough evaluation of home environment.

Recommendation: Discuss family support options and refer to transition planner, case manager, or social worker. Can family assist individual after transition and if so in what capacity? Refer to Home Health nursing for possible teaching and monitoring.

Review Is the plan feasible and safe to individual and family? If not, what other options are available?

- This plan begins on admission and involves individual, family, and other support persons.

Risk for Ineffective Health Management Related to Illness, Medications, Procedures

S T A R	
	Stop
	Think Is this person at risk for injury, falls, medical complications, and/or inability to care for self (activities of daily living)?
	Is there a support person available?
	Is the person competent to manage self-administration of medications, treatment procedures?
	Are additional resources needed?
	Can the person explain how to monitor condition (e.g., blood glucose, sign/symptoms of complications, dietary/mobility restrictions, and when to call his or her primary provider or specialist)?
	Act Contact or provide the appropriate resource (e.g., contacting a support person, home health assessment, additional teaching, printed materials).
	Review Has the problem been addressed? If not, use SBAR to communicate to the appropriate person.

Risk for Ineffective Health Management Related to Insufficient of Knowledge of Disease Process, Treatments, Contraindications, Dietary Management, and Follow-up Care

NOC

Compliance (Engagement) Behavior, Knowledge: Treatment Regimen, Participation in Health Care Decisions, Treatment Behavior: Illness or Injury

NIC

Anticipatory Guidance, Learning Facilitation, Risk Identification, Health Education, Teaching: Procedure/ Treatment, Health System Guidance

Goal

The individual or primary caregiver will describe disease process, causes, and factors contributing to symptoms, and the regimen for disease or symptom control.

Indicators

- Relate the intent to practice health behaviors needed or desired for recovery from illness/symptom management and prevention of recurrence or complications.
- Describe signs and symptoms that need reporting.

Interventions	Rationales
1. Explain any ongoing risks of infection and avoidance strategies post transition. Include instructions in case of any external devices such as an intravenous catheter.	1. Individual and family are more likely to be able to avoid and manage risks if they understand how this pertains to their immediate surroundings.
2. Review all transition medications including purpose, side effects, and how to contact health care personnel for questions or concerns. Reinforce any medications that need to be avoided (e.g., nonsteroidal pain medications may be restricted or contraindicated).	2. Individuals are less likely to stop or change medication regime if they understand the purpose of medications and can obtain rapid assistance with any questions.
3. Provide clear and accurate instructions regarding when, why, and where to report any new or returning symptoms. Example could include fever, change in urine output, and changes in energy or mental status.	3. Individuals and families need ongoing support and clear directions for follow-up of possible problems.

Interventions	*Rationales*
4. Review any dietary recommendations or changes. Elicit concerns regarding ability to follow or access foods for prescribed diet. Consider contacting dietitian for ongoing individual questions or social services for financial concerns.	4. Individuals may need assistance in understanding and incorporating food changes. Financial limitations may hinder prescribed food changes.
5. Provide education, informal or formal, to individual and family with each encounter (e.g., what the medication is and reason for its administration, when procedures are scheduled and approximate length of treatment, clarification of tests and laboratory results that have been reviewed, or availability of outside services). Encourage questions and clarification of data.	5. Engagement can be enhanced with frequent inquires to determine understanding and to clarify personal heath goals (Barnsteiner, Disch, & Walton, 2014).
6. Refer also Hemodialysis and Peritoneal Dialysis care plans.	

Documentation

Vital signs
Respiratory assessment
Weight
Edema (sites, amount)
Specific gravity
Intake and output
Complaints of nausea, vomiting, or muscle cramps
Treatments
Changes in behavior and sensorium
ECG changes

Chronic Kidney Disease

Chronic kidney disease (CKD) refers to the slow, progressive, and irreversible destruction of the kidneys over a period of months to years. CKD can result from a primary renal disorder (e.g., glomerulonephritis or polycystic kidney disease), or as a secondary disorder (e.g., as a complication of diabetes mellitus or hypertension). However, the most common causes of CKD are diabetes, hypertension, and glomerulonephritis, as well as congenital and hereditary factors.

There are five stages of CKD, as outlined in Table III.I. CKD is a progression through an abnormally low and deteriorating glomerular filtration rate, which is usually determined indirectly by the creatinine level in blood serum (Hain & Haras, 2015). When the kidney cannot maintain metabolic, fluid, and electrolyte balance, the result is uremia. As the condition progresses, treatment options include dialysis, transplantation, or palliative care (Hain, & Haras, 2015).

Table III.I   Stages of Chronic Kidney Disease: A Clinical Action Plan

Stage	Description	GFR (mL/min/1.73 m^2)	Action[a]
1	Kidney damage with normal or increased GFR	>90	Diagnosis and treatment; treatment of comorbid conditions; slowed progression; cardiovascular disease (CVD) risk reduction
2	Kidney damage with mild, decreased GFR	60–89	Estimating progression
3	Moderate, decreased GFR	30–59	Evaluating and treating complications
4	Severe, decreased GFR	15–29	Preparation for kidney replacement therapy
5	Kidney failure	<15 (or dialysis)	Replacement (if uremia present)

CKD is defined as either kidney damage or GFR, 60 mL/min/1.73 m^2 for ≥3 months. Kidney damage is defined as pathologic abnormalities or markers of damage including abnormalities in blood or urine tests or imaging studies.

[a]Includes actions from preceding stages

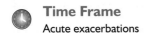

Time Frame
Acute exacerbations

▪▪▪▪ DIAGNOSTIC CLUSTER

Collaborative Problems

Δ Risk for Complications of Fluid Imbalance

▲ Risk for Complications of Anemia

*   Risk for Complications of Hypertension

*   Risk for Complications of Hyperparathyroidism

*   Risk for Complications of Pathological Fractures

Δ Risk for Complications of Hypoalbuminemia

Δ Risk for Complications of Congestive Heart Failure

Δ Risk for Complications of Metabolic Acidosis

Δ Risk for Complications of Pleural Effusion

▲ Risk for Complications of Fluid Overload (refer to Hemodialysis Care Plan)

Nursing Diagnoses

Δ Imbalanced Nutrition related to anorexia, nausea, vomiting, and loss of taste or smell, stomatitis, and unpalatable diet

Δ Powerlessness related to feeling of loss of control and life style restrictions (refer to Unit II)

▲ Risk for Infection related to invasive procedures (refer to Unit II)

Δ Impaired Comfort related to calcium phosphate or urate crystals on skin (refer to Cirrhosis Care Plan)

▲ Risk for Ineffective Health Management related to insufficient knowledge of condition, dietary restrictions, daily recording, pharmacologic therapy, and signs and symptoms of complications, and insufficient resources (e.g., financial, caregiver), follow-up visits, and community resources

Related Care Plans

Hemodialysis

Acute Kidney Failure

Cirrhosis

▲ This diagnosis was reported to be monitored for or managed frequently (75% to 100%).
Δ This diagnosis was reported to be monitored for or managed often (50% to 74%).
* This diagnosis was not included in the validation study.

Transition Criteria

The individual or family will:

1. Describe dietary restrictions, medications, and treatment plan.
2. Maintain contact and follow-up with health care providers (including dialysis, if needed).
3. Keep complete daily records, as instructed.
4. Verbalize available community resources.
5. Relate the intent to comply with agreed-on restrictions and follow-up.
6. State the signs and symptoms that must be reported to a health care professional.
7. Relate the importance of an outlet for feelings and concerns.

Transitional Risk Assessment Plan (TRAP)

Begin this plan on admission.

Implement the Transitional Risk Assessment Plan (TRAP):

* Refer to inside back cover.
* Add each validated risk diagnosis to individual's problem list with the risk code in ( ).
* Refer to Unit II to the individual risk nursing diagnoses/collaborative problems for outcomes and interventions.

R: "Close coordination of care in the post-acute period, early transition follow-up care, enhanced client education and self-management training, proactive end-of-life counseling, and extending the resources and clinical expertise over time via multidisciplinary team management" can lower readmission rates and improve health outcomes (Boutwell & Hwu, 2009, p. 14). Interventions are utilized to activate the individual and family to select changes in their everyday lifestyle choices to improve their health (Hibbard & Greene, 2013).

Collaborative Problems

Risk for Complications of Fluid Imbalance

Risk for Complications of Anemia

Risk for Complications of Hypertension

Risk for Complications of Hyperparathyroidism

Risk for Complications of Pathological Fractures

Risk for Complications of Hypoalbuminemia

Risk for Complications of Congestive Heart Failure

Risk for Complications of Metabolic Acidosis

Risk for Complications of Diabetes

Collaborative Outcomes

The individual will be monitored for early signs and symptoms of (a) fluid imbalance, (b) anemia, (c) hyperparathyroidism, (d) pathologic fractures, (e) hypoalbuminemia, (f) congestive heart failure, (g) metabolic acidosis, (h) hypertension, (i) diabetes, and the individual will receive collaborative interventions if indicated to restore physiologic stability.

Indicators of Physiologic Stability

* Alert, calm, oriented
* Respiration 16 to 20 breaths/min, unlabored respirations with clear breath sounds in all lobes
* Pulse 60 to 100 beats/min with regular rate and rhythm, no palpitations or chest pain
* BP >90/60, <140/90 mm Hg
* Temperature 98.5° F to 99° F
* No or minimal edema (a, f)
* Ideal or desired weight (a, f)
* Urine output >0.5 mL/kg/hr (a, f)
* Red blood cells 4,000,000 to 6,200,000 mm^3 (b)
* White blood cells 48,000 to 100,000 mm^3 (j)
* Hematocrit (b)
  * Male 42% to 50%
  * Female 40% to 48%
* Hemoglobin (b)
  * Male 13 to 18 g/dL
  * Female 12 to 16 g/dL

- Serum albumin 3.5 to 5 g/dL (f)
- Total cholesterol <200 mg/dL (f)
  - Iron 60 to 175 mcg/dL (b)
  - Total iron binding capacity 240 to 450 mcg/dL (b)
- Transferrin saturation 20% to 50% (iron/TIBC × 100%) (b)
- Serum ferritin (b)
  - Males 29 to 438 ng/mL
  - Females 9 to 219 ng/mL
- Serum potassium 3.8 to 5 mEq/L (b, l)
- Serum sodium 135 to 145 mEq/L (a, l)
- Serum calcium 8.5 to 10.5 mg/dL (c, l)
- Serum phosphate 2.7 to 4.6 mg/dL (c, d)
  - Magnesium 1.7 to 3 mEq/L
- Blood urea nitrogen 10 to 20 mg/dL (h, l)
- Creatinine 0.5 to 1.2 ng/mL (h, l)
- Alkaline phosphatase 45 to 150 International Units/L (c)
- Urine sodium 130 to 200 mEq/24 hr (a)
- Creatinine clearance >60 mL/min (f)
- Oxygen saturation (Sao$_2$) >94% (a, h, l)
- Carbon dioxide (Paco$_2$) 35 to 45 mm Hg (a, h)

Interventions	Rationales

1. Monitor for fluid imbalances:
  a. Weight changes
  b. BP changes
  c. Increased pulse
  d. Increased respirations
  e. Neck vein distention
  f. Dependent, peripheral edema
  g. Increased fluid intake
  h. Increased sodium intake
  i. Orthostatic hypotension (decreased fluid volume)
	1. Fluid imbalance, usually hypervolemia, results from failure of kidney to regulate extracellular fluids by decreased sodium and water elimination (Hain & Haras, 2015).

2. Consult with nephrology staff if fluid volume changes. Refer to dialysis care plans for specific fluid management strategies.	2. In advanced CKD, dialysis may be needed to control fluid overload.
3. Frequently monitor vital signs, particularly blood pressure and pulse.	3. Circulating volume must be monitored with CKD to prevent severe hypervolemia.

4. Monitor for anemia:
  a. Dyspnea
  b. Fatigue
  c. Tachycardia
  d. Palpitations
  e. Pallor of nail beds and mucous membranes
  f. Low hemoglobin and hematocrit
  g. Bruising
	4. A decline is directly proportional to the frequency and volume of blood loss associated with phlebotomy-related blood drawing, blood loss during dialysis or other procedures, and a decline in erythropoietin production from the kidney (Hain & Haras, 2015). Decreased hemoglobin indicates fewer RBCs are available to transport oxygen. Shortness of breath, fatigue, tachycardia, and palpitations are common symptoms especially with activity. These may resolve with rest. Cold intolerance also results from fewer RBCs. Pallor is evident where blood flow is close to the skin as in mucous membranes and nail beds. As CKD progresses, RBC survival time decreases due to less erythropoietin production and elevated uremic toxins. Bruising may be more evident.

Interventions	*Rationales*
5. Determine the cause of anemia as:	5. Adequate iron must be available to produce healthy functional RBCs. About 70% of iron is stored in the RBCs and the remainder in the liver and reticuloendothelial system. *Absolute* iron deficiency is indicated by low iron, percent saturation, and ferritin with high TIBC and will respond to iron therapy. *Functional* iron deficiency may have an elevated ferritin indicating an inflammation or infection which blocks iron transfer from for use. Further exploration for a treatable cause is indicated. Individuals who cannot tolerate or are not responsive to oral iron need to be evaluated for intravenous iron. (Hain & Haras, 2015)
a. Assess for blood loss—GI, menses, phlebotomy. See Dialysis Care Plan if indicated.	a. Anemia occurs if blood loss exceeds RBC production. Avoid unnecessary collection of blood specimens by coordinate blood draws. Educate the individual on methods to minimize blood loss (e.g., use a soft toothbrush, avoid vigorous nose blowing, and avoid constipation). Demonstrate how to apply direct pressure over a bleeding site.
b. Evaluate folate and vitamin B_{12} levels	b. Folic acid and B_{12} are absorbed in the intestine. B_{12} is needed to convert folate to the active form and both vitamins are necessary for RBC production and function.
c. Evaluate for possible side effects of medications.	c. Anemia is a side effect of several classes of medication (e.g., immunosuppressant).
d. Evaluate fluid status—see Fluid Management	d. Because of dilution, hemoglobin will appear lower in the presence of fluid overload.
e. Consider hematologic etiology (e.g., myelodyplastic syndrome, thalassemia, malignancy)	e. Disorders of the bone marrow can interfere with RBC production.

6. Evaluate iron status.
   a. Measure serum iron, total iron-binding capacity (TIBC), percentage transferrin saturation (% saturation), and ferritin (see indicators for values).
   b. Correct iron depletion with oral or intravenous iron.
   c. Discuss with the individual any concerns or barriers to taking prescribed oral iron therapy.
   d. Explore possible causes of poor iron absorption (e.g., insufficient dietary iron, poor absorption due to prior GI surgery).
   e. Caution with intravenous iron replacement in severe depletion, intolerance to or poor absorption of oral iron. Monitor for:
      • Symptoms can range from hypotension; dyspnea; chest, back, flank or groin pain; arthralgias/myalgias; fever; and malaise.
      • Individuals need to be monitored and educated on possible side effects including delayed reactions.
      • IV iron needs to be given per the current manufacturer recommendations for each specific product. (Hain & Haras, 2015)

      • All intravenous iron products carry some risk of anaphylactic or anaphylactoid response.

Interventions	*Rationales*
7. Administer bulk-forming laxatives or stool softeners if individual is constipated. Avoid magnesium and phosphate containing laxatives.	7. Constipation is a common side effect of oral iron products. Certain laxatives contain magnesium and phosphate. Individuals with kidney disease already have difficulty excreting usual intake of magnesium and phosphate in foods so need to avoid additional sources of these elements. See Acute Kidney Injury for signs and symptoms of hypermagnesemia and hyperphosphotemia.
8. Provide erythropoiesis-stimulating agent (ESA) therapy as indicated and prescribed **CLINICAL ALERT:** • FDA Black Box Warning for all ESAs. ESAs increase the risk of death, myocardial infarction, stroke, venous thromboembolism, thrombosis of vascular access and tumor progression or recurrence (Hain & Haras, 2015). a. Monitor blood pressure prior to each dose. Dose should be held in presence of uncontrolled hypertension. b. Hemoglobin increases >1 g/dL in less than 2 weeks may contribute to CV events. Goal is to avoid red cell transfusions. Recommendation is to decrease dose if hemoglobin is over 11 g/dL. c. Monitor iron stores—serum iron, percent transferrin saturation, ferritin. d. If the individual on an ESA and/or iron therapy is nonresponsive to therapy or has a drop in hemoglobin evaluate for an underlying cause. e. Assess for underlying causes: • Hyperparathyroidism • Osteitis fibrosa • Hematologic disease • Sudden loss of responsiveness to recombinant human erythropoietin-alfa (rHuEPO)	8. Erythropoietin (EPO) is produced in the kidney. ESAs are genetically engineered EPO administered to maintain hemoglobin levels. Current FDA guidelines for kidney disease recommend not starting ESA therapy until other causes of anemia have been corrected and the hemoglobin level is below 10 g/dL. Hemoglobin levels should not exceed 12 g/dL with active therapy. Dosing depends on the agent used and the laboratory response. Follow the protocols of the institution (Hain & Haras, 2015). a. ESAs increase blood viscosity and can increase blood pressure and possible thrombus formation including stroke. BP medication may be needed. b. Hemoglobin increases >1 g/dL in less than 2 weeks may contribute to CV events. Goal is to avoid red cell transfusions. Recommendation is to decrease dose if hemoglobin is over 11 g/dL. c. Iron stores will be depleted more quickly with ESA therapy. Replete either with oral or intravenous iron before starting ESA and to maintain stores while on ESA. Check quarterly if on maintenance iron or monthly during iron replacement. d. See "Determine the Cause of Anemia" e. Underlying causes of mineral bone disease will need to be diagnosed and corrected.
9. Evaluate aluminum levels and elevated lead levels.	9. Changes in the bone marrow and matrix can affect red blood cell production and bone strength. Loss of renal function alters normal regulation of calcium, phosphorus and parathyroid hormone and elimination of aluminum. Exposure to heavy metals (e.g., aluminum and lead can form deposits in bone which interferes with healthy function). Individuals need to avoid potentially toxic sources including aluminum containing antacids. Referral to hematology may be necessary to further diagnose bone marrow dysfunction (Hain & Haras, 2015).

(continued)

Interventions	*Rationales*

10. Monitor for manifestations of decreased albumin levels:
  a. Serum albumin <3.5 g/dL and proteinuria (>300 mg protein/24 hr)
  b. Edema formation: pedal, facial, sacral
  c. Infection
  d. Hyperlipidemia
  e. Thromboembolism
  f. Signs and symptoms of negative nitrogen balance:
    • Decreased serum cholesterol
    • Decreased caloric intake (<45 kcal/kg)
    • Decreased protein intake (<0.75 g/kg)
    • Delayed wound healing
    • Muscle wasting
	10. When albumin is lost through urinary excretion or peritoneal dialysis, the liver responds by increasing production of plasma proteins. If the loss continues, the liver cannot compensate and hypoalbuminemia increased low-density lipoprotein accumulation, and alterations in the clotting cascade results. Edema formation results from decreased plasma proteins and consequent decreased plasma oncotic pressure that causes a fluid shift from the vascular to the interstitial compartment. Hypovolemia can result from fluid loss, which leads to hemoconcentration and a consequent increase in hemoglobin and hematocrit. If the volume loss becomes great, shock occurs (Deegens & Wetzels, 2011; Grossman & Porth, 2014). A negative nitrogen balance results from protein and caloric malnutrition, leading to an oxygen and nutrient deficit that causes cellular catabolism, cell breakdown, and nitrogen loss. Humoral defenses to infection are depressed owing to protein loss, and general protein reserves are depleted resulting in slowed healing (Brommage, Cotton, Gonyea, Kent, & Stover, 2015).

11. Hold a dietary consultation for nutritional assessment and to provide for the following:
  a. Fluid restrictions (with massive edema)
  b. Low-sodium diet
  c. Adequate calorie intake
  d. Appropriate protein diet with high biological protein (meats, poultry, cheese, milk)
  e. Adjusted phosphate and calcium requirements
	11. Depending on the stage of CKD and the underlying cause protein may be restricted to 0.75 to 1.25 g/kg, with emphasis on high-biological-value protein. High-biological-value proteins supply the essential amino acids necessary for cell growth and repair, but produce less urea nitrogen during metabolism. Calories should be generous (35 to 45 kcal/kg) to allow use of the minerals in protein for tissue maintenance. Tissue catabolism can develop when protein intake is inadequate. Catabolism increases BUN levels, acidosis, and hyperkalemia. A low-sodium diet may be beneficial to prevent additional fluid retention. The individual should be monitored for fluid depletion because of the dangers of hypovolemia and hypotension. Laboratory results will help determine need for phosphate and calcium dietary modifications (Brommage et al., 2015; Clement & Kent, 2015).

12. Evaluate daily:
  a. Weight
  b. Fluid intake and output records
  c. Circumference of the edematous part(s)
  d. Laboratory data: hematocrit, serum potassium, and plasma protein in specific serum albumin
	12. As glomerular filtration rate (GFR) decreases and the functioning nephron mass continues to diminish, the kidneys lose the ability to concentrate urine and to excrete sodium and water; this results in hypervolemia.

13. Monitor for signs and symptoms of congestive heart failure (CHF) and decreased cardiac output:
  a. Gradual increase in heart rate
  b. Increased shortness of breath
  c. Diminished breath sounds, rales
  d. Decreased systolic BP
  e. Presence of or increase in S3 and/or S4
  f. Gallop
  g. Peripheral edema
  h. Distended neck veins
	13. Diminished urinary output causes volume retention that can lead to cardiomegaly and CHF. This results in reduced ability of left ventricle to eject blood and consequent decreased cardiac output and increased pulmonary vascular congestion. This causes fluid to enter the pulmonary tissue, leading to respiratory distress, rales, productive cough, and cyanosis (Walton, 2015).

Interventions	Rationales
14. Encourage engagement to prescribed fluid restrictions. In advanced CKD with decreased urine output the restriction may be 800 to 1,000 mL/24 hr or 24-hour urine output plus 500 mL.	14. An individual who presents with evidence of fluid overload requires fluid restriction based on urine output. In an anuric individual, restriction generally is 800 mL/day, which accounts for insensible losses from metabolism, the GI tract, perspiration, and respiration. Sodium restrictions are usually simultaneously prescribed (Hain & Haras, 2015).
15. Reevaluate and reestablish the individual's optimal "dry" weight—that weight at which an individual is free of any signs or symptoms of overload and maintains a normal blood pressure.	15. An individual with CKD is prone to fluctuations in weight, necessitating frequent reevaluation for optimal fluid balance. Accepted interdialytic weight gain is 1 to 2 lb/24 hr (Hain & Haras, 2015).
16. Collaborate with physician, nurse practitioner, physical assistant, or dietitian in planning an appropriate diet. Encourage adherence to a prescribed-sodium diet (1 to 4 g/24 hr depending on stage of CKD and fluid status).	16. Sodium restrictions should be adjusted based on urine sodium excretion, serial weights, stage of CKD, and current medications (Hain & Haras, 2015; Walton, 2015).

17. Monitor for manifestations of pleural effusion:
  a. Variable dyspnea
  b. Pleuritic pain
  c. Diminished and delayed chest movement on involved side
  d. Bulging of intercostal spaces (in massive effusion)
  e. Decreased breath sounds over site of pleural effusion
  f. Decreased vocal and tactile fremitus
  g. Increased rate and depth of respirations
	17. A pleural effusion is a collection of fluid, either transudates or exudates, in the pleural cavity. Transudates are seen in CKD and result from a rise in pulmonary venous pressure secondary to fluid overload. This transudation also may occur owing to the hypoproteinemia often seen in CKD (Axley, 2015).

18. Monitor for manifestations of pericarditis:
  a. Pericardial friction rub
  b. Elevated temperature
  c. Elevated white blood cell count
  d. Substernal or precordial pain increasing during inspiration
	18. Pericarditis results from irritation by accumulated serum nitrogenous wastes (Axley, 2015).

19. Explain the causes of pain to the individual.	19. The individual may fear that chest pain is signaling a heart attack.

20. Monitor for signs and symptoms of cardiac tamponade:
  a. Rapid decrease in blood pressure
  b. Narrowed pulse pressure
  c. Muffled heart sounds
  d. Distended neck veins
  e. Decreased blood pressure during hemodialysis with intolerance to ultrafiltration
  f. Cardiac arrhythmias
	20. Exaggerated signs and symptoms of effusion implicate worsening pericarditis, pericardial effusion, and slowly developing cardiac tamponade. It can develop at any time in an individual with uremic pericarditis (Axley, 2015).

21. Educate staff and students to report any signs or symptoms of pericarditis or tamponade immediately.	21. Individual will require rapid medical assessment with possible dialysis or surgical intervention (Axley, 2015).

Clinical Alert Report

Advise ancillary staff/student to report to nurse assigned to individual:

- Any changes in mental status such as agitation, lethargy, confusion
- Blood pressure, pulse, or respirations outside of prescribed limits. See "Indicators." Individual parameters may vary depending on individual's medications
- Temperature (oral) 1° F to 2° F over baseline. Uremia suppresses temperature so lower readings may still indicate fever.
- Difficulty breathing or new onset of shortness of breath
- New onset of pain, distended neck veins, decreasing B/P
- Changes in urine from baseline. Fluid management may change during acute illness.
- Any redness, warmth, drainage or tenderness at IV, catheter, or phlebotomy site.

Documentation

Weight (actual, dry)
Vital signs
Laboratory values
Intake and output
Evidence of bleeding (e.g., blood in stool, bruises)
Status of edema
Chest complaints

Nursing Diagnoses

Imbalanced Nutrition Related to Anorexia, Nausea and Vomiting, Loss of Taste or Smell, Stomatitis, and Unpalatable Diet

NOC
Nutritional Status,
Teaching: Nutrition

Goal

The individual will relate the importance of adequate nutritional intake and complying with the prescribed dietary regimen.

NIC
Nutrition Management,
Nutritional Monitoring

Indicators

- Has no nutritional deficiencies
- Has minimal or no edema
- Maintains ideal or desired weight

Interventions	Rationales
1. Establish nutritional goals with the individual/family and a plan of care to achieve them. a. Consult the dietitian for assistance with nutritional assessment, identifying nutritional goals, prescribing diet modifications, and providing nutritional instruction to individual. b. Reinforce the dietary instructions and provide written materials for verbal orders.	1a. A properly prescribed diet is essential in management of CKD to prevent uremic toxicity, fluid and electrolyte imbalances, and catabolism (Brommage et al., 2015) b. Empathy and reinforcement of dietary instructions can increase compliance with diet restrictions (Walton, 2015)
2. Discuss dietary options rather than restrictions.	2. Individuals and families will become discouraged if the diet is too restrictive and unpalatable (Walton, 2015)
3. Encourage the individual to verbalize his or her feelings and frustrations about diet modifications.	3. The individual should be given as much control as possible over his or her diet—for example, have the individual make a list of food and fluid preferences and dislikes and try to incorporate these into the prescribed diet (Brommage et al., 2015).

Interventions	Rationales
4. Provide for and encourage good oral hygiene before and after meals.	4. Proper oral hygiene reduces microorganisms and helps prevent stomatitis.
5. Evaluate, with individual and dietitian, the individual's nutritional status and the diet's effectiveness.	5. Continued evaluation enables alteration of diet according to the individual's specific nutritional needs (Brommage et al., 2015).
6. Explain the need for the individual to eat the maximum protein allowed on the diet.	6. Adequate protein is needed to prevent protein catabolism and muscle wasting (Brommage et al., 2015).
7. Discuss methods for reducing potassium intake, if indicated. a. Drain canned fruits b. Eat cooked vegetables, pasta, and cereals c. Soak fresh vegetables in water before cooking. Use fresh water to cook.	7. Daily potassium intake recommendations for individuals with CKD (not on dialysis) is usually 2 to 4 g/day. Certain foods are lower in potassium. Soaking vegetables removes 50% of the potassium. (Brommage et al., 2015).
8. Prepare for dialysis, as indicated, and monitor for potential complications. Refer to the Hemodialysis and Peritoneal Dialysis care plans for more information.	8. Dialysis is indicated for rising BUN that dietary management cannot control. It also may be necessary to remove excess fluid administered with TPN.
9. Work with the individual to develop a plan to incorporate the diet prescription successfully into her or his daily life.	9. Collaboration provides opportunities for the individual to exert control; this tends to increase compliance (Hain & Haras, 2015; Walton, 2015).

Documentation

Daily weights
Intake (specify food types and amounts)
Output
Mouth assessment
Individual/family teaching
Referrals

> **TRANSITION TO HOME/COMMUNITY CARE**
>
> If indicated, review the risk diagnoses identified for this individual on admission:
> - Is the person still at risk?
> - Can the family reduce the risks?
> - Is the person at higher risk at home?
> - Is a home health nurse assessment needed?
> - Refer to transition planner/case manager/social service.
> - When is this person scheduled for follow-up with primary provider? Specialists? Record dates of appointments.
> - Complete a medication reconciliation prior to transition. Refer to index.

STAR   **Stop**

Think   Think about any new or ongoing issues.
Has degree of kidney function changed, have dietary needs changed, are medications different?
Does individual utilize outside resources (e.g., home health who need updated information)?

Act   Contact or provide the appropriate resource (e.g., contacting a support person, home health assessment, additional teaching, printed materials).

SBAR   *Situation:* Individual is being transitioned home.

Background: Individual lives alone but has had home health nursing twice a month for medication management.

Action: Contact home health with updates medication list and plan.

Recommendation: Home health services may be needed more frequently until individual is stable.

Review   Has the problem been addressed? If not, use SBAR to communicate to the appropriate person.

Risk for Ineffective Health Management Related to Insufficient Knowledge of Condition, Dietary Restrictions, Daily Recording, Pharmacological Therapy, Signs/Symptoms of Complications, Follow-up Visits, and Community Resources

NOC

Compliance Behavior, Knowledge: Treatment Regimen, Participation in Health Care Decisions, Treatment Behavior: Illness

NIC

Anticipatory Guidance, Learning Facilitation, Risk Identification, Health Education, Teaching: Procedure/ Treatment, Health System Guidance

Goal

The goals for this diagnosis represent those associated with transition planning. Refer to the transition criteria.

Interventions	Rationales
1. Develop and implement a teaching plan using techniques and tools appropriate to the individual's understanding. Plan several teaching sessions.	1. Presenting relevant and useful information in an understandable format greatly reduces learning frustration and enhances teaching efforts. Some factors specific to an individual with CKD influence the teaching–learning process (Cahill & Groenhoff, 2015a; Hill, 2015; Longdon, 2015): a. Depressed mentation that necessitates repeating information b. Short attention span that may limit teaching sessions to 10 to 15 minutes c. Altered perceptions that necessitate frequent clarification and reassurance d. Sensory alterations that cause a better response to ideas presented using varied audiovisual formats
2. Implement teaching that includes but is not limited to renal function. a. Normal renal function b. Altered renal function • Disease process • Causes • Physiologic and emotional responses to uremia • Renal replacement therapies	2. Amount and depth of teaching will depend on the individual's present readiness to learn. Several sessions will be needed; include written materials to take home (Cahill & Groenhoff, 2015a, b).
3. Encourage the individual to verbalize anxiety, fears, and questions.	3. Recognizing the individual's fear of failure to learn is vital to successful teaching.
4. Identify factors that may help to predict noncompliance: a. Lack of knowledge b. Noncompliance in the hospital c. Failure to perceive disease's seriousness or chronicity d. Belief that the condition will "go away" on its own e. Belief that the condition is hopeless	4. Openly addressing barriers to compliance may help to minimize or eliminate these barriers.

Interventions	Rationales
5. Include significant others in teaching sessions. Encourage them to provide support without acting as "police."	5. Significant others must be aware of the treatment plan so they can support the individual. "Policing" the individual can disrupt positive relationships.
6. Emphasize to the individual that, ultimately, it is his or her choice and responsibility to comply with the therapeutic regimen.	6. The individual must understand that he or she has control over choices and that his or her choices can improve or impair health (Barnsteiner et al., 2014).
7. If cost of medications is a financial burden for the individual, consult with social services.	7. A referral for financial support can prevent discontinuation because of financial reasons (Kelley & Bednarski, 2015).
8. Assist the individual to identify her or his ideal or desired weight.	8. Establishing an achievable goal may help to improve compliance.
9. Teach the individual to record weight and urinary output daily.	9. Daily weight and urine output measurements allow the individual to monitor her or his own fluid status, and limit fluid intake accordingly.
10. Explain the signs and symptoms of electrolyte imbalances and the need to watch for and report them. (See Collaborative Problems in this entry for more information.)	10. Early detection of electrolyte imbalance enables prompt intervention to prevent serious complications.
11. Teach the individual measures to reduce risk of urinary tract infection: a. Perform proper hygiene after toileting to prevent fecal contamination of urinary tract. b. To prevent urinary stasis, drink the maximum fluids allowed.	11. Repetitive infections can cause further renal damage.
12. Reinforce the need to adhere with diet and fluid restrictions and follow-up care. Consult with the dietitian regarding fluid plan and overall diet.	12. Engagement with diet and fluid restrictions reduces the risk of complications.
13. Teach the individual who has fluid restrictions to relieve thirst by other means: a. Sucking on a lemon wedge, a piece of hard candy, a frozen juice pop, or an ice cube b. Spacing fluid allotment over 24 hours	13. Strategies to reduce thirst without significant fluid intake reduce risk of fluid overload.
14. Encourage the individual to express feelings and frustrations; give positive feedback for adherence to fluid restrictions.	14. Fluid and diet restrictions can be extremely frustrating; positive feedback and reassurance can contribute to continued compliance.
15. Explain importance and risks of erythropoietin stimulating agent (ESA) (e.g., Epoetin alfa therapy and iron supplements).	15. Goal is to avoid red blood cell transfusions and use least amount of therapy needed to maintain hemoglobin in prescribed range, usually 9 to 10 g/dL. Studies have shown incremental improvements in survival, left ventricle hypertrophy, exercise capacity, cognitive function, sleep dysfunction, and overall quality of life with improved hemoglobin. However, studies have also demonstrated potential risks for increased cardiovascular events including stroke. Achieving near normal hemoglobin levels is not a goal for all individuals (Hain & Haras, 2015).

(continued)

Interventions	Rationales
16. Teach the individual to take oral medications with meals whenever possible. If medications must be administered between meals, give with the smallest amount of fluid possible.	16. Planning can reduce unnecessary fluid intake and conserve fluid allowance.
17. Encourage the individual to maintain his or her usual level of activity and continue activities of daily living to the extent possible.	17. Regular activity helps to maintain strength and endurance and promotes overall well-being.
18. Teach the individual and family to watch for and report the following: a. Weight gain or loss greater than 2 lb b. Shortness of breath c. Increasing fatigue or weakness d. Confusion, change in mentation e. Palpitations f. Excessive bruising; excessive menses; excessive bleeding from gums, nose, or cut; blood in urine, stool, or vomitus. g. Increasing oral pain or oral lesions	18. Early reporting of complications enables prompt intervention (Cahill & Groenhoff, 2015b; Hain & Haras, 2015). a. Weight gain greater than 2 lb may indicate fluid retention; weight loss may point to insufficient intake. b. Shortness of breath may be an early sign of pulmonary edema. c. Increasing fatigue or weakness may indicate increasing uremia. d. Confusion or other changes in mentation may point to acidosis or fluid and electrolyte imbalances. e. Palpitations may indicate electrolyte imbalances (K, Ca). f. Excessive bruising, excessive menses, and abnormal bleeding may indicate reduced prothrombin, clotting factors III and VIII, and platelets. g. Oral pain or lesions can result as excessive salivary urea is converted to ammonia in the mouth, which is irritating to the oral mucosa.
19. Discuss with the individual and family any anticipated disease-related stressors: a. Financial difficulties b. Reversal of role responsibilities c. Dependency	19. Discussing the nonphysiologic effects of CKD in family dynamics can help the individual and family to identify effective coping strategies (Cahill & Groenhoff, 2015a, b; Hill, 2015; Kelley & Bednarski, 2015).
20. Provide information about or initiate referrals to community resources (e.g., American Association of Kidney Individuals, National Kidney Foundation, National Kidney Disease Education Program, Kidney School, counseling, self-help groups, peer counseling, Internet information sites, publications).	20. Assistance with home management and dealing with the potential destructive effects on the individual and family may be needed (Cahill & Groenhoff, 2015a, b; Hill, 2015; Kelley & Bednarski, 2015; Longdon, 2015).

Documentation

Individual/family teaching
Referrals, if indicated

NEUROLOGIC DISORDERS

Cerebrovascular Accident (Stroke)

The American Stroke Association (2016a) reports that:

- Cardiovascular disease is the leading global cause of death, accounting for more than 17.3 million deaths/year, a number that is expected to grow to more than 23.6 million by 2030.
- About 795,000 Americans each year suffer a new or recurrent stroke.
- Stroke kills nearly 129,000 people a year. It is the No. 5 cause of death.
- Stroke is a leading cause of disability.
- Stroke is the leading preventable cause of disability.

Cerebrovascular accident (CVA), or stroke, involves a sudden onset of neurologic deficits because of insufficient blood supply to a part of the brain, leading to cellular damage and cellular death (Caplan, 2015). "Unfortunately, neurologic symptoms do not accurately reflect the presence or absence of infarction, and the tempo of the symptoms does not indicate the cause of the ischemia. This is a critical issue because treatment depends upon accurately identifying the cause of symptoms" (Caplan, 2015).

There are two major types of stroke: ischemic stroke and hemorrhagic stroke. Ischemic stroke occurs when a blood vessel that supplies blood to the brain is blocked by a blood clot or plaque. In intracerebral hemorrhage, bleeding occurs directly into the brain parenchyma. The usual mechanism has been described as leakage from small intracerebral arteries damaged by chronic hypertension.

Hypertension is responsible for 60% of hemorrhagic strokes. Other mechanisms include coagulopathies, anticoagulant therapy, thrombolytic therapy for acute myocardial infarction (MI), arteriovenous malformation (AVM), aneurysms, and other vascular malformations (venous and cavernous angiomas), vasculitis, cerebral amyloidosis, alcohol abuse, and illicit drugs such as cocaine, amphetamine, methamphetamine. Hemorrhagic stroke is associated with higher mortality rates than is ischemic stroke (Liebeskind, 2016). Preventing first and recurrent strokes require prompt identification of vulnerable individuals. Some risk factors can be modified including hypertension, cigarette smoking, unhealthy eating habits, sedentary life style, lipid imbalance, poor glycemic control, cocaine use, and alcohol abuse (Wilson, 2015). "Unfortunately, as the 21st century begins, smoking is on the rise in developing countries, even as it declines in the developed countries that have had some success with tobacco control" (Samet, 2015). Exposure to secondhand and/or environmental smoke increases the risk for cardiovascular disease, which includes stroke and respiratory disorders. Electronic cigarettes (e-cigarettes), which do not involve the combustion of tobacco, generate a vapor that almost always contains nicotine (Czogala et al., 2014; Samet, 2015). The nicotine in the vapor could be inhaled by nonsmokers or absorbed across the skin (Samet, 2015).

 Time Frame
Initial diagnosis (Not in Intensive Care Unit)
Recurrent episodes

DIAGNOSTIC CLUSTER

Collaborative Problems

▲ Risk for Complications of Increased Intracranial Pressure

* Risk for Complications of Pneumonia, Atelectasis

▲ Risk for Complications of Adult Respiratory Distress Syndrome

* Risk for Complications of Seizures

* Risk for Complications of Gastrointestinal (GI) Bleeding

* Risk for Complications of Hypothalamic Syndromes

▲ Risk for Complications of Diabetes Incepitus

▲ Risk for Complications of Hyperglycemia

Nursing Diagnoses

▲ Risk for Injury related to visual field, motor, or perception deficits (refer to Unit II)

▲ Risk for Injury related to visual field, motor, or perception deficits (refer to Unit II)

▲ Impaired Physical Mobility related to decreased motor function of (specify) secondary to damage to upper motor neurons (refer to Unit II)

▲ Functional Incontinence related to inability and difficulty in reaching toilet secondary to decreased mobility or motivation (refer to Unit II)

▲ Impaired Swallowing related to muscle paralysis or paresis secondary to damage to upper motor neurons

▲ Self-Care Deficit related to impaired physical mobility or confusion (refer to Immobility or Unconsciousness Care Plan)

△ Unilateral Neglect related to (specify site) secondary to right hemispheric brain damage

△ Total Incontinence related to loss of bladder tone, loss of sphincter control, or inability to perceive bladder cues (refer to Neurogenic Bladder)

* Disuse Syndrome (refer to Immobility/Unconscious Care Plan)

* Risk for Constipation related to Immobility, insufficient IV or PO fluids, low-fiber diet, stress, opiate pain medications (refer to Unit II)

△ Risk for Ineffective Health Regimen Management related to altered ability to maintain self at home secondary to sensory/motor/cognitive deficits and lack of knowledge of caregivers of home care, reality orientation, bowel/bladder program, skin care, signs and symptoms of complications, and community resources

△ Risk for Ineffective Health Regimen Management related to altered ability to maintain self at home secondary to sensory/motor/cognitive deficits and lack of knowledge of caregivers of home care, reality orientation, bowel/bladder program, skin care, signs and symptoms of complications, and community resources

Related Care Plan

Immobility or Unconsciousness

▲ This diagnosis was reported to be monitored for or managed frequently (75% to 100%).
△ This diagnosis was reported to be monitored for or managed often (50% to 74%).
* This diagnosis was not included in the validation study.

Transitional Risk Assessment Plan (TRAP)

Begin this plan on admission.
Implement the Transitional Risk Assessment Plan (TRAP):
- Refer to inside back cover.
- Add each validated risk diagnosis to individual's problem list with the risk code in ( ).
- Refer to Unit II to the individual risk nursing diagnoses/collaborative problems for outcomes and interventions.

  R: *"Close coordination of care in the post-acute period, early transition follow-up care, enhanced client education and self-management training, proactive end-of-life counseling, and extending the resources and clinical expertise over time via multidisciplinary team management" can lower readmission rates and improve health outcomes (Boutwell & Hwu, 2009, p. 14) and are utilized to activate the individual and family to select changes in their everyday lifestyle choices to improve their health (Hibbard & Greene, 2013).*

Transition Criteria

Before transition, the individual or family will:

1. Describe measures for reducing or eliminating selected risk factors.
2. Relate intent to discuss fears and concerns with family members after discharge.
3. Identify methods for management (e.g., of dysphagia, of incontinence).
4. Demonstrate or relate techniques to increase mobility.
5. State signs and symptoms that must be reported to a health care professional.
6. Relate community resources that can provide assistance with management at home.

Collaborative Problems

Risk for Complications of Increased Intracranial Pressure

Risk for Complications of Potential Complication: Pneumonia, Atelectasis

Risk for Complications of Adult Respiratory Distress Syndrome

Risk for Complications of Seizures

Risk for Complications of Stress Ulcers

Risk for Complications of Hypothalamic Syndromes

Risk for Complications of Diabetes Incepitus

Risk for Complications of Hyperglycemia

Collaborative Outcomes

The individual will be monitored for early signs and symptoms of (a) increased intracranial pressure, (b) pneumonia, atelectasis, (c) acute respiratory distress syndrome, (d) seizures, (e) stress ulcers, (f) hypothalamic syndromes, and (g) diabetes incepitus and will receive collaborative interventions if indicated to restore physiologic stability.

Indicators of Physiologic Stability

- Alert, oriented (a, b, c, d)
- Pulse 60 to 100 beats/min (a, b, c, e)
- Respiration 16 to 20 breaths/min (a, b, c,)
- Pupils equal, reactive to light (a, d)
- Temperature 98° F to 99.5° F (c, d)
- Breath sounds equal, no adventitious sounds (a, c)
- Oxygen saturation (pulse oximetry) (Sao_2) >95 (a, b, c)
- Stool negative for occult blood (e)
- Urine specific gravity 1.005 to 1.030 (a, b, e)
- Serum sodium 135 to 145 mEq/L (f)

Interventions	*Rationales*
1. Determine if individual can swallow. If the person is not alert, drooling, and/or has difficulty speaking, do not attempt the test; make the person NPO until a Speech Language Pathologist consult is completed. If those conditions are not present, proceed with the test: "A simple bedside screening evaluation involves asking the individual to sip a teaspoon of water from a cup. If the client can sip and swallow without difficulty, the client is asked to take a large gulp of 60 mL of water and swallow. If there are no signs of coughing or aspiration after 30 seconds, then it is safe for the individual to have a thickened diet until formally assessed by a speech pathologist" (*Massey & Jedlicka, 2002).	1. One of the frequent complications of a stroke is aspiration.

> **CLINICAL ALERT:**
> • "Dysphagia is common after stroke and is a major risk factor for developing aspiration pneumonia. It is important to assess swallowing function prior to administering oral medications or food. Thus, prevention of aspiration in patients with acute stroke includes initial NPO status until swallowing function is evaluated" (Filho, 2015).

2. Consult with speech language pathologist for all individual post-CVA.	

3. Follow protocol for positioning the head of the individual: a. Keep the head in neutral alignment with the body and elevating the head of the bed to 30 degrees for individuals in the acute phase of stroke who are at risk for any of the following problems: • Elevated intracranial pressure (ICP) (i.e., intracerebral hemorrhage, clinical deterioration >24 hours from stroke onset in patients with large ischemic infarction) • Aspiration (e.g., those with dysphagia and/or diminished consciousness) • Cardiopulmonary decompensation or oxygen desaturation (e.g., those with chronic cardiac and pulmonary disease) b. Keep the head of bed flat (0 to 15 degrees head-of-bed position) for individuals in the acute phase (first 24 hours) of ischemic stroke who are not at risk for elevated ICP, aspiration, or worsening cardiopulmonary status.	3. During the acute phase of stroke, the position of the individual and the head of bed should be individualized with respect to the risk of elevated ICP and aspiration, and the presence of comorbid cardiopulmonary disease (Filho, 2015).

4. Determine the last time an individual, diagnosed as post-ischemic stroke, appeared normal. Last seen normal (LSN) is the time noted that the individual seemed normal. This time is critical in order to determine if tissue plasma activator (tPA) can be administered (Filho, 2015).	4. For eligible patients with acute ischemic stroke, we recommend intravenous tissue plasminogen activator (tPA). Therapy, (e.g., alteplase) provided that treatment is initiated within 3 hours of clearly defined symptom onset. For individuals, who cannot be treated in less than 3 hours, it is recommended intravenous alteplase therapy, provided that treatment is initiated within 3 to 4.5 hours of clearly defined symptom onset (Filho, 2015).

Interventions	Rationales

5. Per protocol, regularly assess:
  a. Level of consciousness
  b. Ability to follow commands
  c. Visual fields
  d. Facial and limb weaknesses
  e. Signs/symptoms of aphasia, dysarthria
	5. National Institute of Health recommends the above assessment on admission and every 12 hours for the first 24 hours. Then every 24 hours until individual is discharged. These assessment criteria are elements on the NIH stroke scale with scoring (http://www.ninds.nih.gov/-doctors/NIH_Stroke_Scale.pdf).

6. Monitor BP according to protocol.	6. Both the systolic and diastolic BP are higher after stroke. It appears to rise acutely at the time of stroke. Blood pressure then falls over the next 7 to 10 days, with most of this fall occurring within the first 1 to 2 days. BP elevations after ischemic stroke represent an adaptive response, which helps to maintain the cerebral blood flow and perfusion of the c penumbra (poststroke ischemic tissue of the brain) despite loss of cerebral autoregulation.
7. Discuss with the physician/nurse practitioner/physical assistant the blood pressure goals. CLINICAL ALERT: • Excessive rise in BP could lead to neurologic deterioration from hemorrhage in the presence of a damaged blood–brain barrier. • Excessive reduction in BP can increase cerebral ischemia. • After a stroke, some degree of hypertension may be needed to maintain adequate perfusion of the brain, although very high blood pressure (systolic pressure >200 mm Hg) has been linked to higher mortality rates after stroke (Grise & Adeoye, 2012).	7. Blood pressure reduction is not routinely recommended in individuals with acute ischemic stroke, as it may decrease perfusion and increase cerebral ischemia.

8. Monitor the effectiveness of airway clearance by evaluating
  a. Effectiveness of cough effort
  b. Need for tracheobronchial suctioning
	8. Sixty percent of poststroke pneumonia is the cause by aspiration, and it is usually due to stroke-related dysphagia or to decreased level of consciousness (Ishida, 2015).

9. Monitor for signs and symptoms of increased ICP:
  a. Increasing headache, increased with movement
  b. Changes in cognition, level of consciousness, confusion
  c. New onset or worsening of aphasia
  d. Slowing of pupil respond to pen light
  e. Pulse slowing or increasing (late sign)
  f. Change in respiratory patterns (late sign)
  g. Refer to Unit II Section 2, Risk for Complications of Increased Intracranial Pressure.
	9. Individuals with increased ICP due to hemorrhage, vertebrobasilar ischemia, or bihemispheric ischemia can present with a decreased respiratory drive or muscular airway obstruction. Hypoventilation, with a resulting increase in carbon dioxide, may lead to cerebral vasodilation, which further elevates ICP (Filho, 2015).

10. Monitor temperature and, if indicated, initiate interventions to maintain temperature below 99.5° F. Refer to Unit II Section 2, Risk for Complications of Pneumonia, Atelectasis for additional interventions.	10. "Hyperthermia in the setting of acute cerebral ischemia is associated with increased morbidity and mortality and should be managed aggressively (treat fever >37.5° C [99.5° F])" (Morgenstern et al., 2010).

(continued)

Interventions	*Rationales*

11. Monitor for signs and symptoms of ARDS:
  a. Respiratory discomfort
  b. Noisy tachypnea
  c. Tachycardia
  d. Diffuse rales and rhonchi
	11. Damaged type II cells release inflammatory mediators that increase alveolo-capillary membrane permeability, causing pulmonary edema. Decreased surfactant production decreases alveolar compliance. Respiratory muscles must greatly increase inspiratory pressures to inflate lungs (Filho, 2015).

12. Monitor hydration status by evaluating the following:
  a. Oral intake
  b. Parenteral therapy
  c. Intake and output
  d. Urine specific gravity
	12. A balance must be maintained to ensure hydration to liquefy secretions to maintain euvolemia. Use isotonic solutions (e.g., 0.9% sodium chloride); nonisotonic solutions can worsen cerebral edema, increasing ICP (Filho, 2015). Significantly increased amounts of urine output may indicate diabetes insipidus.

13. Refer to Unit II Section 2, Risk for Complications of Seizures	13. Cerebrovascular disease is the most common known cause of epilepsy in elderly people, causing one-third to one-half of cases. Risk factors for poststroke epilepsy (hemorrhage, cortical involvement, large size) are similar to those for acute symptomatic seizures. Acute symptomatic seizures and recurrent stroke are also risk factors for poststroke epilepsy (Schachter, 2016).
14. Monitor for GI Bleeding.	14. Hypersecretion of gastric juices occurs during periods of stress.
15. Monitor blood sugar.	15. Hyperglycemia, generally defined as a blood glucose level >126 mg/dL (>7.0 mmol/L), is common in individuals with acute stroke and is associated with poor functional outcome. Hyperglycemia may augment brain injury by several mechanisms including increased tissue acidosis from anaerobic metabolism, free radical generation, and increased blood brain barrier permeability (Filho, 2015).

16. Monitor for metabolic dysfunction:
  a. Low serum sodium
  b. Elevated urine sodium
  c. Elevated urine specific gravity
	16. Damage to the hypothalamic region may result in increased secretion of antidiuretic hormone (ADH) (Sterns, 2015).

17. Monitor for diabetes insipidus:
  a. Excess urine output
  b. Extreme thirst
  c. Elevated serum sodium
  d. Low specific gravity
	17. Compression of posterior pituitary gland or its neuronal connections can cause a decrease of ADH (Ramthun, Mocelin, & Delfino, 2011).

Clinical Alert Report

Prior to providing care, advise ancillary staff/student to report the following to the professional nurse assigned to the individual:

- Change in cognitive status
- Oral temperature >99.5° F
- Systolic blood pressure >220 mm Hg or diastolic blood pressure >120 mm Hg
- Systolic BP <90 mm Hg
- Resting pulse >100, <50 beats/min
- Pulse oximetry > 95%
- Respiratory rate >28, <10/min
- Labored or shallow respiration
- Sudden onset of chest pain, leg pain

Documentation

Neurologic assessment
Vital signs
Complaints of vomiting or headache
Changes in status
Swallowing assessment
Intake/output

Nursing Diagnoses

Carp's Cues

After the acute phase of postischemic stroke, the major focus of nursing and other members of the multidiscipline is to reduce and eliminate modifiable risk factors, to assist the individual and family to restore previous functioning as much as possible and to adapt to resultant impaired functioning.

Nursing Diagnosis provides the exact terminology to describe the focus not only for nursing but for other disciplines.

Using Gordon's 11 Functional Health Patterns, the individual/family will be assessed for the presence of compromise functioning and risk factors that can compromise functioning or actual compromised functioning. The nurse in collaboration with the individual and family can determine what priorities are for this individual and family presently. Sometimes, priorities identified by the nurse, are not shared by the individual and/or the family.

Stroke individuals and caregivers are central participants in the rehabilitation process to foster therapy adherence and facilitate optimal community integration and continued quality of life despite residual impairments. With collaborative input from all rehabilitation team members, including stroke survivors and their family, comprehensive and individualized assessment and treatment plans are formulated (Miller, 2015).

"Because stroke is a complex disease process that requires the skills of an interdisciplinary team, nurses frequently play a central role in care coordination throughout the recovery continuum. Furthermore, because across care settings, nurses commonly have the most direct contact with stroke patients and their caregivers, they are often called on to implement management techniques developed by other rehabilitation team members. Consequently, nurses should be familiar with the variety of services and procedures provided by the other disciplines that are central to stroke rehabilitation teams" (Miller, 2015).

Impaired Communication Related to the Effects of Hemisphere (Left or Right) Damage on Language or Speech

NOC
Communication
Ability

Goal

The individual will report improved satisfaction with ability to communicate.

NIC
Communication
Enhancement:
Speech Deficit, Active
Listening, Socialization
Enhancement

Indicators

- Demonstrate improved ability to express self and understand others.
- Report decreased frustration during communication efforts.

Interventions	Rationales
1. Differentiate between language disturbances (dysphagia/aphasia) and speech disturbances (dyspraxia/apraxia).	1. Language involves comprehension and transmission of ideas and feelings. Speech is the mechanics and articulations of verbal expression (Miller, 2015).
2. Collaborate with a speech therapist to evaluate the individual and create a plan (Miller, 2015).	
3. Provide an atmosphere of acceptance and privacy: a. Do not rush. b. Speak slowly and in a normal tone. c. Decrease external noise and distractions. d. Encourage the individual to share frustrations; validate the individual's nonverbal expressions. e. Provide the individual with opportunities to make decisions about his or her care, whenever appropriate. f. Do not force the individual to communicate. g. If the individual laughs or cries uncontrollably, change the subject or activity.	3. Communication is the core of all human relations. Impaired ability to communicate spontaneously is frustrating and embarrassing. Nursing actions should focus on decreasing the tension and conveying an understanding of how difficult the situation must be for the individual.
4. Make every effort to understand the individual's communication efforts: a. Listen attentively. b. Repeat the individual's message back to him or her to ensure understanding. c. Ignore inappropriate word usage; do not correct mistakes. d. Do not pretend you understand; if you do not, ask the individual to repeat. e. Try to anticipate some needs (e.g., Do you need something to drink?).	4. Nurse and family members should make every attempt to understand the individual. Each success, regardless of how minor, decreases frustration and increases motivation.
5. Refer to *Communication Problems After Stroke* at, Complete Guide to Communication; Problems After Stroke. Go to https://www.stroke.org.uk/sites/default/files/complete_guide_to_communication_problems_after_stroke.pdf	

Documentation

Dialogues
Method to use

Risk for Bowel Incontinence Related to Constipation Secondary to Immobility, Side Effects of Medications, Inability to Access Bathroom in Timely Manner

NOC

Tissue Integrity: Skin and Mucous Membranes, Bowel Continence, Bowel Elimination, Hydration

Goal

The individual will report no or fewer episodes of incontinence.

NIC

Perineal Care, Bowel Incontinence Care, Fluid Management, Nutrition Management, Constipation/Impaction Management.

Indicators

• Remove or minimize environmental barriers to bathroom.
• Use proper adaptive equipment to assist with voiding, transfers, and dressing.
• Describe relationship between constipation and bowel incontinence.

Carp's Cues

"Prevalence of fecal incontinence among stroke survivors ranges between 30% and 40% while the patient is in the hospital, 18% at discharge, and between 7% and 9% at 6 months after stroke. During the rehabilitation phase, patients are evaluated to identify and address potential contributing factors (e.g., diet, drug side effects, rectal muscle weakness); however, the strongest independent risk factor for fecal incontinence at 3 months after stroke is needing help getting to the toilet" (Miller et al., 2010).

Interventions	Rationales

1. Explain the causes of bowel incontinence:
  a. Insufficient fluids
  b. Insufficient dietary fiber
  c. Immobility
  d. Constipation	

2. Explain the side effects of anticholinergic medications such as antipsychotics, tricyclic antidepressants, oxybutynin, or antiemetics. These medications predispose toward constipation by reducing contractility of the smooth muscle of the gut and may cause chronic colonic dysmotility with long-term use (*Harari, Coshall, Rudd, & Wolfe, 2003, p. 148).	2. Research "suggests that the potentially modifiable factors of using constipating drugs and of functional difficulties with toilet access are most strongly correlated with new-onset bowel incontinence 3 months after stroke. Disability is a more important factor than age, sex, or stroke-specific factors in causing bowel incontinence in longer-term stroke survivors" (*Harari et al., 2003, p. 148).
3. Explain that fecal incontinence can be prevented and/or corrected. Refer to specific nursing diagnoses in Unit II for interventions that address risk/causative factors such as immobility, dehydration, imbalanced nutrition, impaired physical mobility.	

Impaired Swallowing Related to Muscle Paralysis or Paresis Secondary to Damage to Upper Motor Neurons

NOC
Aspiration Control, Swallowing Status

Goal

The individual will report improved ability to swallow.

NIC
Aspiration Precautions, Swallowing Therapy, Surveillance, Referral, Positioning

Indicators

- Describe causative factors when known.
- Describe rationale and procedures for treatment.

Interventionss	Rationales

1. Determine if individual has swallowing problems and at risk for aspiration:
  a. Assess for the presence of sombulence, drooling, and/or has difficulty speaking, do not attempt the test; make the person NPO until a Speech Language Pathologist consult is completed.
  b. If those conditions are not present, proceed with the test.
	1. Dysphagia (impairment in swallowing) occurs in 30% to 64% of individuals in the acute phase of stroke recovery (Miller et al., 2010)

Interventionss	*Rationales*
c. "A simple bedside screening evaluation involves asking the individual to sip a teaspoon of water from a cup. If the patient can sip and swallow without difficulty, the patient is asked to take a large gulp of 60 mL of water and swallow. If there are no signs of coughing or aspiration after 30 seconds, then it is safe for the individual to have a thickened diet until formally assessed by a speech pathologist" (Jauch et al., 2010; *Massey & Jedlicka, 2002).	
2. Consult with Speech Language Pathologist for all poststroke individuals and a specific plan regarding speech and swallowing (American Heart Association, 2007a).	2. The speech pathologist has the expertise needed to perform the dysphagia evaluation.
3. Post a sign at the bedside to communicate that nothing should be given to eat or drink without first checking with the nurse.	3. The risk of aspiration can be reduced if all visitors/staff/students are alerted.
4. Plan meals for when the individual is well-rested; ensure that reliable suction equipment is on hand during meals. Discontinue feeding if individual is tired.	4. Fatigue can increase the risk of aspiration.
5. Explain the risk for aspiration because of dysphagia. Consult with Speech Language Pathologist, if indicated. a. Before transition, advise to (Tanner &, Culbertson, 2014): • Know how to perform the Heimlich maneuver (individual, other household members). • Sit up straight during all meals and snacking and 30 minutes after. • Take a symptom inventory: Fatigue will contribute to swallowing problems. Think about that if fatigue is present, dysphasia will be worse also. • Mindful eating challenge: Using a fork, place food in mouth. Put your fork down. Chew food very thoroughly, then swallow. Pick up fork again only when mouth is empty. • Do not talk with food in your mouth. • Thicken your liquids. • Eat the right kinds of foods: Avoid hard, crumbly, dry, and crunchy foods. Add gravy for moisture. Eat very soft or pureed foods. • Eat smaller meals (to avoid "swallowing fatigue"). • Alternate liquids and solids: Take a small sip or two of a liquid between bites for moisture. Finish the meal with some liquid.	

Documentation

Intake of foods and fluids
Swallowing difficulties

Unilateral Neglect Related to (Specify Site) Secondary to Right Hemispheric Brain Damage

NOC

Body Image, Body Positioning: Self-Initiated, Self-Care: Activities of Daily Living (ADLs)

Goal

The individual will demonstrate an ability to scan the visual field to compensate for loss of function or sensation in affected limb(s).

NIC

Unilateral Neglect Management, Self-Care Assistance

Indicators

- Describe the deficit and the rationale for treatments.
- Identify safety hazards in the environment.

Interventions	Rationales
1. Monitor for unilateral neglect.	1. Failure to detect or respond to stimuli specifically on the opposite side of brain damage, accurately detects and responds to stimuli on the same side of brain damage.
2. If family is present, explain to the individual/family that unilateral neglect is cluster of attention problems associated with slow and/or inaccurate processing of and responding to stimuli occurring contralateral to the side of the brain damage.	2. Spatial neglect is more commonly associated with lesions of the inferior parietal lobule or temporoparietal region, superior temporal cortex, or frontal lobe. Less common are lesions of the subcortical regions, including the basal ganglia, thalamus, and cingulate cortex (Miller et al., 2010).
3. Reassure the individual that the problem is a result of CVA.	3. Individuals know that something is wrong, but may attribute it to being "disturbed."
4. Initially adapt the individual's environment: a. Take every opportunity, large or small, to help them "tune in" to that side. b. Place the call light, telephone, and bedside stand on the unaffected side. c. Always approach the individual from the center or midline.	4. Interventions are focused on improving awareness of the neglected side (*Davis, 2003). c. This will minimize sensory deprivation initially; however, attempts should be made to have the individual attend to both sides (American Stroke Association, 2016b).
5. Assist the individual with an ADL: a. First, tell person the activity needed, such as "Let's get your fork." b. Take the individual's hand and his or her head automatically turns in that direction and the eyes follow.	5. This intervention reinforces the activity by combining the sense of hearing with the sense of touch.
6. Teach the individual to scan the entire environment, turning the head to compensate for visual field cuts. Remind the individual to scan when ambulating.	6. Scanning can help to prevent injury and increase awareness of entire space.
7. For self-care, instruct the individual to: a. Attend to the affected side first. b. Use adaptive equipment as needed. c. Always check the affected limb(s) during ADLs.	7. The individual may need specific reminders to prevent her or him from ignoring nonfunctioning body parts.

Documentation

Presence of neglect
Individual/family teaching
Response to teaching

> **TRANSITION TO HOME/COMMUNITY CARE**
> If indicated, review the high-risk diagnoses identified for this individual on admission:
> * Is the person still at high risk?
> * Can the family reduce the risks?
> * Is the person at higher risk at home?
> * Is a home health nurse assessment needed?
> * Refer to discharge planner/case manager/social service.
> * When is this person scheduled for follow-up with primary provider? Specialists? Record dates of appointments.
> * Complete a medication reconciliation prior to discharge. Refer to inside back cover.

STAR   **Stop**

Think   Is this person at high risk for injury, falls, medical complications, and/or inability to care for self (ADLs)?
Is there a support person available?
Is the person competent to manage self-administration of medications, treatment procedures? Are additional resources needed?
Can the person explain how to monitor the condition (e.g., blood glucose, sign/symptoms of complications, dietary/mobility restrictions, and when to call his or her primary provider or specialist)?

Act   Contact or provide the appropriate resource (e.g., contacting a support person, home health assessment, additional teaching, printed materials).

Review   Has the problem been addressed? If not, use SBAR to communicate to the appropriate person.

Risk for Ineffective Health Management Related to Altered Ability to Maintain Self at Home Secondary to Sensory/Motor/Cognitive Deficits and Lack of Knowledge of Caregivers of Home Care, Reality Orientation, Bowel/Bladder Program, Skin Care, and Signs and Symptoms of Complications, and Community Resources

NOC

Compliance Behavior, Knowledge: Treatment Regimen, Participation in Health Care Decisions, Treatment Behavior: Illness and Injury, Anticipatory Guidance, Health Education, Risk Management, Learning Facilitation

NIC

Anticipatory Guidance, Risk Identification, Learning Facilitation, Health Education, Teaching: Procedure/Treatment, Health System Guidance

Goal

The goals for this diagnosis represent those associated with transition planning.

Carp's Cues

The effects of a stroke on an individual/family can range from some weakness in one arm to paraplegia to a state of immobility. The ability to perform ADLs, communicate, work, learn, use a phone, access/use the toilet, hold a child, and engage in sexual activity can be unaffected or profoundly compromised. The challenge for nurses is to identify with the individual and family what are their most pressing concerns. These are then addressed prior to transition with the provision of how/where they can seek assistance after transition.

If the individual will be discharged to his or her home, then there will be additional concerns such as caregiving activities, coping, depression, and teaching requirements such as medication compliance, secondary stroke prevention, s/s of complications (diet, smoking, exercising).

Interventions	Rationales
1. Ensure the individual/family has an understanding of stroke, its cause, and treatments prescribed.	1. Understanding can reinforce the need to comply with the treatment regimen (*Schwamm et al., 2005).
2. Explain that the risk of poststroke bladder and bowel dysfunction affects approximately 25% to 50% of stroke survivors.	2. Persistent bladder and bowel difficulties can significantly affect the rehabilitation process (time) and negatively influence stroke survivors' physical and mental health, leading to social isolation and restrictions in subsequent employment and leisure activities.

3. Explain signs and symptoms of complications, and stress the need for immediate evaluation. Go to ER or call 911 (Jauch et al., 2010).
  a. Sudden weakness or numbness in the face, arm, or leg, especially on one side of the body
  b. Difficulty speaking or understanding what is being spoken
  c. Difficulty swallowing
  d. Difficulty in walking or even falling and an inability to get back up
  e. Severe headache
  f. Sudden trouble seeing in one eye or both eyes
  g. Sudden onset of chest pain, leg swelling/redness, shortness of breath
 	
  h. Change in cognitive status, seizures
  i. Oral temperature >99.5° F
  j. Labored or shallow respiration
	3. These may be signs of a cerebral ischemia and an evolving stroke. Time is of the essence because if tissue plasma activator (tPA) is indicated, it must be administered within 3 hours of the onset of symptoms.
	
	  g. Pulmonary embolism risk is highest during the first 3 to 120 days after stroke, with a 50% sudden death rate (Miller et al., 2010).
	  h. These signs and symptoms may indicate increasing ICP or cerebral tissue hypoxia.

4. Discuss with the individual's family the anticipated stressors associated with CVA and its impact on family functioning and role responsibilities. Encourage individual to share concerns when at home with home health nurse and physician/nurse practitioner.	4. The only prediction that can be made of the effects of a family member stroke on the family unit and functioning is that it is unpredictable. Previous family functioning will be challenged and new roles will emerge.

Carp's Cues

For a stroke individual older than 65 years, 6 months after a stroke (Stein, 2008):
- 30% will need assistance when walking.
- 26% will need assistance with ADLs.
- 26% will live in a nursing home.

a. Financial
  b. Changes in role responsibilities
  c. Dependency
  d. Caregiver responsibilities
	
	  d. Refer to Caregiver Role Strain in the index for specific interventions.

(continued)

Interventions	Rationales
5. Explain the possibility of depression poststroke.	5. Depression is one of the most underdiagnosed and undertreated complications after stroke. Its origin may be organic, related to poststroke dysfunction of catecholamine-containing neurons, premorbid, or reactive to the catastrophe of losing function. Although depression has been proposed to influence motor and functional recovery, one study found that its negative impact on functional recovery appeared most significant after hospital discharge rather than during the hospital stay. Poststroke depression is also associated with higher mortality, poorer functional recovery, and less social activity.
6. Advise individual and/or family to consult with primary care provider (PCP) of the following (*Williams et al., 2005): a. Feeling down, depressed, or hopeless b. Trouble falling or staying asleep, or sleeping too much c. Feeling tired or having little energy d. Poor appetite or overeating e. Trouble concentrating on things, such as reading the newspaper or watching television f. Thoughts that you would be better off dead or of hurting yourself in some way	6. Guidelines for treating poststroke depression also recommend screening, assessment, and treatment with an appropriate antidepressant for a period of approximately 6 months.
7. Identify risk factors that can be reduced: a. Hypertension b. Smoking/tobacco use c. Secondhand smoke d. Obesity e. High-fat diet f. High-sodium diet g. Sedentary lifestyle	7. Focusing on factors that can be controlled can improve compliance, increase self-esteem, and reduce feelings of helplessness. a. Hypertension with increased peripheral resistance damages the intima of blood vessels, contributing to arteriosclerosis. b. Tobacco exposure produces tachycardia, raises blood pressure, and constricts blood vessels. The effects of nicotine increase the risk of clot formation with aggregation of platelets and vasoconstriction and deprive tissues of oxygen (CDC, 2014b). c. Low levels of smoke exposure, including exposures to secondhand tobacco smoke, lead to a rapid and sharp increase in dysfunction and inflammation of the lining of the blood vessels, which are implicated in heart attacks and stroke (CDC, 2014b). d. Obesity increases cardiac workload and decrease circulation to peripheral tissues. e. High-fat diet may increase arteriosclerosis and plaque formation. f. Sodium controls water distribution throughout the body. A gain in sodium causes a gain in water, thus increasing the circulating volume. g. Participation in walking and sports has been shown to reduce stroke risk by 20% to 29% (Gallanagh, Quinn, Alexander, & Walters, 2011), and maintain normal glycemic ranges (*Sacco et al., 2006).

Interventions	*Rationales*

8. Provide information about or initiate referrals to community resources; for example:
  a. Counselors, home health agencies
  b. American Heart Association (http://www.americanheart.org)
  c. American Stroke Association (http://www.strokeassociation.org/STROKEORG/)
  d. National Stroke Association (http://www.stroke.org/)
  e. Recovering After a Stroke: A Patient and Family Guide
  f. Consumer Guide Number 16 AHCPR Publication No. 95-0664: May 1995
  g. US Agency for HealthCare Research and Quality (http://www.strokecenter.org/wp-content/uploads/2011/08/Recovering-After-a-Stroke.pdf)
	8. Such resources can provide needed assistance with symptom and home management and help to minimize the potentially destructive effects on the individual and family.

Documentation

Individual/family teaching
Referrals if indicated

Guillain–Barré Syndrome

Guillain–Barré syndrome (GBS) is an acute, rapidly progressing, inflammatory, autoimmune, demyelinating polyneuropathy of the peripheral nervous system, affecting 1 person/100,000 people (National Institute of Neurologic Disorders and Stroke [NINDS], 2016a). Its etiology is unclear, but precipitating events include viral illnesses, immunizations, surgery, and respiratory or gastrointestinal viral or bacterial infection (NINDS, 2016a). There are several subtypes of GBS, but in the most common form, the myelin sheaths surrounding the peripheral nerves are destroyed by an immune reaction, resulting in poor conduction of nerve impulses. GBS can affect muscles, sensory nerves, and cranial nerves, but cognitive function and level of consciousness are not impacted. Early symptoms include weakness and tingling in the extremities, and the disease is characterized by symmetrical, ascending flaccid paralysis and the loss of reflex response. Sensory nerve effects include paresthesias, numbness, and severe pain. Symptom progression may be life-threatening, resulting in quadriplegia, paralysis of facial and respiratory muscles or autonomic involvement causing fluctuating blood pressures, cardiac arrhythmias, paralytic ileus, and other complications (Lemone et al., 2011; NINDS, 2016a). Respiratory failure results in mechanical ventilation for approximately 30% of patients (Andary, Oleszek, Maurelus, & White-McCrimmon, 2016). Manifestations of the disease are variable, with acute progression (1 to 3 weeks) followed by a plateau phase and a recovery stage of slow improvement over weeks to years (NINDS, 2016a). Although it is potentially fatal, most patients with GBS recover with minimal residual disability (NINDS, 2016a). Diagnosis is made based on the individual's history and clinical presentation, as GBS effects develop rapidly, are commonly symmetrical, and deep tendon reflexes are impaired (Bautista & Grossman, 2016). The diagnosis is confirmed by reduced conduction velocity during electromyography (EMG) and nerve conduction studies or abnormal levels of protein in the cerebrospinal fluid (NINDS, 2016a). There is no known cure for GBS, but therapies that lessen the severity of the disease and may accelerate recovery include plasma exchange (plasmapheresis) and intravenous immoglobulin (IVIG) infusion, if initiated early in the disease (Andary et al., 2016). In the acute phase collaborative care focuses on oxygenation, cardiac monitoring, nutritional support, pain management, prevention of complications of immobility, bowel and bladder management, mental status management, and emotional support. Rehabilitation requires interdisciplinary treatment.

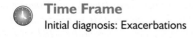

Time Frame
Initial diagnosis: Exacerbations

▪▪▪▪▪ DIAGNOSTIC CLUSTER**

Collaborative Problems

Risk for Complications of Acute Respiratory Failure (ARF)

Risk for Complications of Autonomic Nervous System Failure

Risk for Complications of Peripheral Nervous System Failure

Risk for Complications of Deep Vein Thrombus (refer to Unit II)

Risk for Complications of Decreased Cardiac Output (refer to Unit II)

Risk for Complications of Pneumonia (refer to Unit II)

Nursing Diagnoses

Risk for Ineffective Airway Clearance related to impaired ability to cough (refer to Unit II)

Risk for Impaired Skin Integrity related to immobility, incontinence, sensory-motor deficits (refer to Unit II)

Impaired Swallowing related to swallowing/chewing problems secondary to cranial nerve impairment (refer to Unit II)

Impaired Communication related to muscle weakness and mechanical ventilation (if present) (refer to Mechanical Ventilation Care Plan)

Activity Intolerance related to fatigue and difficulties in performing ADLs (refer to Unit II)

Risk for Self-Care Deficits related to flaccid paralysis, paresis, and fatigue (refer to Unit II)

Risk for Interrupted Family Process related to nature of disorder, role disturbances, and uncertain future (refer to Unit II)

Risk for Ineffective Health Therapeutic Regimen Management related to lack of knowledge of condition, treatments required, stress management, signs and symptoms of complications, and availability of community resources

**This medical condition was not included in the validation study.

TRANSITION TO HOME/COMMUNITY CARE

The individual or family will:

1. Relate intent to discuss fears and concerns with family/trusted friends after discharge.
2. Relate necessity of continuation of therapeutic programs.
3. Relate safety precautions to prevent falls/injury.
4. Identify signs and symptoms that must be reported to a health care professional.

Transitional Risk Assessment Plan (TRAP)

Begin this plan on admission.

Implement the Transitional Risk Assessment Plan (TRAP):

• Refer to inside back cover.
• Add each validated risk diagnosis to individual's problem list with the risk code in ( ).
• Refer to Unit II to the individual risk nursing diagnoses/collaborative problems for outcomes and interventions.

   R: "*Close coordination of care in the post-acute period, early transition follow-up care, enhanced client education and self-management training, proactive end-of-life counseling, and extending the resources and clinical expertise over time via multidisciplinary team management*" can lower readmission rates and improve health outcomes (Boutwell & Hwu, 2009, p. 14). Interventions are utilized to activate the individual and family to select changes in their everyday lifestyle choices to improve their health (Hibbard & Greene, 2013).

Collaborative Problems

Risk for Complications of Acute Respiratory Failure (ARF)

Risk for Complications of Autonomic Nervous System Failure

Risk for Complications of Peripheral Nervous System Failure

Collaborative Outcomes

The individual will be monitored for early signs/symptoms of (a) acute respiratory failure, (b) autonomic nervous system dysfunction, peripheral nervous system failure, and will receive collaborative interventions to stabilize him or her.

Indicators of Physiologic Stability

- Respiration 16 to 20 breaths/min (a)
- Oxygen saturation (pulse oximetry) >95% (a)
- Serum pH 7.35 to 7.45 (a)
- Serum Pco_2 35 to 45 mm Hg (a)
- Cardiac normal sinus rhythm (a)
- Bowel sounds present (b)
- Alert, oriented (a)
- Cranial nerves II to XXII intact (c)
- Urine output >0.5 mL/kg/hr (a)
- Dry, warm skin (b)

Interventions	Rationales
1. Monitor for signs and symptoms of pneumonia and ARF to assist with breathing.	1. Ventilation may become necessary as acute Guillain–Barré progresses, due to paralysis of intercostal and diaphragmatic muscles (Andary et al, 2016). In the acute phase of GBS, ascending paralysis may result in sudden respiratory failure.
a. Auscultate breath sounds.	a. Auscultating breath sounds assesses the adequacy of air flow and detects the presence of adventitious sounds (see Mechanical Ventilation for more information).
b. Assess for secretions: • Encourage the individual to deep breathe and cough. • Position the individual on alternate sides to assist movement of secretions. • Suction if individual is unable to manage secretions. • Reassure individual by maintaining a calm environment.	b. When the respiratory muscles fatigue, cough becomes ineffective, leading to the accumulation of mucus and the formation of mucous plugs in the airway. This accumulation of secretions causes alveolar collapse, leading to ARF.
c. Assess O_2 saturation via pulse oximetry.	c. Pulse oximetry provides ongoing data on O_2 saturation.
d. Assess blood gases: • Monitor for signs of decreased respiratory functions, pH, $Paco_2$, O_2 saturation, and HCO_3.	d. Acid–base imbalance, hypoxemia, hypercarbia, weak cough, ineffective airway clearance, may signify that the individual requires intubation to avoid ARF. Decreased vital capacity and reduced inspiratory or expiratory pressures confirms the need for intubation (Andary et al, 2016).
e. Explain the necessity of intubation to the individual and family if indicated.	e. Intubation is initiated to relieve shortness of breath to avoid ARF, aspiration, and pneumonia.
f. Provide assurance and encouragement for the individual.	f. This will reduce fear of the disease process. Most Guillain–Barré individuals have been healthy, active individuals who suddenly became victims of dependency.
g. Report to the physician/nurse practitioner changes regarding: • Respiratory status and reduced vital capacity and arterial blood gases • GI status	g. Early recognition enables prompt intervention to prevent further complications.

Interventions	Rationales
2. Monitor signs and symptoms of autonomic nervous system dysfunction: a. Blood pressure variations and cardiac arrhythmias	2. Autonomic nervous system dysfunction can develop from involvement of both the sympathetic and para-sympathetic nervous systems. Manifestations include fluctuating blood pressures, hypotension, orthostatic hypotension, abnormal vagal responses (cardiac arrhythmias, heart block, asystole, and syndrome of inappropriate secretion of antidiuretic hormone, para-lytic ileus, urine retention, and diaphoresis) (Andary et al., 2016; NINDS, 2016a).
b. Urinary retention	b. Urinary retention is associated with autonomic nervous system dysfunction.
c. Constipation or paralytic ileus	c. Autonomic dysfunction can decrease bowel motility.
d. Mental status changes that can include sleep disturbances, hallucinations, and delusions.	d. Mental status changes may develop due to auto-nomic dysfunction and occur more frequently in patients with severe symptoms of GBS (Andary et al., 2016).
3. Monitor signs and symptoms of cranial nerve dysfunction.	3. Demyelination of the efferent fibers of the spinal and cranial nerve creates a delay in conduction, resulting in motor weakness or loss of conduction, producing, im-paired sensation, or paralysis (NINDS, 2016a).
4. Monitor for psychological complications such as anxiety and depression.	4. GBS develops rapidly, may result in profound disability which requires extensive medical intervention, and the recovery period may be prolonged. Sudden dependence may precipitate a psychological crisis.

Clinical Alert Report

Prior to providing care, advise ancillary staff/student to report the following to the professional nurse assigned to the individual:

- Change in cognitive status
- Change in swallowing ability
- Oral temperature >100.5° F
- Systolic BP <90 mm Hg
- Resting pulse >100, <50 beats/min
- Respiratory rate >28, <10/min.
- Change in respiratory function (effort)
- Oxygen saturation <90%

Documentation

Vital signs
Intake and output
Neurologic assessment findings
Changes in respiratory status
Response to interventions
Neurologic changes

TRANSITION TO HOME/COMMUNITY CARE

If indicated, review the high-risk diagnoses identified for this individual on admission:

- Is the person still at high risk?
- Can the family reduce the risks?
- Is the person at higher risk at home?
- Is a home health nurse assessment needed?
- Refer to discharge planner/case manager/social service.
- When is this person scheduled for follow-up with primary provider? Specialists? Record dates of appointments.
- Complete a medication reconciliation prior to discharge. Refer to inside back cover.

STAR

Stop

Think   Is this person at high risk for injury, falls, medical complications, and/or inability to care for self (ADLs)?

Is there a support person available?

Is the person competent to manage self-administration of medications, treatment procedures? Are additional resources needed?

Can the person explain how to monitor the condition (e.g., blood glucose, sign/symptoms of complications, dietary/mobility restrictions, and when to call his or her primary provider or specialist)?

Act   Contact or provide the appropriate resource (e.g., contacting a support person, home health assessment, additional teaching, printed materials).

Review   Has the problem been addressed? If not, use SBAR to communicate to the appropriate person.

Nursing Diagnoses

Risk for Ineffective Health Management Related to Lack of Knowledge of Condition, Treatments Required, Stress Management, Signs and Symptoms of Complications, and Availability of Community Resources

NOC

Compliance/ Engagement Behavior, Knowledge: Treatment Regimen, Participation in Health Care Decisions, Treatment Behavior: Illness or Injury

NIC

Anticipatory Guidance, Learning Facilitation, Risk Identification, Health Education, Teaching Procedure/ Treatment, Health System Guidance.

Goal

Refer to discharge criteria.

Interventions	*Rationales*
1. Teach the individual and his or her family the basic pathology of the individual's condition.	1. Understanding can improve compliance and reduce the family unit's frustrations.
2. Assist the individual in identifying realistic short-term goals.	2. Preparation of the individual to set realistic goals for recovery will reduce feelings of depression if goals are not attained.
3. Teach the individual the value of continued ROM (passive or active, dependent on functional ability) and strengthening-stretching exercise programs. Consult physical therapy.	3. Exercise will maintain muscle strength and flexibility and promote circulation in effected extremities (Andary et al., 2016).
4. Teach the individual energy conservation techniques, scheduling planned rest periods, and exercise consistent with tolerance levels.	4. Energy conservation can reduce fatigue (NINDS, 2016a).
5. Teach care of altered body functions: a. Bowel & bladder function: Encourage intake of 2,000 mL of fluid unless contraindicated. b. Nutritional requirements: Provide a diet high in calories and protein. c. Self-care deficits, if necessary. Areas of concern: dressing, grooming, safe ambulation	5. Care instructions: a. Adequate fluid intake promotes bowel and bladder function, prevention of constipation related to reduced activity and peristalsis. b. Protein and calories are required to rebuild muscle mass. c. Encourage maximum individual self-care with ADL activities for purpose of strengthening and increasing independence.
6. Initiate referral to rehabilitation services.	6. Individual will require outpatient or home care multidisciplinary rehabilitation therapy. The recovery period may be as short as a few weeks or may extend to a few years (NINDS, 2016a). A significant percentage of those hospitalized with GBS will require inpatient rehabilitation (Andary et al., 2016).
7. Facilitate referral for psychological counseling and emotional support.	7. GBS often causes sudden paralysis, communication difficulties, and dependence for body functions and ADLs, creating psychological and emotional crisis for individuals and families (NINDS, 2016a).
8. Explain signs and symptoms of complications to report to health care professional. a. Productive cough b. Difficulty with urination, odor to urine c. Prolonged constipation d. Increased weakness or fatigue e. Weight loss	8. Early intervention will minimize complications of the condition.
9. Provide information to assist the individual and family to manage at home. Refer to the following resources: a. Guillain-Barre Syndrome/Chronic Inflammatory Demyelinating Polyneuropathy Foundation International at http://www.gbs-cidp.org b. Case manager/discharge planner referral c. Home health agency	9. Individuals and families who receive community support may cope more effectively with this disease. Functional loss may be significant. Even when deficits are temporary, the individual will require interdisciplinary support during the recovery period.

Multiple Sclerosis

Multiple sclerosis (MS) is the most common autoimmune, inflammatory demyelinating disease of the central nervous system (CNS) (Olek, & Mowry, 2016). It is characterized by acute exacerbations or gradual worsening of neurologic functions and disability (*Ben-Zacharia, 2001; Olek, 2016).

The Multiple Sclerosis Foundation (2016) estimates that more than 400,000 people in the United States and about 2.5 million people around the world have MS. About 200 new cases are diagnosed each week in the United States.

High frequency areas of the world (prevalence of 60/100,000 or more) include all of Europe (including Russia), southern Canada, northern United States, New Zealand, and southeast Australia. In many of these areas, the prevalence is more than 100/100,000; the highest reported rate (300/100,000) is in the Orkney Islands. In the United States, the estimated prevalence is 100/100,000 (0.1%), for a total of at least 250,000 to 300,000 persons with MS (Olek, & Mowry, 2016).

Researchers have reported that the risk of developing MS was significantly reduced for women taking ≥400 International Units/day of vitamin D (Mokry et al., 2015; Salzer et al., 2012)

MRI studies have shown clear evidence that central to the disease process is the gradual destruction of the myelin sheath surrounding nerve cells by autoreactive T-cells (Olek, 2016).

This stripping of nerve fibers interferes with nerve conduction, which leads to various degrees of paralysis and to the other symptoms of the disease (Hickey 2014).

A clinically isolated syndrome (CIS) is the first attack of a disease compatible with MS (e.g., optic neuritis, brainstem syndromes, or transverse myelitis) that exhibits characteristics of inflammatory demyelination but has yet to fulfill MS diagnostic criteria (Olek, 2016)

There are three categories of MS: relapsing-remitting (80% of all cases), secondary progressive, and primary progressive (Hickey, 2014). There are no clinical findings that are unique to MS, but some are highly characteristic of the disease. Common symptoms of MS include sensory symptoms in the limbs or one side of the face, visual loss, acute or subacute motor weakness, diplopia, gait disturbance and balance problems, Lhermitte sign (electric shock-like sensations that run down the back and/or limbs upon flexion of the neck), vertigo, bladder problems, limb ataxia, acute transverse myelitis, and pain. The onset is often polysymptomatic. The most common presenting symptoms are sensory disturbances, followed by weakness and visual disturbances (Olek, 2016; Olek, Narayan, & Frohma, 2016).

When individuals with MS require care in a long-term care facility, they are younger (in their 40s), mentally alert, and have more symptoms of depression. They will reside at the facility for a longer time than the usual resident. They are dependent for much of their care. Caregivers in long-term care facilities are challenged to deliver complex care and provide opportunities to increase mobility and stimulation (*Buchanan, Wang, & Ju, 2002).

Time Frame

Initial diagnosis

Recurrent acute exacerbations

■■■ DIAGNOSTIC CLUSTER**

Collaborative Problems

Risk for Complications of Urinary Tract Infection

Risk for Complications of Seizures

Risk for Complications of Pneumonia

Nursing Diagnoses

Risk for Disturbed Self-Concept related to the effects of prolonged debilitating condition on lifestyle and on achieving developmental tasks and uncertain prognosis

Impaired Comfort related to demyelinated areas of the sensory tract

Risk for Injury related to visual disturbances, vertigo, and altered gait

Risk for Caregiver Role Strain related to unpredictability of care situation or illness course, increasing care needs (refer to Unit II)

Risk for Compromised Family Coping related to the progressive nature of the disorder, role disturbances and uncertain future

Impaired Swallowing related to cerebellar lesions (refer to Cerebrovascular Accident (Stroke) Care Plan)

Impaired Verbal Communication related to dysarthria secondary to ataxia of the muscles of speech (refer to Parkinson Disease Care Plan)

Fatigue related to extremity weakness, spasticity, fear of injury, and stressors (refer to Unit II)

Urinary Retention related to sensorimotor deficits (refer to Neurogenic Bladder Care Plan)

Incontinence (specify) related to poor sphincter control and spastic bladder

Powerlessness related to the unpredictable nature of condition (remission/exacerbation) (refer to Chronic Obstructive Pulmonary Disease Care Plan)

Risk for Ineffective Health Management related to lack of knowledge of condition, treatments, prevention of infection, stress management, aggravating factors, signs and symptoms of complications, and community resources

However, when evaluated with neuropsychological tests, up to 70% of patients have some cognitive impairment. The prevalence of cortical syndromes such as aphasia, apraxia, and agnosia is low.

Related Care Plans

Immobility or Unconsciousness

Corticosteroid Therapy

**This medical condition was not included in the validation study.

TRANSITION TO HOME/COMMUNITY CARE

Before transition, the individual and family will:

1. Relate an intent to share concerns with other family members or trusted friend(s).
2. Identify one strategy to increase independence.
3. Describe actions that can reduce the risk of exacerbation.
4. Identify signs and symptoms that must be reported to a health care professional.

Transitional Risk Assessment Plan (TRAP)

Begin this plan on admission.

Implement the Transitional Risk Assessment Plan (TRAP):

* Refer to inside back cover.
* Add each validated risk diagnosis to individual's problem list with the risk code in ( ).
* Refer to Unit II to the individual risk nursing diagnoses/collaborative problems for outcomes and interventions.

   R: "Close coordination of care in the post-acute period, early transition follow-up care, enhanced client education and self-management training, proactive end-of-life counseling, and extending the resources and clinical expertise over time via multidisciplinary team management" can lower readmission rates and improve health outcomes (Boutwell & Hwu, 2009, p. 14). Interventions are utilized to activate the individual and family to select changes in their everyday lifestyle choices to improve their health (Hibbard & Greene, 2013).

Collaborative Problems

Risk for Complications of Pneumonia

Risk for Complications of Urinary Tract Infections

Risk for Complications of Renal Insufficiency

Risk for Complications of Seizures

Collaborative Outcomes

The (a) urinary tract infections and (b) seizures and (c) pneumonia will receive collaborative interventions if indicated to restore physiologic stability.

Indicators of Physiologic Stability

- Alert, oriented (b, c)
- No abnormal breath sounds (c)
- Oxygen saturation >95% (pulse oximetry) (c)
- Temperature 98° F to 99.5° F (a, c)
- Urine specific gravity 0.005 to 0.030 (a)
- Urine output >0.5 mL/kg/hr (a)
- Clear urine (a)
- No seizure activity (b)

Carp's Cues

The medical treatment and management of multiple sclerosis should be targeted toward relieving symptoms of the disease, treating acute exacerbations, shortening the duration of an acute relapse, reducing frequency of relapses, and preventing disease progression. Many of complications of multiple sclerosis are related to immobility as pneumonia, pressure ulcers, and osteoporosis. Other complications are seizures and those related to medication therapy

Interventions	Rationales
1. Monitor for signs and symptoms of urinary tract infection (UTI):	1. MS exacerbation can be precipitated by any infection (Olek, & Mowry, 2016). MS can cause urinary retention owing to lesions of the afferent pathways from the bladder. Resulting urine stasis contributes to growth of microorganisms. Also, corticosteroid therapy reduces the effectiveness of WBCs against infection.
a. Chills, fever	a. Bacteria can act as a pyrogen by raising the hypothalamic thermostat through the production of endogenous pyrogen that may mediate through prostaglandins. Chills can occur when the temperature setpoint of the hypothalamus changes rapidly.
b. Costovertebral angle (CVA) pain (a dull, constant backache below the 12th rib)	b. CVA pain results from distention of the renal capsule.
c. Leukocytosis	c. Leukocytosis reflects an increase in WBCs to fight infection through phagocytosis.
d. Foul odor or pus in urine	d. Bacteria change the odor and pH of urine.
e. Dysuria, frequent urination	e. Bacteria irritate bladder tissue, causing spasms and frequent urination.

Interventions	Rationales

2. Monitor for pneumonia:
  a. Monitor respiratory status and assess for signs and symptoms of inflammation:
   • Increased respiratory rate (tachypnea), marked dyspnea
   • Fever and chills (sudden or insidious)
   • Productive cough
   • Diminished or absent breath sounds, rales, or crackles
   • Pleuritic chest pain
   • Tachycardia
   • Lethargy
	2. Tracheobronchial inflammation, impaired alveolar capillary membrane function, edema, fever, and increased sputum production disrupt respiratory function and compromise the blood's oxygen-carrying capacity. Reduced chest wall compliance in older adults affects the quality of respiratory effort. In older adults, tachypnea (>26 respirations/min) is an early sign of pneumonia, often occurring 3 to 4 days before a confirmed diagnosis. Delirium or mental status changes are often seen early in pneumonia in older adults (Grossman & Porth, 2014).
	
	    The cause of death in approximately 75% of all multiple sclerosis individuals is usually pneumonia (Olek, & Mowry, 2016).

3. Monitor for seizures. Refer to Care Plan for individual with seizures	3. The effects of demyelination and inflammation on the cortex are increasingly recognized as important in MS, and edema associated with acute MS lesions could also cause cortical hyperexcitability resulting in seizures. Epilepsy occurs in 2% to 3% of individuals with MS. Seizures associated with MS are generally benign and transient, and respond well to antiepileptic drug therapy or require no therapy (Olek, & Mowry, 2016).

Clinical Alert Report

Prior to providing care, advise ancillary staff/student to report the following to the professional nurse assigned to the individual:
* Seizure activity
* Change in cognitive status
* Oral temperature >100.5° F
* Systolic BP <90 mm Hg
* Resting pulse >100, <50 beats/min
* Respiratory rate >28, <10/min
* Oxygen saturation <90%
* Amount of urine output

Documentation

Intake and output
Urine specific gravity

Nursing Diagnoses

Carp's Cues

The medical focus in the treatment of relapsing MS is to reduce the frequency of relapses and limit disease progression. As a result, the clinical assessments often have the sole intention of monitoring for physiologic complications (Correia de Sa et al., 2011).

    The nursing focus for individuals and families coping with MS is to assess their quality of life to identify responses to MS that compromise functioning and increase risks. Using Gordon's 11 Functional Health Patterns, the individual/family will be assessed for the presence of compromised functioning and risk factors that can compromise functioning. The nurse in collaboration with the individual and family can determine what priorities are for this individual and family presently. Sometimes, priorities identified by the nurse are not shared by the individual and/or the family.

Chronic Pain Related to the Demyelinating Process and/or Musculoskeletal in Nature, Secondary to Poor Posture, Poor Balance, or the Abnormal Use of Muscles or Joints as a Result of Spasticity

NOC

Comfort Level, Pain: Disruptive Effects, Pain Control, Depression Control

NIC

Pain Management, Medication Management, Exercise Promotion, Mood Management, Coping Enhancement

Goal

The individual will relate:
- Increased understanding of the causes of their pain and resources/skills needed to cope.
- Will commit to practice at least one noninvasive pain-relief measures such as:
  - Music therapy
  - Stretching exercises, yoga, and/or walking
  - Massage
  - Guided imagery
  - Relaxation therapy
  - Heat/cold therapy

Carp's Cues

The prevalence of pain in individuals with MS is 63.5% (Maloni, 2012). A large, international study reported a lifetime prevalence of pain was 66.5%. The prevalence of the comorbidity of pain and depression was 29.1% (Drulovic et al., 2015). Pain in multiple sclerosis is both a direct consequence of a demyelinating lesion in the central nervous system (*central neuropathic*) or an indirect consequence of the disability associated with MS (*nonneuropathic*) (International Association of the Study of Pain, 2011). Mixed neuropathic and nonneuropathic pain occurs and is typified by headache and painful muscle spasms or spasticity.

Interventions	Rationales
1. Establish a supportive accepting relationship: Acknowledge the pain. Listen attentively their pain experience.	
2. Convey that you are assessing pain because you want to understand it better (not determine if it really exists).	2. Trying to convince health care providers that he/she is experiencing pain will cause the individual anxiety, which compounds the pain. Both are energy depleting.
3. Determine the level of understanding of the individual's condition, causes of pain. Assess the effects of symptoms on quality of life and pain-relieving techniques that he/she uses. Supplement their information and correct misconceptions.	3. "The goal of pain management is recognizing and treating psychological factors of anxiety and depression, enhancing social factors of support and a trusting medical provider relationship and using medications that target pain mechanisms with polypharmacy—that is, combining low doses of several medications to achieve greater efficacy with fewer adverse events" (Maloni, 2012).
4. Explain that the individual's pain may be primary or secondary. a. For a comprehensive resource on pain management for individuals with MS, refer to Maloni (2012). b. Refer also to Unit II Chronic Pain.	4. Primary pain is caused by the demyelinating process and with plaque formation in the spinal cord and brain and is often characterized as having a burning, gnawing, or shooting quality. Secondary pain is caused primarily musculoskeletal in nature, possibly due to poor posture, poor balance, or the abnormal use of muscles or joints as a result of spasticity (Maloni, 2012).

Risk for Injury Related to Visual Disturbances, Vertigo, and Altered Gait

NOC
Risk Control

Goal

The individual will relate fewer injuries.

NIC
Fall Prevention,
Environmental
Management: Safety,
Health Education,
Surveillance: Safety, Risk
Identification

Indicators

- Relate the intent to use safety measures to prevent injury.
- Relate the intent to practice selected prevention measures.

Interventions	Rationales
1. Explain why MS can increase risk for falls.	1. Symptoms including visual impairment, vertigo, impaired proprioception, decreased vibration sense, muscle weakness, and spasticity are the result of progressive damage along neuronal pathways throughout the CNS (Olek et al., 2016).
2. Discuss the consequences of falls (e.g., fracture hips, increased disability).	2. Researchers have documented that approximately 75% of community-dwelling persons with MS who have fallen in the last 6 months self-reported activity restriction due to concerns about falling (Matsuda, Shumway-Cook, Ciol, Bombardier, & Kartin, 2012).
3. Consult with physical therapy for an evaluation	3. Individuals may be resistant to using assistive devices related to issues related to body image. The changing nature of this condition may require an evaluation if their present assistive devise is still safe (e.g., Cane).
4. Refer to Unit II for additional interventions for Risk for Injury.	

TRANSITION TO HOME/COMMUNITY CARE

If indicated, review the high-risk diagnoses identified for this individual on admission:

- Is the person still at high risk?
- Can the family reduce the risks?
- Is the person at higher risk at home?
- Is a home health nurse assessment needed?
- Refer to discharge planner/case manager/social service
- When is this person scheduled for follow-up with primary provider? Specialists? Record dates of appointments.
- Complete a medication reconciliation prior to discharge. Refer to inside back cover.

STAR   **Stop**

Think   Is this person at high risk for injury, falls, medical complications, and/or inability to care for self (ADLs)?
Is there a support person available?
Is the person competent to manage self-administration of medications, treatment procedures? Are additional resources needed?
Can the person explain how to monitor the condition (e.g., blood glucose, sign/symptoms of complications, dietary/mobility restrictions, and when to call his or her primary provider or specialist)?

Act   Contact or provide the appropriate resource (e.g., contacting a support person, home health assessment, additional teaching, printed materials).

Review Has the problem been addressed? If not, use SBAR to communicate to the appropriate person.

Risk for Compromised Family Coping Related to the Progressive Nature of the Disorder, Role Disturbances and Uncertain Future

NOC

Family Coping, Family
Environment: Internal,
Family Normalization,
Parenting

Goal

The family will maintain functional system of mutual support for one another, as evidenced:
- Frequently verbalize feelings to professional nurse and one another.
- Identify appropriate external resources available.

NIC

Family Involvement
Promotion, Coping
Enhancement, Family
Integrity Promotion,
Family Therapy,
Counselling, Referral

Interventions	*Rationales*

1. Assess for risk factors that contribute to marital or relationship dysfunction
  a. Illness-related factors
    • Sudden, unexpected nature of illness
    • Burdensome, chronic problems
    • Potentially disabling nature of illness
    • Decreasing ability to continue home responsibilities
    • Social stigma associated with illness
    • Financial burden
  b. Factors related to behavior of ill family member
    • Refuses to engage in dialogue
    • Isolates self from family
  c. Factors related to overall family functioning
    • Unresolved conflict history (e.g., guilt, blame, hostility, jealousy)
    • Inability to solve problems
    • Ineffective communication patterns among members
    • Changes in role expectations and resulting tension
    • Unclear role boundaries
	1. Research findings show a higher rate of partner abandonment and divorce when the wife was the individual with cancer or multiple sclerosis groups (93 percent and 96 percent respectively, compared to 78 percent women for the primary brain tumor group) (Glantz et al., 2009).

(continued)

Interventions	*Rationales*

2. Promote cohesiveness.
  a. Approach the family with warmth, respect, and support.
    • Keep family members abreast of changes in ill family member's condition when appropriate.
    • Avoid discussing what caused the problem or blaming.
    • Encourage verbalization of guilt, anger, blame, and hostility and subsequent recognition of own feelings in family members.
    • Explain the importance of functional communications, which uses verbal and nonverbal communication to teach behavior, share feelings and values, and evolve decisions about family health practices (Kaakinen, Coelho, Steele, Tabacco, & Hanson, 2015).
	2. It recommend that medical providers be especially sensitive to early suggestions of marital discord in couples affected by the occurrence of a serious medical illness, especially when the woman is the affected spouse and it occurs early in the marriage (Glantz et al., 2009).

3. Assist family to appraise the situation.
  a. What is at stake? Encourage family to have a realistic perspective by providing accurate information and answers to questions. Ensure all family members have input.
  b. What are the choices? Assist family to reorganize roles at home and set priorities to maintain family integrity and reduce stress.
  c. Initiate discussions regarding stressors of home care (physical, emotional, environmental, and financial).
	3. "Family-oriented approaches that include helping a family gain insight and make behavioral changes are most successful" (Halter, 2014).

4. Promote clear boundaries between individuals in family.
  a. Ensure that all family members share their concerns.
  b. Elicit the responsibilities of each member.
  c. Acknowledge the differences.
  d. Explore how each family member engages in leisure activities.
  e. Talking to children.
	4. "Family-oriented approaches that include helping a family gain insight and make behavioral changes are most successful" (Halter, 2014)
	
	  e. Consider the child's age and maturity level and how much he/she can understand the disease. If there is more than one child, talk to them individually. Be aware the children may feel responsible for their parent getting ill. Teens may focus on how their life will change.

5. Explore possible age-related responses with parents (Explore possible age-related responses with parents 2014)
  a. More focus on her/his own body and wellness.
    • Not wanting to spend time with close friends
    • Higher anxiety and stress
    • Trying to act older or younger than she is
    • Behaving badly in public
    • Lying to their friends about your illness
    • Temper tantrums
    • Waiting until you are tired at the end of day to ask for things (such as help with homework)
    • Doing poorly in school
    • Nightmares, bed-wetting, and trouble falling asleep.	

6. Include the child/teen in family decisions.	6. Whether divvying up the household chores or going to the hospital for treatment, it is important to involve the children in some decisions. It will give them sense of control and belonging.

Interventions	Rationales

7. Access age—appropriate children literature as: *Keep S'Myelin*, a newsletter for kids about multiple sclerosis
   a. *Keep S'Myelin* is available online at www.nationalmssociety .org
   b. When a Parent has MS a Teenager's Guide, available at http://www.nationalmssociety.org/NationalMSSociety /media/MSNationalFiles/Brochures/Brochure-When-a-Parent-Has-MS-A-Teenagers-Guide.pdf	

8. If appropriate, discuss the stressors that living with MS can bring to partner relationships. Stress that the individual is still the same individual and that MS symptoms does not have to define the individual,	8. "Early identification and psychosocial intervention might reduce the frequency of divorce and separation, and in turn improve quality of life and quality of care" (Glantz et al., 2009, p. 5242).
9. Suggest the usefulness of counseling for all individuals separately and group.	9. Sexual dysfunction can be the result of multiple problems, including the direct effects of lesions of the motor and sensory pathways within the spinal cord and psychological factors involved with self-image, self-esteem, and fear of rejection from the sexual partner. Mechanical problems created by spasticity, paraparesis, and incontinence further aggravate the problem (Olek & Mowry, 2016).

10. Initiate Health Teaching and Referrals, as necessary
   a. Facilitate family involvement with social supports.
   b. Assist family members to identify reliable positive support parsons (e.g., friends, coworkers); encourage seeking help (emotional, technical) when appropriate.
   c. Enlist help of other professionals (social work, therapist, psychiatrist, school nurse). Only recommend online sources of excellent, practical information for individual and families (e.g., Multiple Sclerosis Association, Multiple Sclerosis Foundation).	

Risk for Ineffective Health Management Related to Lack of Knowledge of Condition, Treatments, Prevention of Infection, Stress Management, Aggravating Factors, Signs and Symptoms of Complications, and Community Resources

NOC

Compliance Behavior, Knowledge: Treatment Regimen, Participation in Health Care Decisions, Treatment Behavior: Illness or Injury

NIC

Anticipatory Guidance, Learning Facilitation, Risk Identification, Health Education, Teaching: Procedure/ Treatment, Health System Guidance

Goal

The goals for this diagnosis represent those associated with transition planning. Refer to the transition criteria.

Carp's Cues

The effect of comorbidities such as depression, urinary incontinence, and symptoms such as spasms, fatigue, vertigo, headaches can have serious ramifications for individuals with MS and their significant others. These comorbidities are barriers to compliance and recovery from relapses. The presence of these additional symptoms can also place a greater burden on careers, family, friends, and other support networks (Correia de Sa et al., 2011).

Interventions	Rationales
1. Evaluate sleep quality at home. Refer to Disturbed Sleep Patterns in Unit II for additional interventions.	1. The prevalence of insomnia in MS is as high as 40%, or several times higher than the prevalence in the general population (Olek & Mowry, 2016). A systematic review of 18 studies has identified the main sleep disorders and their prevalence ranges as (Marrie et al.): 　a. Restless legs syndrome, 14% to 58% (12 studies) 　b. Obstructive sleep apnea, 7% to 58% (5 studies) 　c. Periodic limb movements of sleep, 36% (1 study) 　d. Rapid eye movement sleep behavior disorder, 2% to 3% (2 studies) 　e. Narcolepsy, 0% to 2% (2 studies)
2. Evaluate for the presence of fecal incontinence and constipation. 　a. Explain that constipation can be caused by poor mobility, voluntary fluid restriction to minimize urinary incontinency, anticholinergic drugs taken for concomitant bladder symptoms and poor dietary habits. Refer to Unit II Constipation and Bowel Incontinence for additional interventions.	2. The prevalence of bowel symptoms with MS is over 50%. 　a. Fecal incontinency may arise as a result of diminished perineal and rectal sensation, weak sphincter squeeze pressures, leading to rectal overloading and overflow, or any combination of these factors (Correia de Sa et al., 2011; Olek, 2016).
3. Explain the risk for aspiration because of dysphagia. Consult with Speech Language Pathologist, if indicated. 　a. Advise to (van Schalkwyk, 2012): 　　• Know how to perform the Heimlich maneuver on self and another (individual, other household members). 　　• Sit up straight during all meals and snacking and 30 minutes after. 　　• Take a symptom inventory: Fatigue will contribute to swallowing problems. Think about how if fatigue is present, dysphasia will be worse also. 　　• Mindful eating challenge: Using a fork, place food in mouth. Put your fork down. Chew food very thoroughly, then swallow. Pick up fork again only when mouth is empty. 　　• Do not talk with food in your mouth. 　　• Thicken your liquids. 　　• Eat the right kinds of foods: Avoid hard, crumbly, dry, and crunchy foods. Add gravy for moisture. Eat very soft or pureed foods. 　　• Eat smaller meals, to avoid "swallowing fatigue." 　　• Alternate liquids and solids: Take a small sip or two of a liquid between bites for moisture. Finish the meal with some liquid. 　　• Chin tuck: Tuck your chin downward to the chest slightly while swallowing.	3. Problems with swallowing (dysphagia) in people with MS result from lesions in the brainstem that cause loss of control over the muscles involved in swallowing which can slow swallowing and increase the risk of aspirating food or liquid into the lungs. The effects are delayed swallowing response, reduced pharyngeal peristalsis move food to esophagus, reduced ability of the larynx to close as bolus of food to pass into the esophagus and reduced ability of *the tongue* to manipulate food during chewing and then propelling food back, triggering the swallowing reflex (Multiple Sclerosis. Net, 2016).
4. Assess level of fatigue. Refer to Unit II to Fatigue for interventions for energy conservation, work simplification, scheduled rest periods, and the use of cooling garments (e.g., vest, hat, collar).	4. Fatigue is one of the most common and disabling symptom of MS, occurring in approximately 76% to 92% of MS patients (Correia de Sa et al., 2011).

Interventions	*Rationales*

5. Explain heat intolerance. Fatigue can worsen before and during exacerbations and with increased temperatures.
  a. Advise to manage heat intolerance as follows:
    • Time outside activities for early morning or evening hours to avoid the heat of the day.
    • Spread activities throughout the course of the day to avoid overheating.
    • Use air conditioning in homes and cars, cooling garments, light-colored clothes, and wide-brimmed hats.
    • Avoid exposure to saunas, hot tubs, or even hot showers or baths.
    • Avoid exposure to excessive humidity; dehumidifiers can help indoors.
    • Treat fevers aggressively with around-the-clock antipyretics.
	5. Demyelinated fibers in the central nervous system are very sensitive to even small elevations of core body temperature resulting in conduction delays or even conduction block. The effects of heat exposure are reversed with rest and cooling and do not carry a long-term consequence.

6. Discuss bladder problems. Bladder dysfunction in MS may consist of failure to store, failure to empty, or a combination of the two. Interventions for failure to store include the following:
  a. Scheduled voiding
  b. Limiting fluid intake in the evening
  c. Using anticholinergic medications (e.g., oxybutynin)
  d. Eliminating diuretics (e.g., caffeine)
  e. Refer also to Section II Incontinence	

7. Identify and notify the physician/nurse practitioner/physical assistant of UTI signs and symptoms:
  a. Foul-smelling urine
  b. Increased frequency and urge to urinate
  c. Change in color—dark yellow
  d. Change in consistency—cloudy, sediment, or flecks of blood
	7. Recurrent UTIs are common in MS patients with end-stage bladder disability.

8. Assist in formulating and accepting realistic short- and long-term goals.	8. Mutual goal-setting reinforces the individual's role in improving his or her quality of life.

9. Discuss the factors known to trigger exacerbation (Hickey, 2014):
  a. Undue fatigue or excessive exertion
  b. Overheating or excessive chilling or cold exposure
  c. Infections
  d. Hot environments/hot baths
  e. Fever
  f. Emotional stress
  g. Pregnancy
  h. Cigarette smoking
 	
  i. Alcohol use
	9. This information gives the individual insight into aspects of the condition that can be controlled; this may promote a sense of control and encourage compliance.
	  b. As body temperature rises above the normal range, it blocks conduction across demyelinated regions in the brain and can worsen MS.
	
	  h. Smoking may be a risk factor for transforming a relapsing-remitting clinical course into a secondary-progressive course (*Hernán et al., 2005).
	  i. Since alcohol depresses the central nervous system, it may also have an additive effect with certain medications that are commonly prescribed for MS.

(continued)

Interventions	*Rationales*
10. Stress the importance of the effects of smoking and second-hand smoke has on MS. Refer to index for a few strategies to try and engage the individual to quit.	10. Evidence supports cigarette smoking as an independent risk factor for MS susceptibility and associates smoking with a greater chance of developing progressive disease and accruing more rapid disability (Wingerchuk, 2012). The mechanisms by which smoking might influence the risk of MS and its clinical course are unclear (Wingerchuk, 2012).
11. Teach the importance of constructive stress management and reduction (Hickey, 2014); explain measures such as the following: a. Progressive relaxation techniques b. Self-coaching c. Thought-stopping d. Assertiveness techniques e. Guided imagery f. Exercising (e.g., walking yoga)	11. Managing stress helps the individual to cope and adapt to changes caused by MS. Approaches to stress management include massage therapy, exercise programs, and involvement in religious and social activities.
12. Explain the signs and symptoms that must be reported to a health care professional immediately: a. Worsening of symptoms (e.g., weakness, spasticity, visual disturbances) b. Temperature elevation c. Change in urination patterns or cloudy, foul-smelling urine d. Productive cough with cloudy, greenish sputum	12. Early detection enables prompt intervention to minimize complications. These symptoms may indicate infection (urinary tract or pulmonary).

CLINICAL ALERT:
- Worsening symptoms may herald an exacerbation. Immediate interventions are needed, notify PCP or specialist.

Interventions	*Rationales*
13. Initiate health teaching and Referrals as needed a. Advise to discuss with specialist on cognitive rehabilitation techniques. b. If indicated initiate a PT home visit.	13a. Cognitive training has shown to significantly benefit for three subcategories of cognitive performance: memory span, working memory, and immediate visual memory (Olek, & Mowry, 2016). b. The management of gait problems in MS consists mainly of physical therapy along with the use of mobility aids when they become necessary.
14. Provide information and materials to assist the individual and family to maintain goals and manage at home from sources such as the following: a. National MS Society b. Multiple Sclerosis Society c. American Red Cross d. Jimmie Heuga Center	14. An individual who feels well-supported can cope more effectively with the multiple stressors associated with chronic debilitating disease.

Documentation

Individual/family teaching
Referrals if indicated

Myasthenia Gravis

Myasthenia gravis (MG) is a chronic autoimmune neuromuscular disorder. It is characterized by production of antibodies that block muscle cell receptors for acetylcholine (ACh), the neurotransmitter essential for the stimulation of skeletal muscle contraction (Bautista & Grossman, 2016; *Howard, 2006). Normal amounts of ACh are produced, but due to the lack of functional receptors, skeletal muscle contraction is impaired. In MG individuals, impaired neurotransmission, combined with the normal reduction of ACh released with repeated activity, produces the fatigue and fluctuating weakness of voluntary muscles characteristic of this disorder. Function of affected muscles is usually strongest in the morning. Weakness increases with periods of activity and often improves with periods of rest (NINDS, 2016b). Muscles that control the movement of the eyes and eyelids, facial expression, chewing, speaking, swallowing, and breathing are most commonly affected (NINDS, 2016b).

MG is relatively rare. The estimates of the prevalence of MG in the United States vary widely, from 0.5 to 14 cases/100,000 (Shah & Goldenberg, 2016). MG can occur in any age or ethnic group, but it most commonly occurs in women under 40 and men over 60 years of age (NINDS, 2016b). Individuals often initially report weakness in a single muscle. Onset of symptoms is typically gradual, and the course of the disease is variable. Muscles of the eyes, head, and neck are most frequently affected, and extraocular muscle weakness occurs during the course of the illness in 90% of those affected (Shah & Goldenberg, 2016). Symptom-free periods decrease and muscle weakness increases as the disease progresses. The mechanism leading to immune dysfunction has not been clearly identified (Bautista & Grossman, 2016). Diagnosis of MG is based on patient history and is confirmed through antibody testing and chest computed tomography to evaluate the thymus gland (Shah & Goldenberg, 2016).

Despite there is no cure, individuals may often achieve improvement of their symptoms, and even remission (Shah & Goldenberg, 2016). Treatments focus on reducing, removing, or inhibiting the function of the abnormal antibodies that block the effect of ACh to trigger muscle contraction. These include anticholinesterase inhibitors, intravenous immune globulin, and immunomodulating agents (Shah & Goldenberg, 2016). Surgical removal of the thymus gland (thymectomy) often produces improvement of symptoms, reduced need for medication, or remission (NINDS, 2016b). The thymus gland is located behind the breastbone and has an important role in the development and function of the immune system, but is normally inactive after puberty. Hyperplastic thymus tissue or tumors are frequently found in those with MG (NINDS, 2016b). Plasmapheresis, the removal of abnormal antibodies from the blood plasma, provides relief of symptoms in periods of crisis or when other treatments are ineffective (Bautista & Grossman, 2016). Medications that may exacerbate MG must be avoided (Bautista & Grossman, 2016).

Complications of MG often arise from weakness in the muscle groups affecting swallowing and breathing, causing aspiration, respiratory infection, or respiratory insufficiency (Bautista & Grossman, 2016). Individuals with MG are at risk for two life-threatening complications that can have a similar clinical presentation of extreme weakness and respiratory dysfunction. Myasthenic crisis can be triggered by low ACh levels due to undermedication, incompatible medications, or other triggers such as physical or emotional stress, intercurrent illness, and menstruation. Cholinergic crisis results from excess levels of ACh due to overmedication (Shah & Goldenberg, 2016).

Time Frame
Initial diagnosis
Acute exacerbations
Remissions

■■■■■ DIAGNOSTIC CLUSTER**

Collaborative Problems

Risk for Complications of Respiratory Insufficiency

Risk for Complications of Myasthenic/Cholinergic Crisis

Risk for Complications of Aspiration

Nursing Diagnoses

Risk for Ineffective Airway Clearance related to impaired ability to cough (refer to Chronic Obstructive Pulmonary Disease Care Plan)

Risk for Impaired Swallowing related to neuromuscular weakness (refer to Cerebrovascular Accident [Stroke] Care Plan)

Risk for injury related to visual disturbances, unsteady gait, weakness (refer to Cerebrovascular Accident [Stroke] Care Plan)

Risk for Impaired Verbal Communication related to involvement of muscles for speech (refer to Parkinsonism Care Plan)

Risk for Impaired Skin Integrity related to immobility (refer to Immobility or Unconsciousness Care Plan)

Risk for Activity Intolerance related to fatigue and difficulty in performing ADLs (refer to Unit II)

Risk for Powerlessness related to the unpredictable nature of the condition (remissions/exacerbations)

Risk for Ineffective Therapeutic Regimen Management related to insufficient knowledge of condition, treatments, prevention of infections, stress management, aggravating factors, signs and symptoms of complications, and community resources.

**This medical condition was not included in the validation study.

TRANSITION TO HOME/COMMUNITY CARE

The individual or family will:

1. Verbalize the purpose, schedule, complications, and side effects to report of prescribed medications.
2. Demonstrate safe swallowing techniques if bulbar muscles are affected.
3. Schedule MG medication so peak effect is reached at mealtime.
4. Describe emergency intervention for choking (Heimlich maneuver).
5. Identify strategies to prevent respiratory infection.
6. Identify signs and symptoms of complication or crisis to report to health care provider immediately.
7. Identify the need to consult the neurologist before beginning any medications.
8. State the importance of wearing Medic Alert identification.
9. Relate energy conservation techniques (physical exertion early in day, frequent rest periods).
10. Receive information on community resources, Myasthenia Gravis Foundation (www.myasthenia.org).

Transitional Risk Assessment Plan (TRAP)

Begin this plan on admission.

Implement the Transitional Risk Assessment Plan (TRAP):

- Refer to inside back cover.
- Add each validated risk diagnosis to individual's problem list with the risk code in ( ).
- Refer to Unit II to the individual risk nursing diagnoses/collaborative problems for outcomes and interventions.

R: "Close coordination of care in the post-acute period, early transition follow-up care, enhanced client education and self-management training, proactive end-of-life counseling, and extending the resources and clinical expertise over time via multidisciplinary team management" can lower readmission rates and improve health outcomes (Boutwell & Hwu, 2009, p. 14). Interventions are utilized to activate the individual and family to select changes in their everyday lifestyle choices to improve their health (Hibbard & Greene, 2013).

Collaborative Problems

Risk for Complications of Respiratory Insufficiency

Risk for Complications of Myasthenic/Cholinergic Crisis

Risk for Complications of Aspiration

Collaborative Outcomes

The individual will be monitored for early signs and symptoms of (a) respiratory insufficiency (b) my-asthenic/cholinergic crisis, and (c) aspiration, and will receive collaborative interventions if indicated to restore physiologic stability.

Indicators of Physiologic Stability

- Respiration 16 to 20 breaths/min (a)
- Clear breath sounds with no adventitious sounds (a, c)
- Total lung capacity 5,800 mL (a)
- Vital capacity 4,600 mL (a)
- Intact cough–gag reflex (b, c)
- Heart rate 60 to 100 beats/min (a, b)
- Intact muscle strength (b)
- Dry, warm skin (b)
- BP >90/60, <140/90 mm Hg (a, b)
- No nausea/vomiting (b, c)
- No muscle cramping/twitching (b)
- No continual coughing with swallowing (c)
- Weight maintained at baseline (b, c)

Interventions	Rationales
1. Monitor for sign and symptoms of respiratory distress:	1. The effect of MG on the muscles of the diaphragm and the muscles of respiration may cause an ineffective cough mechanism, decreased movement of the diaphragm, and limited respiratory effort (Bautista & Grossman, 2016).
a. Monitor for changes in respiratory status • Respiratory rate increase • Change in respiratory pattern • Change in breath sounds • Arterial blood gas analyses • Serial vital capacity measurement	a. In MG, antibodies attach to the acetylcholine receptors in voluntary muscles, blocking nerve transmission and muscle contraction. Involvement of respiratory muscles may lead to respiratory insufficiency and failure (NINDS, 2016b). Frequent assessment assists in early identification of ineffective respirations and inadequate oxygenation. Individuals in myasthenic crisis may require mechanical ventilation (Wendell & Levine, 2011).
b. Monitor for increased pulse rate.	b. Increased heart rate may indicate difficulty with air exchange.
c. Do not use pulse oximetry to evaluate respiratory function.	c. Pulse oximetry measures solely oxygenation, not ventilation, and is not a complete measure of respiratory sufficiency. O_2 saturation can be normal while CO_2 is retained; therefore, pulse oximetry is not reliable indicator to determine the amount of paralysis.
d. Elevate head of bed 30 to 40 degrees.	d. Elevation will expand the lungs and enhance diaphragmatic movement.

(continued)

Interventions	Rationales

2. Assess ability to clear airway.
  a. Cough-gag reflex
 	
  b. Suction secretions as necessary
 	
  c. Postural drainage
  d. Position individual side to side
 	
  e. Coughing with swallowing
	2. Ability to clear airway
	  a. In severe MG, function of the muscles involved in these reflexes may be impaired (Wendell & Levine, 2011).
	  b. Inability to swallow saliva and pooling of respiratory sections may require suctioning. Excessive respiratory secretions increase the work of breathing.
	  c. To mobilize secretions.
	  d. Reduces pooling of secretions and prevents pneumonia.
	  e. Coughing with swallowing of liquids or saliva may indicate aspiration.

3. Collaborate with speech therapy to determine if the patient may safely swallow. Institute precautions to reduce aspiration risk:
  a. Plan meal times for peak medication effectiveness.
 	
  b. Plan rest periods prior to meal times.
 	
  c. Have individual eat slowly with small bites.
  d. Teach individual to do Heimlich maneuver on self; also teach caregivers.
	3. Weakness of the laryngeal and pharyngeal muscles involved in swallowing presents risk for aspiration and inadequate nutrition (NINDS, 2016b)
	  a. Meals should be scheduled to provide optimal chewing and swallowing muscle function.
	  b. Chewing and swallowing function is further impaired by fatigue.
	  c. This reduces aspiration risk.
	  d. Knowing emergency management for airway obstruction decreases individual and family anxiety and enhances safety.

4. Assess communication ability.
 	
  a. Anxiety and panic
   • Provide calm, reassuring environment.
   • Provide explanation for treatment.
  b. Increased muscle weakness involving speech
   • Ask questions that require yes or no responses.
   • Encourage individual to use gestures for communication.
   • Allow rest periods between periods of communication.
	4. MG may impair facial mobility and expression, and the muscles controlling speech (dysarthria) (Bautista & Grossman, 2016).
	  a. To reduce anxiety and promote easier respiration.
	
	  b. Establish a method of communication to reduce anxiety or panic.

5. Monitor the individual response to Tensilon testing (edrophonium chloride).	5. This anticholinesterase medication is administered intravenously to differentiate myasthenic from cholinergic crisis. A positive response of rapidly increased muscle strength indicates MG and myasthenic crisis. However, the reliability of this test is questionable, and its use in the clinical setting is decreasing (Bird, 2015).

6. Monitor for signs and symptoms of myasthenic/cholinergic crisis:
  a. Restlessness, anxiety
  b. Dyspnea
  c. Generalized muscle weakness
  d. Increased bronchial secretions/sweating
  e. Difficulty swallowing/speaking
  f. Bradycardia/tachycardia
  g. Hypotension/hypertension
	6. Myasthenic crises result from inadequate amounts of acetylcholine (ACh) due to disease progression, exacerbation, or undermedication. Cholinergic crises are rare but can result from excessive amounts of ACh due to overmedication with anticholinesterase drugs. These are often difficult to distinguish clinically (Bird, 2015).

Interventions	Rationales

7. Monitor for signs and symptoms of adverse effects of cholinergic drugs:
  a. Nausea and vomiting
  b. Diarrhea and abdominal cramping
  c. Sweating
  d. Increased salivation/bronchial secretion
  e. Tachycardia/bradycardia/hypotension
  f. Increased muscle weakness
  g. Increased fatigue
  h. Bronchial relaxation (collapse)
  i. Muscle twitching/cramping
	7. Anticholinesterase drugs increase the strength of muscle contraction by preventing breakdown of acetylcholine at the neuromuscular junction.

8. Assess for ocular manifestations of MG:
  a. Ptosis (drooping of the eyelid)
  b. Diplopia (double vision)
	8. Ocular manifestations are often early and frequent manifestations of MG) (Shah & Goldenberg, 2016).

9. Monitor individual response to thymectomy:
 	
  a. Assess for pulmonary complications.
 	
  b. Pain management with analgesic therapy.
 	
  c. Transient worsening of symptoms in early postoperative period.
  d. Delayed improvement of symptoms.
	9. Thymectomy, surgical removal of the thymus gland, provides improvement or remission in most MG individuals (NINDS, 2016b).
	  a. This major surgery involves a thoracotomy and sternal split or transcervical approach. The individual may have chest tubes and tracheostomy postoperatively.
	  b. Adequate pain relief reduces postoperative complications.
	  c. Surgical stress may exacerbate MG symptoms.
	
	  d. Reduction in symptoms or remission may take months to years to achieve (Bird, 2015).

10. Monitor individual response to plasmapheresis.	10. Removal of acetylcholine receptor antibodies from the blood plasma provides reduction in the manifestations of the disease during periods of crisis or when other treatments are not effective (Bautista & Grossman, 2016). Complications of plasmaperesis in MG patients may include infection or thrombosis of catheter, hypotension due to hypovolemia, electrolyte imbalances, bleeding, allergic, or toxic reaction to the solution utilized in the exchange procedure (Bird, 2015).

Documentation

Vital signs
Neurologic
Change in status
Response to interventions

Nursing Diagnoses

> **TRANSITION TO HOME/COMMUNITY CARE**
>
> If indicated, review the high-risk diagnoses identified for this individual on admission:
> - Is the person still at high risk?
> - Can the family reduce the risks?
> - Is the person at higher risk at home?
> - Is a home health nurse assessment needed?
> - Refer to discharge planner/case manager/social service.
> - When is this person scheduled for follow-up with primary provider? Specialists? Record dates of appointments.
> - Complete a medication reconciliation prior to discharge. Refer to inside back cover.

STAR	
Stop	
Think	Is this person at high risk for injury, falls, medical complications, and/or inability to care for self (ADLs)?
	Is there a support person available?
	Is the person competent to manage self-administration of medications, treatment procedures? Are additional resources needed?
	Can the person explain how to monitor the condition (e.g., blood glucose, signs/symptoms of complications, dietary/mobility restrictions, and when to call his or her primary provider or specialist)?
Act	Contact or provide the appropriate resource (e.g., contacting a support person, home health assessment, additional teaching, printed materials).
Review	Has the problem been addressed? If not, use SBAR to communicate to the appropriate person.

Risk for Ineffective Therapeutic Regimen Management Related to Insufficient Knowledge of Condition, Treatments, Prevention of Infections, Stress Management, Aggravating Factors, Signs and Symptoms of Complications, and Community Resources

NOC
Compliance/ Engagement Behavior, Knowledge: Treatment Regimen, Participation in Health Care Decisions, Treatment Behavior: Illness or Injury

Goals

The goals for this diagnosis represent those associated with transition planning. Refer to the transition criteria.

NIC
Anticipatory Guidance, Learning Facilitation, Risk Identification, Health Education, Teaching: Procedure/ Treatment, Health System Guidance

Interventions	*Rationales*
1. Determine the individual's and his or her family's level of learning. Then explain to them the diagnosis and long-term management of the disease, using methods appropriate to their level of learning.	1. The individual and his or her family must have a good understanding of this chronic disease process to enable them to recognize symptoms leading to complications.
2. Teach the individual the signs and symptoms of myasthenic crisis as distinguished from those of cholinergic crisis: a. Myasthenic crisis • Increased blood pressure • Tachycardia • Restlessness • Apprehension • Increased bronchial secretions, lacrimation, and sweating • Absent cough reflex • Dyspnea • Increased difficulty swallowing • Difficulty speaking b. Cholinergic crisis: • Decreased blood pressure • Bradycardia • Restlessness, apprehension • Increased bronchial secretions, lacrimation, and sweating • Generalized muscle weakness • Fasciculations • Dyspnea • Increased difficulty swallowing • Increased difficulty speaking • Increased blurred vision • Nausea and vomiting • Abdominal cramps and diarrhea	2. A myasthenic crisis results from an insufficiency of acetylcholine, usually induced by a change or withdrawal of medications. Cholinergic crises result from excessive amounts of acetylcholine, usually from overmedication with anticholinesterase medication. The individual needs to know the symptoms of overdose and underdose of his or her medications.
3. Go immediately to the Emergency Room or call 911.	
4. Advise individual/family to become knowledgeable about the medications. a. Correct time—1 hour before meals b. Ask pharmacist of any interactions with food, alcohol, or other medications. c. Advise the individual to keep a medication diary to determine peak medication function.	4. The exact time of an accurate medication dosage coincides with increases in energy demands. Taking medications before meals is essential to provide muscle strength for chewing food.
5. Teach how to manage diplopia and ptosis:	5. Ninety percent of individuals with MG develop ophthalmologic manifestations of the disease. Ptosis is best treated with lid crutches or eyelid tape. Diplopia is managed by attachment of Fresnel prisms attached to glasses, or opaque lens is placed in front of the affected eye or alternating eye patches (Awaad & Ma'Luf, 2015).
6. Advise of the risk for injury and falls. Refer to Risk for Falls for strategies to prevent injuries.	6. Double vision can interfere with one's perception of objects in the environment.
7. Advise of the importance to increase upper/lower extremities strength.	7. Increased strength of large extremities muscles can prevent a fall by allowing the individual to recover their stability if balanced is compromised.

(*continued*)

Interventions	Rationales

8. Teach on strengthening exercise with a demonstration: Stand behind a chair with a high back.
  a. Hold on the back.
  b. Lift your heels to stand on toes.
  c. Repeat this 20 times twice a day.
	8. Stressing the risk for falls and the aftermaths of fractured hips, may motivate the person to incorporate some exercises each day.

9. Advise to consult with neurologist and ophthalmologist to discuss other treatments for ocular manifestations of MG (Awaad & Ma'Luf, 2015).
  a. Fresnel prisms
  b. Strabismus surgery
 	
  c. Blepharoptosis surgery
	9a. Incorporated into a lens to correct diplopia
	  b. Successful muscle surgery for selected individuals with a stable course of MG and persistent diplopia has been reported.
	  c. Ptosis surgery may be indicated for individuals with a stable ptosis, with unsatisfactory response to medical therapy for MG.

10. Instruct on strategies to increase nutritional intake and prevent aspiration,
  a. Rest before eating and between bites.
    • Advise if they are very tired or swallowing is difficult, advise the individual not to eat or drink at all until symptoms improve.
  b. Choose foods that are easy to chew and swallow (e.g., thickened liquids, viscous foods).
  c. Advise to take small sips of liquids.
  d. Avoid foods that require a lot of chewing (e.g., sticky foods, steak, very hot, spicy, dry, and gritty).
  e. Eat small frequent meals; eat slowly.
  f. Try to eat larger meals in morning rather than evening.
  g. Plan meals ½ hour after cholinesterase inhibitor dose.
  h. Advise, when eating, to sit in an upright position with head bent slightly forward.
  i. Instruct family member how to do the Heimlich maneuver and the individual how to perform the maneuver if alone. This emergency maneuver can displace an aspirated piece of food.
	10. In situations where swallowing is too difficult, then the myasthenic may be advised. Swallowing difficulties make the individual at high risk for aspiration. Individuals with myasthenia usually do well at the beginning of a meal but tire at the end, making swallowing too difficult. At some point, there can be a total loss of ability to chew and swallow.
	
	  d. Foods that require a lot of chewing effort can tire out the myasthenic and cause difficulty in swallowing. Hot foods tend to increase muscle weakness.
	  f. Muscles will be stronger in the morning.
	  g. This provides optimal effects of the medicine on muscle function.
	  h. This position will create a gravity force for the downward motion of food.

11. Teach energy conservation. Refer to Unit II Fatigue.	11. Rest periods should be scheduled when medication peaks are low. The individual should learn to space tasks. Teach the family the importance of vital rest periods and planning activities.

12. Teach stress management strategies:
  a. Use of relaxation tapes
  b. Guided imagery
  c. Referral to community resource for stress management course
	12. Uncontrolled stress factors can lead to an acute exacerbation of the disease. Stress is also fatiguing and some stress is not avoidable. Stress management provides an outlet for unavoidable stress.

Interventions	Rationales

13. Inform the individual of factors that are known to trigger exacerbations:
  a. Excessive weakness
  b. Increased stressors
  c. Upper respiratory infection
  d. Exposure to ultraviolet light
  e. Surgery
  f. Pregnancy
  g. Hot and cold temperatures
	13. This information can provide the individual with insight of the disease and promote a sense of personal control. If the individual is pregnant or considering a pregnancy, she should consult with her physician/nurse practitioner as the course of pregnancy with MG is unpredictable, and she will require close observation.

14. Explain signs and symptoms that must be reported to a health care professional:
  a. Increased muscle weakness
  b. Progressive symptoms of visual disturbance. Difficulty breathing, chewing and swallowing, and sweating
  c. Productive cough
	14. Early intervention can minimize pending complications. These symptoms can be warnings of a crisis.

15. Provide information and literature to assist the individual and her or his family to manage long-term goals at home. Resources are as follows:
  a. Myasthenia Gravis Foundation (www.myasthenia.org)
  b. Home health agency
  c. Case manager referral
	15. The individual and family who receive community support will cope more effectively with this progressive chronic disease.

Documentation

Individual/family teaching
Referrals if indicated

Parkinson's Disease

Parkinson's disease (PD) is a chronic, slow, progressive neurodegenerative disease resulting in the depletion of dopaminergic neurons in the basal ganglia, also known as the subcortical motor nuclei of the cerebrum. The basal ganglia is composed of the substantia nigra, striatum, globus pallidus, subthalamic nucleus, and red nucleus. The neurotransmitter dopamine is produced and stored in the substantia nigra. Symptoms of PD are usually seen when there is cell loss in the substantia nigra, resulting in a reduction of striatal dopamine (Hickey, 2014). Lewy bodies, intracellular protein deposits, are also seen and considered a pathologic hallmark of PD.

The classic signs and symptoms of PD include resting tremors, rigidity of muscles, akinesia/bradykinesia, postural disturbances, and loss of postural reflexes. Secondary symptoms include difficulty with fine motor function, soft monotone voice, mask-like face, generalized weakness and muscle fatigue, cognitive impairments/dementia, sleep disturbances, and autonomic manifestations which include the following: drooling, seborrhea, dysphagia, excessive perspiration, constipation, orthostatic hypotension, urinary hesitation and frequency, urgency, nocturia, urge incontinence, and erectile dysfunction and impotence (Hickey, 2014). PD typically affects 1% of people over the age of 65 years with the average age of onset being 60 years with prevalence higher in Caucasian men. Early onset of PD has affected people as young as 20. Genetics have also been linked to the development of PD; specifically, 10 autosomal dominant and recessive genes (Hickey, 2014). Depression is the most common psychiatric syndrome, with prevalence in PD as high as 42% (Tanzy, 2015a).

 Time Frame
Secondary diagnosis (hospitalization not usual)

■■■■■ DIAGNOSTIC CLUSTER**

Collaborative Problems

Risk for Complications of Long-Term Levodopa Treatment Syndrome

Risk for Complications of Dysphasia (leading to malnutrition or aspiration)

Risk for Complications of Pneumonia (refer to Unit II)

Risk for Complications of Urinary Tract Infections (refer to Unit II)

Risk for Complications of Sensory Abnormalities (leading to pain and paresthesias)

Nursing Diagnoses

Impaired Verbal Communication related to dysarthria secondary to ataxia of muscles of speech

Impaired Physical Mobility related to effects of muscle rigidity, tremors, and slowness of movement on ADLs

Risk for Constipation related to decreased peristalsis secondary to impaired autonomic system (refer to Unit II Section 1)

Impaired swallowing related to difficulty with bolus propulsion and clearance secondary to weak esophageal peristalsis, decrease in upper esophageal sphincter opening diameter, decreased anterior laryngeal motion, and impaired pharyngeal motility

Risk for Injury related to Orthostatic Hypotension (refer to Unit II)

Disturbed Sleep Patterns related to multifactorial elements as nocturnal motor disturbances, nocturia, depressive symptoms, and medication use

Risk for Ineffective Health Management related to lack of knowledge of condition, treatments required, stress management, signs and symptoms of complications, and availability of community resources

Related Care Plan

Neurogenic Bladder

**This medical condition was not included in the validation study.

Transition Criteria

Before transition, the individual and family will:

1. Relate the intent to share concerns with another family member or a trusted friend.
2. Identify one strategy to increase independence.
3. Describe measures that can reduce the risk of exacerbation.
4. Identify signs and symptoms that must be reported to a health care professional.
5. Make sure the individual and his or her family know what community resources are available to them, such as the Parkinson's Disease Foundation (http://www.pdf.org).

Transitional Risk Assessment Plan (TRAP)

Begin this plan on admission.

Implement the Transitional Risk Assessment Plan (TRAP):

- Refer to inside back cover.
- Add each validated risk diagnosis to individual's problem list with the risk code in ( ).
- Refer to Unit II to the individual risk nursing diagnoses/collaborative problems for outcomes and interventions.

  R: "Close coordination of care in the post-acute period, early transition follow-up care, enhanced client education and self-management training, proactive end-of-life counseling, and extending the resources and clinical expertise over time via multidisciplinary team management" can lower readmission rates and improve health outcomes (Boutwell & Hwu, 2009, p. 14). Interventions are utilized to activate the individual and family to select changes in their everyday lifestyle choices to improve their health (Hibbard & Greene, 2013).

Collaborative Problems

Risk for Complications of Long-Term Levodopa Treatment Syndrome

Risk for Complications of Aspiration Pneumonia

Risk for Complications of Urinary Tract Infections

Risk for Complications of Sensory Abnormalities (Leading to Pain and Paresthesias)

Collaborative Outcomes

The individual will be monitored for early signs and symptoms of (a) long-term levodopa treatment syndrome and (b) aspiration/pneumonia, (c) urinary tract infections, (d) sensory abnormalities, and receive collaborative intervention to restore physiologic stability.

Indicators of Physiologic Stability

- Less or no fluctuations between involuntary movements (tics, tremors, rigidity, and repetitive, bizarre movements) and bradykinesia (slowed movements) (a)
- Intact cough–gag reflexes (b)
- Intact muscle strength (b)
- No continual coughing with swallowing (b)
- Dizziness, lightheadedness, and possible fainting with standing (d)
- Sudden decrease in blood pressure when sitting or standing (d)
- Respiration 16 to 20 breaths/min (b)
- Respiration relaxed and rhythmic (b)
- Breath sound present all lobes (b)
- No rales or wheezing (b)
- Extremity pain, numbness, or tingling (d)
- Urinary urgency, urinary frequency, and nocturia (c)
- Pain on voiding (burning) (c)
- Fever (c)

Interventions	Rationales
1. Explain long-term levodopa treatment syndrome to the individual and family.	1. A substantial number of individuals with PD develop levodopa-induced complications occur in at least 50% of individuals after 5 to 10 years of treatment (Tarsy, 2015a). However, several observational studies have noted that motor complications are more common in individuals with young-onset PD compared with older onset (Tarsy, 2015). Kumar, Van Gerpen, Bower, and Ahlskog (*2005) reported in a population-based study that compared individuals, who were 40 to 59 years of age at PD onset with those who were older than 70 years of age at PD onset, the corresponding 5-year incidence of dyskinesia was 50% vs. 16% percent.
2. Explain symptoms of the levodopa-induced complications (Tarsy, 2015b). a. Motor fluctuations (the wearing-off phenomenon) b. Involuntary movements known as dyskinesia c. Abnormal cramps and postures of the extremities and trunk known as dystonia. d. Fluctuates between being symptom-free and severe Parkinson symptoms. e. Symptoms may last minutes or hours.	2. "The increase in motor fluctuations over time is most likely due to progressive degeneration of nigrostriatal dopamine terminals, which increasingly limits the normal physiologic uptake and release of dopamine" (Tarsy, 2015a).

Interventions	Rationales
3. Evaluate swallowing effectiveness. Refer to Impaired Swallowing.	3. "Swallowing problems are frequent in PD. Research has shown that self-report of 'no difficulty' is not a reliable indicator of swallowing ability" (Kalf, de Swart, Bloem, & Munneke, 2012).
4. Monitor ability to cough and the effectiveness of airway clearance. Ensure a consult with speech therapy to evaluate cough effectiveness to: a. Effectiveness of cough effort b. Need for tracheobronchial suctioning	4. Pneumonia and dementia are the leading causes of death in individuals with PD (Lethbridge, Johnston, & Turnbull, 2013). a. Fontana and Widdicombe (2007) and Ebihara et al. (*2003) reported significant decrement in cough function with PD, including decreased peak electromyogram amplitude of abdominal muscles during both reflexive and voluntary cough, and decreases in cough sensitivity necessary for activation of a reflexively induced cough. These changes contribute to aspiration (Pitts et al., 2009).
5. Monitor individual for signs and symptoms of urinary retention and UTI. a. Chills and fever b. Leukocytosis c. Bacteria and pus in urine d. Dysuria and frequency e. Bladder distention f. Urine overflow (30 to 60 mL of urine every 15 to 30 minutes)	5. Autonomic failure that occurs with PD causes urinate retention and subsequent UTIs (Grossman & Porth, 2014).
6. Monitor for signs and symptoms of respiratory distress, and position to assist with breathing: a. Report immediately any change in respiratory or ability to swallow b. Auscultate breath sounds. c. Assess for secretions: • Encourage the individual to breathe deep and cough. • Position individual side to side to assist movement of secretions. • Suction if individual is unable to manage secretions. • Reassure individual by maintaining a calm environment. d. Assess O_2 saturation via pulse oximetry.	6. PD affects basal ganglia dysfunction resulting in "weakness of the facial, oropharyngeal, and laryngeal muscles can result in a compromised swallow and secretion clearance. Weakness of these muscles can also compromise the airway due to physical obstruction, particularly when lying flat. The cough reflex is diminished due to weakness of the abdominal muscles, increasing the risk of aspiration" (Mangera, Panesar, & Makker, 2012).

Clinical Alert Report

Prior to providing care, advise ancillary staff/student to report the following to the professional nurse assigned to the individual:
- Change in cognitive status
- Oral temperature >100.5° F
- Systolic BP <90 mm Hg
- Resting pulse >100, <50 beats/min
- Respiratory rate >28, <10/min

Documentation

Changes in symptoms

Nursing Diagnoses

Impaired Verbal Communication Related to Dysarthria Secondary to Ataxia of Muscles of Speech

NOC
Communication:
Expressive Ability

Goal

The individual will demonstrate improved ability to express self.

NIC
Active Listening,
Communication
Enhancement: Speech
Deficit

Indicator

• Demonstrate techniques and exercises to improve speech and strengthen muscles.

Interventions	Rationales
1. Explain the disorder's effects on speech.	1. Understanding may promote compliance with speech improvement exercises.
2. Explain the benefits of daily speech improvement exercises.	2. Daily exercises help to improve the efficiency of speech musculature and increase rate, volume, and articulation.
3. Refer the individual to a speech pathologist to design an individualized speech program, as recommended by the American Parkinson's Disease Association.	3. These exercises improve muscle tone and control and speech clarity.

Documentation

Assessment of speech
Exercises taught
Referrals, if indicated

Impaired Swallowing Related to Difficulty With Bolus Propulsion and Clearance Secondary to Weak Esophageal Peristalsis

NOC
Aspiration Control,
Swallowing Status

Goal

The individual will report improved ability to swallow.

NIC
Aspiration Precautions,
Swallowing Therapy,
Surveillance, Referral,
Positioning

Indicators

• Describe causative factors when known.
  • Discuss the effects of eating problems have on nutrition
  • Explore feeling associated with dining with others, in public, at work
• Describe rationale and procedures for treatment.

Interventions	Rationales

> **CLINICAL ALERT:**
> • It is a myth that dysphagia is only a problem in late-stage PD. Dysphagia can occur at ANY stage (Ciucci & Busch, 2014). Dysphagia in individuals with PD is caused by residue in pharynx, abnormal airway soma-sensory function, decrease in upper esophageal opening, and relaxation and silent aspiration (Walshe, 2014).

Interventions	*Rationales*

1. Determine if individual has swallowing problems and is at risk for aspiration:
   a. If the person is not alert, drooling, and/or has difficulty speaking, do not attempt the test.
   b. Do not rely on the individual's reports of not having difficulty swallowing, as the sole assessment data.
	1. Assessment of dysphagia should not be confined to questioning because the person with reduced sensation and cognitive function may be unaware of their swallowing difficulties and even in those with normal cognition and sensation consider difficulties as part of aging and the disease process (Walshe, 2014). A meta-analysis revealed that subjective dysphagia occurs in one-third of community-dwelling PD patients (Kalf, 2012). When measured objectively dysphagia rates were much higher, with 4 out of 5 individuals being affected. This suggests that dysphagia is common in PD, but patients do not always report swallowing difficulties unless asked. This underreporting calls for a proactive clinical approach to dysphagia, particularly in light of the serious clinical consequences (Kalf, 2012).

2. Make the person NPO until a Speech Language Pathologist consult is completed. Post a sign at the bedside to communicate that nothing should be given to eat or drink without first checking with the nurse.	2. The risk of aspiration can be reduced if all visitors/staff/students are alerted.
3. If those conditions are not present, proceed with the test if there will be a delay in the Speech Language Pathologist consult. "A simple bedside screening evaluation involves asking the individual to sip a teaspoon of water from a cup. If the person can sip and swallow without difficulty, the person is asked to take a large gulp of 60 mL of water and swallow. If there are no signs of coughing or aspiration after 30 seconds, then it is safe for the individual to have a thickened diet until formally assessed by a speech pathologist" (*Massey & Jedlicka, 2002; Jauch et al., 2010).	3. "Assessment requires a multidisciplinary approach with nurses and caregivers trained in detecting the signs of oropharyngeal dysphagia at mealtime with further more detailed assessment provided by speech language pathologists (SLPs), radiologist with onward referral to other specialists (e.g. gastroenterologists, otolaryngologists, pulmonary physicians, dietitians, physical therapists, occupational therapists etc." (Walshe, 2014). If there will be a delay in the evaluation that prevents the individual from drinking or eating, the nurse can perform a simple bedside screening evaluation.
4. Consult with Speech Language Pathologist for all individuals with PD and a specific plan regarding speech and swallowing (Walshe, 2014). **CLINICAL ALERT:** • "Oropharyngeal dysphagia can have a negative impact not only for the individual but for carers, families and others. Oropharyngeal dysphagia also causes considerable discomfort for the individual with choking episodes which are anxiety provoking" (Walshe, 2014). "For people with Parkinson's disease (PD) the additional discomfort of excess saliva, e.g., drooling resulting from a decreased ability to swallow is considerable."	4. The speech pathologist has the expertise needed to perform the dysphagia evaluation.
5. Explore how their swallowing problems have affected their lives.	5. Quality of life is significantly impacted by the presence of dysphagia with decreased quality of life as the disease progresses. Social activities and dining with others (Pitts et al., 2009). Oropharyngeal dysphagia can affect social activities and reduce participation in society as the swallowing difficulty limits the ability to eat out socially (Walshe, 2014).
6. Follow plan for dysphagia from the speech therapist. Refer also to Impaired Swallowing in Unit II Section 1.	

Disturbed Sleep Patterns Related to Multifactorial Elements as Nocturnal Motor Disturbances, Nocturia, Depressive Symptoms, and Medication Use

NOC
Rest, Sleep, Well-Being

NIC
Energy Management, Sleep Enhancement, Environmental Management

Goal

The individual will report a satisfactory balance of rest and activity as evidenced by the following indicators:
- Complete at least four sleep cycles (100 minutes each) undisturbed.
- State factors that increase or decrease the quality of sleep.

Interventions	Rationales
CLINICAL ALERT: • Sleep disorders associated to PD include insomnia, daytime sleepiness with sleep attacks, restless legs syndrome, and rapid eye movement. Sleep disorders affect between 55% and 80% of individuals with PD (Chou, 2016a).	
1. Initiate a dialogue regarding their sleep habits, quality, and complaints.	1. Sleep problems are ranked as one of the most troublesome nonmotor symptoms in a survey of individuals with both early- and late-stage PD (Politis et al., 2010). The most common sleep disturbances in PD are sleep fragmentation (frequent awakening throughout the night) and early morning awakening (Chou, 2016a).
2. Consult with the physician/nurse practitioner/physical assistant for a pharmacological agent if indicated.	
3. Refer to Disturbed Sleep Patterns in Unit II Section 1.	

Impaired Physical Mobility Related to Effects of Muscle Rigidity, Tremors, and Slowness of Movement on Activities of Daily Living

NOC
Ambulation: Walking, Joint Movement: Active Mobility Level

NIC
Exercise Therapy: Joint Mobility, Exercise Promotion: Strength Training, Exercise Therapy: Ambulation, Positioning, Teaching: Prescribed Activity/ Exercise

Goal

The individual will describe measures to increase mobility.

Indicators

- Demonstrate exercises to improve mobility.
- Demonstrate a wide-base gait with arm swinging.
- Identify one strategy to increase independence.
- Relate intent to exercise at home.

Interventions	Rationales

> **CLINICAL ALERT:**
> • "It is not clear if exercise can slow the progression of Parkinson disease. However, it can help patients to feel better, both physically and mentally. Aerobic exercise may have a positive effect on disease status while improving quality of life and socialization. Favorable studies have appeared in the medical literature on exercises to improve balance, flexibility, and strength (including dance and Tai Chi)."

Interventions	Rationales
1. Explain the causes of the symptoms.	1. The individual's understanding may help to promote compliance with an exercise program at home.
2. Teach the individual to walk erect while looking at the horizon, with feet separated and arms swinging normally.	2. Conscious efforts to simulate normal gait and posture can improve mobility and minimize loss of balance.
3. Suggest a. Simple strengthening and stretching exercises. b. Aerobic exercises, such as walking (outdoors or on a treadmill, with support), riding a stationary bicycle, swimming, or water aerobics are easy to perform and usually energizing.	3. Exercise can help to prevent some of the complications of PD caused by rigidity and flexed (or bent) posture, such as shoulder, hip, and back pain. The benefits of exercise will persist as long as exercise continues. Many patients who participate in an exercise program feel more confident and gain a sense of control over their disease.
4. Consult with physical therapy for a specific exercise program. Explain that even short bouts of physical activity are also beneficial.	4. An exercise program of range of motion and aerobic exercise (tailored to the person's ability) can help to preserve muscle strength and coordination. Exercise programs should begin with low intensity activities, and gradually intensify (National Parkinson Foundation, 2016).
5. Stress to the individual that compliance with the exercise program is ultimately his or her choice.	5. Promoting the individual's feelings of control and self-determination may improve compliance with the exercise program.
6. Refer to the Fatigue nursing diagnosis in the index for additional interventions.	

> **TRANSITION TO HOME/COMMUNITY CARE**
> If indicated, review the risk diagnoses identified for this individual on admission:
> • Is the person still at risk?
> • Can the family reduce the risks?
> • Is the person at higher risk at home?
> • Is a home health nurse assessment needed?
> • Refer to transition planner/case manager/social service.
> • When is this person scheduled for follow-up with primary provider? Specialists? Record dates of appointments.
> • Complete a medication reconciliation prior to transition. Refer to index.

STAR   **Stop**

Think   Is this person at risk for injury, falls, medical complications, and/or inability to care for self (ADLs)?

Is there a support person available?

Is the person competent to manage self-administration of medications, treatment procedures? Are additional resources needed?

Can the person explain how to monitor the condition (e.g., blood glucose, sign/symptoms of complications, dietary/mobility restrictions, and when to call his or her primary provider or specialist)?

Act   Contact or provide the appropriate resource (e.g., contacting a support person, home health assessment, additional teaching, printed materials).

Review   Has the problem been addressed? If not, use SBAR to communicate to the appropriate person.

Risk for Ineffective Health Management Related to Lack of Knowledge of Condition, Treatments Required, Stress Management, Signs and Symptoms of Complications, and Community Resources

NOC

Compliance Behavior, Knowledge: Treatment Regimen, Participation in Health Care Decisions, Treatment Behavior: Illness or Injury

Goals

Refer to transition criteria.

NIC

Anticipatory Guidance, Learning Facilitation, Risk Identification, Health Education, Teaching Procedure/ Treatment, Health System Guidance

Interventions	Rationales
1. Teach the individual and his or her family the basic pathology of the individual's condition.	1. Understanding can improve compliance and reduce the family unit's frustrations.
2. Assist in identifying realistic short-term goals.	2. Setting realistic goals for recovery can reduce feelings of depression if goals are not attained.
3. Teach the individual energy conservation techniques, scheduling planned rest periods, and exercise consistent with tolerance levels. Refer to Unit II Section 1 Fatigue for specific interventions.	3. Energy conservation can reduce fatigue (NINDS, 2007).
4. Ensure referrals to multidiscipline services, speech therapy, nationalist, professional nurses.	4. Individual/family will require outpatient or home care of a multidisciplinary team.
5. Facilitate referral for psychological counseling and emotional support.	5. PD often causes sudden paralysis, communication difficulties, and dependence for body functions and ADLs creating psychological and emotional crisis for individuals and families (NINDS, 2011).

Interventions	Rationales

6. Explain signs and symptoms of complications to report to health care professional.
  a. Difficulty swallowing
  b. Productive cough
  c. Difficulty with urination, odor to urine
  d. Prolonged constipation
  e. Increased weakness or fatigue
  f. Weight loss
	6. Early intervention will minimize complications of the condition.

7. Provide information to assist with management at home. Refer to the following resources:
  a. National Parkinson's Foundation (http://www.parkinson.org/site)
  b. Case manager/transition planner referral
  c. Home health agency
    • Printed information: Patient information: PD treatment options—education, support, and therapy (Beyond the Basics). In *UpToDate*. Retrieved from http://www.uptodate.com/contents/parkinson-disease-treatment-options-education-support-and-therapy-beyond-the-basics?source=search_result&search=exercise++and+parkinson%27s&selectedTitle=4~150
    • National Parkinson Foundation under neuroprotective benefits of exercise. Retrieved from http://www.parkinson.org/understanding-parkinsons/treatment/Exercise/
	7. Individuals and families who receive community support may cope more effectively with this disease. Functional loss may be significant. Even when deficits are temporary, the individual will require interdisciplinary support during the recovery period.

Documentation

Condition on transition
Referrals, if indicated

Seizure Disorders

Carp's Cues

If a seizure disorder has not been confirmed, refer to Unit II Risk for Complications of Seizures instead of this care plan.

Seizure disorders constitute a chronic syndrome in which a neurologic dysfunction in cerebral tissue produces recurrent paroxysmal episodes, which are referred to as seizures. A seizure is defined as an uncontrolled electrical discharge of neurons in the brain that interrupts normal functions, such as disturbances of behavior, mood, sensation, perception, movement, and/or muscle tone.

Seizures are diagnosed as epileptic or reactive. Epilepsy is a chronic neurologic condition, usually with an underlying condition (as permanent brain injury) that affects the delicate systems that govern how electrical energy behaves in the brain, making the brain susceptible to recurring seizures (Epilepsy Foundation, 2007; *Lewis et al., 2004). Reactive seizures are single or multiple seizures resulting from a transient systemic problem (e.g., fever, infection, alcohol withdrawal, tumors, stroke, and toxic or metabolic disturbances).

Alcohol abuse is one of the most common causes of adolescent- and adult-onset seizures. Seizures, nearly always generalized tonic–clonic, occur in about 10% of adults during withdrawal. Multiple seizures happen in about 60% of these individuals. The first seizure occurs 7 hours to 2 days after the last drink, and the time between the first and last seizure is usually 6 hours or less (Hoffman & Weinhouse, 2015). Less than one-half of epilepsy cases have an identifiable cause (Schachter, 2015).

Carp's Cues

Alcohol abuse is one of the most common causes of adolescent- and adult-onset seizures. Seizures, nearly always generalized tonic/clonic, occur in about 10% of adults during withdrawal. Multiple seizures happen in about 60% of these individuals. The first seizure occurs 7 hours to 2 days after the last drink, and the time between the first and last seizure is usually 6 hours or less (Hoffman & Weinhouse, 2015).

Seizures are classified into two main categories: partial-onset (focal) seizures begin in a focal area of the cerebral cortex, whereas generalized-onset seizures have an onset recorded simultaneously in both cerebral hemispheres (Berg et al., 2010). Generalized seizures are further classified into the following categories: (a) absence, (b) myoclonic, (c) tonic/clonic, (d) tonic, and (e) atonic seizures (International League against Epilepsy, 2007).

 Time Frame

Initial diagnosis

Recurrent acute episodes

▪▪▪■ DIAGNOSTIC CLUSTER

Collaborative Problems

Risk for Complications of Status Epilepticus

Nursing Diagnoses

▲ Risk for Ineffective Airway Clearance related to relaxation of tongue and gag reflexes secondary to disruption in muscle innervations.

Anxiety related to fear of embarrassment secondary to having a seizure in public

Δ Risk for Ineffective Health Management related to insufficient knowledge of condition, medication, and care during seizures, environmental hazards, and community resources.

▲ This diagnosis was reported to be monitored for or managed frequently (75% to 100%).

Δ This diagnosis was reported to be monitored for or managed often (50% to 74%).

Transition Criteria

Before transition, the individual or family will:

1. State the intent to wear medical identification.
2. Relate activities to be avoided.
3. Relate the importance of complying with the prescribed medication regimen.
4. Relate the side effects of prescribed medications.
5. State situations that increase the possibility of a seizure.
6. State signs and symptoms that must be reported to a health care professional.
7. Ensure that the individual and her or his family are aware of community resources for epilepsy, such as http://www.ilae-epilepsy.org/ and http://www.epilepsyfoundation.org.
8. Make sure that the individual has understood all required follow-up appointments prior to transition.

Transitional Risk Assessment Plan (TRAP)

Begin this plan on admission.

Implement the Transitional Risk Assessment Plan (TRAP):

* Refer to inside back cover.
* Add each validated risk diagnosis to individual's problem list with the risk code in ( ).
* Refer to Unit II to the individual risk nursing diagnoses/collaborative problems for outcomes and interventions.

R: *"Close coordination of care in the post-acute period, early transition follow-up care, enhanced client education and self-management training, proactive end-of-life counseling, and extending the resources and clinical expertise over time via multidisciplinary team management" can lower readmission rates and improve health outcomes (Boutwell & Hwu, 2009, p. 14).*

Collaborative Problems

Risk for Complications of Status Epilepticus

Collaborative Outcomes

The individual will be monitored for early signs and symptoms of status epilepticus and will receive collaborative interventions if indicated to restore physiologic stability.

Indicators of Physiologic Stability

* Heart rate 60 to 100 beats/min (a, b)
* BP >90/60, <140/90 mm Hg (a, b)
* No seizure activity (a, b)
* Serum pH 7.35 to 7.45 (a, b)
* Serum Pco_2 35 to 45 mm Hg (a, b)
* Pulse oximetry (Sao_2) >95 (a, b)

Interventions	Rationales
1. Determine whether the individual senses an aura before onset of seizure activity. If so advise him or her to immediately report to nursing staff/student and if standing to sit or lie down.	1. This can prevent injuries from falling or hitting head on an object.
2. If seizure activity occurs, observe or acquire details from those who witnessed it and document the following (Hickey, 2014): a. Behavior prior to seizure b. Site of onset of seizure c. Progression and sequencing of activity d. Type of movements: clonic (jerking), tonic (stiffening) • Twitching, head turning, dystonia (muscle spasms and twisting of limbs) • Parts of body involved (symmetry, unilateral, bilateral) e. Changes in pupil size or position (open, rolling, deviation) f. Skin changes (color, temperature, perspiration) g. Urinary or bowel incontinence h. Duration i. Unconsciousness (duration) j. Behavior after seizure k. Weakness, paralysis after seizure l. Sleep after seizure (postictal period)	2. An accurate, comprehensive description of a seizure can assist the physician/nurse practitioner with appropriate anticonvulsant and optimal seizure management (Hickey, 2014; *South Carolina Department of Disabilities and Special Needs, 2006). b. Site of onset and order of progression are important in diagnosing causation. c. Progression of seizure activity may assist in identifying its anatomic focus.

Interventions	Rationales
3. In older adults, assess for presence of atypical signs/symptoms of seizures (Austin & Abdulla, 2013): a. Strange feelings, staring b. Minor behavioral changes, memory lapses c. Unaccountable loss of time d. Transient confusion	3. Age-related changes in the brain produce seizures that preset differently in older adults. Only 25% of older adults with epilepsy present with tonic/clonic seizures (Austin, 2013).
4. During seizure activity, take measures to ensure adequate ventilation (e.g., loosen clothing). *Do not* try to force an airway or tongue blade through clenched teeth.	4. Strong clonic–tonic movements can cause airway occlusion. Forced airway insertion can cause injury.
5. Provide privacy during and after seizure activity.	5. To protect the individual from embarrassment
6. During seizure activity, gently guide movements to prevent injury. Do not attempt to restrict movements.	6. Physical restraint could result in musculoskeletal injury.
7. If the individual is sitting when seizure activity occurs, ease him or her to the floor and place something soft under his or her head.	7. These measures help prevent injury.
8. After seizure activity subsides, position individual on the side.	8. This position helps prevent aspiration of secretions.
9. Allow person to sleep after seizure activity; reorient on awakening. **CLINICAL ALERT:** • Call Rapid Response Team if seizure continues more than two (2) consecutive minutes or the individual experiences two (2) or more generalized seizures without full recovery of consciousness between seizures (Hickey, 2014).	9. The person may experience amnesia; reorientation can help him or her regain a sense of control and can help reduce anxiety.
10. Initiate protocol: a. Establish airway. b. Suction p.r.n. c. Administer oxygen through nasal catheter. d. Initiate an IV line.	10. Status epilepticus is a medical emergency with a 10% mortality rate. Impaired respiration can cause systemic and cerebral hypoxia. IV administration of a rapid-acting anticonvulsant (e.g., diazepam) is indicated (Hickey, 2014).
11. Keep the bed in a low position with the side rails up, and pad the side rails with blankets.	11. These precautions help prevent injury from fall or trauma.
12. If appropriate, question individual when stable about: a. Any strange feelings, smells, movements that precede a seizure, time of day. b. Reports of fatigue, confusion.	
13. If the individual's condition is chronic, refer to Nursing Care Plan for Seizure Disorder in Unit III.	

Clinical Alert Report

Prior to providing care, advise ancillary staff/student to report the following to the professional nurse assigned to the individual:
- Any signs of seizure activity
- Intermittent, nonresponsive, blank stares
- Provide with a written cheat sheet with what to observe if seizure activity is witnessed. Write it as soon as possible.
- If the individual is older, advise to observe for new onset, intermittent or temporary change in behavior (e.g., staring, blank looks, memory, transient confusion, and reports of vague/strange feelings).

Documentation

Abnormal findings
Seizure activity flow sheet

Nursing Diagnoses

Anxiety Related to Fear of Embarrassment Secondary to Having a Seizure in Public

NOC
Anxiety Level, Coping, Impulse Control

Goal

The individual will relate an increase in psychological and physiologic comfort.

NIC
Anxiety Reduction, Impulse Control Training, Anticipatory Guidance

Indicators

- Use effective coping mechanisms.
- Describe his or her anxiety and perceptions.

 Carp's Cues

Living with epilepsy presents challenges affecting many aspects of life, including relationships with family and friends, school, employment, and leisure activities. While medications and other treatments help manage seizures, more than 1 million people continue to have seizures that impact their daily activities.

Interventions	Rationales
1. Provide opportunities for the individual and significant others to express their feelings alone and with each other.	1. Witnessing a seizure is terrifying for others and embarrassing for the individual prone to them. This shame and humiliation contributes to anxiety, depression, hostility, and secrecy. Family members also may experience these feelings. Frank discussions may reduce feelings of shame and isolation.
2. Allow opportunities for the individual to share concerns regarding seizures in public.	2. Stigma associated with epilepsy is a huge concern for people living with epilepsy. An individual with epilepsy may tend to separate him or herself from family, friends, and society (*Lewis et al., 2004).
3. Provide support and validate that individual's concerns are normal.	3. Possible losses related to epilepsy are loss of control, independence, employment, self-confidence, transportation, family, and friends. When a person feels listened to and understood, his or her loss is validated and normalized (*Lewis et al., 2004).

Interventions	Rationales
4. Assist the individual in identifying activities that are pleasurable and nonhazardous.	4. Fear of injury may contribute to isolation.
5. Stress the importance of adhering to the treatment plan.	5. Adherence to the medication regimen can help to prevent or reduce seizure episodes.
6. Discuss sharing the diagnosis with family members, friends, coworkers, and social contacts.	6. Open dialogue with others forewarns them of possible seizures; this can reduce the shock of witnessing a seizure and possibly enable assistive action.
7. Discuss situations through which the individual can meet others in a similar situation: a. Support groups b. Epilepsy Foundation of America	7. Sharing with others in a similar situation may give the individual a more realistic view of the seizure disorder and of societal perception of it (Epilepsy Foundation, 2007).

Documentation

Individual's concerns
Interaction with individual

STAR **Stop**

Think Is this person at risk for injury, falls, medical complications, and/or inability to care for self (ADLs)?
Is there a support person available?
Is the person competent to manage self-administration of medications, treatment procedures? Are additional resources needed?
Can the person explain how to monitor the condition (e.g., blood glucose, signs/symptoms of complications, dietary/mobility restrictions, and when to call his or her primary provider or specialist)?

Act Contact or provide the appropriate resource (e.g., contacting a support person, home health assessment, additional teaching, printed materials).

Review Has the problem been addressed? If not, use SBAR to communicate to the appropriate person.

Risk for Ineffective Health Management Related to Insufficient Knowledge of Condition, Medications, Care during Seizures, Environmental Hazards, and Community Resources

NOC
Compliance Behavior, Knowledge: Treatment Regimen, Participation in Health Care Decisions, Treatment Behavior: Illness or Injury

Goals

The goals for this diagnosis represent those associated with transition planning. Refer to the transition criteria.

NIC
Anticipatory Guidance, Learning Facilitation, Risk Identification, Health Education, Health System Guidance

Interventions	Rationales
1. Teach the individual and her or his family about seizure disorders and treatment; correct any misconceptions. Ask if they know anyone with a seizure disorder.	1. The individual and family's understanding of seizure disorders and the prescribed treatment regimen strongly influences compliance with the regimen.
2. If the individual is on medication therapy, teach the following information: a. Never discontinue a drug abruptly b. Side effects and signs of toxicity c. The need to have drug blood levels monitored, if indicated d. The need for periodic complete blood counts, if indicated e. The effects of Dilantin, if ordered, on gingival tissue and the need for regular dental examinations.	2a. Abrupt discontinuation can precipitate status epilepticus. b. Early identification of problems enables prompt intervention to prevent serious complications. c. Drug blood levels provide a guide for adjusting drug dosage. d. Long-term use of some anticonvulsive drugs, such as hydantoins (e.g., phenytoin [Dilantin]), can cause blood dyscrasias. e. Long-term phenytoin therapy can cause gingival hyperplasia.
3. Provide information regarding situations that increase the risk of seizure (*Bader & Littlejohns, 2004): a. Excess stimulation b. Alcohol ingestion c. Excessive caffeine intake d. Excessive stress e. Febrile illness f. Flashing lights g. Noisy environment h. Poorly adjusted television screen i. Excessive fatigue, sedentary activity level, lack of sleep j. Hypoglycemia k. Constipation l. Diarrhea	3. Certain situations have been identified as increasing seizure episodes, although the actual mechanisms behind them are unknown (*Bader & Littlejohns, 2004). i. Regular activity and exercise are important. Activity tends to inhibit rather than increase seizures. Fatigue and hyperventilation should be avoided.
4. Advise not to use alcohol, recreational, or street drugs.	4. All are stimulants and can cause seizure if withdrawal occurs.
5. Practice safety measure associated with an activity: a. Swim with a "buddy."	
6. Advise to discuss the use of supplements with PCP.	6. Anticonvulsant drugs may cause low levels of calcium, vitamin D, and vitamin K; calcium supplements can interfere with anticonvulsant drugs.
7. Discuss why certain activities are hazardous and should be avoided: a. Swimming alone b. When riding bicycles, rollerblades, or using scooters without a helmet c. Driving (unless seizure-free for the period determined by state laws) d. Operating potentially hazardous machinery e. Mountain climbing f. Occupations in which the individual could be injured or cause injury to others	

Interventions	Rationales
8. Discuss with PCP, prior to using herbs/essential oils	8. Some herbs increase the risk of seizure or interact with a medication for epilepsy such as ginkgo, primrose oil, St. John's wort, and white willow. Some essential oils should also be avoided, such as eucalyptus, fennel, hyssop, and pennyroyal tansy.
9. Refer the individual to the Epilepsy Foundation website for information regarding employment issues: http://www.epilepsyfoundation.org/livingwithepilepsy/employmenttopics/index.cfm	9. There are a few occupations that the federal government has barred individual with epilepsy from engaging in (e.g., pilots, commercial truck drivers). Generally an individual prone to seizures should avoid any activity that could place him, her, or others in danger should a seizure occur.
10. Teach the individual how to recognize the warning signals of a seizure and what to do to minimize injury (*Bader & Littlejohns, 2004; *Lewis et al., 2004).	
11. Refer the individual and family to community resources and reference material for assistance with management (e.g., Epilepsy Foundation of America, counseling, occupational rehabilitation).	11. Such resources may provide additional information and support.

Documentation

Individual/family teaching
Referrals if indicated

HEMATOLOGIC DISORDERS

Sickle Cell Disease

Sickle cell disease (SCD) is an incurable genetic disorder affecting approximately 100,000 Americans. SCD occurs among about 1 out of every 365 Black or African American births. SCD occurs among about 1 out of every 16,300 Hispanic American births. About 1 in 13 Black or African American babies is born with sickle cell trait (SCT).

The life expectancy of persons with sickle cell anemia is reduced. Some individuals, however, can remain without symptoms for years, while others do not survive infancy or early childhood. The average life expectancy in America has improved. It is now in the mid-40 years of age range (Sickle Cell Disease Association of America, 2016).

Vaso-occlusive phenomena and hemolysis are the clinical hallmarks of SCD, an inherited disorder due to homozygosity for the abnormal hemoglobin, hemoglobin S (HbS). Vaso-occlusion results in recurrent painful episodes (previously called sickle cell crisis) and a variety of serious organ system complications that can lead to lifelong disabilities and/or early death (Vichinsky, 2014).

Under certain conditions, this hemoglobin leads to anemia and acute and chronic tissue damage secondary to the "sickling"—that is, turning into the sickle form—of the abnormal red cells. HbS molecules tend to bond to one another and to hemoglobin A, forming long aggregates or tactoids. These aggregates increase the viscosity of blood, causing stasis in blood flow. The low oxygen tension concentration of HbS causes the cells to assume a sickle rather than a biconcave shape. This hemoglobin damages erythrocyte membranes, leading to erythrocyte rupture and chronic hemolytic anemia (Grossman & Porth, 2014).

Symptoms of sickle cell anemia result from thrombosis and infarction, leading to vaso-occlusive crises (VOCs). The incidence of sickle cell crises varies among individuals. Some report an incident once a year, whereas others report more than one a week.

⏱ Time Frame
Acute sickling crisis

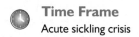

DIAGNOSTIC CLUSTER

Collaborative Problems

△   Risk for Complications of Acute Chest Syndrome

△   Risk for Complications of Infection

*   Risk for Complications of Anemia

*   Risk for Complications of Vaso-Occlusive Crisis

*   Risk for Complications of Aplastic Crisis

*   Risk for Complications of Leg Ulcers

*   Risk for Complications of Neurologic Dysfunction

*   Risk for Complications of Splenic Dysfunction

*   Risk for Complications of Avascular Necrosis of Femoral/Humeral Heads

*   Risk for Complications of Priapism

Nursing Diagnoses

▲ Acute Pain related to viscous blood and tissue hypoxia

Δ Risk for Ineffective Health Management related to insufficient knowledge of disease process, risk factors for sickling crisis, pain management, signs and symptoms of complications, genetic counseling, and family planning services

▲ This diagnosis was reported to be monitored for or managed frequently (75% to 100%).

Δ This diagnosis was reported to be monitored for or managed often (50% to 74%).

* This diagnosis was not included in the validation study.

Transition Criteria

Before transition, the individual or family will:

1. Identify precipitating factors of present crisis, if possible.
2. Plan one change in life style to reduce crisis or to improve health.
3. Describe signs and symptoms that must be reported to a health care professional.
4. Describe necessary health maintenance and follow-up care.

Transitional Risk Assessment Plan (TRAP)

Begin This Plan on Admission

Implement the Transitional Risk Assessment Plan (TRAP)

- Refer to front/back inside covers
- Add each validated High-Risk Diagnosis to Individual's Problem List with the risk code in ( ).
- Refer to Section II to the individual high-risk nursing diagnoses/collaborative problems for outcomes and interventions

R: "Close coordination of care in the post-acute period, early discharge follow-up care, enhanced patient education and self-management training, proactive end-of-life counseling, and extending the resources and clinical expertise over time via multidisciplinary team management" can lower readmission rates and improve health outcomes (Boutwell & Hwu, 2009, p. 14). Interventions are utilized to activate the individual and family to select changes in their everyday lifestyle choices to improve their health (Hibbard & Greene, 2013).

Collaborative Problems

Potential Complication: Anemia

Potential Complication: Sickle Cell Crisis

Potential Complication: Acute Chest Syndrome

Potential Complication: Infection

Potential Complication: Leg Ulcers

Potential Complication: Neurologic Dysfunction

Potential Complication: Splenic Dysfunction

Potential Complication: Osteonecrosis

Collaborative Outcomes

The individual will be monitored for early signs and symptoms of (a) anemia, (b) vaso-occlusive crisis, (c) acute chest syndrome, (d) aplastic anemia, (e) infection, (f) leg ulcers, (g) neurologic dysfunction, (h) splenic dysfunction, (i) priapism, and (j) osteonecrosis (femoral/humeral heads) and will receive collaborative interventions if indicated to restore physiologic stability.

Indicators of Physiologic Stability

- Hemoglobin (a, b, d)
  - Males: 13 to 18 gm/dL
  - Females: 12 to 16 gm/dL
- Hematocrit (a, b, d)
  - Males: 42% to 50%
  - Females: 40% to 48%
- Red blood cells (a, b, d)
  - Males: 4.6 to 5.9 million/mm^3
  - Females: 4.2 to 5.4 million/mm^3
- Platelets 150,000 to 400,000/mm^3 (e)
- White blood cells 4,300 to 10,800/mm^3 (e)
- Oxygen saturation >95% (a, b, c, d)
- No or minimal bone pain (b, e, j)
- No or minimal abdominal pain (b, e, h)
- No or minimal chest pain (c)
- No or minimal fatigue (a, b, e)
- Pinkish, ruddy, brownish, or olive skin tones (a, b)
- No or minimal headache (b, g)
- Clear, oriented (b, g)
- Clear speech (b, g)
- Pulse rate 60 to 100 beats/min (a, b, c, g, h)
- Respirations 16 to 20 breaths/min (b, c, e, g)
- BP >90/60, <140/90 mm Hg (a, b, c, g, h)
- Temperature 98° F to 99.5° F (b, a, e, f, j)
- Urine output >0.5 mL/kg/hr (b, c, h)
- Urine specific gravity 1.005 to 1.030 (b, c, h)
- Flaccid penis (i)

Interventions	Rationales
1. Monitor for signs and symptoms of anemia: a. Lethargy b. Weakness c. Fatigue d. Increased pallor e. Dyspnea on exertion	1. Because anemia is common with most of these individuals, low hemoglobins are relatively tolerated; therefore, changes should be described in reference to an individual's baseline or acute symptoms (Grossman & Porth, 2014).
2. Monitor laboratory values, including complete blood cell count (CBC) with reticulocyte count.	2. Elevated reticulocytes (normal level about 1%) indicate active erythropoiesis. Lack of elevation with anemia may represent a problem (Grossman & Porth, 2014).
3. Monitor for vaso-occlusive phenomena (VOC): a. Sudden onset of pain in any body part. It often involves the abdomen, bones, joints, and soft tissue, acute joint necrosis or avascular necrosis, or acute abdomen (National Institutes of Health [NIH], 2015a).	3. Often, no precipitating cause can be identified. However, because deoxygenated HbS becomes semisolid, the most likely physiologic trigger of VOCs is hypoxemia. The crisis may last several hours to several days and terminate as abruptly as it began.
4. Monitor: a. Oxygen saturation with pulse oximetry. b. Hydration status (urine output, specific gravity) c. Level of consciousness	4a. O$_2$ should be administered only if oxygen saturation is less than 95%. b. Dehydration can contribute to vaso-occlusion c. Change in consciousness can be due to a cerebral infarction.

Interventions	Rationales
5. Aggressively hydrate (1.5× maintenance volume). Avoid IV therapy, if possible.	5. Hydration can disrupt the clustered cells and improve hypoxemia.

6. Monitor for signs and symptoms of acute chest syndrome (Field & DeBaun, 2015):
  a. Sudden onset of:
    • Chest pain
    • Pain in the arms and legs
    • Rib and sternal pain
  b. Other findings:
    • Temperature ≥38.5° C
    • >2% decrease in Spo_2 (O_2 saturation) from a documented steady-state value on room air ($Fio_2 = 0.21$)
    • Pao_2 <60 mm Hg
    • Tachypnea (per age-adjusted normal)
    • Intercostal retractions, nasal flaring, or use of accessory muscles of respiration
    • Cough, wheezing
    • Rales
	6. Acute chest syndrome is the term used to represent this group of symptoms, namely, acute pleuritic chest pain, fever, leukocytosis, and infiltrates on chest X-ray seen in SCD. Acute chest syndrome (ACS) is a leading cause of death for individuals with SCD (Field & DeBaun, 2015). This represents a medical emergency is the result of bone marrow or fat emboli leading to pulmonary infarction (Field & DeBaun, 2015). Initiate protocols (e.g., intravenous access).

7. Monitor for signs and symptoms of infection:
  a. Fever
  b. Pain
  c. Chills
  d. Increased white blood cells
	7. Bacterial infection is one major cause of morbidity and mortality. Decreased functioning of the spleen (asplenia) results from sickle cell anemia. The loss of the spleen's ability to filter and to destroy various infectious organisms increases the risk of infection (Field & DeBaun, 2015).

8. Monitor for splenic sequestration (Field, Vichinsky, & DeBaun, 2016)
  a. Splenic enlargement, often tender
  b. A drop in hemoglobin concentration of at least 2 g/dL
  c. Thrombocytopenia
  d. Reticulocytosis
	8. Splenic sequestration is a potentially life-threatening complication of SCD that requires admission to the hospital for maintenance of hemodynamic stability (Field et al., 2016).

9. Monitor for aplastic crisis:
  a. Increased fatigue
  b. Pallor (may replace the typical jaundice of SCD)
  c. Activity intolerance
  d. Shortness of breath
	9. An aplastic crisis is characterized by the transient arrest of erythropoiesis, leading to abrupt reductions in hemoglobin concentration and red cell precursors in the bone marrow, and a markedly reduced number of reticulocytes in the peripheral blood. Causes may be viruses as Epstein–Barr virus or bacterial infections as streptococcal, salmonella as well as use of hydroxyurea (Vichinsky, 2014).

10. Monitor for early signs and symptoms of leg ulcers:
  a. Hyperpigmentation
  b. Skin wrinkling
  c. Pruritus, tenderness
	10. Leg ulcers are a frequent complication in SCD, causing significant physical disability and a negative psychologic and social impact, occurring usually after the age of 10 (Minniti, Eckman, Sebastiani, Steinberg, & Ballas, 2010).

(continued)

Interventions   *Rationales*

> **CLINICAL ALERT:**
> • Leg ulcers are painful and often disabling complications of SCD. They tend to be indolent, intractable, and heal slowly over months to years. The pain may be severe, excruciating, penetrating, sharp, and stinging in nature (Minniti et al., 2010).

11. Monitor for changes in neurologic function:
    a. Cognitive change
    b. Speech disturbances
    c. Sudden headache
    d. Numbness, tingling

> **CLINICAL ALERT:**
> • The Cooperative Study of Sickle Cell Disease found that 24% of individuals with sickle cell anemia experienced a clinical overt stroke by age 45 (Vichinsky, 2014).

11. Cerebral infarction and intracranial hemorrhage are complications of SCD. Occlusion of nutrient arteries to major cerebral arteries causes progressive wall damage and eventual occlusion of the major vessel. Intracerebral hemorrhage may be secondary to hypoxic necrosis of vessel walls (Grossmam & Porth, 2014).

12. Recognize and explain priapism.
    a. Low flow from ischemic, veno-occlusive events causes stasis, hypoxia, and acidosis of venous blood during a normal erection, resulting in sickling of erythrocytes within the venous sinusoids of the corpus cavernosa (Field, Vemulakonda, & DeBaun, 2014).
    b. Educate individual to report a sustained unwanted, erection over 30 minutes.
    c. Risk factors for developing priapism with SCD include full bladder, prolonged sexual activity, fever or dehydration, exposure to alcohol, marijuana, or cocaine, or use of psychotropic agents, sildenafil, or testosterone.

12. Priapism is a sustained penile erection in the absence of sexual activity or desire. The definition of "sustained" in this setting is unclear, but priapism is generally defined as an unwanted erection lasting more than 2 to 4 hours (Field et al., 2014).

13. If priapism occurs, instruct to (Field et al., 2014; Olujohungbe & Burnett, 2013)
    a. Use oral analgesics for pain control
    b. Attempt to urinate as soon as priapism begins.
    c. Anecdotal evidence has also suggested that exercise, warm compresses, and masturbation may also be beneficial.

13. "Prompt recognition and appropriate treatment of a priapism episode in males with sickle cell disease (SCD) is critical, as the end result of prolonged and/or repeated episodes of priapism can be ischemia and fibrosis in the corpus cavernosa of the penis, potentially leading to impaired sexual function and impotence" (Field et al., 2014).

14. Monitor for osteonecrosis and vaso-occlusive pain episodes. Instruct to report any of the following:
    a. Mild erythema and warmth, as well as local tenderness on palpation
    b. Fever
    c. Limited movement
    d. Acute onset of deep-seated pain

14. Vaso-occlusive pain episodes can lead to bone infarcts, necrosis, and, over time, degenerative changes in marrow-containing bone. Many individuals with SCD also suffer from the long-term consequences of vaso-occlusive pain episodes in the musculoskeletal system, such as avascular necrosis of the femoral heads or collapsed vertebral bodies, leading to a chronic state of pain in addition to the more acute painful episodes (George & DeBaun, 2016).

Although the long bones are affected most commonly, children and adults can present with vaso-occlusive pain episodes of virtually any bony structure containing red (erythropoietic) marrow, including ribs, sternum, vertebral bodies, and skull.

Clinical Alert Report

Prior to providing care, advise ancillary staff/student to report the following to the professional nurse assigned to the individual:

- New onset/worsening of pain
- Decreased urine output <0.5 mL/kg/hr
- Change in cognitive status
- Oral temperature >100.5° F
- Systolic BP <90 mm Hg
- Resting pulse >100, <50 beats/min
- Respiratory rate >28, <10/min
- Oxygen saturation <90%

Documentation

Skin assessment
Neurologic
Vital signs
Abnormal findings
Interventions
Evaluation

Nursing Diagnoses

Acute Pain Related to Viscous Blood and Tissue Hypoxia

NOC

Comfort Level, Pain Control

NIC

Pain Management, Medication Management, Emotional Support, Teaching: Individual, Heat/Cold Application, Simple Massage

Goal

The individual will report decreased pain after pain-relief measures.

Indicators

- Relate factors that increase pain
- Relate factors that can precipitate pain

Interventions

CLINICAL ALERT:
- New epidemiological findings redefine pain in SCD as being more often a chronic manifestation than was previously thought, although acute pain is still the hallmark of the disease. SCD pain intensity, the number of painful locations, and the frequency of hospitalizations due to SCD pain may worsen with age (Smith & Scherer, 2010).

1. Ask the individual if the painful episode is "typical" or "unusual." (Most individuals have a distinctive, unique pattern of pain.)

Rationales

1. Changes may indicate another complication (e.g., infection, abdominal surgical emergency).

(continued)

Interventions	Rationales
2. Assess for any signs of infection (e.g., respiratory, urinary, vaginal). (Painful events often occur with infection.)	
3. Aggressively manage acute pain episodes. Consult with physician or advanced practice nurse.	3. The pain of SCD, like the pain of cancer, should be treated based on individual's tolerance and discretion.
4. Avoid all ice and cold compresses.	4. Cold products should be avoided because they may precipitate sickling (DeBaun & Vichinsky, 2015). Refer to Acute/Chronic Pain in Unit II Section 1 for management of pain utilizing cardinal principles as outlined by the American Pain Society (APS) and an evidence-based guideline from the National Heart, Lung, and Blood Institute (NHLBI) at the National Institutes of Health (NIH).

Documentation

Type, route, and dosage of all medications
Status of pain
Degree of relief from pain-relief measures

> ### TRANSITION TO HOME/COMMUNITY CARE
> - If indicated, Review the high-risk diagnoses identified for this individual on admission:
>   - Is the person still at high risk?
>   - Can the family/reduce the risks?
>   - Is the person at higher risk at home?
>   - Is a home health nurse assessment needed?
>   - Refer to Discharge Planner/Case Manager/Social Service.
> - When is this person scheduled for follow-up with primary provider? Specialists? Record dates of appointments.
> - Complete a medication reconciliation prior to discharge > Refer to front/back cover.

STAR

Stop

Think Is this person at high risk for injury, falls, medical complications, and/or inability to care for self (activities of daily living)?
Is there a support person available?
Is the person competent to manage self-administration of medications, treatment procedures?
Can the person explain how to monitor condition (e.g., blood glucose, sign/symptoms of complications, dietary/mobility restrictions) and when to call his/her primary provider or specialist? Are additional resources needed?

Act Contact or provide the appropriate resource (e.g., contacting a support person, home health assessment, additional teaching, printed materials)

Review Has the problem been addressed? If not use SBAR to communicate to the appropriate person.

Risk for Ineffective Health Management Related to Insufficient Knowledge of Disease Process, Risk Factors for Vaso-Occlusive, Pain Management, Signs and Symptoms of Complications, Genetic Counseling, and Family Planning Services

NOC

Compliance Behavior, Knowledge: Treatment Regimen, Participation in Health Care Decisions, Treatment Behavior: Illness or Injury

NIC

Anticipatory Guidance, Risk Identification, Health Education, Learning Facilitation

Goals

The goals for this diagnosis represent those associated with transition planning. Refer to the transition criteria.

Interventions	Rationales
CLINICAL ALERT: • Emotional distress, including symptoms of depression and anxiety, may adversely affect the course and complicate the treatment of chronic physical conditions (Treadwell, Barreda, Kaur, & Gildengorin, 2015). Researchers reported "that barriers to health care were correlated with depression and anxiety symptoms, mental HRQL, and greater ED utilization support the need to view SCD care within a biobehavioral framework" (Treadwell et al., 2015, p. 17). Health care provider negative attitudes and lack of knowledge were the most frequently cited barriers for adults in our study, particularly in the context of ED and inpatient care (Treadwell et al., 2015).	
1. Review present situation, disease process, and treatment.	1. Even though the individual has had the disease since childhood, the nurse should evaluate present knowledge

2. Discuss precipitating factors
   a. High altitude (more than 7,000 feet above sea level)
   b. Unpressurized aircraft
   c. Dehydration (e.g., diaphoresis, diarrhea, vomiting)
   d. Strenuous physical activity
   e. Cold temperatures (e.g., iced liquids)
 	
   f. Infection (e.g., respiratory, urinary, vaginal), fever
   g. Ingestion of alcohol
   h. Cigarette smoking
	2a,b. Decreased oxygen tension can cause red blood cells to sickle.
	   c,d. Any situation that causes dehydration or increases blood viscosity can precipitate sickling.
	   e. Cold causes peripheral vasoconstriction, which slows circulation.
	   f. The exact mechanism is unknown.
	   g. Alcohol use promotes dehydration.
	   h. Nicotine interferes with oxygen exchange.

3. Emphasize the need to drink at least 16 cups (8 oz) of fluid daily and to increase to 24 to 32 cups during a painful crisis or when at risk for dehydration.	3. Dehydration must be prevented to prevent a sickling crisis. Discuss the importance of maintaining optimal health.

(continued)

Interventions	Rationales

4. Explain components of a healthy lifestyle
   a. Regular health care professional examinations (e.g., oph-thalmic, general)
   b. Good nutrition
   c. Stress reduction methods
   d. Dental hygiene
   e. Daily vitamin without iron
	4. Adhering to a health maintenance plan can reduce risk factors that contribute to crisis. This replaces some of the vitamins and micronutrients commonly reported to be deficient in these individuals, including zinc, vitamin D, vitamin E, vitamin C, vitamin A, magnesium, selenium, carotenoids, and flavonoids. Excessive iron stores and oxidative injury may contribute to the depletion of antioxidant vitamins (Field et al., 2016).

5. Explain the importance of an eye examination every 6 to 12 months.	5. SCD can cause retinopathy by plugging small retinal vessels and causing neovascularization (Grossmam & Porth, 2014).

6. Stress the importance of reporting signs and symptoms of infection early.
   a. Persistent cough
   b. Fever
   c. Foul-smelling vaginal drainage
   d. Cloudy, reddish, or foul-smelling urine
   e. Increased redness of wound
   f. Purulent drainage from wound
	6. Early recognition of an infection and treatment may prevent a crisis.

7. After crisis, help to identify some warning signs that occur days or hours before a crisis. Advise to increase fluid intake and to take nonsteroidal anti-inflammatory drugs (NSAIDs) or acetaminophen if kidneys are affected per instructions of primary care provider (PCP) (NIH, 2015a).	7. Some individuals with SCD experience a prodromal stage (a gradual buildup of symptoms for days before a crisis). More commonly, however, symptoms begin less than 1 hour before a crisis) (NIH, 2015a).
8. Instruct to access prompt treatment of cuts, insect bites, and other sources for infection.	8. Decreased peripheral circulation increases the risk of infection.
9. Explain to monitor for leg ulcers especially at ankles and to report early signs.	9. Leg ulcers occur in areas with less subcutaneous fat, thin skin, and with decreased blood flow. The commonest sites are the medial and lateral malleoli (ankles), often becoming circumferential if not controlled early; the medial malleolus is more commonly involved than the lateral malleolus. Less common sites are the anterior tibial area, dorsum of the foot, and Achilles tendon (Minniti et al., 2010).
10. Teach to avoid sources of infection such as sick individuals and high-risk sexual activity.	
11. Advise of the importance of immunizations (e.g., influenza [yearly], pneumonia vaccines, age-appropriate [e.g., HPV, Zoster, pertussis *Neisseria meningitidis*, *Haemophilus influenzae* (type B), and hepatitis A & B virus]) (Field et al., 2016).	11. Immunizations are a cornerstone of infection prevention in SCD (Field et al., 2016).

12. Teach to seek medical care in certain situations, including the following:
   a. Persistent fever (>38.3° C)
   b. Chest pain, shortness of breath, nausea, and vomiting
   c. Abdominal pain with nausea and vomiting
   d. Persistent headache not experienced previous
	12. These signs and symptoms can indicate infection, thrombosis and infarction, leading to vaso-occlusive crises (VOCs). Immediate medical attention is required.

Interventions	Rationales
13. Refer to Living Well with Sickle Cell Disease at http://www.cdc.gov/ncbddd/sicklecell/documents/livingwell-with-sickle-cell-disease_self-caretoolkit.pdf for a comprehensive source for helping individual's/families cope with SCD.	
14. Explore the individual/partner's knowledge regarding the genetic aspects of the disease. Refer to appropriate resource (e.g., genetic counseling).	14. This disease is hereditary. If both parents have the SCT, the chance that a child will have SCD is 25%. If one parent is carrying the trait and the other actually has disease, the odds increase to 50% that their child will inherit the disease. Screening and genetic counseling theoretically have the potential to drastically reduce the prevalence of SCD (Maakaron, 2013). The incidence of offspring inheriting SCD is related to parents as carriers or noncarriers of the hemoglobin genotype AS.

Documentation

Transition summary record
Individual/family teaching
Outcome achievement
Referrals if indicated

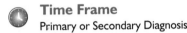

INTEGUMENTARY DISORDERS

Pressure Ulcers

Pressure ulcers are among the most common conditions encountered in acutely hospitalized individuals (0% to 46%), in critical care (13.1% to 45.5%) or those requiring long-term institutional care (4.1% to 32.2%). An estimated 2.5 million pressure ulcers are treated each year in acute care facilities in the United States alone (National Pressure Ulcer Advisory Panel, European Pressure Ulcer Advisory Panel, 2014).

Pressure ulcers are localized areas of cellular necrosis that tend to occur from prolonged compression of soft tissue between a bony prominence and a firm surface, most commonly as a result of immobility. Injury ranges from nonblanchable erythema of intact skin to deep ulceration extending to the bone. Extrinsic factors that exert mechanical force on soft tissue include pressure, shear, friction, and maceration. Intrinsic factors that determine susceptibility to tissue breakdown include malnutrition, anemia, loss of sensation, impaired mobility, advanced age, decreased mental status, incontinence, and infection. Extrinsic and intrinsic factors interact to produce ischemia and necrosis of soft tissue in susceptible persons (National Pressure Ulcer Advisory Panel, European Pressure Ulcer Advisory Panel, 2014).

Time Frame
Primary or Secondary Diagnosis

■■■■ DIAGNOSTIC CLUSTER

Collaborative Problems

Risk for Complications of Infection (Sepsis and Osteomyelitis)

Nursing Diagnoses

▲ Pressure Ulcer related to mechanical destruction of tissue secondary to pressure, shear, and/or friction

▲ Impaired Physical Mobility related to imposed restrictions, deconditioned status, loss of motor control, or altered mental status (refer to Unit II)

▲ Imbalanced Nutrition related to insufficient oral intake sufficient for wound healing (refer to Unit II and Generic Care Plan for Surgical Conditions > Altered Nutrition)

▲ Risk for Infection related to loss of skin integrity, and exposure of ulcer base to fecal/urinary drainage

△ Risk for Ineffective Health Management related to insufficient knowledge of etiology, prevention, wound care adaption, and home care

Related Care Plan

Immobility or Unconsciousness

▲ This diagnosis was reported to be monitored for or managed frequently (75% to 100%).
△ This diagnosis was reported to be monitored for or managed often (50% to 74%).

Transition Criteria

Before transition, the individual or family will:

1. Identify factors that contribute to ulcer development.
2. Demonstrate the ability to perform skills necessary to prevent and treat pressure ulcers.
3. State the intent to continue prevention and treatment strategies at home (e.g., activity, nutrition).

Transitional Risk Assessment Plan (TRAP)

Begin this plan on admission.

Implement the Transitional Risk Assessment Plan (TRAP):

* Refer to inside back cover (Braden Scale)
* Add each validated risk diagnosis to individual's problem list with the risk code in ( ).
* Refer to Unit II to the individual risk nursing diagnoses/collaborative problems for outcomes and interventions.

> *R:* *"Close coordination of care in the post-acute period, early transition follow-up care, enhanced client educa-tion and self-management training, proactive end-of-life counseling, and extending the resources and clinical expertise over time via multidisciplinary team management" can lower readmission rates and improve health outcomes (Boutwell & Hwu, 2009, p. 14). Interventions are utilized to activate the individual and family to select changes in their everyday lifestyle choices to improve their health (Hibbard & Greene, 2013).*

Collaborative Problems

Risk for Complications of Systemic Inflammatory Response Syndrome (SIRS)/Sepsis/Osteomyelitis

Collaborative Outcomes

The individual will be monitored for early signs and symptoms of acute wound infection and will receive collaborative interventions if indicated to restore physiologic stability, promote wound healing, and prevent infection.

Indicators of Physiologic Stability and Wound Healing

* Temperature 98° F to 99.5° F
* Heart rate 60 to 100 beats/min
* Blood pressure >90/60, <140/90 mm Hg
* Respiration 16 to 20 breaths/min
* Urine output >0.5 mL/kg/hr
* Pink, healthy wound tissues
* Negative blood culture
* White blood count 4,300 to 10,800 cells/mm^3
* Oriented, alert

Interventions	*Rationales*
CLINICAL ALERT: • Would healing is delayed and/may be abnormal when pressure ulcer have a significant bacterial burden and infection (Advisory Panel, European Pressure Ulcer Advisory Panel, 2014, p. 162).	

1. Monitor for signs of infection in pressure ulcer (Armstrong & Meyr, 2016):
   a. Wound drainage
   b. Discoloration
   c. Delayed healing
   d. Friable granulation tissue
   e. Increasing pain and increased temperature
   f. Malodor
   g. Pocketing and bridging
	1. Necrotic tissue contains high levels of both anaerobic and aerobic bacteria (Grossman & Porth, 2014).

(continued)

Interventions	Rationales
2. Monitor for signs and symptoms of wound infection > SIRS > sepsis > osteomyelitis: a. Temperature >101° F or <98.6° F or <36° C or >38° C b. Tachycardia (>90 beats/min) and tachypnea (>20 breaths/min) c. Pale, cool skin d. Decreased urine output e. WBCs and bacteria in urine (remove) Lactate >4 mmol/L f. Positive blood culture, wound and bone cultures g. Elevated white blood count >12,000 cells/mm^3 or decreased WBC <4,000 cells/mm^3 h. Confusion, changes in mentation i. Refer to Unit II for interventions for sepsis. j. Chronically elevated platelets (>370) and CRP (>10) levels for osteomyelitis Refer to Unit II Section 2—Risk for Complications of Sepsis/SIRS.	2. Gram-positive and gram-negative organisms can invade open wounds; debilitated individuals are more vulnerable. Response to sepsis results in massive vasodilation and hypovolemia, resulting in tissue hypoxia and decreased renal function and cardiac output. This in turn triggers a compensatory response of increased heart rate and respirations to correct hypoxia and acidosis. Bacteria in urine or blood indicate infection (National Pressure Ulcer Advisory Panel, European Pressure Ulcer Advisory Panel, 2014). j. Elevated platelets and CRP levels indicate acute/chronic inflammatory response and may be monitored to guide efficacy of treatment.

Clinical Alert Report

Prior to providing care, advise ancillary staff/student to report the following to the professional nurse assigned to the individual:

* Temperature <36° C or >38° C
* Respiratory rate >20 breaths/min
* Heart rate >90 beats/min
* Acute mental status changes
* Unusual warmth and redness at or around the wound
* Urine output <0.5 mL/kg/hr
* Increased foul wound drainage
* Increased wound size
* Gray or black tissues
* Exposed muscle/bone
* Increased wound pain in sensate individuals or increased spasticity (indicator of pain) in paralyzed individuals.

Documentation

Pressure Ulcer Risk Assessment at admission and daily
Wound Documentation Record (per institutional policy)
Skin Assessment Tool at admission and daily, with documentation of lesions

Nursing Diagnosis

Pressure Ulcer Related to Mechanical Destruction of Tissue Secondary to Pressure, Shear, and/or Friction

 NOC
Risk Control: Infectious Process, Mobility, Nutrition Status, Hydration, Immobility Consequences: Physiological

Goal

The individual will demonstrate progressive healing of tissues, and no new skin injury.

Pressure Ulcer Care,
Fluid Management,
Nutrition Management,
Infection Protection,
Teaching: Individual,
Skin Surveillance,
Wound Care

Indicators

- Participates in risk assessment.
- Expresses willingness to participate in prevention of pressure ulcers.
- Describes etiology and prevention measures.
- Explains rationale for interventions.

> **Carp's Cues**
>
> The following interventions focus on prevention of additional or worsening of pressure ulcer(s), promotion of healing, and treatment of the pressure ulcer(s).

Interventions	*Rationales*
1. Assess dependent skin areas with every position turn. a. Use finger or transparent disk to assess whether skin is blanchable or nonblanchable.	1. "Blanchable erythema is visible skin redness that become white when pressure is applied and reddens when pressure relieved" (National Pressure Ulcer Advisory Panel, European Pressure Ulcer Advisory Panel, 2014, p. 63). It may result from normal reactive hyperemia that should disappear within several hours or it may result from inflammatory erythema with intact capillary bed. Nonblanchable erythema is visible redness that persists with the application of pressure, which indicates structural damage to microcirculation (p. 63). This represents Category/Stage I pressure ulcer (National Pressure Ulcer Advisory Panel, European Pressure Ulcer Advisory Panel, 2014).
2. Assess skin temperature, edema, and change in tissue consistency as compared to surrounding tissue.	2. Localized heat. Edema and change in tissue consistency as induration/hardness as compared to surrounding tissue are warning signs for pressure ulcer development.
3. Observe the skin for pressure damage caused by medical devices (e.g., catheters and [National Pressure Ulcer Advisory Panel, European Pressure Ulcer Advisory Panel, 2014] cervical collars). **CLINICAL ALERT:** • Do not wear gloves when assessing skin temperature and changes in tissue consistency. As indicated, cleanse skin prior to assessing and follow usual hand-washing procedures.	
4. Document all skin assessments, noting details of any pain possibly related to pressure damage.	4. The frequency of inspection may need to be increased in response to any deterioration in overall condition.
5. Ask the individual if they have any areas of discomfort or pain that could be attributed to pressure damage.	5. Studies reported that pain over the site was a precursor to tissue breakdown (National Pressure Ulcer Advisory Panel, European Pressure Ulcer Advisory Panel, 2014).
6. Access the wound specialist, if there are changes in skin assessment (e.g., nonblanchable erythema).	6. Researchers have reported that the failure to identify early stages of pressure damage results in greater numbers of people with darkly pigmented skin developing more severe forms of pressure damage (National Pressure Ulcer Advisory Panel, European Pressure Ulcer Advisory Panel, 2014). Early identification and initiation of corrective measure are critical for all types of skin tones.

(continued)

Interventions	*Rationales*
7. For individuals with darkly pigmented skin, consider (*Bennett, 1995; Clark, 2010, p. 17): a. The color of intact dark pigmented skin may remain unchanged (does not blanch) when pressure is applied over a bony prominence. b. Local areas of intact skin that are subject to pressure may feel either warm or cool when touched. This assessment should be performed without gloves to make it easier to distinguish differences in temperature after any body fluids are cleansed before making this direct contact. c. Areas of skin subjected to pressure may be purplish/ bluish/violet in color. This can be compared with the erythema seen in people with lighter skin tones. d. Complains of, or indicate, current or recent pain or discomfort at body sites where pressure has been applied.	7. Stage I pressure ulcers are underdetected in individuals with darkly pigmented skin. Visual cues for changes in skin appearance may be relatively easy to observe in Caucasian skin but with darker pigmentation it may be harder to spot visual signs of early changes due to pressure damage (Clark, 2010, National Pressure Ulcer Advisory Panel, European Pressure Ulcer Advisory Panel, 2014).
8. Increase frequency of the turning schedule if any non-blanchable erythema is noted. Consult with prescribing professional for the utilization of pressure-dispersing devices and microclimate manipulation devices in addition to repositioning.	8. Principles of pressure ulcer prevention include reducing or rotating pressure on soft tissue. If pressure on soft tissue exceeds intracapillary pressure (approximately 32 mm Hg), capillary occlusion and resulting hypoxia can cause tissue damage. The greater the duration of immobility, the greater the likelihood of the development of small vessel thrombosis and subsequent tissue necrosis (National Pressure Ulcer Advisory Panel, European Pressure Ulcer Advisory Panel, 2014).

> **CLINICAL ALERT:**
> - Peterson, Gravenstein, Schwab, van Oostrom, and Caruso. (2013) reported using pressure mapping devices to measure pressure on skin/tissue, when high-risk individuals were positioned on their back, left side, and right side. "Bedridden individuals at risk for pressure ulcer formation exhibit high skin-bed interface pressures on specific skin areas that are likely always at risk (i.e., triple-jeopardy and always-at-risk areas) for the vast majority of the time they are in bed despite routine repositioning care. Triple jeopardy were skin area that were consistently compressed in all three positions. Health care providers are unaware of the actual tissue-relieving effectiveness (or lack thereof) of their repositioning interventions, which may partially explain why pressure ulcer mitigation strategies are not always successful. Relieving at-risk tissue is a necessary part of pressure ulcer prevention, but the repositioning practice itself needs improvement" (Peterson et al., 2013).

Interventions	*Rationales*
9. Place the individual in normal or neutral position with body weight evenly distributed. Use 30 degrees laterally inclined position when possible. Avoid postures that increase pressure, such as the 90-degree side-lying position, or the semirecumbent position.	9. Pressure is a compressing downward force on a given area. If pressure against soft tissue is greater than intracapillary blood pressure (approximately 32 mm Hg), the capillaries can be occluded, and the tissue can be damaged as a result of hypoxia. Heel protection devices should elevate the heel completely (offload them) in such a way as to distribute the weight of the leg along the calf without putting pressure on the Achilles tendon.

Interventions	Rationales
10. Use transfer aids to reduce friction and shear. Lift—do not drag—the individual while repositioning.	10. Shear is a parallel force in which one layer of tissue moves in one direction and another layer moves in the opposite direction. If the skin sticks to the bed linen and the weight of the body makes the skeleton slide down inside the skin (as with semi-Fowler's positioning), the subepidermal capillaries may become angulated and pinched, resulting in decreased perfusion of the tissue (Grossman & Porth, 2014). Friction is the physiologic wearing away of tissue. If the skin is rubbed against the bed linens, the epidermis can be denuded by abrasion.
11. Avoid positioning the individual: a. Directly onto medical devices, such as tubes or drainage systems. b. On bony prominences with existing nonblanchable erythema. c. With head-of-bed elevation or a slouched position that places pressure and shear on the sacrum and coccyx.	11. Reposition the individual in such a way that pressure is relieved or redistributed.
12. Instruct to: a. Lift self-using chair arms every 10 minutes, if possible, or assist in rising up off the chair at least every hour, depending on risk factors present b. Not elevate the legs unless calves are supported to reduce the pressure over the ischial tuberosities c. Pad the chair with pressure-relieving cushion	12. Pressure ulcer can result from soft tissue compression between a bony prominence and an external surface for a prolonged period of time (Berlowitz, 2014a).
13. Use of support surfaces to prevent pressure ulcers a. Use a pressure-redistributing seat cushion for individuals sitting in a chair whose mobility is reduced. b. Limit the time an individual spends seated in a chair without pressure relief. c. Use alternating-pressure active support overlays or mattress as indicated.	13. A pressure-reducing surface must not be able to be fully compressed by the body. To be effective, a support surface must be capable of first being deformed and then redistributing the weight of the body across the surface. Comfort is not a valid criterion for determining adequate pressure reduction. A hand check should be performed to determine if the product is effectively reducing pressure. The palm is placed under the pressure-reducing mattress; if the individual can feel the hand or the caregiver can feel the individual, the pressure is not adequate (National Pressure Ulcer Advisory Panel, European Pressure Ulcer Advisory Panel, 2014).
14. Attempt to modify contributing factors to lessen the possibility of a pressure ulcer developing (National Pressure Ulcer Advisory Panel, European Pressure Ulcer Advisory Panel, 2014). a. Incontinence of urine or feces b. Determine the etiology of the incontinence c. Maintain sufficient fluid intake for adequate hydration (approximately 2,500 mL daily, unless contraindicated), check oral mucous membranes for moisture, and check urine specific gravity. d. Establish a schedule for emptying the bladder (begin with every 2 hours). e. If the individual is confused, determine what his or her incontinence pattern is and intervene before incontinence occurs. f. Explain the problem; secure his or her cooperation for the plan.	14. Maceration is a mechanism by which the tissue is softened by prolonged wetting or soaking. If the skin becomes waterlogged, the cells are weakened and the epidermis is easily eroded. Bowel incontinence is more damaging than urinary incontinence due to the additional digestive enzymes found in stool. Care must be taken to prevent excoriation (National Pressure Ulcer Advisory Panel, European Pressure Ulcer Advisory Panel, 2014).

(continued)

Interventions	*Rationales*

g. When incontinent, wash the perineum with a liquid soap.

h. Apply a protective barrier to the perineal region (incontinence film barrier spray or wipes).

i. Check frequently for incontinence when indicated.

j. For additional interventions, refer to *Impaired Urinary Elimination in Unit II Section 1.*

---

15. Whenever possible, do not turn the individual onto a body surface that is still reddened from a previous episode of pressure loading.	
a. Do not use massage for pressure ulcer prevention or do not vigorously rub skin that is at risk for pressure ulceration.	15a. Massage is contraindicated in the presence of acute inflammation and where there is the possibility of damaged blood vessels or fragile skin.
b. Use skin emollients to hydrate dry skin in order to reduce risk of skin damage. Protect the skin from exposure to excessive moisture with a barrier product.	b. Excessive moisture will contribute to maceration when tissues are softened by prolonged wetting, which breaks down the protective layer of epidermis/dermis.
c. Avoid use of synthetic sheepskin pads; cutout, ring, or donut-type devices; and water-filled gloves.	c. These products are irritating and create pressure, which compromises circulation day.

---

16. Ensure a nutritional assessment is completed by a registered dietician/nutritionist using the Mini Nutritional Assessment (MNA) if possible.	16. MNA is the only nutritional screening tool that has been specifically validated in individuals with pressure ulcers (National Pressure Ulcer Advisory Panel, European Pressure Ulcer Advisory Panel, 2014).

---

17. Consult with wound specialist for a plan for treating pressure ulcers using moist wound healing principles, as follows:	17. Expert and timely guidance to promote wound healing with the most appropriate interventions following standards of care and facility formulary. When wounds are semi-occluded and the wounds surface remains moist, epidermal cells migrate more rapidly over the surface (National Pressure Ulcer Advisory Panel, European Pressure Ulcer Advisory Panel, 2014).
	Blisters indicate stage II pressure ulcers; the fluid contained in the blister provides an environment for formation of granulation tissue.
a. Avoid breaking blisters	a. Irrigation with normal saline solution may aid in removing dead cells and reducing bacterial count. Forceful irrigation should not be used in the presence of granulation tissue and new epithelium.
b. Flush ulcer base with sterile saline solution. If it is infected, use forceful irrigation. Wipe out wound with clean gauze to remove debris.	b. These products may be cytotoxic to tissue.
c. Avoid using wound cleansers and topical antiseptics (Hydrogen peroxide, betadine, or bleach solutions) (National Pressure Ulcer Advisory Panel, European Pressure Ulcer Advisory Panel, 2014).	c. A necrotic tissue promotes bacterial growth and does not heal until the necrotic tissue is removed.
d. Consult with wound specialist or surgeon to debride necrotic tissues enzymatically, mechanically, or surgically.	d. Moist wounds heal faster (National Pressure Ulcer Advisory Panel, European Pressure Ulcer Advisory Panel, 2014). Optimal dressing will absorb exudates adequately and protect the wound from contamination and injury.
e. Cover pressure ulcers (remove that have broken skin) with a semi-occlusive dressing that maintains a moist environment.	e. Stable eschar serves as a natural biologic cover for wound.
f. Stable (dry, adherent, intact, without erythema or movement) eschar on heels should not be removed except after vascular inflow has been evaluated as normal and by a wound specialist or surgeon.	

Interventions	Rationales
18. Consult with a wound specialist for treatment of deep or infected pressure ulcers.	18. Expert consultation may be needed for more specific interventions. a. Notify interdisciplinary team to generate appropriate referrals.
19. Determine the nutritional status. Consult with a nutritionist.	19. Wound healing requires increased protein and CHO intake to prevent weight loss and promote healing.

Documentation

Pressure Ulcer Risk Assessment at admission and daily (National Pressure Ulcer Advisory Panel, European Pressure Ulcer Advisory Panel, 2014)
Wound Documentation Record (per institutional policy)
Skin Assessment Tool at admission and daily, with documentation of lesions

Risk for Infection Related to Exposure of Ulcer Base to Fecal/Urinary Drainage

NOC

Infection Severity, Wound Healing: Primary Intention, Immune Status

Goal

The individual will verbalize risk factors associated with infection, and the precautions needed.

NIC

Infection Control, Wound Care, Incision Site Care, Health Education

Indicators

- Demonstrate meticulous hand-washing and skin hygiene technique by the time of care transition.
- Describe methods of infection transmission.
- Describe the influence of nutrition on infection prevention.

Interventions	Rationales
1. Consult with Wound Nursing Specialist for specific guidelines to prevent infection.	1. Expert and timely guidance to promote wound healing with the most appropriate interventions following standards of care and facility formulary.
2. Teach the importance of good skin hygiene and protection from contamination. Use emollients if skin is dry, but do not leave skin "wet" from too much lotion or cream.	2. Dry skin is susceptible to cracking and infection. Excessive emollient use can lead to maceration.
3. Protect the skin from exposure to urine/feces. a. Cleanse the skin thoroughly after each incontinent episode, using mild soap and water. Apply skin sealant, cream, or emollient to act as a barrier to urine and feces. b. Collect feces and urine in an appropriate containment device (e.g., condom catheter, fecal incontinence pouch, polymer-filled incontinent pads).	3. Contact with urine and stool can cause skin maceration. Feces may be more ulcerogenic than urine, owing to bacteria and toxins in stool. Incontinent individuals are five times at greater risk for pressure ulcers. Use barrier creams after each incontinent episode (Berlowitz, 2014b).
4. Consider using occlusive dressings on clean superficial ulcers, but never on deep ulcers.	4. Occlusive dressings protect superficial wounds from urine and feces, but can trap bacteria in deep wounds. These are not effective when urine soaked or liquid feces (National Pressure Ulcer Advisory Panel, European Pressure Ulcer Advisory Panel, 2014).
5. Monitor for signs of local wound infection (e.g., purulent drainage, cellulitis). Promptly report changes in wound condition.	

Documentation

> Skin condition (e.g., redness, maceration, denuded areas)
> Wound appearance (size, depth, tissue colors—pink, red, black, etc.)
> Amount and frequency of incontinence
> Skin care and hygiene measures
> Containment devices used
> Change in skin condition

TRANSITION TO HOME/COMMUNITY CARE

If indicated, review the risk diagnoses identified for this individual on admission:

- Is the person still at risk?
- Can the family reduce the risks?
- Is the person at higher risk at home?
- Is a home health nurse assessment needed?
- Refer to transition planner/case manager/social service.
- Is a referral to a wound clinic needed?
- When is this person scheduled for follow-up with primary provider? Specialists? Record dates of appointments.
- Complete a medication reconciliation prior to transition. Refer to index.

STAR

Stop

Think   Is this person at risk for injury, falls, medical complications, and/or inability to care for self (activities of daily living)?

Is there a support person available?

Is the person competent to manage self-administration of medications, treatment procedures? Are additional resources needed?

Can the person explain how to monitor the condition (e.g., blood glucose, signs/symptoms of complications, dietary/mobility restrictions, and when to call his or her primary provider or specialist)?

Act   Contact or provide the appropriate resource (e.g., contacting a support person, home health assessment, additional teaching, printed materials).

Review   Has the problem been addressed? If not, use SBAR to communicate to the appropriate person.

Risk for Ineffective Health Regimen Management Related to Insufficient Knowledge of Etiology, Prevention, Treatment, and Home Care

NOC

Compliance Behavior, Knowledge: Treatment Regimen, Participation in Health Care Decisions, Treatment Behavior: Illness or Injury

NIC

Anticipatory Guidance, Risk Identification, Learning Facilitation, Learning Readiness Enhancement

Goals

The goals for this diagnosis represent those associated with transition planning. Refer to the transition criteria.

Interventions	Rationales

1. Teach the individual/family measures to prevent additional pressure ulcers (National Pressure Ulcer Advisory Panel, European Pressure Ulcer Advisory Panel, 2014). Optimal nutrition—provide dietary literature.
  a. Mobility—use of wheel chair and transfer techniques
  b. Turning and pressure relief
  c. Shifts in body weight every 20 minutes
  d. Active and passive range of motion
  e. Skin care
  f. Skin protection from urine and feces
  g. Recognition of tissue damage, what to do and who to contact
	1. Preventing pressure ulcers is much easier than treating them. Early intervention for tissue injury can prevent progression to a pressure ulcer.

2. Teach the individual methods of treating pressure ulcers (National Pressure Ulcer Advisory Panel, European Pressure Ulcer Advisory Panel, 2014).
  a. Use of pressure ulcer prevention principles
  b. Wound care specific to each ulcer
  c. How to evaluate effectiveness of current treatment
	2. These specific instructions help the individual and family learn to promote healing and prevent infection.
	
	  a. Instruct in how, when, and who to contact for wound supplies and concerns.

3. Ask family members to determine the amount of assistance they need in caring for the individual.	3. This assessment is required to determine if the family can provide necessary care and if referrals are indicated.
4. Consult with wound specialist to determine equipment and supply needs (e.g., pressure relief devices, wheelchair cushion, dressings). Consult with social services, if necessary, for assistance in obtaining needed equipment and supplies.	4. Provide medical orders, prescriptions a. Check that individual insurance will cover needed items.
5. Ensure that the individual and family have a referral to a wound clinic, home health agency.	5. Ongoing assessment and teaching will be necessary to sustain the complex level of care.
6. Report to prescribing provider when food and/or fluid intake is decreased.	6. Fortified foods and/or high calorie. High-protein oral nutrition supplements between meals may be needed (National Pressure Ulcer Advisory Panel, European Pressure Ulcer Advisory Panel, 2014).

7. Advise family/friends the importance of nutritionally dense foods/beverages vs. calories dense foods/beverages.
  a. Calorie-dense foods, also called energy-dense foods, contain high levels of calories per serving in fat and carbohydrates. Many processed foods are considered calorie dense, such as cakes, cookies, snacks, donuts, and candies.
  b. Nutrient-dense foods contain high levels of nutrients, such as protein, carbohydrates, fats, vitamins, and minerals, but with less calories. Some nutrient-dense foods are fresh fruits, vegetables, berries, melons, dark-green vegetables, sweet potatoes, tomatoes and whole grains, including quinoa, barley, bulger, and oats. Lean beef and pork are high in protein and contain high levels of zinc, iron, and B-vitamins.
	7. Individuals with pressure ulcers need 30 to 35 kcal/kg body weight, 1.25 to 1.5 g protein/kg of body weight daily and vitamins and minerals. Calorie-dense foods do not provide the needed nutrients and can replace the needed nutrient-dense foods when the individual's appetite is poor (National Pressure Ulcer Advisory Panel, European Pressure Ulcer Advisory Panel, 2014).

8. Refer to Imbalance Nutrition for interventions related to promoting optimal intake of required nutrients.	

Documentation

Individual/family teaching
Referrals, if indicated

MUSCULOSKELETAL AND CONNECTIVE TISSUE DISORDERS

Fractures

Fractures are breaks in the continuity of a bone. They result from external pressure greater than the bone can absorb. When a fracture displaces a bone, it also damages surrounding structures—muscles, tendons, nerves, and blood vessels. Closed fractures do not penetrate the skin; open fractures do.

Traumatic injuries cause most fractures. Fractures are classified according to location, type, and pattern of the fracture. Fractured bones can be repositioned (reduced) by closed manipulation or surgical (open) reduction (Grossman & Porth, 2014). Some fractures can have anatomic alignment maintained by a splint or cast. Other fractures require hardware to accomplish internal fixation (e.g., pins, screws, plates).

Posttraumatic osteomyelitis accounts for up to 47% of cases (Schmitt, 2015). Open fractures are at greater risk, with infection rates reported to range from 2% to 50% (Schmitt, 2015). The extent of soft tissue injury from the trauma is the most significant risk factor. With open fracture, copious irrigation and fracture stabilization are critical for reducing the risk of infection (Schmitt, 2015).

Fracture incidence peaks in youth and the elderly. Among youth, long-bone fractures predominate and are more common among males. After the age of 35, fracture incidence climbs precipitously, as bone density declines pathologic fractures, however, occur even without trauma in bones weakened from excessive demineralization. Refer to Unit II to Risk for Complications of Pathologic Fractures.

Time Frame
Initial diagnosis

▮▮▮▮▮ DIAGNOSTIC CLUSTER

Collaborative Problems

▲ Risk for Complications of Neurologic/Vascular Injury

* Risk for Complications of Compartment Syndrome

▲ Risk for Complications of Fat Embolism

▲ Risk for Complications of Hemorrhage/Hematoma Formation

▲ Risk for Complications of Thromboembolism (refer to Unit II)

Nursing Diagnoses

▲ Acute pain related to tissue trauma secondary to fracture (refer to Acute Pain in Unit II)

▲ Self-Care Deficit (specify) related to limitation of movement secondary to fracture (refer to Casts Care Plan)

▲ Risk for Ineffective Respiratory Function related to immobility secondary to traction or fixation devices (refer to Immobility or Unconsciousness Care Plan)

Δ Risk for Ineffective Health Management related to insufficient knowledge of condition, signs and symptoms of complications, activity restrictions

Related Care Plan

Casts

▲ This diagnosis was reported to be monitored for or managed frequently (75% to 100%).
Δ This diagnosis was reported to be monitored for or managed often (50% to 74%).
* This diagnosis was not included in the validation study.

Transition Criteria

Before transition, the individual or family will:

1. Describe necessary precautions during activity.
2. State signs and symptoms that must be reported to a health care professional.
3. Demonstrate the ability to provide self-care or report available assistance at home.

Transitional Risk Assessment Plan (TRAP)

Begin this plan on admission.

Implement the Transitional Risk Assessment Plan (TRAP):

• Refer to inside back cover.
• Add each validated risk diagnosis to individual's problem list with the risk code in ( ).
• Refer to Unit II to the individual risk nursing diagnoses/collaborative problems for outcomes and interventions.

> *R: "Close coordination of care in the post-acute period, early transition follow-up care, enhanced client education and self-management training, proactive end-of-life counseling, and extending the resources and clinical expertise over time via multidisciplinary team management" can lower readmission rates and improve health outcomes (Boutwell & Hwu, 2009, p. 14). Interventions are utilized to activate the individual and family to select changes in their everyday lifestyle choices to improve their health (Hibbard & Greene, 2013).*

Collaborative Problems

Risk for Complications of Neurologic/Vascular Injury

Risk for Complications of Compartment Syndrome

Risk for Complications of Fat Embolism

Risk for Complications of Hemorrhage/Hematoma Formation

Risk for Complications of Osteomyelitis

Risk for Complications of Thromboembolism

Risk for Complications of Nonunion and Malunion

Collaborative Outcomes

The individual will be monitored for early signs and symptoms of (a) neurologic/vascular injury, (b) compartment syndrome, (c) fat embolism, and (d) cardiovascular alterations, and will receive collaborative interventions if indicated to restore physiologic stability.

Indicators of Physiologic Stability

• Pedal pulses 2+, equal (a, b, d)
• Capillary refill <3 seconds (a, b, d)
• Warm extremities (a, b, d)
• No complaints of paresthesia, tingling (a, b, d)
• Pain relieved by medications (b)
• Minimal swelling (a, b, d)
• Ability to move toes or fingers (b)
• BP >90/60, <140/90 mm Hg (d)
• Pulse 60 to 100 beats/min (d)
• Respiration 16 to 20 breaths/min (d)
• Temperature 98° F to 99.5° F (c)
• Oriented, calm, alert (c, d)
• Urine output >0.5 mL/kg/hr (c, d)
• No evidence of petechiae

CLINICAL ALERT:
- "Certain fractures can cause severe hemorrhage or predispose to other life-threatening complications. Femur fractures that disrupt the femoral artery or its branches are potentially fatal. Pelvic fractures can damage pelvic arteries or veins causing life-threatening hemorrhage; the more displaced the pelvic fracture, the greater the potential blood loss. Hip fractures, particularly in the elderly, may prevent ambulation, resulting in potentially life-threatening complications, such as pneumonia, thromboembolic disease, and possibly rhabdomyolysis, if there is a prolonged period of immobility. Individuals with multiple rib fractures are at substantial risk for pulmonary contusion and related complications" (Howe, 2016).

Interventions	*Rationales*

1. Monitor for signs and symptoms of neurologic/vascular injury, comparing findings on the affected limb to those of the other limb:
  a. Diminished or absent pedal pulses in affected limb
  b. Numbness or tingling
  c. Capillary refill time >3 seconds
  d. Pallor, blanching, cyanosis, coolness
  e. Inability to flex or extend extremity
	1. Trauma causes tissue edema and blood loss that reduces tissue perfusion. Inadequate circulation and edema damage peripheral nerves, resulting in decreased sensation, movement, and circulation (Grossman & Porth, 2014).

2. Assess for specific signs of compartment syndrome (Grossman & Porth 2014; Stracciolini & Hammerberg, 2014).
 	
  a. Complaints of tingling or burning sensations > numbness
  b. Pain is out of proportion to the injury, unrelieved by narcotics.
  c. Pain with passive stretch of muscles in the affected compartment or hyperextension of digits (toes or fingers) (early finding). A new and persistent deep ache in an arm or leg.
  d. Electricity-like pain in the limb
  e. Increases with the elevation of the extremity
  f. Involved compartment or limb will feel tense and warm on palpation.
  g. Skin is tight and shiny
  h. Late signs/symptoms
  i. Diminished or absent pulse
  j. Pallor, cool skin
  k. Pale, grayish, or whitish tone to skin
  l. Prolonged capillary refill (>3 seconds)
  m. Complaints of weakness when moving affected limb
  n. Progresses to inability to move joint or fingers/toes
  o. Pulselessness
	2. The muscle groups of limbs are divided into sections, or compartments, formed by strong, potentially unyielding, fascial membranes (Howe, 2016). Acute compartment syndrome (ACS) occurs when increased pressure within a compartment compromises the circulation and function of tissues within that space. With fractures, bleeding or swelling within a fascial compartment creates the increased pressure. (Stracciolini & Hammerberg, 2014).
	    Early symptoms and signs can include pain out of proportion to the apparent injury, persistent deep ache or burning pain, paresthesias, and pain with passive stretching of muscles in the affected compartment (Stracciolini & Hammerberg, 2014).
	2a. Sensory deficits typically precede motor deficits and manifest distal to the involved compartment.
	
	2c. Passive stretching of muscles decreases muscle compartment, thus increasing pain. Pain in response to passive stretching of muscles within the affected compartment is widely described as a sensitive early sign of ACS (Stracciolini & Hammerberg, 2014).

3. Examine laboratory findings of compartment syndrome
  a. Elevated white blood cell (WBC) count and erythrocyte sedimentation rate (ESR)
  b. Lowered serum pH	

Interventions	Rationales
c. Elevated temperature d. Elevated serum potassium	
4. Assess neurovascular function at least every hour for first 24 hours.	4. A delay in diagnosis is the most important determinant of a poor individual outcome.
5. Instruct to report unusual, new, or different sensations (e.g., tingling, numbness, and/or decreased ability to move toes or fingers).	5. Early detection of compromise can prevent serious impairment.
6. When the individual is unconscious or heavily sedated and unable to complain or report sensations, intensive assessment is required.	6. Permanent nerve injury can occur within 12 to 24 hours of nerve compression.
7. If pain medications become ineffective, consider compartmental syndrome.	7. Opioids are ineffective for neurovascular pain (Pasero & McCaffery, 2011).
8. If signs of compartment syndrome occur: a. Discontinue excessive elevation and ice applications. b. Keep the body part below the level of the heart. c. Remove restrictive dressings, splints.	8b. This will to improve blood flow into the compartment. c. Elevation and external devices will impede perfusion.
9. Initiate nasal oxygen	9. This will improve oxygenation to compromised tissue.
10. Immediately, advise physician, physical assistant/nurse practitioner of the need for the evaluation of the neurovascular changes assessed or reported by the individual.	10. Immediate medical assessment will determine what specific interventions are needed (e.g., measurement of compartment pressures, emergency surgery [fasciotomy], removal of cast, splints).
11. Monitor and document compartment pressures according to protocol. Report elevated pressures promptly.	11. A delay in diagnosis is the most important determinant of a poor individual outcome. Early detection of compromise can prevent serious impairment. Permanent nerve injury can occur within 12 to 24 hours of nerve compression.
12. Monitor for signs and symptoms of fat embolism (Howe, 2016; Weinhouse, 2016): a. Respiratory hypoxia (tachypnea, dyspnea, and cyanosis) b. Cerebral changes (nonspecific, ranging from acute confusion to drowsiness, rigidity, seizures, or coma) c. Petechial rash (pinpoint, flat, round red spots under the skin surface caused by intradermal hemorrhage [bleeding into the skin]). Petechiae are quite tiny (less than 3 mm in diameter) and do not blanch when pressed upon.	12. Fat embolism syndrome (FES) is a difficult diagnosis because it is gradual. It is associated with closed long-bone fractures of the lower extremity, most commonly involving the femoral shaft. FES typically manifests 24 to 72 hours after injury (Howe, 2016). a. Hypoxemia, dyspnea, and tachypnea are the most frequent early findings (Weinstien, 2016). b. Neurologic abnormalities usually occur after the development of respiratory distress. Seizures and focal deficits also have been described. The neurologic findings are transient and fully reversible in most cases (Weinstein, 2016). c. The characteristic petechial rash may be the last component of the triad to develop. It occurs in only 20% to 50% of cases. It appears found most often on the head, neck, anterior thorax, axillae, and subconjunctiva. The petechiae result from the occlusion of dermal capillaries by fat emboli, leading to extravasation of erythrocytes (no abnormalities of platelet function have been documented). The rash resolves in 5 to 7 days (Weinstien, 2016).

(continued)

Interventions	*Rationales*
13. Monitor lab results for changes in arterial blood gases and for a sudden inexplicable drop in hematocrit or platelet values.	13. Blood gases will show hypoxia, with a Pao_2 of less than 60 mm Hg along with the presence of respiratory acidosis (hypercapnia). A decrease in hematocrit occurs within 24 to 48 hours and is attributed to intra-alveolar hemorrhage.
14. Monitor for elevated temperature (>103° F <38.5° C)	14. Temperature increases are a response to circulating fatty acids. Infection will also cause an increase in temperature.

15. Identify individual at higher risk for infection and osteomyelitis (Schmitt, 2015)
  a. Severity of fracture
  b. Severity of soft tissue injury
  c. Degree of bacterial contamination
  d. Presence of underlying vascular insufficiency (e.g., peripheral vascular disease or diabetes)
  e. Adequacy of surgical debridement
	15. Complications of surgical intervention include local infection in the form of cellulitis or osteomyelitis and systemic infection in the form of sepsis. Posttraumatic osteomyelitis accounts for up to 47% of cases. Open fractures are at greater risk, with infection rates reported to range from 2% to 50%. The extent of soft tissue injury at presentation appears to be the most significant risk factor (Howe, 2016).
	
	  The tibia is the bone most frequently affected by posttraumatic osteomyelitis, probably because it is the most common site of open fracture due its lack of muscle covering and limited anastomotic blood supply (Schmitt, 2015).

16. Monitor for infection/osteomyelitis (Schmitt, 2015):
  a. Nonunion of the fracture
  b. Poor wound healing after wound closure
  c. Fever
  d. Local wound drainage
  e. Erythema, warmth, swelling
  f. Pain	

17. Minimize movement of a fractured extremity for the first 3 days after the injury.	17. Immobilization minimizes further tissue trauma, reduces the risk of embolism dislodgment, infection, and rhabdomyolysis.

18. Monitor for early signs and symptoms of hemorrhage/shock:
  a. Increasing pulse rate with normal or slightly decreased blood pressure
  b. Decreasing urine output
  c. Restlessness, agitation, change in mentation
  d. Increasing respiratory rate
	18. Bone is very vascular; blood loss can be substantial, especially with multiple fractures and fractures of the pelvis and femur. The compensatory response to decreased circulatory volume involves increasing blood oxygen by raising heart and respiratory rates, and decreasing circulation to the extremities (marked by decreased pulses, cool skin). Diminished cerebral oxygenation can cause altered mentation (Grossman & Porth, 2014).

Clinical Alert Report

Advise ancillary staff/student to report:
- Unrelieved or increasing pain
- Pain with passive stretch movement or flexion of toes or fingers
- Skin changes (mottled or cyanotic skin, rash)
- Complaints of numbness (paresthesia)
- Inability to move toes or fingers
- Change in cognitive status
- Oral temperature >100.5° F
- Systolic BP <90 mm Hg
- Resting pulse >100, <50 beats/min
- Respiratory rate >28, <10 breaths/min
- Oxygen saturation <90%
- Temperature
- Dyspnea

Documentation

Vital signs
Pulses, color, warmth, sensation, movement of distal areas
Intake and output
Unusual complaints

Risk for Ineffective Health Management Related to Insufficient Knowledge of Condition, Signs and Symptoms of Complications, and Activity Restrictions

NOC

Compliance Behavior, Knowledge: Treatment Regimen, Participation in Health Care Decisions, Treatment Behavior: Illness or Injury

NIC

Risk Identification, Health Education, Teaching: Procedure/ Treatment

Goals

The goals for this diagnosis represent those associated with transition planning. Refer to the transition criteria.

Interventions	Rationales
1. Teach to watch for and to call physician/nurse practitioner/ physical assistant and report the following immediately: a. Severe pain b. Tingling, numbness c. Skin discoloration/rash d. Cold extremities e. Change in orientation f. Change in appearance of alignment	1. These signs may indicate neurovascular compression, a condition requiring immediate medical intervention.
2. Explain the risks of infection and the signs of osteomyelitis (Chills, high fever) a. Rapid pulse b. Malaise c. Painful, tender extremity not relieved with medication, rest, ice, and elevation	
3. Explain activity restrictions. Weight-bearing status is dependent upon stability of the fracture or internal fixation devices. Explain cast care.	3. Resting the affected limb reduces displacement of fractures.
4. Explain nonunion and malunion—Incomplete healing of a fracture where the cortices of the bone fragments do not reconnect is called a nonunion. When a fracture heals with a deformity (e.g., angulation, rotation, incongruent joint surface), this is called a malunion. A subset of fractures is more susceptible to these complications.	4. Nonunions commonly present with persistent pain, swelling, or instability beyond the time when healing should normally have occurred. Individuals with increased risk risks as those with diabetes, smokers, osteoporosis, malnutrition, or neuropathy, must be reevaluated frequently (usually weekly or every other week).
5. Explain the importance of keeping follow-up appointments.	

Documentation

Individual/family teaching
Outcome achievement or status

Osteomyelitis

Osteomyelitis is an infection of the bone and surrounding tissues. Osteomyelitis can occur as a result of contiguous spread of infection to bone from adjacent soft tissues and joints, hematogenous seeding, or direct inoculation of infection into the bone as a result of trauma or surgery (Lalani, 2015). The infection may result from a blood-borne infection from other sites (e.g., infected tonsils, pressure ulcer, inner ear infection) or may be due to direct bone contamination, as with an open fracture, trauma, or surgery. Other risk factors include diabetes, hemodialysis, poor blood supply, from the presence of indwelling fixation or prosthetic devices, use of illegal injected drugs and individuals who have had their spleen removed. In adults, the feet, spine bones (vertebrae), and hips (pelvis) are most commonly affected.

Acute osteomyelitis may develop over several days to weeks. Chronic osteomyelitis may occur from acute osteomyelitis after months.

Time Frame
Initial or secondary diagnosis

▮▮▮▮▮ DIAGNOSTIC CLUSTER**

Collaborative Problems

Risk for Complications of Bone Abscess

Risk for Complications of Sepsis (refer to Unit II Risk for Complications of Sepsis)

Nursing Diagnoses

Pain related to soft tissue edema secondary to infection (refer to Pain in Unit II)

Impaired Physical Mobility related to limited range of motion of affected bone (refer to Impaired Physical Mobility in Unit II)

Risk for Ineffective Health Management related to insufficient knowledge of condition, etiology, course, pharmacologic therapy, nutritional requirements, pain management, and signs and symptoms of complications

**This medical condition was not included in the validation study.

Transition Criteria

Before transition, the individual or family will do the following:

1. Identify factors that contribute to osteomyelitis.
2. Relate the signs and symptoms that must be reported to a health care professional.
3. Verbalize an intent to implement lifestyle changes needed for healing.

Transitional Risk Assessment Plan (TRAP)

Begin this plan on admission.
Implement the Transitional Risk Assessment Plan (TRAP):
- Refer to inside back cover.
- Add each validated risk diagnosis to individual's problem list with the risk code in ( ).
- Refer to Unit II to the individual risk nursing diagnoses/collaborative problems for outcomes and interventions.

> *R: "Close coordination of care in the post-acute period, early transition follow-up care, enhanced client education and self-management training, proactive end-of-life counseling, and extending the resources and clinical expertise over time via multidisciplinary team management" can lower readmission rates and improve health outcomes (Boutwell & Hwu, 2009, p. 14). Interventions are utilized to activate the individual and family to select changes in their everyday lifestyle choices to improve their health (Hibbard & Greene, 2013).*

Collaborative Problems

Risk for Complications of Bone Abscess

Risk for Complications of Chronic Osteomyelitis

Collaborative Outcomes

The individual will be monitored for early signs and symptoms of bone abscesses and sepsis, and collaboratively intervene to stabilize the individual and will receive collaborative interventions if indicated to restore physiologic stability.

Indicators of Physiologic Stability

- Temperature 98° F to 99.5° F
- Heart rate 60 to 100 beats/min
- Respiratory rate 16 to 20 breaths/min
- WBC count >12,000 cells/mm^3, <4,000 cells/mm^3

Interventions	Rationales

1. Monitor for fever and chills
  a. Bone pain (with and without movement)
  b. Increasing tenderness
  c. Warmth
  d. Swelling
  e. Erythema
	1. As pus accumulates, the pressure increases, causing ischemia in the bone compartment.
	
	    Acute osteomyelitis typically presents with gradual onset of symptoms over several days. Individuals usually present with dull pain at the involved site, with or without movement. Local findings (tenderness, warmth, erythema, and swelling) and systemic symptoms (fever, rigors) may also be present. However, individuals with osteomyelitis involving sites such as the hip, vertebrae, or pelvis tend to manifest few signs or symptoms other than pain (Lalani, 2015). Subacute osteomyelitis generally presents with mild pain over several weeks, with minimal fever and few constitutional symptoms (Lalani, 2015).

Clinical Alert Report

Prior to providing care, advise ancillary staff/student to report the following to the professional nurse assigned to the individual immediately:
- Chills, fever, temperature >100.5° F
- New onset inability to move the limb or joint
- Reports of increased pain in the affected joint, especially with movement
- Increased swelling (increased fluid within the joint)
- Red and warm joint

Documentation

Vital signs
Pulses, color, warmth, sensation, and movement of distal areas
Complaints of increasing pain, immobility
Change in orientation
Unusual complaints

Nursing Diagnosis

> **TRANSITION TO HOME/COMMUNITY CARE**
>
> If indicated, review the risk diagnoses identified for this individual on admission:
> - Is the person still at risk?
> - Can the family reduce the risks?
> - Is the person at higher risk at home?
> - Is a home health nurse assessment needed?
> - Refer to transition planner/case manager/social service.
> - When is this person scheduled for follow-up with primary provider? Specialists? Record dates of appointments.
> - Complete a medication reconciliation prior to transition. Refer to index.

STAR

Stop

Think   Is this person at risk for injury, falls, medical complications, and/or inability to care for self (activities of daily living)?

Is there a support person available?

Is the person competent to manage self-administration of medications, treatment procedures? Are additional resources needed?

Can the person explain how to monitor the condition (e.g., blood glucose, signs/symptoms of complications, dietary/mobility restrictions, and when to call his or her primary provider or specialist)?

Act   Contact or provide the appropriate resource (e.g., contacting a support person, home health assessment, additional teaching, printed materials).

Review   Has the problem been addressed? If not, use SBAR to communicate to the appropriate person.

Risk for Ineffective Health Management Related to Insufficient Knowledge of Condition, Etiology, Course, Pharmacologic Therapy, Nutritional Requirements, Pain Management, and Signs and Symptoms of Complications

NOC

Compliance/ Engagement Behavior, Knowledge: Treatment Regimen, Participation in Health Care Decisions, Treatment Behavior: Illness or Injury

NIC

Anticipatory Guidance, Risk Identification, Learning Facilitation, Health Education, Health System Guidance

Goals

The goals for this diagnosis represent those associated with transition planning. Refer to the transition criteria.

Interventions	Rationales

1. Determine the individual's knowledge of condition, prognosis, and treatment.
  a. Review proper handling techniques of pin sites or external fixation, if applicable.
	1. The individual's understanding contributes to improved compliance and reduced risk.
	  a. Occlusion at pin site can engender growth of microorganisms.

Interventions	Rationales

2. Teach the individual infection control for drains and wounds:
   a. Use proper aseptic techniques for dressing changes and care of pins/external fixates.
   b. Ensure strict hand-washing before and after wound care.
   c. Use proper techniques for disposal of soiled dressing.
	2. These measures help to prevent the introduction of additional microorganisms into the wound; they also reduce the risk of transmitting infection to others.

3. Avoid describing foods as bad or good. Explain nutrient density of foods (*Hunter & Cason, 2006).
   a. Foods that are nutrient dense:
     • Fruits and vegetables that are bright or deeply colored
     • Foods that are fortified
     • Lower fat versions of meats*, milk, dairy products, and eggs
   b. Foods that are less nutrient dense:
     • Be lighter or whiter in color (e.g., pasta and white rice)
     • Contain a lot of refined sugar (e.g., cake and ice cream)
     • Be refined products (white bread as compared to whole grains)
     • Contain high amounts of fat for the amount of nutrients compared to similar products (fat-free milk vs. ice cream)
     • For example:
       • Apple is a better choice than a bag of pretzels with the same number of calories, but apple provides fiber, vitamin C, and potassium.
       • An orange is better than orange juice because it has fiber.
	3a. Nutrient dense foods give the most nutrients for the fewest amount of calories.
	
	b. Foods that less nutrient dense are usually high in calories in fat or carbohydrates and low in protein.

4. Ensures a consult with dietician. Reinforce nutritional requirements and dietary sources (Lutz, Mazur, & Litch, 2015).
 	
   a. Calories/day: 2,500 to 3,000; protein sources: dairy, meat, poultry, fish, and legumes.
   b. B-complex vitamins; sources: meat, nuts, and fortified cereals.
   c. Vitamin C: 75 to 300 mg; sources: green vegetables and citrus fruit.
   d. Vitamin A; sources: meat, fish, eggs, dairy products.
 	
   e. Phosphorus, magnesium, and vitamin D; sources: multivitamins
	4. Inadequate protein-calorie nutrition can impair normal wound-healing mechanisms. For healthy adults, daily nutritional requirements are approximately 1.25 to 1.5 g of protein/kg of body weight and 25 to 30 kcal/kg. These requirements can increase, however, for individuals with sizeable wounds.
	
	b. B-complex vitamins are required for metabolism of carbohydrates, fat, and protein.
	c. Vitamin C is required for the hydroxylation of proline and subsequent collagen synthesis for healing.
	d. Vitamin A deficiency reduces fibronectin on the wound surface, reducing cell chemotaxis, adhesion, and tissue repair.
	e. Vitamin D is essential for bone metabolism by increasing the absorption of calcium and phosphorus.

5. Explain the need for supplements (e.g., milkshakes and puddings).	5. Supplements may be needed to ensure the daily caloric requirement.
6. Discuss techniques to manage pain. Refer to index under acute or chronic pain.	
7. Explain that antibiotics are taken for at least 4 to 6 weeks, often through an IV at home if indicated.	7. "Most experts favor continuing parenteral antimicrobial therapy at least until debrided bone has been covered by vascularized soft tissue, which is usually at least six weeks from the last debridement. Antimicrobial therapy may be administered on an outpatient basis via a long-term intravenous catheter with close monitoring" (Lalani, 2015).

(continued)

Interventions	Rationales
8. Explain the importance continuing laboratory tests as indicated by the specific antibiotic.	8. Depending on the antibiotic agent, monitoring may include weekly serum drug levels, renal function, liver function, and/or hematologic function (Lalani, 2015).

9. Teach the individual to monitor and
  a. Call 911 right away if you have any of the following:
   • Chest pain
   • Shortness of breath
  b. Call your doctor immediately if you have any of the following:
   • Increasing pain in an arm or leg
   • Pain that is not relieved by medication
   • Pain or swelling in the infected area
   • Fever above 100.4° F (38° C) or shaking chills
   • Redness, warmth, and swelling of a joint or bony area
   • Muscle spasms
   • Nausea or vomiting
	9. Infection that begins in the bone can spread into the joint quickly, leading to septic arthritis (Lalani, 2015).

10. Ensure follow-up is scheduled with:
    a. Home health nursing agency
    b. Specialist

Documentation

Individual/family teaching
Referrals

Inflammatory Joint Disease (Rheumatoid Arthritis, Infectious Arthritis, or Septic Arthritis)

Rheumatoid arthritis (RA) is a chronic inflammatory disease, characterized by uncontrolled proliferation of synovial tissue and a wide array of multisystem comorbidities. It presents as a characteristic inflammation with destructive synovitis in multiple diarthrodial joints. A diarthrodial joint is a joint in which the opposing bony surfaces are covered with a layer of hyaline cartilage or fibrocartilage as knees, fingers, wrist, hip, vertebra, and shoulder (Firestein, 2016).

RA is characterized by cycles of exacerbations and remission.

Many organs other than the exocrine glands may be affected in individuals with Sjögren syndrome (SS); these include the skin and joints; the lungs, heart, and gastrointestinal tract, including the pancreas and liver; the kidneys, bladder, and gynecologic system; and both the peripheral nervous system (PNS) and central nervous system (CNS) (Baer, 2016).

Approximately, 15% to 20% of individuals have intermittent disease with periods of exacerbation and a relatively good prognosis. At 20 years, over 60% of individuals with RA belong to functional class III (significantly impaired, self-caring, using aids, requiring joint replacements) or class IV (loss of independence requiring daily care) (Venables & Maini, 2016).

Genetic susceptibility is evident, with incidence of the disease in immediate and extended families of individuals with RA is high. Women who smoked at least 25 cigarettes a day for more than 20 years had a relative risk of 1.4 for developing RA compared with those who had never smoked. Smoking (current or prior) is a major trigger for RA (Wasserman, 2011).

Bacteria can travel through the bloodstream from another site of active infection, resulting in hematogenous seeding of the joint. Organisms can also be introduced through trauma or surgical incision. Septic arthritis due to bacterial infection is often a destructive form of acute arthritis. In most cases, bacterial arthritis arises from hematogenous spread to the joint.

The etiology of septic arthritis is unknown, but research has been able to piece together the predisposing factors such as age >80 years, diabetes mellitus, RA, presence of prosthetic joint, recent joint surgery, skin infection, intravenous drug abuse, alcoholism, and prior intra-articular corticosteroid injection (Gabriel & Crowson, 2015;

Goldenberg & Sexton, 2015). Precise diagnosis is made by aspiration of the joint (arthrocentesis) and culture of the synovial fluid. Blood cultures for aerobic and anaerobic organisms should also be obtained. Septic arthritis is a medical emergency that requires prompt diagnosis and treatment to prevent joint destruction and systemic inflammatory response syndrome (SIRS) (Goldenberg & Sexton, 2015; Horowitz et al., 2011).

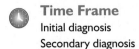

Time Frame
Initial diagnosis
Secondary diagnosis

■■■■ DIAGNOSTIC CLUSTER**

Collaborative Problems

Risk for Complications of Septic Arthritis

Risk for Complications of Sjögren Syndrome

Risk for Complications of Neuropathy

Risk for Complications of Anemia, Leukopenia (refer to Inflammatory Bowel Disease in Unit II)

Risk for Complications of Avascular Necrosis

Risk for Complications of Cardiopulmonary Effects (pericarditis, pericardial effusion, cardiomyopathy, pleurisy, pleural effusions, and congestive heart failure) (refer to Unit II)

Risk for Complications of Systemic inflammatory response syndrome (SIRS) (refer to Unit II)

Nursing Diagnoses

Fatigue related to decreased mobility, stiffness (refer to Fatigue in Unit II)

Risk for Impaired Oral Mucous Membrane related to effects of medications or Sjögren syndrome

Disturbed Sleep Pattern related to pain or secondary to fibrositis (refer to Disturbed Sleep Pattern in Unit II)

Impaired Physical Mobility related to pain and limited joint motion (refer to Impaired Physical Mobility in Unit II)

Chronic Pain related to inflammation of joints and juxta-articular structures

Interrupted Family Processes related to difficulty/inability of ill individual to assume role responsibilities secondary to fatigue and limited motion (refer to Multiple Sclerosis Care Plan)

Powerlessness related to physical and psychological changes imposed by the disease (refer to Chronic Obstructive Pulmonary Disease Care Plan)

Risk for Ineffective Health Management related to insufficient knowledge of condition, pharmacologic therapy, home care, stress management, and quackery

Related Care Plans

Raynaud Disease

Congestive Heart Failure

Diabetes Mellitus

**This medical condition was not included in the validation study.

Transition Criteria

Before transition the individual or family will:

1. Identify components of a standard treatment program for inflammatory arthritis.
2. Relate proper use of medications and other treatment modalities.

3. Identify factors that restrict self-care and home maintenance.
4. Relate signs and symptoms that must be reported to a health care professional.

Transitional Risk Assessment Plan (TRAP)

Begin this plan on admission.
Implement the Transitional Risk Assessment Plan (TRAP):
- Refer to inside back cover.
- Add each validated risk diagnosis to individual's problem list with the risk code in ( ).
- Refer to Unit II to the individual risk nursing diagnoses/collaborative problems for outcomes and interventions.

   R: *"Close coordination of care in the post-acute period, early transition follow-up care, enhanced client education and self-management training, proactive end-of-life counseling, and extending the resources and clinical expertise over time via multidisciplinary team management" can lower readmission rates and improve health outcomes (Boutwell & Hwu, 2009, p. 14). Interventions are utilized to activate the individual and family to select changes in their everyday lifestyle choices to improve their health (Hibbard & Greene, 2013).*

Collaborative Problems

Risk for Complications of Septic Arthritis

Risk for Complications of Sjögren Syndrome

Risk for Complications of Neuropathy

Risk for Complications of Avascular Necrosis

Collaborative Outcomes

The individual will be monitored for early signs and symptoms of (a) septic arthritis, (b) Sjögren syndrome, (c) neuropathy, (d) anemia, and (e) avascular necrosis, and will receive collaborative interventions if indicated to restore physiologic stability.

Indicators of Physiologic Stability

- Temperature 98° F to 99.5° F (a, h)
- No change in usual level of pain (a)
- Moist mucous membranes (b)
- No complaints of paresthesias and numbness (c)
- Hemoglobin (d)
  - Male: 14 to 18 g/dL
  - Female: 12 to 16 g/dL
- WBC count 4,300 to 10,800 cells/mm³ (a)
- Joint pain with weight-bearing (e)
- Limited to no range of movement (e)

Interventions	Rationales
1. Monitor for signs and symptoms of septic arthritis (Goldenberg & Sexton, 2015): a. Chills, fever, temp >100.5° F b. Inability to move the limb with the infected joint c. New onset severe pain in the affected joint, especially with movement d. Swelling (increased fluid within the joint) e. Warmth (the joint is red and warm to touch because of increased blood flow)	1. Septic arthritis which causes joint inflammation resulting from a viral, bacterial, or fungal organism invading the synovium and synovial fluid. Bacteria travel through the bloodstream from another site of active infection, resulting in hematogenous seeding of the joint. Inflammation of a joint cavity causes severe pain, erythema, and swelling. Because infection often spreads from a primary site elsewhere in the body, fever or shaking chills often accompany articular manifestations (Goldenberg & Sexton, 2015).

Interventions	*Rationales*
f. New onset or worsening of swelling, pain, fever, and chills needs an urgent evaluation.	f. "Prompt diagnosis and treatment of infectious arthritis can help prevent significant morbidity and mortality. The acute onset of monoarticular joint pain, erythema, heat, and immobility should raise suspicion of sepsis" (Horowitz et al., 2012).

2. Monitor for signs and symptoms of Sjögren syndrome:
  a. Dry mucous membranes (mouth, vagina)
  b. Nasal crusting and epistaxis
  c. Decreased salivary and lacrimal gland secretions
  d. Salivary gland enlargement
	2. Sjögren syndrome is a systemic chronic inflammatory disorder characterized by lymphocytic infiltrates in glandular/exocrine organs. Most individuals with Sjögren syndrome present with sicca symptoms, such as xerophthalmia (dry eyes), xerostomia (dry mouth), and parotid gland enlargements can affect extraglandular organ systems including the skin, lung, heart, kidney, neural, and hematopoietic systems.

3. Monitor for respiratory complications of Sjogren syndrome (Carvalho, Deheinzelin, & Kairalla, 2016):
  a. Cough (usually nonproductive)
  b. Chest pain
  c. Dyspnea
	3. Respiratory complications of Sjogren syndrome include airway mucosal dryness (also known as xerotrachea), a variety of interstitial lung diseases (ILDs), non-Hodgkin lymphomas, pleural thickening or effusion, and, rarely, thromboembolic disease or pulmonary hypertension (Carvalho et al., 2016).

4. Monitor for symptoms of neuropathy:
  a. Paresthesias
  b. Numbness
	4. Swelling and actual joint changes can cause nerve entrapment.

5. Monitor for signs and symptoms of avascular necrosis:
  a. Joint pain increasing over time and unrelieved with analgesia
  b. Increased limited range of movement and weight-bearing capability
	5. Osteonecrosis, also known as aseptic necrosis, avascular necrosis (AVN), atraumatic necrosis, and ischemic necrosis, is a pathologic process that has been associated with numerous conditions and therapeutic interventions. Avascular necrosis can occur when the circulation to the bone is impaired (e.g., joint edema). Immune complexes isolated from synovial fluids may stimulate the production of tumor necrosis factor (TNF) from monocytes/macrophages. TNF promotes the destruction of bone by increasing the number of osteoclasts and decreasing the number of osteoblasts at the site of inflammation (Firestein, 2016).

6. Monitor for signs and symptoms of cardiopulmonary involvement.
  a. Arrhythmias
  b. Shortness of breath on exertion or rest
  c. Rales on auscultation
  d. Chest pain
  e. Dry or moist cough
  f. Friction rub with respirations
	6. There is a large body of epidemiologic evidence linking RA with the premature development of cardiovascular disease. This relates, at least in part, to the systemic inflammatory burden in RA, which has been shown to predispose to the development of premature atherosclerosis. The leading cause of death in individuals with RA is cardiovascular disease (Baer, 2016).

Clinical Alert Report

Prior to providing care, advise ancillary staff/student to report the following to the professional nurse assigned to the individual immediately:

- Chills, fever, temp >100.5° F
- New onset inability to move the limb or joint
- Reports of increased pain in the affected joint, especially with movement
- Increased swelling (increased fluid within the joint)
- Red and warm joint
- Chest pain
- New dry or moist cough
- Complaints of shortness of breath

Documentation

Changes in range of motion
Complaints, evaluation, responses

Nursing Diagnosis

Impaired Comfort Related to Dry eyes, Dry Mouth Secondary to Effects of Medications or Sjögren Syndrome

NOC
Symptom Control, Comfort Status

Goal

The individual will report an improvement in eye and mouth dryness.

NIC
Oral Health Restoration, Oral Health Maintenance, Environmental Management: Comfort

Indicators

- Identify factors that contribute to mucus membrane dryness.
- Relate the need to report oral ulcers or stomatitis to a health care provider.
- Identify strategies for maintaining moist oral and eye mucosa.
- Relate the need for frequent, regular dental care for Sjögren syndrome sequelae.

Interventions	*Rationales*
1. Teach the individual to inspect the mouth during daily oral hygiene activities and to report ulcers or stomatitis to a health care provider.	1. Early detection of these problems enables prompt intervention to prevent serious complications.
2. Teach the individual to drink adequate amounts of non-sugared liquids.	2. Well-hydrated oral tissue is more resistant to breakdown.
3. Teach the individual the importance of regular dental care and topical fluoride treatments (Zero et al., 2016).	3. Secondary Sjögren syndrome can result in excessively dry oral mucosa and predispose the individual to tooth decay and gum disease (Zero et al., 2016).

4. Advise for dry mouth:
  a. Chew sugarless gum or suck on sugarless, sour hard candies (especially grape or lemon).
  b. Avoid extremely hot or cold foods.
  c. Try sucking on a nonnutritive object (such as a cherry pit).
  d. Avoid mouthwashes that contain alcohol. Instead, rinse your mouth with water several times a day.
  e. Brush your teeth gently with a fluoride nonfoaming toothpaste after every meal and before going to bed.
	4a. This will stimulate saliva production.
	
	  b. These are irritating to mucosal.
	  c. This can stimulate increase salivation.
	
	  d. Alcohol can cause drying of tissue.
	
	  e. Nonfoaming toothpastes are less drying.

Interventions	Rationales
f. Avoid sugary foods and snacks. When sugary foods are eaten, immediately brush or rinse your teeth.	f. This will help prevent tooth decay.
g. If you wear dentures, disinfect them often.	g. This will help prevent infection.
h. Look at your mouth every day to check for sores and redness that could signal an infection.	
5. Advise for dry eyes to (Foulks et al., 2015):	5. All attempts should be made to decrease dry eyes from evaporation and sources of infection
a. Blink several times a minute while reading or working on the computer. Lower the computer monitor below eye level.	a. This can decrease the width of the eyelid opening and help conserves tears.
b. Protect your eyes from windy or breezy conditions.	
c. Use humidifiers in the rooms where you spend much of your time, including your bedroom. Use distilled water in areas with hard water.	
d. Do not smoke, and stay away from smoky rooms.	
e. If you wear eye makeup, apply only to the upper eyelids and to the tips of your eyelashes to keep it out of your eyes.	
f. Eyeglasses fitted with moisture shields can decrease evaporation.	
g. Swim or ski goggles are also effective in decreasing evaporation, but wrap-around sunglasses are generally more useful.	
h. Use of contact lens can aggravate dry-eye symptoms, and its use is also associated with infections.	

Documentation

Oral assessments
Eye assessments

Chronic Pain Related to Inflammation of Joints and Juxta-articular Structures

NOC
Comfort Level, Pain: Disruptive Effects, Pain Control, Depression Level

Goal

The individual will relate improvement of pain and, when possible, increase daily activities.

NIC
Pain Management, Medication Management, Exercise Promotion, Mood Management, Coping Enhancement

Indicators

- Receive validation that pain exists.
- Practice selected noninvasive pain relief measures to manage pain.
- Relate improvement of pain and, when possible, increase daily activities.

Interventions	Rationales
1. Teach the individual to differentiate between joint pain and stiffness.	1. When there is joint pain, techniques for joint protection are instituted. When flares are diminished, active ROM exercises are indicated.
2. If joints are inflamed, let the individual rest and avoid activities that stress joints. Gentle ROM exercises may be tried.	2. ROM exercises can prevent contractures but inflamed joints are at risk for injury.

Interventions	*Rationales*
3. Apply local heat or cold to affected joints for approximately 20 to 30 minutes three to four times a day. Check the temperature of warm soaks or covering a cold/ice pack with a towel.	3. Avoid temperatures likely to cause skin or tissue damage.
4. Encourage a warm bath or shower first thing in the morning to reduce morning stiffness.	4. Treatment of inflammatory joint pain focuses on the reduction of discomfort and inflammation by the use of local comfort measures, joint rest, and the use of anti-inflammatory or disease-modifying medication.
5. Advise to balance rest with exercise (Schur, Ravinder, Maini, & Gibofsky, 2014)	5. Pain and stiffness often lead individuals to avoid using affected joints. This lack of use can result in loss of joint motion, contractures, and muscle atrophy, thereby decreasing joint stability and producing a further increase in fatigue (Schur et al., 2014).

6. Encourage the use of adjunctive pain control measures:
  a. Progressive relaxation
  b. Transcutaneous electrical nerve stimulation (TENS)
  c. Biofeedback
  d. Imagery/music/acupuncture
	6. Pain is a subjective, multifactorial experience that can be modified by the use of cognitive and physical techniques to reduce the intensity or perception of pain (Pasero & McCaffery, 2011).

Documentation

Assessment of affected joints: pain, swelling, warmth, erythema
Response to pain relief measures

TRANSITION TO HOME/COMMUNITY CARE

If indicated, review the risk diagnoses identified for this individual on admission:

* Is the person still at risk?
* Can the family reduce the risks?
* Is the person at higher risk at home?
* Is a home health nurse assessment needed?
* Refer to transition planner/case manager/social service.
* When is this person scheduled for follow-up with primary provider? Specialists? Record dates of appointments.
* Complete a medication reconciliation prior to transition. Refer to index.

STAR   **Stop**

Think   Is this person at risk for injury, falls, medical complications, and/or inability to care for self (activities of daily living)?

Is there a support person available?

Is the person competent to manage self-administration of medications, treatment procedures? Are additional resources needed?

Can the person explain how to monitor the condition (e.g., blood glucose, sign/symptoms of complications, dietary/mobility restrictions, and when to call his or her primary provider or specialist)?

Act   Contact or provide the appropriate resource (e.g., contacting a support person, home health assessment, additional teaching, printed materials).

Review   Has the problem been addressed? If not, use SBAR to communicate to the appropriate person.

Risk for Ineffective Health Management Related to Insufficient Knowledge of Condition, Pharmacologic Therapy, Home Care, Stress Management, and Quackery

NOC

Compliance/ Engagement Behavior, Knowledge: Treatment Regimen, Participation in Health Care Decisions, Treatment Behavior: Illness or Injury

NIC

Anticipatory Guidance, Learning Facilitation, Risk Identification, Health Education, Teaching: Procedure/ Treatment, Health System Guidance

Goals

The goals for this diagnosis represent those associated with transition planning. Refer to the transition criteria.

Interventions	Rationales

1. Explain inflammatory arthritis using teaching aids appropriate to the individual's and family members' levels of understanding. Explain the following:
a. Inflammatory process
b. Joint function and structure
c. Effects of inflammation on joints and juxta-articular structures
d. Extra-articular manifestations of the disease process
e. Chronic nature of the disease
f. Disease course (remission/exacerbation)
g. Low incidence of significant or total disability
h. Components of the standard treatment program:
  • Medications (e.g., aspirin, nonsteroidal anti-inflammatory drugs, disease-modifying agents, cytotoxic agents, corticosteroids)
  • Local comfort measures
  • Exercise/rest
  • Joint protection/assistive devices
  • Consultation with other disciplines
	1. Inflammatory joint disease is a chronic illness. Education should emphasize a good understanding of the inflammatory process and actions the individual can take to manage symptoms and minimize their impact on his or her life.

2. Teach to identify characteristics of quackery: a. "Secret" formulas or devices for curing arthritis b. Advertisements using "case histories" and "testimonials" c. Rejection of standard components of a treatment program d. Claims of persecution by the "medical establishment"	2. An accurate and full understanding of inflammatory joint disease and its treatment lessens the individual's susceptibility to quackery.
3. Explain that some medications will worsen the symptoms of Sjögren syndrome (dry mouth, dry eyes) a. Antihistamines, decongestants, antidepressants, diuretics (water pills), tranquilizers, some blood pressure medications, some diarrhea medications, some antipsychotic medications	

Interventions	Rationales
4. Teach the individual to take prescribed medications properly and to report symptoms of side effects promptly.	4. Adhering to the schedule may help to prevent fluctuating drug blood levels and can reduce side effects. Prompt reporting of side effects enables intervention to prevent serious problems.
5. Explain the relationship of stress to inflammatory diseases. Discuss stress management techniques: a. Progressive relaxation b. Guided imagery c. Regular exercise	5. Stressful events may be associated with an increase in disease activity. Effective use of stress management techniques can help to minimize the effects of stress on the disease process.
6. Reinforce the importance of routine follow-up care.	6. Follow-up care can identify complications early and help to reduce disabilities from disuse.
7. Advise of community resources. a. Arthritis Foundation (http://www.arthritis.org /living-with-arthritis/tools-resources/) b. American College of Rheumatology (ACR) c. National Institute of Arthritis and Musculoskeletal and Skin Diseases (NIAMS) http://www.nih.gov/niams/ d. Sjogren's Syndrome Foundation https://www.sjogrens .org/home/member-community	7. Such resources can provide specific additional information to enhance self-care.

Documentation

Individual/family teaching
Status on transition
Referrals, if indicated

INFECTIOUS AND IMMUNODEFICIENT DISORDERS

Human Immunodeficiency Virus/Acquired Immunodeficiency Syndrome

An infection caused by the human immunodeficiency virus (HIV), acquired immunodeficiency syndrome (AIDS) was first reported in the United States in 1981. AIDS represents the end-stage of a continuum of HIV infection and its sequelae. Major modes of infection transmission include sexual activity with an infected person and exposure to infected needles or drug paraphernalia, blood, or blood products. If the mother is not on antiviral therapy, a fetus can contract HIV infection from an infected mother perinatally. HIV infects primarily the T4-cell lymphocytes; this interferes with cell-mediated immunity. Without antiviral therapy the clinical consequences of this progressive immune deficiency are opportunistic infections (OIs) and malignancies. Beginning in the 1990s, the increased number of available medications has slowed the course of HIV dramatically. Individuals, who are compliant with their antiviral therapy, are living well to become senior citizens.

Time Frame
Initial diagnosis
Recurrent acute episodes

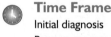

DIAGNOSTIC CLUSTER

Collaborative Problems

▲ Risk for Complications of Opportunistic Infections

△ Risk for Complications of Malignancies

▲ Risk for Complications of Sepsis (refer to Unit II Section 2 Risk for Complications of Sepsis)

* Risk for Complications of Myelosuppression (refer to Leukemia Care Plan)

* Risk for Complications of Peripheral Neuropathy

* Risk for Complications of HIV-Related Nephropathy

Nursing Diagnoses

▲ Risk for Impaired Oral Mucous Membrane related to compromised immune system

▲ Risk for Infection Transmission related to the infectious nature of blood and body fluids (refer to Unit II Section 1 Risk for Infection Transmission)

* Risk for Imbalanced Nutrition related to HIV infection, opportunistic infections/malignancies associated with AIDS (refer to Unit II Section 1 Imbalanced Nutrition)

* Risk for Ineffective Coping related to situational crisis (i.e., new HIV diagnosis or AIDS diagnosis, first hospitalization)

△ Anxiety related to perceived effects of illness on life style and unknown future (refer to Cancer: Initial Diagnosis Care Plan)

△ Grieving related to loss of body function and its effects on life style (refer to Cancer: Initial Diagnosis Care Plan)

▲ Risk for Infection related to increased susceptibility secondary to compromised immune system (refer to Leukemia Care Plan)

▲ Fatigue related to effects of disease, stress, chronic infections, and nutritional deficiency

▲ Risk for Ineffective Health Management related to insufficient knowledge of HIV, its transmission, prevention, treatment, and community resources

* Risk for Caregiver Role Strain related to AIDS-associated shame/stigma, and uncertainty about course of illness and demands on caregiver

Related Care Plan

Palliative Care Plan

▲ This diagnosis was reported to be monitored for or managed frequently (75% to 100%).

Δ This diagnosis was reported to be monitored for or managed often (50% to 74%).

* This diagnosis was not included in the validation study

Transition Criteria

Before transition, the individual or family will:

1. Relate the implications of the diagnosis.
2. Describe the prescribed medication regimen.
3. Identify modes of HIV transmission.
4. Identify infection-control measures.
5. Describe signs and symptoms that must be reported to a health care professional.
6. Identify available community resources.

Transitional Risk Assessment Plan (TRAP)

Begin This Plan on Admission

Implement the Transitional Risk Assessment Plan (TRAP)

- Refer to Front/back inside covers.
- Add each validated High Risk Diagnosis to Individual's Problem List with the risk code in ().
- Refer to Section II to the individual high-risk nursing diagnoses/collaborative problems for outcomes and interventions.

  R: *"Close coordination of care in the post-acute period, early discharge follow-up care, enhanced patient education and self-management training, proactive end-of-life counseling, and extending the resources and clinical expertise over time via multidisciplinary team management" can lower readmission rates and improve health outcomes (Boutwell & Hwu, 2009, p. 14). Interventions are utilized to activate the individual and family to select changes in their everyday lifestyle choices to improve their health (Hibbard & Greene, 2013).*

Collaborative Problems

Risk for Complications of Opportunistic Infections

Risk for Complications of Malignancies

Risk for Complications of Sepsis

Risk for Complications of Peripheral Neuropathy

Risk for Complications of HIV-Related Nephropathy

Collaborative Outcomes

The individual will be monitored for early signs and symptoms of (a) opportunistic infections (pneumonia, encephalitis, enteritis, cytomegalovirus, herpes simplex, herpes zoster, stomatitis, esophagitis, meningitis), (b) malignancies, (c) sepsis, and (d) HIV-associated peripheral neuropathy, and will receive collaborative interventions if indicated to restore physiologic stability.

Indicators of Physiologic Stability

- Temperature 98° F to 99.5° F (a, c)
- Respirations 16 to 20 breaths/min (a, c)
- Sao$_2$ arterial oxygen saturation (pulse oximeter >95%) (c)
- Paco$_2$ arterial carbon dioxide 35 to 45 mm Hg (c)
- Urine output >5 mL/kg/hr (c)
- No proteinuria (c)
- Creatinine 0.2 to 0.8 ng/mL (c)
- Serum albumin 3.5 to 5 g/dL (c)
- Blood urea nitrogen 10 to 20 mg/dL (c)
- Alert, oriented (a)
- No seizures, no headaches (a)
- Regular, formed stools (a)
- No herpetic or zoster lesions (a)
- Swallows with no difficulty (a)
- No change in vision (a)
- No weight loss (b)
- No new lesions (b)
- No lymphadenopathy (b)
- No leg pain, burning, or paresthesia (d)

 Carp's Cues

Individuals with undiagnosed HIV infections can often present with OIs, which leads to the diagnosis of AIDS.

Interventions	Rationales

1. Monitor for OIs:
  a. Protozoal:
    • *Pneumocystis carinii* pneumonia (dry, nonproductive cough, fever, dyspnea)
    • *Toxoplasma gondii* encephalitis (headache, lethargy, seizures)
    • *Cryptosporidium enteritis* (watery diarrhea, malaise, nausea, abdominal cramps)
	1. Severe immune deficiencies with CD4 <200% cause OI and malignancies. Antiretroviral therapy (ART) has dramatically reduced OIs. Early treatment can often prevent serious complications (e.g., sepsis) and increases the chance of a favorable response to treatment.

b. Viral:
    • Genital herpes simplex (cluster of blister-like lesions, pain), herpes simplex (Single blister-like lesion or cluster, pain), perirectal abscesses (severe pain, bleeding, rectal discharge)
    • Cytomegalovirus (CMV) retinitis, colitis, pneumonitis, encephalitis, or other organ disease
    • Progressive multifocal leukoencephalopathy (headache, decreased mentation)
    • *Varicella zoster*, disseminated (shingles) (a tract (horizontal pattern) of blisters-like lesions, painful, reddened)
	b. Herpes simplex is common and painful. The CMV infections are responsible for significant morbidity (e.g., blindness).

c. Fungal: (Fungal can be chronic, with relapses.)
    • *Candida albicans* oral, stomatitis, and esophagitis (exudate, complaints of unusual taste in mouth, discomfort with hot drinks)
    • *Cryptococcus neoformans* meningitis (fever, headache, blurred vision, stiff neck, confusion)
    • *Mycobacterium aviumintracellulare* disseminated
    • *Mycobacterium tuberculosis* extrapulmonary and pulmonary
	c. Fungal infections frequently affect the pulmonary system.

(continued)

Interventions	Rationales

CLINICAL ALERT:
- Emphasize the need to report symptoms early. Advise that if the individual is severely compromised, some symptoms will not be present (e.g., increased temperature).

---

2. Administer medications for OIs, as prescribed. Consult a pharmacological reference for specific nursing implications (Arcangelo & Peterson, 2016; National Institute of Health [NIH], 2015b).

2. Some treatments for OIs are life-long to prevent reoccurrences.

---

3. Monitor for malignancies:

   a. Kaposi sarcoma: Painless, palpable lesions (purplish, pinkish, or red) frequently on trunk, neck, arms, and head.
   b. Extracutaneous lesions in gastrointestinal (GI) tract, lymph nodes, buccal mucosa, and lungs
   c. Pruritus, weight loss
   d. Lymphoma (non-Hodgkin, Burkitt):
      - Painless lymphadenopathy (an early site at neck, axilla, inguinal area)

3. The malignancies that affect AIDS individuals are related to immunosuppression.
   a. Kaposi sarcoma is cancer of the lymphatic vessel (endothelial wall). It is not skin cancer.

   - Non-Hodgkin lymphomas can progress into the bone marrow, liver, spleen, gastrointestinal, and nervous systems.

---

4. Monitor for signs and symptoms of sepsis/SIRS. Refer to Unit II Section 2, Collaborative Problems—Risk for Complications of Sepsis/SIRS

---

5. Monitor and support use of prescribed prophylactic medication for OIs. Refer to NIH (2015b)

CLINICAL ALERT:
- In the era prior to potent ART, DSPN usually occurred in the setting of advanced immunosuppression, for example CD4 range 26 to 275 in one study. In most studies, the incidence of HIV-associated DSPN appears to have decreased in the era of potent ART. Other factors associated with DSPN include aging, longer duration of HIV infection, host factors such as diabetes, hypertriglyceridemia, nutritional deficiencies, mitochondrial polymorphisms, substance use, and the use of older nucleoside reverse transcriptase inhibitors such as didanosine and stavudine (Nardin & Freeman, 2015).

Interventions	*Rationales*

6. Monitor for distal symmetrical polyneuropathy (DSPN)
  a. Bilateral tingling, and numbness in the toes; gradually spreads proximally in the lower extremities
  b. Neuropathic pain is common and may be the presenting symptom.
  c. Sensory loss to all sensory modalities (vibration, pinprick, temperature) in a stocking distribution
  d. Reduced deep tendon reflexes or absent at the ankles
  e. Sensory findings in the hands are associated with drug toxicity.
  f. Ensure that a specialist has been consulted if DSPN is not evaluated.
	6. Viral antigens play in provoking immune activation and inducing a microenvironment that is toxic to the peripheral nerve and is associated with a reduction in mitochondrial DNA content and changes in morphology. In addition, HIV impairs reinnervation limiting the ability of the peripheral nervous system to heal itself (Nardin & Freeman, 2015).

Clinical Alert Report

Prior to providing care, advise ancillary staff/student to report the following to the professional nurse assigned to the individual:

- New onset or worsening of headaches
- New lesions (skin, oral mucosa)
- Change in cognitive status
- Oral temperature >100.5° F
- Systolic BP <90 mm Hg
- Resting pulse >100, <50 beats/min
- Respiratory rate >28, <10 breaths/min
- Oxygen saturation <90%

Documentation

Lesions (number, size, locations)
Respiratory assessment
Neurologic assessment (mentation, orientation, affect)
Mouth assessment

Risk for Infection Transmission Related to the Infectious Nature of the Individual's Blood and Body Fluids[7]

NOC

Infection Severity, Risk Control, Risk Detection

Goal

The individual will take necessary steps to prevent infection transmission.

NIC

Teaching: Disease Process, Infection Protection

Indicators

- Describe the factors that contribute to HIV transmission
- Describe how to disinfect infected objects or surfaces

---

[7]This diagnosis is not currently on the NANDA list, but has been included for clarity and usefulness.

Interventions	Rationales
1. Adhere to universal precautions. Wash hands before and after contact with all individuals in care situations.	1. Universal precautions are to prevent the transmission of blood-borne pathogens from individual to caregiver. They are taken with all individuals regardless of diagnosis, age, or sexual orientation of the individual. The particular precautions taken with each individual client are dependent on the potential of transmission related to the care to be rendered and not to the individual's diagnosis. Handwashing is one of the most important means of preventing the spread of infection
2. Identify candidates for preexposure prophylaxis (CDC, 2014d): a. A man or woman who sometimes has sex without using a condom, especially if one has a sex partner who you know has HIV infection b. If one does know whether their partner has HIV infection and their partner is engaged in risk behavior (e.g., inject drugs, having sex with other people) c. If the person or partner has been diagnosed recently with a sexually transmitted infection d. If their partner has HIV infection. e. To help protect from getting HIV infection while one tries to get pregnant, during pregnancy, or while breastfeeding.	
3. Explain preexposure prophylaxis: a. Fixed-dose combination of tenofovir disoproxil fumarate (TDF) and emtricitabine (FTC) b. Everyday dosing	
4. Advise individuals to discuss preexposure prophylaxis with the HIV specialist or primary care provider (PCP).	4. The HIV epidemic in the United States is growing. About 50,000 people get infected with HIV each year. More of these infections are happening in some groups of people and some areas of the country than in others (CDC, 2016h).

CLINICAL ALERT:
* Recent findings from several clinical trials have demonstrated safety and a substantial reduction in the rate of HIV acquisition for men who have sex with men (MSM), men and women in heterosexual discordant couples, and heterosexual men and women recruited as individuals who were prescribed daily oral antiretroviral preexposure prophylaxis (PrEP) with a fixed-dose combination of tenofovir disoproxil fumarate (TDF) and emtricitabine (FTC). Refer to Unit II Section 1 nursing diagnosis Risk for Infection Transmission for specific interventions (CDC, 2016h).

Risk for Ineffective Coping Related to Situational Crisis (i.e., New HIV or AIDS Diagnosis and/or First Hospitalization)

NOC

Coping, Self-Esteem, Social Interaction Skills

Goal

The individual will make decisions and follow through with appropriate actions to change provocative situations in his or her personal environment.

NIC
Coping Enhancement, Counseling, Emotional Support, Active Listening, Assertiveness Training, Behavior Modification

Indicators

- Verbalize feelings related to emotional state.
- Focus on the present.
- Identify response patterns and the consequences of resulting behavior.
- Identify personal strengths and accept support through the nursing relationship.

Interventions	Rationales
1. If this is a new diagnosis (AIDS, 2015) Focus on a. Finding an HIV care provider, even if you do not feel sick.	1. Your HIV care provider will be the person who partners with you to manage your HIV. He or she will monitor your health on an ongoing basis and work with you to develop a treatment plan.

2. Before one decides to tell people that are HIV-positive, explore (AIDS.gov):
  a. Who could you talk with about this?
  b. Think about the people you rely on for support, like family, friends, or coworkers.
  c. What kind of relationship do you have with them? What are the pros and cons of telling them you are living with HIV?
  d. Are there particular issues a person might have that will affect how much he or she can support you?
  e. What is that person's attitude and knowledge about HIV?
  f. Why do you want to disclose to this person? What kind of support can this person provide?
  g. For each person you want to tell, ask yourself if the person needs to know now—or if it is better to wait.
  h. If the individual are not ready to tell other people about their HIV diagnosis, advise them that this is ok. Identify community resources and professional organizations that offer support groups for newly diagnosed people, one-on-one counseling, peer counselors, or health educators.
	2. Disenfranchised grief occurs when social stigma is associated with a death or illness (e.g., suicide, AIDS); the person may be alone, emotionally isolated, or fearful of public expressions of grief (*Bateman, 1999; Lemming & Dickson, 2010). Gay men who have experienced multiple AIDS-related losses (e.g., loss of friends and community, disintegrating family structures, and social networks) may receive little understanding from heterosexuals (*Cotton et al., 2006; *Mallinson, 1999).

> **CLINICAL ALERT:**
> - It is very important that current and past sexual partners are advised of the risk exposure as also if exposure is from shared needles. If desired, the health department can notify sexual or needle-sharing partners that they may have been exposed to HIV without giving the name of the source.

Interventions	Rationales
3. Encourage expression of anxiety, anger, and fear. Listen attentively and nonjudgmentally.	3. Listening is credited as a helpful strategy to assist individuals coping with AIDS. Anger at AIDS-associated prejudice or lack of understanding of others occurs commonly among the HIV-infected.
4. Encourage to share her or his feelings regarding the multiple fears associated with AIDS (e.g., death, friends, community, family structure, and social networks).	4. Complex social issues of morality, sexuality, contagion, and shame are associated with AIDS-related losses and interfere with grieving and coping (*Cotton et al., 2006; *Mallison, 1999).

(continued)

Interventions	Rationales
5. Encourage and provide exercise, recreation, diversional activities, and independent activities-of-daily-living (ADLs) performance.	5. Diversional activities can provide opportunities of rest from mental and emotional distress. Maximal independence and participation in activities can increase self-confidence and self-esteem.
6. Instruct on the benefits stress management techniques (e.g., distraction, relaxation imagery), as appropriate.	6. Stress reduction techniques can assist the individual in dealing with personal fears and anxieties.

TRANSITION TO HOME/COMMUNITY CARE
- If indicated, review the high-risk diagnoses identified for this individual on admission:
  - Is the person still at high risk?
  - Can the family/ reduce the risks?
  - Is the person at higher risk at home?
  - Is a home health nurse assessment needed?
  - Refer to discharge planner/case manager/social service.
- When is this person scheduled for follow-up with primary provider? Specialists? Record dates of appointments.
- Complete a medication reconciliation prior to discharge > Refer to front/back cover.

STAR

Stop

Think Is this person at risk for injury, falls, medical complications, and/or inability to care for self (activities of daily living)?

Is the person competent to manage self-administration of medications, treatment procedures? Are additional resources needed?

Can the person explain how to monitor condition (e.g., sign/symptoms of complications, and when to call his or her primary provider or specialist)?

Act Use SBAR to notify the appropriate professional.

SBAR *Situation:* Mr. Smith will be scheduled to be transitioned to his home.

Background: Mr. Smith lives alone. He (state his disabilities, self-care needs, treatments.)

Action: A more thorough reevaluation of where he can be transitioned is needed.

Recommendation: Referral to social service/transition planner/case manager.

Review Is the response/solution the right option for the individual? If not, discuss the situation with the appropriate person, department, and/or agency (using SBAR).

Risk for Ineffective Health Management Related to Insufficient Knowledge of HIV, Its Transmission, Prevention, Treatment, Health Promotion Activities, and Community Resources

NOC

Compliance Behavior, Knowledge: Treatment Regimen, Participation in Health Care Decisions, Treatment Behavior: Illness or Injury

Goals

The goals for this diagnosis represent those associated with transition planning. Refer to the transition criteria.

Anticipatory Guidance,
Risk Identification,
Health Education,
Learning Facilitation

Interventions	Rationales
1. Present HIV-positive status as a condition, which is life-long but treatable as a chronic disease. With health promotion, medication adherence and healthy lifestyle choices are important. Stress to comply with age-related recommendations as immunizations, cancer screening, etc.	1. Prior to antiviral therapy an HIV-positive test represented a terminal illness.
2. Teach about the basic pathophysiology of HIV infection and concepts of the immune system.	2. Understanding of HIV and its effects on the body is the basis of all further learning.
3. Teach HIV routes of transmission and preventive measures/risk reduction activities.	3. The importance of efforts to prevent HIV transmission to infected persons as well as prevention of reinfection by a resistant strain of HIV or with other sexually transmitted diseases (STDs), if a person is already infected cannot be overstated.
4. Discuss the importance of adhering to medication schedule daily.	4. Strict adherence to ART is key to sustained HIV suppression, reduced risk of drug resistance, improved overall health, quality of life, and survival, as well as decreased risk of HIV transmission (Cohen et al., 2011).
5. Assess for behavioral, structural, and psychosocial barriers to adherence: a. Psychosocial (depression and other mental illnesses, neurocognitive impairment) b. Behavioral (low health literacy, high levels of alcohol consumption, active substance use, nondisclosure of HIV serostatus, denial, stigma, adolescent/young adults' failure to adopt practices that facilitate adherence, such as linking medication taking to daily activities or using a medication reminder system or a pill organizer) c. Structural (homelessness, poverty, and inconsistent access to medications)	5. Advise the PCP and/or specialist of these barriers and to consider delaying starting antiviral therapy. Failure to adhere to combination ART will create viral resistance to therapy and resistant HIV strains. Failure to suppress HIV viral loads can increase transmission if one engages in risk behaviors (Cohen et al., 2011).
6. Instruct that individuals with AIDS (e.g., CD4+ count <200 cells/μL) should avoid untreated water sources (well water, lakes, streams, swimming pools)	6. Viable oocysts (cryptosporidium) in feces can be transmitted directly through contact with infected humans or animals, particularly those with diarrhea. Oocysts can contaminate recreational water sources (e.g., swimming pools, lakes) and public water supplies and might persist despite standard chlorination. Person-to-person transmission is common, especially among sexually active men who have sex with men (MSM). Young children with cryptosporidial diarrhea might infect adults during diapering and cleaning after defecation (NIH, 2015b).
7. Explain the factors that impinge on the attainment of health-related goals as: a. Unsafe sexual practices b. Substance abuse.	7a. Sexually transmitted infection further compromises the immune system. b. Heroin, cocaine, alcohol (ETOH), marijuana, and amphetamines are all possible factors in immune suppression. Substance abuse also interferes with adherence to medication regimen.

Interventions	Rationales
c. Tobacco use	c. The detrimental effects of nicotine addiction are well known (e.g., circulatory, respiratory).
d. Lack of adherence to therapy	d. Strict adherence to combination ART is necessary to prevent subtherapeutic levels of medication conducive to the emergence of viral resistance and consequent disease progression

8. For individual with peripheral neuropathy:
  a. Avoid ill-fitting shoes.
 	
  b. Keep feet and hands cool.
	8a. Too tight shoes will cause throbbing, cramps, and irritations. Too loose shoes will not provide sufficient support.
	  b. Individuals with peripheral neuropathy report pain is worse in the summer and under the covers at night.

9. Initiate health teaching and referrals as indicated a. Advise to access information on a variety of HIV-related topics at https://aidsinfo.nih.gov/	9. Provide information and encourage appropriate utilization of community resources supportive of persons living with HIV and their significant others.

Documentation

Individual/family teaching
Referrals, if indicated

For Advanced/End-Stage AIDS

Risk for Caregiver Role Strain Related to AIDS-Associated Shame/Stigma, and Uncertainty about the Course of Illness and Demands on the Caregiver

NOC
Caregiver Well-Being, Role Performance, Care-Giving Endurance Potential, Family Coping, Family Integrity

Goals

The caregiver will relate a plan on how to continue social activities despite caregiving responsibilities.

NIC
Caregiver Support, Respite Care, Coping Enhancement, Family Mobilization, Mutual Goal Setting, Support System Enhancement, Anticipatory Guidance

Indicators

• Identify activities that are important for self.
• Relate intent to enlist the help of at least two people.

CLINICAL ALERT:
• Pirraglia et al. (*2005) reported "that the burden of caregiving was strongly and independently associated with depression in the informal caregiver of HIV-infected individuals. In addition, medical comorbidity besides HIV in the informal caregiver, illicit drug use by the informal caregiver, having others to help besides the HIV patient, spending all day together, and duration of the HIV patient's diagnosis were also associated with greater depression in the informal caregiver. Of all other characteristics of the informal caregiver, of the relationship between the informal caregiver and HIV patient, or of the HIV patient, none was independently associated with depression in the informal caregiver."

Interventions	Rationales
1. Explore the meanings and beliefs that caregivers hold regarding the individual's HIV infection.	1. The caregiver's feelings of shame or guilt regarding the individual's HIV infection or life style may prohibit optimal caregiving. The caregiver may need help in expressing his or her feelings regarding these traditionally taboo topics (*Brown & Powell-Cope, 1991; *Pirraglia et al., 2005; Powell-Cope & Brown, 1992).
2. Encourage the caregiver's consistent acknowledgment of, and support for, the caregiving role.	2. AIDS caregivers often receive little to no support for their caregiving role. Their fear of discrimination and ambivalent feelings toward themselves or the individual stops them from disclosing their situation. This leads to feelings of isolation (*Brown & Powell-Cope, 1991; *Powell-Cope & Brown, 1992).
3. Assist the caregiver with anticipating the uncertainty, role changes, and unpredictability of their caregiving role, and course of the HIV infection itself.	3. Uncertainty is a common concern in caregivers of persons with life-threatening illnesses. The ability to anticipate certain events or changes can allay some anxiety for caregivers (*Brown & Powell-Cope, 1991).
4. Assist the caregiver with decision-making regarding whom to tell about his or her AIDS caregiving role.	4. Fear of rejection and isolation can make the decision of whom to tell anxiety-provoking and overpowering to AIDS caregivers (*Powell-Cope & Brown, 1992).
5. Assist the caregiver with the "staging" method of disclosure of the AIDS caregiving role, if they desire.	5. Disclosure by "staging" of the information is less anxiety-provoking than full disclosure (e.g., Stage I: "My son is sick." Stage II: "My son is under a doctor's care and needs to stay with me until he is back on his feet." Stage III: "My son has AIDS and needs my help.") (*Powell-Cope & Brown, 1992).
6. Reinforce the caregivers' knowledge of HIV transmission, infection-control precautions for the home, and so on. Provide written information on same and be available for questions.	6. Fear of HIV transmission to self and other members of their household is a major concern of AIDS caregivers (*Brown & Powell-Cope, 1991).
7. Identify and assist—with help of community resources supportive of AIDS caregivers, such as community case management services—AIDS caregivers' support groups, day care, respite care, and the like.	7. AIDS caregivers need support that recognizes their unique needs, and support should be used to reinforce their caregiving.

> **CLINICAL ALERT:**
> - Pirraglia et al. (*2005) reported "that the relationship between depression and caregiver burden appears to be unaffected by HIV severity. The burden of care may be related to the medical comorbidity and social disadvantages common among HIV patients and their informal caregivers."
> - Refer to Unit II Section I nursing diagnosis Caregiver Role Strain for additional interventions if indicated.

Systemic Lupus Erythematosus

Systemic lupus erythematosus (SLE) is a chronic, occasionally life-threatening, multisystem disorder. Individuals may present with a wide array of symptoms, signs, and laboratory findings and have a variable prognosis that depends upon the disease severity and type of organ involvement (Wallace, 2015).

SLE can affect any organ system. SLE can affect pleural and pericardial membranes, joints, skin, blood cells, and nervous and glomerular tissue. Symptoms vary from person to person. Almost everyone with SLE has joint pain and swelling. This chronic disease follows a relapsing and remitting course.

Accelerated atherosclerosis, pulmonary hypertension, and antiphospholipid syndrome, as well as osteopenia or osteoporosis, are among the comorbid conditions, which can be treated and for which screening tests are appropriately used.

The major causes of death in the first few years of illness are active disease (e.g., central nervous system [CNS] and renal disease) or infection due to immunosuppression, while causes of late death include complications of SLE (e.g., end-stage renal disease), treatment complications, and cardiovascular disease.

The frequency of SLE varies by race and ethnicity. A new analysis of medical records obtained through the United States Indian Health Service estimates that the prevalence of lupus US American Indians and Alaska Natives (AI/AN) are among the highest for any group previously reported, including rates previously reported for African Americans (Ferucci et al., 2014). Following American Indians and Alaska Natives are African Americans, Asians, and Hispanics.

The female preponderance of lupus individuals is 10:1, with males. Incidence is higher in first-degree relatives. The Lupus Foundation of American estimates prevalence to be up to 1.5 million cases (Lupus Foundation of America, 2013).

Time Frame
Initial diagnosis
Secondary diagnosis
Severe SLE flare

▪▪▪▪ DIAGNOSTIC CLUSTER**

Collaborative Problems

Risk for Complications of Sepsis

Risk for Complications of Septic Arthritis (refer to Inflammatory Joint Disease Care Plan)

Risk for Complications of Pericarditis

Risk for Complications of Hematological abnormalities

Risk for Complications of Pulmonary Dysfunction

Risk for Complications of Neuropsychiatric Disorders

Risk for Complications of Nephritis

Risk for Complications of Sjögren Syndrome (refer to Inflammatory Joint Disease Care Plan)

Nursing Diagnoses

Fatigue related to decreased mobility joint pain and effects of chronic inflammation (refer to Inflammatory Joint Disease Care Plan)

Risk for Disturbed Self-Concept related to inability to achieve developmental tasks secondary to disabling condition and changes in appearance (refer to Unit II Section 1 nursing diagnosis Disturbed Self-Concept)

Risk for Injury related to increased dermal vulnerability secondary to disease process

Risk for Ineffective Health Management related to insufficient knowledge of condition, rest versus activity requirements, pharmacologic therapy, signs and symptoms of complications, risk factors, and community resources

Related Care Plan

Corticosteroid Therapy

**This medical condition was not included in the validation study.

Transition Criteria

Before transition, the individual or family will:

1. Identify components of a standard treatment program.
2. Relate proper use of medications.
3. Describe actions to reduce the risk of exacerbations.
4. Identify signs and symptoms that must be reported to a health care professional.

Transitional Risk Assessment Plan (TRAP)

Begin this plan on admission.
Implement the Transitional Risk Assessment Plan (TRAP).
- Refer to front/back inside covers.
- Add each validated high-risk diagnosis to individual's problem list with the risk code in ( ).
- Refer to Unit II to the individual high-risk nursing diagnoses/collaborative problems for outcomes and interventions,

    R: "Close coordination of care in the post-acute period, early discharge follow-up care, enhanced patient education and self-management training, proactive end-of-life counseling, and extending the resources and clinical expertise over time via multidisciplinary team management" can lower readmission rates and improve health outcomes (Boutwell & Hwu, 2009, p. 14). Interventions are utilized to activate the individual and family to select changes in their everyday lifestyle choices to improve their health (Hibbard & Greene, 2013).

Collaborative Problems

Risk for Complications of Sepsis

Risk for Complications of Septic Arthritis

Risk for Complications of Pericarditis

Risk for Complications of Hematological Abnormalities

Risk for Complications of Pulmonary Dysfunction

Risk for Complications of Neuropsychiatric Disorders

Risk for Complications of Nephritis

Risk for Complications of Sjögren Syndrome

Collaborative Outcomes

The individual will be monitored for early signs and symptoms of (a sepsis) (b) septic arthritis (c) pericarditis, (d) hematological abnormalities, (e) pulmonary dysfunction, (f) neuropsychiatric disorders, and (g) nephritis and will receive collaborative interventions if indicated to restore physiologic stability.

Indicators of Physiologic Stability

- Oriented, calm (a, f)
- No new complaints of pain (a, b)
- No complaints of headache (f)
- No complaints of chest pain, dyspnea (c)
- Intact sensation and motor function (b, c, f)
- Blood pressure >90/60 mm Hg (a, c, f)
- Pulse 60 to 100 beats/min (a, c, e)
- Respirations 16 to 20 breaths/min (a, b, c, f)
- Breath sounds throughout (a, d, f)
- Temperature 98° F to 99.5° F (a, b)
- Capillary refill <3 seconds (a, c e)

- Liver function tests
  - Alanine aminotransferase (ALT) (d)
  - Aspartate aminotransferase (AST) (d)
  - Bilirubin total D.1 to 1.2 mg/dL (d)
  - Prothrombin time 9.5 to 12 seconds (d)
  - Partial prothrombin time 20 to 45 seconds (d)
  - Bleeding time 1 to 9 minutes (d)
- Stool for occult blood: negative (d)
- Arterial blood gases
  - Oxygen saturation (Sao$_2$) 94% to 100% (a, b, c)
  - Carbon dioxide (Paco$_2$) 35 to 45 mm Hg (ac, g)
  - Serum pH 7.35 to 7.45 (c)
- Renal function (g)
  - Creatinine 0.7 to 1.4 mg/dL
  - Blood urea nitrogen 10 to 20 mg/dL
  - Prealbumin
  - Urine creatinine clearance
- Complete blood count (d)
  - Hemoglobin: Male 13 to 18 gm/dL; Female 12 to 16 g/dL
  - Hematocrit: Male 42% to 50%; Female 40% to 48%
  - Red blood cells: Male 4.6 to 5.9 million/mm^3; Female 4.2 to 5.4 million/mm^3
  - White blood cells 5,000 to 10,800/mm^3 (a, b, d)
  - Platelets 100,000 to 400,000/mm^3
- No seizures (f)

CLINICAL ALERT:

Poor prognostic factors for survival in SLE include (Sutton, Davidson, & Bruce 2013; Wallace, 2015):

- Renal disease (especially diffuse proliferative glomerulonephritis)
- Hypertension
- Male sex
- Young age
- Older age at presentation
- Low socioeconomic status
- Black race, which may primarily reflect low socioeconomic status
- Presence of antiphospholipid antibodies
- Antiphospholipid antibody syndrome
- High overall disease activity

Interventions	Rationales

1. Monitor for a flare (Wallace, 2015):
   a. Mild SLE flare—new onset low-grade fevers, a malar rash, arthralgias, with increasingly fatigued mild leukopenia.
   b. Moderate SLE flare—new onset pleuritic chest pain and a swollen elbow. Laboratory evaluation reveals elevated acute phase reactants. Right-sided pleural effusion per X-ray.
   c. Severe SLE flare—new onset renal insufficiency and significant proteinuria due to lupus nephritis. Laboratory evaluation is notable for a low C3, C4, elevated dsDNA antibodies, and elevated acute phase reactants.
	1. The clinical course of SLE is variable and may be characterized by unpredictable disease flares and remissions. The most useful laboratory tests to predict an SLE flare (particularly lupus nephritis) are the onset of an increased serum titer of anti-dsDNA antibodies and hypocomplementemia (especially CH50, C3, and C4) (Wallace, 2015).

Interventions	Rationales
2. Monitor for sepsis Refer to Unit II Section 2, Collaborative Problems—Risk for Complications of SIRS/Sepsis	2. Damage to cell membranes can provide sites for gram-positive and gram-negative organisms.

3. Monitor for signs and symptoms of pulmonary complications as including pleurisy, pleural effusion, pneumonitis, pulmonary hypertension, and interstitial lung disease.
    a. Acute onset of respiratory symptoms
    b. Fever
    c. Inspiratory crackles
    d. Hypoxemia
    e. Cough and hemoptysis
    f. Decreased exercise tolerance
 	
 CLINICAL ALERT:
• Hemoptysis may indicate diffuse alveolar hemorrhage (DAH), a rare, acute, life-threatening pulmonary complication of SLE (Dellaripa & Danoff, 2016).
	3. At some time during their course, most individuals with SLE show signs of involvement of the lung, pulmonary vasculature, pleura, and/or diaphragm (Dellaripa & Danoff, 2016). SLE may lead to multiple pulmonary complications, which may manifest acutely or slowly. Pleurisy with pleuritic chest pain with or without pleural effusions is the most common feature of acute pulmonary involvement in SLE (Dellaripa & Danoff, 2016).

4. Monitor for pericarditis:
    a. Pericarditis, with or without an effusion, is the most common cardiac manifestation of SLE occurring in approximately 25% of patents at some point during their disease course (Gladman, 2015).
    b. Chest pain beneath left clavicle and in the neck and left scapular region; aggravated by movement or deep breaths, relieved by leaning forward.
    c. Pericardial rub
    d. Temperature >101° F
	4. Excessive autoantibodies combine with antigens to form immune complexes. These complexes are deposited in vascular and tissue surfaces, triggering an inflammatory response and eventually local tissue injury. Thus, SLE can affect any organ system (Grossman & Porth, 2014).

5. Monitor for hematologic disorders:
    a. Hemolytic anemia
    b. Leukopenia
    c. Lymphopenia
    d. Thrombocytopenia
	5. This vasculopathy is characterized by a small to moderate perivascular accumulation of mononuclear cells, without destruction (e.g., fibrinoid necrosis) of the blood vessel. There may be small infarcts due to luminal occlusion (Schur, 2015). Antibodies against red blood cells result in hemolytic anemia. Antibodies against platelets result in thrombocytopenia. B-lymphocyte production is regulated by a balance of CD4+ and CD8+ lymphocytes (T cells). This balance is disrupted by SLE (Grossmam & Porth, 2014).

6. Teach the individual to report purpura and ecchymosis.	6. These are manifestations of platelet deficiencies.
7. Monitor for thromboembolic disease. Refer to Unit II Section 2 to Risk for Complications of Deep Vein Thrombosis	7. Thromboembolic disease can complicate SLE, particularly in the context of antiphospholipid antibodies. Although the precise mechanism is unknown, thromboembolic disease can affect both the venous and arterial circulations (Gladman, 2015).

8. Monitor for renal involvement:
    a. Increasing serum creatinine
    b. Decreasing glomerular filtration rate
    c. Proteinuria of 1.0 g/24 hr
    d. Elevated BP
	8. Approximately 50% of SLE individuals have renal involvement, and it is a significant cause of morbidity and mortality (Danila et al., 2009). Thus, periodic screening or the presence of lupus nephritis with urinalyses, quantitation of proteinuria, and estimation of the glomerular filtration rate is an important component of the ongoing management of SLE individuals (Gladman, 2015).

(continued)

Interventions	*Rationales*

9. Monitor for neuropsychiatric involvement
  a. Psychiatric manifestations
    • Psychosis, which may be due to SLE or to glucocorticoid treatment
    • Depression, anxiety, and mania
  b. Neurological
    • Cognitive dysfunction, headache
    • Organic brain syndromes
    • Delirium, seizures
    • Peripheral neuropathies
	9. SLE may affect the nervous system at multiple levels, with differing neuropathology (Schur, 2015).

CLINICAL ALERT:
- Prospective studies suggest that from 50% to 78% of neurologic episodes are caused by secondary factors (Hanly et al., 2009), including:
  - Infections associated with immunosuppressive therapy
  - Metabolic complications of other organ system failure, such as uremia
  - Hypertension
  - Toxic effects of therapy (particularly corticosteroids)

Clinical Alert Report

Prior to providing care, advise ancillary staff/student to report the following to the professional nurse assigned to the individual:
- Any changes in mental status such as orientation, agitation, lethargy, confusion
- Blood pressure, pulse, or respirations outside of prescribed limits. See "Indicators." Individual parameters may vary depending on individual's medications
- Temperature (oral) 1° F to 2° F over baseline
- Difficulty breathing or new onset of shortness of breath
- New onset of pain (chest, joint, head)
- Changes in urine from baseline.
- Chills, fever, temperature >100.5° F
- New onset inability to move the limb or joint
- Reports of increased pain in the affected joint, especially with movement
- Increased swelling (increased fluid within the joint)
- Red and warm joint
- Chest pain
- Complaints of shortness of breath

Documentation

Vital signs
Peripheral pulses
Complaints
Responses to treatment

Nursing Diagnosis

High Risk for Injury Related to Increased Dermal Vulnerability Secondary to Disease Process

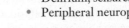

Goal

The individual will identify causative factors that may increase disease activity (e.g., sun exposure).

NIC

Fall Prevention,
Environmental
Management: Safety,
Health Education,
Surveillance: Safety, Risk
Identification

Indicators

- Identify measures to reduce damage to skin by the sun.
- Identify strategies to manage skin damage should it occur.
- Identify signs and symptoms of cellulitis.

Interventions	*Rationales*
CLINICAL ALERT: • Photosensitivity is an abnormal cutaneous response to ultraviolet radiation (UVR) and, in some individuals, visible light. Depending upon the type of photosensitivity disease, the abnormal response can manifest as macular erythema, papules, plaques, vesicles, bullae, telangiectasias, or eczematous patches. For some photosensitivity diseases, the rash may result in scarring.	

1. Explain the relationship between sun exposure and disease activity. Identify strategies to limit sun exposure:
  a. Avoidance of midday sun (between 10 a.m. and 4 p.m.)
  b. Protective clothing: long sleeved shirts and pants, broad brim hats
  c. Window films that block UVR for cars and homes
  d. Broad spectrum sunscreen (protects against both UVA and UVB)
  e. Do not use tanning beds
	1. Through an unknown mechanism, exposure to ultraviolet light can precipitate an exacerbation of both skin and systemic diseases. The individual's understanding of this relationship should encourage him or her to limit sun exposure.
	
	Sun avoidance and protective clothing should be emphasized as important measures of photoprotection for individuals with photosensitivity disorders. Sunscreen alone is not sufficient and should be used as an adjunct to other methods of sun protection (Elmets, 2015).

2. Explain the need to avoid fluorescent lighting or a too-hot stove.	2. Like sunlight, fluorescent lighting produces ultraviolet rays.
3. Advise of the effects of tobacco use on their disorder. Refer to index for strategies to promote smoking cessation.	3. Discoid lupus seems to be more severe in people who smoke. Plus, smoking seems to make certain medicines for discoid lupus less effective (Elmets, 2015).
4. Each the individual to recognize signs and symptoms of vasculitis and to report them promptly to a health care professional as tenderness, swelling, warmth, redness.	4. Vascular inflammation of the smallest blood vessels, capillaries, and venules can cause occlusion.
5. Advise that special cosmetic products can make the skin changes less obvious in men and women, for example, brand names, Dermablend and Covermark (Elmets, 2015).	

Documentation

Skin assessment

> ### TRANSITION TO HOME/COMMUNITY CARE
> - If indicated, review the high-risk diagnoses identified for this individual on admission:
>   - Is he person still at high risk?
>   - Can the family/reduce the risks?
>   - Is the person at higher risk at home?
>   - Is a home health nurse assessment needed?
>   - Refer to Discharge Planner/Case Manager/Social Service
> - When is this person scheduled for follow-up with primary provider? Specialists? Record dates of appointments.
> - Complete a medication reconciliation prior to discharge > Refer to front/back cover.

STAR

Stop

Think   Is this person at risk for injury, falls, medical complications, and/or inability to care for self (activities of daily living)?

Is there a support person available?

Is the person competent to manage self-administration of medications, treatment procedures?

Are additional resources needed?

Can the person explain how to monitor condition (e.g., sign/symptoms of complications, and when to call his or her primary provider or specialist?

Act   Contact or provide the appropriate resource (e.g., contacting a support person, home health assessment, additional teaching, printed materials).

Review   Has the problem been addressed? If not, use SBAR to communicate to the appropriate person.

Risk for Ineffective Health Management Related to Insufficient Knowledge of Condition, Rest versus Activity Requirements, Pharmacologic Therapy, Signs and Symptoms of Complications, Risk Factors, and Community Resources

NOC

Compliance Behavior, Knowledge: Treatment Regimen, Participation in Health Care Decisions, Treatment Behavior: Illness or Injury

Goals

The goals for this diagnosis represent those associated with transition planning. See the transition criteria.

NIC

Anticipatory Guidance, Risk Identification, Learning Facilitation, Support Group

---

Interventions	*Rationales*
1. Instruct to seek medical care for evaluation of new symptoms, including fever. Advise them regarding their heightened risks for infection and cardiovascular disease. Educate individuals with SLE regarding aggressive lipid and blood pressure goals to minimize the risk of coronary artery disease.	
2. Instruct to avoid exposure to sunlight and ultraviolet light. Refer to High Risk for Injury in this Care Plan.	

Interventions	*Rationales*
3. Advise that pregnancies should be planned. Explain that active SLE at the time of conception is a strong predictor of adverse maternal and obstetrical outcomes (Bermas & Smith, 2015).	3. However, pregnancy in women with SLE carries a higher maternal and fetal risk compared with pregnancy in healthy women. The prognosis for both mother and child is best when SLE has been quiescent for at least 6 months prior to the pregnancy (Bermas & Smith, 2015).

4. Explain SLE in terms appropriate for their levels of understanding. Discuss the following:
  a. The inflammatory process
  b. Organ systems at risk of involvement (see Potential Complications in this Care Plan for more information)
  c. Chronic nature of disease (remission/exacerbation)
	4. Understanding can help to improve engagement and self-manage (refer to Risk for Compromised Engagement in Unit II Section 1).

5. Teach the need to balance activity and rest. (Refer to the Inflammatory Joint Disease Care Plan for specific strategies.)	5. The chronic fatigue associated with SLE necessitates strategies to prevent exhaustion and maintain the highest level of independent functioning (*Albano & Wallace, 2001).
6. Teach the need for meticulous, gentle mouth care.	6. Vasculitis can increase the risk of mouth lesions and injury.

7. Teach Warning Signs of a Flare and to contact their specialist or PCP
  a. Increased fatigue
  b. Pain
  c. Rash
  d. Fever
  e. Abdominal discomfort
  f. Headache
  g. Dizziness
	7. Early treatment of a flare can reduce the severity of the flare and damage to joints, etc.

8. Explain the relationship of stress and autoimmune disorders. Discuss stress management techniques:
  a. Progressive relaxation
  b. Guided imagery
  c. Regular exercise (e.g., walking, swimming)
  d. Refer the individual to a counselor and psychiatrist, as appropriate
	8. Stress may be associated with an increase in disease activity. Stress management techniques can reduce the stress and fatigue associated with unmanaged conflicts (*Albano & Wallace, 2001).

9. Discuss complementary therapies that may help to reduce inflammation of joints and tissues (*Shirato, 2005) as massage, acupuncture.	9. Studies have shown benefits (*Shirato, 2005).

10. Initiate referrals to appropriate community/resources:
  a. Arthritis Foundation, http://www.arthritis.org
  b. Lupus Foundation of America, http://www.lupus.org/
  c. National Institute of Arthritis and Musculoskeletal and Skin Diseases (NIAMS) http://www.niams.nih.gov/
	10. Additional self-help information may be very useful for self-care. Provide excellent support and education for the individual and family.

Documentation

Individual/family teaching
Referrals, if indicated

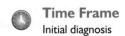 NEOPLASTIC DISORDERS

Cancer: Initial Diagnosis

Cancer involves a disturbance in normal cell growth in which abnormal cells arise from normal cells, reproduce rapidly, and infiltrate tissues, lymph, and blood vessels. The destruction caused by cancer depends on its site, whether or not it metastasizes, its obstructive effects, and its effects on the body's defense system (e.g., nutrition, hematopoiesis). Cancer is classified according to the cell of origin: malignant tumors from epithelial tissue are called *carcinomas* and those from connective tissue are known as *sarcomas*. Treatment varies depending on classification, cancer stage, and other factors.

The American Cancer Society (2015) reported that 1,658,370 new cancer cases were diagnosed in 2015. In 2015, about 589,430 Americans are expected to die of cancer, or about 1,620 people/day. Nearly 14.5 million Americans with a history of cancer were alive on January 1, 2014. Cancer death rates for individuals with the least education are more than twice those of the most educated. The elimination of educational and racial disparities could potentially have avoided about 37% (60,370) of the premature cancer deaths among individuals aged 25 to 64 years (Siegel et al., 2011).

Time Frame
Initial diagnosis

■■■■■ DIAGNOSTIC CLUSTER

Nursing Diagnoses

▲ Anxiety related to unfamiliar hospital environment, uncertainty about outcomes, feelings of helplessness and hopelessness, and insufficient knowledge about cancer and treatment

▲ Interrupted Family Processes related to fears associated with recent cancer diagnosis, disruptions associated with treatments, financial problems, and uncertain future

▲ Grieving related to potential loss of body function and the perceived effects of cancer on lifestyle (refer to Grieving in Unit II)

Δ Risk for Spiritual Distress related to conflicts centering on the meaning of life, cancer, spiritual beliefs, and death (refer to Palliative Care Plan)

▲ Risk for Ineffective Health Management related to complexity and cost of therapeutic regimen, complexity of health care system, shortened length of stay, insufficient knowledge of treatment, and barriers to comprehension secondary to language barriers, cognitive deficits, hearing and/or visual impairment, anxiety, and lack of motivation

Related Care Plans

Chemotherapy

Radiation Therapy

▲ This diagnosis was reported to be monitored for or managed frequently (75% to 100%).
Δ This diagnosis was reported to be monitored for or managed often (50% to 74%).

Transition Criteria

Before transition, the individual or family will:

1. Relate the intent to share concerns with a trusted confidante.
2. Describe early signs of family dysfunction.
3. Identify signs and symptoms that must be reported to a health care professional.
4. Identify available community resources.

Transitional Risk Assessment Plan (TRAP)

Begin this plan on admission.

Implement the Transitional Risk Assessment Plan (TRAP):

- Refer to inside back cover.
- Add each validated risk diagnosis to individual's problem list with the risk code in ( ).
- Refer to Unit II to the individual risk nursing diagnoses/collaborative problems for outcomes and interventions.

  R: "Close coordination of care in the post-acute period, early transition follow-up care, enhanced client education and self-management training, proactive end-of-life counseling, and extending the resources and clinical expertise over time via multidisciplinary team management" can lower readmission rates and improve health outcomes (Boutwell & Hwu, 2009, p. 14). Interventions are utilized to activate the individual and family to select changes in their everyday lifestyle choices to improve their health (Hibbard & Greene, 2013).

Collaborative Problems

The collaborative problems caused by cancer depend on its site, whether it metastasizes, its obstructive effects, and its effects on the body's defense system (e.g., white blood cell count, renal insufficiency). For example, cancer of the breast can metastasize to the brain, lung, liver, and bone. In this case, the collaborative problems Risk for Complications of Increased Intracranial Pressure, Risk for Complications of Hepatic Insufficiency, Risk for Complications of Respiratory Insufficiency, and Risk for Complications of Pathological Fractures would be appropriate. Refer to the collaborative problems in Unit II for specific collaborative problems.

Nursing Diagnoses

Anxiety Related to Unfamiliar Hospital Environment, Uncertainty about Outcomes, Feelings of Helplessness and Hopelessness, and Insufficient Knowledge about Cancer and Treatment

NOC
Anxiety Self-Control, Family Coping, Family Normalization

Goal

The individual will report increased psychological comfort.

NIC
Anxiety Reduction, Anticipatory Guidance, Family Involvement Promotion, Coping Enhancement, Family Integrity Promotion

Indicators

- Share concerns regarding the cancer diagnosis.
- Identify one strategy that reduces anxiety.

CLINICAL ALERT: Cancer remains a feared diagnosis that many individuals continue to link to death despite recent and continuing advances in early detection, treatment, and survival. A cancer diagnosis affects not only the individual, but also their family and friends. They may feel scared, uncertain, or angry about the unwanted changes cancer will bring to their lives and theirs. Individuals may feel numb or confused. Individuals may have trouble listening to, understanding, or remembering what people tell them during this time. This is especially true when they are first that they have cancer. It's not uncommon for people to shut down mentally once they hear the word "Cancer" (American Cancer Society, 2014).

Interventions	Rationales
1. Provide opportunities for the individual and family members to share feelings (anger, guilt, loss, and pain): a. Initiate frequent contacts and provide an atmosphere that promotes calm and relaxation. b. Convey a nonjudgmental attitude and listen attentively. c. Explore own feelings and behaviors. d. When you first learn that you have cancer, you may feel as if your life is out of control. This could be because: • You wonder if you are going to live. • Your normal routine is disrupted by doctor visits and treatments. • People use medical terms that you do not understand. • You feel like you cannot do the things you enjoy. • You feel helpless and lonely.	1. Frequent contact by caregiver indicates acceptance and may facilitate trust. The individual may be hesitant to approach the staff/student because of negative self-concept. The nurse should not make assumptions about an individual's or family member's reaction; validating the individual's particular fears and concerns helps to increase awareness. The nurse who can talk openly about life after a cancer diagnosis offers encouragement and hope (*Barsevick, Much, & Sweeney, 2000).
2. Promote balanced communication, which occurs when nurses meet jointly with individuals and their family/support persons (Northouse, Williams, Given, & McCorkle, 2012). a. Avoid "privileged communication", which is direct communication between the professional and the family not including the individual. b. Avoid "filtered communication", which occurs when information is given to the individual but not to family/support persons.	2. Balanced communication allows for both the individual and family/support systems to meet concurrently with the professional. It allows for open communication and offers each person a greater understanding of the other. Although not as common today, the negative consequences of privileged communication are that some topics are seem to be difficult to discuss openly, it disrupts professional/family communication, encourages avoiding certain topic and that the individual is unable to cope with the information. Filtered communications reduce direct communication with the family/support persons. It relies on the individual to communicate what they heard, understand or remember. It lacks direct communication with the family, which prevents them from asking questions or sharing their concerns. It also prevents the family/support persons from being present for support. It is a realistic appraisal of a person's illness or situation with a belief that they will cope and experience some positive outcome from the experience. Even when cure is not possible, other outcomes can be positive, extended remission, better pain control, participation in meaningful activities (Northouse, 2011).
3. Encourage an open discussion of cancer, their feelings including their experiences of others.	3. Sharing feelings will allow each individual a better understanding of one another's feelings and thus provide support.
4. Allow the individual's family and support persons to share their feelings regarding the diagnosis and actual or anticipated effects (anger, rage, depression, or guilt).	4. Cancer can have a negative impact on the family financially, socially, and emotionally. All family members are affected by a cancer diagnosis, including children. This stressor on the children must be addressed; support groups are available (Northouse, 2011).
5. Promote an optimistic outlook that is realistic for their situation.	5. Optimism is not false sense of hope or denial. (Northouse, 2011).

Interventions	Rationales

6. Identify those at risk for unsuccessful adjustment:
  a. Poor ego strength
  b. Ineffective problem-solving ability
  c. Poor motivation
  d. History of pre-existing relationship problems.
  e. Poor overall health
  f. Lack of positive support systems
  g. Unstable economic status
  h. Rejection of counseling (shipes, 1987)
	6. An individual identified at risk may need referrals for counseling. Successful adjustment is influenced by factors such as previous coping success, achievement of developmental tasks, extent to which the disorder and treatment interfere with goal-directed activity, sense of self-determination and control, and realistic perception of the disorder.

7. Promote physical activity and exercise. Appropriate for individual. Assist the individual to determine the level of activity advisable (e.g., slow walk in park).	7. Physical activity provides diversion and a sense of normalcy. Individuals who exercise may improve their quality of life. Refer to Getting Started to Increase Activity on thePoint.
8. Recommend this excellent, no-cost resource for individuals and families facing new cancer diagnosis or living with cancer: Taking Time Support for People With Cancer from National Cancer Institute (Retrieved at http://www.cancer.gov/publications/individual-education/takingtime.pdf). The introduction reads; This book was written for you—the person with cancer. Where are you in this challenge? You may have just learned that you have cancer. Or you may be in treatment. At every point, most likely you have a range of feelings. It is important to try to accept these feelings and learn how to live with them as best as you can. Feelings about your cancer may be with you for a long time. This book is for you, but it can also be helpful to those people who are close to you. It may help them better understand what you are going through. And even if you have no close relatives or live far away from your family, you may have friends who you think of as your "family." Whatever "family" means to you, share this book with those who love and care about you.	

Documentation

Present emotional status
Interventions utilized

Interrupted Family Processes Related to Fears Associated with Recent Cancer Diagnosis, Disruptions Associated With Treatments, Financial Problems, and Uncertain Future

NOC

Family Coping, Family Normalization, Parenting Performance

Goal

The family will maintain a functional system of mutual support.

NIC

Family Involvement Promotion, Coping Enhancement, Family Integrity Promotion

Indicators

- Verbalize feelings regarding the diagnosis and prognosis.
- Identify signs of family dysfunction.
- Identify appropriate resources to seek, when needed.

Interventions	Rationales
1. Explore family members' perceptions of the situation. Explore their fears.	1. Verbalization can provide an opportunity for clarification and validation of feelings and concerns; this contributes to family unity. Spouses report increased anxiety prior to transition from hospital and anger at the individual for egocentricity during home-care period.
2. Determine if present coping mechanisms are effective.	2. If needed, refer families to community resources (e.g., counseling). This can help to maintain the existing family structure and its function as a supportive unit. Cancer challenges one's values and beliefs; this can result in changed cognitive, affective, and behavioral responses.
3. Encourage the family to call on its social network (e.g., friends, relatives, church members) for emotional and other support.	3. Outside assistance may help to reduce the perception that the family must "go it alone."
4. Explain that adjustment to cancer is an ongoing process. Common periods of crisis and significant challenge include the following (National Cancer Institute, 2015): a. Diagnosis b. Treatment (surgery, radiation, and chemotherapy) c. Posttreatment and remission d. Recurrence and palliative care e. Survivorship	4. "Adjustment or psychosocial adaptation to cancer has been defined as an ongoing process in which the individual tries to manage emotional distress, solve specific cancer-related problems, and gain mastery or control over cancer-related life events" (National Institute of Cancer, 2015). Adjustment to cancer is not a unitary, single event but rather a series of ongoing coping responses to the multiple tasks associated with living with cancer. Individual are faced with many challenges that vary with the clinical course of the disease (National Institute of Cancer, 2015).
5. Identify dysfunctional coping mechanisms: a. Substance abuse b. Continued denial c. Exploitation of one or more family members d. Separation or avoidance. Refer for counseling, as necessary.	5. A family with a history of unsuccessful coping may need additional resources. A family with unresolved conflicts before diagnosis is at risk.
6. Direct to community agencies and other sources of assistance (e.g., financial, housekeeping, direct care, childcare), as needed.	

STAR

Stop

Think Does individual understand treatment options? Benefits? Risks?

Act Contact the physician/nurse practitioner.

Situation: I am calling about Mr. Aidol. In discussing his treatment decisions, he has asked some questions about his choices.

Background: With his new diagnosis of pancreatic cancer, he is questioning if surgery is the best option.

Assessment: I think the problem is that Mr. Aidol does not understand the risks/benefits of surgery and other treatment options as chemotherapy, radiation, palliative care.

Recommendation: I would recommend that you (his oncologist) meet with him and his family to discuss all the treatment options available.

Review Has the problem been addressed? If not, use SBAR to communicate to the manager, department head.

Documentation

Present emotional status
Interventions
Response to nursing interventions
Referrals as needed

> **TRANSITION TO HOME/COMMUNITY CARE**
> If indicated, review the risk diagnoses identified for this individual on admission:
> * Is the person still at risk?
> * Can the family reduce the risks?
> * Is the person at higher risk at home?
> * Is a home health nurse assessment needed?
> * Refer to transition planner/case manager/social service.
> * When is this person scheduled for follow-up with primary provider? Specialists? Record dates of appointments.
> * Complete a medication reconciliation prior to transition. Refer to index.

STAR

Stop

Think   Is this person at risk for injury, falls, medical complications, and/or inability to care for self (activities of daily living)?

Is there a support person available?

Is the person competent to manage self-administration of medications, treatment procedures? Are additional resources needed?

Can the person explain how to monitor the condition (e.g., blood glucose, signs/symptoms of complications, dietary/mobility restrictions, and when to call his or her primary provider or specialist)?

Act   Contact or provide the appropriate resource (e.g., contacting a support person, home health assessment, additional teaching, printed materials).

Review   Has the problem been addressed? If not, use SBAR to communicate to the appropriate person.

Risk for Ineffective Health Management Related to Complexity and Cost of Therapeutic Regimen, Complexity of Health Care System, Shortened Length of Stay, Insufficient Knowledge of Treatment, and Barriers to Comprehension Secondary to Language Barriers, Cognitive Deficits, Hearing and/or Visual Impairment, Anxiety and Lack of Motivation

Refer to Generic Medical care Plan in Unit III.

CLINICAL SITUATIONS

Alcohol Dependency

Alcohol use in the United States (Substance Abuse and Mental Health Services Administration [SAMHSA], 2014):

- Prevalence of Drinking: In 2014, 87.6% of people ages 18 or older reported that they drank alcohol at some point in their lifetime; 71.0% reported that they drank in the past year; 56.9% reported that they drank in the past month.
- Prevalence of Binge Drinking and Heavy Drinking: In 2014, 24.7% of people ages 18 or older reported that they engaged in binge drinking in the past month; 6.7% reported that they engaged in heavy drinking in the past month.
  - Adults (ages 18+): 16.3 million adults ages 18 and older (6.8% of this age group) had an alcohol use disorder (AUD) in 2014. This includes 10.6 million men (9.2% of men in this age group) and 5.7 million women (4.6% of women in this age group).
  - Youth (ages 12 to 17): In 2014, an estimated 679,000 adolescents ages 12 to 17 (2.7% of this age group) had an AUD. This number includes 367,000 females (3.0% of females in this age group) and 311,000 males (2.5% of males in this age group).
- An estimated 55,000 adolescents (18,000 males and 37,000 females) received treatment for an alcohol problem in a specialized facility in 2014.
- It is estimated that one in every four or five hospitalized persons is an alcohol abuser (Hoffman & Weinhouse, 2015; *McKinley, 2005). Problem drinking is classified as at-risk drinking, abuse, and dependency (alcoholism). Refer to Box III.I for signs/symptoms of problem drinking. At-risk individuals consume quantities of alcohol that put them at risk of dependence.

Clinically, only one of every 10 alcoholics is diagnosed, and clinicians do not ask about alcohol use unless it is obvious. It is critical to identify people who abuse alcohol to prevent potentially fatal withdrawal symptoms. Surgical individuals are at risk for alcohol withdrawal syndrome because of the preprocedural

---

Box III.I DIFFERENTIATION OF AT-RISK DRINKING, ALCOHOL ABUSE, AND ALCOHOL DEPENDENCE

"At-Risk Drinking" is defined for healthy adults in general, drinking more than these single day or weekly limits is considered "at-risk" or "heavy" drinking (SAMHSA, 2014):
- **Men:** More than four drinks on any day or 14/week
- **Women:** More than three drinks on any day or 7/week

"Alcohol abuse is a drinking pattern that results in significant and recurrent adverse consequences. Alcohol abusers may fail to fulfill major school, work, or family obligations. They may have drinking-related legal problems, such as repeated arrests for driving while intoxicated. They may have relationship problems related to their drinking."
Some examples are:
- Had times when you ended up drinking more, or longer than you intended?
- More than once wanted to cut down or stop drinking, or tried to, but couldn't?
- Spent a lot of time drinking? Or being sick or getting over the after effects? Experienced craving—a strong need, or urge, to drink?
- Found that drinking—or being sick from drinking—often interfered with taking care of your home or family? Or caused job troubles? Or school problems?
- Continued to drink even though it was causing trouble with your family or friends?
- Had to drink much more than you once did to get the effect you want? Or found that your usual number of drinks had much less effect than before?
- Found that when the effects of alcohol were wearing off, you had withdrawal symptoms, such as trouble sleeping, shakiness, irritability, anxiety, depression, restlessness, nausea, or sweating?

"Alcohol dependence" (alcoholism) has four signs/symptoms:
- Craving, strong urge to drink,
- Loss of control, inability to stop,
- Physical dependence with withdrawal symptoms (irritability, mood changes, craving, muscle cramps), and
- The need to drink greater amounts to get "High."

and postoperative fasting. Most signs and symptoms are caused by the rapid removal of the depressant effects of alcohol on the central nervous system. The focus of medical and nursing care is to prevent, not to observe for, the complications of alcohol withdrawal). Prevention includes aggressive management of early withdrawal and close monitoring of the individual's response (Hoffman, & Weinhouse, 2015).

Time Frame
Secondary diagnosis

■ ■ ■ ■ DIAGNOSTIC CLUSTER**

Collaborative Problems

Risk for Complications of Delirium Tremens

Risk for Complications of Autonomic Hyperactivity

Risk for Complications of Seizures (refer to Risk for Complications of Seizures in Unit II)

Risk for Complications of Alcohol Hallucinosis

Risk for Complications of Hypovolemia (refer to Risk for Complications of Hypovolemia in Unit II)

Risk for Complications of Hypoglycemia (refer to Risk for Complications of Hypo/Hyperglycemia in Unit II)

Nursing Diagnoses

Risk for Violence related to (examples) impulsive behavior, disorientation, tremors, or impaired judgment

Ineffective Denial related to acknowledgment of alcohol abuse or dependency

Risk for Ineffective Health Management related to insufficient knowledge of condition, treatments available, at-risk situations, and community resources

**This clinical situation was not included in the validation study.

Transition Criteria

Before transition, the individual or family will:

1. Recognize that alcoholism is a disease.
2. Acknowledge the negative effects of alcoholism in their lives.
3. Identify community resources available for treatment of alcoholism.

Transitional Risk Assessment Plan (TRAP)

Begin this plan on admission.
Implement the Transitional Risk Assessment Plan (TRAP):
- Refer to inside back cover.
- Add each validated risk diagnosis to individual's problem list with the risk code in ( ).
- Refer to Unit II to the individual risk nursing diagnoses/collaborative problems for outcomes and interventions.

  R: "Close coordination of care in the post-acute period, early transition follow-up care, enhanced client education and self-management training, proactive end-of-life counseling, and extending the resources and clinical expertise over time via multidisciplinary team management" can lower readmission rates and improve health outcomes (Boutwell & Hwu, 2009, p. 14). Interventions are utilized to activate the individual and family to select changes in their everyday lifestyle choices to improve their health (Hibbard & Greene, 2013).

Collaborative Problems

Risk for Complications of Delirium Tremens

Risk for Complications of Autonomic Hyperactivity

Risk for Complications of Alcohol Hallucinosis

Collaborative Outcomes

The individual will be monitored for early signs and symptoms of (a) delirium tremens, (b) autonomic hyperactivity, (c) seizures, (d) alcohol hallucinosis, (e) hypovolemia, and (f) hypoglycemia, and will receive collaborative interventions if indicated to restore physiologic stability.

Indicators of Physiologic Stability

- No seizure activity (a, b, c)
- Calm, oriented (a, b, d)
- Temperature 98° F to 99.5° F (d)
- Pulse 60 to 100 beats/min (a, b, d)
- BP >90/60, <140/90 mm Hg (a, b, d)
- No reports of hallucinations (a, d)

Carp's Cues

It is estimated that one in five individuals admitted to a hospital suffers from an AUD such as alcohol abuse or dependence (Elliott, Geyer, Lionetti & Doty, 2012). It is very common for individuals and their families to deny or under-report alcohol consumption. The nurse must routinely assess all individuals and their families for patterns of alcohol consumption. Five percent (5%) of individuals with alcohol withdrawal progress to delirium tremors; 5% of individuals with delirium tremors die.

CLINICAL ALERT: The National Institute on Alcohol Abuse and Alcoholism (NIAAA, 2007) in the United States estimates amounts of alcohol that increase health risks below. Specifying these thresholds is an inexact science based on epidemiological evidence. Amounts are based on a "standard drink," which is defined as 12 g of ethanol, 5 ounces of wine, 12 ounces of beer, or 1.5 ounces of 80 proof spirits.
  Unhealthy drinking is defined as (NIAAA, 2007; Saitz, 2015):
- For men under age 65—more than 14 standard drinks/week on average.
- For woman, and adults 65 years and older, more than seven standard drinks/week on average
- More than three drinks on any day
- More than four drinks on any day

Interventions	Rationales
1. Carefully attempt to determine if the individual abuses alcohol on admission and during routine encounters. Consult with the family regarding perception of alcohol consumption. Explain why accurate information is necessary.	1. "In patients who are physically dependent on alcohol, the central nervous system adapts to the presence of alcohol and loses the ability to function normally in its absence. Signs and symptoms of AWS reflect declining blood alcohol levels. These usually appear within a few hours to a few days after cessation of alcohol consumption, although in some patients symptoms may develop up to 10 days after the last drink" (Elliott et al., 2012).
2. In a matter-of-fact manner, obtain history of drinking patterns from the individual or significant others (*Kappas-Larson & Lathrop, 1993): a. When did the individual have his or her last drink? b. How much was consumed on that day? c. On how many days of the last 30 did the individual consume alcohol? d. What was the average intake? e. What was the most consumed?	2. Alcoholics tend to underestimate alcohol consumed; therefore, multiply the amount a man tells you by two to three drinks and for a woman by four to five drinks (*Smith-DiJulio, 2001).

Interventions	Rationales
3. Determine the individual's attitude toward drinking by asking the CAGE questions: a. Have you ever thought you should cut down your drinking? b. Have you ever been annoyed by criticism of your drinking? c. Have you ever felt guilty about your drinking? d. Do you drink in the morning (i.e., "Eye-opener") (*Ewing, 1984)?	3. These questions can be used to identify possible defensiveness and similar attitudes about drinking.
4. Obtain history of previous withdrawals, as applicable: a. Delirium tremens (DTs): Time of onset, manifestation b. Seizures: Time of onset, type	4. Withdrawal symptoms usually present within 6 hours after cessation of drinking. Withdrawal can occur in individuals who are considered "social drinkers" (6 ounces of alcohol daily for 3 to 4 weeks). Withdrawal-associated seizures usually occur within 12 to 48 after the last drink, but can occur after on two hours of abstinence (Hoffman & Weinhouse, 2015).
5. Monitor for signs/symptoms of alcohol withdrawal (American Psychiatric Association, 2014): a. Two or more of the following, developing within several hours to a few days after cessation or reduction of heavy and prolonged alcohol use. • Autonomic hyperactivity • Increased hand tremor • Insomnia • Nausea or vomiting • Transient hallucinations or illusions • Psychomotor agitation • Anxiety • Grand mal seizures **CLINICAL ALERT:** • Among surgical individuals with unhealthy drinking, individuals who experience perioperative alcohol withdrawal have higher levels of morbidity than individuals without withdrawal (Gordon, 2016).	5. The diagnostic criteria also specify that signs and symptoms cause "clinically significant" distress or impairment, that they are not due to another medical condition, and that they "are not better accounted for by another mental disorder" (American Psychiatric Association, 2014).
6. When surgery is anticipated, notify the surgeon/anesthesiologist/nurse anesthetist if alcohol abuse is confirmed or suspected.	6. Individuals with alcohol-related health problems (e.g., malnourished, hepatic disorders, immune deficiency, withdrawal) are at risk for perioperative and postoperative complications. "Chronic alcohol use increases dose requirements for general anesthetic agents. These increased anesthetic requirements can exacerbate the risk of cardiovascular instability in patients who may be suffering from cardiomyopathy, heart failure, or dehydration. Chronic heavy alcohol use is associated with a twofold to fivefold increase in postoperative complications. Depletion of coagulation factors and thrombocytopenia increase the incidence of postoperative bleeding. Immune deficiency as a result of leucopoenia and altered cytokine production increase the risk of postoperative infection (especially, surgical wounds, respiratory system, or urinary tract). Electrolyte disturbances or periods of relative hypotension exacerbate the risk. Alcohol use is an independent risk factor for the development of acute confusion or delirium after operation" (Gordon, 2016).

(continued)

Interventions	Rationales
7. Obtain complete history of prescription, over-the-counter and "street" drugs taken. **CLINICAL ALERT:** • "Between 12 and 24 hours after alcohol cessation, some patients may experience visual, auditory, or tactile hallucinations which usually end within 48 hours. Most patients are aware that the unusual sensations aren't real" (Elliott et al., 2013). The most severe form of alcohol withdrawal is DTs, characterized by altered mental status and severe autonomic hyperactivity that may lead to cardiovascular collapse. These signs and symptoms occur 48 to 96 hours after the last drink. If untreated, death can occur from respiratory and cardiovascular collapse (Elliott et al., 2013).	7. Benzodiazepine or barbiturate withdrawal may mimic alcohol withdrawal and will complicate the picture. Substance abusers tend to cross-abuse substances (Elliott et al., 2013).

8. Monitor all persons suspected of, or identified as, risk for alcohol withdrawal syndrome for alcohol withdrawal signs/symptoms using the Clinical Institute Withdrawal Assessment for Alcohol (*Sullivan, Sykora, Schneiderman, Naranjo, & Sellers, 1989).
  a. Nausea and Vomiting—Ask "Do you feel sick to your stomach? Have you vomited?"
  b. Tremor—Arms extended and fingers spread apart.
  c. Paroxysmal sweats
  d. Anxiety—Ask "Do you feel nervous?"
  e. Agitation
  f. Tactile disturbances—Ask "Have you any itching, pins and needles sensations, any burning, any numbness, or do you feel bugs crawling on or under your skin?"
  g. Auditory disturbances—Ask "Are you more aware of sounds around you? Are they harsh? Do they frighten you? Are you hearing anything that is disturbing to you? Are you hearing things you know are not there?"
  h. Visual disturbances—Ask, "Does the light appear to be too bright? Is its color different? Does it hurt your eyes? Are you seeing anything that is disturbing to you? Are you seeing things you know are not there?"
  i. Headache, fullness in head—Ask, "Does your head feel different? Does it feel like there is a band around your head?" Do not rate for dizziness or lightheadedness. Otherwise, rate severity.
  j. Orientation and clouding of sensorium—Ask "What day is this? Where are you? Who am I?"
 	
 CLINICAL ALERT:
• The most severe form of alcohol withdrawal is DTs, characterized by altered mental status and severe autonomic hyperactivity that may lead to cardiovascular collapse. Only about 5% of individuals with alcohol withdrawal progress to DTs, but about 5% of these individuals die (Hoffman & Weinhouse, 2015).
	8. The Clinical Institute Withdrawal Assessment for Alcohol, revised (CIWA-Ar) is the gold standard withdrawal assessment rating scale in both hospital and outpatient settings (Elliott et al., 2013; *Sullivan et al., 1989).
	
	This evidence-based, validated objective observer-rated assessment tool is designed to maintain consistency in individual assessment and treatment (Elliott et al., 2013).
	
	"Clinicians use the CIWA-Ar tool to rate 10 signs and symptoms on numeric scales to determine their severity. The total score can range from 0 (no symptoms) to a maximum of 67" (Elliott et al., 2013, p. 40). Any score over 18 indicates severe withdrawal (*Sullivan et al., 1989).
	
	The tool takes about 5 minutes to administer (Elliott et al., 2013).
	
	"The CIWA-Ar provides a measure of withdrawal severity and helps to guide treatment, enabling clinicians to intervene early in withdrawal to prevent poor patient outcomes" (Elliott et al., 2013, p. 40).

Interventions	Rationales
9. Consult with physician/nurse practitioner/physical assistant regarding the individual's risk and the initiation of benzodiazepine therapy, with dosage determined by assessment findings.	9. Benzodiazepine requirements in alcohol withdrawal are highly variable and individual-specific. Fixed schedules may oversedate or undersedate (Elliott et al., 2013).
10. Explain to the individual and family what is occurring. Observe for desired effects of benzodiazepine therapy: a. Relief from withdrawal symptoms b. Individual sleeping peacefully, but can be roused	10. Family members may not be aware of the individual's alcohol abuse. Information regarding the situation is confidential and may be prohibited is the individual does not consent.
11. Monitor for and intervene promptly in cases of status epilepticus. Call Rapid Response team and follow the institution's emergency protocol.	11. Benzodiazepine is the drug of choice in controlling withdrawal symptoms. Neuroleptics cause hypotension and lower seizure threshold. Barbiturates may effectively control symptoms of withdrawal but have no advantages over benzodiazepines (Elliott et al., 2013). Several studies have demonstrated that phenytoin (Dilantin) is ineffective in the treatment of alcohol withdrawal seizures and the drug should not be used for this purpose (Hoffman & Weinhouse, 2015). Status epilepticus is life threatening if not controlled immediately with IV benzodiazepine.
12. Monitor and restore fluid and electrolyte balances.	12. Fluid and electrolyte losses from vomiting, profuse perspiration, and decreased antidiuretic hormone (from alcohol ingestion) cause dehydration. Increased neuromuscular activity can deplete magnesium and IV glucose administration can cause intracellular shift of magnesium (Grossman & Porth, 2014).
13. Monitor for hypoglycemia.	13. Alcohol depletes liver glycogen stores and impairs gluconeogenesis. Alcoholics are also malnourished (Grossman & Porth, 2014).
14. Monitor vital signs every 30 minutes initially.	14. Individuals in withdrawal will have elevated heart rate, respirations, and fever. Those experiencing DTs can be expected to have a low-grade fever. A rectal temperature greater than 99.9° F, however, is a clue to possible infection. Hypotension may be associated with pneumonia and a clue to infection (Grossman & Porth, 2014).
15. Monitor laboratory values: White blood cell (WBC) count, liver function studies, serum glucose, occult blood, albumin, prealbumin, serum alcohol level, electrolytes.	15. Laboratory values may indicate alcohol-related conditions. Alcohol abuse causes a range of immunopathologic events. In alcoholic liver disease, albumin is lowered because of decreased synthesis by liver and malnutrition (Grossman & Porth, 2014).
16. Observe for side effects or overmedication of benzodiazepine therapy: a. Oversedation b. Slurred speech c. Ataxia d. Nystagmus	16. All medications have a therapeutic window and are not without their side effects.
17. Maintain the individual IV, running continuously.	17. Necessary for fluid replacement, dextrose, thiamin bolus, benzodiazepine, and magnesium sulfate administrations. Chlordiazepoxide and diazepam should not be given intramuscularly because of unpredictable absorption (Elliott et al., 2013).

Documentation

Vital signs
Alcohol withdrawal symptoms

Nursing Diagnoses

Ineffective Denial Related to Acknowledgment of Alcohol Abuse or Dependency

NOC

Anxiety Level, Coping, Social Support, Substance Addiction Consequences, Knowledge: Substance Abuse Control, Knowledge: Disease Process

Goal

The individual will acknowledge an alcohol/drug abuse problem.

NIC

Coping Enhancement, Anxiety Reduction, Counseling, Mutual Goal Setting, Substance Abuse Treatment, Support System Enhancement, Support Group

Indicators

- Explain the psychological and physiologic effects of alcohol or drug use.
- Abstain from alcohol/drug use.

Interventions	*Rationales*

1. Assist in understanding addiction
  a. Be nonjudgmental. Explain addiction is a disorder with choices.
  b. Assist the individual to gain an intellectual understanding that this is an illness, not a moral problem.
  c. Have the individual identify triggers for their addiction. Discuss how to avoid.
  d. Provide opportunities to perform successfully; gradually increase responsibility.
  e. Provide educational information about the progressive nature
	1. Denial is a major response in people with addictions. It is the inability to accept one's loss of control over the addictive behavior or severity of the associated consequences (Boyd, 2012).

2. Help the individual to understand that alcoholism is an illness, not a moral problem. Explain that addiction "does not cure itself" and that it requires abstinence and treatment of the underlying issues (Halter, 2014).	2. Historically alcoholics have been viewed as immoral and degenerate. Acknowledgment of alcoholism as a disease can increase the individual's sense of trust.
3. Assist the individual to examine how drinking has affected relationships, work, and so on. Ask how he or she feels when not drinking.	3. During alcohol-related health problems, the individual may be more likely to acknowledge his or her drinking problem.

4. Separately, allow family members as individuals and a group to share pent-up feelings.
  a. Validate feelings as normal.
  b. Correct inaccurate beliefs.
	4. Alcoholism disturbs family communication. Sharing feelings is uncommon because of a history of disappointment. Diminished sharing and silence can maintain disturbed families for long periods. Communication focuses mainly on family members trying to control the other individual's drinking behavior (The National Council on Alcoholism and Drug Dependence [NCADD], 2016).

Interventions	Rationales
5. Emphasize that family members are not responsible for the individual's drinking (*Carson & Smith-DiJulio, 2006; *Starling & Martin, 1990). 　a. Explain that emotional difficulties are relationship-based rather than "psychiatric." 　b. Instruct that their feelings and experiences are associated frequently with family alcoholism.	5. "The potential value of reaching the alcoholic individual by first assisting family members should not be underestimated" (*Grisham & Estes, 1982, p. 257). The family and health care professional must accept that no certain outcome can be promised for the alcoholic, even when the family gets help (NCADD, 2016).
6. Assist the family to gain insight into behavior. Discuss ineffective methods families use such as: 　a. Hiding alcohol or car keys 　b. Anger, silence, threats, crying 　c. Making excuses for work, family, or friends 　d. Bailing the individual out of jail	
7. Explain how these behaviors do not stop drinking, increase family anger, remove the responsibility for drinking from the individual, and prevent the individual from suffering the consequences of his or her drinking behavior (*Smith-DiJulio, 2006).	7. Interventions focus on assisting the family to change their ineffective communication and response patterns (*Smith-DiJulio, 2006).
8. Emphasize that helping the alcoholic means first helping themselves. 　a. Focus on the effects of their response. 　b. Allow the individual to be responsible for his or her drinking behavior. 　c. Describe activities that will improve their lives, as individuals and a family. 　d. Initiate one stress management technique (e.g., aerobic exercise, assertiveness course, meditation).	8. Family members use denial to avoid admitting the problem and dealing with their contribution to it, and in the hope that the problem will disappear if not disclosed (*Collins, Leonard, & Searles, 1990).
9. Discuss with family that recovery will dramatically change usual family dynamics. 　a. The alcoholic is removed from the center of attention. 　b. All family roles will be challenged. 　c. Family members will have to focus on themselves instead of on the alcoholic individual. 　d. Family members will have to assume responsibility for their behavior, rather than blaming others. 　e. Behavioral problems of children serve a purpose for the family.	9. Ending the drinking behavior threatens the family integrity because the family functioning is centered around the alcoholism (Haber et al., 2010).
10. Initiate health teaching regarding community resources and referrals as indicated. 　a. Al-Anon 　b. Alcoholics anonymous family therapy 　c. Individual therapy 　d. Self-help groups	10. The family is the unit of treatment when one member is an alcoholic. Referrals are needed for long-term therapy.

Documentation

Dialogues

> **TRANSITION TO HOME/COMMUNITY CARE**
> If indicated, review the risk diagnoses identified for this individual on admission:
> * Is the person still at risk?
> * Can the family/reduce the risks?
> * Is the person at higher risk at home?
> * Is a home health nurse assessment needed?
> * Refer to transition planner/case manager/social service.
> * When is this person scheduled for follow-up with primary provider? Specialists? Record dates of appointments.
> * Complete a medication reconciliation prior to transition. Refer to inside back cover.

STAR **Stop**

Think   Is this person at risk for injury, falls, medical complications, and/or inability to care for self (activities of daily living)?

Is there a support person available?

Is the person competent to manage self-administration of medications, treatment procedures? Are additional resources needed?

Can the person explain how to monitor the condition (e.g., blood glucose, signs/symptoms of complications, dietary/mobility restrictions, and when to call his or her primary provider or specialist)?

Act   Contact or provide the appropriate resource (e.g., contacting a support person, home health assessment, additional teaching, printed materials).

Review Has the problem been addressed? If not, use SBAR to communicate to the appropriate person.

Risk for Ineffective Health Management Related to Insufficient Knowledge of Condition, Treatments Available, Risk Situations, and Community Resources

NOC

Compliance Behavior, Knowledge: Treatment Regimen, Participation in Health Care Decisions, Treatment Behavior: Illness or Injury

NIC

Substance Use Prevention, Substance Use Treatment, Behavior Modification, Support System Enhancement, Health System Guidance

Goals

The goals for this diagnosis represent those associated with transition planning. Refer to the transition criteria.

> **CLINICAL ALERT:** "Addiction is a family disease that stresses the family to the breaking point, impacts the stability of the home, the family's unity, mental health, physical health, finances, and overall family dynamics.
>
> Living with addiction can put family members under unusual stress. Normal routines are constantly being interrupted by unexpected or even frightening kinds of experiences that are part of living with alcohol and drug use. What is being said often doesn't match up with what family members sense, feel beneath the surface or see right in front of their eyes. The alcohol or drug user as well as family members may bend, manipulate and deny reality in their attempt to maintain a family order that they experience as gradually slipping away. The entire system becomes absorbed by a problem that is slowly spinning out of control. Little things become big and big things get minimized as pain is denied and slips out sideways" (NCADD, 2016).

Interventions	Rationales
1. Educate the individual regarding the disease of alcoholism and its effects on self, family, job, and finances: loss of control, social problems, legal problems, family problems, employment difficulties.	1. Acknowledging alcoholism's effects on one's life can motivate an individual to change behavior. It may be especially useful to do this after the person experiences the discomforts of withdrawal (Lander, Howsare, & Byrne, 2013).

Interventions	Rationales
2. Encourage open dialogue with all individuals in the family. Explore impact on children and extended family.	2. Encourage involved persons to share their feelings related to their experiences in the family is important as it helps them to break the silence so often associated with living with an substance use disorder and it can also increase their awareness about cognitive and behavioral patterns that contribute to the SUD (Lander et al., 2013).
3. Teach the individual to recognize and respond to the various alcohol-related medical conditions that are present.	3. Continued alcohol abuse will lead to varying alcohol-related medical conditions as described in the collaborative problems.
4. Provide treatment referrals for family, members (children, spouses, adult parents) where appropriate (Lander et al., 2013). a. Family therapy, couples therapy b. Play therapy, social skills training c. Parent training d. Psychiatric services	4. The disease of addiction prevents individuals from learning adaptive social and other coping skills.
5. Inform about AA, NA for the individual with an SUD and Al-Anon, Nar-Anon, Alateen for family members. Provide location and times of meetings in their area.	5. Family functioning and individuals is compromised from the disorder of alcoholism. Issues of individual family safety and well-being must be addresses.
6. If there are safety issues with regard to children or the elderly, Child Protective Services or Elder Protective Services referral may be needed.	
7. Ask questions about if the current living situation is physically safe or if there have been past or present incidences of domestic violence.	

Documentation

Referrals

Teaching

Immobility or Unconsciousness

A progressive mobility activity protocol (PMAP) is a nursing and interdisciplinary team approach to increase an individual's movement through a series of progressive steps from passive range of motion to ambulating independently as their medical stability increases (American Association of Critical Care Nurses, 2012; Hopkins & Spuhler, 2009).

"The act of lying down shifts 11% of the total blood volume away from the legs, with most going to the chest. Within the first 3 days of bed rest, an 8% to 10% reduction in plasma volume occurs, with the loss stabilizing to 15% to 20% by the fourth week. These changes result in increased cardiovascular workload, elevated resting heart rate, and a decrease in stroke volume with a reduction in cardiac output" (Vollman, 2012, p. 70). In 12 healthy older adults after 10 days of bed rest, deconditioning has a significant effect on the skeletal muscles used in standing and walking and has been linked to falls, functional decline, increased frailty, and immobility (Gillis, MacDonald, & MacIssac, 2008).

"Observation of 45 hospitalised medical patients indicated that, on average, 83% of the hospital stay was spent lying in bed. The amount of time spent standing or walked ranged from 0.2–21%. In several studies of missed nursing care, defined as required nursing care that is omitted or significantly delayed, ambulation of patients was identified as the most frequently missed element of inpatient nursing care, missed 76.1–88.7% of the time" (Kalisch, Lee, & Dabney, 2014).

Inexperienced intensive care unit (ICU) nurses may believe that increased mobility contributes to falls or disruption of equipment integrity (e.g., ventilators, parenteral therapy). A shift is needed in the culture that individuals in ICU on complete bed rest is not acceptable routine (Winkelman & Peereboom, 2010).

"Sarcopenia, a loss of muscle mass, can begin after only 2 days of bed rest, decreasing muscle strength by 1%–3% per day. One week of bed rest can result in a 20% decrease in muscle strength and an additional 20% muscle strength loss for each week on bed rest" (De Jonghe et al., 2007 cited in King, 2012).

Winkelman and Peereboom (2010) studied the perceived barriers and facilitators of ICU nurses to increase in-bed and out-of-bed movement. They reported the factor that facilitated success with in-bed or out-of-bed mobilization as

- The presence of a protocol in the institution, which guided decisions about readiness for increased activity
- Glasgow coma score greater than 10
- Beds that provided a chair position
- Prescriber's order
- Expert mentor (nurse, physical therapist)

Winkelman and Peereboom (2010) reported barriers as:

- Absence of the above facilitators
- Nurse's perception of the individual nonreadiness for increased activity
- Physical therapy is not consulted

This care plan addresses the needs of individuals who are immobile and either unconscious or conscious. All of these collaborative problems and nursing diagnoses can be found in other sections of this book. In addition to the following diagnostic cluster, refer to the specific coexisting medical disease or condition (e.g., renal failure and cancer).

DIAGNOSTIC CLUSTER

Collaborative Problems

▲ Risk for Complications of Pneumonia, Atelectasis (refer to Unit II)

▲ Risk for Complications of Fluid/Electrolyte Imbalance (refer to Unit II)

▲ Risk for Complications of Sepsis (refer to Unit II)

▲ Risk for Complications of Thrombophlebitis (refer to Unit II)

△ Risk for Complications of Renal Calculi (refer to Unit II)

Nursing Diagnoses

△ Disuse Syndrome related to effects of immobility on body systems (refer to Unit II)

▲ (Specify) Self-Care Deficit related to immobility (refer to Unit II)

△ Powerlessness related to feelings of loss of control and the restrictions placed on lifestyle (refer to Unit II)

▲ Risk for Pressure Ulcer related to mechanical destruction of tissue secondary to pressure, shear, and/or friction (refer to Unit II)

▲ Risk for Ineffective Airway Clearance related to stasis of secretions secondary to inadequate cough and decreased mobility (refer to Chronic Obstructive Pulmonary Disease Care Plan)

▲ Total Incontinence related to unconscious state (refer to Neurogenic Bladder Care Plan)

△ Risk for Impaired Oral Mucous Membrane related to immobility to perform own mouth care and pooling of secretions (refer to Unit II)

▲ This diagnosis was reported to be monitored for or managed frequently (75% to 100%).
△ This diagnosis was reported to be monitored for or managed often (50% to 74%).

Palliative Care

Both hospice care and palliative care have the same principles of comfort and support (National Cancer Institute [NCI], 2010). Hospice care is provided to individuals with terminal illness with a likelihood of dying in 6 months or less. Palliative care is offered earlier in the disease process than hospice care for someone with a life-threatening disease at the time of diagnosis or anytime throughout the course of illness. Hospice care is usually defined as "When cure is no longer realistic, the aim is to achieve the best death and dying process possible in the circumstances" (Australian Department of Health & Human Services [Australian DHHS], 2007a, p. 2).

In 2002, the World Health Organization (WHO) defined palliative care as " an approach that improves the quality of life of patients and their family facing the problems associated with life-threatening illness, through the prevention and relief of suffering by means of early identification and impeccable assessment and treatment of pain and other problems, physical, psychosocial and spiritual." Palliative care is a multidisciplinary medical specialty dedicated to the care of individuals with serious, life-threatening illnesses such as cancer, cardiac disease, chronic obstructive pulmonary disease (COPD), kidney failure, Alzheimer's, HIV/AIDS, and amyotrophic lateral sclerosis (ALS). The focus of palliative care is symptom management—relief from pain, shortness of breath, anxiety, fatigue, constipation, nausea, loss of appetite, and difficulty sleeping. The goal is to improve the quality of life for both the individual and the family. It is appropriate at any age and can be provided along with curative treatment at any stage of an illness. The goal is accomplished through interventions that maintain physical, social, and spiritual well-being; improve communication and coordination of care, and ensure culturally appropriate care that is consistent with the values and preferences of the individual. A holistic approach is necessary in palliative care to encompass the wide range of human responses to serious illness (Jacqueline Finerson, personal communication, September 2013; World Health Organization, 2016).

The Support Study's findings are as follows (*Support Study, 1995):

A 2-year prospective observational study "of 9,105 adults hospitalized with one or more of nine life-threatening diagnoses; and overall 6-month mortality rate of 47%, was designed to improve end-of-life decision making and reduce the frequency of a mechanically supported, painful, and prolonged process of dying."

"The phase I observation documented shortcomings in communication, frequency of aggressive treatment, and the characteristics of hospital death: only 47% of physicians knew when their patients preferred to avoid CPR; 46% of do-not-resuscitate (DNR) orders were written within 2 days of death; 38% of patients who died spent at least 10 days in an intensive care unit (ICU); and for 50% of conscious patients who died in hospital, family members reported moderate to severe pain at least half the time."

In phase II, "Physicians in the intervention group received estimates of the likelihood of 6-month survival for every day up to 6 months, outcomes of cardiopulmonary resuscitation (CPR), and functional disability at 2 months. A specially trained nurse had multiple contacts with the client, family, physician, and hospital staff/student to elicit preferences, improve understanding of outcomes, encourage attention to pain control, and facilitate advance care planning and client–physician communication."

"During the phase II intervention, patients experienced no improvement in client–physician communication (e.g., 37% of control patients and 40% of intervention patients discussed CPR preferences) or in the five targeted outcomes, i.e., incidence of timing of written DNR orders (adjusted ratio, 1.02; 95% confidence interval [CI], 0.90 to 1.15) physicians' knowledge of their patients' preferences not to be resuscitated (adjusted ratio, 1.22; 95% CI, 0.99 to 1.49), number of days spent in an ICU, receiving mechanical ventilation, or comatose before death (adjusted ratio, 0.97; 95% CI, 0.87 to 1.07), or level of reported pain (adjusted ratio, 1.15; 95% CI, 1.00 to 1.33). The intervention also did not reduce use of hospital resources (adjusted ratio, 1.05; 95% CI, 0.99 to 1.12)."

The researchers concluded "The phase I observation of SUPPORT confirmed substantial shortcomings in care for seriously ill hospitalized adults." The phase II intervention failed to improve care of client outcomes. Enhancing opportunities for more client–physician communication, although advocated as the major method for improving client outcomes, may be inadequate to change established practices. To improve the experience of seriously ill and dying patients, greater individual and societal commitment and more proactive and forceful measures may be needed.

Carp's Cues

Eighteen years later, how far have we come? A systematic analysis of the nursing literature (from 1996 to 2011) concerning the nurse's roles and strategies in end-of-life (EOL) decision making concluded with a promising trend (Adams et al., 2011). Nurses have three roles in EOL decision making: information brokers, supporters, and advocates. Of most significant, "whereas earlier literature indicated that nurses were involved in an indirect manner, recent literature indicates that nurses are more actively engaged as advocates in EOL decision making with both physicians and family members, challenging the status quo and helping all of the parties see the big picture" (Adams et al., 2011). The researchers reported that the "literature suggests that when nurses are actively engaged with family members by interpreting and explaining to them what is happening and explaining prognoses, family members are more satisfied and able to move forward in their acceptance and decision-making" (Adams et al., 2011). Through their roles as information brokers, supporters, and advocates, nurses were "a voice to speak up" (Baggs, 2007, p. 504) coaching, challenging, and arguing for individuals to have a "good death" (Adams et al., 2011).

In contrast, our physician colleagues have not progressed as well. Sixty percent of oncologists prefer to wait until there are no more treatments to give before they will discuss advanced medical directives, hospice care, or code status. Unfortunately, 50% of individuals with lung cancer, when referred to hospice, are within 2 months of their death (Huskamp et al., 2009). Physicians continue to hesitate to discuss poor prognostic outcomes and EOL issues with individuals and their families (Mack & Smith, 2012). Reasons given for their failure to disclose are that this information is depressing, takes away hope, unsure of prognosis, and that these discussions are difficult. The literature disputes all of these reasons except the last (Mack & Smith, 2012).

Physicians, especially specialists, have limited relationships with individuals and their families. Their time to disclose is limited and thus the encounter of disclosure, if it occurs, is often the individual/family listening, with little dialogue occurring.

Nurses have the privilege of having multiple opportunities to dialogue with individuals and their families. They know them. They can explore what and how much information the individual desires. Their presence as the physician discloses the diagnosis and prognosis can be very beneficial for all involved. Nurse expertise can lend support to physician colleagues, who do not have the nurses' expertise nor the time. Specialists are particularly vulnerable because of their limited relationship with the individual/family. With subsequent encounters, nurses can explore with individuals and families the meaning of this information and their perceptions of its impact on their lives. More discussions, feelings, and questions will surface and that is the goal: meaningful dialogue.

■■■■■ DIAGNOSTIC CLUSTER**

Collaborative Problems

Risk for Complications of Hypercalcemia

Risk for Complications of Delirium

Risk for Complications of Pleural Effusions

Risk for Complications of Opioid-Induced Side Effects Toxicity

Risk for Complications of Pathologic Fractures

Risk for Complications of Spinal Cord Compression

Risk for Complications of Superior Vena Cava Obstruction

Risk for Complications of Bowel Obstruction

Risk for Complications of End-Stage Medical Condition (e.g., CHF, COPD, AIDS, Renal Failure) (refer to the related care plan in index)

Risk for Complications of Chemotherapy (refer to Chemotherapy Care Plan)

Risk for Complications of Radiation Therapy (refer to Radiation Therapy Care Plan)

Nursing Diagnoses

Risk for Compromised Human Dignity related to multiple factors associated with end-of-life treatments and decision making
Altered Comfort related to breathlessness (e.g., pleural effusion, severe anemia, agitation) or pruritus (e.g., liver failure, skin problems)
Death Anxiety related to (specify the unknown, uncertainty, fears, conflicts, suffering, and the impact on others as perceived by the individual and significant others)
Anticipatory Grieving related to losses associated with illness, disabilities and impending death and their effects on loved ones
Acute/Chronic Pain related to disease process (refer to Unit II)
Constipation related to the effects of disease and/or opioids on intestinal function, inactivity, and/or low fiber intake (refer to Unit II)
Nausea/Vomiting related to the effects of medications and disease process (refer to Unit II)
Fatigue related to the effects of disease activity, complications, nausea, anemia, and the presence of comorbidities (refer to Unit II)
Risk for Disturbed Sleep Patterns related to multiple factors/discomforts (refer to Unit II)
Acute Confusion related to (e.g., fever, infection, electrolyte disturbances, dehydration) (refer to Unit II)
Risk for Caregiver Role Strain related to multiple care responsibilities and to caregivers stress and sorrow (refer to Unit II).
Risk for Spiritual Distress related to challenge to spiritual beliefs secondary to terminal illness (refer to Unit II)
Risk for Ineffective Health Management related insufficient knowledge of actions needed for exacerbated symptoms or sudden onset of new symptoms, home management, resources available

**This medical condition was not included in the validation study.

Transition Criteria

Before transition, the individual or family will:

1. Report a reduction in symptom(s) as (specify)
2. Describe his or her personal wishes/decisions
3. Reports an increase in family interactions
4. Plan for transition to establish care in a new setting if anticipated
5. Report the acceptable level of burden from symptom(s) as (specify)

Transitional Risk Assessment Plan (TRAP)

Begin this plan on admission.
Implement the Transitional Risk Assessment Plan (TRAP):
- Refer to inside back cover.
- Add each validated risk diagnosis to individual's problem list with the risk code in ( ).
- Refer to Unit II to the individual risk nursing diagnoses/collaborative problems for outcomes and interventions.

  R: "Close coordination of care in the post-acute period, early transition follow-up care, enhanced client education and self-management training, proactive end-of-life counseling, and extending the resources and clinical expertise over time via multidisciplinary team management" can lower readmission rates and improve health outcomes (Boutwell & Hwu, 2009, p. 14). Interventions are utilized to activate the individual and family to select changes in their everyday lifestyle choices to improve their health (Hibbard & Greene, 2013).

Collaborative Problems

Risk for Complications of Hypercalcemia

Risk for Complications of Delirium

Risk for Complications of Pleural Effusions

Risk for Complications of Ascites

Risk for Complications of Opioid-Induced Side Effects Toxicity

Risk for Complications of Pathologic Fractures

Risk for Complications of Spinal Cord Compression

Risk for Complications of Superior Vena Cava Obstruction

Risk for Complications of Bowel Obstruction

Collaborative Outcomes

The individual will be monitored for early signs and symptoms of (a) hypercalcemia, (b) delirium, (c) malignant effusions (pleural ascites pericardial), (d) opioid-induced side effects, (e) pathologic fractures, (f) spinal cord compression, (g) superior vena cava syndrome, and (h) bowel obstruction, and will receive collaborative interventions if indicated to restore physiologic stability.

Indicators of Physiologic Stability[8]

- Alert, oriented (a, b, d, g)
- No new onset of a change or fluctuations of impairments in attention span, cognition, concentration, alertness, and/or consciousness (a, c, f)
- EKG: Normal sinus rhythm (a)
- No seizures (a)
- No new onset nausea or vomiting (a, h)
- No new onset constipation (a, h)
- Pulse 60 to 100 beats/min (b, d)
- Respirations 16 to 20 breaths/min (b, d)
- No complaints of breathlessness (c, d)
- No pleuritic pain (b)
- Full breath sounds in all quadrants (b, c)
- No increase in abdominal girth (c)
- No visual or conjunctival changes (g)
- No hoarseness or stridor (g)
- No bone pain (e)
- No new complaints of band of pain encircling body (f)
- No new complaints of stiffness, tingling, numbness (f)
- No new complaints of retention/incontinence (f)
- Normal bowel movements (f, h)
- No venous distention (c, g)
- Serum magnesium 1.3 to 2.4 mEq/L (c)
- Serum sodium 135 to 145 mEq/L (c)
- Serum potassium 3.8 to 5 mEq/L (c)
- Corrected serum calcium <2.6 mmol/L (a)
- Serum albumin 3.5 to 5 g/dL (c)
- Serum prealbumin 20 to 50 g/dL (c)
- Serum protein 6 to 8 g/dL (c)
- Partial thromboplastin time (PTT) 20 to 45 seconds (c)

---

[8]These indicators take on a different significance as the individual progresses to end-stage disease and death.

- Hemoglobin (c)
  - Male: 13 to 18 g/dL
  - Female: 12 to 16 g/dL
- Hematocrit (c)
  - Male: 42% to 50%
  - Female: 40% to 48%
- Platelets 100,000 to 400,000/mm^3 (c)

Interventions	Rationales

CLINICAL ALERT:
- Emergencies in palliative care, when death is expected, are different from those in other medical situations, when if left untreated will immediately threaten life.
- In palliative care, if the condition left untreated seriously threatens the quality of remaining life, interventions may be indicated.
- Discussions regarding options available must be initiated by the physician/nurse practitioner with the ill individual/or significant others prior to occurrences.

1. Monitor for medication-induced side effects (Dahlin, 2013):
   a. Risk for complication of opioid-induced side effects:
      - Sedation
      - Nausea/vomiting
      - Constipation
      - Delirium
      - Hyperalgesia
      - Urinary retention
      - Seizures
      - Respiratory depression
      - Hallucinations
      - Myoclonus
      - Pruritus
   b. Consult physician/nurse practitioner for differential diagnoses and if indicated management of opioid administration. Consult with pain management if indicated.

1. Some intervention options are changing the route of administration, reducing the systemic dose; add a non-opioid analgesic, regional analgesia/anesthesia (Cherney et al., 2001).

   Avoid polypharmacy, experience on drug–drug interactions concerning opioids are limited (Kotlinska-Lemieszek, Klepstad, & Haugen, 2015)

2. Explain palliative sedation to individual and/or significant others (e.g., prevalent indications for sedation were dyspnea and/or delirium).
   a. Statement on palliative sedation (*American Association of Hospice and Palliative Care Medicine, 2006):
      - Palliative care seeks to relieve suffering associated with disease. Unfortunately, not all symptoms associated with advanced illness can be controlled with pharmacologic or other interventions. Individuals need and deserve assurance that suffering will be effectively addressed, as both the fear of severe suffering and the suffering itself add to the burden of terminal illness.
      - Ordinary sedation: The ordinary use of sedative medications for the treatment of anxiety, agitated depression, insomnia, or related disorders, in which the goal of treatment is the relief of the symptom without reducing the individual's level of consciousness.

2. "Palliative sedation, when appropriately indicated and correctly used to relieve unbearable suffering, does not seem to have any detrimental effect on survival of individuals with terminal cancer. In this setting, palliative sedation is a medical intervention that must be considered as part of a continuum of palliative care" (Maltoni, Scarpi, Rosati, Derni, & Fabbri, 2012, p. 1378). Controlled sedation is successful in dying individuals with untreatable symptoms, did not hasten death, and yielded satisfactory results for relatives.

(continued)

Interventions	Rationales
• Palliative sedation: The use of sedative medication at least in part to reduce individual awareness of distressing symptoms that are insufficiently controlled by symptom-specific therapies. The level of sedation is proportionate to the individual's level of distress, and alertness is preserved as much as possible. • Palliative sedation to unconsciousness: The administration of sedatives to the point of unconsciousness, when less extreme sedation has not achieved sufficient relief of distressing symptoms. This practice is used only for the most severe, intractable suffering at the very end of life.	

Carp's Cues

The fact that dying people require symptom relief does not mean that symptom relief causes death. Studies demonstrate that symptom relief near death does not hasten death (Maltoni et al., 2012; Mercadante, Intravaia, Ferrera, Villari, & David, 2009). To the contrary, untreated symptoms such as pain, stress, and anxiety lead to worsening strain and exhaustion in individuals and family members alike. Intractable pain itself, in fact, may hasten death.

Health care providers have a responsibility to do no harm and to relieve suffering. This is as true with palliative sedation as with any other aspect of medical treatment. In the United States, Supreme Court rulings (*Vacco v. Quill*, 1997; *Washington v. Glucksberg*, 1997) supported the concept of sedation when used to relieve intractable suffering.

Interventions	Rationales
3. Monitor for calcium levels and for signs and symptoms of hypercalcemia:	3. Severe hypercalcemia is life threatening. Hypercalcemia is the most common life-threatening metabolic complication occurring in an estimated 20% to 30% of all adults with cancer, with an incidence of 40% to 50% with breast cancer and malignant myeloma (Horwitz, 2012). These symptoms accompany mild hypercalcemia. They are distressing to the individuals and carers. Treatment can improve remaining quality of life even when time is limited if desired (Australian DHHS, 2007b).
a. Corrected serum calcium level range 2.10 to 2.55 b. Nausea c. Anorexia and vomiting d. Constipation e. Thirst, polyuria f. Altered mental status, confusion > coma g. Arrhythmias (shortened QT interval and widened T wave) h. Numbness or tingling in fingers and toes i. Severe dehydration	a. Serum calcium >2.6 is diagnostic. Mild hypercalcemia <3 mmol/L is usually asymptomatic.
4. If the decision is made to treat hypercalcemia, rehydration with intravenous fluids will be initiated and possibly bisphosphonate infusion. Following bisphosphonate infusions, the serum calcium will fluctuate up and down giving an unreliable reading until 48 hours after infusion (Australian DHHS, 2007b).	4. Bisphosphonate inhibits osteoclast resorption and thus reduces the amount of serum calcium (Grossman & Porth, 2014).

Interventions	Rationales

5. Monitor for signs and symptoms of pleural effusion:
  a. Dyspnea
  b. Cough
  c. Chest pain
  d. Decreased breath sounds
	5. A pleural effusion may be caused by cancer of lung, breast, lymphoma, and leukemia, or by cancer treatments such as radiation and chemotherapy. Some individuals with cancer have other conditions that can cause pleural effusion such as congestive heart failure, pneumonia, pulmonary embolus, and malnutrition.

6. Notify physician/nurse practitioner for an evaluation of symptoms (e.g., chest X-ray, CT scan). If the decision is made to treat pleural effusion, for example, thoracentesis will be initiated.	6. Removal of the fluid may help to relieve severe symptoms for a short time.

7. Monitor for signs and symptoms of ascites:
  a. Abdominal distension
  b. Discomfort
  c. Shortness of breath
  d. Diminished appetite
  e. Fatigue
  f. Nausea
  g. Pain
  h. Immobility
  i. Lower extremity oedema
	7. Refractory ascites is common in individuals with end-stage malignancy. It has been suggested that about 50% of individuals with cancer have malignant ascites (Ayantunde & Parsons 2007; *Rosenberg, 2006). Prognosis is mainly determined by the origin of the primary cancer especially, individuals with ovarian, endometrial, breast, and gastrointestinal are at risk of developing ascites (*Rosenberg, 2006; Walton & Nottingham 2007).
	
	When symptomatic relief is not achieved by causal cancer management, paracentesis is performed frequently. This procedure provides relief in up to 90% of individuals and has a low complication rate. However, it frequently requires multiple procedures, often in an outpatient hospital setting. Permanent percutaneous drainage of refractory malignant ascites is a safe and satisfying intervention which enables individuals to drain ascites before symptoms worsen (Courtney et al., 2008; Mercadante et al., 2008; *O'Neill, Weissleder, Gervais, Hahn, & Mueller, 2001).

8. Monitor for signs and symptoms of pathologic fracture:
  a. Localized pain that becomes continuous and unrelenting
  b. Visible bone deformity
  c. Crepitation on movement
  d. Loss of movement or use
  e. Localized soft tissue edema
  f. Skin discoloration
  g. Tenderness to percussion over involved spine
	8. Pathologic fractures can be caused by any type of bone tumor, but the majority of pathologic fractures in the elderly are secondary to metastatic carcinomas. Metastatic cancer deposits in the proximal femur may weaken the bone and cause a pathologic hip fracture. Bones most susceptible to tumor invasion are those with the greatest bone marrow activity and blood flow—the vertebrae, pelvis, ribs, skull, and sternum. The most common sites for long-bone metastasis are the femur and humerus (*Lindqvist, Widmarkt, & Rasmussen, 2006).

9. Maintain alignment and immobilize the site if fracture is suspected.	9. Immobilization helps reduce soft tissue damage from dislocations.
10. Notify physician/nurse practitioner for evaluation of possible fracture (e.g., X-ray and treatment).	10. The goal of treatment of impending or pathologic fracture is to provide pain relief and a functionally stable immobilization device.

11. Monitor for signs and symptoms of spinal cord compression (SCC):
 	
  a. Back pain
    • Localized at first
    • Described as belt-like pain at the level of the compression
    • Worse when lying down, coughing, sneezing, or moving
	11. SCC occurs when a spinal cord tumor or metastatic tumor grows in the spine and destroys the bony vertebral body that surrounds the cord, or wraps around the spinal cord and its nerve roots. This can cause the vertebral body to collapse and compress the spinal cord.
	  a. The most common area for spinal cord metastases is the thoracic spine (70%). Back pain is caused by irritation of the nerve roots by the tumor.

(continued)

Interventions	*Rationales*
b. Neurologic symptoms: • Complaints of muscle weakness, heaviness or stiffness of limbs • Change in gait • Change in or loss of sensation (e.g., numbness and tingling) • Change in bowel or urinary habits (e.g., constipation or inability to urinate)	b. If untreated, SCC may progress to cause serious neurologic problems such as paralysis. Fewer than 25% of people who are paralyzed at the time they are diagnosed with SCC will regain their ability to walk after treatment.
12. Notify physician/nurse practitioner for an evaluation of possible SCC (e.g., imaging tests [X-rays, MRI, or myelogram]) and treatment (e.g., steroids, palliative chemotherapy, radiation).	12. Goals of treatment are to relieve compression, which will reduce or control pain, and to stabilize the spine. Individuals in final stage of terminal illness will likely have corticosteroid therapy.
13. Monitor for signs and symptoms of superior vena cava obstruction (SVCO) (Nickloes, 2012): a. Early signs: • Facial, trunk, upper extremity edema • Pronounced venous pattern on trunk • Shortness of breath b. Late signs: • Hoarseness, stridor • Engorged conjunctiva, visual disturbances • Headache, dizziness • Decreased cardiac output • Flushed edematous face • Tachypnea, orthopnea c. Raise the head of the bed	13. The most common cause of superior vena cava syndrome is cancer. Primary or metastatic cancer in the upper lobe of the right lung can compress the superior vena cava. Lymphoma or other tumors located in the mediastinum can also cause compression of the superior vena cava. a. These symptoms are caused by the inability of the blood to return to the heart. b. SVCO occurs when the superior vena cava becomes occluded by a tumor or thrombus. Commonly associated with lung cancer, breast cancer, and lymphomas, SVCS causes impaired venous return from the head and upper extremities, resulting in upper body edema and prominent collateral circulation (Nickloes, 2012). c. Individuals with clinical superior vena cava syndrome (SVCO) can have significant symptomatic improvement with elevation of the head of the bed and supplemental oxygen (Nickloes, 2012).
14. Notify physician/nurse practitioner for an evaluation of possible SVCO (e.g., imaging tests [X-rays, MRI, or myelogram]) and treatment (e.g., steroids, palliative chemotherapy, radiation) (Nickloes, 2012).	14. Goals of treatment are to relieve compression, which will reduce or control pain, and to stabilize the spine. Individuals in final stage of terminal illness will likely have corticosteroid therapy.
15. Explain palliative chemotherapy (Weissman, 2009).	15. Palliative chemotherapy can shrink cancer tumors and improve or eliminate distressing symptoms for a period of time, such as dyspnea, pain.
16. Ensure that the individual/family understand the median duration of response. If not, access oncologist for this information (Bruera, 2012).	16. The median duration of response is how long the individual's cancer can be expected to respond to chemotherapy. The number ranges from 3 to 12 months. Individuals and family need this information to evaluate if the benefits outweigh the side effects of chemotherapy (Bruera, 2012).

Clinical Alert Report

Prior to providing care, advise ancillary staff/student to report the following to the professional nurse assigned to the individual:

* Change in cognitive status
* Oral temperature >100.5° F
* Systolic BP <90 mm Hg
* Resting pulse >100, <50 beats/min
* Respiratory rate >28, <10 breaths/min
* Complaints of new onset:
  * Back pain
  * Numbness
  * Edema
  * Shortness of breath
  * Localized bone pain
  * Inability to defecate, urinate

Nursing Diagnoses

Risk for Compromised Human Dignity Related to Potential Barriers to a Peaceful End-of-Life Transition

 Carp's Cues

Determine if the agency has a policy for prevention of compromised human dignity. This type of policy or standard may be titled differently. Agency policies can assist the nurse when problematic situations occur; however, the moral obligation to protect and defend the dignity of individuals or groups does not depend on the existence of a policy.

NOC

Abuse Protection, Comfort Level, Knowledge: Illness Care, Self-Esteem, Dignified Dying, Spiritual Well-Being, Information Processing

Goal

The individual/significant others will report respectful and considerate care according to their EOL wishes.

NIC

Individual Rights Protection, Anticipatory Guidance, Counseling, Emotional Support, Preparatory Sensory Information, Family Support, Humor, Mutual Goal Setting, and Teaching: Procedure/ Treatment, Touch

Indicators

* Respect for privacy
* Facilitate shared decision-making process
* Priority to individual's or designated surrogate decision maker requests/decisions
* Clear, accurate, timely explanations with options
* Optimal control of distressful symptoms

 Carp's Cues

The ANA's (2010a) position statement on *Registered Nurses' Roles and Responsibilities in providing Expert Care and Counseling at the End of Life* states:

"Nurses are leaders and vigilant advocates for the delivery of dignified and humane care. Nurses actively participate in assessing and assuring the responsible and appropriate use of interventions in order to minimize unwarranted or unwanted treatment and patient suffering" (ANA, 2010a, pp. 7–8). "Nursing interventions are intended to produce beneficial effects, contribute to quality outcomes, *and—above all—do no harm*" (ANA, 2010b, p. 15).

Do not participate in lying, do not ignore it for any reason, and if what you are witnessing is just wrong, speak up.

Interventions	*Rationales*

1. Determine and accept your own moral responsibility. Be "a voice to speak up" (Bach, Plooeg, & Black, 2009, p. 504).
  a. If the nurse is a student or inexperienced in navigating the issues and potential conflicts in providing care to individuals/significant others, consultation with a nurse competent with EOL conflicts is imperative.
  b. Attempts to go it alone can be responsible for interventions/interactions that are problematic and even worse than harmful to individuals and significant others.
	1. Nurses have reported feelings of powerlessness within the work environment because of not addressing unacceptable care conditions and their own moral distress (*Hamric, 2000).

2. Provide care to each individual and family as you would expect or demand for your family, partner, child, friend, or colleague.	2. Setting this personal standard can spur you to defend the individual/group, especially when they do not belong to the same socioeconomic group as you.
3. Explore "how well the client and family understand the patient's relevant medical conditions and what their expectations, hopes, and concerns are."	3. "This listening phase can provide insight into the patient's values and goals and how much the patient and family want to engage in these discussions."
4. Allow the individual an opportunity to share his or her feelings after a difficult situation and maintain privacy for the individual's information and emotional responses.	4. Allowing the individual to share his or her feelings can help him or her maintain or regain dignity. Recognition of the individual as a living, thinking, and experiencing human being enhances dignity (*Walsh & Kowanko, 2002).

5. Advocate for the individual/family with their physician/nurse practitioner before conflicts arise:
  a. Elicit the individual's and/or family's perception of the situation
  b. Explore everyone's expectations.
  c. Explore if the individual's and/or family's expectations are realistic.
  d. Offer your observations of the individual/family understanding of the situation to involved health care professionals (e.g., manager, nurse colleagues, physicians, nurse practitioners).
	5. Being less than truthful and/or unrealistic is a barrier to providing appropriate care and eventually a "good death" (*Beckstrand, Callsiter, & Kirchhoff, 2006).

6. Seek to accompany the physician/nurse practitioner when he or she is going to disclose the diagnosis, prognosis, and/or treatment plan.	6. Knowing exactly what the individual/family has been told will help the nurse continue dialogue and to provide clarity when questions arise.

7. Explore with individual and family what their understanding of the situation is:
  a. What did your physician/nurse practitioner tell you?
  b. Is there anything else that you want to know?
  c. Does the family want to restrict information to the individual?
  d. If needed, instruct individual or family to write down specific questions for physician/nurse practitioner.
	7. Individuals have the right to access as much or as little information that they can manage at this time. Individuals will vary regarding how much information they desire. Despite what the nurse believes an individual should know, all discussions regarding diagnosis and prognosis must be carefully approached.
	  Some individuals do not want to know their prognosis. Some are overwhelmed with the information and cannot cope with the reality at the present time.

Interventions	Rationales

8. If the individual is in the last stages of EOL, engage in a dialogue with the individual and family separately regarding their assumptions of the individual's prognosis (*Murray, Boyd, & Sheikh, 2005).
  a. Consider how the individual and/or significant others would respond to the following theoretical questions:
    • If death is approaching, would they be surprised if the individual were to die in a few hours or days?
    • If death is not imminent but expected, would they be surprised if the individual were to die in 6 months, a year?
  b. If their actions/discussions indicate that they are unaware or unable to deal with the EOL reality, consult with an expert nurse and/or specialist in ethics for assistance.
	8. Survival estimates are not viewed with an emphasis of when someone will die, but instead to provide information to allow all involved to be aware of the transition as needed as the individual deteriorates. The process of dying has many uncertainties and is unstable with the individual's condition oscillating from day to day with eventual deterioration.

9. Avoid giving a specific time for the expected time of death. "It is helpful to give a range of time, such as 'hours to days,' 'days to weeks' or 'weeks to months'" (Yarbro, Wujeck, & Gobel, 2011, p. 1836).	9. Family members and friends will be able to better plan their time spent with their loved one with this information (Yarbro et al., 2011).

10. Develop strategies to transition individuals from acute care to palliative care. Explain the difference between acute care and palliative care. Address:
  a. Change for a focus from curing to caring
    • The focus of care must be solely to relieve suffering. Painful treatments to prolong dying are inhumane and unethical.
    • "Appropriately negotiated treatment abatement and symptom relief does not constitute causing death" (Australian DHHS, 2007a, p. 2).
    • "By working in harmony of the reality of the situation, health care professionals can improve the journey considerably, but failure to recognize the dying process can make it worse, and prevent the timely deployment of appropriate palliative care" (Australian DHHS, 2007a, p. 2).
    • "The best possible pain and symptom relief in the clinical circumstances is both the patient's right and the clinician's duty" (Australian DHHS, 2010a, p. 2).
	10. "Neither patients nor persons responsible can insist on treatment that is futile and therefore medically contraindicated in the circumstances, nor can they insist on actions that are illegal or contrary to professional ethics" (Australian DHHS, 2007a, p. 3).

11. Access physician/nurse practitioner to discuss the options for treatment. Emphasize that the persons involved in the decision making (individuals, significant others) can change their minds anytime.	11. The options for the treatment plan must be discussed with the benefits and hazards of each option. If the individual is capable of decision making, his or her wishes are priority. If not capable, the designated decision making should honor what the individual would choose if he or she could.
12. Ensure that all members of the health care team understand the individual/significant others decisions. Document clearly. Alert the next nurse at the handover.	12. In the moment of an emergency, panic can cause undesirable decisions that create only more pain and suffering.
13. Enlist the services of hospice when indicated.	13. Hospice organizations have the expertise and resources for palliative care.

14. Seek if possible to transfer individual out of the ICU and out of the hospital.
  a. If feasible, plan to transition or transfer the individual out of the hospital.
  b. Explore the Going Home Initiative at Baystate Medical Center, Springfield, Massachusetts (Lusardi et al., 2011).
	14. ICU environments have many barriers to a palliative care environment (e.g., noise, frequent interruptions, close quarters, futile treatments).

(continued)

Interventions	Rationales
15. When extreme measures that are futile are planned or are being provided for an individual, initiate STAR:	15. "Extreme measures, when futile, are an infringement of the basic respect for the dignity innate in being a person" (*Walsh & Kowanko, 2002, p. 146). "Practice expecting that honoring and protecting the dignity of individual/groups is not a value but a way of being" (*Söderberg, Gilje, & Norberg, 1998).

STAR   **Stop**

     Think   Is this situation wrong

     Act   Discuss situation with instructor/ another nurse/manager/physician/ nurse practitioner using SBAR

     SBAR

       Situation: Invasive treatments, increased pain, no improvement

       Backgound: Terminal status, previous treatments

       Assessment: Individual's desire to stop present treatments. Family "wants to try everything."

       Recommendation: Family conference with nurse, physician/nurse practitioner, and/or ethics consultant to discuss the situation (futility, pain) vs. palliative care

     Review

Interventions	Rationales
16. Discuss with involved personnel an incident that was disrespectful to an individual or family. Report any incident that may be a violation of an individual's dignity to the appropriate person.	16. Professionals have a responsibility to practice ethically and morally and to address situations and personnel that compromise human dignity.
17. Advocate for EOL decision dialogues with all individuals and their families and your friends and relatives, especially when the situation is not critical. Direct them to create written documents of their decisions and to advise family of the document.	17. Exploring EOL decisions when there are no imminent threats to survival provide the most optimal setting for discussions. Decisions that are viewed as well-thought-out may assist the family with honoring their loved one's decision.

> ### Clinical Alert Report
> Advise ancillary staff/student to report any questions or concerns that the individual/family ask in regard to condition, prognosis, treatments immediately.

Documentation

Significant discussions

Incident report, if indicated for unacceptable staff/student behavior.

Impaired Comfort Related to Episodes of Breathlessness, Agitation, and/or Pruritus

NOC

Symptom Control;
Comfort Status,
Dignified Life Closure,
Personal Autonomy

Goal

The individual/significant others will report preservation of individual dignity, comfort, and safety and a reduction of stress and distress in individual/significant others.

NIC

Symptom Management,
Pruritus Management,
Fever Treatment,
Environmental
Management: Comfort,
Dying Care

Indicators

- Modification of agitation and aggressive behaviors
- Improvement in sleep quality
- Reduction in anxiety in individual/significant others

Interventions	Rationales
1. Assess for sources of discomfort: a. Pruritus > Refer to Cirrhosis Care Plan b. Breathlessness c. Delirium (hypoactive/hyperactive [agitation])	

2. For breathlessness, ensure that the individual's breathlessness has been fully evaluated, if indicated:
a. Provide interventions to reduce breathlessness, acknowledge fears (Australian DHHS, 2007c).
• Sit individual up, avoid abdominal or chest compressions, avoid restrictive clothing.
• Provide cool airflow over face (e.g., fan).
• Teach controlled diaphragmatic breathing.
• Engage in distractions that are enjoyed (e.g., music, company, massage).
b. Evaluate if supplemental oxygen is beneficial with a trial. Evaluate the risks versus benefits (Australian DHHS, 2007c)
• Benefits: Individuals with oxygen saturation <90% may have benefit.
• Adverse effects
  • Dependency on equipment can increase anxiety if equipment problems occur.
  • Initially perceived benefits can be placebo and when this effect diminishes, anxiety can increase.
  • Causes nasal dryness, crusting, bleeding, trauma to nares
  • Irritates upper airways > cough
  • Increases risk for tripping/falls (tether line)
  • Noisy day and night
c. Consult with physician/nurse practitioner for pharmacologic management (e.g., opioids, antianxiety, dexamethasone).
	2. Some causes of breathlessness such as pain, anxiety, infection, pleural effusion, airway obstruction, and anemia may be corrected.
	
	b. Supplemental oxygen is often used to quickly solve episodes of breathlessness. It is thought to be benign, when in fact it comes with risks. Individuals with COPD will benefit: while individuals with cancer probably will not.
	
	c. Certain medications can reduce the perception of dyspnea.

Interventions	*Rationales*
3. For delirium (agitation): "When deciding whether to investigate and treat underlying causes if present consider if this would be" (Australian DHHS, 2007d, p. 4): a. Appropriate to the goals of care and stage of illness b. Realistic and reasonably likely to be achievable c. Likely to improve quality of life d. Overly burdensome e. Consistent with individual's understanding and wishes/advances directives f. If indicated, ensure that hyperactive behavior has been fully evaluated.	 f. Some causes of hyperactive behavior are treatable as sleep deprivation, nicotine withdrawal, multiple medications, hypercalcemia, infection, oversedation, pain, constipation, urinary retention, and drug/alcohol withdrawal.
g. Provide interventions to reduce agitation, acknowledge fears of significant others (Australian DHHS, 2007d). • Attempt to keep immediate environment familiar. • Encourage familiar objects (e.g., pictures). • Reduce unnecessary noise/stimulation (e.g., loud talking, disturbing TV shows). • Approach individual slowly in a quiet voice. Reorient individual with each encounter. • Use simple, brief sentences. • Ensure frequent rest periods. h. Allow significant others to express their fears and concerns. i. Consult with physician/nurse practitioner for pharmacologic management (e.g., opioids, antianxiety, dexamethasone).	g. Interventions should focus on calming the environment to reduce stressors. h. Witnessing confusion/agitation in a loved one is one of the most distressing situations. i. Certain medications can reduce the perception of dyspnea.

Clinical Alert Report

Advise ancillary staff/student to report:

• Any questions or concerns that the individual/family ask in regard to condition, prognosis, treatments immediately
• Increase/decrease in activity
• Change in cognition

Documentation

Exacerbation of symptoms
Interventions
Response

Death Anxiety Related to (Specify the Unknown, Uncertainty, Fears, Conflicts, Suffering and the Impact on Others as Perceived by the Individual and Significant Others)

NOC

Dignified Life Closure, Fear Self-Control, Individual Satisfaction, Decision Making, Family Coping

Goal

The individual will report or show diminished anxiety or fear.

NIC

Limit Setting, Individual
Rights Protection,
Family Support,
Dying Care, Coping
Enhancement, Active
Listening, Emotional
Support, Spiritual
Support

Indicators

- Share feelings regarding dying.
- Identify specific requests that will increase psychological comfort.

Interventions	Rationales

1. For an individual with a new or early diagnosis of a potentially terminal condition:
  a. Allow the individual and family separate opportunities to discuss their understanding of the condition. Correct misinformation.
  b. Access valid information regarding condition, treatment options, and stage of condition from primary provider (physician, nurse practitioner).
  c. Ensure a discussion of the prognosis if known.
	1. With a diagnosis of a potential terminal illness, individuals and families should be given opportunities to talk about treatments, cures, and goals regarding quality of life (e.g., curative vs. symptomatic comfort care).

2. For the individual experiencing a progression of a terminal illness:
  a. Explore with the individual his or her understanding of the situation and feelings.
 	
  b. Ensure that the primary physician or nurse practitioner initiate a discussion regarding the situation and options desired by the individual.
 	
  c. Discuss with family and individual palliative care and strategies that can be used for dyspnea, pain, and other discomforts (Yabro et al., 2011).
 	
  d. Elicit from the individual and individual's family specific requests for EOL care.
	2a. It is important to determine the individual's understanding of the situation and personal preferences or requests.
	  b. These discussions provide insight into the individual's understanding and directs treatment decisions. Research reports that only 31% of persons with terminal conditions reported EOL discussions with a physician (Wright, Wood, Lynch, & Clark, 2008).
	  c. During the final stage of life, anxiety for the individual and family is highly correlated with the presence or fear of other symptoms such as dyspnea, pain, and fear of the unknown (Yabro et al., 2011).
	  d. Persons with advanced cancer identified their priorities as protection of dignity, sense of control, pain control, inappropriate prolongation of dying, and strengthening relationships (*Singer et al., 1999; Volker, 2004).
	  e. According to Ellershaw and Wilkinson (*2003), possible signs and symptoms of a disturbed dying in individuals are expressions of agitation or fear, loss of dignity, and expressions of concerns about sharing the dying phase with relatives. Relatives may complain about exhaustion or express their concerns about the relief of symptoms.

3. Provide opportunities for the person to discuss EOL decisions. Be direct and empathetic.	3. Clover, Carter, and Whyte. (*2004) found that a person's readiness to participate in EOL decisions depends on the skills of the professional nurse to encourage the individual to share his or her wishes.

(continued)

Interventions	*Rationales*
4. Encourage the individual to reconstruct his or her worldview: 　a. Allow the individual to verbalize feelings about the meaning of death. 　b. Advise the individual that there are no right or wrong feelings. 　c. Advise the individual that responses are his or her choice. 　d. Acknowledge struggles. 　e. Encourage dialogue with a spiritual mentor or trusted friend.	4. When an individual is facing death, reconstructing a world view involves balancing thoughts about the painful subject with avoiding painful thoughts.
5. Allow significant others opportunities to share their perceptions and concerns. Advise them that sadness is expected and normal.	5. Clarification is needed to determine if their concerns regarding EOL care is consistent with the individual. "It is normal and healthy to feel sad at the end of life, to grieve the impending loss of everything a person holds dear" (Coombs-Lee, 2014, p. 12).
6. Encourage difficult but truthful conversations (e.g., sorrow, mistakes, disagreements). 　a. Use questions or statements to encourage expression of thoughts, feelings, and concerns; for example, tell: "I see it's difficult for you" (facilitate open communication to promote sharing). 　b. Use silence/listening to encourage the expression of feelings, thoughts, and concerns. 　c. Be a listener for the relatives by spending designated time.	6. "Avoiding truthful conversations does not bring hope and comfort: it brings isolation and loneliness" (Coombs-Lee, 2014, p. 12).
7. To foster psycho-spiritual growth, open dialogue with the individual specifically (*Yakimo, Kurlowicz, & Murray, 2004, p. 700): 　a. If your time is indeed shortened, what do you need to get done? 　b. Are there people whom you need to contact in order to resolve feelings or unfinished business? 　c. What do you want to do with the time you have left?	
8. If appropriate, offer to help the individual to contact others to resolve conflicts (old or new) verbally or in writing. Validate that forgiveness is not a seeking reconciliation, "but a letting go of a hurt" (*Yakimo, 2006). 　a. The nurse through listening can help the individual with personal growth.	8. "Asking for or providing forgiveness is a powerful healing tool" (*Yakimo, 2006).
9. Explain preparatory depression and associated behaviors to significant others (*Yakimo, 2006). 　a. Realization of impending death 　b. Reviewing what their life has meant 　c. Reflections on life review and sorrow of impeding losses	9. Preparatory depression is when the person realizes his or her approaching death and desires to be released from suffering (*Yakimo, 2006).
10. Encourage significant others to allow for life review and sorrow and not to try and cheer him or her up. Encourage the individual to: 　a. Tell life stories, journaling, and reminisce. 　b. Discuss leaving a legacy: Donation, personal articles, or taped messages.	10. Strategies that help the individual find meaning in failures and successes can reduce anxiety and depression. Acceptance of the final separation in life is not reached until the dying individual's life review and sorrow is listened to (*Yakimo, 2006).

Interventions	*Rationales*
11. Respect the dying individual's wishes (e.g., few or no visitors, modifications in care, no heroic measures, or food or liquid preferences). a. Encourage reflective activities such as personal prayer, meditation, and journal writing. b. Return to a previously pleasurable activity. Examples include painting, music, woodworking, and quilting. c. Return the gift of love to others by listening, praying for others, sharing personal wisdom gained from illness, and creating legacy gifts.	11. If the person is ready to release life and die, and others expect him or her to want to continue to live, that person's own depression, grief, and turmoil are increased (*Yakimo, 2006). b. Promoting and restoring interests, imagination, and creativity enhance quality of life (*Brant, 1998).
12. Aggressively manage unrelieved symptoms such as nausea, pruritus, pain, vomiting, and fatigue.	12. Serious unrelieved symptoms can cause a distressing death and needless added suffering for families (*Nelson et al., 2000). Fatigue and pain consume excess energy and reduce energy needed for optimal dialogue (*Matzo & Sherman, 2001).
13. Prepare significant others for changes in their loved one that may occur as death nears: a. Early: Sleep more, eat/drink less, trouble swallowing, become more confused. have less pain, withdraw from others, trouble hearing b. Moaning sounds, moist breathing sounds, long periods without breathing followed by several quick, deep breaths, cool hands, arms, feet or legs, turning blue around nose, mouth, fingers, toes (Hospice and Palliative Nurse's Association, 2016; Yarbro et al., 2011).	13. Clear, direct discussions can reduce the family's anxiety when these signs and symptoms occur and reduce attempts to reduce these signs and symptoms such as trying to force fluids (Yarbro et al., 2011).
14. Avoid giving a specific time for the expected time of death. "It is helpful to give a range of time, such as 'hours to days,' 'days to weeks' or 'weeks to months'" (Yarbro et al., 2011, p. 1836).	14. Family members and friends will be able to better plan their time spent with their loved one with this information (Yarbro et al., 2011).

Documentation

Significant discussions

Anticipatory Grieving Related to Losses Associated with Illness, Disabilities and Impending Death and their Effects on Loved Ones

NOC

Coping, Family Coping, Grief Resolution, Psychosocial Adjustment: Life Change

Goal

Individual/family will identify expected loss and grief reactions will be freely expressed.

Indicators

* Participate in decision making for the future.
* Share concerns with significant others.

NIC

Family Support, Grief Work Facilitation, Coping Enhancement, Anticipatory Guidance, Emotional Support

Interventions	*Rationales*
1. Assess for causative and contributing factors of anticipated or potential loss (e.g., terminal illness, role changes, financial burden, loss of relationships, physical changes).	
2. Assess individual response: a. Denial b. Shock c. Rejection d. Anger e. Bargaining f. Depression g. Isolation h. Guilt i. Helplessness/hopelessness j. Fear k. Sadness l. Anxiety	
3. Encourage the individual to share concerns: a. Use open-ended questions and reflection b. Acknowledge the value of the individual and his or her grief by using touch, sitting with him or her, and verbalizing your concern. c. Recognize that some people may choose not to share their concerns, but convey that you are available if they desire to do so later.	3a. "What are your thoughts today?" "How do you feel?" b. "This must be very difficult." "What is most important to you now?" c. "What do you hope for?"
4. Assist the individual and family to identify strengths: a. "What do you do well?" b. "What are you willing to do to address this issue?" c. "Is religion/spirituality a source of strength for you?" d. "Do you have close friends?" e. "Whom do you turn to in times of need?" f. "What does this person do for you?" g. "What sources of strength have you called upon successfully in the past?"	
5. Promote integrity of the individual and family by acknowledging strengths: a. "Your brother looks forward to your visit." b. "Your family is so concerned for you."	
6. Support the individual and family with grief reactions: a. Prepare them for possible grief reactions. b. Explain possible grief reactions. c. Focus on the current situation until the individual or family indicates the desire to discuss the future.	

Interventions	Rationales

7. Promote family cohesiveness:
a. Identify availability of a support system:
  • Meet consistently with family members.
  • Identify family member roles, strengths, and weaknesses.
b. Identify communication patterns within the family unit:
  • Assess positive and negative feedback, verbal and nonverbal communication, and body language.
  • Listen and clarify messages being sent.
c. Provide for the concept of hope:
  • Supply accurate information.
  • Resist the temptation to give false hope.
  • Discuss concerns willingly.
  • Help the family reframe hope (i.e., for a peaceful death).
d. Promote group decision making to enhance group autonomy:
  • Establish consistent times to meet with the individual and family.
  • Encourage members to talk directly with and to listen to one another.
	7. Mourners who were busy with the practical and necessary caregiving tasks of the dying individual may not address the impending loss and, therefore, are at risk for delayed grieving response (*Worten, 2002).

8. For the dying individual with young children or siblings of a dying child/adolescent.
a. Communicate in an honest and open manner with the individual and with the child.
b. Provide guidance on how to grief together instead of in isolation.
c. Encourage conversation with the partner or relatives about the children's/siblings future.
d. Encourage honesty in conversations about the impending death toward the child/sibling (although the amount of information may differ per age, even a young child can understand simple explanations for instance the body not working any more (Warnick, 2015).
e. Seek for activities the individual can maintain performing with his/her children/siblings.
f. Provide professional support (e.g., psychologist, school nurse, family bereavement program).
g. Support parents to inform the child's/siblings' social environment about the situation.
	8. The death of a parent or sibling is the most difficult thing a child can experience. Parents need support in such a situation.
	    "The perspective of individuals who have experienced the dying or death of an immediate family member as youth are finally being engaged and reflected in the literature. This represents a significant advancement in the field of child and adolescent grief. Whether experiencing the illness or dying of a parent or sibling, many of the themes they expressed involved a desire to be included in honest conversations about the illness, treatment, and prognosis" (Warnick, 2015).
	    "Youth articulate a clear need for early notification of an impending death to allow them time to process their thoughts and feelings, ask questions, and participate in final conversations when they are ready to do so" (Warnick, 2015).

9. Provide for expression of grief:
a. Encourage emotional expressions of grieving.
b. Caution the individual about use of sedatives and tranquilizers, which may prevent or delay expressions.
c. Encourage verbalization by individuals of all age groups and families.
  • Support family cohesiveness.
  • Promote and verbalize strengths of the family group.
d. Encourage the individual and family to engage in life review:
  • Focus and support the social network relationships.
  • Reevaluate past life experiences and integrate them into a new meaning.
  • Convey empathic understanding.
  • Explore unfinished business.	

(continued)

Interventions	Rationales
10. Provide health teaching and referrals, as indicated:	10. The knowledge that no further treatment is warranted and that death is imminent may give rise to feelings of powerlessness, anger, profound sadness, and other grief responses. Open, honest discussions can help the individual and family members accept and cope with the situation and their response to it (O'Mallon, 2009).
a. Refer the individual with potential for dysfunctional grieving responses for counseling (psychiatrist, nurse therapist, counselor, psychologist).	a. Research validates that professional interventions and professionally supported voluntary and self-help services are capable of reducing the risk of psychiatric and psychoanalytic disorders resulting from bereavement (Bonnano & Lillenfied, 2008).

b. Explain what to expect:
  • Sadness
  • Rejection
  • Feelings of aloneness
  • Anger
  • Guilt
  • Labile emotions
  • Fear
  • Feeling of "going crazy"
c. Teach the individual and family signs of resolution:
  • Grieving individuals no longer lives in the past but establishes new goals for life.
  • Grieving individuals redefine relationship with the lost object/person.
  • Grieving individuals begin to resocialize.
d. Teach signs of complicated responses and referrals needed:
  • Defenses used in uncomplicated grief work that become exaggerated or maladaptive responses
  • Persistent absence of any emotion
  • Prolonged intense reactions of anxiety, anger, fear, guilt, and helplessness
e. Identify agencies that may enhance grief work:
  • Self-help groups
  • Widow-to-widow groups
  • Parents of deceased children
  • Single-parent groups
  • Bereavement groups

Documentation

Significant discussions

TRANSITION TO HOME/COMMUNITY CARE

If indicated, review the risk diagnoses identified for this individual on admission:
• Is the person still at risk?
• Can the family reduce the risks?
• Is the person at higher risk at home?
• Is a home health nurse assessment needed?
• Refer to transition planner/case manager/social service.
• When is this person scheduled for follow-up with primary provider? Specialists? Record dates of appointments.
• Complete a medication reconciliation prior to transition. Refer to index.
• Is the family capable to care for the individual at home, are they not overburdened?

STAR	Stop	
	Think	Is this person at risk for injury, falls, medical complications, and/or inability to care for self (activities of daily living)?

STAR **Stop**

Think   Is this person at risk for injury, falls, medical complications, and/or inability to care for self (activities of daily living)?

Is there a support person available?

Is the person competent to manage self-administration of medications, treatment procedures? Are additional resources needed?

Can the person explain how to monitor the condition (e.g., blood glucose, signs/symptoms of complications, dietary/mobility restrictions, and when to call his or her primary provider or specialist)?

Act   Contact or provide the appropriate resource (e.g., contacting a support person, home health assessment, additional teaching, printed materials).

Review   Has the problem been addressed? If not, use SBAR to communicate to the appropriate person.

Risk for Care Giver Role Strain Related to the Multiple Changes/Stressors Associated with Transition to Palliative Home Care

NOC

Caregiver Well-Being, Caregiver Lifestyle Disruption, Caregiver Emotional Health, Caregiver Role Endurance Potential, Family Coping, Family Integrity, Caregiver Performance: Direct Care, Caregiver Performance: Indirect Care, Care giver Role Endurance

Goals

The caregiver will:

- Relate what needs to be completed prior to transition to home care
- Identify the services to expect from palliative/hospice agencies
- Share frustrations regarding caregiving responsibilities
- Identify one source of support
- Identify two changes that would improve daily life if implemented
- Be honest about limits to his or her caregiving abilities according to his or her own grief

The family will:

- Relate two strategies to increase weekly support or help
- Convey empathy to caregiver regarding daily responsibilities

NIC

Caregiver Support, Respite Care, Coping Enhancement, Family Mobilization, Mutual Goal Setting, Support System Enhancement, Anticipatory Guidance, Discharge Planning, Case Management, Teaching, Telephone Follow-up, Telephone Consultation

Interventions	Rationales
1. Educate yourself regarding palliative/hospice services in the home.	1. To prepare individuals and their families for care at home, nurses need to clearly understand what they will experience during the time between care provided by the "sending" (hospital) and "receiving" (home hospice) providers (Does, Rhudy, Holland, & Olson, 2011).

Interventions	Rationales
2. Ensure that family understand the services that will be provided at home (e.g., when, what, how often).	2. Failure to prepare individuals/family for transition to home care has proven to result in suboptimal outcomes, the development of new or worsening symptoms, unplanned rehospitalizations, medical errors, and other adverse events (Does et al., 2011).
3. Elicit from caregivers their concerns, fears.	3. Does et al. (2011) reported that many family members were not yet comfortable with their new roles as caregivers, were not sure what to expect, and identified feeling scared. Lack of clarity regarding hospice care entailed a tension between "hospice will take care of everything" and uncertainty over what exactly was meant by "everything" (p. 400).
4. Elicit for the individual his or her expectations, concerns, fears.	4. For many individuals at end of their life "going home" is the most important task remaining to achieve (Does et al., 2011).
5. Access palliative/hospice specialist to clarify the type and timing of services to be provided. Request that they instruct them on management of "emergencies."	5. Lack of clarity causes a tension during the transition from hospital to home hospice: "The period between leaving the hospital and the first home hospice visit is one in which the individual and family are particularly vulnerable" (Does et al., 2011). Frank discussions are needed to differentiate on managing deterioration, impending death, and emergencies (e.g., when to call 911, when not to).
6. Allow the family to share their expectation of home care. Clarify their understanding of: a. Necessary supplies (e.g., dressings, hospital bed, commode) b. Current medication regimen available for doses needed (e.g., same day after transition at home) c. Knowledge of management of pain, other symptoms d. Ability to manage treatments (e.g., wounds, catheters) e. Who to call for advice f. Manage medication regimen	6. Managing care transitions require clear communication among providers to prevent complications in home care. In addition, hospital staff/student frequently overestimate individual/family knowledge and capabilities or inadequately assess their abilities to provide care, and clinicians may not be as attuned to specialized EOL care deemed critical by individuals and their families.
7. If prescribed, initiate a discussion regarding acquiring a hospital bed and its placement prior to bringing the family member home. a. Ordering the bed for delivery prior to transition b. Criteria for selecting and preparing the space	7 Families have reported difficulty accessing equipment prior to transition. Optimal placement of the bed should permit interactions with visitors and ease of access to care (Does et al., 2011).
8. Explain the disruptions that will occur and that their home life will be different than before. "Going home on palliative/hospice services is different from just going home" (Does et al., 2011, p. 396).	8. This home will now become an "Open House," with numerous persons coming into the house (Does et al., 2011).
9. Encourage conversation about caregivers (dis)abilities in entertaining in care activities.	9. Caregivers may feel pressed to perform care activities they not actually feel comfortable with. This might occur due to feelings of guilt and obligation toward the dying relative or due to lack of professional health care professionals. The uncertainty of the length of the dying phase is also of impact.

Documentation

Individual/family teaching
Referrals

Sexual Assault

Department of Justice's National Crime Victimization Survey (NCVS)—there is an average of 293,066 victims (age 12 or older) of rape and sexual assault each year (U.S. Department of Justice, 2014). Females knew their offenders in almost 70% of violent crimes committed against them; males knew their offenders in 45% of violent crimes committed against them (Bureau of Justice, 2010). Rape is a crime using sexual means to humiliate, dominate, and degrade the victim (*Symes, 2000). Sexual assault is forced and violent oral, vaginal, or anal penetration of a person without his or her consent. This care plan focuses on nursing for an individual who has been sexually assaulted and is hospitalized for injuries.

Individuals, who have been sexually assaulted may be reluctant, to report the assault to law enforcement and to seek medical attention for a variety of reasons as (U.S. Department of Justice, 2014)

- Blame themselves for the sexual assault and feel embarrassed
- Fear of retaliation from assailant(s)
- Worry about whether they will be believed
- May lack the ability or emotional strength to access services
- May not have their own transportation or access to public transportation
- May also not speak English well
- Fear that reporting the assault may jeopardize their immigration status
- May lack health insurance and may not be aware that, as a crime victim, they are eligible for financial reimbursements for certain services
- May perceive the medical forensic examination as yet another violation
- Because of its extensive and intrusive nature in the immediate aftermath of the assault. Rather than seek assistance, a sexual assault victim may simply want to go somewhere safe, clean up, and try to forget the assault ever happened.

Carp's Cues

The word rape has a history of being viewed as a crime of passion not a crime of violence. Women were (or are) asked what they were wearing or doing prior to the rape. Sexual assault is defined as any sexual activity involving a person who does not or cannot (due to alcohol, drugs, or some sort of incapacitation) consent. The phrase sexual assault denotes unprovoked violence, which defines the perpetrator as the criminal and the victim as a "victim of a crime." Rape/Sexual Assault can be defined differently by each state.

As an nurse practitioner, this author has interacted with numerous girls and women who have shared their sexual assaults with me; some for the first time in their lives. Two themes were woven into their stories: (1) Guilt that they contributed to the assault and (2) profound disappointment with their mother's response. Many mothers blame their daughter for the event and sometimes refuse to believe their daughter if a relative or paramour is involved; or they suggest that their daughter provoked the event.

Perhaps that was the only reaction her mother could have at the time, for whatever reason. I discuss forgiveness with these girls/women. Forgiveness never means you accept what happened, only that you are going to release the pain from yourself. Stop carrying it around with you. Forgiveness is a gift you give yourself (Carpenito-Moyet, 2017, p. 485).

Girls and women shared stories that the rape would not have happened if they had not:

Worn that short skirt

Drank too much

Walked home in the dark

Had engaged in kissing and hugging

Had not went somewhere alone with him

Kevin Caruso wrote, "And remember that all rapists are cowards, criminals, and losers and belong in prison." "There never is an excuse for rape, and it is always a very serious crime." Accessed at http://www.suicide.org/rape-victims-prone-to-suicide.html

Time Frame

Coexisting with (trauma requiring hospitalization)

▪▪▪▪▪▪ DIAGNOSTIC CLUSTER**

Collaborative Problems

Risk for Complications of Sexually Transmitted Infection (STI)

Risk for Complications of Unwanted Pregnancy

Collaborative Problems associated with physical injuries sometimes caused by sexual assault include fractures, head injuries, abdominal injuries, and burns (refer to the collaborative problem index for specific problems)

Nursing Diagnoses

Rape Trauma Syndrome

**This situation was not included in the validation study.

Transition Criteria

Before transition, the individual or family will:

1. Share feelings.
2. Describe rationales and treatment procedures.
3. Identify what needs to be done now and take steps toward the goals.
4. Relate the intent to seek professional help after transition.
5. Identify members of support system available.

Transitional Risk Assessment Plan (TRAP)

Begin this plan on admission.
Implement the Transitional Risk Assessment Plan (TRAP):
- Refer to inside back cover.
- Add each validated risk diagnosis to individual's problem list with the risk code in ( ).
- Refer to Unit II to the individual risk nursing diagnoses/collaborative problems for outcomes and interventions.

R: "Close coordination of care in the post-acute period, early transition follow-up care, enhanced client education and self-management training, proactive end-of-life counseling, and extending the resources and clinical expertise over time via multidisciplinary team management" can lower readmission rates and improve health outcomes (Boutwell & Hwu, 2009, p. 14). Interventions are utilized to activate the individual and family to select changes in their everyday lifestyle choices to improve their health (Hibbard & Greene, 2013).

Collaborative Problems

Risk for Complications of Sexually Transmitted Infection

Risk for Complications of Unwanted Pregnancy

Collaborative Outcomes

The individual will be advised of measures to prevent and/or treat (a) STIs and (b) unwanted pregnancy.

Indicators of Physiologic Stability

- Evidence of treatment for chlamydia
- Evidence of treatment for gonorrhea

- Prophylactic treatment for pregnancy
- Negative results for trichomonal infection or evidence of treatment
- Negative results on rapid plasma reagin test (RPR) or evidence of treatment
- Evidence of postexposure prophylaxis for HIV

CLINICAL ALERT: State laws differ regarding mandatory reporting of abuse or assaults on adults. Some states require reporting of elder abuse to Adult Protective Services (APS) and/or the police. Some states require mandatory reporting of visible evidence of domestic violence. It is important to understand that a health care professional can report a suspicion of abuse or neglect to the appropriate agency. An investigation will determine if the suspicion is valid. Suspicions should be reported: It is better to be proven wrong rather than for unreported abuse to continue.

The following statistics are reported about sexual assault: U.S. Department of Justice, *National Crime Victimization Study: 2009 to 2013* (Rape, Abuse and Incest National Network [RAINN], 2016)

- 44% of victims are under age 18
- 80% are under age 30
- Approximately 4/5 of assaults are committed by someone known to the victim
- 47% of rapists are a friend or acquaintance
- 5% are a relative
- Approximately 50% of all rape/sexual assault incidents were reported by victims to have occurred within 1 mile of their home or at their home.

Nursing Diagnoses

Rape Trauma Syndrome

In this care plan, nursing diagnoses will appear prior to the Collaborative Problems due to the nature of the situation

NOC

Abuse Protection, Abuse Recovery Status, Coping

NIC

Abuse Protection, Support, Coping Enhancement, Rape Trauma Treatment, Support Group, Anxiety Reduction, Presence, Emotional Support, Calming, Technique, Active Listening, Family Support, Grief Work, Facilitation

Goals

Refer to transition criteria.

CLINICAL ALERT: Various agencies have reported out of every 100 rapes, of the 32 get reported

- Seven lead to arrest.
- Three are referred to prosecutors.
- Two lead to a felony conviction.
- Two rapists will spend a single day in prison.
- The other 98 will walk free.

Sources: Justice Department, National Crime Victimization Survey: 2008–2012. FBI, Uniform Crime Reports, Arrest Data: 2006–2010, FBI, Uniform Crime Reports, Offenses Cleared Data: 2006–2010. Department of Justice, Felony Defendents in Large Urban Counties: 2009. Department of Justice, Felony Defendents in Large Urban Counties: 2009. Retrieved from https://rainn.org/get-information/statistics/reporting-rates

Interventions	*Rationales*

CLINICAL ALERT:
* One in 5 women and one in 71 men will be raped at some times in their lives (Black, et al.2011). Male-on-male rape has been heavily stigmatized. According to psychologist Dr. Sarah Crome, fewer than 1 in 10 male–male rapes are reported. As a group, male rape victims reported a lack of services and support, and legal systems are often ill-equipped to deal with this type of crime (RAINN, 2009).

---

1. Provide interventions to decrease anxiety. Ask the person > How can I help you?

   a. Limit people to whom the individual must describe assault.

   b. Do not leave individual alone.
   c. Maintain a nonjudgmental attitude.
   d. Explore the available support systems.

   e. Create a plan to increase sense of safety. Be specific.

1. Sexual assault is a crime of violence against a person's body and will. Sex offenders use physical and/or psychological aggression or coercion to victimize, in the process threatening a victim's sense of privacy, safety, autonomy, and well-being (U.S. Department of Justice, 2014).

   a. Repeatedly relating the incident increases shame and anxiety.
   b. Isolation can increase anxiety.
   c. Support system provides some stability and safety.
   d. The individual should not be transitioned from the facility without a support person with them.

Carp's Cues

I share with each individual this scenario. "Instead of being sexually assaulted, imagine that you were hit over the head with a shovel. Would it matter what you were wearing, how much alcohol you drank or what you were saying or doing at the time? Sexual assault is not sex; it is a violent act, like hitting someone on the head with a shovel. I suggest that the next time they have self-blame, they think of the shovel."

---

2. If the individual expresses that she is at fault for the assault as:
   a. Worn too sexy clothes
   b. Drank too much
   c. Walked home after dark
   d. Had engaged in kissing and hugging
   e. Went with him alone to another place

2. Most victims of sexual assault blame themselves for the assault (*Carson & Smith-DiJulio, 2006).

---

3. Explain the Legal Issues and Police Investigation (*Heinrich, 1987).
   a. Explain that the choice to report the rape is the victim's. Explore pros and cons of reporting.
   b. Explain briefly the police protocol.
   c. Explain the medical legal examination.
   d. Refer to Standard of Care or SANE Nurse for guidance in the postassault care.

3. The evidentiary examination is especially distressing because it can be reminiscent of the assault (*Ledray, 2001). The medical–legal examination serves to assess the condition of the victim and to gather documentary evidence. It consists of a general examination; oral, pelvic, and rectal examinations; a culture for sperm and sexually transmitted diseases; serum pregnancy test; blood typing; and a drug and alcohol screen. Obvious debris is placed in separate envelopes. Dried sperm is collected. The victim's pubic hair and head hair are combed, and samples are placed in separate envelopes. Fingernail scrapings are placed in separate envelopes for each hand (*Heinrich, 1987).

Interventions	Rationales
4. Assist the individual to identify major concerns (psychological, medical, and legal) and his or her perception of needed help.	4. Sexual assault is always associated with coercion and threatened or actual violence. It is by this means the assailant takes control from the victim. Involving the victim in decision making begins reestablishing a sense of control (*Carson & Smith-DiJulio, 2006).
5. Whenever possible, provide crisis counseling within 1 hour of rape trauma event: a. Ask permission to contact the rape crisis counselor.	5. Victim empowerment is the primary antidote to the trauma of sexual assault (*Carson & Smith-DiJulio, 2006).

6. Promote a trusting relationship by providing emotional support with unconditional positive regard and acceptance:
 	
  a. Stay with the individual during acute stage, or arrange for other support.
  b. Brief the individual on police and hospital procedures during acute stage.
  c. Assist during medical examination and explain all procedures in advance.
  d. Help the individual to meet personal needs (bathing after examination and after evidence has been acquired).
  e. Listen attentively to the individual's requests.
  f. Maintain unhurried attitude toward the individual and her or his family.
  g. Avoid rescue feelings toward the individual.
  h. Maintain nonjudgmental attitude.
  i. Support the individual's beliefs and value system; avoid labeling.
  j. Reassure the individual that the symptoms are normal responses that will lessen and improve with time.
	6. Providing immediate and ongoing empathy and support prepares victims for referral to more in-depth psychological counseling. Main issues in the acute stage are being in control, fearing being left alone, and having someone to listen (*Carson & Smith-DiJulio, 2006).
	a–i. Victims are vulnerable to any statement that can be construed as blaming. Their normal defenses are weakened. When asked too many questions, individuals can feel "grilled." This interferes with the rapport between helper and individual.
	
	  j. The victim needs to understand that a wide range of behavior and emotional responses is normal.

7. Explain the care and examination she or he will experience:
 	
  a. Maintaining eye contact, conduct the examinations in an unhurried manner.
 	
  b. Explain every detail slowly before action.
  c. Make every attempt to provide privacy, draping body parts, limit exposure.
	7. Because the victim's right to deny or consent has been violently violated, it is important to seek permission for subsequent care (*Heinrich, 1987). It is important to tell the individual as much as is practical or possible about what is happening and why. Even in life-threatening situations, any sense of control given to the individual is helpful.
	  a. Unhurried and confident actions, eye contact, and affirming the victim is safe help to calm and assure that he or she is alive and worthy.
	  b. Cognitive dysfunction impairs short-term memory.
	  c. The victim of rape needs to understand the common reactions to this experience. Any exposure or loss of privacy is especially distressing because it can be reminiscent of the assault (*Ledray, 2001).

8. Provide interventions to assist with regaining control (*Smith-DiJulio, 2001):
  a. Listen, listen, listen.
 	
  b. "How can I help you?"
	8a. Probably the best response is simply for the nurse to listen without judgment and ask more than once what to do to support the individual recovery (*Carosella, 1995).
	  b. Many traumatized people repeat their stories over and over. This is part of the healing and diminishes with time.

(continued)

Interventions	Rationales
9. Reassure that feelings and reactions are normal responses and accept where the individual is in the recovery process.	9. Emotional care must aim to convey respect and understanding; communicate empathy, reassurance, and support; encourage ventilation of feelings; preserve dignity; empower the victim; provide anticipatory guidance; and ensure adequate follow-up.
10. Explore available support systems. Involve significant others: a. Share with family and friends the victim's immediate needs for love and support. b. Refer to counseling services. c. Encourage the individual and their support persons to read, Voices of Courage: Inspiration from Survivors of Sexual Assault. Can be retrieved at http://www.datesafeproject.org/wp-content/uploads/2015/08/voices_of_courage_ebook_2013.pdf	10b. Postponing professional help may lengthen the time reactions persist and lengthens recovery. c. Voices of Courage exposes the reality of sexual assault but more importantly taking back one's control of their lives.

For Prevention of Pregnancy and Sexually Transmitted Infections

Interventions	Rationales
CLINICAL ALERT: • HIV seroconversion has occurred in persons whose only known risk factor was sexual assault or sexual abuse, but the frequency of this occurrence likely is low. In consensual sex, the per-act risk for HIV transmission from vaginal intercourse is 0.1% to 0.2%, and for receptive rectal intercourse, 0.5% to 3% (Centers for Disease Control and Prevention [CDC], 2015c).	
1. The Centers for Disease Control and Prevention recommend (CDC, 2015c): a. An empiric antimicrobial regimen for chlamydia, gonorrhea, and trichomonas. b. Determine if the individual is at risk for pregnancy and if ECP is indicated • No contraceptive use • No surgical sterilization • History of infertility • Postmenopausal emergency contraception. c. Explain ECP and that it can cause nausea and vomiting from high estrogen content. d. Postexposure hepatitis B vaccination (without HBIG) if the hepatitis status of the assailant is unknown and the survivor has not been previously vaccinated. If the assailant is known to be HBsAg-positive, unvaccinated survivors should receive both hepatitis B vaccine and HBIG.	1a. This measure should be considered when the assault could result in pregnancy in the survivor. Emergency contraceptive pill (ECP) delays ovulation and interferes with tubal transport of egg or sperm (Arcangelo & Peterson, 2016). b. Considered when the assault could result in pregnancy in the survivor. ECP delays ovulation and interferes with tubal transport of egg or sperm (Arcangelo & Peterson, 2016). c. ECP delays ovulation and interferes with tubal transport of egg or sperm (Arcangelo & Peterson, 2016). d. The vaccine and HBIG, if indicated, should be administered to sexual assault survivors at the time of the initial examination, and follow-up doses of vaccine should be administered 1 to 2 and 4 to 6 months after the first dose. Survivors who were previously vaccinated but did not receive postvaccination testing should receive a single vaccine booster dose (see Hepatitis B).

Interventions	Rationales
e. HPV vaccination is recommended for female survivors aged 9 to 26 years and male survivors aged 9 to 21 years. For MSM with who have not received HPV vaccine or who have been incompletely vaccinated, vaccine can be administered through age 26 years.	e. The HPV vaccine should be administered to sexual assault survivors at the time of the initial examination, and follow-up dose administered at 1 to 2 months and 6 months after the first dose.

> **CLINICAL ALERT:**
> • The CDC and other expert groups recommend preventive treatment if the mouth, vagina, anus, or nonintact skin (e.g., a cut) was exposed to the assailant's blood or bodily fluids that is visibly contaminated with blood (CDC, 2015c).

2. The CDC (2015c) recommendations for HIV postexposure prophylaxis are individualized according to risk as: a. Exposure was less or equal to 72 hours b. Substantial exposure risk c. Known or unknown HIV status of assailant	2. The anguish after an assault also might prevent the survivor from accurately weighing exposure risks and benefits of nPEP and from making an informed decision regarding initiating therapy, even when such therapy is considered warranted by the health care provider. In this instance, the survivor can be provided a 3- to 5-day supply of nPEP and scheduled for follow-up at a time that allows for provision of the remaining 23 days of medication (if nPEP has been initiated by the survivor) without interruption in dosing. A follow-up visit also creates opportunity for additional counseling as needed (CDC, 2015c).
3. If nPEP is offered, the following information should be discussed with the survivor: a. The necessity of early initiation of nPEP to optimize potential benefits (i.e., as soon as possible after and up to 72 hours after the assault); b. The importance of close follow-up; c. The benefit of adherence to recommended dosing; and taking every dose increases its effectiveness. d. Potential adverse effects of antiretrovirals. Providers should emphasize that severe adverse effects are rare from nPEP (CDC, 2015c).	3. The importance of taking the medications every day and for the duration of treatment is critical to prevent HIV infection. Clinical management of the survivor should be implemented according to the HIV nPEP guidelines and in collaboration with specialists (CDC, 2015c).

> ### *Clinical Alert Report*
> Prior to providing care, advise ancillary staff/student to report the following to the professional nurse assigned to the individual:
> • Any change in levels of anxiety
> • Increase in distress
> • Distressful visitors

Documentation

• Injuries
• Emotional state
• Documentation protocol for sexual assault

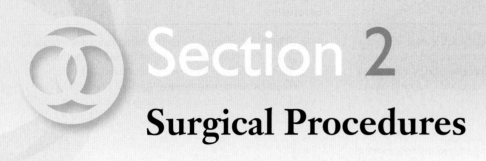

Section 2

Surgical Procedures

Generic Care Plan for an Individual Experiencing Surgery

This care plan presents nursing diagnoses and collaborative problems that commonly apply to individuals (and their significant others) experiencing all types of surgery. Nursing diagnoses and collaborative problems specific to a surgical procedure (e.g., for total knee replacement, cholecystectomies are presented in the care plan for that procedure). Basic postoperative nursing care will not be repeated in the specific surgical procedure care plans.

 Time Frame
Preoperative and postoperative periods

 Carp's Cues
Before any planned surgery, the majority of individuals arrive the morning of surgery. It is the responsibility of the nursing staff/students in the presurgical unit and surgical suite to provide simple explanations before interventions and some teaching on what to expect after surgery. High levels of anxiety will impair the individual's level of comprehension.

■■■■■ DIAGNOSTIC CLUSTER

Nursing Diagnoses

Preoperative

Anxiety/Fear related to surgical experience, loss of control, unpredictable outcome, and insufficient knowledge of preoperative routines, postoperative exercises and activities, and postoperative changes and sensations

Postoperative

Collaborative Problems

Risk for Complications of Bleeding

Risk for Complications of Hypovolemia/Shock

Risk for Complications of Evisceration/Dehiscence

Risk for Complications of Paralytic Ileus

Risk for Complications of Infection (Peritonitis, Incision)

Risk for Complications of Urinary Retention

Risk for Complications of Deep Vein Thrombosis (DVT)

Nursing Diagnoses

Risk for Ineffective Respiratory Function related to immobility secondary to postanesthesia state and pain

Risk for (Surgical Site) Infection related to access for organism invasion secondary to surgery

Acute Pain related to surgical interruption of body structures, flatus, and immobility

Risk for Imbalanced Nutrition related to increased protein and vitamin requirements for wound healing and decreased intake secondary to pain, nausea, vomiting, and diet restrictions

Risk for Delayed Surgical Recovery related to factors that can inhibit wound healing, optimal national intake, and mobilization necessary for *recuperation*

Risk for Constipation related to decreased peristalsis secondary to immobility and the effects of anesthesia and narcotics

Impaired Physical Mobility related to pain and weakness secondary to anesthesia, tissue hypoxia, and insufficient fluid and nutrient intake

Risk for Ineffective Health Management related to insufficient knowledge of care of operative site, restrictions (diet, activity), medications, signs and symptoms of complications, and follow-up care

Transition Criteria

Before transition, the individual and/or family will:

1. Describe any at-home activity restrictions.
2. Describe at-home wound and pain management.
3. Discuss fluid and nutritional requirements for proper wound healing.
4. List the signs and symptoms that must be reported to a health care professional.
5. Describe necessary follow-up care.

Transitional Risk Assessment Plan (TRAP)

Begin this plan on admission.
Implement the Transitional Risk Assessment Plan (TRAP):
- Refer to inside back cover.
- Add each validated risk diagnosis to individual's problem list with the risk code in ( ).
- Refer the individual risk nursing diagnoses/collaborative problems for outcomes and interventions in Unit II.

> *R:* "*Close coordination of care in the post-acute period, early transition follow-up care, enhanced client educa-tion and self-management training, proactive end-of-life counseling, and extending the resources and clinical expertise over time via multidisciplinary team management*" *can lower readmission rates and improve health outcomes (Boutwell & Hwu, 2009, p. 14). Interventions are utilized to activate the individual and family to select changes in their everyday lifestyle choices to improve their health (Hibbard & Greene, 2013).*

Preoperative: Nursing Diagnosis

Anxiety/Fear Related to Surgical Experience, Loss of Control, Unpredictable Outcome, and Insufficient Knowledge of Preoperative Routines, Postoperative Exercises and Activities, and Postoperative Changes and Sensations

NOC
Anxiety Reduction, Coping, Impulse Control

Goal

The individual will communicate feelings regarding the surgical experience, including the limitations and restrictions, and discuss any therapeutic medical devices (e.g., braces, crutches, plasters), that will apply postoperatively.

NIC

Anxiety Reduction, Impulse Control Training, Anticipatory Guidance

Indicators

- Verbalize, if asked, what to expect regarding routines, environment, and sensations.
- Demonstrate postoperative exercises, splinting, and respiratory regimen.

Carp's Cues

Please refer to the Generic Care Plan for the Surgical Individual for detailed interventions for managing all surgical conditions. This care plan addresses specific additional interventions associated with any type of surgery performed.

Interventions	*Rationales*
CLINICAL ALERT: • Although research has shown preoperative teaching to be an essential nursing activity, it has become increasing difficult to accomplish. Increased outpatient surgery and morning admission on the day of surgery have reduced time available for assessment and preparation activities including teaching (*Yount & Schoessler, 1991).	

1. Address the five dimensions of preoperative teaching (*Yount & Schoessler, 1991):
  a. Psychosocial support
  b. Situational information
  c. Individual role
  d. Expected sensations—discomforts
  e. Skills training	

2. Provide emotional support and encouragement to share her or his feelings/fears. Ask what are you most concerned about right now? Correct any misconceptions and inaccurate information.	2. Modifiable contributing factors to anxiety include incomplete and inaccurate information. Providing accurate information and correcting misconceptions may help to reduce fears and reduce anxiety.

3. Allow and encourage family members and significant others to share their fears and concerns. Correct inaccurate information.
  a. Explain all interventions before providing them.
  b. Explain what to expect in the operating room and recovery room.
	3. Effective support from family members, other relatives, and friends can help the individual to cope with surgery and recovery.

4. Notify the physician/nurse practitioner if the individual exhibits severe or panic anxiety.	4. Immediate notification enables prompt assessment and possible pharmacologic intervention.
5. Notify the physician/nurse practitioner/physical assistant if the individual needs any further explanations about the procedure.	5. The physician/nurse practitioner/physical assistant is responsible for explaining the surgery to the individual and family; the nurse, for determining their level of understanding and then notifying the physician/nurse practitioner of the need to provide more information, if necessary.

Documentation

Vital signs
Medications administered

Postoperative: Collaborative Problems

Risk for Complications of Bleeding

Risk for Complications of Hypovolemia/Shock

Risk for Complications of Evisceration/Dehiscence

Risk for Complications of Paralytic Ileus

Risk for Complications of Infection (Peritonitis, Incision)

Risk for Complications of Urinary Retention

Risk for Complications of Thrombophlebitis

Collaborative Outcomes

The individual will be monitored for early signs and symptoms of (a) bleeding, (b) hypovolemia/shock, (c) evisceration/dehiscence, (d) paralytic ileus, (e) infection, (f) urinary retention, and (g) thrombophlebitis and will receive collaborative interventions if indicated to restore physiologic stability.

Indicators of Physiologic Stability

- Respirations 16 to 20 breaths/min, relaxed and rhythmic (a, b)
- Breath sound present in all lobes (a, b)
- No rales or wheezing (a, b)
- Pulse 60 to 100 beats/min (a, b)
- BP >90/60, <140/90 mm Hg (a, b)
- Capillary refill <3 seconds (a, b)
- Peripheral pulses full, equal (a, b)
- Temperature 98.5° F to 99° F (a, b, e)
- Urine output >0.5 mL/kg/hr (a, b)
- No bladder distention (f)
- No difficulty voiding (f)
- Surgical wound intact (c, e)
- Minimal serosanguineous drainage (e)
- Bowel sounds present (b, d)
- No nausea and vomiting (b, d)
- No abdominal distention (b, d)
- No calf tenderness, warmth, or edema (g)
- White blood cells 4,000 to 10,000/mm^3 (e)
- Hemoglobin (a)
  - Male 14 to 18 g/dL
  - Female 12 to 16 g/dL
- Hematocrit (a)
  - Male 42% to 52%
  - Female 37% to 47%
- Oxygen saturation (Sao$_2$) >94% (a, b)

Interventions	Rationales
1. Monitor for signs and symptoms of bleeding/hypovolemia/shock (when fluid volume decreases, the body responds to compensate) (Grossman & Porth, 2014):	1. The compensatory response to decreased circulatory volume aims to increase blood oxygen through increased heart and respiratory rates and decreased peripheral circulation (manifested by diminished peripheral pulses and cool skin).
a. Urine output <0.5 mL/kg/hr (early sign)	a. The kidney responds to decreased fluid volume by increasing the release of the antidiuretic hormone, which increases sodium retention and reduces urine production (Grossman & Porth, 2014).

Interventions	*Rationales*
b. Thirst c. Increased pulse rate with normal or slightly decreased blood pressure d. Increased capillary refill >3 seconds e. Decreased oxygen saturation <94% (pulse oximetry) f. Increased respiratory rate g. Diminished peripheral pulses h. Cool, pale, or cyanotic skin i. Restlessness, agitation, decreased mentation (late sign)	i. Decreased oxygen to the brain results in altered mentation.
2. Determine the risk status of the individual for postoperative hypovolemia (oliguria). a. Causes of oliguria can be divided into three categories: prerenal (blood flow related), renal (intrinsic kidney disorders), and postrenal (outlet obstruction)	2a. Prerenal causes can be fluid loss during surgery and as a result of nothing-by-mouth (NPO) status can disrupt fluid balance in a high-risk individual. Stress can cause sodium and water retention. Postoperative decreased urine output can be caused by hypovolemia (bleeding, fluid loss, NPO status, inadequate fluid replacement). Postrenal causes can be blocked urinary catheter or postoperative urinary retention.

3. Institute hourly urine output monitoring according to protocol and individual risks:
   a. Intake (parenteral and oral)
   b. Output and other losses (urine, drainage, and vomiting)	

4. Palpate for bladder distention and evaluate patency of urinary catheter.
   a. The kidneys respond to changes in blood volume and hypoxemia by reducing urine production.
   b. Decreased urine output is an earlier sign of hypovolemia than changes in pulse and blood pressure.
   c. Promptly report decreasing urine output.
	4. This will assess for outlet obstruction and blocked urinary catheter.

5. Monitor surgical site for the signs/symptoms of dehiscence and evisceration:
   a. Serosanguineous seepage from wound
   b. Inadequate incisional closure
	5. Wound dehiscence is the partial or complete separation of the outer layers of the joined incision and evisceration. Evisceration is the protrusion of the intestines through the open incision. The seepage of serosanguineous fluid through a closed abdominal wound is an early sign of abdominal wound dehiscence with possible evisceration.

> **CLINICAL ALERT:**
> • "A wound is a disruption of the normal structure and function of the skin and underlying soft tissue. Acute wounds in normal, healthy individuals heal through an orderly sequence of physiological events that include hemostasis, inflammation, epithelialization, fibroplasia, and maturation. When this process is altered or stalled, a chronic wound may develop and this is more likely to occur in patients with underlying disorders such as peripheral artery disease, diabetes, venous insufficiency, nutritional deficiencies, and other disease states" (Armstrong & Meyr, 2014).

Interventions	*Rationales*

6. Monitor for signs of paralytic ileus:
  a. Absent bowel sounds
  b. Nausea, vomiting
  c. Abdominal distention
	6. Intraoperative manipulation of abdominal organs and the depressive effects of narcotics and anesthetics on peristalsis can cause paralytic ileus, usually between the third and fifth postoperative day. Pain typically is localized, sharp, and intermittent.

7. Monitor for sepsis and systemic inflammatory response syndrome (Halloran, 2009):
  a. Urine output <0.5 mL/kg/hr
 	
  b. Body temperature greater than 38° C or less than 36° C
  c. Heart rate greater than 90/min
 	
  d. Hyperkalemia
 	
  e. Decreasing blood pressure
  f. Respiratory rate greater than 20/min
 	
  g. Hyperglycemia
 	
  h. White blood cell count greater than 12,000/µL or less than 4,000/µL or presence of 10% immature neutrophils
	7a. Urine output is decreased when sodium shifts into the cells, which pulls water into cells. Decreased circulation to kidneys reduces their ability to detoxify the toxins that result from anaerobic metabolism.
	
	  c. Decreased blood flow to brain, heart, and kidneys triggers baroreceptors and release of catecholamines, increasing heart rate/cardiac output and further increasing vasoconstriction.
	  d. Potassium moves into the cell with the sodium, impairing nervous, cardiovascular, and muscle cell function.
	  e. Movement of water into the cell causes hypovolemia.
	  f. Anaerobic metabolism decreases circulating oxygen. The body attempts to increase oxygenation by increasing respiratory rate.
	  g. The liver and kidneys produce more glucose in response to the release of epinephrine, norepinephrine, cortisol, and glucagon. Anaerobic metabolism reduces the effects of insulin. Insulin resistance contributes to multiple organ failure, nosocomial infection, and renal injury (Ball, deBeer, Gomm, Hickman, & Collins, 2007).
	  h. Increased white cells indicate an infectious process

8. Ensure blood culture is done before the start of any antibiotic. Culture any suspected infection sites (urine, sputum, invasive lines). **CLINICAL ALERT:** • Blood culture obtained after antibiotic therapy has been initiated can be inaccurate. • Research of individuals with septic shock demonstrated that the time to initiation of appropriate antimicrobial therapy was the strongest predictor of mortality (Schmidt & Mandel, 2012). • Microorganisms can be introduced into the body during surgery or through the incision. • Circulating pathogens trigger the body's defense mechanisms: WBCs are released to destroy some pathogens, and the hypothalamus raises the body temperature to kill others. Wound redness, tenderness, and edema result from lymphocyte migration to the area.	8. "Poor outcomes are associated with inadequate or inappropriate antimicrobial therapy (i.e., treatment with antibiotics to which the pathogen was later shown to be resistant in vitro). They are also associated with delays in initiating antimicrobial therapy, even short delays (e.g., an hour)" (Schmidt & Mandel, 2012).

9. Monitor for signs of urinary retention:
  a. Bladder distention and unrelieved associated pain (*Wagner, Johnson, & Kidd, 2006)
  b. Urine overflows (30 to 60 mL, or urine every 15 to 30 minutes)
	9. Anesthesia relaxes the muscles, affecting the bladder. As muscle tone returns, spasms of the bladder sphincter prevent urine outflow, causing bladder distention. When urine retention increases the intravesical pressure, the sphincter releases urine and control of flow is regained. Pain medications interfere with the perception of bladder fullness and urge to void.

(continued)

Interventions	*Rationales*
10. Instruct the individual to report bladder discomfort or inability to void.	10. Bladder discomfort and failure to void may be early signs of urinary retention.
11. If the individual does not void within 8 to 10 hours after surgery or complains of bladder discomfort, do the following: a. Warm the bedpan. b. Encourage the individual to get out of bed to use the bathroom, if possible. c. Instruct a male individual to stand when urinating, if possible. d. Run water in the sink as the individual attempts to void. e. Pour warm water over the individual's perineum.	11. These measures may help to promote relaxation of the urinary sphincter and facilitate voiding.
12. If the individual still cannot void, follow the protocols for straight catheterization, as ordered.	12. Straight catheterization is preferable to indwelling catheterization, because it carries less risk of urinary tract infection from ascending pathogens.
13. Monitor the status of DVT, noting: a. Diminished or absent peripheral pulses b. Unusual warmth and redness or coolness and cyanosis, increased leg swelling c. Increasing leg pain	13. Avoid performing Homans' sign (dorsiflexion *of the foot*) (Numerous studies have documented the unreliability of Homans' sign). Urbano (*2001) reported "Estimates of the accuracy of Homans' sign range from it being positive in 8% to 56% of cases of proven DVT and positive in greater than 50% of symptomatic clients without DVT" (p. 23). a. Insufficient circulation causes pain and diminished peripheral pulses. b. Unusual warmth and redness point to inflammation; coolness and cyanosis indicate vascular obstruction. c. Leg pain results from tissue hypoxia.
14. Monitor for signs and symptoms of pulmonary embolism: a. Acute, sharp chest pain b. Acute dyspnea, restlessness, cyanosis, decreased mental status or anxiety c. Cool, moist, and/or bluish-colored skin d. Tachycardia e. Tachypnea (Shaughnessy, 2007) f. Neck vein distention g. Crackles **CLINICAL ALERT:** • Call a code or rapid response team if sudden, severe chest pain, increased dyspnea, tachypnea occur. • Begin emergency care, as indicated (e.g., bag-mask ventilation, IV access).	14. Occlusion of pulmonary arteries impedes blood flow to the distal lung, producing a hypoxic state (Grossman & Porth, 2014).
15. Consult with physician/nurse practitioner for intermittent pneumatic compression devices or graduated compression stockings.	15. These should be used for individuals who are bleeding or at risk for it.
16. Evaluate hydration status based on urine specific gravity, intake/output, weights, and serum osmolality. Take steps to ensure adequate hydration.	16. Increased blood viscosity and coagulability and decreased cardiac output may contribute to thrombus formation.
17. Encourage individual to perform isotonic leg exercises.	17. They promote venous return.

Interventions	*Rationales*
18. Ambulate as soon as possible with at least 5 minutes of walking each waking hour. Avoid prolonged chair sitting with legs dependent. Explain risk of DVT and PE. If individual is resistant, evaluate the reason for pain.	18. Walking contracts leg muscles, stimulates the venous pump, and reduces stasis.
19. Elevate the affected extremity above the level of the heart unless contraindicated (e.g., CHF).	19. This positioning can help reduce interstitial swelling by promoting venous return.
20. Explain the effects of nicotine (cigarettes, cigars, smokeless tobacco) on circulation. Refer to Getting Started to Quit Smoking on thePoint.	20. Nicotine can cause vasoconstriction and hypercoagulable state, which contributes to poor circulation and clot formation (Giardina, 1999).

Clinical Alert Report

Before providing care, advise ancillary staff/student to report the following to the professional nurse assigned to the individual:

- Change in cognitive status
- Sudden restlessness, agitation, decreased mentation
- Oral temperature >100.5° F
- Systolic BP <90 mm Hg
- Resting pulse >100, <50
- Respiratory rate >28, <10/min
- Oxygen saturation <90%
- A report of leg pain, soreness. Increased leg swelling
- Diminished peripheral pulses
- Unusual warmth and redness
- Cool, pale, moist, or cyanotic skin
- Increased immobility (e.g., refusal to ambulate)
- Urine output <0.5 mL/kg/hr
- Increased drainage for wound
- Increased tenderness/complaints of pain

Documentation

Vital signs (pulses, respirations, blood pressure, and temperature)
Circulation (color, peripheral pulses)
Intake (oral, parenteral)
Output (urinary, tubes, specific gravity)
Bowel function (bowel sounds, defecation, distention)
Wound (color, drainage)
Unusual complaints or assessment findings

Postoperative: Nursing Diagnoses

Risk for Ineffective Respiratory Function Related to Immobility Secondary to Postanesthesia State and Pain

NOC
Aspiration Control, Respiratory Status

Goal

The individual will exhibit clear lung fields.

NIC
Airway Management, Cough Enhancement, Respiratory Monitoring, Positioning

Indicators

- Breath sounds present in all lobes
- Clear breath sounds in all lobes (no wheezes or congestion)
- Relaxed rhythmic respirations

Interventions	Rationales
1. Monitor respiratory status: Vital signs, pulse oximetry.	
2. Auscultate lung fields for diminished and abnormal breath sounds.	2. Presence of rales indicates retained secretions. Diminished breath sounds may indicate atelectasis.
3. Take measures to prevent aspiration. Position the individual on his or her side, with pillows supporting the back and knees slightly flexed.	3. In the postoperative period, decreased sensorium and hypoventilation contribute to increased risk of aspiration.
4. Reinforce preoperative individual teaching about the importance of turning, coughing, deep breathing, and leg exercises every 1 to 2 hours.	4. Postoperative pain may discourage compliance; reinforcing the importance of these measures may improve compliance.
5. Promote the following as soon as the individual returns to the unit: a. Deep breaths b. Coughing (except if contraindicated) c. Frequent turning d. Early ambulation e. Incentive spirometry every hour (10 breaths each time, or as ordered) (*Wagner et al., 2006).	5. Exercises and movement promote lung expansion and mobilization of secretions. Incentive spirometry promotes deep breathing by providing a visual indicator of the effectiveness of the breathing effort. Coughing assists in dislodging mucus plugs. Coughing is contraindicated in individuals who have had a head injury, intracranial surgery, eye surgery, or plastic surgery, because it increases intracranial and intraocular pressure and tension on delicate tissues (plastic surgery).
6. Encourage adequate oral fluid intake, as indicated.	6. Adequate hydration liquefies secretions, which enables easier expectoration and prevents stasis of secretions that provide a medium for microorganism growth. It also helps to decrease blood viscosity, which lowers the risk of clot formation.

Documentation

Temperature
Respiratory rate and rhythm
Breath sounds
Respiratory treatments and individual responses

Risk for (Surgical Site) Infection Related to Access for Organism Invasion Secondary to Surgery

NIC
Infection Control, Wound Care, Incision Site Care, Health Education

Goal

The individual will demonstrate healing of wound.

NOC
Infection Status, Wound Healing: Primary Infection, Immune Status

Indicators

- No abnormal drainage
- Intact, approximated wound edges

Interventions	Rationales
1. Identify individuals at risk for delayed wound healing: a. Malnourishment b. Tobacco use c. Obesity d. Anemia e. Diabetes f. Cancer	1. Delayed wound healing can allow microorganisms to enter the wound. "Surgical Site Infection (SSI) remains a substantial cause of morbidity, prolonged hospitalization, and death. SSI is associated with a mortality rate of 3%, and 75% of SSI-associated deaths are directly attributable to the SSI" (Centers for Disease Control and Prevention [CDC], 2015a).

Interventions	Rationales
g. Corticosteroid therapy h. Renal insufficiency i. Hypovolemia j. Hypoxia k. Surgery >3 hours l. Night or emergency surgery m. Zinc, copper, magnesium deficiency n. Immune system compromise	
2. Closely monitor the surgical sites in obese individuals.	2. A literature search reported that obesity compromises wound healing owing to inherent anatomic features of adipose tissue, vascular insufficiencies, cellular and composition modifications, oxidative stress, alterations in immune mediators, and nutritional deficiencies. These deficiencies may result in decreased collagen synthesis, decreased capacity to fight infection, and decreased ability to support the necessary mechanisms of the healing cascade (Pierpont et al., 2014)
3. Monitor normal wound healing by noting the following (Armstrong & Meyr, 2014; Mercandetti, 2013): a. Evidence of intact, approximated wound edges (primary intention). Within 48 hours after surgery, fibrin and epithelial cells, as well as strands of collagen fill in the gaps and seal the incision. b. Slight swelling, slight scabbing around sutures or staples and wound edges, and some redness and warmth. c. Expected drainage (1 to 5 days after surgery: sanguineous (bloody) to serosanguineous/watery mixture of serum and blood to serous (yellowish, clear). d. By day 5, a "healing ridge" of granulation tissue can be palpated directly under the incision and extending approximately 1 cm on both sides of the wound.	3. These observations are the normal inflammatory reaction triggered by the surgical procedure. Any deviations from this normal healing process—especially between post-op days 5 and 10—could spell trouble. Most dehiscence occurs 4 to 14 days after surgery (Mercandetti, 2013).

> **CLINICAL ALERT:**
> - A surgical wound with edges approximated by sutures usually heals by primary intention.
> - Granulation tissue is not visible and scar formation is minimal.
> - In contrast, a surgical wound with a drain or an abscess heals by secondary intention or granulation and has more distinct scar formation.
> - A restructured wound heals by third intention and results in a wider and deeper scar.

Interventions	Rationales
4. Maintain normothermia. Monitor temperature every 4 hours; notify physician/nurse practitioner if temperature is greater than 100.8° F	4. Hypothermia also increases the risk of surgical wound infection; hypothermia directly impairs immune function including T-cell-mediated antibody production. Thermoregulatory vasoconstriction decreases subcutaneous oxygen tension and increases the risk of wound infection (Seamon et al., 2012; Sessler, 2016).
5. Monitor for inadequate tissue oxygen in risk individuals (e.g., pulse oximetry): a. Advise smokers that the risk of wound infection is tripled in smokers (*Sessler, 2006).	5. Deceased tissue oxygen impairs tissue repair (*Sessler, 2006).

(continued)

Interventions	*Rationales*
b. Monitor for hyperglycemia in diabetic and nondiabetic individuals.	b. SSIs have been found to double in both diabetic and nondiabetic individuals and postcardiac surgical individuals when blood glucose exceeds 200 mg/dL in the first 48 hours (*Sessler, 2006).
c. Consult with physician/nurse practitioner for interventions to achieve rigorous postoperative glucose control.	c. Aggressive insulin infusion protocol has been shown to reduce wound infections, multiple organ failure, sepsis, and mortality in critical care individuals (*Sessler, 2006).
d. Aggressively manage postoperative pain using prevention vs. p.r.n. medication administration.	d. Postoperative pain provokes an autonomic response that produces arteriolar vasoconstriction and reduces circulation needed for wound healing (*Sessler, 2006).
e. Prevent hypovolemia.	e. Small-volume deficits can substantially reduce peripheral circulation (*Sessler, 2006).
6. Assess wound site every 24 hours and apply dressing if indicated; report any abnormal findings (e.g., increased redness, change in drainage, failure for edges to seal).	6. Wound healing by primary intention requires a dressing to protect it from contamination until the edges seal (usually 24 hours). Wound healing by secondary intention requires a dressing to maintain adequate hydration; the dressing is not needed after wound edges seal.
7. Monitor for signs and symptoms of wound infection: a. Increased swelling and redness b. Wound separation c. Increased serosanguineous or purulent drainage d. Prolonged subnormal temperature or significantly elevated temperature	7. Tissue responds to pathogen infiltration with increased blood and lymph flow (manifested by edema, redness, and increased drainage) and reduced epithelialization (marked by wound separation). Circulating pathogens trigger the hypothalamus to elevate the body temperature; certain pathogens cannot survive at higher temperatures.
8. Explain when a dressing is indicated for a wound healing by primary intention, and for one healing by secondary intention.	8. A wound healing by primary intention requires a dressing to protect it from contamination until the edges seal (usually by 24 hours). A wound healing by secondary intention requires a dressing to maintain adequate hydration; the dressing is not needed after wound edges seal.
9. Teach and assist the individual in the following: a. Supporting the surgical site when moving b. Splinting the area when coughing, sneezing, or vomiting	9. A wound typically requires 3 weeks for strong scar formation. Stress on the suture line before this occurs can cause disruption.
10. If indicated, consult an enterostomal or clinical nurse specialist for specific skin care measures.	10. Management of a complex wound or impaired healing requires expert nursing consultation.

Documentation

Status of wound
Signs and symptoms of infection
Temperature

Risk for Delayed Surgical Recovery Related to Factors That Can Inhibit Wound Healing, Optimal National Intake, and Mobilization Necessary for Recuperation

NOC
Wound healing::primary intention, Mobility. Surgical Recovery: Convalescence/ Immediate Postoperative

NIC
Incision site care, Pain management, Nutrition management, Self-Care assistance

Goals

The individual will:
- Have surgical site that shows evidence of healing. Preexisting...
- Increase mobility and participation in self-care activities
- Report if pain is relieved to their satisfaction
- Resume presurgery intake

Interventions	*Rationales*
1. Assess for the following risk factors: Add up the number of risk factors (from 1 to 10) in the (). The higher the score, the greater their risk. For example, an individual who smokes, has diabetes mellitus, and is obese has a total score of 15. The diagnosis can be written as *High Risk for Delayed Surgical Healing* (15) or add the risk factors, for example, as *High Risk for Delayed Surgical Healing related to obesity, diabetes mellitus, and tobacco use.*	
a. Infection colonization of microorganisms (1)	a. Preoperative nares colonization with *Staphylococcus aureus* noted in 30% of most healthy populations, especially methicillin-resistant *S. aureus* (MRSA), predisposes individuals to higher risk of SSI (Price et al., 2008).
b. Preexisting remote body site infection (1) c. Preoperative contaminated or dirty wound (e.g., posttrauma) (1)	b, c. Preoperative nares colonization with *S. aureus* noted in 30% of most healthy populations, especially methicillin-resistant *S. aureus* (MRSA), predisposes individuals to higher risk of SSI (Price et al., 2008)The Risk of SSI is influenced by the amount and virulence of the microorganism and the ability of the individual to resist it (Pear, 2007).
d. Glucocorticoid steroids (2)	d. Glucocorticoid steroids delay healing via global anti-inflammatory effects and suppression of cellular wound responses, including fibroblast proliferation and collagen synthesis. Systemic steroids cause wounds to heal with incomplete granulation tissue and reduced wound contraction (Armstrong & Meyr, 2014; Franz, Steed, & Robson, 2007; Guo & DiPietro, 2010).
e. Tobacco use (3)	e. Smoking has a transient effect on the tissue microenvironment and a prolonged effect on inflammatory and reparative cell functions, leading to delayed healing and complications. Quitting smoking 4 weeks before surgery restores tissue oxygenation and metabolism rapidly (Sørensen, 2012)
f. Malnutrition (4)	f. Malnourished individuals have been found to have less competent immune response to infection and decreased nutritional stores that will impair wound healing (Armstrong & Meyr, 2014; Speaar, 2008).
g. Obesity (5)	g. An obese individual may experience a compromise in wound healing owing to poor blood supply to adipose tissue. In addition, antibiotics are not absorbed well by adipose tissue. Despite excessive food intake, many obese individuals have protein malnutrition, which further impedes the healing (*Cheadle, 2006; Pierpont et al., 2014).
h. Perioperative hyperglycemia (6)	h. There are two primary mechanisms that place individuals experiencing acute perioperative hyperglycemia at increased risk for SSI. The first mechanism is the decreased vascular circulation that occurs, reducing tissue perfusion and impairing cellular-level functions. A clinical study by Akbari et al. (*1998) noted that when healthy, nondiabetic subjects ingested a glucose load, the endothelial-dependent vasodilatation in both the micro- and macrocirculations were impaired, similar to that seen in diabetic individuals. The second affected mechanism is the reduced activity of the cellular immunity functions of chemotaxis, phagocytosis, and killing of polymorphonuclear cells as well as monocytes/macrophages that have been shown to occur in the acute hyperglycemic state (Kwon, Thompson, & Dellinger, 2013)

Interventions	Rationales
i. Diabetes mellitus (7)	i. Postsurgical adverse outcomes related to diabetes mellitus are believed to be related to the preexisting complications of chronic hyperglycemia, which include vascular atherosclerotic disease and peripheral as well as autonomic neuropathies (Armstrong & Meyr, 2014; Geerlings & Hoepelman, 1999).
j. Altered immune response (8)	j. Suppression of the immune system by disease, medication, or age can delay wound healing (*Cheadle, 2006).
k. Chronic alcohol use/acute alcohol intoxication (9)	k. Chronic alcohol exposure causes impaired wound healing and enhanced host susceptibility to infections. Wounds from trauma in the presence of acute alcohol exposure have a higher rate of postinjury infection owing to decreased neutrophil recruitment and phagocytic function (Guo & DiPietro, 2010).
2. Explain the effects of nicotine (cigarettes, cigars, smokeless tobacco) on circulation 　a. If the individual quits smoking before the surgery, stress the importance of continued smoking cessation to reduce the risk of infection. Refer to Getting Started to Quit Smoking on thePoint at and print guidelines for the individual.	2. Nicotine can cause vasoconstriction and hypercoagulable state that contributes to poor circulation and clot formation (Giardina, 1999). Smoking cessation for at least 4 weeks before surgery reduces SSIs, but not other healing complications.
3. Refer to specific nursing diagnoses to reduce the risk factors if amenable to nursing care as: 　a. Imbalanced Nutrition 　b. Obesity 　c. Risk-Prone Behaviors, for example, alcohol, tobacco use 　d. Ineffective Health Management related to .... as evidenced by uncontrolled glucose levels 　e. Nonengagement related to .... as evidenced by inadequate management of disease (specify)	
4. Initiate health teaching and referrals as needed 　a. Demonstrate wound care, observe a relative or the individual doing wound care. 　b. Refer to drug/alcohol program if indicated. 　c. Arrange for home nursing consultation. 　d. Refer to diabetic education program.	

Acute Pain Related to Surgical Interruption of Body Structures, Flatus, and Immobility

NOC
Comfort Level, Pain Control

Goal

An individual will report progressive reduction of pain and an increase in activity.

NIC
Pain Management, Medication Management, Emotional Support, Teaching: Individual, Hot/Cold Application, Simple Massage

Indicators

• Relate factors that increase pain.
• Report effective interventions.

Interventions	Rationales
1. Collaborate with the individual to determine effective pain-relief interventions.	1. An individual experiencing pain may feel a loss of control over his or her body and life. Collaboration can help minimize this feeling.
2. Teach the individual to splint the surgical wound with a pillow when coughing, sneezing, or vomiting.	2. Splinting reduces stress on the suture line by equalizing pressure across the wound.
3. Listen attentively to complaints, and convey that you are assessing the pain because you want to understand it better, not because you are trying to determine if it really exists.	3. An individual who feels the need to convince health care providers that she or he actually is experiencing pain is likely to have increased anxiety that can lead to greater pain.

4. Provide optimal pain relief with prescribed analgesics:
  a. Determine the preferred administration route—by mouth, intramuscular, intravenous, or rectal. Consult with the physician or advanced practice nurse.
 	
  b. Assess vital signs—especially respiratory rate—before and after administering any narcotic agent.
  c. Take a preventive approach to pain medication; that is, administer medication before an activity (e.g., ambulation) to enhance participation (but be sure to evaluate the hazards of sedation); instruct the individual to request pain medication as needed before pain becomes severe.
  d. After administering the pain medication, return in ½ hour to evaluate its effectiveness.
	4a. The proper administration route optimizes the efficacy of pain medications. The oral route is preferred in most cases; for some drugs, the liquid dosage form may be given to an individual who has difficulty swallowing. If frequent injections are necessary, the intravenous (IV) route is preferred to minimize pain and maximize absorption; however, IV administration may produce more profound side effects than other routes.
	  b. Narcotics can depress the respiratory center of the brain.
	  c. The preventive approach may reduce the total 24-hour dose as compared with the p.r.n. approach; it also provides a more constant blood drug level, reduces the individual's craving for the drug, and eliminates the anxiety associated with having to ask for and wait for p.r.n. relief.
	  d. Each individual responds differently to pain medication; careful monitoring is needed to assess individual response (*Lehne, 2004; Lewis et al., 2011).

5. Explain and assist with noninvasive and nonpharmacologic pain-relief measures (e.g., splinting the incision site, proper positioning, heat or cold application). Refer to Acute Pain for additional interventions in Unit II Section 1.	5. These measures can help to reduce pain by substituting another stimulus to prevent painful stimuli from reaching higher brain centers. In addition, relaxation reduces muscle tension and may help enhance the individual's sense of control over pain.

6. Teach the individual to expel flatus by the following measures:
  a. Walking as soon as possible after surgery
  b. Changing positions regularly, as possible (e.g., lying prone, assuming the knee–chest position)
	6. Postoperatively, sluggish peristalsis results in accumulation of nonabsorbable gas. Pain occurs when unaffected bowel segments contract in an attempt to expel this accumulated gas. Activity speeds the return of peristalsis and the expulsion of flatus; proper positioning helps cause the gas to rise and be expelled.

Documentation

Type, route, and dosage schedule of all prescribed medications
Unsatisfactory relief from pain-relief measures

Risk for Imbalanced Nutrition: Related to Increased Protein and Vitamin Requirements for Wound Healing and Decreased Intake Secondary to Pain, Nausea, Vomiting, and Diet Restrictions

NOC
Nutritional Status,
Teaching: Nutrition

Goal

The individual will resume ingestion of the daily nutritional requirements.

NIC
Nutrition Management,
Nutritional Monitoring

Indicators

- Selections from the four basic food groups, taking into account cultural preferences and allergies (*Lewis et al., 2004).
- 2,000 to 3,000 mL of fluids.
- Adequate fiber, vitamins, and minerals.

Interventions	Rationales
1. Start clear liquids when signs of bowel function return.	1. Clear liquid diets supply fluid and electrolytes in a form that requires minimal digestion and little stimulation of the gastrointestinal tract.
2. If oral intake does not progress from clear fluids, consult with dietician.	
3. Restrict fluids before meals and large amounts of fluids at any time; instead, encourage the individual to ingest small amounts of ice chips or sip cool, clear liquids (e.g., dilute tea, Jell-O water, flat ginger ale, or cola) frequently, unless vomiting persists.	3. Gastric distention from fluid ingestion can trigger the vagal visceral afferent pathways that stimulate the medulla oblongata (vomiting center) (*Wagner et al., 2006).
4. Teach the individual to move slowly.	4. Rapid movements stimulate the vomiting center by triggering vestibulocerebellar afferents.
5. Reduce or eliminate unpleasant sights and odors.	5. Noxious odors and sights can stimulate the vomiting center.
6. Provide good mouth care after the individual vomits.	6. Good oral care reduces the noxious taste.
7. Instruct the individual to avoid lying down flat for at least 2 hours after eating. An individual who must rest should sit or recline with her or his head at least 4 inches higher than the feet.	7. Pressure on the stomach can trigger vagal visceral afferent stimulation of the vomiting center in the brain.
8. Teach the individual to practice relaxation exercises during episodes of nausea. Refer also to Nausea in Unit II Section 1.	8. Concentrating on relaxation activities may help to block stimulation of the vomiting center.
9. Maintain good oral hygiene at all times.	9. A clean, refreshed mouth can stimulate the appetite.
10. Administer an antiemetic agent before meals, if indicated. If individual is unable or unwilling to drink, notify physician/nurse practitioner/physical assistant for antiemetics or parenteral fluids.	10. Antiemetics prevent nausea and vomiting.

Documentation

Intake and output (amount, type, time)
Vomiting (amount, description)
Multidisciplinary individual education record

Risk for Constipation Related to Decreased Peristalsis Secondary to Immobility and the Effects of Anesthesia and Narcotics

NOC
Bowel Elimination,
Hydration, Symptom
Control

Goal

The individual will resume effective preoperative bowel function.

NIC
Bowel Management,
Fluid Management,
Constipation/Impaction
Management

Indicators

- No bowel distention
- Bowel sounds in all quadrants

Interventions	Rationales
1. Monitor for bowel sounds, abdominal distention, and bowel movements. After surgery, opioid pain medications, anticholinergic, anesthesia, decreased oral intake, and immobility can cause constipation.	1. Manipulation of the bowel during surgery can decrease peristalsis. Decreased oral intake and decreased activity the first few days after the surgery will decrease bowel motility.
a. Explain that a bowel movement should occur 2 to 3 days after surgery. Drink 6 to 8 glasses of water daily.	
b. Assess bowel sounds to determine when to introduce liquids. Advance diet as tolerated.	b. Bowel sounds indicate the return of peristalsis.
2. Explain the effects of daily activity on elimination. Assist with ambulation when possible.	2. Activity influences bowel elimination and expelling of gas by improving abdominal muscle tone and stimulating appetite and peristalsis.
3. Promote factors that contribute to optimal elimination.	
a. Balanced diet: Review a list of foods high in bulk (e.g., fresh fruits with skins, bran, nuts and seeds, whole grain breads and cereals, cooked fruits and vegetables, and fruit juices).	3a. A well-balanced diet high in fiber content stimulates peristalsis.
b. Encourage intake of fluids at least 8 to 10 glasses (about 2,000 mL) daily, unless contraindicated.	b. Sufficient fluid intake is necessary to maintain bowel patterns and promote proper stool consistency.
4. Notify the physician/nurse practitioner/physical assistant if bowel sounds do not return within 6 to 10 hours, or if elimination does not return within 2 to 3 days postoperatively.	4. Absence of bowel sounds may indicate paralytic ileus; absence of bowel movements

Documentation

Bowel movements
Bowel sounds

Impaired Physical Mobility Related to Pain and Weakness Secondary to Anesthesia, Tissue Hypoxia, and Insufficient Fluid and Nutrient Intake

NOC
Ambulation, Fall Prevention, Mobility

Goal

The individual will increase tolerance to activities of daily living (ADLs).

NIC
Ambulation, Energy Management, Exercise Promotion, Mutual Goal Setting, Teaching: Prescribed Activity

Indicators

- Progressive ambulation
- Ability to perform ADLs

Interventions	Rationales
1. Encourage progress in the activity level during each shift, as indicated:	1. A gradual increase in activity allows the individual's cardiopulmonary system to return to its preoperative state without excessive strain.
a. Allow the individual's legs to dangle first; support the individual from the side.	a. Dangling the legs first helps to minimize orthostatic hypotension.
b. Place the bed in high position and raise the head of the bed.	b. Raising the head of the bed helps to reduce stress on suture lines.
c. Encourage the individual to increase activity when pain is at a minimum or after pain-relief measures take effect.	
2. If ambulation is problematic, refer to Activity Intolerance for specifics in Progressive Ambulation Protocol.	

(*continued*)

Interventions	Rationales

3. Assess for abnormal responses to increased activity:
  a. Decreased pulse rate
  b. Decreased or unchanged systolic blood pressure
  c. Excessively increased or decreased respiratory rate
  d. Confusion or vertigo
	3. Activity tolerance depends on the individual's ability to adapt to the physiologic requirements of increased activity. The expected immediate physiologic responses to activity are increased blood pressure and increased respiratory rate and depth. After 3 minutes, the pulse rate should decrease to within 10 beats/min of the individual's usual resting rate. Abnormal findings represent the body's inability to meet the increased oxygen demands imposed by activity.

Documentation

Ambulation (time, amount)

Abnormal or unexpected response to increased activity

> **TRANSITION TO HOME/COMMUNITY CARE**
>
> If indicated, review the risk diagnoses identified for this individual on admission:
> - Is the person still at risk?
> - Can the family reduce the risks?
> - Is the person at higher risk at home?
> - Is a Home Health Nurse assessment needed?
> - Refer to transition planner/case manager/social service
> - When is this person scheduled for follow-up with primary provider? Specialists? Record dates of appointments.
> - Complete a medication reconciliation before transition. Refer to index.

STAR

Stop

Think   Is this person at high risk for injury, falls, medical complications, and/or inability to care for self (activities of daily living) at home?

    Is there a support person available?

    Is the person competent to manage self-administration of medications, treatment procedures? Are additional resources needed?

    Can the person explain how to monitor the condition (e.g., blood glucose, signs/symptoms of complications, dietary/mobility restrictions, and when to call his or her primary provider or specialist)?

Act   Contact or provide the appropriate resource (e.g., contacting a support person, home health assessment, additional teaching, printed materials).

Review   Has the problem been addressed? If not, use SBAR to communicate to the appropriate person.

Risk for Ineffective Health Management Related to Insufficient Knowledge of Care of Operative Site, Restrictions (Diet, Activity), Medications, Signs and Symptoms of Complications, and Follow-Up Care

NOC

Compliance (Engagement)
Behavior, Knowledge:
Treatment Regimen,
Participation: Health-Care
Decisions, Treatment
Behavior: Illness or Injury

Goals

The goals for this diagnosis represent those associated with transition planning. Refer to the transition criteria.

NIC

Anticipatory Guidance,
Learning Facilitation,
Risk Management,
Health Education,
Teaching: Procedures/
Treatments, Health
System Guidance

Interventions	Rationales
1. Explain the process of normal wound healing by noting the following (Armstrong & Meyr, 2014; Beattie, 2007): a. Within 48 hours the wound edges are together. b. Slight swelling, slight scabbing around sutures or staples and wound edges with some redness and warmth is normal. c. Some drainage (1 to 5 days after surgery, bloody to watery rose colored to pink to yellowish/clear). d. By day 5, a "healing ridge" of scar tissue can be palpated directly under the incision and extending on both sides of the wound. e. Advise to report to surgeon/primary care provider if the condition of the wound or drainage changes.	1. Teaching what is expected will prepare the person to identify abnormal signs and the need to report. These observations are the normal inflammatory reaction triggered by the surgical procedure. Any deviations from this normal healing process—especially between post-op days 5 and 10—can indicate infection or dehiscence. Most dehiscence occurs 4 to 14 days after surgery.
2. As appropriate, explain and demonstrate care of an uncomplicated surgical wound: a. Washing with soap and water b. Dressing changes using clean technique	2. Uncomplicated wounds have sealed edges after 24 hours and therefore do not require aseptic technique or a dressing; however, a dressing may be applied if the wound is at risk for injury.
3. As appropriate, explain and demonstrate care of a complicated surgical wound.	3. Aseptic technique is necessary to prevent wound contamination during dressing changes. Hand-washing helps to prevent contamination of the wound and the spread of infection. Proper handling and disposal of contaminated dressings helps to prevent infection transmission. Daily assessment is necessary to evaluate healing and detect complications.
4. If a home health nurse is needed for wound care, initiate a referral.	
5. Teach the individual about factors that can delay wound healing: a. Keep wound covered until the wound is sealed to prevent dehydrated wound tissue b. Wound infection c. Inadequate nutrition and hydration d. Compromised blood supply e. Increased stress or excessive activity	5a. Epithelial migration is impeded under dry crust; movement is three times faster over moist tissue (Grossman & Porth, 2014). b. The exudates in infected wounds impair epithelialization and wound closure. c. To repair tissue, the body needs increased protein and carbohydrate intake and adequate hydration for vascular transport of oxygen and wastes. d. Blood supply to injured tissue must be adequate to transport leukocytes and remove wastes. e. Increased stress and activity result in higher levels of chalone, a mitotic inhibitor that depresses epidermal regeneration.
6. Reinforce activity restrictions, as indicated (e.g., bending, lifting). Advise to ask surgeon at post-op office visit regarding activity restrictions.	6. Avoiding certain activities decreases the risk of wound dehiscence before scar formation (usually after 3 weeks).
7. Explain that a bowel movement should occur 2 to 3 days after surgery. Advise to: a. Drink 6 to 8 glasses of water daily b. Eat light meals c. Keep urine clear or a pale yellow	7. Optimal bowel elimination requires good hydration/urine color is a good measure of hydration (e.g., pale = well hydrated)
8. Explain that a well-balanced diet is needed to meet the body's needs for surgical wound healing (Lutz, Mazur, & Litch, 2015).	8. To support proper wound healing, your body needs adequate intake of calories, protein, iron, vitamin A, vitamin C, zinc, and adequate hydration for vascular transport of oxygen and wastes.

(continued)

Interventions	Rationales
a. Iron: The practice of avoiding transfusions owing to risks and shorter postoperative stays results in individuals leaving hospital after surgery with lower hemoglobin (Hb) than previously. Iron is needed to replenish red blood cells decreased with the blood loss during surgery.	a. Iron-rich foods include meat, shellfish, baked potato with skin, legumes, chickpeas, kidney beans, peas, apricots, egg, whole grain bread, tamarind, iron-fortified cereals.
b. Vitamin A: Cellular differentiation, proliferation, epithelialization, collagen synthesis (scar tissue) counteract catabolic effect of steroids with renal failure owing to greater potential for toxicity.	b. Vitamin A-rich foods include fish,* dairy products,* grape fruit, cantaloupe, mango, peaches, papaya, collard greens,* sweet potatoes, carrots, kale,* spinach.*
c. Vitamin C: Collagen synthesis (scar tissue). Not for individuals with renal failure owing to risk for renal oxalate stone formation.	c. Vitamin C-rich foods include oranges, melons, strawberries, papaya, broccoli, bell peppers, baked potato, tomato, cauliflower.
d. Zinc: Protein synthesis, cellular replication, collagen formation; large wounds, chest tubes, and wound drains contribute to further zinc losses.	d. Zinc-rich foods include meat, pork, seafood, dark poultry, dairy products, beans

9. Teach the individual and family to watch for and report signs and symptoms of possible complications: a. Persistent temperature elevation b. Difficulty breathing, chest pain c. Change in sputum characteristics d. Increasing weakness, fatigue, pain, or abdominal distention e. Wound changes (e.g., separation, unusual or increased drainage, increased redness or swelling) f. Voiding difficulties, burning on urination, urinary frequency, or cloudy, foul-smelling urine g. Pain, swelling, and warmth in calf	9. Early detection and reporting danger signs and symptoms enable prompt intervention to minimize the severity of complications.

> **CLINICAL ALERT:**
> • Instruct to promptly report any of the above signs/symptoms to surgeon for an evaluation of complications such as infections, DVT, urinary retention or go to the ER.

*Also rich in iron

Documentation

Transition instructions
Individual leaving the hospital
Status at transition (pain, activity, wound healing)

Abdominal Aortic Aneurysm Repair

"Approximately 15,000 deaths annually in the United States are attributed to abdominal aortic aneurysm (AAA)" (Collins, 2015). Elective AAA repair before the development of symptoms is the most effective means to prevent rupture (Collins, 2015).

In spite of improvements in prehospital care, cardiovascular anesthesia, and critical care, postoperative mortality following repair of ruptured AAA remains about 40% to 50% (Collins, 2015). "Mortality can be as high as 90 percent in individuals who suffer rupture of an AAA prehospital. However, the survival rate is good in the subset of, individuals who are not in severe shock and who receive timely, expert surgical intervention" (Pearce, 2011). "Mortality in elective AAA repair is drastically lower than that associated with rupture. Consequently, the emphasis must be on early detection and repair free from complications" (Dillavou, 2015; Pearce, 2011).

The major risk factors or accelerators for AAA include age 60 or older, male gender, positive family history of aneurysm, cardiovascular disease, a history of ever smoking, and hypertension (Collins, 2015).

The two primary methods of AAA repair are open and endovascular. Open AAA repair requires direct access to the aorta through an abdominal or retroperitoneal approach.

Endovascular aneurysm repair (EVAR) is an important advance in the treatment of abdominal aortic aneurysm (AAA). EVAR is performed by inserting graft components folded and compressed within a delivery sheath through the lumen of an access vessel, usually the common femoral artery" (Chaer, 2015).

"Upon deployment, the endograft expands, contacting the aortic wall proximally and iliac vessels distally to exclude the aortic aneurysm sac from aortic blood flow and pressure" (Chaer, 2015). "Compared with open AAA repair, EVAR is associated with a significant reduction in perioperative mortality, primarily because EVAR does not require operative exposure of the aorta or aortic clamping" (Chaer, 2015).

Time Frame
Preoperative
Postoperative periods

▪▪▪■■ DIAGNOSTIC CLUSTER

Postoperative Period

Collaborative Problems

Risk for Complications of Endoleaks

Risk for Complications of Distal Vessel Thrombosis or Emboli

Risk for Complications of Renal Failure

Risk for Complications of Mesenteric Ischemia/Thrombosis

Risk for Complications of Spinal Cord Ischemia

Risk for Complication of Acute Inflammatory Syndrome

Nursing Diagnoses

▲ Risk for Infection related to location of surgical incision (refer to Arterial Bypass Graft)

▲ Risk for Ineffective Health Management related to insufficient knowledge of home care, activity restrictions, signs and symptoms of complications, and follow-up care

Related Care Plan

General Surgery Generic Care Plan

▲ This diagnosis was reported to be monitored for or managed frequently (75% to 100%).
▲ This diagnosis was reported to be monitored for or managed often (50% to 74%).

Transition Criteria

Before transition, the individual or family will:

1. State wound care measures to perform at home.
2. Verbalize precautions regarding activities.
3. State signs and symptoms that must be reported to a health care professional.

Transitional Risk Assessment Plan (TRAP)

Begin this plan on admission.

Implement the Transitional Risk Assessment Plan (TRAP):

* Refer to inside back cover.
* Add each validated risk diagnosis to individual's problem list with the risk code in ( ).
* Refer to Unit II to the individual risk nursing diagnoses/collaborative problems for outcomes and interventions in Unit II.

R: "Close coordination of care in the post-acute period, early transition follow-up care, enhanced client education and self-management training, proactive end-of-life counseling, and extending the resources and clinical expertise over time via multidisciplinary team management" can lower readmission rates and improve health outcomes (Boutwell & Hwu, 2009, p. 14). Interventions are utilized to activate the individual and family to select changes in their everyday lifestyle choices to improve their health (Hibbard & Greene, 2013).

Collaborative Outcomes

The individual will be monitored for early signs and symptoms of (a) rupture of aneurysm (preoperative), (b) distal vessel thrombosis/emboli, (c) renal failure, (d) mesenteric ischemia/thrombosis, and (e) spinal cord ischemia, and will receive collaborative interventions if indicated to restore physiologic stability.

Indicators of Physiologic Stability

* Calm, oriented (a, d)
* All pulses palpable and strong (a, b, e)
* No abdominal, pelvic, chest pain (a, b)
* Nontender abdomen (a, b, d)
* Capillary refill <3 seconds (b)
* No numbness of extremities (b, e)
* Urine output >0.5 mL/kg/hr (c, e)
* Blood urea nitrogen 5 to 25 mg/dL (c)
* Serum creatinine
  * Male 0.6 to 1.5 g/dL
  * Female 0.6 to 1.1 g/dL
* Sensory/motor functions intact (e)
* Bowel sounds present 5 to 30 times/min (d)
* Flatus present (d)
* Soft-formed bowel movements (d)

 Carp's Cues

Please refer to the Generic Care Plan for the Surgical Client for detailed interventions for managing all surgical conditions. This care plan addresses specific additional interventions associated with the type of surgery performed.

Interventions	Rationales
1. Monitor all pulses (carotid, brachial, radial, ulnar, femoral, popliteal, dorsalis pedis, and posterior tibial) and blood pressure.	1. A carotid bruit must be evaluated preoperatively to rule out risk of stroke during the operation. Assessing upper extremity pulses establishes a baseline for follow-up after arterial lines are in place and arterial punctures are made for blood gas analysis. Assessing lower extremity pulses establishes a baseline for postoperative assessment. A potential complication of aneurysm repair is thrombosis or embolus of distal vessels. Also, individuals with abdominal aneurysm have a higher incidence of popliteal aneurysm than the general population.

Interventions	Rationales
2. If before surgery, monitor for signs and symptoms of aneurysm rupture: **CLINICAL ALERT:** • If there is a sudden change in the individual's hemodynamic status, complaints of acute abdominal pain with intense back, chest, or pelvic pain, pain sometimes described as "tearing," call Rapid Response Team. • Pain results from massive tissue hypoxia and profuse bleeding into the abdominal cavity (*Beese-Bjurstrom, 2004). a. Tender, pulsating abdomen b. Restlessness c. Shock	3. The larger the aneurysm, the greater the risk of rupture. Risk of rupture increases significantly when aneurysm size is >5 cm. a. Abdominal pulsations and tenderness result from rhythmic pulsations of the artery and tissue hypoxia, respectively. b. Restlessness is a response to tissue hypoxia. c. Shock may result from massive blood loss and tissue hypoxia.

Postoperative: Collaborative Problems

Risk for Complications of Distal Vessel Thrombosis or Emboli

Risk for Complications of Renal Failure

Risk for Complications of Mesenteric Ischemia/Thrombosis

Risk for Complications of Spinal Cord Ischemia

Risk for Complications of Aortoenteric Fistula

Risk for Complications of Endoleak

Risk for Complication of Acute Inflammatory Syndrome

Interventions	Rationales
1. Monitor for complications of anticoagulant therapy. Refer to Risk for Complications of Anticoagulant Therapy.	1. Heparin is utilized intraoperatively to prevent thrombosis formation.
2. Monitor for signs of ischemic complications (Chaer, 2015).	2. Ischemic complications are the result of thrombosis, embolization, endoleaks, or malpositioning of graft. The diagnosis of endoleak is made on follow-up imaging, usually computed tomography (CT), that demonstrates blood outside the bounds of the endograft (Chaer, 2015).
3. Monitor for deep vein thrombosis (DVT): a. Diminished distal pulses, increased capillary refill time (>3 seconds) b. Pallor or darkened patches of skin c. Refer to Risk for Complications of DVT in Unit II for specific complications.	
4. Assess for access site complications such as hematoma, acute thrombosis of the accessed vessel, distal embolization, dissection, pseudoaneurysm, and arteriovenous fistula (Chaer, 2015).	4. Access site complications are among the most common problems after endovascular aortic repair, occurring in 9% to 16% of patients following endovascular AAA repair (Chaer, 2015).

(continued)

Interventions	*Rationales*

> **CLINICAL ALERT**
> * "Ischemia may be due to arterial thrombosis, embolism, arterial dissection, or arterial obstruction as a result of the endograft positioning" (Chaer, 2015).
> * "Ischemia may affect any arterial bed in the immediate vicinity of the endograft or distal to it, including the kidneys, intestines, pelvic muscles or organs, and lower extremities" (Chaer, 2015).

5. Monitor for colinic ischemia: a. Decreased bowel sounds. b. Constipation or diarrhea (may be bloody) (*Beese-Bjurstrom, 2004). c. Increasing abdominal pain or girth (*Beese-Bjurstrom, 2004). d. New-onset nausea/vomiting.	5. The mesenteric artery, like the renal artery, is at risk for thrombosis. b. A liquid bowel movement before the third postoperative day may point to bowel ischemia; may be bloody. c. Postoperative pain normally decreases each day.
6. Monitor for spinal cord ischemia: a. Urinary retention or incontinence b. Complaints of numbness of legs, feet c. Change in sensation or ability to move toes	6. Inadequate perfusion above the second lumbar vertebra (L2) can result in bladder dysfunction.
7. Monitor for renal dysfunction: a. Urinary retention or incontinence b. Decreased urine output	7. Severe renal dysfunction after elective endovascular repair may be related to renal ischemia or the administration of intravenous contrast (Chaer, 2015). Thrombosis can cause renal artery compromise.
8. Monitor for limb occlusion: a. Lower extremity pulses b. Complaints of pain in legs with ambulation	8. Kinking of graft or poor outflow supplying the leg results in a cool, pale, numb, tingling, or painful sensation.

> **CLINICAL ALERT:**
> * Any change in clinical assessment data indicating possible thrombosis or impaired circulation requires immediate notification of surgeon.

9. If the individual complains of pain, assess its location and characteristics.	9. It is important to differentiate pain of surgical manipulation from ischemic pain. Microembolization from the aneurysm to the distal skin causes skin infarctions manifested by point discomfort at the infarct and a dark pink-purple discoloration.
10. Monitor for abdominal compartment syndrome in individuals post ruptured repair. Refer to Index for Risk for Complications of Abdominal Compartment Syndrome.	10. The risk of abdominal compartment syndrome is increased in individuals with ruptured AAA owing to the extent of fluid resuscitation, and the volume effect of the retroperitoneal hematoma.
11. Monitor for acute inflammatory syndrome: a. Fever b. Leukocytosis c. Elevated serum C-reactive protein (CRP) concentration, perigraft air	11. Between 13% and 60% of individuals experience a transient acute flu-like inflammatory syndrome following aortic endograft placement that can delay the usually quick recovery following EVAR. It can occur during the first week to 10 days after implantation. The etiology is unknown.
12. Carefully monitor intake, output, and hydration and renal status (e.g., central venous pressure/hemodynamic monitoring every hour for the first 24 hours postoperatively) (*Anderson, 2001).	12. Hypovolemia can cause thrombosis of graft and decrease renal perfusion. Cross-clamping during surgery will disrupt blood flow to the renal arteries.

Interventions	Rationales
13. Monitor blood pressure and report elevations from baseline.	13. Hypertension can result from vasoconstrictor and can potentiate graft rupture.
14. Monitor for retroperitoneal bleeding (Dillavou, 2015): a. Decreased hematocrit b. Hypotension c. Tachycardia d. Back pain e. Gray Turner sign (ecchymotic [bluish] discoloration in flank area)	14. Retroperitoneal bleeding can occur after endovascular surgery (Dillavou, 2015).
15. Monitor for intra-abdominal bleeding (Dillavou, 2015): a. Increased abdominal girth b. Decreased hematocrit c. Hypotension d. Tachycardia	15. Intra-abdominal bleeding can occur during the first 24 hours postoperatively.
16. Palpate or Doppler peripheral pulses every hour for the first 24 hours.	16. Early detection of graft failure can prevent limb loss.
17. Monitor for signs of infection. Refer to Risk for Infection in Unit II Section 1.	17. Wound and endovascular graft infections can occur.

Clinical Alert Report

Before providing care, advise ancillary staff/student to report the following to the professional nurse assigned to the individual:

- Change in cognitive status
- New-onset abdominal/back pain
- Oral temperature >100.5° F
- Systolic BP <90 mm Hg
- Resting pulse >100, <50
- Respiratory rate >28, <10/min
- Oxygen saturation <90%
- Decreased/absent bowel sounds
- Urine output <0.5 mg/kg/hr

Documentation

Vital signs
Circulation (distal, pulses, color)
Bowel sounds, presence of occult blood
Lower extremities (sensation, motor function)
Urine (output, occult blood)
Characteristics of pain
Unrelieved pain
Interventions, response to interventions

Postoperative: Nursing Diagnoses

TRANSITION TO HOME/COMMUNITY CARE

If indicated, review the risk diagnoses identified for this individual on admission:

- Is the person still at risk?
- Can the family reduce the risks?
- Is the person at higher risk at home?
- Is a Home Health Nurse assessment needed?
- Refer to transition planner/case manager/social service
- When is this person scheduled for follow-up with primary provider? Specialists? Record dates of appointments.
- Complete a medication reconciliation before transition. Refer to index.

STAR   **Stop**

Think   Is this person at high risk for injury, falls, medical complications, and/or inability to care for self (activities of daily living)?

Is there a support person available?

Is the person competent to manage self-administration of medications, treatment procedures? Are additional resources needed?

Can the person explain how to monitor the condition (e.g., blood glucose, signs/symptoms of complications, dietary/mobility restrictions, and when to call his or her primary provider or specialist)?

Act   Contact or provide the appropriate resource (e.g., contacting a support person, home health assessment, additional teaching, printed materials).

Review   Has the problem been addressed? If not, use SBAR to communicate to the appropriate person.

Risk for Ineffective Health Management Related to Insufficient Knowledge of Home Care, Activity Restrictions, Signs and Symptoms of Complications, and Follow-Up Care

NOC

Compliance (Engagement) Behavior, Knowledge: Treatment Regimen, Participation: Health Care Decisions, Treatment Behavior: Illness or Injury

NIC

Anticipatory Guidance, Risk Identification, Health Education, Learning Facilitation

Goal

The goals for this diagnosis represent those associated with transition planning. Refer to the transition criteria.

Interventions	Rationales
1. For wound care measures and rationale, refer to the General Surgery Care Plan.	
2. If an aorto-bifemoral graft was performed, reinforce the need for a slouched position when sitting.	2. A slouched position helps to prevent graft kinking and possible occlusion.
3. Reinforce activity restrictions (e.g., car riding, stair climbing, lifting). Specifically ask surgeon how long to continue restrictions at postop office visit.	3. About 5 to 6 weeks after abdominal surgery for an individual in good nutritional status, the collagen matrix of the wound becomes strong enough to withstand stress from activity. The surgeon may prefer to limit activity for a longer period, because certain activities place tension on the surgical site (Walker et al., 2010). The period of activity restriction is significantly less with endovascular repair, as incisions are smaller.
4. Advise relatives that the recommendation for screening for AAA are: a. Men 60 years of age or older and who are either siblings or offspring of individuals with AAAs should undergo physical examination and ultrasound screening. b. Men who are 65 to 75 years of age who have ever smoked should undergo a physical examination and one-time ultrasound screening.	4. The United States Preventive Services Task Force (USPSTF) has made these recommendations so that if an aneurysm is found, it can be monitored and surgically removed if more than 5.5 cm rather than risking a rupture (LeFevre, 2014). Elective surgery for AA has a mortality rate between 1% and 5%, whereas the mortality rate for ruptured AAA is 60% in the community and 40% of those that make it to surgery (Eidt, 2015)
5. If the individual smokes, reinforce the health benefits of quitting, and refer the individual to a smoking cessation program, if available. Refer to Getting Started to Quit Smoking on thePoint.	5. Tobacco acts as a potent vasoconstrictor that increases stress on the graft.

Interventions	Rationales
6. Stress the importance of managing hypertension, if indicated.	6. Hypertension can cause false aneurysms at the anastomosis site.
7. Instruct to immediately call the surgeon if: a. Any changes in color, temperature, or sensation in the legs. b. Blood in stools or darkening of stools. c. New-onset diarrhea/constipation	7a. These signs and symptoms may indicate thrombosis or embolism that requires immediate evaluation. b. Duodenal bleeding may be a sign of erosion of the aortic graft into the duodenum.
8. Explain acute inflammatory syndrome or postimplantation syndrome (PIS): a. Fever b. Leukocytosis c. Elevated serum CRP concentration.	8. Between 13% and 60% of individuals experience a transient acute flu-like inflammatory syndrome after aortic endograft placement that can delay the usually quick recovery following EVAR. It can occur during the first week to 10 days after implantation. The type of the endograft's material seems to play a role in the inflammatory response. It is generally a benign condition, though in some individuals it may negatively affect outcome as sepsis (Arnaoutoglou et al., 2015).
9. Seek emergency treatment if (call 911 if needed): a. Complaints of sudden chest/abdominal/back pain b. Change in cognitive status c. Sudden increasing pulse rate, respirations d. New-onset cool, pale, numb, tingling, or painful lower limb(s) e. New-onset urinary retention/incontinence	
10. Refer to a publication on AAA and surgical repair from the Society of Vascular Nursing, access at http://www .svnnet.org/wp-content/uploads/2015/09/SVN-Abdominal-Aortic-Aneurysms-Endovascular-Repair.pdf	

Documentation

Teaching/instructions given
Referrals, if indicated

Amputation

In the United States, approximately 185,000 amputations are performed annually. There were an estimated in 2005, that there were an 1.6 million individuals living with the loss of a limb; these estimates are expected to more than double to 3.6 million such individuals by the year 2050 (Ertl, 2012).

Amputation is the surgical severing and removal of a limb. Amputations are caused by accidents (23%), disease (74%), and congenital disorders (3%). The most common reason for amputation is peripheral vascular disease, especially for those more than 50 years old (Mills et al., 2014). Lower extremity amputation is about 15 to 20 times greater in people with diabetes (Calvert, Penner, Younger, & Wing, 2007). Lower limb constitutes 80% to 85% of all amputations, with nearly two-thirds related to diabetes (Philbin, DeLuccia, Nitsch, & Maurus, 2007). Of dysvascular amputations, 15% to 28% of individuals undergo contralateral limb amputations within 3 years.

The following factors will affect the outcome of amputation: the individual's nutritional status, age, tissue perfusion, smoking habits, presurgery infection, and the presence of coexisting diseases such as diabetes, anemia, and renal failure.

Time Frame
Preoperative and postoperative periods

▪▪▪▪▪ DIAGNOSTIC CLUSTER

Preoperative Period

Nursing Diagnoses

▲ Anxiety related to insufficient knowledge of postoperative routines, postoperative sensations, and crutch-walking techniques

Related Care Plan

▲ General Surgery Generic Care Plan

Postoperative Period

Collaborative Problems

▲ Risk for Complications of Edema of Stump

▲ Risk for Complications of Wound Hematoma

▲ Risk for Complications of Hemorrhage

* Risk for Complications of Delayed Wound Healing

Nursing Diagnoses

△ Risk for Disturbed Body Image related to perceived negative effects of amputation and response of others to appearance

▲ Risk for Impaired Physical Mobility related to limited movement secondary to pain

▲ Grieving related to loss of limb and its effects on lifestyle

▲ Acute/Chronic Pain related to phantom limb sensations secondary to peripheral nerve stimulation and abnormal impulses to central nervous system

▲ Risk for Falls related to altered gait and hazards of assistive devices (refer to Risk for Falls in Unit II)

▲ Risk for Ineffective Health Management related to insufficient knowledge of activity of daily living (ADL) adaptations, stump care, signs/symptoms of complications, gait training, and follow-up care

▲ This diagnosis was reported to be monitored for or managed frequently (75% to 100%).
△ This diagnosis was reported to be monitored for or managed often (50% to 74%).

Transition Criteria

Before transition, the individual and family will:

1. Share their fear and concerns regarding the effects of amputation.
2. Describe daily stump care.
3. Explain phantom sensations and interventions to reduce them.
4. Describe measures to protect the stump from injury.
5. Identify what to report to surgeon after transition.
6. Demonstrate self-care activities correctly and safely for physical therapists.

Transitional Risk Assessment Plan (TRAP)

Begin this plan on admission.
Implement the Transitional Risk Assessment Plan (TRAP):

• Refer to inside back cover.
• Add each validated risk diagnosis to individual's problem list with the risk code in ().
• Refer to the individual risk nursing diagnoses/collaborative problems for outcomes and interventions in Unit II.

R: *"Close coordination of care in the post-acute period, early transition follow-up care, enhanced client educa-tion and self-management training, proactive end-of-life counseling, and extending the resources and clinical expertise over time via multidisciplinary team management" can lower readmission rates and improve health outcomes (Boutwell & Hwu, 2009, p. 14). Interventions are utilized to activate the individual and family to select changes in their everyday lifestyle choices to improve their health (Hibbard & Greene, 2013).*

Preoperative: Nursing Diagnosis

Anxiety Related to Insufficient Knowledge of Postoperative Routines, Postoperative Sensations, and Crutch-Walking Techniques

NOC
Anxiety Control, Coping, Impulse Control

Goal

NIC
Anxiety Reduction, Impulse Control Training, Anticipatory Guidance

Indicators

- Ask questions.
- Express concerns.

 Carp's Cues

Please refer to the Generic Care Plan for the Surgical Client for detailed interventions for managing all surgical conditions. This care plan addresses specific additional interventions associated with the type of surgery performed.

Interventions	Rationales
1. Explore the individual's feelings about the impending surgery. a. Allow the individual to direct discussion. b. Do not assume or project how the individual feels.	1. Some individuals may perceive amputation as a devastating event, while others will view the surgery as an opportunity to eliminate pain and improve quality of life.
2. Help to establish realistic expectations.	2. Successful prosthetic rehabilitation requires cooperation, coordination, tremendous physical energy and fitness, and a well-fitting, comfortable prosthesis (*Chin, Sawamura, & Shiba, 2006; *Piasecki, 2000; *Yetzer, 1996).
3. Consult with other team members (e.g., physical therapy) to see the individual preoperatively.	3. Preoperative instructions on postoperative activity help the individual to focus on rehabilitation instead of on the surgery; this may help to reduce anxiety.
4. Discuss postoperative expectations, including the following: a. Appearance of the stump b. Positioning c. Phantom pain	4. These explanations help to reduce fears associated with unknown situations and to decrease anxiety. a,b. The stump will be elevated for 24 hours after surgery to prevent edema. The individual will be assisted into the prone position three to four times a day to prevent hip contractures (*Piasecki, 2000). c. Research suggests that 85% of amputees have phantom limb pain ranging from daily to weekly to yearly (*Richardson, Glenn, Nurmikko, & Horgan, 2006).
5. Explain that immediately after surgery, the individual will perceive the amputated limb as if it were still intact and of the same shape and size as before surgery.	5. Immediately after surgery, most amputees feel the phantom limb as it was before surgery.

Documentation

Assessment of learning readiness and ability
Individual teaching
Response to teaching

Postoperative: Collaborative Problems

Risk for Complications of Edema of Stump

Risk for Complications of Wound Hematoma

Risk for Complications of Tissue Necrosis

Risk for Complications of Infection

Risk for Complications of Delayed Wound Healing

Collaborative Outcomes

The individual will be monitored for early signs and symptoms of (a) edema of stump, (b) wound hematoma, (c) tissue necrosis, and (d) infection and will receive collaborative interventions if indicated to restore physiologic stability.

Indicators of Physiologic Stability

- Diminishing edema (a)
- No evidence of boggy tissue, discoloration, skin changes (c)
- Approximated suture line (a, b, d)
- No point tenderness (b, c)
- Temperature 98° F to 99.5° F (d)
- White blood cells 4,300 to 10,800 mm^3 (d)

Interventions	Rationales
1. Closely monitor cardiac, pulmonary, and renal function **CLINICAL ALERT:** • Individuals requiring amputations have comorbidities such as diabetes or cardiac, vascular, respiratory, or renal disease, which increase the risk of developing postoperative complications after amputation.	1. Myocardial infarction is the most common cause of death after lower extremity amputation in individuals with peripheral artery disease. Pulmonary complications, including atelectasis and pneumonia, result in 5% of major lower extremity amputations. The incidence of new-onset renal failure after a lower extremity major amputation is 0.6% to 2.6%. Renal failure is associated with increased operative and long-term mortality (*Aulivola et al., 2004; Subedi & Grossberg, 2011).
2. Elevate the stump with calf tilted 15 degrees as prescribed, usually for the first 24 hours only.	2. Elevation for the first 24 hours will reduce edema and promote venous and lymphatic return. Elevation of the limb more than 15 degrees can cause flexion contractions (Toy, 2012)
3. Aggressively, monitor the incision for the following: a. Edema along suture lines b. Ruddy color changes c. Oozing dark blood d. Point tenderness on palpation	3. Peripheral vascular disorders are the major cause of lower limb amputations. After amputation, peripheral vascular disorders continue and thus increase the risk for infection and tissue necrosis. Individuals with diabetes are 5 times more at risk for postsurgical infections (*Harker, 2006; Kalapatapu, 2016).
4. Monitor for tissue necrosis: a. Dusky skin changes b. Mottled/purple discoloration c. Dry or wet gangrene d. Sloughy tissue (necrotic tissue separating from healthy tissue) e. Cool tissue, very painful	4. Poor tissue perfusion before surgery increases the risk of tissue necrosis postoperatively (Grossman & Porth, 2014).

Interventions	Rationales

CLINICAL ALERT:
- Any sign of necrosis must be reported immediately.

Interventions	Rationales
5. Monitor for edema along suture line and signs of delayed healing (Calvert et al., 2007).	5. Traumatized tissue responds with lymphedema. Excessive edema must be detected to prevent tension on the suture line that can cause bleeding. Tissue compression from edema can compromise circulation (Kalapatapu, 2016). Delayed wound healing is the most common complication, especially among diabetics (Calvert et al., 2007).
6. Monitor for signs of hematoma: Contact surgeon with findings. a. Unapproximated suture line b. Ruddy color changes of skin along suture line c. Oozing dark blood from suture line d. Point tenderness on palpation	6. Individuals with stump hematoma causing pain and stump swelling with or without drainage will have the wound opened partially, the hematoma evacuated, and the wound washed out and packed with a moist saline dressing. Hematoma may compromise flap healing and delay rehabilitation (Kalapatapu, 2016).
7. The stump site should be cleaned and dried thoroughly before reapplying the dressing, ensuring the dressing is not too tight or too loose (Virani, Werunga, Ewashen, & Green, 2015).	7. Tight dressings can cause ischemia of the stump, while loose dressings can prevent the stump from forming the conical shape that assists prosthesis fitting (Virani et al., 2015).

Clinical Alert Report

Before providing care, advise ancillary staff/student to report the following to the professional nurse assigned to the individual:
- Oral temperature >100.5° F
- Appearance of wound. The nurse supervising the student and/or ancillary staff should ask to be notified when the dressing is removed, to perform a detailed assessment.

Documentation

Appearance of suture line
Appearance of skin around suture line
Drainage
Abnormal findings

Postoperative: Nursing Diagnoses

Risk for Disturbed Body Image Related to Perceived Negative Effects of Amputation and Response of Others to Appearance

NOC

Body Image, Child Development: (specify age), Grief Resolution, Psychosocial Adjustment: Life Change, Self-Esteem

Goal

The individual will communicate feelings about his or her changed appearance.

Indicators

- Express an interest in dress and grooming.
- Discuss feelings with family.

NIC

Self-Esteem Enhancement, Counseling, Presence, Active Listening, Body Image Enhancement, Grief Work Facilitation, Support Group, Referral

Carp's Cues

"We all get older. Unfortunately, many of us have to deal with amputation at the same time. Though we don't have much control over aging, we do have some power over the way we see ourselves" (Saberi, 2012). This quote is from a three-page article from the National Limb Loss Information Center: Coping With Aging and Amputation: *How Changing the Way You Think Could Change Your Health* (http://www.amputee-coalition.org/senior_step/coping_aging.html).

    I would recommend that the nurse/student read this before giving care to an individual who has had or is approaching a limb amputation. This would also be very appropriate to give the individual and family. Don't be surprised if you find it meaningful for your life and practice, even though you have both your legs.

Interventions	*Rationales*
1. Contact the individual frequently to inquire about condition or requests. **CLINICAL ALERT:** • "An amputation induces several limitations in performing professional, leisure and social activities. It disturbs the integrity of the human body and lowers the quality of life (QoL) due to reduced mobility, pain and physical integrity. Patients are affected psychologically and socially. Psychological issues range from depression, anxiety and to suicide in severe cases. The loss of a body part also affects the perception of someone's own body and its appearance" (Holzer et al., 2014).	1. Frequent contact by the caregiver indicates acceptance and may facilitate trust. The individual may be hesitant to approach staff/student because of negative feelings; the nurse must reach out (*Dudas, 1997). Holzer et al. (2014) reported that individuals with lower-limb amputations have lower levels of body image perception and quality of life. However, levels of self-esteem were reported to be similar in both study groups.
2. Encourage the individual to verbalize feelings about appearance and perceptions of lifestyle impacts. What are you most concerned about? Validate the individual's perceptions and assure him or her that they are normal and appropriate.	2. Expressing feelings and perceptions increases the individual's self-awareness and helps the nurse to plan effective interventions to address the individual's needs. Validating perceptions provides reassurance and can decrease anxiety (*Dudas, 1997).
3. Assist the individual in identifying personal attributes and strengths.	3. These can help the individual to focus on the positive characteristics that contribute to the whole concept of self, rather than only on the change in body image. The nurse should reinforce these positive aspects and encourage the individual to reincorporate them into his or her new self-concept (*Dudas, 1997). Body image is strongly related to depression, perception of poor quality of life, low self-esteem, increased general anxiety, lower levels of satisfaction with prosthetic, participation in activity, and social isolation (Gallagher, Horgan, Franchignoni, Giordano, & MacLachlan; 2007; Yazicioglu, Taskaynatan, Guzelkucuk, & Tugcu, 2007).
4. Encourage optimal hygiene, grooming, and other self-care activities. What leisure activities are enjoyed?	4. Participation in self-care and planning promotes positive coping with the change. Holzer et al. (2014) reported the most common strategies to maintain a specific leisure activity was seeking instrumental help and determination.
5. Encourage the to perform as many activities as possible unassisted.	5. Nonparticipation in self-care and overprotection by caregivers tend to promote feelings of helplessness and dependence.
6. When appropriate, discuss the anticipated changes in lifestyle. Convey that adaptive goal pursuit and goal adjustment strategies in response to goal disruptions after limb loss can foster positive outcomes (Dunne, Coffey, Gallagher, & Desmond, 2014).	6. Dunne et al. (2014) reported that the most common adjustments were accepting limitations, emotional support from friends and family), and adjusting goals to constraints.

Interventions	Rationales

Carp's Cues

To review research findings that identified characteristics of individuals who adapt successfully to limb amputation access "If I can do it I will do it, if I can't, I can't": a study of adaptive self-regulatory strategies after lower limb amputation.

Interventions	Rationales
7. Prepare the individual's family and significant others for physical and emotional changes.	7. Support can be given more freely and more realistically if others are prepared (*Dudas, 1997).
8. Refer an individual to counseling, as appropriate.	8. Professional counseling is indicated for an individual postamputation.

Documentation

Present emotional status
Dialogues

Risk for Impaired Physical Mobility Related to Limited Movement Secondary to Pain

NOC
Ambulation: Walking, Joint Movement: Active, Mobility Level

Goal

The individual will report increased use of affected limb.

Indicators

- Demonstrate safe use of adaptive devices.
- Use safety measures to prevent injury.

NIC
Exercise Therapy: Joint Mobility, Exercise Promotion: Strength Training, Exercise Therapy: Ambulation, Positioning, Teaching: Prescribed Activity/Exercise, Teaching: Assistive Device, Teaching: Strategy

Interventions	Rationales
1. Implement the activity and exercise plan as prescribed by physical therapist.	1. Exercises are indicated for muscle strengthening and to prevent abduction and flexion contractures (Kalapatapu, 2016; Virani et al., 2015).
2. Assist the individual into a prone position three to four times a day for at least 15 minutes. Encourage the individual to sleep in this position.	2. Abdominal lying places the pelvic joints in an extended position that extends the extensor muscles and prevents contractures (Kalapatapu, 2016).
3. Elevate the stump by raising the foot of the bed or by placing a rolled towel under the stump; the use of a pillow under the stump should be discouraged (Society for Vascular Nursing, 2014).	3. These methods prevent contractures.
4. Avoid prolonged sitting.	4. Prolonged sitting can cause hip flexion contractures.
5. Emphasize progress with all activities, no matter how small. Convey that the individual can successfully manage adaptation to the prosthesis.	5. Other people's belief that they can successfully cope increases one's own confidence (*Bandura, 1982).

Documentation

> Exercises
> Range of motion

Nursing Diagnosis

Grieving Related to Loss of a Limb and Its Effects on Lifestyle

NOC
Coping, Family Coping,
Grief Resolution,
Psychosocial
Adjustment: Life Change

Goal

The individual will describe the meaning of the loss.

NIC
Anticipatory Guidance,
Risk Management,
Health Education,
Learning Facilitation

Indicators

- Express grief.
- Report an intent to discuss feelings with family members or significant others.

Interventions	*Rationales*
1. Provide opportunities for the individual and family members to ventilate feelings, discuss the loss openly, and explore the personal meaning of the loss. Explain that grief is a common and healthy reaction.	1. "Limb amputation may bring about life-altering effects, such as altered body image, disability, loss of employment, chronic pain, anxiety and depression that negatively affect quality of life and psychosocial adjustment" (Virani et al., 2015).

> **CLINICAL ALERT:**
> - "Immediate reactions to the prospect of amputation vary; they depend on whether the amputation was planned, occurred within the context of a chronic medical illness, or was necessitated by the sudden onset of infection or trauma. The context for amputation affects the psychological sequelae during the rehabilitation phase as well. When there is time to think about impending loss, classic stages of grief may be experienced" (Bhuvaneswar, Epstein, & Stern, 2007).

2. Discuss the reality of everyday emotions such as anger, guilt, and jealousy; relate the hazards of denying these feelings.	2. A positive response by individual's family or significant others is one of the most important factors in the individual's own acceptance of the loss (*Butler, Turkal, & Seidl, 1992).
3. Refer the individual to amputee support group. Determine if a trained amputee visitor can see the individual, if indicated.	3. This allows the individual and his or her family the opportunity to ventilate and ask questions.
4. Refer to Grieving in Unit II.	

Documentation

> Present emotional status
> Interventions
> Response to interventions

Acute/Chronic Pain Related to Phantom Limb Sensations Secondary to Peripheral Nerve Stimulation and Abnormal Impulses to Central Nervous System

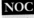

NOC
Comfort Level, Pain:
Disruptive Effects, Pain
Control, Symptom
Control

Goal

The individual will differentiate between surgical pain and phantom pain and will report decreased phantom pain.

NIC
Pain Management,
Medication
Management, Emotional
Support, Symptom
Control

Indicators

- Describe the difference between surgical pain and phantom pain
- State the reasons for phantom sensation.
- Demonstrate techniques for managing phantom sensation.

Carp's Cues

The incidence of post-op phantom limb pain/sensation has been reported to be 72% to 84%; at 6 months it is 67% to 90%. The incidence of preamputation pain increases the incidence of phantom pain. For some amputees, intense preoperative pain may be a predictor of postoperative phantom limb pain (PLP), which is similar in nature to preamputation pain (*Flor, 2002). This can be explained by the proprioceptive theory.

Preamputation pain memories stored in the brain continue to send constant pain signals that mimic the quality and location of preamputation pain (Weeks, Anderson-Barnes, & Tsao, 2010).

Interventions	Rationales
1. Explain and assess for the two types of pain that may be present postamputation: a. The pain of surgery is dull, throbbing, or aching. b. The pain resulting from severed nerves is sharp, shooting, tingling, or burning (phantom pain).	1. The differentiation of surgical pain from phantom pain is important since the treatment for each is different (Melsom & Danjoux, 2011).

2. Review proposed theoretical mechanisms to explain phantom limb pain.
a. Peripheral mechanism
  • Stump and neuroma hyperactivity
b. Central neural mechanisms
  • Spinal cord sensitization and changes
  • Cortical reorganization and cortical-motor sensory dissociation
  • Body schema, neuromatrix, and neurosignature hypothesis
c. Psychogenic mechanism
	2. PLP was traditionally thought to be primarily a psychiatric illness. With evidence from research over the past decades, the paradigm has shifted more toward changes at several levels of the neural axis, especially the cortex (*Flor, Nikolajsen & Jensen, 2006; Subedi & Grossberg, 2011).

3. Explain that the phantom limb pain sensations are normal and encourage to report them. Sensations are physiologic, not psychological in origin. Individuals prefer personal education regarding phantom sensations rather than reading about it.	3. The individual may be hesitant to discuss phantom sensations for fear of appearing abnormal. Nearly 100% of individuals with amputations report phantom pain sensation of varying degree during their first 6 months. Education reduces anxiety and opens lines of communication.
4. Explain phantom sensations. a. Phantom sensations are nonpainful sensations that may manifest as sensations of position of the amputated limb (proprioception or kinesthetic); of movement (kinetic); of feelings within the missing limb (exteroceptive) such as paresthesia, tickling, itching, warmth or cold, something touching the phantom limb, or numbness; or sensations as if an object, such as a ring, watch, or shoe, is still on the limb (superadded). b. Phantom pain is any sensation so intense it manifests as pain (Bosmans et al., 2007; *Richardson et al, 2006). Phantom sensations occur in 29% to 78% of individuals with amputations; phantom pain occurs in 49% to 83% of individuals (Bosmans et al., 2007).	4. Phantom sensations are caused by stimulation of the nerve proximal to the amputation that previously extended to the limb. The individual perceives the stimulation as originating from the absent limb. There is no agreement on the exact cause of phantom limb pain. Stimulus of peripheral nerves proximal to the amputation is thought to be a cause. Another explanation is that severed nerves may send impulses that are perceived by the brain as abnormal.
5. Describe some techniques used to reduce or alleviate phantom pain after the surgical site has healed. Consult with physical therapist: a. Wrapping the residual limb in a warm, soft towel, heating pad	5. Stimulation causing a second sensation may serve to override the phantom sensation (Kalapatapu, 2016; Subedi & Grossberg, 2011).

(continued)

Interventions	Rationales

b. Wrapping the residual limb in a cold pack or applying a cooling cream or gel

c. Soaking in a warm bath or using the shower to massage the residual limb

d. Massaging the residual limb with both hands

e. Transcutaneous electrical nerve stimulation (TENS)

f. Mentally exercising the missing limb in the area where the pain occurs

g. Mentally relaxing the missing limb and the residual limb

h. Tightening the muscles in the residual limb and slowly releasing them

i. For people with a prosthesis, putting it on and taking a short walk

j. Increase the time walking on prosthesis

k. Changing position, moving around, or standing up

l. Biofeedback

6. For management of incisional pain related to surgical wound, refer to Generic Care Plan for the Surgical Client.

Documentation

Reports of pain
Interventions
Response to interventions

TRANSITION TO HOME/COMMUNITY CARE

If indicated, review the risk diagnoses identified for this individual on admission:

- Is the person still at risk?
- Can the family reduce the risks?
- Is the person at higher risk at home?
- Is a Home Health Nurse assessment needed?
- Refer to transition planner/case manager/social service
- When is this person scheduled for follow-up with primary provider? Specialists? Record dates of appointments.
- Complete a medication reconciliation before transition. Refer to index.

STAR

Stop

Think   Is this person at high risk for injury, falls, medical complications, and/or inability to care for self (activities of daily living)?

Is there a support person available?

Is the person competent to manage self-administration of medications, treatment procedures? Are additional resources needed?

Can the person explain how to monitor the condition (e.g., blood glucose, signs/symptoms of complications, dietary/mobility restrictions, and when to call his or her primary provider or specialist)?

Act   Contact or provide the appropriate resource (e.g., contacting a support person, home health assessment, additional teaching, printed materials).

Review   Has the problem been addressed? If not, use SBAR to communicate to the appropriate person.

Risk for Ineffective Health Management Related to Insufficient Knowledge of Activity of Daily Living (ADL) Adaptations, Stump Care, Signs/Symptoms of Complications, Gait Training, and Follow-Up Care

NOC
Compliance Behavior, Knowledge: Treatment Regimen, Participation: Health Care Decisions, Treatment Behavior: Illness or Injury

NIC
Anticipatory Guidance, Risk Identification, Health Education, Learning Facilitation, Amputation Care

Transition Goal

The goals for this diagnosis represent those associated with transition planning. Refer to the transition criteria.

Interventions	Rationales

1. Reinforce the importance of preventing injury to the remaining foot with:
  a. Daily inspection for corns, calluses, blisters, and signs of infection
  b. Wearing sturdy slippers or shoes
  c. Prompt reporting of early signs of infection (e.g., a minor cut that does not heal in 1 to 2 days)
	1. Daily care is necessary to deflect or prevent injury, especially if a circulatory disorder was a contributing factor to amputation.

2. Instruct the individual to place a chair or other large object next to the bed at home to prevent him or her from getting out of bed at night and attempting to stand on the stump when not fully awake.	2. Phantom sensations include a kinesthetic awareness of the absent limb. A half-asleep individual arising during the night may fall and damage the healing stump (Kalapatapu, 2016).
3. To assist an individual to decide to quit smoking, refer to Care Plan for Chronic Obstructive Pulmonary Disease for strategies to motivate an individual to quit tobacco use. Refer also to Getting Started to Quit Smoking on thePoint (printable to give to individual)	3. Nicotine in tobacco constricts arterial vessels, which decreases blood flow to the healing stump. If amputation was related to atherosclerosis, tobacco use may threaten the stump's survival (CDC, 2015b).
4. Ensure the individual/family can properly clean, examine, and bandage the stump.	4. It is necessary to regularly examine the stump for expected changes (e.g., muscle and scar atrophy) and unexpected changes (e.g., skin breakdown, redness, tenderness, increased warmth or coolness, numbness or tingling).

5. Explain the risks for infection and the need to report immediately to surgeon:
  a. Fever (oral temperature of 100.5° F or greater)
  b. Increased pain
  c. Increased swelling, boggy tissue
  d. Dusky skin changes
  e. Mottled/purple discoloration
  f. Increased wound drainage
  g. Cool tissue
	5. Hematomas of the wound contribute to infection. Coexisting diabetes mellitus reduces resistance to bacteria and causes diminished circulation. Tissue necrosis also can result from decreased circulation, chronic swelling, and infection. These changes should be reported.

6. Explain what to expect in the healing process (American Academy of Orthotists and Prosthetics, 2014): a. This stage begins with hospital discharge and extends 4, 6, or even 8 weeks after surgery. During this time one recovers from surgery, wound healing continues, and rehabilitation begins. Frequently, end points of this stage are characterized as the point of wound healing and the point of being ready for prosthetic fitting.	6. Specific explanations of what to expect can reduce anxiety and alert the individual.

(continued)

Interventions	Rationales
b. The immediate recovery period begins with the healing of the wound and usually extends 4 to 6 months from the healing date.	
7. Explain the transition to a rehabilitative facility.	7. The sooner the individual engages in rehabilitation, the more successful the prosthetic ambulation.
8. Recommend an online publication such as Lower Extremity Amputations from the *Education Committee of the Society for Vascular Nursing*, which addresses living with an amputation, access at http://www.svnnet.org/wp-content /uploads/2015/09/LE-Amps-2014-	

Documentation

Individual/family teaching
Response to teaching
Referrals, if indicated

Arterial Bypass Grafting in the Lower Extremity

"Peripheral artery disease (PAD) results from the build-up of plaque (atherosclerosis) in the arteries of the legs. For most people with PAD, symptoms may be mild or absent, and no treatment of the artery blockages is required. However as these blockages become more extensive, clients may experience pain and disability that limits their walking, and in the most advanced cases individuals may be at risk for loss of the limb unless circulation is improved. For these clients with severe PAD, attempts to improve blood flow in the leg are usually indicated. The goals of improving blood flow to the limb are to reduce pain, improve functional ability and quality of life, and to prevent amputation" (Conte & Farber, 2015). For individuals with combined inflow and outflow disease in whom symptoms of critical limb ischemia or infection persist after inflow revascularization, an outflow revascularization procedure should be performed (ACCF/AHA Task Force on Practice Guidelines, 2011).

Surgical treatments for PAD can be minimally invasive as angioplasty or stenting or arterial bypass surgery, depending on the severity and location of the arterial blockage (Conti & Farber, 2015). Bypass surgery is immediately successful in 90% to 95%percent of cases (Conti & Farber, 2015). The short- and long-term success of the procedure is linked to two factors: (1) the material employed for the bypass graft itself and (2) the quality of the arteries in the lower leg to which the graft is attached (Conti & Farber, 2015).

This general approach may differ in very young individuals (<40 years of age) with claudication. Symptoms in this group of individuals are typically owing to a far more aggressive atherosclerotic disease process than that experienced by the majority of older individuals with claudication. van Goor and Boontje (*1995) found unsatisfactory outcomes in individuals <40 years of age including initial vascular reconstructions failed in 72%, only 25% of survivors were asymptomatic, and average mortality rate at 10 years after initial surgery was 31%.

 Time Frame
Postoperative periods

▪▪▪■■■DIAGNOSTIC CLUSTER

Collaborative Problems

*   Risk for Complications of Deep Vein Thrombosis/Pulmonary Embolism (refer to Risk for Complications of DVT/PE in Unit II)

Δ   Risk for Complications of Thrombosis of Graft

Δ   Risk for Complications of Compartment Syndrome

△ Risk for Complications of Lymphocele

▲ Risk for Complications of Disruption of Anastomosis or Puncture Site

▲ Risk for Complications of Renal Failure (refer to Risk for Complications of Renal Insufficiency in Unit II)

Nursing Diagnoses

▲ Acute Pain related to increased tissue perfusion to previous ischemic tissue

△ Risk for Ineffective Health Management related to insufficient knowledge of wound care, signs and symptoms of complications, activity restrictions, and follow-up care

Related Care Plans

▲ General Surgery Generic Care Plan

▲ Abdominal Aortic Aneurysm Resection

▲ This diagnosis was reported to be monitored for or managed frequently (75% to 100%).
△ This diagnosis was reported to be monitored for or managed often (50% to 74%).

Transition Criteria

Before transition, the individual and/or family will:

1. Demonstrate proper wound care.
2. Demonstrate correct pulse palpation technique.
3. State the signs and symptoms that must be reported to a health care professional.

> **Transitional Risk Assessment Plan (TRAP)**
>
> Begin this plan on admission.
> Implement the Transitional Risk Assessment Plan (TRAP):
> * Refer to inside back cover.
> * Add each validated risk diagnosis to individual's problem list with the risk code in ( ).
> * Refer to the individual risk nursing diagnoses/collaborative problems for outcomes and interventions in Unit II.
>
> *R: "Close coordination of care in the post-acute period, early transition follow-up care, enhanced client education and self-management training, proactive end-of-life counseling, and extending the resources and clinical expertise over time via multidisciplinary team management" can lower readmission rates and improve health outcomes (Boutwell & Hwu, 2009, p. 14). Interventions are utilized to activate the individual and family to select changes in their everyday lifestyle choices to improve their health (Hibbard & Greene, 2013).*

Collaborative Problems

Risk for Complications of Thrombosis of Graft

Risk for Complications of Compartment Syndrome

Risk for Complications of Lymphocele

Risk for Complications of Disruption of Anastomosis or Puncture Site

Collaborative Outcomes

The individual will be monitored for early signs and symptoms of (a) thrombosis of graft, (b) compartment syndrome, (c) lymphocele, and (d) disruption of anastomosis and will receive collaborative interventions if indicated to restore physiologic stability.

Indicators of Physiologic Stability

* Capillary refill <3 seconds (a, b, d)
* Peripheral pulses: full, present (a)

- Warm, not mottled limbs (a, b)
- Intact sensation (a, b)
- Minimal limb edema (b)
- No pain with passive stretching (a, b)
- Intact muscle tension (a, b)
- Increasing wound drainage (c)
- Increasing local swelling (b, c)
- No bounding pulsation over graft (d)
- Can move toes (b)

Carp's Cues

Please refer to the Generic Care Plan for the Surgical Client for detailed interventions for managing all surgical conditions. This care plan addresses specific additional interventions associated with this type of surgery performed.

Interventions	Rationales
1. Monitor graft patency, palpate a graft patency, palpate a graft near the skin surface, and assess distal pulses for changes from the baseline (e.g., Doppler pressure).	1. Graft patency is essential to arterial circulation.
2. Monitor peripheral circulation hourly initially per protocol, compare extremities (pulses, sensation, capillary refill, skin color, temperature). a. Sudden decrease in arterial flow, indicating thrombosed graft, is an emergency requiring immediate surgical exploration of the graft (*Edwards, Abullarade, & Turnbull, 1996). b. Report any changes, which may indicate thrombolic occlusion of the graft, immediately.	2. A sudden change in temperature, drop in pressure, or absence of pulses indicates graft thrombosis. Changes in sensation or motor function can indicate arterial thrombosis or compartment syndrome (*Edwards et al., 1996).
3. Maintain bed rest as prescribed, usually1 to 2 days.	3. Bed rest helps to prevent graft trauma from injury.
4. Keep the limb warm but do not use electric heating pads or hot water bottles.	4. Peripheral nerve ischemia causes diminished sensation. High temperatures of heating devices may damage tissue without the individual feeling discomfort.
5. Instruct the individual to sit in a "slouched" position and not to cross legs. If leg elevation is ordered, elevate the entire leg and pelvis to heart level unless contraindicated.	5. Sharp flexion and pressure on the graft must be avoided to prevent graft damage (*Edwards et al., 1996).

> **CLINICAL ALERT:**
> - Revascularization procedures and treatments, such as extremity bypass surgery, embolectomy, and thrombolysis, increase the risk for acute compartment syndrome (ACS). This phenomenon is known as postischemic compartment syndrome and is owing to tissue swelling from reperfusion. The syndrome can occur from a few hours after the procedure up to several days later. Residual effects from anesthesia and postoperative sedation can make early detection of ACS more difficult immediately after surgery (Stracciolini & Hammerberg, 2014).

Interventions	Rationales
6. Monitor for signs and symptoms of ACS: a. Edema of revascularized limb b. Complaints of pain with passive stretching of the muscle c. weakness of toe flexion and pain with passive extension of the toes	6. After a period of ischemia comes a period of increased capillary wall permeability. Restoration of arterial flow causes plasma and extracellular fluid to flow into the tissues, producing massive swelling in the calf muscles. The edema compresses the blood vessels and nerves within the nonexpanding fascia . The nerves become anoxic,

Interventions	Rationales
d. Decreased sensation, motor function, or paresthesias of the distal limb e. Increased tension and firmness of muscle **CLINICAL ALERT:** • Postoperative edema is expected in the new revascularized limb. • Careful assessment alerts the nurse to edema severe enough to cause compartment syndrome. • Access surgeon for an evaluation when excess edema is suspected (*Edwards et al., 1996).	causing paresthesias and motor deficits. Urgent fasciotomy is required to relieve pressure and preserve the limb (Sieggreen, 2007; Stracciolini & Hammerberg, 2014).

7. Monitor for signs and symptoms of lymphocele:
   a. Discomfort accompanied by local swelling
   b. Large amounts of clear or pink-tinged drainage
      • Contact the surgeon.
	7. A major lymphatic channel courses through the inner thigh area. If the lymphatic chain is lacerated during the operation, drainage may occur. The large amount of accumulated fluid seeks the path of least resistance and usually drains through the incision (Grossman & Porth, 2014).

8. Monitor for disruption of anastomosis:
   a. Decrease in perfusion of distal extremity
   b. Bounding aneurysmal pulsation over the anastomosis site. If bleeding occurs, apply firm, constant pressure over the site and notify the physician/nurse practitioner/physical assistant .
	8. Hemorrhage from anastomotic disruption is an emergency requiring immediate surgical intervention.

 Clinical Alert Report

Before providing care, advise ancillary staff/student to report the following to the professional nurse assigned to the individual:
- Capillary refill >3 seconds
- Decreased peripheral pulses
- Cool, mottled limbs
- Decreased sensation
- Increasing limb edema
- New complaints of pain, difficulty in moving toes
- Increasing wound drainage

Documentation

Vital signs
Distal pulses
Circulatory status
Presence and description of pain
Unusual events, actions, responses
Wound drainage and appearance

Nursing Diagnoses

Acute Pain Related to Increased Tissue Perfusion to Previous Ischemic Tissue

 NOC
Comfort Level, Pain Control

Goal

The individual will report pain relief after interventions.

NIC

Pain Management,
Medication Management,
Emotional Support,
Teaching: Individual,
Heat/Cold Application,
Simple Massage

Indicators

- State the reason for the pain.
- Relate signs and symptoms of ischemia.

Interventions	Rationales
1. Monitor the "Six P's" of acute ischemia related to arterial occlusion: pain, coolness, pulselessness, pallor, paresthesia, and paralysis (begins with generic motor deficits) (Sieggreen, 2007).	1. Acute ischemia related to arterial occlusion needs early identification to prevent permanent damage.
2. Explain the source of pain and reassure the individual that the sensation is temporary and will decrease each day.	2. Pain results from the reperfusion of previously ischemic sensory nerve endings. Pain lessens as reperfusion progresses.
3. Assess carefully to differentiate between the pain of reperfusion and the pain of ischemia (reperfused tissue is warm and edematous; ischemic tissue is cool). Notify the surgeon immediately if ischemia is suspected.	3. Ischemic pain may indicate graft failure and warrants immediate evaluation.
4. Refer to the nursing diagnosis Acute Pain in the General Surgery Care Plan for additional interventions.	

Documentation

Unrelieved pain
Interventions
Response to interventions

TRANSITION TO HOME/COMMUNITY CARE

If indicated, review the risk diagnoses identified for this individual on admission:

- Is the person still at risk?
- Can the family reduce the risks?
- Is the person at higher risk at home?
- Is a Home Health Nurse assessment needed?
- Refer to transition planner/case manager/social service
- When is this person scheduled for follow-up with primary provider? Specialists? Record dates of appointments.
- Complete a medication reconciliation before transition. Refer to index.

STAR

Stop

Think   Is this person at high risk for injury, falls, medical complications, and/or inability to care for self (activities of daily living)?

Is there a support person available?

Is the person competent to manage self-administration of medications, treatment procedures? Are additional resources needed?

Can the person explain how to monitor the condition (e.g., blood glucose, signs/symptoms of complications, dietary/mobility restrictions, and when to call his or her primary provider or specialist)?

Act   Contact or provide the appropriate resource (e.g., contacting a support person, home health assessment, additional teaching, printed materials).

Review   Has the problem been addressed? If not, use SBAR to communicate to the appropriate person.

Risk for Ineffective Health Management Related to Insufficient Knowledge of Wound Care, Signs and Symptoms of Complications, Activity Restrictions, and Follow-Up Care

NOC

Compliance Behavior,
Knowledge: Treatment
Regimen, Participation:
Health Care Decisions,
Treatment Behavior:
Illness or Injury

NIC

Anticipatory Guidance,
Risk Management,
Health Education,
Learning Facilitation

Goals

The goals for this diagnosis represent those associated with transitional planning. Refer to the transition criteria.

Interventions	Rationales
1. Teach the individual and family the proper wound care techniques. (Refer to the nursing diagnosis Risk for Ineffective Therapeutic Regimen Management in the General Surgery Care Plan, Appendix II, for specific measures.)	1. Proper wound care can prevent infection that delays healing (*Edwards et al., 1996).

2. Reinforce teaching regarding activity restrictions and mobility (Macon Vascular Institute, 2014)
  a. No lifting more than 5 lb (1/2 gallon of milk) for 2 weeks.
  b. Slowing increases activity. Walk short distances on flat surfaces at first then increase distance as tolerated. Avoid exercising in extreme temperatures.
  c. Leg swelling after bypass surgery is common and may occur for a few months after the surgery. When you are sitting or resting elevate your legs above the level of your heart. If you have been asked to wear compression stockings, put them on first thing in the morning and remove them at night.
  d. Limit stair climbing to two times a day for the week after your surgery.
  e. You may ride in a car. No driving until after the first post-op visit.
  f. Sexual intercourse should be avoided for 2 weeks, avoid positions that will cause strain on the incision area for 2 to 3 weeks.
	2. The individual's understanding may encourage compliance with the therapeutic regimen.
	
	  b. Activity should be increased gradually to promote circulation and reduce loss of strength.
	
	  c. Dependent positioning of the legs increases postoperative swelling. Positions of hip–knee flexion impede venous return.
	
	  d. Early ambulation is recommended to restore muscle activity and enhance venous blood return.

3. Teach the individual and family or support persons how to assess graft patency.
  a. Assess pulses and capillary refill.
  b. Palpate the graft for pulsations, if near the surface.
	3. Monitoring circulatory status must be continued at home.

4. Teach to recognize signs and symptoms of problems and report them immediately.
  a. Sudden onset of shortness of breath (call 911)
  b. Absence of pulses
  c. Change in temperature of the leg or foot
  d. Paresthesias and other changes in sensation
  e. Increased pain
  f. Increased swelling
  g. Wound or sore in the affected leg
  h. Changes in the incision site (e.g., redness, drainage)
  i. Fever (>100.5° F)
	4. Reporting these signs of compromised circulation, infection, or possible graft failure promptly enables intervention to prevent serious complications. Diminished circulation impedes healing; infection can cause graft failure (*Hirsch et al., 2006).

5. Reinforce teaching regarding foot care and prevention of injury to the leg. Refer to Peripheral Arterial Care Plan for specific teaching.	5. Continued care and precautions are necessary at home.

Carp's Cues

Refer to Getting Started to Quit Smoking, Getting Started to Increase Activity, and Getting Started to Healthy Eating on the Point for printable handouts to give to individual.

Documentation

Individual/family teaching
Response to teaching

Breast Surgery (Lumpectomy, Mastectomy)

The primary treatment for breast cancer is removal of the cancerous tissue. The type of surgery is based on the type of tumor, size of tumor, grade of tumor, estrogen and progesterone receptors, and individual preference. Mastectomy is indicated for individuals who are not candidates for breast- conserving therapy, for example, two or more primary tumors in separate quadrants of the breast, persistently positive resection margins and individuals who prefer mastectomy (Feigelson et al., 2013), and for prophylactic purposes to reduce the risk of breast cancer (Kwong, 2016). With either a lumpectomy or a mastectomy, one or several axillary lymph nodes may be examined and/or removed. *Lumpectomy*, also known as breast-conserving surgery or partial mastectomy, is the removal of the cancerous tissue and a small amount of adjacent tissue with overlying skin left in place. Axillary nodes may be dissected through a separate incision. Lumpectomy is not usually recommended for tumors larger than 5 cm. However, women with a strong desire to save their breast may opt for chemotherapy or hormone therapy given before surgery to shrink the tumor. Lumpectomy followed by radiation therapy is currently the standard of care, and research has shown lumpectomy to be equally as effective as mastectomy for early- stage breast cancer (Giuliano & Hurvitz, 2012). A nipple-areolar sparing mastectomy (NSM) preserves the dermis and epidermis of the nipple but removes the major ducts from within the nipple lumen (Kwong, 2016).

Post mastectomy individuals can choose breast reconstruction with implant, reconstruction with their own tissue, or choose to wear prostheses. Nipple-areolar complex is a plastic surgery technique.

Axillary lymph node removal is important in staging, preventing axillary recurrence, and treatment planning. More common, sentinel node biopsy is done intraoperatively; if negative for spread of disease, axillary dissection may be omitted. Surgery may be followed by radiation, chemotherapy, hormonal therapy, or combinations of these.

 Time Frame

Each breast cancer case is individualized based on a number of factors, including treatment decisions and tumor characteristics. With each case, careful consideration includes the kind of surgery, the desire for reconstruction of the breast, genetic profile of likelihood of recurrence, targeted therapy, and hormonal therapy. Balance must be placed on the characteristic and staging of the cancer inclusive of the individual's wishes and impact on quality of life. Hospital stay is routinely not needed for a lumpectomy, and a 1- to 2- day hospital stay for mastectomy.

Preoperative and Postoperative Periods

Individuals should be offered a consultation with a reconstructive plastic surgeon to discuss options and ensure *preoperatively* they understand and have made informed decisions on treatment and reconstruction. "Accumulating data support the view that immediate breast reconstruction provides substantial psychosocial benefits over delayed reconstruction and preserves normal perceptions of body image in women undergoing mastectomy" (Nahabedia, 2015).

▪▪▪▪▪ DIAGNOSTIC CLUSTER

Nursing Diagnoses

Preoperative Period

Refer to Generic Surgical Care Plan

Postoperative Period

Collaborative Problems

Risk for Complications of Neurovascular Compromise

Risk for Complications of Deep Vein Thrombosis

Risk for Complications of Seroma Formation

Nursing Diagnoses

▲ Anxiety/Fear related to perceived effects of surgery (immediate: pain, nausea, vomiting; post transition: relationships, edema, work) and prognosis

Risk for Injury related to compromised lymph drainage and motor and sensory function in affected arm

Risk for Ineffective Health Therapeutic Regimen Management related to insufficient knowledge of wound care, exercises, breast prosthesis, signs and symptoms of complications, hand/arm precautions, community resources, and follow-up care

Related Care Plan

General Surgery Generic Care Plan

Transition Criteria

Before transition, the individual and family will:

1. Demonstrate hand and arm exercises.
2. Verbalize understanding of ways to reduce the risk of lymphedema (i.e., wear loose clothes or jewelry on the surgical side, elevate surgical arm to a point higher than the heart when resting, do not let arm hang down, do not apply heat to limb).
3. Demonstrate breast self-examination.
4. State care measures to perform at home.
5. Discuss strategies for performing activities of daily living.
6. State necessary precautions.
7. State the signs and symptoms that must be reported to a health care professional.
8. Verbalize an intent to share feelings and concerns with significant others.
9. Identify available community resources and self-help groups.

> **Transitional Risk Assessment Plan (TRAP)**
>
> Begin this plan on admission.
> Implement the Transitional Risk Assessment Plan (TRAP):
> - Refer to inside back cover.
> - Add each validated risk diagnosis to individual's problem list with the risk code in ( ).
> - Refer to the individual risk nursing diagnoses/collaborative problems for outcomes and interventions in Unit II.
>
> *R:* "*Close coordination of care in the post-acute period, early transition follow-up care, enhanced client education and self-management training, proactive end-of-life counseling, and extending the resources and clinical expertise over time via multidisciplinary team management" can lower readmission rates and improve health outcomes (Boutwell & Hwu, 2009, p. 14). Interventions are utilized to activate the individual and family to select changes in their everyday lifestyle choices to improve their health (Hibbard & Greene, 2013).*

Collaborative Problems

Risk for Complications of Neurovascular Compromise

Risk for Complications of Deep Vein Thrombosis

Risk for Complications of Seroma Formation

Collaborative Outcomes

The individual will be monitored for early signs and symptoms of neurovascular compromise and will receive collaborative interventions if indicated to restore physiologic stability.

NIC
Fall Prevention, Environmental Management: Safety, Health Education, Surveillance: Safety, Risk Identification

Indicators of Physiologic Stability

- Radial pulses full, bounding
- No numbness or tingling of hand
- Capillary refill <3 seconds
- Warm, not mottled extremity
- Intact finger flexion and extension

>> **Carp's Cues**

Please refer to the Generic Care Plan for the Surgical Client for detailed interventions for managing all surgical conditions. This care plan addresses specific additional interventions associated with the type of surgery performed.

Interventions	Rationales
1. Monitor for signs and symptoms of neurovascular compromise by comparing findings between limbs: a. Diminished or absent radial pulse b. Numbness or tingling in hand c. Capillary refill time >3 seconds d. Pallor, blanching, or cyanosis and coolness of extremity e. Inability to flex or extend fingers	1. Significant edema of the arm occurs in 10% to 30% of individuals after axillary dissection (Yarbro, Wujcik, & Gobel, 2011).
2. Maintain compression devices and promote early ambulation.	2. Sequential compression devices rather than systemic prophylaxis is recommended for low-risk individuals because the rate of deep vein thrombosis after breast surgery is low and systemic prophylaxis is associated with a high risk of wound hematoma (Kwong, 2016).
3. Monitor skin flap sites for drainage. Assure drains are patent.	3. Seroma formation, a collection of serous fluid under the skin flaps, often occurs after breast and axillary surgery (Kwong, 2016). Untreated seroma formation results in delayed wound healing, wound infection, wound dehiscence, flap necrosis, delayed recovery, and poor cosmetic outcome (*Agrawal, Ayantunde, & Cheung, 2006). Seromas are more likely to occur after mastectomy than with breast-conserving surgery (*Hashemi et al., 2004; Kwong, 2016).

Documentation

Radial pulse assessment
Affected arm: color, sensation, capillary refill time, movement

> **CLINICAL ALERT:**
> - Notify surgeon for:
>   - Complaints of numbness or tingling of hand
>   - Capillary refill >3 seconds
>   - Cool, mottled extremity
>   - Diminished finger flexion and extension

Nursing Diagnosis

Anxiety/Fear Related to Perceived Effects of Surgery (Immediate: Pain, Edema; Post transition: Relationships, Work) and Prognosis

NOC
Anxiety Reduction, Coping, Impulse Control

Goal

The individual will share concerns regarding the surgery and its outcome. A clear explanation of expectations during the hospital stay should be explained during preoperative counseling.

NIC
Anxiety Reduction, Impulse Control Training, Anticipatory Guidance

Indicators

- Describe actions that can help to reduce postoperative edema and immobility.
- State the intent to share feelings with family, significant others, or friends.

> **CLINICAL ALERT:**
> - Research has shown levels of preoperative stress and worries about outcomes directly relate to the incidence of postsurgical nausea, fatigue, pain, and discomfort (*Montgomery & Bowbjerg, 2004).

Interventions	Rationales
1. Encourage the individual to verbalize their concerns and fears. Stay with them as much as possible and convey empathy and concern.	1. After facing a cancer diagnosis and undergoing a mastectomy, your patient needs a great deal of teaching and support.
2. Explore with individual sources of his or her distress. **CLINICAL ALERT:** • Individuals are at an increased risk of distress with fear and worry about the future. • Individual may express anger, fear, and feeling out of control. • Physical symptoms may include poor sleep, appetite, concentration, preoccupation with thoughts of illness and death, and concerns of role changes (National Comprehensive Cancer Network [NCCN], 2014).	2. Distress is a multifactorial unpleasant emotional experience of psychological (cognitive, behavioral, emotional), social, and/or spiritual nature that may interfere with the ability to cope effectively with cancer, its physical symptoms, and its treatment. Distress extends along a continuum, ranging from common normal feelings of vulnerability, sadness, and fears to problems that can become disabling, such as depression, anxiety, panic, social isolation, and existential and spiritual crisis (NCCN, 2014).
3. The following suggestions for talking and supporting someone with cancer are excerpted from spouses, partners, family (retrieved from The Breast Care site.com) a. For partners, friends, and other support persons, meet them alone: • Convey "Chances are pretty good that you are the person the individual leans on most for emotional support. And chances are equally good that you play the same role for them. That's why it is especially important for you to be sensitive to the physical and psychological changes your loved one is undergoing or has undergone" (The Breast Care site.com, 2011). • Share "If you are a friend or family member of a breast cancer survivor, you should keep in mind that the goal is to help your friend or loved one feel that you are there for them and that they are not isolated in their experience." • Examples of how to initiate sharing of feelings as open-ended questions: "How are you doing with it?" (If you say "How are you ," your friend or loved one may only answer "Fine" and then the conversation may stop.) If you are not sure whether someone wants to talk, you can ask directly, "Do you want to talk?"	3. Individuals/family who are empowered with knowledge, resources, and a sense of control will ultimately manage their care to reduce risk of side effects, to make informed treatment decisions, and to receive the follow-up care needed. • Research has shown that satisfaction with partner support and support from other adults positively affects the woman's adjustment (Hoskins et al., 2016). Partners may feel unsure of how to show support and affection (Susan B. Komen for the Cure, 2007b). • An open-ended question allows the person to say how she is feeling. Sometimes your loved one may want to talk and sometimes she may not want to talk. Both are okay. • Accept both the person's thoughts and feelings. A good listener lets the speaker know that she has been heard.

Interventions	*Rationales*
• Clarify that the message to their loved one is "I am here for you." Avoid trying to give solutions, just Listen. Give the gift of acceptance and permission to share their feeling.	• Validating someone's experience is comforting. It helps them feel more normal as they are going through a situation that is not at all normal for them.

Documentation

Dialogues
Interventions

Risk for Injury Related to Compromised Lymph Drainage, Motor and Sensory Function in Affected Arm

NOC

Risk Control, Safety Status: Falls Occurrence

Goal

The individual will report no injuries to the affected arm.

NIC

Fall Prevention, Environmental Management: Safety, Health Education, Surveillance: Safety, Risk Identification

Indicators

• Relate the factors that contribute to lymphedema.
• Describe activities that are hazardous to the affected arm.

Interventions	*Rationales*
CLINICAL ALERT: • Unfortunately, there is no accepted definition of clinically significant lymphedema, and as a result it is difficult to advise the woman of the amount of lymphedema post breast cancer surgery (Koul et al., 2007).	

1. Instruct to avoid positioning the limb in a gravity-dependent position for prolonged time periods; this includes prolonged standing, sitting, or crossing legs. Monitor for signs and symptoms of sensorimotor impairment:
  a. Impaired joint movement
  b. Muscle weakness
  c. Numbness or tingling
	1. Simple elevation of a lymphedematous limb may reduce swelling, particularly in the early stage of lymphedema. However, elevation alone is not an effective long-term therapy.

2. Monitor regular measurements of arm circumference for changes. Instruct to promptly report any changes in size, sensation, color, temperature, or skin condition.	2. Individuals should be taught how to monitor their lymphedema, including serial measurement of limb circumference.
CLINICAL ALERT: • Rarely, edema may be severe enough to interfere with the use of the limb. • Consult with provider if edema persists or worsens. • Mild diuretic, compressor pump, manual compression, or use of a lymphedema sleeve may be indicated.	

Interventions	Rationales
3. Monitor for increase in lymphedema, as more aggressive therapy may be indicated.	3. Late or secondary edema can develop years after treatment; individual should be evaluated by provider to rule out infection or recurrence of disease.
4. Teach the individual to avoid the following: a. Vaccines, blood samples, injections, and blood pressure measurements on affected arm b. Constrictive jewelry and clothing c. Carrying a shoulder bag or heavy object with the affected arm d. Brassieres with thin shoulder straps (use wide-strap or no-strap brassieres instead) e. Lifting objects weighing more than 5 to 10 lb; leaning on arm	4a, b. It is hypothesized that limb constriction (no matter how brief) can increase pressure in the limb increasing lymph production, potentially leading to stenosis and fibrosis of the lymphatic vessels (Mohler & Mehrara, 2016).
5. Teach precautions to prevent trauma to the affected arm and hand: a. Using long-gloved potholders b. Avoiding cuts, scratches, and bruises (e.g., using a thimble when sewing) c. Avoiding injections and venipunctures of any kind d. Avoiding strong detergents or other chemical agents e. Wearing heavy gardening gloves and avoiding gardening in thorny plants f. Using electric razor under arms g. Protecting from sunburn and avoiding excessive heat (e.g., saunas, hot tubs, or tanning beds) h. Keeping skin clean and well moisturized i. Not cutting cuticles j. Promptly treating infections of hand and arm (National Cancer Institute, 2007; Susan B. Komen for the Cure, 2007a)	5. Skin care is a priority with lymphedema. The body has a difficult time clearing bacteria in tissue affected with lymphedema, resulting in a higher risk of infection to the area (*Cheville & Gergich, 2004).
6. Teach the individual to cleanse arm or hand wounds promptly, and to observe carefully for early signs of infection (e.g., redness, increased warmth). Stress the need to report any signs promptly.	6. Compromised lymph drainage weakens the body's defense against infection; this necessitates increased emphasis on infection prevention. Studies show that prophylactic antibiotics significantly reduce the incidence of surgical site infection, lowering potential morbidity (*Cunningham, Bunn, & Handscomb, 2006).
7. Teach the individual to keep the wrist higher than the elbow and the elbow higher than the heart whenever possible.	7. This will reduce edema.
8. Stress importance to keep physical therapy appointments.	8. Randomized trials support physiotherapy to improve arm mobility to limit the development of lymphedema (Mohler & Mehrara, 2016). Complete decongestive physiotherapy exercise (e.g., opening and closing the hand), manual lymphatic drainage (a specific type of massage), and physical therapy have been shown to reduce swelling and lymphedema-related infection (Susan B. Komen for the Cure, 2007a).
9. Advise the purpose of compression garments that will be initiated in physiotherapy	9. In early stages of lymphedema, external compression is used to diminish ultrafiltration and is achieved with repetitively applied, multilayered padding materials and short-stretch (also called low-stretch) bandages. Combined therapy was approximately twice as effective in reducing limb volume (Mohler & Mehrara, 2016).

Documentation

Individual/family teaching

> **TRANSITION TO HOME/COMMUNITY CARE**
>
> If indicated, review the risk diagnoses identified for this individual on admission:
> * Is the person still at risk?
> * Can the family reduce the risks?
> * Is the person at higher risk at home?
> * Is a Home Health Nurse assessment needed?
> * Refer to transition planner/case manager/social service
> * When is this person scheduled for follow-up with primary provider? Specialists? Record dates of appointments.
> * Complete a medication reconciliation before transition. Refer to index.

STAR		
	Stop	
	Think	Is this person at high risk for injury, falls, medical complications, and/or inability to care for self (activities of daily living)?
		Is there a support person available?
		Is the person competent to manage self-administration of medications, treatment procedures?
		Are additional resources needed?
		Can the person explain how to monitor the condition (e.g., blood glucose, sign/symptoms of complications, dietary/mobility restrictions, and when to call his or her primary provider or specialist)?
	Act	Contact or provide the appropriate resource (e.g., contacting a support person, home health assessment, additional teaching, printed materials).
	Review	Has the problem been addressed? If not, use SBAR to communicate to the appropriate person.

Risk for Ineffective Health Management Related to Insufficient Knowledge of Wound Care, Exercises, Breast Prosthesis, Signs and Symptoms of Complications, Hand/Arm Precautions, Community Resources, and Follow-Up Care

NOC

Compliance Behavior, Knowledge: Treatment Regimen, Participation: Health Care Decisions, Treatment Behavior: Illness or Injury

NIC

Anticipatory Guidance, Risk Identification, Health Education, Learning Facilitation

Goals

The goals for this diagnosis represent those associated with transition planning. Refer to the transition criteria.

Interventions	Rationales
1. Teach the individual breast self-examination techniques; instruct her to examine both breasts periodically.	1. Periodic, careful breast self-examination can detect problems early; this improves the likelihood of successful treatment (*Nettina, 2006).
2. Teach the individual wound care measures (refer to Generic Care Plan for the Surgical Client for details) and to avoid using strong deodorants and shaving of axilla for 2 weeks after surgery (Yarbro et al., 2011).	2. Proper wound care is essential to reduce risk of infection. Irritation of the axilla should be avoided to decrease risk of infection (Yarbro et al., 2011).

Interventions	Rationales
3. Explain "phantom breast syndrome," which is the sensation of residual breast tissue persisting for years after surgery. Individual may experience pain, but itching, nipple sensation, erotic sensations, and premenstrual-type breast soreness are also described (*Jamison, Wellisch, Katz, & Pasnau, 1979; Kwong, 2016).	3. Explanations may help to relieve individual anxiety if symptoms develop and may even reduce the frequency of this syndrome (Kwong, 2016).
4. Access information about breast prostheses for the individual.	4. A prosthesis of optimal contour, size, and weight provides normal appearance, promotes good posture, and helps to prevent back and shoulder strain.
5. Explain the benefits of strengthening and aerobic exercises.	5. Strengthening exercises increase lymph flow with muscle-pumping action. Aerobic activity elevates the heart and respiratory rates; this stimulates the lymphatic transport (Yarbro et al., 2011).
6. Explain the use of a compression sleeve, if ordered.	6. Compression increases lymphatic return and reduces edema.
7. Explain to expect fatigue in the months after surgery (*Badger, Braden, & Michel, 2001).	7. Fatigue has been found to be the most frequently reported side effect (*Badger et al., 2001).
8. Instruct to report promptly any signs and symptoms of complications, including these: a. Pain that is not relieved by medication b. Fever more than 100° F or chills c. Excessive bleeding, such as a bloody dressing d. Excessive swelling e. Redness outside the dressing f. Discharge or bad odor from the wound g. Allergic or other reactions to medication(s) h. Constipation i. Increasing anxiety, depression, trouble sleeping	8. These signs and symptoms point to increasing lymphedema, which can lead to impaired sensorimotor function or infection.
9. Initiate health teaching and referrals as needed a. Provide written instructions on activity limitations, exercises, wound care, and follow-up appointments b. Refer to rehabilitation services as needed to improve shoulder function and reduce the risk of lymphedema c. Discuss available community resources (e.g., Reach for Recovery, ENCORE). Encourage contact and initiate referrals, if appropriate. Home health care may be helpful owing to short length of hospitalization after surgery (*Nettina, 2006). d. Contact the American Cancer Society (ACS) for a prosthesis product list for your area.	9. Personal sources of information have been found to be more important than written materials.

Documentation

Individual/family teaching
Referrals, if indicated

Carotid Endarterectomy

A Multidisciplinary Consensus Statement from the American Heart Association concluded that carotid endarterectomy, performed in medical centers with documented combined perioperative morbidity and mortality for asymptomatic endarterectomy of less than 3%, in conjunction with aggressive modifiable risk factor management is beneficial for individuals who have an asymptomatic stenosis exceeding 60% diameter reduction confirmed by angiography (Jauch et al., 2013).

Symptomatic occlusion indicates the occurrence of a transient ischemic attack (TIA) or cerebral vascular accident (*Greelish, Mohler, & Fairman, 2006b). The procedure may be performed under general or local anesthesia; local anesthesia significantly reduces morbidity and mortality.

Time Frame
Postoperative periods

▪▪▪■■ DIAGNOSTIC CLUSTER

Postoperative Period

Collaborative Problems

Circulatory

▲ Risk for Complications of Thrombosis

▲ Risk for Complications of Hyperperfusion Syndrome

▲ Risk for Complications of Labile Hypertension

▲ Risk for Complications of Hemorrhage

Neurologic

▲ Risk for Complications of Cerebral Infarction

▲ Risk for Complications of Cranial Nerve Impairment

▲ Risk for Complications of Respiratory/Airway Obstruction

Nursing Diagnoses

▲ Risk for Injury or Falls related to syncope secondary to vascular insufficiency (refer to Risk for Falls in Unit II)

△ Risk for Ineffective Health Management related to insufficient knowledge of home care, signs and symptoms of complications, risk factors, activity restrictions, and follow-up care

Related Care Plan

General Surgery Generic Care plan

▲ This diagnosis was reported to be monitored for or managed frequently (75% to 100%).

Transition Criteria

Before transition, the individual and family will:

1. Describe wound care techniques.
2. State activity restrictions for home care.
3. Demonstrate range-of-motion (ROM) exercises.
4. State the signs and symptoms that must be reported to a health care professional.
5. Identify risk factors and describe their relationship to arterial disease.

Transitional Risk Assessment Plan (TRAP)

Begin this plan on admission.
Implement the Transitional Risk Assessment Plan (TRAP):
* Refer to inside back cover.
* Add each validated risk diagnosis to individual's problem list with the risk code in ( ).
* Refer to the individual risk nursing diagnoses/collaborative problems for outcomes and interventions in Unit II.

R: "*Close coordination of care in the post-acute period, early transition follow-up care, enhanced client education and self-management training, proactive end-of-life counseling, and extending the resources and clinical expertise over time via multidisciplinary team management*" can lower readmission rates and improve health outcomes (Boutwell & Hwu, 2009, p. 14). Interventions are utilized to activate the individual and family to select changes in their everyday lifestyle choices to improve their health (Hibbard & Greene, 2013).

Collaborative Problems

Risk for Complications of Circulatory Problems, Thrombosis, Hyperperfusion Syndrome, Labile Hypertension, Hemorrhage, Cerebral Infarction

Risk for Complications of Neurologic Problems, Cerebral Infarction, Cranial Nerve Impairment, Local Nerve Impairment

Risk for Complications of Respiratory/Airway Obstruction

Collaborative Outcomes

The individual will be monitored for early signs and symptoms of (a) vascular problems, (b) neurologic deficits, and (c) respiratory obstruction and will receive collaborative interventions if indicated to restore physiologic stability.

Indicators of Physiologic Stability

- Respirations—quiet, regular, unlabored (a, b, c)
- Respirations 16 to 20 breaths/min (a, b, c)
- BP >90/60, <140/90 mm Hg (a, b)
- Pulse 60 to 100 beats/min (a, b, c)
- Temperature 98° F to 99.5° F (a)
- Alert, oriented (b)
- Pupils, equal, reactive to light (b)
- Intact motor function (b)
- Clear speech (b)
- Swallowing reflex intact (b)
- Facial symmetry (b)
- Full ROM upper/lower limbs (b)
- Urine output >0.5 mL/kg/hr (a, b, c)
- Oxygen saturation (Sao_2) 94 to 100 mm Hg (a, b, c)
- Partial pressure of carbon dioxide ($Paco_2$) 35 to 45 mm Hg (a, b, c)
- pH 7.35 to 7.45 (a, b, c)
- Hemoglobin
  - Male 13 to 15 g/dL (a, b, c)
  - Female 12 to 10 g/dL (a, b, c)
- Hematocrit
  - Male 42% to 50% (a, b, c)
  - Female 40% to 48% (a, b, c)
- Mean arterial pressure 60 to 160 mm Hg (a, b, c)
- White blood count 4,000 to 10,800 mm³ (a, b, c)

 Carp's Cues

Please refer to the Generic Care Plan for the Surgical Client for detailed interventions for managing all surgical conditions. This care plan addresses specific additional interventions associated with the type of surgery performed.

Interventions	Rationales
1. Monitor for the following: a. Respiratory obstruction (check trachea for deviation from midline; listen for respiratory stridor)	1a. The risks associated with respiratory compromise secondary to neck hematomas or recurrent laryngeal nerve injury, A postoperative neck hematoma can be catastrophic and result in abrupt loss of the airway (Mohler & Fairman, 2015).
b. Blood pressure lability—monitor closely for the first 24 hours c. Peri-incisional swelling or bleeding	b. Frequent difficulty with blood pressure control after manipulation of the carotid sinus. Because blood pressure lability is common in the first 12 to 24 hours postoperatively, it is standard care for individual postcarotid endarterectomy (CEA) to be placed in a monitored setting with an arterial line in place (Fairman, 2016).
2. Monitor status of headache. Report promptly if headache is worsening. Use a scale of 0 to 10 to monitor for changes. **CLINICAL ALERT:** • "Neurologic changes in the patient after CEA must be considered to be related to problems at the endarterectomy site (e.g., thrombosis, intimal flap) until proven otherwise" (Mohler & Fairman, 2015).	2. Minor headache is common after CEA, but increasing or severe headache in the postoperative period may be an indicator of cerebral hyperperfusion syndrome or intracranial hemorrhage. A CT scan is warranted (Fairman, 2016).

3. Monitor for changes in neurologic function (Fairman, 2016):
   a. Level of consciousness
   b. Pupillary response
   c. Motor/sensory function of all four extremities (check hand grasps and ability to move legs)
	3. Stroke is the second most common cause of death after CEA. Manifestations of cerebral infarction include neuromuscular impairment of the contralateral body side (Mohler & Fairman, 2015).

4. Monitor for cranial nerve dysfunction (Fairman, 2016):	4. The surgical procedure can temporarily or permanently disrupt cranial nerve functions (Faitrman, 2016; *National Library of Medicine, 2006). Most cranial nerve injuries resolve over a few months; permanent injuries are rare (Faitrman, 2016). Nerve damage affects around 8% of people but is usually temporary and disappears within a month.

a. Difficulty with speech
   b. Dysphagia
   c. Upper airway obstruction
   d. Upward protrusion of lower lip
   e. Sagging shoulder
   f. Difficulty raising arm or shoulder
   g. Loss of gag reflex
   h. Hoarseness
   i. Asymmetrical movements of vocal cords
   j. Numbness/weakness of face on the surgical side
	a. The hypoglossal nerve controls intrinsic and extrinsic muscles for tongue movement.
	
	   d. The facial nerve controls facial motor function and taste.
	   e. The accessory nerve controls the trapezius and sternocleidomastoid muscles.
	   g. The vagus nerve regulates movements of swallowing and sensation to the pharynx and larynx. Laryngeal nerve (branches of vagus nerve) damage may cause unilateral vocal cord paralysis (Faitrman, 2016). Stimulation of the glossopharyngeal nerve may cause hypotension and bradycardia. Dissection of trigeminal nerve may lead to sensory loss in the affected area.

5. Monitor for hyperperfusion syndrome (Mohler & Fairman, 2015): a. Headache ipsilateral (same side) to the revascularized internal carotid, typically improved in upright posture, may herald the syndrome in the first week after endarterectomy.	5. Before surgery, to maintain sufficient cerebral blood flow, small vessels compensate with chronic maximal dilatation. The dilated vessels may be unable to vasoconstrict sufficiently to protect the capillary bed (Mohler & Fairman, 2015). Breakthrough perfusion pressure then causes edema and hemorrhage, which in turn result in the clinical manifestations. Hypertension is a frequent predecessor of the syndrome, underscoring the importance of good perioperative blood pressure control.

Interventions	*Rationales*

b. Alert the individual and significant others to monitor for this type of headache. Immediately call surgeon with the information

CLINICAL ALERT:
- Hyperperfusion syndrome is probably the cause of most postoperative intracerebral hemorrhages and seizures in the first 2 weeks after CEA.

Clinical Alert Report

Before providing care, advise ancillary staff/student to report the following to the professional nurse assigned to the individual:
- Change in cognitive status
- Change in voice
- Difficulty swallowing
- Oral temperature >100.5° F
- Systolic BP <90 mm Hg
- Resting pulse >100, <50
- Respiratory rate >28, <10/min
- Oxygen saturation <90%

Documentation

Vital signs
Patency of the temporal artery on the operative side
Level of consciousness
Pupillary response
Motor function (hand grasp, leg movement)
Cranial nerve function
Wound assessment

Nursing Diagnoses

TRANSITION TO HOME/COMMUNITY CARE

If indicated, review the risk diagnoses identified for this individual on admission:
- Is the person still at risk?
- Can the family reduce the risks?
- Is the person at higher risk at home?
- Is a Home Health Nurse assessment needed?
- Refer to transition planner/case manager/social service
- When is this person scheduled for follow-up with primary provider? Specialists? Record dates of appointments.
- Complete a medication reconciliation before transition. Refer to index.

S T A R

Stop

Think Is this person at high risk for injury, falls, medical complications, and/or inability to care for self (activities of daily living)?

Is there a support person available?

Is the person competent to manage self-administration of medications, treatment procedures? Are additional resources needed?

Can the person explain how to monitor the condition (e.g., blood glucose, signs/symptoms of complications, dietary/mobility restrictions, and when to call his or her primary provider or specialist)?

Act Contact or provide the appropriate resource (e.g., contacting a support person, home health assessment, additional teaching, printed materials).

Review Has the problem been addressed? If not, use SBAR to communicate to the appropriate person.

Risk for Ineffective Health Management Related to Insufficient Knowledge of Home Care, Signs and Symptoms of Complications, Risk Factors, Activity Restrictions, and Follow-Up Care

NOC
Compliance Behavior, Knowledge: Treatment Regimen, Participation: Health Care Decisions, Treatment Behavior: Illness or Injury

NIC
Anticipatory Guidance, Risk Management, Health Education, Learning Facilitation

Goals

The goals for this diagnosis represent those associated with transition planning. Refer to the transition criteria.

Interventions	Rationales
1. Advise the individual will have neck pain and difficulty swallowing for a few days. Advise to eat soft foods.	
2. Advise to seek emergency care if: a. Numbness or weakness of the face, arms, or legs, especially on one side of the body b. Confusion and trouble speaking or understanding speech c. Trouble seeing in one or both eyes d. Dizziness, trouble walking, loss of balance or coordination, and unexplained falls. e. Increasing headache with no clear cause f. Increased swelling in neck g. Headache ipsilateral (same side) to the revascularized internal carotid, typically improved in upright posture	2a–e. These signs and symptoms can indicate cerebral ischemia. Stroke is the second most common cause of death after CEA. Rates range from less than 0.25% to more than 3% depending upon the indication for CEA and other factors, including the experience of the surgeon (Mohler & Fairman, 2015). g. This type of headache may indicate and may herald hyperperfusion syndrome in the first week after endarterectomy
3. Teach the individual and family to watch for and report the following to their surgeon: a. Swelling of, or drainage from, the incision b. Temperature >100.5° F	3. These signs are indicative of infection.
4. Teach the individual and family about the vascular disease process and prevention of further arterial occlusions (Sieggreen, 2007).	4. The development of atherosclerosis is influenced by heredity and also by lifestyle factors, such as dietary habits and levels of exercise.
5. Teach about the risk factors for atherosclerosis that can be modified or eliminated: a. Elevated blood cholesterol and triglycerides b. Hypertension c. Tobacco use or exposure to tobacco smoke d. Diabetes, types 1 and 2 e. Obesity f. Inactivity, lack of exercise Refer to How Can Atherosclerosis Be Prevented or Delayed? accessed at ttps://www.nhlbi.nih.gov/health/health-topics/topics/atherosclerosis/prevention Refer to Getting Started to Quit Smoking, Getting Started to Increase Activity, and Getting Started to Healthy Eating on thePoint.	5. Addressing risk factors and encouraging regular follow-up with the physician/nurse practitioner/physical assistant can inhibit worsening of atherosclerotic vascular disorders (e.g., myocardial infarction, stroke) (Wilson, 2015).

Documentation

Individual/family teaching
Referrals, if indicated

Colostomy

A colostomy is an opening between the colon and the abdominal wall. The proximal end of the colon is sutured to the skin. A colostomy is performed when it is imperative to bypass or remove the distal colon, rectum, or anus, and it is either inadvisable or not feasible to restore gastrointestinal continuity. If the distal rectum and anorectal sphincter mechanism are removed, the colostomy is permanent; however, if the sphincter mechanism is preserved, there is the potential for ostomy reversal (Francone, 2015)

Clinical settings that may warrant construction of a permanent colostomy include abdominal perineal resection for rectal cancer, fecal incontinence- related anal outlet dysfunction or perianal sepsis, total abdominal proctocolectomy for severe Crohn colitis or total abdominal proctocolectomy for severe ulcerative colitis (Francone, 2015).

There are different names for colostomies, which are dependent on where the stoma is created. There is the *ascending colostomy*, which has an opening created from the ascending colon, and is found on the right abdomen. Because the stoma is created from the first section of the colon, stool is more liquid and contains digestive enzymes that irritate the skin. This type of colostomy is the least common (Francone, 2015).

The *transverse colostomy* may have one or two openings in the upper abdomen, middle, or right side, which are created from the transverse colon. If there are two openings in the stoma (called a double-barrel colostomy), one is used to pass stool and the other, mucus. The stool has passed through the ascending colon, so it tends to be liquid to semiformed. This method is mostly used for temporary colostomies (Francone, 2015).

In a *descending or sigmoid colostomy*, the descending or sigmoid colon is used to create the stoma, typically on the left lower abdomen. This is the most common type of colostomy surgery and generally produces stool that is semiformed to well-formed because it has passed through the ascending and transverse colon (Francone, 2015).

 Time Frame
Preoperative and postoperative periods

■■■■■ DIAGNOSTIC CLUSTER

Collaborative Problems

▲ Risk for Complications of Peristomal Tissue

▲ Risk for Complications of Stoma

* Risk for Complications of Intra-abdominal sepsis

* Risk for Complications of Large Bowel Obstruction

* Risk for Complications of Perforation of Genitourinary Tract

Nursing Diagnoses

▲ Risk for Disturbed Self-Concept related to effects of ostomy on body image and lifestyle

Δ Risk for Loneliness related to fears associated with possible odor and leakage from appliance in public.

Δ Grieving related to implications of cancer diagnosis, refer to: Cancer: Initial Diagnosis.

▲ Risk for Ineffective Health Regimen Management related to insufficient knowledge of stoma pouching procedure, colostomy irrigation, peristomal skin care, perineal wound care, and incorporation of ostomy care into activities of daily living (ADLs).

Related Care Plan

General Surgery Generic Care Plan

▲ This diagnosis was reported to be monitored for or managed frequently (75% to 100%).

Δ This diagnosis was reported to be monitored for or managed often (50% to 74%).

* This diagnosis was not included in the validation study.

Transition Criteria

Before transition, the individual and family will:

1. Elicit concerns or problems with ostomy care at home, including stoma, pouching, irrigation, and skin care.
2. State signs and symptoms that must be reported to a health care professional.
3. Verbalize intent to share with significant others' feelings and concerns related to ostomy.
4. Identify available community resources and self-help groups:
   a. Home health nurse
   b. United Ostomy Association
   c. American Cancer Foundation

Transitional Risk Assessment Plan (TRAP)

Begin this plan on admission.
Implement the Transitional Risk Assessment Plan (TRAP):
* Refer to inside back cover.
* Add each validated risk diagnosis to individual's problem list with the risk code in ( ).
* Refer to the individual risk nursing diagnoses/collaborative problems for outcomes and interventions in Unit II.

R: *"Close coordination of care in the post-acute period, early transition follow-up care, enhanced client education and self-management training, proactive end-of-life counseling, and extending the resources and clinical expertise over time via multidisciplinary team management" can lower readmission rates and improve health outcomes (Boutwell & Hwu, 2009, p. 14). Interventions are utilized to activate the individual and family to select changes in their everyday lifestyle choices to improve their health (Hibbard & Greene, 2013).*

Preoperative Period: Collaborative Problem

Risk for Impaired Tissue Integrity Related to Anatomical Barriers to Precise Placement of Stoma During Surgery

NOC
Tissue integrity: Skin and mucous membrane (stoma)

Goal

The individual will have site selection and marking of stoma placement before surgery

NIC
Teaching, Surveillance

Indicators

* An ostomy nurse specialist will evaluate for site selection and will mark site or
* If the situation is emergent, a nurse or physician, who has expertise in site selection, should be accessed.

Interventions	Rationales
1. When it is first known that an individual may have an ostomy, access the ostomy nurse specialist	1. The sooner the specialist is activated the more likely that the expert will be available to do the site election. Multiple studies indicate that individuals who have their stoma site marked preoperatively by a trained clinician have fewer ostomy-related complications (e.g., peristomal dermatitis) (Francone, 2015; Wound, Ostomy and Continence Nurses Society, 2014).

Interventions	Rationales
2. When it known that the specialist will not be available for site selection, notify the health profession known for competence in site selection. **CLINICAL ALERT:** • Site selection should never be done casually. Every attempt should be made to have the individual with the most expertise complete the site selection. The stoma site should be selected to avoid fat folds, scars, and bony prominences (Wound, Ostomy and Continence Nurses Society, 2014). The quality of life of this individual can be seriously impaired if incorrect placement results in leaking and peristomal dermatitis. "In retrospective reviews, proper site selection is essential for minimizing postoperative complications and achieving a good postoperative quality of life" (Francone, 2015).	2. Stoma site marking should be performed by an Enterostomal Nurse (ETN), Rectal Surgeon or a health care professional who has been trained in the principles of stoma site marking and is aware of the implications of ostomy care and poor stoma site marking (Wound, Ostomy and Continence Nurses Society, 2014).
2. Site selection should take place not in the operating room if at all possible. The following criteria may be useful in situations when an expert is not available (Wound, Ostomy and Continence Nurses Society, 2014, pp. 3, 4): a. Physical considerations: Large/protruding/pendulous abdomen, abdominal folds, wrinkles, scars/suture lines, other stomas, rectus abdominis muscle, waist line, iliac crest, braces, pendulous breasts, vision, dexterity, and the presence of a hernia. b. Examine the individual's exposed abdomen in various positions (e.g., standing, lying, sitting, and bending forward) to observe for creases, valleys, scars, folds, skin turgor, and contour. c. With the individual lying on his or her back, identify the rectus abdominis muscle. This can be done by having the individual do a modified sit up (i.e., raise the head up and off the bed) or by having the individual cough. Palpate the edge of the rectus abdominis muscle. Expert opinion suggests that placement of the stoma within the rectus abdominis muscle may help prevent a peristomal hernia and/or a prolapse. d. The mark should initially be made with a sticker or ink pen that can be removed if this is not the optimal spot. e. It may be desirable to mark sites on the right and left sides of the abdomen to prepare for a change in the surgical outcome, and number the first choice as #1. f. Have the person assume sitting, bending, and lying positions to assess and confirm the best choice. g. It is important to have the individual confirm they can see the site. However, the critical consideration should be a flat pouching surface.	2. Principles of proper stoma site selection, including placement of the stoma within the rectus abdominis muscle, use of multiple t positions to identify appropriate stoma sites, avoidance of folds and scars, and consideration of the clothing/beltline. This could make the difference between an ostomy pouch leaking or not for the person's lifetime. Types of skin damage included erosion, maceration, erythema, and irritant dermatitis (Wound, Ostomy and Continence Nurses Society, 2014).

Collaborative Problems

Risk for Complications of Peristomal Tissue

Risk for Complications of Stoma

Risk for Complications of Intra-abdominal Sepsis

Risk for Complications of Large Bowel Obstruction

Risk for Complications of Perforation of Genitourinary Tract

Collaborative Outcomes

The individual will be monitored for early signs and symptoms of (a) peristomal complications, (b) stomal complications, (c) intra-abdominal sepsis, (d) large bowel obstruction, and (e) perforation of genitourinary tract and will receive collaborative interventions if indicated to restore physiologic stability.

Indicators of Physiologic Stability

- Intact bowel sounds in all quadrants (d)
- Intact peristomal muscle tone (a, b)
- Free-flowing ostomy fluid (a, b)
- No evidence of bleeding (a, b)
- No evidence of infection (c)
- No complaints of nausea/vomiting/hiccups (c, d)
- Nondistended abdomen (d)
- Perineal wound intact (if sutured) (c)
- Temperature 98° F to 99.5° F; no chills (c)
- BP >90/60, <140/90 mm Hg (c)
- Pulse 60 to 100 beats/min (c)
- Respirations 16 to 20 breaths/min
- Urine output >0.5 mL/kg/hr (e, j)

 Carp's Cues

Please refer to the Generic Care Plan for the Surgical Client for detailed interventions for managing all surgical conditions. This care plan addresses specific additional interventions associated with this type of surgery performed.

Interventions	Rationales
1. Monitor for early stomal complications:	1. The most early common complications were stomal retraction, stomal bleeding, necrosis, mucocutaneous separation, and peristomal skin problems (Landmann, 2015).
a. Stomal bleeding	a. Stomal bleeding—usually indicates either a stomal laceration from a poorly fitting appliance or the presence of peristomal varices in the individual with portal hypertension.
b. Stomal retraction	b. Stomal retraction is defined as a stoma that is 0.5 cm or more below the skin surface within 6 weeks of construction, typically as a result of tension on the stoma. Stomal retraction leads to leakage and difficulties with pouch adherence, resulting in peristomal skin irritation.

 CLINICAL ALERT:
- Obesity (defined as a body mass index 0.25 kg/m^2) has been associated with stomal (retraction, prolapse, and necrosis) and peristomal skin problems in multiple studies.

c. Necrosis (death of stomal tissue with impaired local blood flow)	c. The incidence of stomal necrosis in the immediate postoperative period is as high as 14%. Adequate mobilization of the bowel, preservation of the blood supply to the stoma, and an adequate trephine size are important factors for avoiding this complication.
d. Mucocutaneous separation, retraction (disappearance of normal stomal protrusion in line with or below skin level)	d. Mucocutaneous separation refers to the separation of the ostomy from the peristomal skin. Mucocutaneous separation results in leakage and skin irritation. It occurs in 12% to 24% of individuals early in the postoperative period.
e. Stenosis, fistula, trauma	

Interventions	Rationales

2. Monitor the following:
   a. Color, size, and shape of the stoma; and mucocutaneous separation
   b. Color, amount, and consistency of ostomy effluent
 	
   c. Complaints of cramping abdominal pain, nausea and vomiting, and abdominal distention
   d. Fit of ostomy appliance and appliance belt
	2a. These changes can indicate inflammation, retraction, prolapse, or edema.
	   b. These changes can indicate bleeding or infection. Decreased output can indicate obstruction.
	   c. These complaints may indicate obstruction.
	
	   d. An improperly fitting appliance or belt can cause mechanical trauma to the stoma

3. If mucocutaneous separation occurs, notify wound/ostomy nurse specialist or surgeon.	3. Special techniques are needed to prevent fecal contamination.
4. Monitor perineal wound for signs and symptoms of infection, bleeding, and drainage.	

5. Monitor for intra-abdominal sepsis (Minkes, 2013)
   a. Complaints of nausea, hiccups
   b. Spiking fevers, chills
   c. Tachycardia
   d. Elevated WBC	

CLINICAL ALERT:
- Immediately notify surgeon.
- Leakage of GI fluid into the peritoneal cavity (e.g., a leak at the anastomotic site) can cause serious infections (e.g., staphylococcal).

6. Monitor for intestinal obstruction (Minkes, 2013):
   a. Increasing pain
   b. Decreased/absent bowel sounds or hyperperistalsis
   c. Clinical evidence of hypovolemia
	6. "Intestinal obstruction is also common. Stoma strictures can occur at the skin level, fascial level, or both. Partial obstruction can result in hyperperistalsis and hypersecretion; massive fluid losses through the stoma may result in dehydration. Other causes of obstruction include luminal plugging caused by ingested food, adhesive intestinal obstruction, internal hernia, and volvulus" (Minkes, 2013).

7. Monitor for large bowel obstruction; notify the physician/nurse practitioner, if detected:
   a. Decreased bowel sounds
   b. Nausea, vomiting
   c. Abdominal distention
	7. Intraoperative manipulation of the abdominal organs and the depressive effects of anesthesia and narcotics can cause decreased peristalsis.

8. Monitor for perforation of bladder:
   a. Acute pelvic pain
   b. Nausea, vomiting, malaise
   c. Abdominal distention
   d. Costovertebral angle tenderness, ileus, fever, flank pain
	8. Intraoperatively, the bladder can be punctured during the colon resection. Urine leakage into perineum will cause infection.

CLINICAL ALERT:
- Call Rapid Response Team if signs of bladder perforation occur.

Clinical Alert Report

Before providing care, advise ancillary staff/student to report the following to the professional nurse assigned to the individual:
- Change in cognitive status
- Oral temperature >100.5° F

- Systolic BP <90 mm Hg
- Resting pulse >100, <50
- Respiratory rate >28, <10/min
- Oxygen saturation <90%
- New- onset pelvic pain
- Nausea/vomiting
- Change in stoma appearance
- Urine output <0.5 mL/kg/hr

Documentation

Intake and output
Bowel sounds
Wound status
Stoma condition

Postoperative: Nursing Diagnoses

Risk for Disturbed Self-Concept Related to Effects of Ostomy on Body Image and Lifestyle

NOC
Anxiety Reduction,
Coping, Impulse
Control

Goal

The individual will communicate feelings about the ostomy and will share their perceptions of the effects on their daily lives.

NIC
Hope Instillation,
Mood Management,
Values Clarification,
Counseling, Referral,
Support Group, Coping
Enhancement

Indicators

- Acknowledge changes in body structure and function.
- Participate actively in stoma care
- Seek out information on self-care

 ### Carp's Cues

"The average period of time needed to resolve the psychological distress produced by ostomy surgery and restore optimal quality of life is not known, but existing evidence suggests that this process requires 12 months or longer" (Registered Nurses' Association of Ontario, 2009). Long-term recovery is characterized initially by taking control of ostomy care, followed by seeking to recover a sense of normalcy and reestablishing work-related and social activities (Registered Nurses' Association of Ontario, 2009). "The individual must adapt to new patterns of fecal elimination and to their altered body and image of themselves. Successful adaptation requires the individual to master new skills and to deal effectively with the many emotional issues associated with their altered anatomy and with altered continence" (Landmann, 2015).

Interventions	Rationales
1. Contact the individual frequently and treat him or her with warm, positive regard.	1. Frequent contact by caregiver indicates acceptance and may facilitate trust. The individual may be hesitant to approach staff/student because of a negative self-concept (Colwell & Beitz, 2007).
2. Incorporate emotional support into technical ostomy self-care sessions. Encourage the individual to perform as much self-care as possible.	2. Nursing interventions that enable individual s to increase self-efficacy in ostomy management act as enablers as they struggle to reestablish a sense of normalcy after ostomy surgery. Impaired body image is associated with symptoms of weakness, fragility, unattractiveness, and feelings of stigma (Registered Nurses' Association of Ontario, 2009).
3. Assess if individual looks at and touches the stoma.	3. Persson and Helstrom (2002) reported that postostomy, individuals emphasized the initial shock and emotional distress they experienced when the stoma was first visualized.

Interventions	Rationales
	The nurse should not make assumptions about a individual's reactions to ostomy surgery. The individual may require help in accepting the reality of the altered body appearance and function, or in dealing with an overwhelming situation (Richbourg, Thorpe, & Rapp, 2007).
4. Encourage the individual to verbalize feelings (both positive and negative) about the stoma and perceptions of its anticipated effects on his or her lifestyle (Registered Nurses' Association of Ontario, 2009).	4. "The assessment of self-esteem in ostomized people is becoming increasingly important and necessary, because when subjected to this surgery, these people start living a different experience, where their standard of living and rhythm of life begin to change. Their desires and values are often not fulfilled nor respected; they feel rejected, seeking seclusion because of the odor and elimination of feces through the abdomen" (Salomé, de Almeida, & Silveira, 2014).
5. Validate the individual's perceptions and reassure that such responses are normal and appropriate.	5. Validating the individual's perceptions promotes self-awareness and provides reassurance. Sharing gives the nurse an opportunity to identify and dispel misconceptions and allay anxiety and self-doubt (Registered Nurses' Association of Ontario, 2009).
6. Ensure that support persons have been included in learning ostomy care principles. Assess the individual's interactions with support persons.	6. Other people's response to the ostomy is one of the most important factors influencing acceptance of it.
7. Encourage to reestablish his or her preoperative socialization pattern. Help the individual through such measures as progressively increasing his or her socializing time in the hospital, role-playing possible situations that may cause anxiety, and encouraging him or her to visualize and anticipate solutions to "worst-case scenarios" for social situations.	7. Encouraging and facilitating socialization help to prevent isolation. Role-playing can help to identify and learn to cope with potential anxiety-causing situations in a nonthreatening environment.
8. Encourage the individual/partner to initiate future discussions regarding effects on their relationship with primary care provider and/or ostomy nurse specialist.	8. Future discussions will be needed; however, when the nurse postoperatively initiates the discussion, it gives the concerned individuals permission for future dialogue.

Documentation

Present emotional status
Interventions
Response to interventions

> **TRANSITION TO HOME/COMMUNITY CARE**
>
> If indicated, review the risk diagnoses identified for this individual on admission:
> - Is the person still at risk?
> - Can the family reduce the risks?
> - Is the person at higher risk at home?
> - Is a Home Health Nurse assessment needed?
> - Refer to transition planner/case manager/social service
> - When is this person scheduled for follow-up with primary provider? Specialists? Record dates of appointments.
> - Complete a medication reconciliation before transition. Refer to index.

STAR		
	Stop	
	Think	Is this person at high risk for injury, falls, medical complications, and/or inability to care for self (activities of daily living)?
		Is there a support person available?
		Is the person competent to manage self-administration of medications, treatment procedures? Are additional resources needed?
		Can the person explain how to monitor the condition (e.g., blood glucose, sign/symptoms of complications, dietary/mobility restrictions, and when to call his or her primary provider or specialist)?
	Act	Contact or provide the appropriate resource (e.g., contacting a support person, home health assessment, additional teaching, printed materials).
	Review	Has the problem been addressed? If not, use SBAR to communicate to the appropriate person.

Risk for Ineffective Health Management Related to Insufficient Knowledge of Stoma Poaching Procedure, Colostomy Irrigation, Peristomal Skin Care, Perineal Wound Care, and Incorporation of Ostomy Care into Activities of Daily Living (ADLs)

NOC

Compliance Behavior, Knowledge: Treatment Regimen, Participation: Health Care Decisions, Treatment Behavior: Illness or Injury

NIC

Anticipatory Guidance, Ostomy Care, Learning Facilitation, Risk Management, Health Education

Goals

The goals for this diagnosis represent those associated with transition planning. Refer to the transition criteria.

Interventions	Rationales
1. Continuously assess the individual's ability to manage colostomy care. Consult/refer ostomy nurse specialist as indicated.	1. The details of ostomy management are taught by the nurse specialist. The unit nurse is responsible for evaluating the individual's competency.
2. Observe the condition of the stoma and peristomal skin during pouch changes.	2. Regular observation enables early detection of skin problems.
3. Watch for and report signs and symptoms of infection or abscess (e.g., pain or purulent drainage).	
4. Review methods for reducing odor learned from wound care/ostomy specialist.	4. Minimizing odor improves self-confidence and can permit more effective socialization. Bacterial proliferation in retained effluent increases odor with time. A full pouch also puts excessive pressure on seals, which increases risk of leakage.
5. Ensure that a consult with nutritionist has occurred. a. Ensure there is access to an enterostomal nurse specialist when at home.	5. The colonoscopy affects absorption and use of nutrients. a. An expert should be available to answer questions as the individual assumes more self-care.
6. Discuss community resources/self-help groups, including: a. Home health nurse b. United Ostomy Associations, www.uoaa.org c. National Foundation for Ileitis and Colitis (800-343-3637) d. American Cancer Foundation e. Community suppliers of ostomy equipment f. Financial reimbursement for ostomy equipment	6. Personal sources of information have been found to be more important than written materials (Richbourg et al., 2007).

Documentation

Individual/family teaching
Response to teaching as well as achieved outcomes or the status of each goal

Coronary Artery Bypass Grafting

Coronary artery bypass graft (CABG) surgery is recommended for individuals with obstructive coronary artery disease whose survival will be improved compared to medical therapy or percutaneous coronary intervention (PCI) (Aranki & Aroesty, 2016).

Surgery most often involves a median sternotomy incision with cardiopulmonary bypass, or extracorporeal circulation, to circulate and oxygenate the blood while diverting it from the heart and lungs to provide a bloodless operative field for the surgeon. The saphenous vein is the most common venous graft used for bypassing the coronary circulation (Aranki & Aroesty, 2016). Most individuals receive both arterial and venous grafts during CABG and long-term graft patency is significantly better with the former.

Saphenous vein graft (SVG) occlusion occurs within 30 days of CABG surgery in approximately 10% of grafts (Aranki & Aroesty, 2015). Potential consequences of graft failure (loss of patency) include the development of angina, myocardial infarction, or cardiac death (Aranki & Aroesty, 2016).

The number of off-pump CABG operations continues to decrease, since expected benefits have been largely marginal or absent, with the possible exception of individuals with predicted very high-risk surgical scores for whom the risk of stroke was lower with off-pump CABG (Aranki & Aroesty, 2016; Marui et al., 2012). There are studies that have suggested a significant superiority for on-pump CABG with regard to SVG patency when compared to off-pump surgery (Aranki & Aroesty, 2016).

Time Frame
Postoperative periods (not intensive care period)

▪▪▪▪ DIAGNOSTIC CLUSTER

Postoperative Period

Collaborative Problems

* Risk for Complications of Saphenous vein graft (SVG) occlusion

▲ Risk for Complications of Cardiovascular Insufficiency

▲ Risk for Complications of Respiratory Insufficiency

▲ Risk for Complications of Renal Insufficiency

* Risk for Complications of Postcardiotomy Delirium

Nursing Diagnoses

Δ Fear related to transfer from intensive environment of the critical care unit and potential for complications

Δ Interrupted Family Processes related to disruption of family life, fear of outcome (death, disability), and stressful environment (ICU) (refer to Interrupted Family Processes in Unit II Section 1)

▲ Impaired Comfort related to surgical incisions, chest tubes, and immobility secondary to lengthy surgery (refer to General Surgery Care Plan)

Δ Risk for Ineffective Therapeutic Regimen Management related to insufficient knowledge of incisional care, pain management (angina, incisions), signs and symptoms of complications, condition, pharmacologic care, risk factors, restrictions, stress management techniques, and follow-up care

Related Care Plans

General Surgery Generic Care Plan

(continued)

Thoracic Surgery

▲ This diagnosis was reported to be monitored for or managed frequently (75% to 100%).

Δ This diagnosis was reported to be monitored for or managed often (50% to 74%).

* This diagnosis was not included in the validation study.

Transition Criteria

Before transition, the individual and family will:

1. Demonstrate insertion site care.
2. Relate at-home restrictions and follow-up care.
3. State signs and symptoms that must be reported to a health-care professional.
4. Relate a plan to reduce risk factors, as necessary.

> ### **Transitional Risk Assessment Plan (TRAP)**
>
> Begin this plan on admission.
> Implement the Transitional Risk Assessment Plan (TRAP):
> * Refer to inside back cover.
> * Add each validated risk diagnosis to individual's problem list with the risk code in ( ).
> * Refer to the individual risk nursing diagnoses/collaborative problems for outcomes and interventions in Unit II.
>
> *R:* *"Close coordination of care in the post-acute period, early transition follow-up care, enhanced client education and self-management training, proactive end-of-life counseling, and extending the resources and clinical expertise over time via multidisciplinary team management" can lower readmission rates and improve health outcomes (Boutwell & Hwu, 2009, p. 14). Interventions are utilized to activate the individual and family to select changes in their everyday lifestyle choices to improve their health (Hibbard & Greene, 2013).*

Postoperative: Collaborative Problems

Risk for Complications of Cardiovascular Insufficiency

Risk for Complications of Respiratory Insufficiency

Risk for Complications of Renal Insufficiency

Risk for Complications of Postcardiotomy Delirium

Collaborative Outcomes

The nurse will detect early signs and symptoms of (a) cardiovascular insufficiency, (b) respiratory insufficiency, (c) renal insufficiency, (d) hyperthermia, and (e) postcardiotomy delirium and will collaboratively intervene to stabilize the individual.

Indicators of Physiologic Stability

* Oriented, calm (a, b, c, d, e)
* No change in vision (a)
* Normal sinus rhythm (EKG) (a, b)
* Heart rate 60 to 100 beats/min (a, b)
* BP >90/60, <140/90 mm Hg (a, b)
* No complaints of syncope, palpitations (a, b)
* Mean arterial pressure 70/90 mm Hg (a, b)
* Pulmonary artery wedge pressure 4 to 12 mm Hg (a, b)
* Cardiac output/index >2.4 (a, b)
* Pulmonary artery systolic pressure 20 to 30 mm Hg (a, b)

- Pulmonary artery diastolic pressure 10 to 15 mm Hg (a, b)
- Hematocrit (a)
  - Males 42% to 50%
  - Females 40% to 48%
- Temperature 98° F to 99.5° F (d)
- Minimal change in pulse pressure (a, b)
- Respirations 16 to 20 breaths/min (a, b)
- Urine output >0.5 mL/kg/hr (a, b, c)
- Capillary refill <3 seconds (a, b)
- Skin warm, no pallor, cyanosis, or grayness (a, b)
- No complaints of palpitations, syncope, chest pain (a, b)
- No neck vein distention (a, b)
- Cardiac enzymes (a)
  - Myoglobin up to 85 mg/mL
  - Creatine phosphokinase (CK)
    - Males 50 to 325 mU/mL
    - Females 50 to 250 mU/mL
  - Troponin complex (C, I, T)
  - Hemoglobin (a)
    - Males 13 to 18 g/dL
    - Females 12 to 16 g/dL
- Partial thromboplastin time (PTT) 20 to 45 seconds (a)
- International normalized ratio (INR) 1.0 (a)
- Platelets 100,000 to 400,000/mm^3 (a)
- Prothrombin time (PT) >20 seconds (a)
- Urine specific gravity 1.005 to 1.025 (a, b, c)
- Blood urea nitrogen 8 to 20 mg/dL (a, b, c)
- Creatinine 0.6 to 1.2 mg/dL (c)
- Potassium 3.5 to 5.0 mEq/L (c)
- Magnesium 1.84 to 3.0 mEq/L (c)
- Sodium 135 to 145 mEq/L (c)
- Calcium 8.5 to 10.5 mg/dL (c)
- Oxygen saturation (Sao_2) 4 to 100 mm Hg (a, b)
- Carbon dioxide ($Paco_2$) 35 to 45 mm Hg (a, b)
- pH 7.35 to 7.45 (a, b)
- Relaxed, regular, deep, rhythmic respirations (a, b)
- No rales, crackles, wheezing (b)
- Wound approximated, minimal drainage (d)
- Chest tube drainage <200 mL/hr (d)
- Full, easy to palpate pulses (a, b)
- No evidence of petechiae (pinpoint round, reddish lesions) or ecchymoses (bruises) (a)
- No seizure activity (a, d, e)

CLINICAL ALERT:
- "The Northern New England Cardiovascular Disease Study Group's (NNECDSG) undertook a quality improvement effort to reduce mortality for urgent patients undergoing CABG surgery by optimizing a patient's readiness for surgery during the preoperative period. The interventions were grouped into a bundle called the 'readiness bundle' that included 7 interventions: use of aspirin (within 7 days), use of a β-blocker (within 24 hours), use of a statin type lipid-lowering agent (within 24 hours), preoperative hematocrit greater than 30%, 6 AM glucose level less than 150 mg/dL (to convert to millimoles per liter, multiply by 0.0555) on the day of surgery, delaying surgery a minimum of 3 days after an acute myocardial infarction, and induction heart rate less than 80/min" (Chaisson et al., 2014).
- The major complications associated with CABG are death, myocardial infarction, stroke, wound infection, prolonged requirement for mechanical ventilation, acute kidney injury, and bleeding requiring transfusion

or reoperation. Acute kidney injury (AKI, previously called acute renal failure) is a potential complication of CABG surgery that can arise from a variety of causes, including intraoperative hypotension, postoperative cardiac complications that impair renal perfusion, hemolysis, atheroemboli, and exposure to contrast media. Deep venous thrombosis (DVT) and pulmonary embolism (PE) may be difficult to recognize after CABG surgery and are therefore likely to be underdiagnosed. Acute kidney injury is a potential complication of CABG that can arise from a variety of causes, including intraoperative hypotension, postoperative cardiac complications that impair renal perfusion, hemolysis, atheroemboli, and exposure to contrast media (Aranki & Aroesty, 2016; Aranki, Aroesty, & Suri, 2015).

Interventions	Rationales
1. Monitor for the following as per unit standard (Aranki, & Aroesty, 2015; Aranki et al., 2015): a. Arrhythmias: abnormal rate or conduction b. ECG changes: ST segment depression or elevation; T-wave changes; PR, QRS, or QT interval changes c. Peripheral pulses (pedal, tibial, popliteal, femoral, radial, brachial) d. Blood pressure (arterial, left atrial, pulmonary artery) e. Pulmonary artery diastolic pressure (PAD) f. Pulmonary artery wedge pressure (PAWP) g. Cardiac output/index h. Cardiac enzymes daily (e.g., creatine phosphokinase, troponin complex) i. Urine output j. Skin color, temperature k. Capillary refill l. Palpitations m. Syncope n. Cardiac emergencies (e.g., arrest or ventricular fibrillation)	1. Arrhythmias are a known complication after cardiac surgery. Both tachyarrhythmias and bradyarrhythmias can present in the postoperative period. Atrial fibrillation is the most common heart rhythm disorder. However, ventricular arrhythmias and conduction disturbances can also occur. Sustained ventricular arrhythmias in the recovery period after cardiac surgery may warrant acute treatment and long-term preventive strategy in the absence of reversible causes (Peretto, Durante, Limite, Cianflone, 2014).
2. Monitor for signs and symptoms of hypovolemia, hypotension/hypertension, and low cardiac output (refer to General Surgical Care Plan for interventions/rationale).	2. Postoperative hypertension is common; it can cause decreased stroke volume and increased myocardial oxygen demand (Silvestry, 2016).
3. Monitor for respiratory complication (Silvestry, 2016): a. Pleural effusion • Pneumonia • Atelectasis • Decreased thoracic compliance • Diaphragmatic dysfunction • Acute lung injury	3. Pleural effusions are common postoperative findings in individuals who undergo various cardiac surgical procedures. Most follow a benign course. Pleural effusions may also occur with postcardiac injury syndrome (PCIS) or may be the initial manifestation of a potentially serious complicating event. Sternotomy and thoracotomy incisions produce pain, which impairs the ability to cough and breathe deeply. This increases the risk for pneumonia. Atelectasis occurs in up to 70% of individuals after cardiac surgery, usually as a result of single lung ventilation and intentional lung collapse during the surgery. Chest wall and lung compliance decrease postoperatively (Silvestry, 2016). Phrenic nerve injury during surgery is rare, but may cause diaphragmatic dysfunction or paralysis if it occurs.

Interventions	*Rationales*
4. Monitor for signs and symptoms of respiratory insufficiency: a. Increased respiratory rate b. Dyspnea c. Use of accessory muscles of respiration d. Cyanosis e. Increasing crackles or wheezing f. Increased Pco_2, decreased O_2 saturation, decreased pH g. Decreased Svo_2 h. Restlessness i. Decreased capillary refill time >3 seconds	4. Monitoring respiratory function can detect early signs/symptoms of respiratory complication
5. Monitor for signs and symptoms of hemorrhage or hypovolemia: a. Incisional bleeding b. Chest tube drainage >200 mL/hr c. Increased heart rate, decreased blood pressure, increased respirations d. Weak or absent peripheral pulses e. Cool, moist skin f. Dizziness g. Petechiae h. Ecchymoses i. Bleeding gums j. Decreased hemoglobin and hematocrit k. Increased PT, PTT, INR, and decreased platelet count l. Decreased urine output (<0.5 mL/kg/hr)	5. Bleeding is usually owing to incomplete surgical hemostasis, residual heparin effect after cardiopulmonary bypass, clotting factor depletion, hypothermia, postoperative hypotension, hemodilution (dilutional thrombocytopenia and coagulopathy), and/or platelet abnormalities (platelet dysfunction and thrombocytopenia) (Silvestry, 2016).

CLINICAL ALERT:
- "The best preventive strategy is to optimize renal perfusion (i.e., avoid hypotension and hypovolemia) and to avoid potentially nephrotoxic agents (e.g., aminoglycoside antibiotics, angiotensin converting enzyme inhibitors, and radiologic contrast agents) in the immediate postoperative period" (Silvestry, 2016).

Interventions	*Rationales*
6. Monitor for signs and symptoms of acute renal injury/failure (Silvestry, 2016): a. Elevated BUN, creatinine, and potassium b. Decreased urine output (<0.5 mL/kg/hr) c. Elevated urine specific gravity (>1.030) d. Weight gain e. Elevated CVP and PAP	6. Acute renal injury/failure occurs in up to 30% of individuals who have undergone cardiac surgery, when defined as a 50% increase in the serum creatinine concentration above baseline. Acute kidney injury (AKI) can arise from a variety of causes, including intraoperative hypotension, postoperative cardiac complications that impair renal perfusion, hemolysis, ather oemboli, and exposure to contrast (Silvestry, 2016).
7. Monitor for signs and symptoms of cerebrovascular accident stroke, cognitive dysfunction, and peripheral neuropathy: a. Unequal pupil size and reaction b. Paralysis or paresthesias in extremities c. Decreased level of consciousness d. Dizziness e. Blurred vision f. Slurred speech g. Confusion h. Altered motor and sensory function	7. The major neurologic problems are stroke, neuropsychiatric abnormalities such as cognitive dysfunction, and peripheral neuropathy.

(continued)

Interventions	Rationales

 Carp's Cues

It is important that the nurse know this individual's pre-surgery baseline cognitive status before surgery in order to determine if changes have occurred.

Interventions	Rationales

8. Monitor for signs and symptoms of postcardiotomy delirium:
  a. Disturbances in attention
  b. Disturbances in cognition
  c. Hypoactive
  d. Hyperactive
  e. Disorientation
  f. Confusion
	8. Postoperative delirium usually develops on postoperative days 1 through 3 and resolves within hours to days. The complication has various clinical manifestations and can be classified as a hyperactive, hypoactive, and mixed delirium. One study reported postoperative delirium occurred in 24.5% of individuals with significantly longer stays (and greater prevalence of falls) than did individuals without delirium. Individuals with delirium also had a significantly greater likelihood for discharge to a nursing facility (Mangusan, Hooper, Denslow, Travis, 2015). This disorder may result from surgery-related microemboli, sensory overload or deprivation, altered sleep pattern, prolonged mechanical ventilation duration hypoxia, medications, metabolic disorders, or hypotension.

Documentation

Vital signs
Cardiac rhythm
Peripheral pulses
Skin color, temperature, moisture
Neck vein distention
Respiratory assessment
Neurologic assessment
Intake (oral, IVs, blood products)
Incisions (color, drainage, swelling)
Output (chest tubes, nasogastric tube)
Bowel function (bowel sounds, distention)
Sputum (amount, tenaciousness, color)
Change in physiologic status
Interventions
Response to interventions

Nursing Diagnoses

Fear Related to Transfer From Intensive Environment of the Critical Care Unit and Potential for Complications

NOC
Anxiety Control, Fear Control

Goal

The individual will report a decreased level of anxiety or fear.

NIC
Anxiety Reduction, Coping Enhancement, Presence, Counseling

Indicators

• Verbalize any concerns regarding the completed surgery, possible complications, and the critical care environment.
• Verbalize the intent to share fears with one person after transition.

CLINICAL ALERT:
- "During the past few decades the numbers of ICUs and beds has increased significantly, but so too has the demand for intensive care. Currently large, and increasing, numbers of critically ill patients require transfer between critical care units. Inter-unit transfer poses significant risks to critically ill patients, particularly those requiring multiple organ support (Droogh, Smit, Absalom, Ligtenberg, Zijlstra, 2015).

Interventions	*Rationales*
1. Expect concerns/questions about the transfer. Use clinical data to support rationale for the transfer.	1. "Individuals sometimes struggle with feelings of abandonment, vulnerability, helplessness, and unimportance. Ambivalent feelings about the upcoming transfers are also shown to be common; both positive and negative emotions have been reported" (Häggström & Bäckström, 2014).
2. Take steps to reduce the individual's levels of anxiety and fear: a. Reassure that you or other nurses are always close by and will respond promptly to requests. b. Convey a sense of empathy and understanding. c. Minimize external stimuli (e.g., close the room door, dim the lights, speak in a quiet voice, decrease the volume level of equipment alarms, and position equipment so that alarms are diverted away from the individual). d. Plan care measures to provide adequate periods of uninterrupted rest and sleep. e. Promote relaxation; encourage regular rest periods throughout the day. f. Explain each procedure before performing it.	2. This sharing allows the nurse to correct any erroneous information the individual may believe and to assure the individual that concerns and fears are normal; this may help to reduce anxiety (Häggström & Bäckström, 2014).

TRANSITION TO HOME/COMMUNITY CARE
If indicated, review the risk diagnoses identified for this individual on admission:
- Is the person still at risk?
- Can the family reduce the risks?
- Is the person at higher risk at home?
- Is a Home Health Nurse assessment needed?
- Refer to transition planner/case manager/social service
- When is this person scheduled for follow-up with primary provider? Specialists? Record dates of appointments.
- Complete a medication reconciliation before transition. Refer to index.

STAR **Stop**

Think Is this person at high risk for injury, falls, medical complications, and/or inability to care for self (activities of daily living)?
Is there a support person available?
Is the person competent to manage self-administration of medications, treatment procedures? Are additional resources needed?
Can the person explain how to monitor the condition (e.g., blood glucose, signs/symptoms of complications, dietary/mobility restrictions, and when to call his or her primary provider or specialist)?

Act Contact or provide the appropriate resource (e.g., contacting a support person, home health assessment, additional teaching, printed materials).

Review Has the problem been addressed? If not, use SBAR to communicate to the appropriate person.

Risk for Ineffective Health Management Related to Insufficient Knowledge of Incisional Care, Pain Management (Angina, Incisions), Signs and Symptoms of Complications, Condition, Pharmacologic Care, Risk Factors, Restrictions, Stress Management Techniques, and Follow-Up Care

NOC

Compliance/
Engagement Behavior,
Knowledge: Treatment
Regimen, Participation:
Health-Care Decisions,
Treatment Behavior:
Illness or Injury

NIC

Anticipatory Guidance,
Risk Identification,
Health Education,
Learning Facilitation

Goal

The goals for this diagnosis represent those associated with transition planning. Refer to the transition criteria.

Interventions	Rationales

1. Explain and demonstrate care of uncomplicated surgical incisions:
  a. Wash with soap and water (bath and shower, as permitted; use lukewarm water).
  b. Wear loose clothing until incision areas are no longer tender.
	1. Correct technique is needed to reduce the risk of infection.

2. Provide instruction for pain management:
  a. For incision pain (sore, sharp, stabbing):
    • Take pain medication as prescribed and before activities that cause discomfort.
    • Continue to use the splinting technique, as needed.
 	
  b. For angina (tightness, squeezing, pressure, pain, or mild ache in chest; indigestion; choking sensation; pain in jaw, neck, and between shoulder blades; numbness, tingling, and aching in either arm or hand):
    • Stop whatever you are doing and sit down.
    • Take nitroglycerin, as prescribed (e.g., one tablet every 5 minutes sublingually until pain subsides or a maximum of three tablets have been taken).
    • If pain is unrelieved by three nitroglycerin tablets, call 911 for immediate transportation to the emergency room.
	2a. Adequate instruction in pain management can reduce the fear of pain by providing a sense of control. Combining analgesics and nonsteroidal anti-inflammatory agents may increase the effectiveness of pain management (*Martin & Turkelson, 2006).
	
	b. Angina is a symptom of cardiac tissue hypoxia. Immediate rest reduces the tissues' oxygen requirements. Nitroglycerin causes coronary vasodilation, which increases coronary blood flow in an attempt to increase myocardial oxygen supply.

3. Provide instruction regarding the individual's condition and reduction of risk factors:
  a. Reinforce the purpose and outcome of CABG surgery.
  b. Explain the risk factors that need to be eliminated or reduced (e.g., obesity, smoking, high cholesterol, sedentary lifestyle, regular heavy alcohol intake, excessive stress, hypertension, or uncontrolled diabetes mellitus).
  c. Refer to index for intervention s to address the above risk factors
	3. Surgery does not replace the need to reduce risk factors.
	
	a. Preoperative anxiety may have interfered with retention of preoperative teaching.
	b. Emphasizing those risk factors that can be reduced may decrease the individual's sense of powerlessness regarding those factors that cannot be reduced, such as heredity.

4. Consult a dietitian, and refer the individual to appropriate community resources.	4. Weight reduction reduces peripheral resistance and cardiac output.
5. Teach about a low-fat, high-fiber, low-cholesterol diet; consult with a dietitian.	5. A low-fat, high-fiber, and low-cholesterol diet can reduce or prevent arteriosclerosis in some individuals.

Interventions	*Rationales*
6. Provide instruction in a progressive activity program: a. Increase activity gradually.	6a. Progressive regular exercise increases cardiac stroke volume, thus increasing the heart's efficiency without greatly altering the rate.
b. Consult with a physical therapist and cardiac rehabilitation specialist.	b. These professionals can provide specific guidelines.
c. Schedule frequent rest periods throughout the day for the first 6 to 8 weeks. Balance periods of activity with periods of rest.	c. Rest periods reduce myocardial oxygen demands.
d. Consult with the physician before resuming work, driving, strenuous recreational activities (e.g., jogging, golfing, and other sports), and travel (airplane or automobile).	d. Avoid heavy lifting and extremes of shoulder movement (e.g., as in tennis, baseball, and golf) for 6 to 8 weeks after surgery to allow for complete healing of the breast bone (sternum) (Aroesty, 2016).
e. Try to get 8 to 10 hours of sleep each night.	e. Sleep allows the body restorative time.
f. Avoid isometric exercises (e.g., lifting anything more than 10 lb). Avoid pushing anything weighing more than 10 lb (e.g., vacuum cleaner, grocery cart) for 6 to 8 weeks.	f. Isometric exercises and straining increase cardiac workload and peripheral resistance. They also place stress on the healing sternum.
g. Limit stair climbing to once or twice a day.	g. Stair climbing increases cardiac workload.
7. Consult with the physician about when sexual activity can be resumed.	7. In the first 2 weeks after an uncomplicated heart attack, most people are at high risk of heart-related problems during sex as a result of a rise in the heart rate and blood pressure. However, this risk becomes much smaller by 6 weeks after the heart attack (Aroesty, 2016).
8. Provide instructions regarding prescribed medications (i.e., purpose, dosage and administration techniques, and possible side effects).	8. Understanding can help to improve compliance and reduce the risk of overdose and morbidity.

9. Teach the individual and family to report these signs and symptoms of complications to the surgeon:
  a. Fever greater than 100.4° F (38° C)
  b. Reddened skin, bleeding, or pus-like drainage from the incision
  c. Weight gain exceeding 3 lb in 1 day or 5 lb in 1 week
	9. Early reporting of complications enables prompt interventions to minimize their severity.

10. Advise to call 911 if they experience :
  a. New or worsened pain in the chest or around the incision
  b. A rapid heart rate
  c. Calf swelling, tenderness, warmth, or pain
  d. Difficulty breathing
	10. Immediate medical evaluation to determine if a serious complication is occurring (e.g., deep vein thrombosis, arrhythmia, myocardial infarction)

11. Provide information regarding community organizations (e.g., American Heart Association, "Mended Hearts Club").	11. Community resources after discharge can assist with adaptation and self-help strategies.

12. Ensure appointments have been scheduled with:
  a. Surgeon
  b. Primary care provider
  c. Home health nursing agency
  d. Cardiac rehabilitation
	12. "Follow-up care is of great importance since individuals, who have had bypass surgery have a significantly increased risk of more cardiac events, including recurrent chest pain, heart attack, heart failure, and an increased risk of dying. The risk of these problems is greatly reduced by closely following a clinician's recommendations for rehabilitation, follow-up visits, and treatments" (Aroesty, 2016).

Documentation

Individual/family teaching
Response to teaching
Referrals, if indicated

Fractured Hip and Femur

International Osteoporosis Foundation (2015) and the Centers for Disease Control and Prevention [CDC] (2016a) report that:

* Each year at least 280,000 older people—those 65 and older—are hospitalized for hip fractures in the United States (International Osteoporosis Foundation, 2015).
* More than 95% of hip fractures are caused by falling, usually by falling sideways (CDC, 2016d).
* One out of five individuals who fracture a hip will die within a year of their injury in the United States (CDC, 2016a).
* Worldwide, nearly 75% of hip, spine, and distal forearm fractures occur among patients 65 years or over (International Osteoporosis Foundation, 2015).
* Osteoporosis affects an estimated 75 million people in Europe, the United States, and Japan (International Osteoporosis Foundation, 2015).
* Approximately 1.6 million hip fractures occur worldwide each year, by 2050 this number could reach between 4.5 million and 6.3 million (International Osteoporosis Foundation, 2015).

Elderly individuals are more vulnerable to hip fractures because of osteoporosis, mobility, Vision, and deconditioning problems.

The type of surgery for hip fractures depends on the location of the break and bone fragments and the age of the individual. Surgery may include internal fixation (screws, rods, or plates) to stabilize broken bones or hip replacement (partial or total) (American Academy of Orthopaedic Surgeons, 2014).

Carp's Cues

Please refer to the Generic Surgical Care Plan for detailed interventions for managing all surgical conditions. This care plan addresses specific additional interventions associated with the type of surgery performed.

Time Frame
Postoperative periods

■■■■■ DIAGNOSTIC CLUSTER

Postoperative Period

Collaborative Problems

▲ Risk for Complications of Fat Emboli (refer to unit II)

▲ Risk for Complications of Displacement of Hip Joint

▲ Risk for Complications of Compartment Syndrome (refer to Unit II)

▲ Risk for Complications of Peroneal/Sciatic Nerve Palsy

△ Risk for Complications of Venous Stasis/Thrombosis (refer to Unit II)

△ Risk for Complications of Avascular Necrosis of Femoral Head (refer to Inflammatory Joint Disease)

△ Risk for Complications of Sepsis (refer to Unit II)

Risk for Complications of Hemorrhage/Shock (refer to Generic Care Plan for the Surgical Client)

Risk for Complications of Pulmonary Embolism (refer to Generic Care Plan for the Surgical Client)

Nursing Diagnoses

▲ Acute Pain related to trauma and muscle spasms

▲ Risk for Constipation related to immobility (refer to Unit II)

▲ Risk for Pressure Ulcer related to immobility and urinary incontinence secondary to inability to reach toilet quickly enough between urge to void and need to void (refer to Unit II)

▲ Risk for Ineffective Health Management related to insufficient knowledge of activity restrictions, assistive devices, home care, follow-up care, and supportive services

Related Care Plan

General Surgery Generic Care Plan

▲ This diagnosis was reported to be monitored for or managed frequently (75% to 100%).
Δ This diagnosis was reported to be monitored for or managed often (50% to 74%).

Transition Criteria

Before transition, the client and family will:

1. Demonstrate care of the surgical site and use of assistive devices.
2. Relate at-home restrictions and follow-up care.
3. State the signs and symptoms that must be reported to a health care professional.
4. Demonstrate a clear understanding of medications.

> **Transitional Risk Assessment Plan (TRAP)**
>
> Begin this plan on admission.
> Implement the Transitional Risk Assessment Plan (TRAP):
> • Refer to inside back cover.
> • Add each validated risk diagnosis to client's problem list with the risk code in ( ).
> • Refer to the individual risk nursing diagnoses/collaborative problems for outcomes and interventions in Unit II.
>
> *R:* *"Close coordination of care in the post-acute period, early transition follow-up care, enhanced client education and self-management training, proactive end-of-life counseling, and extending the resources and clinical expertise over time via multidisciplinary team management" can lower readmission rates and improve health outcomes (Boutwell & Hwu, 2009, p. 14). Interventions are utilized to activate the individual and family to select changes in their everyday lifestyle choices to improve their health (Hibbard & Greene, 2013).*

Postoperative: Collaborative Problems

Risk for Complications of Fat Emboli

Risk for Complications of Peroneal/Sciatic Nerve Palsy

Risk for Complications of Hip Joint Displacement

Collaborative Outcomes

The individual will be monitored for early signs and symptoms of (a) fat emboli, (b) compartment syndrome, (c) peroneal/sciatic nerve palsy, (d) hip joint displacement, (e) venous stasis/thrombosis, (f) avascular necrosis of femoral head, and (g) sepsis and will receive collaborative interventions if indicated to restore physiologic stability.

Indicators of Physiologic Stability

• Alert, calm, oriented (g)
• Temperature 98.5° F to 99° F (a, f, g)
• Heart rate 60 to 100 beats/min (a, g)
• Respirations 16 to 20 breaths/min (a, g)

- BP >90/60, <140/90 mm Hg (a, g)
- Peripheral pulses: full, equal, strong (b)
- Sensation intact (b)
- No pain with passive dorsiflexion (calf, toes) (b)
- Pain relieved by analgesics (b)
- No tingling in legs (b, c)
- Can move legs (b, c, d)
- No calf or thigh redness, warmth (e)
- Affected extremity aligned (d)
- No petechiae (upper trunk, axilla) (a)
- Urine output >0.5 mL/kg/hr (a, g)
- White blood cells 4,000 to 10,800 (g)
- Oxygen saturation 94% to 100% (a, g)
- Capillary refill <3 seconds (b)

 Carp's Cues

Please refer to the Generic Care Plan for the individual experiencing surgery for detailed interventions for managing all surgical conditions. This care plan addresses specific additional interventions associated with the type of surgery performed.

Interventions	Rationales
CLINICAL ALERT: • "Among the reasons that FES is difficult to diagnose is that it can complicate widely disparate clinical conditions and may vary in severity. Management is supportive, with an estimated mortality rate of 5 to 15 percent" (Weinhouse, 2016).	
1. Monitor for signs and symptoms of fat embolism (Weinhouse, 2016):	1. Fat emboli may be the result of fat globules entering the bloodstream through tissue (usually bone marrow or adipose tissue) that has been disrupted by trauma or, alternatively, via production of the toxic intermediaries of plasma-derived fat (e.g., chylomicrons or infused lipids). Fat emboli, unlike other emboli, are gradual, with respiratory and neurological signs/symptoms of hypoxemia, fever, and a petechial rash. Fat embolism syndrome (FES) typically manifests 4 to 72 hours after the initial insult, but may rarely occur as early as 12 hours or as late as 2 weeks after the inciting event (Weinhouse, 2016).
a. Respiratory hypoxia (tachypnea, dyspnea, and cyanosis)	a. Hypoxemia, dyspnea, and tachypnea are the most frequent early findings. Fat droplets act as emboli, becoming impacted in the pulmonary microvasculature and other microvascular beds such as in the brain. Embolism begins rather slowly and attains a maximum in about 48 hours.
b. Cerebral changes (nonspecific, ranging from acute confusion to drowsiness, rigidity, convulsions, or coma) **CLINICAL ALERT:** • Before surgery, approximately 25% of individuals have moderate to severe cognitive impairment and 15.25% have mild cognitive impairments (Clarke & Santy-Tomilinson, 2014). Thus, presurgical cognitive status must be considered in postoperative assessment.	b, c. Cerebral changes are seen in 86% of clients with FES. It occurs in up to 60% of cases and is due to embolization of small dermal capillaries leading to extravasation of erythrocytes. This produces a petechial rash in the conjunctiva, oral mucous membrane, and skin folds of the upper body, especially in the neck and axilla.
c. Petechial rash	

Interventions	Rationales
2. Monitor for hypoxemia with pulse oximetry.	2. Pulmonary dysfunction is the earliest sign of fat embolism to manifest and is seen in 75% of clients; it progresses to respiratory failure in 10% of the cases. Hypoxemia may be detected hours before the onset of respiratory complaints.
3. Sciatic peroneal nerve palsy (Baima & Krivickas, 2008; Wolf et al., 2014): a. Decreased sensation to light touch (numbness and tingling at the top of the foot) b. Inability to distinguish between sharp and dull sensations c. Paralysis d. Foot drop e. Walking abnormalities (e.g., toes drag while walking) f. Pain	3. In a retrospective review of over 2,200 consecutive individuals treated for hip fractures, 0.7% of individuals were identified to have sciatic nerve palsy postoperatively; the duration of preoperative traction was associated with greater likelihood of sciatic nerve palsy, suggesting that the preoperative traction may lead to sciatic nerve palsy (*Kemler, de Vries & van der Tol, 2006).
4. Prevent dislocation during turning by placing a pillow between the client's legs.	4. The pillow will maintain abduction and alignment.
5. Monitor for signs and symptoms of hip joint displacement: a. External rotation of affected extremity b. Affected extremity shorter than unaffected extremity c. Increased pain	5. The overall incidence of dislocation in primary total hip arthroplasty ranges from 0% to 2%. The majority of dislocations occur posteriorly, typically with flexion, adduction, and internal rotation of the limb. Anterior dislocations are less frequent and typically occur with extension, adduction, and external rotation of the limb (Foster, 2015).

Clinical Alert Report

Before providing care, advise ancillary staff/student to report the following to the professional nurse assigned to the client:

- Change in cognitive status
- New onset of rash
- Oral temperature >100.5° F
- Systolic BP <90 mm Hg
- Resting pulse >100, <50
- Respiratory rate >28, <10/min
- Oxygen saturation <90%
- Complaints of decreased sensation to light touch (numbness and tingling at the top of the foot)
- External rotation of affected extremity
- Affected extremity shorter than unaffected extremity
- Complaints of increased pain

Documentation

Vital signs
Distal limb sensation, paresthesias, circulation
Intake (oral, parenteral)
Output (urine, urine specific gravity)
Wound (color, drainage, swelling, rate of health)

Postoperative: Nursing Diagnoses

Acute Pain Related to Trauma and Muscle Spasms

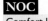
NOC
Comfort Level, Pain Control

Goal

The individual will report satisfactory relief as evidenced by the indicators listed below.

NIC

Pain Management, Medication Management, Emotional Support, Teaching: Individual, Hot/Cold Application, Simple Massage

Indicators

- Increased participation in activities of recovery.
- Reduction in reported pain using 0 to 10 pain scale.

Interventions	Rationales
1. Assess for nonverbal indications of pain in cognitively compromised individuals as grimacing, restlessness, agitation, reluctance to move (Clarke & Santy-Tomilinson, 2014).	1. Cognitively impaired individuals may be unable to report pain.
2. Position the individual in proper alignment. Handle the individual gently, supporting the leg with your hands or a pillow.	2. Optimal alignment reduces pressure on nerves and tissues; this reduces pain. Muscle spasms accompany movement.
3. Use a trochanter roll to support the involved extremity in the neutral position (Clarke & Santy-Tomilinson, 2014).	3. The trochanter roll prevents or minimizes external rotation.
4. Preoperatively, roll only on affected side with pillow between legs (Clarke & Santy-Tomilinson, 2014).	4. This prevents dislocation or further displacement.
5. Refer to the General Surgery Care Plan for general pain relief interventions.	

Documentation

Participation in self-care

> **TRANSITION TO HOME/COMMUNITY CARE**
> If indicated, review the risk diagnoses identified for this individual on admission:
> - Is the person still at risk?
> - Can the family reduce the risks?
> - Is the person at higher risk at home?
> - Is a Home Health Nurse assessment needed?
> - Refer to transition planner/case manager/social service
> - When is this person scheduled for follow-up with primary provider? Specialists? Record dates of appointments.
> - Complete a medication reconciliation before transition. Refer to index.

S T A R   **Stop**

Think   Is this person at high risk for injury, falls, medical complications, and/or inability to care for self (activities of daily living)?
Is there a support person available?
Is the person competent to manage self-administration of medications, treatment procedures? Are additional resources needed?
Can the person explain how to monitor the condition (e.g., blood glucose, signs/symptoms of complications, dietary/mobility restrictions, and when to call his or her primary provider or specialist)?

Act   Contact or provide the appropriate resource (e.g., contacting a support person, home health assessment, additional teaching, printed materials).

Review   Has the problem been addressed? If not, use SBAR to communicate to the appropriate person.

Risk for Ineffective Health Management Related to Insufficient Knowledge of Activity Restrictions, Assistive Devices, Home Care, Follow-Up Care, and Supportive Services

NOC

Compliance/
Engagement Behavior,
Knowledge: Treatment
Regimen, Participation:
Health Care Decisions,
Treatment Behavior:
Illness or Injury

NIC

Anticipatory Guidance,
Risk Management,
Learning Facilitation,
Health Education,
Teaching: Procedure/
Treatment, Health
System Guidance

Goals

The goals for this diagnosis represent those associated with transition planning. Refer to the transition criteria.

Interventions	Rationales
CLINICAL ALERT: • Postoperatively, the stress of surgery and immobility contribute to serious problems of malnutrition, dehydration, constipation, pressure ulcers, delirium, functional decline, and death (Clarke & Santy-Tomilinson, 2014).	
1. Ensure that the individual's ability to ambulate and perform ADLs has been evaluated.	1. The individual's self-care abilities before transition need to be assessed to determine the need for referrals.
2. Evaluate mental status and presence of depression and/or confusion.	2. Individuals with confusion and depressive symptomatology have very high risk for prolonged disability and death.
3. Consult with a specialist for management of depression, as necessary.	3. Early detection and treatment of depression can reduce hospital stay and long-term disabilities.
4. Ensure written instructions are provided for exercises and activity restrictions.	4. These measures may help to reduce risk of injury.
5. Advise to report any changes in gait and an increase in pain.	5. This may indicate a dislocation.
6. Explain the importance of progressive care (i.e., from early non–weight-bearing ambulation to self-care within the client's abilities).	6. The risk of complications increases with each day of immobility, particularly in an elderly client (Clarke & Santy-Tomilinson, 2014).

7. Teach to watch for and report subtle signs of infection:
  a. Increased temperature chills
  b. Malaise
  c. Pain unrelieved with analgesia (*Lewis et al., 2004)
	7. Hip fracture typically affects elderly individuals, who have a decreased ability to compensate for physiologic and immunologic system changes that may mask pronounced signs and symptoms of infection.

8. Teach to watch for and report subtle signs of DVT and to seek medical evaluation. a. Change in sensation in leg (aching, warmer, pain)	8. The risk for DVT continues after surgery for 3 months.
9. Teach the importance of avoiding immobility. Stress the importance of participating aggressively in physical therapy and with exercises at home	9. Studies support that intensive exercise training administered by physical therapy to patients after discharge from hospital care improves functional outcomes, leg strength, and health status (American Academy of Orthopaedic Surgeons, 2014).

(continued)

Interventions	Rationales
10. Ensure that a dietician consult occurs. Stress the critical nature of dietary protein for healing and prevention of complications. Stress the importance of taking the prescribed calcium and vitamin D every day and probably for their lifetime.	10. Studies report that protein energy malnutrition is an important determinant of outcome in older patients with hip fracture (American Academy of Orthopaedic Surgeons, 2014). Studies show benefits of either supplemental calcium, vitamin D, or both to reduce fall risk and prevent fractures in the elderly. There is a high prevalence of vitamin D deficiency among hip fracture patients (Bischoff-Ferrari et al., 2010) and hip fracture patients have a 5 to 10× increased risk of a second hip fracture and other fragility fractures (*Harwood et al., 2006) reported by the American Academy of Orthopaedic Surgeons (2014).
11. Explain the possibility of delirium and contributing factors (electrolyte imbalances, metabolic abnormalities, infection, hypoxia, pain, medications, unfamiliar environment. Refer to Acute Confusion if indicated in Unit II.	
12. Ensure appointments are scheduled for home assessments (nursing, physical therapy, occupational therapy, social services) (American Academy of Orthopaedic Surgeons, 2014).	12. For follow-up for any hospitalization, appointment-keeping behavior is enhanced when the inpatient team schedules outpatient medical follow-up before transition. Ideally, the inpatient care providers or case managers/transition planners will schedule follow-up visit(s) with the appropriate professionals, including primary care provider and specialist (American Diabetes Association, 2015).

Documentation

Individual/ family teaching and return demonstration of understanding of education
Outcome achievement or status
Referrals, if indicated

Hysterectomy

A hysterectomy is a surgery to remove a woman's uterus for a variety of reasons such as (Walters, 2016):

- Uterine leiomyomas
- Abnormal uterine bleeding
- Pelvic organ prolapse
- Pelvic pain or infection (e.g., endometriosis, pelvic inflammatory diseases)
- Malignant and premalignant disease

Hysterectomy can be performed vaginally, abdominally, laparoscopically, or with robot-assisted laparoscopy. Hysterectomy can also be performed by combining two of these four routes, such as in laparoscopically assisted vaginal hysterectomy or laparoscopic hysterectomy combined with a minilaparotomy to remove the uterine specimen from the peritoneal cavity. "Hysterectomy has been associated with improvements in physical and mental quality-of-life measures, body image, and aspects of sexual activity, with few differences among surgical route" (Walters, 2016).

The choice of hysterectomy route is individualized to the woman. Important factors include (Walters, 2016):

- Extent of gynecologic pathology—What is the best access to appropriately treat the disease?
- Relative risks and benefits of hysterectomy route—Which technique is associated with the lowest risk of complications for this individual?
- Need to perform additional procedures—What is the best access for management of concomitant pathology?
- The woman's preferences—Is there a preference for hysterectomy approach?
- Surgeon's competence, preference, and available support facilities.

Vaginal hysterectomy is associated with better outcomes and fewer complications than other approaches, e.g., faster return to normal activities by approximately 12 days, shortened hospital stays by approximately 1 day. Outcomes that were worse for laparoscopic hysterectomy compared with abdominal hysterectomy include twofold increased risk of urinary tract (bladder or ureter) injuries and approximately 30 minutes longer operative time (Walters, 2016).

Contraindications to laparoscopic hysterectomy are significant cardiopulmonary disease with intolerance to increased intraperitoneal pressure and suspicion of malignancy when division and removal in small pieces (as of a tumor) would be required (American Association of Gynecologic Laparoscopists, 2011).

Time Frame
Postoperative periods

■■■DIAGNOSTIC CLUSTER

Postoperative Period

Collaborative Problems

▲ Risk for Complications of Uterine, Ureter, Bladder, Bowel Trauma

▲ Risk for Complications of Vaginal Bleeding

▲ Risk for Complications of Deep Vein Thrombosis

▲ Risk for Complications of Neurological Deficits Secondary to Epidural Therapy

Nursing Diagnoses

△ Risk for Disturbed Self-Concept related to perceived effects on sexuality and feminine role

△ Risk for Ineffective Health Management related to insufficient knowledge of perineal/incisional care, signs of complications, activity restrictions, loss of menses, hormone therapy, and follow-up care

▲ This diagnosis was reported to be monitored for or managed frequently (75% to 100%).
△ This diagnosis was reported to be monitored for or managed often (50% to 74%).

Transition Criteria

Before transition, the individual and family will:

1. State wound care procedures to follow at home, especially ensuring that the individual can monitor for wound infection and separation, if the abdominal approach is used.
2. Verbalize precautions to take regarding activities, especially the lifting restrictions of no more that 5 lb until cleared by doctor (usually after 6 weeks).
3. State the signs and symptoms that must be reported to a health care professional, such as fever, drainage, redness, swelling, unresolved pain, and transition associated with itching and bad smelling odors.
4. Verbalize an intent to share feelings and concerns with significant others.

Transitional Risk Assessment Plan (TRAP)

Begin this plan on admission.
Implement the Transitional Risk Assessment Plan (TRAP):
* Refer to inside back cover.
* Add each validated risk diagnosis to individual's problem list with the risk code in ( ).
* Refer to the individual risk nursing diagnoses/collaborative problems for outcomes and interventions in Unit II.

R: "Close coordination of care in the post-acute period, early transition follow-up care, enhanced client education and self-management training, proactive end-of-life counseling, and extending the resources and clinical expertise over time via multidisciplinary team management" can lower readmission rates and improve health outcomes (Boutwell & Hwu, 2009, p. 14). Interventions are utilized to activate the individual and family to select changes in their everyday lifestyle choices to improve their health (Hibbard & Greene, 2013).

Postoperative: Collaborative Problems

Risk for Complications of Uterine Ureter, Bladder, Bowel Trauma

Risk for Complications of Vaginal Bleeding

Risk for Complications of Deep Vein Thrombosis

Risk for Complications of Neurological Deficits Associated With Epidural Injection

Collaborative Outcomes

The individual will be monitored for early signs and symptoms of (a) uterine, ureter, bladder, and bowel trauma, (b) vaginal bleeding, (c) deep vein thrombosis, (d) infection, (e) hemodynamic instability, and (f) neurologic and neuromuscular deficits and will receive collaborative interventions if indicated to restore physiologic stability.

Indicators of Physiologic Stability

- Urine output >0.5 mL/kg/hr (a)
- Clear urine (a)
- Intact bowel sounds all quadrants (a)
- Flatus present (a)
- No leg pain (c)
- No leg edema (c)
- Light-colored vaginal drainage (b)
- No headache (particularly, spinal headache owing to epidural therapy) (e, f) (*Lehne, 2004)
- Monitor signs of hypotension (owing to epidural therapy) (e, f) (*Lehne, 2004)
- No fever (d)
- No cardiac arrhythmias (e, f)
- No decreased level of consciousness (e, f)

Carp's Cues

Please refer to the Generic Care Plan for the Surgical Client for detailed interventions for managing all surgical conditions. This care plan addresses specific additional interventions associated with the type of surgery performed.

Interventions	*Rationales*
CLINICAL ALERT: • Extensive gynecologic surgery often entails meticulous dissection near the bladder, rectum, ureters, and great vessels of the pelvis. Complications of gynecologic surgery include hemorrhage, infection, thromboembolism, and visceral damage (Mann, 2015).	

1. Monitor for signs and symptoms of uterine ureter, bladder, or rectal trauma:
  a. Urinary retention
  b. Prolonged diminished bowel sounds
  c. Bloody, cloudy urine
  d. Absence of flatus
	1. Proximity of these structures to the surgical site may predispose them to atony because of edema or nerve trauma.

2. Identify the level of DVT risk for this individual (American College of Obstetricians and Gynecologists [ACOG], 2012):
  a. Low: Surgery lasting <30 minutes in individuals <40 years old without additional risk factors. Refer to Risk Factors for CVT (Box III.2).
  b. Moderate:
    • Surgery lasting <30 minutes in individuals with additional risk factors; surgery lasting <30 minutes in	

individuals aged 40 to 60 years with no additional risk factors; major surgery in individuals <40 years with no additional risk factors.

- Surgery lasting <30 minutes in individuals >60 years or with additional risk factors; major surgery in individuals >40 years or with additional risk factors.

c. Highest: Major surgery in individuals >60 years plus prior VTE, cancer, or molecular hypercoagulable state.

2. Without thromboprophylaxis, individuals who undergo major gynecologic surgery have a prevalence of DVT in the range of 15% to 40%. Asymptomatic DVT is also highly associated with the development of significant PE. Because most PE-associated fatalities occur within 30 minutes of onset, leaving a very narrow window for medical intervention, clinicians must identify those at high risk for VTE and administer effective thromboprophylaxis to minimize the occurrence of this potentially preventable cause of death (Pai & Douketis, 2016).

3. Monitor for signs and symptoms of deep-vein thrombosis (DVT).
   a. Refer to Risk for Complications of DVT in Unit II Section 2 for interventions.

4. Perform leg exercises every hour while in bed. Ambulate as early, as indicated, then mobilize as ordered (ACOG, 2012).

4. Leg exercises and ambulation contract leg muscles, stimulate the venous pump, and reduce stasis. Movement reduces stasis and vascular pooling in legs; pressure under knees can interfere with peripheral circulation.

5. If the surgical route is vaginal, monitor vaginal bleeding every 2 to 4 hours:
   a. Monitor vaginal drainage. Record amount and color.
   b. If packing is used, notify the surgeon if packing is saturated or clots are passed.
   c. Notify the physician/nurse practitioner if perineal pad is saturated.

5. Slight bloody drainage is expected. You will probably have some vaginal discharge that will gradually become white/yellow, usually still be present at your post-op visit.
   a. Frank vaginal bleeding, if it occurs, should be light.
   b, c. Packing is used if hemostasis is a problem during surgery. Excess bleeding or clots can indicate abnormal bleeding.

6. If the route is abdominal, monitor for incisional and vaginal bleeding every 2 hours.

6. The female pelvis has an abundant supply of blood vessels, creating a risk for bleeding (Grossman & Porth, 2014).

Box III.2   RISK FACTORS FOR DEEP VEIN THROMBOSIS (ACOG, 2012; *Geerts et al., 2004; National Institutes of Health, 2011)

- Surgery
- Trauma (major or lower extremity)
- Immobility, paresis
- Malignancy
- Cancer therapy (hormonal, chemotherapy, or radiotherapy)
- Previous venous thromboembolism
- Increasing age
- Pregnancy and the postpartum period
- Estrogen-containing oral contraception or hormone therapy
- Selective estrogen receptor modulators
- Acute medical illness

- Heart or respiratory failure
- Inflammatory bowel disease
- Myeloproliferative disorders
- Paroxysmal nocturnal hemoglobinuria
- Nephrotic syndrome
- Obesity
- Smoking
- Varicose veins
- Central venous catheterization
- Inherited or acquired thrombophilia

Clinical Alert Report

Before providing care, advise ancillary staff/student to report the following to the professional nurse assigned to the individual:

- Change in cognition/consciousness
- Oral temperature >100.5° F
- Systolic BP <90 mm Hg
- Resting pulse >100, <50
- Respiratory rate >28, <10/min
- Oxygen saturation <90%
- Bright red bleeding

Documentation

Vital signs (including adverse reactions to epidural therapy)
Perineal drainage
Intake and output
Turning, ambulation

Postoperative: Nursing Diagnoses

Risk for Disturbed Self-Concept Related to Significance of Loss

NOC

Quality of Life,
Depression Level, Self-
Esteem, Coping

Goal

The individual will acknowledge change in body structure and function.

NIC

Hope Instillation,
Mood Management,
Values Clarification,
Counseling, Referral,
Support Group, Coping
Enhancement

Indicators

• Communicate feelings about the hysterectomy.
• Participate in self-care within the restricted guidelines set by surgeon.

Interventions	Rationales
CLINICAL ALERT: • Hysterectomy carries the stress of surgery and potential postoperative complications and has been associated with anxiety, depression, changes in self-esteem, and sexual functioning. "Early work in the area of depression post hysterectomy confirmed the notion that women were more depressed after hysterectomy than other kinds of surgery" (Cohen, Linenberger, Wehry, & Welz, 2011). Lindemann (1941) found a 40% rate of depression in women post hysterectomy, and this increase in depression was corroborated by Melody (1962). • Research has proven these beliefs to be invalid (Cohen et al., 2011). Cohen et al. (2011) reported positive levels of anxiety, depression, changes in self-esteem, and sexual functioning in a longitudinal study with interviews at 1 week, 8 weeks, 6 months, and 1 year post hysterectomy.	
1. Contact frequently and treat her with warm, positive regard. Ask her "How do you think this surgery will affect you?"	1. Frequent contact by the caregiver indicates acceptance and may facilitate trust. The individual may be hesitant to approach staff because of her fears. A direct question can facilitate her sharing and reduce the nurse's thinking "I know what she is afraid of ." The purpose is to promote sharing not necessarily trying to eliminate her fears or concerns. Sharing concerns and ventilating feelings provide an opportunity for the nurse to correct any misinformation.
2. Discuss the surgery and her concerns of the effects on functioning with family members or significant others; correct any misconceptions. Encourage her to share her feelings and perceptions with her partner.	2. Open dialogue is often critical to acknowledgment of concerns as mutual sharing.

Documentation

Present emotional status
Response to interventions

> **TRANSITION TO HOME/COMMUNITY CARE**
> If indicated, review the risk diagnoses identified for this individual on admission:
> * Is the person still at risk?
> * Can the family reduce the risks?
> * Is the person at higher risk at home?
> * Is a Home Health Nurse assessment needed?
> * Refer to transition planner/case manager/social service.
> * When is this person scheduled for follow-up with primary provider? Specialists? Record dates of appointments.
> * Complete a medication reconciliation before transition. Refer to index.

STAR

Stop

Think   Is this person at high risk for injury, falls, medical complications, and/or inability to care for self (activities of daily living)?
Is there a support person available?
Is the person competent to manage self-administration of medications, treatment procedures? Are additional resources needed?
Can the person explain how to monitor the condition (e.g., blood glucose, signs/symptoms of complications, dietary/mobility restrictions, and when to call his or her primary provider or specialist)?

Act   Contact or provide the appropriate resource (e.g., contacting a support person, home health assessment, additional teaching, printed materials).

Review   Has the problem been addressed? If not, use SBAR to communicate to the appropriate person.

Risk for Ineffective Health Management Related to Insufficient Knowledge of Perineal/Incisional Care, Signs of Complications, Activity Restrictions, Loss of Menses, Hormone Therapy, and Follow-Up Care

NOC
Compliance/
Engagement Behavior,
Knowledge: Treatment
Regimen, Participation:
Health Care Decisions,
Treatment Behavior:
Illness or Injury

Goals

The goals for this diagnosis represent those associated with transition planning. Refer to the transition criteria.

NIC
Anticipatory Guidance,
Health Education, Risk
Management, Support
Group, Learning
Facilitation

Interventions	Rationales
1. Explain care of an uncomplicated wound (abdominal hysterectomy). Refer to Generic Care Plan for Individual experiencing surgery.	1. Proper wound care helps to reduce microorganisms at the incision site and prevent infection.
2. Explain perineal care (vaginal hysterectomy); teach the individual to do the following: a. Wash thoroughly with soap and water. b. Change the peripad frequently. c. After elimination, wipe from the front to back using a clean tissue for each front-to-back pass.	2. Proper perineal care reduces microorganisms around the perineum and minimizes their entry into the vagina.

(continued)

Interventions	*Rationales*
3. Explain the need to increase activity, as tolerated, while maintaining restrictions such as no lifting greater than 5 lb for 6 weeks after the surgery.	3. Physical activity, especially early and frequent ambulation, can help to prevent or minimize abdominal cramps, a common complaint during recovery from abdominal hysterectomy and prevent deep vein thrombosis.
4. Teach to watch for and report the following: a. Temperature greater than 100° F (37.7° C) b. Vaginal bleeding that is greater than a typical menstrual period or is bright red c. Urinary incontinence, urgency, burning, or frequency d. Severe abdominal pain e. New- onset leg pain or swelling	4. Because of the abundance of blood vessels in the female pelvis, hysterectomy carries a higher risk of postoperative bleeding than most other surgeries. Bleeding most often occurs within 24 hours after surgery, but risk also occurs on the fourth, ninth, and 21st postoperative days, when the sutures dissolve. A small amount of pink, yellow, or brown serous drainage or even minor frank vaginal bleeding (no heavier than normal menstrual flow) is normal and expected. e. Leg pain and/or edema may indicate a DVT.
5. Ensure a follow-up appointment is scheduled. Reinforce the importance of keeping scheduled appointments.	

Documentation

Individual/family Teaching
Outcome achievement or status

Ileostomy

An ileostomy (temporary or permanent) is performed when it is necessary to remove or bypass the entire colon and rectum, or to protect a distal colorectal, coloanal, or ileoanal anastomosis. An ileostomy can be constructed either as a diverting loop stoma or end-stoma, with or without a continent reservoir (Francone, 2015).

Ileostomy is the surgical creation of an opening between the ileum and the abdominal wall for the purpose of fecal diversion. An ileostomy is typically indicated for individuals with pathologic small bowel conditions, such as ulcerative colitis, cancer complications, Crohn's disease, and familial polyposis (*Hyland, 2002; Wound, Ostomy and Continence Nurses Society, 2014). The entire colon, rectum, and anus are removed or bypassed with a permanent ileostomy. With a temporary ileostomy, all or part of the colon is removed, but part or all of the rectum is left intact (Wound, Ostomy and Continence Nurses Society, 2014).

Loop ileostomies are usually temporary and are formed to (Adkins, 2015):

- Protect a distal anastomosis;
- Protect the anastomosis of an ileal-anal pouch or a colo-anal pouch during the healing process;
- Aid healing in Crohn's disease, which affects the colon and the anus;
- Aid healing of fistula tracts (the result of underlying pathology; e.g., abscess, malignancy, Crohn's disease, trauma, sepsis).

 Time Frame
Postoperative periods

▌▌▌▌▌▌ DIAGNOSTIC CLUSTER

Preoperative Period

Risk for Impaired Tissue Integrity related to anatomical barriers to precise placement of stoma during surgery.

Postoperative Period

Collaborative Problems

▲ Risk for Complications of Peristomal Ulceration/Herniation

▲ Risk for Complications of Stomal Necrosis, Retraction Prolapse, Stenosis, Obstruction

▲ Risk for Complications of Fluid and Electrolyte Imbalances

△ Risk for Complications of Ileal Reservoir Pouchitis (Kock Pouch)

△ Risk for Complications of Failed Nipple Valve (Kock Pouch)

△ Risk for Complications of Ileoanal Kock Pouchitis

△ Risk for Complications of Cholelithiasis

△ Risk for Complications of Urinary Calculi

Nursing Diagnoses

▲ Risk for Disturbed Self-Concept related to effects of ostomy on body image and lifestyle.

△ Anxiety related to lack of knowledge of ileostomy care and perceived negative effects on lifestyle (refer to Colostomy Care Plan)

△ Risk for Ineffective Health Management related to insufficient knowledge of stoma pouching procedure, peristomal skin care, perineal wound care, and incorporation of ostomy care into activities of daily living (ADLs)

Related Care Plan

Generic Care Plan for the Surgical Client

▲ This diagnosis was reported to be monitored for or managed frequently (75% to 100%).
△ This diagnosis was reported to be monitored for or managed often (50% to 74%).

Transition Criteria

Before transition, the individual and family will:

1. Discuss and give return demonstration in relation to ostomy care at home, including stoma, pouching, irrigation, skin care.
2. Discuss strategies for incorporating ostomy management into ADLs.
3. Verbalize precautions for medication use and food intake.
4. State signs and symptoms that must be reported to a health care professional.
5. Verbalize an intent to share feelings and concerns related to ostomy with significant others.
6. Identify available community resources and self-help groups.

Transitional Risk Assessment Plan (TRAP)

Begin this plan on admission.
Implement the Transitional Risk Assessment Plan (TRAP):
- Refer to inside back cover.
- Add each validated risk diagnosis to individual's problem list with the risk code in ( ).
- Refer to the individual risk nursing diagnoses/collaborative problems for outcomes and interventions in Unit II.

> R: "Close coordination of care in the post-acute period, early transition follow-up care, enhanced client education and self-management training, proactive end-of-life counseling, and extending the resources and clinical expertise over time via multidisciplinary team management" can lower readmission rates and improve health outcomes (Boutwell & Hwu, 2009, p. 14). Interventions are utilized to activate the individual and family to select changes in their everyday lifestyle choices to improve their health (Hibbard & Greene, 2013).

Preoperative Period

Risk for Impaired Tissue Integrity Related to Anatomical Barriers to Precise Placement of Stoma During Surgery

NOC
Tissue integrity: Skin and mucous membrane (stoma)

Goal

The individual will have site selection and marking of stoma placement before surgery

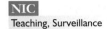

Indicators

- An ostomy nurse specialist will evaluate for site selection and will mark site or
- If the situation is emergent, a nurse of physician, who has expertise in site selection, should be accessed.

Interventions	Rationales
1. When it is first known that an individual may have an ostomy, access the ostomy nurse specialist	1. The sooner the specialist is activated the more likely that the expert will be available to do the site selection. Multiple studies indicate that individuals who have their stoma site marked preoperatively by a trained clinician have fewer ostomy-related complications (e.g., peristomal dermatitis) (Francone, 2015; Wound, Ostomy and Continence Nurses Society, 2014).
2. When it known that the specialist will not be available for site selection, notify the health professional known for competence in site selection.	2. "Stoma site marking should be performed by an Enterostomal Nurse (ETN), Rectal Surgeon or a health care professional who has been trained in the principles of stoma site marking and is aware of the implications of ostomy care and poor stoma site marking."

> **CLINICAL ALERT:**
> - Site selection should never be done casually. Every attempt should be made to have the individual with the most expertise complete the site selection. The stoma site should be selected to avoid fat folds, scars, and bony prominences (Wound, Ostomy and Continence Nurses Society, 2014). The quality of life of this individual can be seriously impaired if incorrect placement results in leaking and peristomal dermatitis. "In retrospective reviews, proper site selection is essential for minimizing postoperative complications and achieving a good postoperative quality of life" (Francone, 2015).

3. Site selection should take place not in the operating room if at all possible. The following criteria may be useful in situations when an expert is not available (Wound, Ostomy and Continence Nurses Society, 2014, pp. 3, 4):
   a. Physical considerations: Large/protruding/pendulous abdomen, abdominal folds, wrinkles, scars/suture lines, other stomas, rectus abdominis muscle, waist line, iliac crest, braces, pendulous breasts, vision, dexterity, and the presence of a hernia.
   b. Examine the individual's exposed abdomen in various positions (e.g., standing, lying, sitting, and bending forward) to observe for creases, valleys, scars, folds, skin turgor, and contour.
   c. With the individual lying on his or her back, identify the rectus abdominis muscle. This can be done by having the individual do a modified sit-up (i.e., raise the head up and off the bed) or by having the individual cough. Palpate the edge of the rectus abdominis muscle. Expert opinion suggests that placement of the stoma within the rectus abdominis muscle may help prevent a peristomal hernia and/or a prolapse.
   d. The mark should initially be made with a sticker or ink pen that can be removed if this is not the optimal spot.
   e. It may be desirable to mark sites on the right and left sides of the abdomen to prepare for a change in the surgical outcome, and number the first choice as #1.
   f. Have the person assume sitting, bending, and lying positions to assess and confirm the best choice.
   g. It is important to have the individual confirm they can see the site. However, the critical consideration should be a flat pouching surface.

3. Principles of proper stoma site selection include placement of the stoma within the rectus abdominis muscle, use of multiple positions to identify appropriate stoma sites, avoidance of folds and scars, and consideration of the clothing/beltline. This could make the difference between an ostomy pouch leaking or not for the person's lifetime. Types of skin damage include erosion, maceration, erythema, and irritant dermatitis (Wound, Ostomy and Continence Nurses Society, 2014).

Postoperative: Collaborative Problems

Risk for Complications of Intra-abdominal Hypertension (Refer to Unit II)

Risk for Complications of Peristomal Ulceration/Herniation

Risk for Complications of Stomal Necrosis, Retraction, Prolapse, Stenosis, Obstruction

Risk for Complications of Fluid and Electrolyte Imbalances

Risk for Complications of Pouchitis

Risk for Complications of Failed Nipple Valve

Risk for Complications of Cholelithiasis

Risk for Complications of Urinary Calculi

Collaborative Outcomes

The individual will be monitored for early signs and symptoms of peristomal complications such as (a) peristomal ulceration/herniation; (b) stomal necrosis, retraction; (c) prolapse, stenosis, obstruction; (e) pouchitis; (f) fluid and electrolyte imbalances; (g) cholelithiasis; (h) urinary calculi and will receive collaborative interventions if indicated to restore physiologic stability.

Indicators of Physiologic Stability

* Intact peristomal muscle tone (a)
* No stomal ulceration (a)
* No complaints of abdominal cramping or pain (b, e,)
* No abdominal or flank pain (g, h)
* No nausea or vomiting (b, g, e)
* No abdominal distention (b, h, f)
* Urine output >0.5 mL/hr (g, e, h)
* Minimal or no weight loss (e, f)
* Clear, pale urine (e, f, h)
* Urine specific gravity 1.005 to 1.030 (e, f)
* No change in stool color (e, f)
* No epigastric fullness (g)
* No jaundice (g)
* Temperature 98.5° F to 99° F (e, f)

 Carp's Cues

Please refer to the Generic Care Plan for the Surgical Client for detailed interventions for managing all surgical conditions. This care plan addresses specific additional interventions associated with the type of surgery performed.

Interventions	Rationales
CLINICAL ALERT: • Complications after stoma creation surgery can occur shortly after surgery, in 10 days, 3 to 6 months, and 1 to 2 years with a rate of 0% to 22%.	
1. Monitor for early stomal complications	1. The most early common complications were stomal retraction, stomal bleeding, necrosis, mucocutaneous separation, and peristomal skin problems (Landmann, 2015).
a. Stomal bleeding	a. Stomal bleeding—usually indicates either a stomal laceration from a poorly fitting appliance or the presence of peristomal varices in the individual with portal hypertension

(continued)

Interventions	*Rationales*
b. Stomal retraction	b. Stomal retraction is defined as a stoma that is 0.5 cm or more below the skin surface within 6 weeks of construction, typically as a result of tension on the stoma. Stomal retraction leads to leakage and difficulties with pouch adherence, resulting in peristomal skin irritation.
c. Necrosis (death of stomal tissue with impaired local blood flow)	c. The incidence of stomal necrosis in the immediate postoperative period is as high as 14%. Adequate mobilization of the bowel, preservation of the blood supply to the stoma, and an adequate trephine size are important factors for avoiding this complication.
d. Mucocutaneous separation, retraction (disappearance of normal stomal protrusion in line with or below skin level) e. Stenosis, fistula, trauma **Clinical Alert:** • Obesity (defined as a body mass index 25 kg/m²) has been associated with stomal (retraction, prolapse, and necrosis) and peristomal skin problems in multiple studies	d. Mucocutaneous separation refers to the separation of the ostomy from the peristomal skin. Mucocutaneous separation results in leakage and skin irritation. It occurs in 12% to 24% of individuals early in the postoperative period.
2. Monitor for stomal necrosis, prolapse, retraction, stenosis, and obstruction. Assess the following: a. Color, size, and shape of stoma b. Color, amount, and consistency of ostomy effluent c. Complaints of cramping, abdominal pain, nausea and vomiting, and abdominal distention d. Ostomy appliance and appliance belt fit	2. Daily assessment is necessary to detect early changes in stoma condition: a. These changes can indicate inflammation, retraction, prolapse, or edema. b. These changes can indicate bleeding or infection. Decreased output can indicate obstruction. c. These complaints may indicate obstruction. d. Contributing factors are the acid content in the small bowel, high intestinal effluent, excessive tension, necrosis, retraction, or mucocutaneous separation. Improperly fitting appliance or belt can cause mechanical trauma to the stoma. Early detection of ulcerations and herniation can prevent serious tissue damage (Wound, Ostomy and Continence Nurses Society, 2014).
3. Monitor for bulging around the stoma.	3. This finding may indicate herniation, which is caused by loops of intestine protruding through the abdominal wall.
4. Monitor for obstruction: a. Crampy abdominal pain and may feel bloated b. Pain very severe and constant c. Loss of appetite, and nausea and/or vomiting d. Very liquid output, no solids, explosive force (partial obstruction) e. No liquid, solid, or gas output (complete obstruction) **Clinical Alert:** • Notify surgeon immediately	4. A partial obstruction will allow fluid but no solids to pass leading to complete obstruction.
5. Monitor for ischemia: a. Stoma narrows or contracts at the skin or fascia b. Decrease effluent from stoma	5. Factors that contribute to ischemia are excessive tension, necrosis, retraction, mucocutaneous separation.
6. Monitor for signs and symptoms of ileal reservoir or ileo-anal pouchitis (Minkes, 2013): a. Acute increase in effluent flow b. Evidence of dehydration	6. Pouchitis or ileitis involves inflammation of the internal pouch. The cause is unknown, but bacterial growth in the pouch is a suspected causative factor. Insufficiently frequent pouch emptying increases the risk of infection.

Interventions	Rationales
c. Abdominal pain and bloating, nausea and vomiting d. Fever	
7. Monitor output closely. Consult with surgeon or wound/ostomy specialist for treatment.	7. Insertion of an indwelling catheter may be indicated to permit continuous straight drainage.

8. Monitor for signs of fluid and electrolyte imbalance:
  a. High volume of watery ostomy output (more than five 1/3- to ½-filled pouches or >1,000 mL daily)
  b. Decreased serum sodium, potassium, magnesium levels
  c. Weight loss
  d. Nausea and vomiting, anorexia, abdominal distention
	8. Disturbances in the major determinants of intestinal fluid absorption negatively impact the ability to reabsorb this large fluid load. The major determinants include intestinal mucosal surface area, the health or integrity of the mucosa, the status of small bowel motility, and the osmolarity of solutes in the intestinal lumen. Postileostomy, individuals who are left with insufficient small bowel absorptive surface area develop malabsorption, malnutrition, diarrhea, and electrolyte abnormalities. The subset of individuals with clinically significant malabsorption and malnutrition are said to have developed short-bowel syndrome (Cagir, 2015).

9. Administer fluid and electrolyte replacement therapy, as ordered. Monitor fluid status cautiously.	9. Replacement therapy may be needed to prevent serious electrolyte imbalance or fluid deficiency, and cardiac arrhythmias (ventricular ectopic, ventricular tachycardia, and Torsades de pointes) (*Lewis et al., 2004; *Wagner, Johnson, & Kidd, 2006). "In contrast aggressive postoperative fluid resuscitation may distort the ostomy, resulting in retraction and necrosis if the stoma is under tension" (Butler, 2009).

10. Monitor for cholelithiasis (gallstones):
  a. Epigastric fullness
  b. Abdominal distention
  c. Vague pain
  d. Very dark urine
  e. Grayish or clay-colored stools
  f. Jaundice
  g. Elevated cholesterol
	10. Changes in absorption of bile acids postoperatively increase cholesterol levels and can cause gallstones (Minkes, 2015).

11. Monitor for urinary calculi (stones):
  a. Lower abdominal pain
  b. Flank pain
  c. Hematuria
  d. Decreased urine output
  e. Increased urine specific gravity
	11. Individuals with ileostomies were found to have significantly lower urinary pH and volume; higher concentrations of calcium, oxalate, and uric acid; and increased risk of forming uric acid and calcium stones. In addition, small bowel resection combined with an ileostomy increased the ileostomy output, lowered the urinary volume more, and reduced urinary calcium excretion. The concentration of urinary oxalate increased and the risk of both uric acid and calcium stones was high (Evan, Lingeman, & Coe, 2009).

12. Consult with surgeon if the above signs and symptoms occur.

Clinical Alert Report

Before providing care, advise ancillary staff/student to report the following to the professional nurse assigned to the individual:

- Change in cognitive status
- Oral temperature >100.5° F
- Systolic BP <90 mm Hg
- Resting pulse >100, <50
- Respiratory rate >28, <10/min
- Oxygen saturation <90%
- Change in effluent, amount, presence of blood
- No effluent
- Complaints of nausea, abdominal pain

Risk for Disturbed Self-Concept Related to Effects of Ostomy on Body Image

NOC

Quality of Life, Coping, Depression, Self-Esteem

NIC

Hope Instillation, Mood Management, Values Clarification, Counseling, Referral, Support Group, Coping Enhancement

Goal

The individual will communicate feelings about the ostomy and will share their perceptions of the effects on their daily lives.

Indicators

- Acknowledge changes in body structure and function
- Participate actively in stoma care
- Seeks out information on self-care

 Carp's Cues

"The average period of time needed to resolve the psychological distress produced by ostomy surgery and restore optimal quality of life is not known, but existing evidence suggests that this process requires 12 months or longer" (Registered Nurses' Association of Ontario, 2009). Long-term recovery is characterized initially by taking control of ostomy care, followed by seeking to recover a sense of normalcy and reestablishing work-related and social activities (Registered Nurses' Association of Ontario, 2009). "The individual must adapt to new patterns of fecal elimination and to their altered body and image of themselves. Successful adaptation requires the patient to master new skills and to deal effectively with the many emotional issues associated with their altered anatomy and with altered continence" (Landmann, 2015).

Interventions	Rationales

1. Connect with the individual frequently. Ask, what are you most concerned about?
   a. Nurses are often fearful of asking a question to which they may not know how to respond to the individual's response.
   b. This fear creates dialogue that is superficial and meaningless.
   c. Your response could acknowledge the situation: "I am sorry you are in this situation" or "Tell me more about this."
   d. Then just listen. Listening to someone pour out his or her soul to you never means you take away the fears, BUT you can listen to them.
   e. If there are some answers to the individual's concerns that someone else, such as an ostomy nurse specialist, is better qualified to address, consult that specialist.
   f. Nurses must learn to be comfortable sitting in a dark cave with individuals without talking about the light.
	1. Frequent contact by the caregiver indicates acceptance and may facilitate trust. This question will help the nurse focus on the concern of the individual, not what "we think the concerns are."

2. Encourage the individual to verbalize feelings (both positive and negative) about the stoma and perceptions of its anticipated effects on his or her lifestyle (Registered Nurses' Association of Ontario, 2009).	2. "The assessment of self-esteem in ostomized people is becoming increasingly important and necessary, because when subjected to this surgery, these people start living a different experience, where their standard of living and rhythm of life begin to change. Their desires and values are often not fulfilled nor respected; they feel rejected, seeking seclusion because of the odor and elimination of feces through the abdomen" (Salomé, de Almeida, & Silveira, 2014).
3. Validate the perceptions and reassure that such responses are normal and appropriate.	3. Validating perceptions promotes self-awareness and provides reassurance. Sharing gives the nurse an opportunity to identify and dispel misconceptions and allay anxiety and self-doubt (Registered Nurses' Association of Ontario, 2009).

Interventions	Rationales
4. Ensure that support persons have been included in learning ostomy care principles. Assess the interactions with support persons.	4. Other people's response to the ostomy is one of the most important factors influencing acceptance of it.
5. Encourage to reestablish his or her preoperative socialization pattern. Help the individual through such measures as progressively increasing his or her socializing time in the hospital, role-playing possible situations that may cause anxiety, and encouraging him or her to visualize and anticipate solutions to "worst-case scenarios" for social situations.	5. Encouraging and facilitating socialization help to prevent isolation. Role-playing can help to identify and learn to cope with potential anxiety-causing situations in a non-threatening environment.
6. Encourage the individual/partner to initiate future discussions regarding effects on their relationship with primary care provider and/or ostomy nurse specialist.	6. Future discussions will be needed; however, when the nurse postoperatively initiates the discussion, it gives the concerned individuals permission for future dialogue.
7. Incorporate emotional support into technical ostomy self-care sessions. Richbourg, Thorpe, and Rapp (2007) have identified four stages of psychological adjustment that ostomy individuals may experience: a. Narration. The individual recounts his or her illness experience and reveals understanding of how and why he or she finds self in this situation. b. Visualization and verbalization. The individual looks at and expresses feelings about his or her stoma. c. Participation. The individual progresses from observer to assistant, then to independent performer of the mechanical aspects of ostomy care. d. Exploration. The individual begins to explore methods of incorporating the ostomy into her or his lifestyle.	
8. Involve support persons in learning ostomy care principles. Assess the interactions with support persons.	8. Other people's response to the ostomy is one of the most important factors influencing the individual's acceptance of it.
9. Encourage the individual to discuss plans for incorporating ostomy care into his or her lifestyle. Is the individual concerned about a specific situation (e.g., travel, eating out)? Share the individual's concerns with the nurse specialist.	9. Evidence that the individual will pursue his or her goals and resume lifestyle reflects positive adjustment (*Junkin & Beitz, 2005).
10. Suggest to meet with a person from the United Ostomy Associations (UOA) who can share similar experiences.	10. In addition to the professional nurse's clinical expertise, the individual may choose to take advantage of a UOA visitor's actual experience with an ostomy

Documentation

Present emotional status
Discussions

> **TRANSITION TO HOME/COMMUNITY CARE**
> If indicated, review the risk diagnoses identified for this individual on admission:
> * Is the person still at risk?
> * Can the family reduce the risks?
> * Is the person at higher risk at home?
> * Is a Home Health Nurse assessment needed?
> * Refer to transition planner/case manager/social service
> * When is this person scheduled for follow-up with primary provider? Specialists? Record dates of appointments.
> * Complete a medication reconciliation before transition. Refer to index.

STAR   **Stop**

         Think   Is this person at high risk for injury, falls, medical complications, and/or inability to care for self (activities of daily living)?

Is there a support person available?

Is the person competent to manage self-administration of medications, treatment procedures? Are additional resources needed?

Can the person explain how to monitor the condition (e.g., blood glucose, signs/symptoms of complications, dietary/mobility restrictions, and when to call his or her primary provider or specialist)?

         Act   Contact or provide the appropriate resource (e.g., contacting a support person, home health assessment, additional teaching, printed materials).

         Review Has the problem been addressed? If not, use SBAR to communicate to the appropriate person.

Risk for Ineffective Health Management Related to Insufficient Knowledge of Stoma Pouching Procedure, Peristomal Skin Care, Perineal Wound Care, and Incorporation of Ostomy Care into Activities of Daily Living (ADLs)

NOC

Compliance Behavior,
Knowledge: Treatment
Regimen, Participation:
Health Care Decisions,
Treatment Behavior:
Illness or Injury

Goals

The goals for this diagnosis represent those associated with transition planning. Refer to the transition criteria.

NIC

Ostomy Care,
Anticipatory Guidance,
Risk Identification,
Learning Facilitation,
Health Education

Interventions	Rationales
CLINICAL ALERT: • Most clinical nurses are not responsible for the specific teaching of ostomy care and its implications on lifestyle and function. • The wound care/ostomy specialist will provide an organized teaching plan. • However, since nurses are responsible for care 24/7, each nurse needs to be confident in basic ostomy care. • A good method to learn this care is to watch the nurse specialist provide/teach ostomy care.	
1. When providing care, explore fears and concerns. Identify and dispel any misinformation or misconceptions the individual/significant others has regarding ileostomy (Richbourg et al., 2007).	1. Replacing misinformation with facts can reduce anxiety.

2. Emphasize the importance of adequate fluid and salt intake; explain also risk situations for dehydration such as:
   a. Hot weather
   b. Exercising in hot weather
   c. Episodes of diarrhea
   d. When intake is reduced (e.g., illness)
	2. Loss of the reabsorptive surface of the large bowel increases the amount of water and sodium loss in the stool. If the ileostomy is high (more proximal in the ileum), additional potassium losses may also occur.

Interventions	Rationales

3. Advise to:
  a. Drink enough fluid to have at least 1 quart of ostomy output daily and pale urine
  b. Drink more fluids and consume extra salt in hot weather
  c. Eat foods high in potassium (e.g., bananas, oranges)	

4. Discuss signs and symptoms of fluid and electrolyte imbalances:
  a. Extreme thirst
  b. Dry skin and oral mucous membrane
  c. Dark yellow urine output
  d. Weakness, fatigue
  e. Muscle cramps
  f. Orthostatic hypotension (feeling faint when suddenly changing positions)	

5. Ensure that a consult with nutritionist/wound/ostomy nurse specialist has occurred.	5. The nutritionist or wound/ostomy nurse specialist will review foods to avoid controlling odor and preventing food blockage.

6. Teach signs/symptoms of food blockage: abdominal cramping
  a. Swelling of the stoma
  b. Absence of ileostomy output for more than 4 to 6 hours	

7. Advise to call surgeon/wound/ostomy specialist if self-care measures taught to relieve blockage are not effective.	

> **CLINICAL ALERT:**
> - An individual with a stoma is at increased risk for peristomal skin breakdown.
> - Factors that influence skin integrity include composition, quantity, and consistency of the ostomy effluent; allergies; mechanical trauma; the underlying disease and its treatment (including medications); surgical construction and location of the stoma; the quality of ostomy and periostomal skin care; availability of proper supplies; nutritional status; overall health status; hygiene; and activity level.

Interventions	Rationales

8. Ensure that supplies/prescriptions are provided as:
  a. Stoma supplies as wafers and pouches, and ostomy accessories, such as pastes, powder, rings, etc.
  b. Gloves, dressing tape
	8. Information on medication changes, pending tests and studies, and follow-up needs must be accurately and promptly communicated to outpatient primary care provider. Transition summaries should be transmitted to the primary care provider as soon as possible after transition.

9. Ensure appointments have been scheduled for primary care provider, specialists, home nursing assessment, diagnostic tests.	9. Appointment-keeping behavior is enhanced when the inpatient team schedules outpatient medical follow-up before discharge. Ideally, the inpatient care providers or case managers/transition planners will schedule follow-up visit(s) with the appropriate professionals, including primary care provider, endocrinologist, and diabetes educator.
10. Discuss community resources/self-help groups: a. United Ostomy Associations of America, Inc. (UOAA), www.uoaa.org. For local support group information, the interactive website includes discussion boards.	

(continued)

Interventions	*Rationales*

b. International Ostomy Association (IOA), www.ostomy international.org. Advocates for and outlines the rights of ostomates.

c. Wound, Ostomy and Continence Nurses Society (WOCN), www.wocn.org

d. Community suppliers of ostomy equipment

Clinical Alert Report

- Before providing care, advise ancillary staff/student to report the following to the professional nurse assigned to the individual:
- Any questions regarding home care, self-care.

Documentation

Individual/family teaching
Outcome achievement or status

Nephrectomy

Nephrectomy is the surgical procedure of removing a kidney or a section of a kidney. A nephrectomy is performed on individuals with cancer of the kidney (renal cell carcinoma); a disease in which cysts (sac-like structures) displace healthy kidney tissue (polycystic kidney disease); massive trauma to the kidney, serious kidney infections, and renal failure. It is also used to remove a healthy kidney from a donor for the purposes of kidney transplantation (National Kidney Foundation, 2015; Santucci, 2015).

The removal of the kidney can be classified in various ways: a *simple nephrectomy* is the removal of the kidney, while a *radical nephrectomy* is removal of the kidney and possibly the surrounding perinephric fat, Gerota's fascia, and lymph nodes. Laparoscopic techniques are also utilized for *partial nephrectomies*, which are referred to as a nephron-sparing nephrectomy (Santucci, 2015).

Time Frame
Preoperative and postoperative periods

▪▪▪▪▪ DIAGNOSTIC CLUSTER

Preoperative Period

Collaborative Problems

▲ Risk for Complications of Hemorrhage/Shock

▲ Risk for Complications of Paralytic Ileus

▲ Risk for Complications of Renal Insufficiency

△ Risk for Complications of Pyelonephritis

△ Risk for Complications of Pneumothorax Secondary to Thoracic Approach Thoracic

Surgery

Nursing Diagnoses

▲ Risk for Ineffective Health Management related to insufficient knowledge of hydration requirements, nephrostomy care, and signs and symptoms of complications

△ Acute Pain related to distention of renal capsule and incision (refer to General Surgery)

▲ Risk for Ineffective Respiratory Function related to pain on breathing and coughing secondary to location of incision (refer to General Surgery)

Related Care Plans

General Surgery Generic Care Plan

Cancer (Initial Diagnosis)

▲ This diagnosis was reported to be monitored for or managed frequently (75% to 100%).
Δ This diagnosis was reported to be monitored for or managed often (50% to 74%).

Transition Criteria

Before discharge, the individual and family will:

1. Demonstrate nephrostomy tube care.
2. State measures for at-home wound care.
3. Share feelings regarding loss of kidney.
4. State signs and symptoms that must be reported to a health care professional.
5. Explain the difference between incisional pain and the pain of infection.

Transitional Risk Assessment Plan (TRAP)

Begin this plan on admission.
Implement the Transitional Risk Assessment Plan (TRAP):
- Refer to inside back cover.
- Add each validated risk diagnosis to individual's problem list with the risk code in ( ).
- Refer to the individual risk nursing diagnoses/collaborative problems for outcomes and interventions in Unit II.

   R: "Close coordination of care in the post-acute period, early transition follow-up care, enhanced client education and self-management training, proactive end-of-life counseling, and extending the resources and clinical expertise over time via multidisciplinary team management" can lower readmission rates and improve health outcomes (Boutwell & Hwu, 2009, p. 14). Interventions are utilized to activate the individual and family to select changes in their everyday lifestyle choices to improve their health (Hibbard & Greene, 2013).

Postoperative: Collaborative Problems

Risk for Complications of Hemorrhage/Shock

Risk for Complications of Paralytic Ileus

Risk for Complications of Renal Insufficiency

Risk for Complications of Pyelonephritis

Collaborative Outcomes

The individual will be monitored for early signs and symptoms of (a) hemorrhage/shock, (b) paralytic ileus, (c) renal insufficiency (partial nephrectomy), and (d) pyelonephritis (partial nephrectomy) and will receive collaborative interventions if indicated to restore physiologic stability.

Indicators of Physiologic Stability

- Calm, oriented, alert (a)
- Pulse 60 to 100 beats/min (a)
- Respirations 16 to 20 breaths/min (a)
- BP >90/60, <140/90 mm Hg (a) (James et al., 2014)
- No chills (d)

- Temperature 98.5° F to 99° F (d)
- Urine specific gravity 1.005 to 1.030 (c, d)
- Urine output >0.5 mL/hr (a, c, d)
- Full peripheral pulses (a)
- Capillary refill <3 seconds (a)
- Dry, warm skin (a)
- Hemoglobin (a)
  - Male 13 to 18 g/dL
  - Female 12 to 16 g/dL
- Hematocrit (a)
  - Male 42% to 50%
  - Female 40% to 48%
- Bowel sounds present, all quadrants (b)
- No abdominal distention (b)
- White blood cells 5,000 to 10,000/mm^3 (d)
- Urine sodium 130 to 200 mEq/24 hr (c)
- Blood urea nitrogen 10 to 20 mg/dL (c)
- Potassium 3.8 to 5 mEq/L (c)
- Serum sodium 135 to 145 mEq/L (c)
- Phosphorus 2.5 to 4.5 mg/dL (c)
- Creatinine clearance 100 to 150 mL of blood cleared per mm (c)
- No costovertebral angle (CVA) tenderness (d)
- Urine is negative for bacteria (d)
- No complaints of dysuria or frequency (d)
- No bladder distention (d)

Carp's Cues

Please refer to the Generic Care Plan for the Surgical Client for detailed interventions for managing all surgical conditions. This care plan addresses specific additional interventions associated with the type of surgery performed.

Interventions	Rationales

1. Monitor for signs and symptoms of hemorrhage/shock every hour for the first 24 hours, then every 4 hours:
  a. Increasing pulse rate with normal or slightly decreased blood pressure
  b. Decreased oxygen saturation (pulse oximetry) <94%
  c. Urine output <0.5 mL/kg/hr (normal value for urine output is 0.5 to 1.0 mL/kg/hr) (Dutka & Szromba, 2015)
  d. Restlessness, agitation, change in mentation
  e. Increasing respiratory rate
  f. Diminished peripheral pulses
  g. Cool, pale, or cyanotic skin
  h. Thirst
	1. Because the renal capsule is very vascular, massive blood loss can occur. The compensatory response to decreased circulatory volume is to increase blood oxygen by increasing the heart and respiratory rates and decreasing circulation to extremities (manifested by decreased pulses and cool skin). Diminished cerebral oxygenation can cause changes in mentation. Decreased oxygen to kidneys results in decreased urine output.

2. Monitor fluid status hourly: Accurate daily assessment of body weight is more reliable in measuring fluid loss than intake-vs-output, because it accounts for water loss during fever, diaphoresis, and respiration: 1 L (1,000 mL) of water weighs 1 kg or 2.2 lb (Dutka & Szromba, 2015).
  a. Intake (parenteral, oral)
  b. Output and loss (urinary, drainage, vomiting)
  c. Weigh daily at same time in same clothes, if needed
	2. Fluid loss owing to surgery and nothing-by-mouth (NPO) status can disrupt fluid balance in some individuals. Stress can produce sodium and water retention.

3. Monitor surgical site for bleeding, dehiscence, and evisceration.	3. Frequent monitoring enables early detection of complications. Hypotension and vasospasm during surgery can cause temporary hemostasis and can result in delayed bleeding.

Interventions	Rationales
4. Teach the individual to splint the incision site with a pillow when coughing and deep breathing (to decrease/prevent occurrences of postoperative pneumonia secondary to the inability to breathe deeply owing to pain).	4. Splinting reduces stress on suture lines by equalizing the pressure across the incision site.

5. Monitor for signs and symptoms of paralytic ileus:
  a. Decreased or absent bowel sounds
  b. Abdominal distention
  c. Abdominal discomfort
6. Do not initiate fluids until bowel sounds are present. Begin with small amounts. Note the individual's response and the type and amount of emesis, if any.
	5, 6. Reflex paralysis of intestinal peristalsis and manipulation of the colon to gain access place the individual at risk for ileus. The depressive effects of narcotics, and anesthetics on peristalsis, as well as the handling of the bowel during surgery can also cause paralytic ileus. Ileus can occur between the third and fifth postoperative day. Pain can be localized, sharp, and intermittent (Kalff, Wehner, & Litkouhi, 2015).

7. Monitor for early signs and symptoms of renal insufficiency:
 	
  a. Sustained elevated urine specific gravity
  b. Elevated urine sodium level
 	
  c. Sustained insufficient urine output (<30 mL/hr)
  d. Elevated blood pressure
 	
  e. Elevated BUN and serum creatinine, potassium, phosphorus, and ammonia; decreased creatinine clearance
	7. Renal insufficiency can result from edema caused by surgical manipulation (partial nephrectomy) or by a nonpatent nephrostomy tube.
	a, b. Ability of renal tubules to reabsorb electrolytes results in increased urine sodium levels and urine specific gravity.
	c, d. Decreased glomerular filtration rate eventually leads to insufficient urine output and increased renin production, resulting in elevated blood pressure in the body's attempt to increase renal blood flow.
	e. These changes result from decreased excretion of urea and creatinine in urine.

8. Monitor the individual for signs and symptoms of infection:
 	
  a. Chills and fever
 	
  b. Change in the type of pain
 	
  c. Costovertebral angle (CVA) pain (a dull, constant backache below the 12th rib)
  d. Leukocytosis
 	
  e. Bacteria and pus in urine
 	
  f. Dysuria and frequency
	8. Microorganisms can be introduced into the body during surgery or through the incision. Urinary tract infections can be caused by urinary stasis (e.g., from a nonpatent nephrostomy tube) or by irritation of tissue by calculi.
	a. Endogenous pyrogens are released and they reset the hypothalamic setpoint to febrile levels. The body temperature is sensed as "too cool"; shivering and vasoconstriction result, to generate and consume heat. The core temperature rises to the new setpoint level, resulting in fever. The leukocytes (WBCs) are the circulating cells of the immune system; although their quantities are limited, they are an extremely quick and powerful defense system and respond immediately to foreign invaders by going to the site of involvement (Porat & Dinarello, 2015). Wound redness, tenderness, and edema result from lymphocyte migration to the area (Mizell, 2014).
	b. An individual may experience considerable discomfort in the area around the incision and may need to be taught the difference between incisional pain and infection pain. Incisional pain will decrease each day, while infection pain will increase and is usually accompanied by fever (Mariano, 2015).
	c. CVA pain results from distention of the renal capsule.
	d. Leukocytosis reflects an increase in WBCs to fight infection through phagocytosis.
	e. Bacteria and pus in urine indicate a urinary tract infection.
	f. Bacteria irritate bladder tissue, causing spasms, and frequency.

(continued)

Interventions	*Rationales*

9. Monitor for signs of urinary retention:
  a. Bladder distention
  b. Urine overflow (30 to 60 mL of urine every 15 to 30 minutes)
	9. Trauma to the detrusor muscle and injury to the pelvic nerves during surgery can inhibit bladder function. Anxiety and pain can cause spasms of the reflex sphincters. Bladder neck edema can also cause retention. Sedatives and narcotics can affect the central nervous system and the effectiveness of the smooth muscles (Mueller, 2016).

10. Instruct the individual to report bladder discomfort or inability to void.	10. Overdistention of the bladder can aggravate an individual's ability to empty the bladder (Mueller, 2016).

Clinical Alert Report

Before providing care, advise ancillary staff/student to report the following to the professional nurse assigned to the individual:

- Please add data that need to be reported for the collaborative problems. Most often this is applicable to physiologic problems such as significant change in vital signs, change in cognition, skin, new onset of pain, etc.

Documentation

Vital signs
Circulatory status
Intake (oral, parenteral)
Output (urinary drainage color, clarity, sediment, drainage tubes)
Bowel function (bowel sounds, defecation pattern, abdominal distention)
Wound status (color, drainage, pain around incision, tenderness)

TRANSITION TO HOME/COMMUNITY CARE

If indicated, review the risk diagnoses identified for this individual on admission:

- Is the person still at risk?
- Can the family reduce the risks?
- Is the person at higher risk at home?
- Is a Home Health Nurse assessment needed?
- Refer to transition planner/case manager/social service
- When is this person scheduled for follow-up with primary provider? Specialists? Record dates of appointments.
- Complete a medication reconciliation before transition. Refer to index.

STAR

Stop

Think   Is this person at high risk for injury, falls, medical complications, and/or inability to care for self (activities of daily living)?
Is there a support person available?
Is the person competent to manage self-administration of medications, treatment procedures? Are additional resources needed?
Can the person explain how to monitor the condition (e.g., blood glucose, signs/symptoms of complications, dietary/mobility restrictions, and when to call his or her primary provider or specialist)?

Act   Contact or provide the appropriate resource (e.g., contacting a support person, home health assessment, additional teaching, printed materials).

Review   Has the problem been addressed? If not, use SBAR to communicate to the appropriate person.

Postoperative: Nursing Diagnosis

Risk for Ineffective Therapeutic Regimen Health Management Related to Insufficient Knowledge of Hydration Requirements, Nephrostomy Care, and Signs and Symptoms of Complications

NOC
Compliance Behavior, Knowledge: Treatment Regimen, Participation: Health Care Decisions, Treatment Behavior: Illness or Injury

NIC
Anticipatory Guidance, Risk Identification, Health Education, Learning Facilitation

Goals

The goals for this diagnosis represent those associated with discharge planning. Refer to the discharge criteria.

Interventions	Rationales
1. Explain the need to maintain optimal hydration.	1. Optimal hydration reduces urinary stasis, decreasing the risk of infection and calculi formation.
2. Teach and have the individual perform a return demonstration of nephrostomy care measures, including: a. Aseptic technique b. Skin care c. Tube stabilization	2. Proper techniques can reduce the risk of infection. Movement of the tube can cause dislodgement or tissue trauma.
3. Teach the individual to use pillows to support the back when lying on side.	3. Certain positions will decrease tension on the incisional area.
4. Explain why the pain is severe, as well as other discomforts. Teach the individual to avoid lifting any weight more than 10 lb for 6 weeks.	4. The individual's position of and the incision's size cause severe pain. The individual's position on the operating room table will cause muscular aches and pains.
5. Teach the individual to report the following: a. Decreased urine output b. Fever or malaise c. Purulent, cloudy drainage from or around the tube	5. Early detection enables prompt intervention to prevent serious complications such as renal insufficiency and infection.
6. Refer the individual and family to a home health-care agency for follow-up care.	6. A home care nurse evaluates the individual/family's ability for home care and provides periodic assessment of renal function and development of infection.

Documentation

Transition summary record
Teaching and clarification of understanding toward education
Outcome achievement or status
Referrals

Radical Prostatectomy

The American Cancer Society's estimates for prostate cancer in the United States for 2016 are about 180,890 new cases of prostate cancer and about 26,120 deaths from prostate cancer. Prostate cancer is the second leading cause of cancer death in American men, behind only lung cancer. About 1 man in 39 will die of prostate cancer (American Cancer Society, 2016a, 2016b).

Standard management options for men with clinically localized prostate cancer include radical prostatectomy, radiation therapy (RT), including external beam RT and/or brachytherapy, and for appropriately selected individuals, active surveillance. Radical prostatectomy is a treatment option for individuals with localized prostate cancer, along with external beam radiation therapy, brachytherapy, and in some cases active surveillance. Radical prostatectomy is not indicated for individuals with distant metastases or when there is tumor fixation to adjacent structures (Klein, 2016).

Radical prostatectomy can be performed using either an open approach or via a minimally invasive (robotic or laparoscopic) technique. Compared with an open technique, minimally invasive approaches use a smaller incision. Analyses of large databases indicate that the usage of robotic surgery has increased rapidly and now constitutes a majority of radical prostatectomies (Klein, 2016).

Time Frame
Postoperative periods

■ ■ ■ ■ ■ ■ DIAGNOSTIC CLUSTER

Collaborative Problems

▲ Risk for Complications of Hemorrhage

▲ Risk for Complications of Clot Formation

△ Risk for Complications of Thrombophlebitis

Nursing Diagnoses

▲ Acute Pain related to bladder spasms; clot retention; and back, leg, and incisional pain

△ Risk for Ineffective Sexuality Patterns related to fear of impotence resulting from surgical intervention

▲ Risk for Ineffective Health Management related to insufficient knowledge of fluid restrictions, catheter care, activity restrictions, urinary control, and signs and symptoms of complications

Related Care Plan

General Surgery Generic Care Plan

▲ This diagnosis was reported to be monitored for or managed frequently (75% to 100%).
△ This diagnosis was reported to be monitored for or managed often (50% to 74%).

Transition Criteria

Before transition, the individual and family will:

1. Identify the need for increased oral fluid intake.
2. Demonstrate care of the indwelling (Foley) catheter.
3. Demonstrate wound care for home care.
4. Verbalize necessary precautions for activity and urination.
5. State the signs and symptoms that must be reported to a health care professional.
6. Verbalize an intent to share feelings and concerns related to sexual function with significant others and the surgeon.

Transitional Risk Assessment Plan (TRAP)

Begin this plan on admission.
Implement the Transitional Risk Assessment Plan (TRAP):
• Refer to inside back cover.
• Add each validated risk diagnosis to individual's problem list with the risk code in ( ).
• Refer to the individual risk nursing diagnoses/collaborative problems for outcomes and interventions in Unit II.

R: "Close coordination of care in the post-acute period, early transition follow-up care, enhanced client education and self-management training, proactive end-of-life counseling, and extending the resources and clinical expertise over time via multidisciplinary team management" can lower readmission rates and improve health outcomes (Boutwell & Hwu, 2009, p. 14). Interventions are utilized to activate the individual and family to select changes in their everyday lifestyle choices to improve their health (Hibbard & Greene, 2013).

Postoperative: Collaborative Problems

Risk for Complications of Hemorrhage

Risk for Complications of Clot Formation

Risk for Complications of Urinary Leak from Anastomosis Site

Risk for Complications of Thrombophlebitis (Refer to Generic Surgical Care Plan)

Collaborative Outcomes

The individual will be monitored for early signs and symptoms of (a) hemorrhage, (b) clot formation, (c) urinary retention, and (d) urinary leak at anastomosis site and will receive collaborative interventions if indicated to restore physiologic stability.

Indicators of Physiologic Stability

- Calm, oriented, alert (a)
- Pulse 60 to 100 beats/min (a)
- Respirations 16 to 20 breaths/min (a)
- BP >90/60, <140 to 90 mm Hg (a)
- Temperature 98° F to 99.5° F
- Urine output >0.5 mL/hr (a)
- Pink or clear red urine in the first 24 hours (a)
- Amber pink urine after 24 hours (a)
- Warm, dry skin (a)
- Hemoglobin (a)
  - Male 13 to 18 g/dL
  - Female 12 to 16 g/dL
- Hematocrit (a)
  - Male 42% to 50%
  - Female 40% to 48%
- Continuous flowing bladder irrigation (b, c)
- No bladder distention (c)
- No increase in drainage from JP drain (d)

Carp's Cues

Please refer to the Generic Care Plan for the Surgical Client for detailed interventions for managing all surgical conditions. This care plan addresses specific additional interventions associated with the type of surgery performed.

> **CLINICAL ALERT:**
> - An increase in operative time of 30 or 60 minutes was associated with 1.6 and 2.8 times increased VTE risks. A 5-point increase in body mass index and need for blood transfusion were also associated with increased risk of VTE (Abel et al., 2014).

Interventions	Rationales

1. Monitor for signs and symptoms of hemorrhage and notify surgeon at first sign of bleeding.
   a. Abnormal urine characteristics (e.g., highly viscous, clots, bright red, or burgundy color)
   b. Increased pulse rate
   c. Urine output <0.5 mL/kg/hr
   d. Restlessness, agitation
   e. Cool, pale, or cyanotic skin
   f. Hemoglobin and hematocrit values
	1. Significant bleeding after endoscopic prostatic surgery is still a potentially life-threatening complication. Prophylactic measures have been employed to reduce perioperative bleeding but persistent bleeding postendoscopic prostatic surgery should be treated promptly to prevent the risk of rapid deterioration (Lynch, Sriprasad, Subramonian, & Thompson, 2010).
	   The prostate gland is highly vascular, receiving its blood supply from the internal iliac artery. Elderly individual s and those who have had prolonged urinary retention are vulner

(continued)

Interventions	Rationales
	able to rapid changes in bladder contents and fluid volume. During the first 24 hours after surgery, urine should be pink or clear red, gradually becoming amber to pink-tinged by the fourth day. Bright red urine with clots indicates arterial bleeding. Burgundy-colored urine indicates venous bleeding, which usually resolves spontaneously. Clots are expected; their absence may point to blood dyscrasias. Hemoglobin and hematocrit values decline if significant postoperative bleeding occurs (Grossman & Porth, 2014).
2. Monitor dressings, catheters, and drains that vary depending on the type of surgery performed: a. Suprapubic approach: • Urethral catheter • Suprapubic tube • Abdominal drain b. Retropubic approach: • Urethral catheter • Abdominal drain c. Perineal approach: • Urethral catheter • Perineal drain	2. Heavy venous bleeding is expected the first 24 hours for all approaches except the perineal approach. Blood loss can occur from the catheter or incision.
3. Instruct to do the following: a. Avoid straining for bowel elimination. b. Do not sit in a firm, upright chair. c. Recline slightly while on the toilet.	3. Increased pressure on the rectum can trigger bleeding and perforated rectal tissue.
4. Provide bladder irrigation as prescribed; maintain aseptic technique: a. Continuous (closed) b. Manual: Using a bulb syringe, irrigate the catheter with 30 to 60 mL normal saline solution every 3 to 4 hours, as needed.	4. "The surgical outcome of prostate surgery (TURP and open prostatectomy) has definitely improved over the years. Improved laser surgical techniques have been introduced. With these improvements, especially in the area of surgical hemostasis, it is certainly time to reconsider the routine use of CBI, which has been an integral part of prostate surgery and might have been more relevant during the evolving stages of these surgeries" (Okorie, 2015).
5. Ensure adequate fluid intake (oral, parenteral).	5. Optimal hydration dilutes urine and prevents clot formation.
6. Monitor for urine leak from anastomosis site (high-volume Jackson-Pratt (JP) drain output)	6. A JP drain is placed at the anastomosis site between the bladder neck and urethra. If hemostasis is disrupted, urine can leak into the site and drain. Increased wound drainage may suggest a urine leak, lymph leak, or pelvic bleeding.
7. Notify surgeon of possible urine leak for assessment (e.g., testing the drainage fluid for the presence of creatinine, cystogram) and treatment (e.g., urinary catheter is placed on traction).	7. Traction will allow the leak site to heal. If drainage fluid is positive for creatinine, a leak is confirmed. Cystogram can confirm the location and extent of leak.

Clinical Alert Report

Before providing care, advise ancillary staff/student to report the following to the professional nurse assigned to the individual:

• Change in cognitive status
• Oral temperature >100.5° F
• Systolic BP <90 mm Hg
• Resting pulse >100, <50

- Respiratory rate >28, <10/min
- Oxygen saturation <90%
- Increase in drainage
- Decreased urine output
- New-onset bloody urine
- New complaints of leg pain

Documentation

Vital signs
Intake and output
Urine (color, viscosity, presence of clots)
Drains
Continuous irrigations/manual irrigations (times, amounts)

Postoperative: Nursing Diagnoses

Acute Pain Related to Bladder Spasms; Clot Retention; and Back, Leg, and Incisional Pain

NOC
Comfort Level, Pain Control

NIC
Pain Management, Medication Management, Emotional Support, Teaching: Individual, Heat/Cold Application, Simple Massage

Goal

The individual will report decreased pain after pain relief interventions.

Indicators

- Can do leg exercises.
- Increase activity progressively.

Interventions	Rationales
1. Monitor for intermittent suprapubic pain: bladder spasms, burning sensation at the tip of the penis.	1. Irritation from an indwelling catheter can cause bladder spasms and pain in the penis.
2. Monitor for persistent suprapubic pain: bladder distention with sensations of fullness and tightness, inability to void.	2. Catheter obstruction can cause urinary retention, leading to increased bladder spasms and increased risk of infection.
3. Monitor for lower back and leg pain. Provide gentle massage to the back, and heat to the legs, if necessary.	3. During surgery, the individual lies in the lithotomy position that can stretch and aggravate muscles that normally may be underused.
4. Anchor the catheter to the leg with a catheter leg strap.	4. Pressure from a dangling catheter can damage the urinary sphincter, resulting in urinary incontinence after catheter removal. Catheter movement also increases the likelihood of bladder spasms.
5. Monitor for testicular pain.	5. Clipping the vas deferens causes congestion of seminal fluid and blood. This congestion takes several weeks to resolve.
6. Administer medication, as ordered, for pain and spasms.	6. Antispasmodic medications (e.g., opioids and belladonna suppositories) prevent bladder spasms. Analgesic medications diminish the incisional pain.
7. Encourage adequate oral fluid intake (at least 2,000 mL/day, unless contraindicated).	7. Adequate hydration dilutes urine that helps to flush out clots.

(continued)

Interventions	Rationales
8. Manually irrigate the indwelling catheter only when prescribed.	8. Each time the closed system is opened for manual irrigation, risk of bacterial contamination increases.
9. Monitor output of wound drains (*Rigdon, 2006).	
10. Refer to Generic Surgical Care Plan for pain management strategies.	

Documentation

Type, dose, route of all medications
Complaints of pain (type, site, duration)
Unsatisfactory pain relief

Risk for Ineffective Sexuality Patterns Related to Fear of Impotence Resulting From Surgical Intervention

NOC

Body Image, Self-Esteem, Role Performance, Sexual Identity: Acceptance

Goals

The individual will discuss his feelings and concerns regarding the effects of surgery on sexuality and sexual functioning.

NIC

Behavior Management: Sexual, Sexual Counseling, Emotional Support, Active Listening, Teaching: Sexuality

Indicators

• Engages in discussions on fears and concern regarding sexual activity after discharge from hospital.
• Explains effects of surgery on sexual function and expected course of resolution.

> **CLINICAL ALERT:**
> Sexuality problems (e.g., poor erections, difficulty with orgasm) were a moderate or big problem in 59% of men after 2 months in a series of 603 individuals who had undergone radical prostatectomy. Although there was some gradual improvement with time, 43% still reported such problems 2 years after prostatectomy. The likelihood of regaining potency after radical prostatectomy decreases with increasing age. In one series, the potency rate after surgery was 86% in men in their 40s, and 80%, 60%, and 42% for men in their 50s, 60s, and 70s, respectively.
> Penile sensation and the ability to have an orgasm are preserved even if the erectile nerves are removed during radical prostatectomy.

Interventions	Rationales
1. Explain the effects of surgery on sexual function (orgasms, erections, fertility, ejaculations). Potency can be preserved in many men with normal preoperative erectile function who undergo bilateral nerve-sparing radical prostatectomy.	1. Damage to the urinary sphincter can lead to urinary incontinence after radical prostatectomy. However, complete urinary incontinence is uncommon after retropubic radical prostatectomy. However, the majority of men do experience some degree of urinary incontinence after radical prostatectomy, particularly stress incontinence. If one or both nerve bundles responsible for erections are spared during surgery, erections will return. Orgasms will occur without ejaculations. It may take more than a year after wound healing and all edema from surgery subsides for full function to return. Men older than 70 years probably

Interventions	Rationales
	will not regain erections; ejaculate will be reduced but will still contain sperm. Robot-assisted laparoscopic approaches report 90% return to good sexual function after surgery. The frequency of impotence depends upon multiple factors, including age, pretreatment sexual functioning, and type of surgery (nerve-sparing vs. nonnerve-sparing). A validated model that may be useful in counseling individuals has been developed to help predict the probability of erectile function 2 years after radical prostatectomy (Klein, 2016).
2. Explore previous sexual function before surgery. Use familiar terms, when possible, and explain unfamiliar terms.	2. Previous patterns of functioning need to be considered as they do influence postsurgical functioning. Unfamiliar medical terminology may cause confusion and misunderstanding.
3. Explain that the surgeon's permission to resume sexual activity is needed. Clearly state that cancer of the prostate is not transmitted sexually.	3. Complete healing is needed to prevent bleeding and to resolve edema, which usually takes 6 weeks to 3 months.
4. Provide opportunities for the partner to share concerns and questions.	4. Partners are crucial to the recovery process. They manage their own anxiety and also assist their partner in managing his (*Maliski, Heilemann, & McCorkle, 2001). Cultural and religious beliefs may affect the spouse's participation and queries (Sublett, 2007).
5. Encourage the individual to continue to discuss concerns with significant others and professionals postdischarge.	5. At some point postdischarge, PDE5 inhibitors (e.g., sildenafil, tadalafil) may be prescribed to stimulate erections if not medically contraindicated. The success rate in men who have undergone prostate cancer surgery is between 25% and 30%.

TRANSITION TO HOME/COMMUNITY CARE

If indicated, review the risk diagnoses identified for this individual on admission:

- Is the person still at risk?
- Can the family reduce the risks?
- Is the person at higher risk at home?
- Is a Home Health Nurse assessment needed?
- Refer to transition planner/case manager/social service
- When is this person scheduled for follow-up with primary provider? Specialists? Record dates of appointments.
- Complete a medication reconciliation before transition. Refer to index.

STAR

Stop

Think Is this person at high risk for injury, falls, medical complications, and/or inability to care for self (activities of daily living)?

Is there a support person available?

Is the person competent to manage self-administration of medications, treatment procedures? Are additional resources needed?

Can the person explain how to monitor the condition (e.g., blood glucose, signs/symptoms of complications, dietary/mobility restrictions, and when to call his or her primary provider or specialist)?

Act Contact or provide the appropriate resource (e.g., contacting a support person, home health assessment, additional teaching, printed materials).

Review Has the problem been addressed? If not, use SBAR to communicate to the appropriate person.

Documentation

Expressed concerns

Client teaching

Risk for Ineffective Health Management Related to Insufficient Knowledge of Fluid Restrictions, Catheter Care, Activity Restrictions, Urinary Control, and Signs and Symptoms of Complications

NOC

Compliance Behavior, Knowledge: Treatment Regimen, Participation: Health Care Decisions, Treatment Behavior: Illness or Injury

NIC

Anticipatory Guidance, Risk Identification, Health Education, Learning Facilitation

Goals

The goals for this diagnosis represent those associated with transition planning. Refer to the transition criteria.

Interventions	Rationales
1. Reinforce the need for adequate oral fluid intake (at least 2,000 mL/day, unless contraindicated).	1. Optimal hydration helps to reestablish bladder tone after catheter removal by stimulating voiding, diluting urine, and decreasing susceptibility to urinary tract infections and clot formation.
2. Explain that scrotal/penile swelling and bruising are normal and are strategies to reduce symptoms (*Starnes & Sims, 2006). a. Elevate scrotum with a small towel or washcloth when sitting or lying down. b. Wear supportive briefs or an athletic support.	2. Scrotal/penile swelling, resulting from trauma during surgery, will resolve in 7 to 10 days.

3. Teach indwelling catheter care:
a. Explain that the duration for needing the urinary catheter will be 1 to 3 weeks. Gently, wash the urinary meatus with soap and water twice a day. If it becomes irritated, apply antibiotic cream to the irritated area twice a day.
b. Increase the frequency of cleansing if drainage is evident around the catheter insertion site.
c. Instruct individual/family member on use of:
  • Leg collection bag:
    • Observe individual applying, removing, and connecting equipment.
    • Instruct to reposition every 4 to 6 hours
  • Urinary drainage bag:
    • Observe individual applying, changing, and connecting equipment.
    • Advise not to use, leg bag when frequent emptying is not possible, care trip, nighttime.
d. Always keep any type of collection bag below the level of the bladder.
	3. The indwelling catheter provides a route for bacteria that are normally found on the urinary meatus to enter the urinary tract. These measures help to reduce risk of urinary tract infection.
	
	• Repositioning to other leg or lower or higher on the leg will prevent prolonged pressure to skin/tissues.

4. Instruct on care of pelvic drain at home, if needed.	4. This drain is usually removed the first day postoperatively; however, sometimes it is left in a week or more (University of Michigan Health System, 2007).

Interventions	*Rationales*

5. Reinforce activity restrictions that may include the following:
  a. Avoid straining with bowel movements; increase intake of dietary fiber or take stool softeners, if indicated.
  b. Do not use suppositories or enemas.
  c. Avoid sitting with legs dependent.
  d. Avoid heavy lifting and strenuous activity or sport for 4 weeks.
  e. Please refrain from driving for 1 week after your surgery.
  f. Avoid activities (running, golf, exercising, horseback riding, motorcycles, bicycling) for 6 weeks after surgery.
  g. Avoid climbing stairs as a form of exercise.
  h. Avoid sitting still in one position for too long (more than 45 minutes).
  i. Avoid bathtubs, swimming pools, hot tubs, or otherwise submerging yourself in water for as long as the catheter is in place. Showering is fine as soon as you go home.
  j. Avoid sexual intercourse until the physician/nurse practitioner advises otherwise.
	5. These restrictions are necessary to reduce the risk of internal bleeding. These activities can stress the surgical site and impede healing of surgical site.

> **CLINICAL ALERT:**
>
> There are three major types of incontinence (American Cancer Society, 2016):
>
> • Men with *stress incontinence* might leak urine when they cough, laugh, sneeze, or exercise. Stress incontinence is the most common type after prostate surgery. It is usually caused by problems with the valve that keeps urine in the bladder (the bladder sphincter). Prostate cancer treatments can damage the muscles that form this valve or the nerves that keep the muscles working.
>
> • Men with *overflow incontinence* have trouble emptying their bladder. They take a long time to urinate and have a dribbling stream with little force. Overflow incontinence is usually caused by blockage or narrowing of the bladder outlet by scar tissue.
>
> • Men with *urge incontinence* have a sudden need to urinate. This problem occurs when the bladder becomes too sensitive to stretching as it fills with urine.

6. Explain that urinary continence will return in phases after the catheter is removed (University of Michigan Health System, 2007):
Phase 1—You are dry when you are lying down at night.
Phase 2—You have periods of good urinary control in the early morning.
Phase 3—Urinary control lasts for longer intervals and later into the afternoon and evening.
  a. Dribbling, frequency, and urgency may occur initially, but will gradually subside over weeks.
	6. Continence will return gradually in phases from a few weeks to several months. Continence returns sooner after robotic surgery.
	
	  a. Difficulty resuming normal voiding patterns may be related to bladder neck trauma, urinary tract infection, or catheter irritation. While the indwelling catheter is in place, constant urine drainage decreases muscle control and increases flaccidity.

Interventions	*Rationales*
7. Teach exercises to strengthen perineal muscles: explain that when you tighten your pelvic muscles to stop the flow of urine or prevent the passing of gas, you are performing a Kegel exercise. a. Tighten and tense buttocks, hold for 10 seconds, then relax for 10 seconds; repeat 10 times. b. Tighten only the pelvic muscles; keep your abdominal, thigh, and buttock muscles relaxed. c. Do exercises frequently (6 to 12 times a day; 10 at a time). d. Advise that Kegel exercises can be performed while sitting or standing, anywhere and anytime.	7. Kegel exercises for men can strengthen the pelvic floor muscles, which support the bladder and bowel and affect sexual function. Regular contracture of the sphincter muscles will strengthen the pelvic floor muscles and decrease incontinence in 4 to 6 weeks. Use of biofeedback or anal electrical stimulation may help prevent continued incontinence (Mayo Clinic, 2016).
8. Advise to: a. Avoid drinking fluids near bedtime b. Avoiding caffeine and alcohol can help to prevent problems. c. Wear a pants liner or incontinent pants initially, if needed.	8. Caffeine acts as a mild diuretic and makes it more difficult to control urine. Alcohol may increase the burning sensations on urination.
9. Instruct to call 911 or to go to the nearest emergency room if there are any signs of pulmonary embolus (blood clot from pelvis that has gotten into the blood circulation of the lung): a. Sudden-onset chest pain b. New onset of difficulty breathing or worsening of usual breathlessness c. Sensation of heart racing	

10. Instruct on the signs and symptoms to report to surgeon without delay:
a. Signs of a blood clot in the legs or pelvis (deep vein thrombosis)
  • Pain in the back of the thigh, calf, or groin
  • Swelling of the leg
  • Red streaking color or warmth of the leg
b. Problems with the surgical incision
  • Redness and/or warmth around incision
  • Pus draining from the incision
  • Separation of the skin at the incision line
c. Problems with the urethral catheter
  • Urine not draining
  • Red blood that does not clear soon after resting and increasing fluid intake
  • Urethral catheter inadvertently pulled out from the bladder or penis
d. Other
  • Fever with temperature by mouth greater than 101° F
  • Nausea, vomiting, or severe abdominal bloating
  • Pain not relieved by prescribed medications
  • Inability to urinate after catheter removal
  • Decreased force of stream and sensation of incomplete emptying after catheter removal	

11. Ensure appointments are scheduled for home assessments (nursing, physical therapy, occupational therapy, social services) and surgeon.	11. For follow-up for any hospitalization, appointment-keeping behavior is enhanced when the inpatient team schedules outpatient medical follow-up before transition. Ideally, the inpatient care providers or case managers/transition planners will schedule follow-up visit(s) with the appropriate professionals, including primary care provider, surgeon (Barnsteiner, Disch, & Walton, 2014).

Interventions	Rationales
12. Initiate a discussion regarding a healthier lifestyle to prevent cardiovascular, pulmonary, and musculoskeletal complications. Emphasize the damaging effects of: a. Overweight/obesity on multiple body systems and occurrence of chronic diseases (e.g., diabetes mellitus). Refer to thePoint for a printout of "Getting Started to a healthy weight." b. Sedentary life style. Refer to thePoint for a printout of "Getting Started to Moving More." c. Tobacco use. Refer to "Getting Started to Stop Smoking."	12. Motivation to improve an unhealthy lifestyle is often increased when individuals are experiencing a health problem, acutely (Barnsteiner et al., 2014).

Documentation

Individual/family teaching
Referrals, if indicated

Lumbar Spinal Surgery

Surgery of the spine is performed for several reasons, such as trauma, removal of tumors/lesions, spinal stenosis, and for disc disease when diagnostic tests reveal a herniation that is not responding to conservative treatment.

Only a small minority of individuals suffering from low back pain ever require surgery. However, rates of surgical procedures are rising in the United States, particularly for spinal fusion in individuals with nonspecific back pain (Chou, 2016b; *Weinstein et al., 2006). More intense interdisciplinary rehabilitation is more effective than surgery and less intense interdisciplinary rehabilitation (Chou, 2016b).

For the small minority of low back pain individuals with severe or progressive motor weakness, or signs and symptoms of cauda equina syndrome, urgent evaluation by a neurosurgeon or orthopedic surgeon with experience in back surgery is indicated (Chou, 2016b).

Lumbar spinal stenosis (LSS) refers to an anatomic condition that includes narrowing of the intarsia (central) canal, lateral recess, and/or neural foramina. Spondylosis, or degenerative arthritis affecting the spine, is the most common cause of LSS and typically affects individuals over the age of 60 years (Hickey, 2014).

Several different surgical approaches may be used; however, this is dependent on the on the type of disease or site of injury for which surgical intervention is indicated. Types of spinal surgery are:

- *Spinal Fusion*: Spinal fusion is the most common surgery for back pain. In a spinal fusion, a surgeon joins spinal bones, called vertebrae, together. This restricts motion between the bones of the spine. Fusion also limits the stretching of nerves.
- *Laminectomy*: In a laminectomy, a surgeon removes parts of the bone, bone, or ligaments in the back. This relieves pressure on spinal nerves that may be causing pain or weakness.
  A laminectomy, however, can cause the spine to be less stable. To help prevent the spinal bones from becoming unstable, a spinal fusion may be performed. Spinal fusion can be done at the same time as laminectomy.
- *Foraminotomy*: During a foraminotomy, a surgeon cuts away bone at the sides of vertebrae to widen the space where nerve roots exit the spine. The enlarged space may relieve pressure on the nerves, thereby relieving pain.
- *Discectomy*: A bulging or "slipped" disc may press on a spinal nerve and cause back pain. In a discectomy, the surgeon removes all or part of the disc. A discectomy can be done through a large incision or through a smaller incision using tools from outside the body. A discectomy may be part of a larger surgery that includes laminectomy, foraminotomy, or spinal fusion.
- *Disc Replacement*: In artificial disc replacement, a surgeon removes a damaged spinal disc and inserts an artificial disc between the vertebrae.

Minimally invasive spine surgery (MISS) fusions and decompression procedures (such as discectomy and laminectomy) are performed with special tools called tubular retractors. During the procedure, a small incision is made and the tubular retractor is inserted through the skin and soft tissues down to the spinal column. This creates a tunnel to the small area where the problem exists in the spine. The tubular retractor holds the muscles open and is kept in place throughout the procedure. Some techniques employ lasers to vaporize parts of the disc or automated techniques for removing portions of the disc. They have the potential advantage of quicker recovery from surgery compared to standard open discectomy or microdiscectomy.

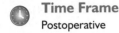

Time Frame
Postoperative

DIAGNOSTIC CLUSTER

Postoperative Period

Collaborative Problems

▲ Risk for Complications of Paralytic Ileus

▲ Risk for Complications of Neurological Sensory and Motor Impairments

▲ Risk for Complications of Cauda Equina

▲ Risk for Complications of Cerebrospinal Fluid Fistula/Pseudomeningocele

▲ Risk for Deep Vein Thrombosis/Pulmonary Embolism (refer to Risk for Complications of Deep Vein Thrombosis/Pulmonary Embolism in Unit II Section 2)

Nursing Diagnoses

▲ Acute Pain related to muscle spasms (back, thigh) secondary to nerve irritation during surgery, edema, skeletal malalignment, or bladder distention

▲ Risk for Falls related to altered mobility secondary to gait unsteadiness and lumbar instability (refer to Unit II Section 1)

▲ Risk for Ineffective Health Management related to insufficient knowledge of home care, activity restrictions, and exercise program

Related Care Plan

General Surgery Generic care plan

▲ This diagnosis was reported to be monitored for or managed frequently (75% to 100%).

Transition Criteria

Before transition, the individual or family will:

1. Describe proper wound care and techniques to prevent infection at home
2. Verbalize necessary activity precautions, including those regarding time frames for sitting, standing, no lifting, bending, or twisting
3. Lifting, and twisting restrictions. Reinforce the following: no lifting, bending, or twisting; no sitting for long periods of time
4. State signs and symptoms that must be reported to the surgeon

Transitional Risk Assessment Plan (TRAP)

Begin this plan on admission.
Implement the Transitional Risk Assessment Plan (TRAP):
• Refer to inside back cover.
• Add each validated risk diagnosis to individual's problem list with the risk code in ( ).
• Refer to the individual risk nursing diagnoses/collaborative problems for outcomes and interventions in Unit II.

R: "Close coordination of care in the post-acute period, early transition follow-up care, enhanced client education and self-management training, proactive end-of-life counseling, and extending the resources and clinical expertise over time via multidisciplinary team management" can lower readmission rates and improve health outcomes (Boutwell & Hwu, 2009, p. 14). Interventions are utilized to activate the individual and family to select changes in their everyday lifestyle choices to improve their health (Hibbard & Greene, 2013).

Collaborative Problems

Risk for Complications of Neurological Sensory and/or Motor Impairment

Risk for Complications of Cauda Equina

Risk for Complications of Paralytic Ileus

Risk for Complications of Cerebrospinal Fluid Fistula/Pseudomeningocele

Collaborative Outcomes

The individual will be monitored for early signs and symptoms of (a) sensory and/or motor impairment, (b) urinary retention, (c) paralytic ileus, and (d) cerebrospinal fistula and collaboratively intervene to stabilize the individual.

Indicators of Physiologic Stability

- Motor function equal and intact (a)
- Sensory function equal and intact (a)
- Strength equal and intact (a)
- Urinary output >0.5 mL/kg/hr (a, b)
- Can verbalize bladder fullness (a, b)
- No complaints of lower abdominal pain (a, b)
- Bowel sounds present and all quadrants (c)
- Reports flatus (c)
- Bowel movement by third day (c)
- Minimal or no drainage (d)
- Negative glucose test of drainage (d)
- No complaints of headache (d)

> **CLINICAL ALERT:**
> - The complication incidence for prospective thoracolumbar studies is (20.4%) Medical comorbidities, advanced individual age, and body mass index can contribute to complication incidence.

Interventions	Rationales
1. Monitor symmetry of sensory and motor function in extremities (Hickey, 2014): a. To touch, light pin scratch b. Strength (have the individual push your hands away with his or her soles, then pull his or her feet up against resistance) c. Compare findings from right side to left side and preoperative baseline	1. Cord or nerve root edema, pressure on a nerve root from herniated disc fragments, or hematoma at the operative site can cause or exacerbate deficits in motor and sensory functions postoperatively. Surgical manipulation can result in nerve damage causing paresthesias, paralysis, and possibly respiratory insufficiency (Hickey, 2014).

(continued)

Interventions	Rationales
2. Monitor for (Duncan & Bailey, 2011; Hickey, 2014) ability to sense bladder fullness perineal numbness, urinary retention or incontinence, progressive motor weakness and progressively decreasing sensation in the lower extremities	2. The cauda equina is a collection of dorsal and ventral lumbar and sacral nerve roots, typically L1–L5 and S1. Cauda equina syndrome (CES) is usually characterized as an acute compressive neuropathy with a symptom complex that commonly presents as perineal (saddle) numbness, urinary retention or incontinence, and bilateral leg pain and weakness, typically after lumbar disc herniation. The incidence of postoperative urinary retention is 8%. Of those 2.8% accounts for cauda equina syndrome (Duncan & Bailey, 2011).
3. If possible, stand a male individual 8 to 12 hours after surgery to void (mobilize as soon as possible either by nursing staff or physical therapy)	3. Urination, especially when the individual lies flat, may be owing to difficulty voiding in a horizontal position, the depressant effects of perioperative drugs, or sympathetic fiber stimulation during surgery (Hickey, 2014).

4. Monitor bowel function:
  a. Bowel sounds in all quadrants returning within 24 hours of surgery
  b. Flatus and defecation resuming by the second or third postoperative day
	4. Surgery on the lumbosacral spine decreases innervation of the bowels, reducing peristalsis and possibly leading to transient paralytic ileus.

5. Monitor for signs and symptoms of cerebrospinal fluid fistula and pseudomeningocele (Kalfas, Lobo, & McCormack, 2012):
  a. A watery discharge is assumed to be CSF, particularly if leakage is augmented by upright posture or Valsalva maneuver or is associated with postural headaches.
    Or
  If the leaking fluid produces a clear halo that surrounds a central pink stain on an absorbent surface (e.g., sheets or cotton gauze), the fluid is most likely CSF. If the leaking fluid produces a clear halo that surrounds a central pink stain on an absorbent surface (e.g., sheets or cotton gauze), the fluid is most likely CSF.
  b. Severe headache, which becomes worse when sitting up and gets better while lying down, light sensitivity, nausea, and complaints of neck stiffness.
Report findings to surgeon at once.
	5. Cerebrospinal fluid (CSF) fistulas and pseudomeningoceles are relatively rare complications of spine surgery. CSF leakage that occurs after satisfactory wound healing can lead to the development of a pseudomeningocele in the paraspinal tissues. Incomplete closure of the dura causes CSF drainage (Kalfas et al., 2012).

6. Monitor and report incisional dressing for drainage. Note color, consistency, odor, and amount and notate if erythema or edema is present. If incision appears to be unapproximated, suspect wound dehiscence. Report immediately.	6. Drainage should be minimal and if drainage does occur, suspect cerebrospinal fluid leakage.

Documentation

Vital signs (hemodynamics, neurologic, and neurovascular)
Intake and output (strict)
Circulation (color, peripheral pulses)
Neurologic sensory and motor status (reflexes, sensory, and motor function)
Bowel function (bowel sounds, defecation)
Wound condition (color, drainage, swelling, amount of drainage, if any)
Changes in status
Worsening pain

Nursing Diagnoses

Acute Pain Related to Muscle Spasms (Back or Thigh) Secondary to Nerve Irritation During Surgery, Edema, Skeletal Misalignment, or Bladder Distention

NOC
Comfort Level, Pain Control

Goal

The individual will report progressive pain reduction and/or alleviation after pain relief interventions.

NIC
Pain Management, Medication Management, Emotional Support, Teaching: Individual, Heat/Cold Application, Simple Massage

Indicators

- Describe and/or demonstrate pharmacologic and nonpharmacologic techniques to reduce pain.
- Report movements to avoid, ensuring that the individual and family understand the limitations and expectations required postsurgery.

Interventions	Rationales
1. Ask to rate pain from 0 to 10 before and after medication administration. Consult with the physician/nurse practitioner/physical assistant if relief is unsatisfactory. Also, be sure to observe for visual cues and facial expressions showing that the individual appears to be in pain. Unsatisfactory pain relief will deter movement in bed and early mobilization.	1. An objective rating scale can help to evaluate the subjective experience of pain. Pain management is critical to prevent immobility which can cause thrombus formation, pneumonia, and pressure ulcers.
2. Teach the importance of complying with the brace regimen.	2. Wearing a brace can prevent future hardware failure and pseudarthrosis. Individuals should mobilize quickly unless ordered differently owing to complication (e.g., CSF leak).
3. Evaluate if brace fits properly and is correctly aligned.	3. Mobilizing devices can cause sustained pressure on tissues leading to ischemia and tissue necrosis.
4. Instruct and help to roll to side and bring legs down while simultaneously rising up with the torso from the bed. Teach the individual to use arms and legs to transfer weight properly when getting out of bed.	4. This minimizes twisting at the waist. Instruct and help individual to rise from a chair using the legs, rather than pushing off with the back. Using the stronger muscles of the arms and legs can reduce strain on the back.
5. Encourage walking, standing, and sitting for short periods from the first postoperative day or as soon as possible after surgery, ensuring that the individual understands that the nurse or physical therapist will ambulate him or her the first time and continue to do so until he or she is deemed at low risk for falls. Assess carefully in the first few days after surgery to ensure proper use of body mechanics and to detect any gait or posture problems.	5. Activity goals depend on the individual's pain level and functional ability. Gait or posture problems can contribute to pain on walking, standing, or sitting. Ensure that the individual is wearing brace, if prescribed.
6. Teach the individual the following precautions to maintain proper body alignment (Hickey, 2014). a. Use the log-rolling technique to turn and reposition in bed. (Refer to the nursing diagnosis Risk for Injury in this care plan for details.) b. Avoid stress or strain on the operative site. c. Use the side-lying position in bed with the legs bent up evenly and the abdomen and back supported by pillows. d. Teach the individual to keep her or his spine straight and when on side to place a pillow between the legs. Place pillow to support upper arm as well and to prevent the shoulder from sagging.	6. Proper body alignment avoids tension on the operative site and reduces spasms. Techniques are taught to keep the lower spine as flat as possible and prevent twisting, flexing, or hyperextending (Hickey, 2014).

(continued)

Interventions	Rationales

    e. Sit with knees higher than hips.
    f. When standing, regularly shift weight bearing from one foot to the other.

7. Refer to the General Surgery Care Plan for general pain-relief techniques.

Documentation

Type, dose, route, frequency of all medications

Pain scale reassessment (30 minutes after narcotics have been administered, reassess pain level and 1 hour for all others)

Activity level

Individual's response to pain medication

Risk for Ineffective Health Management Related to Insufficient Knowledge of Home Care, Activity Restrictions, and Exercise Program

NOC

Compliance Behavior, Knowledge: Treatment Regimen, Participation: Health Care Decisions

Goals

The goals for this diagnosis represent those associated with transition planning. Refer to the transition criteria.

NIC

Anticipatory Guidance, Learning Facilitation, Risk Management, Health Education, Teaching: Procedure/Treatment, Health System Guidance

Interventions	Rationales
1. Teach the individual the proper use of a back brace, if indicated.	1. The decision whether to use a brace and the type of brace used varies widely. The decision is dependent on the surgery performed, bone quality, and physician preference. If braces are ordered, the individual should be given specific guidelines regarding use (American Association of Neuroscience Nurses, 2015).

2. Teach recovery precautions, such as the following:
  a. Sleeping on a firm mattress
  b. Maintaining proper body mechanics
  c. Wearing only moderately high-heeled shoes
  d. Sitting in a straight-backed chair with feet on a stool and knees flexed slightly higher than the hips
  e. For at least 3 weeks postsurgery, limit sitting time to 15 to 20 minutes
	2. Techniques that reduce stress and strain on the lumbosacral spine can decrease spasms and help to prevent disruption of surgical site and hardware.

3. Review activity restrictions and exercise program (American Association of Neuroscience Nurses, 2015): a. Avoid heavy lifting (anything heavier than a gallon of milk) for the first 4 to 6 weeks.	

Interventions	Rationales
b. Reinforce alternative planning and problem solving for everyday activities (e.g., vacuuming, doing laundry, and performing child care). c. Avoid prolonged sitting or standing for the first 4 to 6 weeks, including long car trips. d. Individual should begin a walking program that includes progressively longer distances two to three times/day. e. Continue an exercise program prescribed by the physical therapist.	3. It is important to stress limitations. For example, individuals with small children will not be able to lift them. Activities, such as loading the dishwasher and dryer, which require considerable bending, and vacuuming, which requires twisting, will not be possible. It is recommended that an individual have a caregiver attending to them for a minimum of 24 to 36 hours after discharge. Activity will improve pain tolerance and decrease muscle spasms (American Association of Neuroscience Nurses, 2015).
4. Review incision care. Refer to Generic Surgical Care Plan in Unit III Section 2.	
5. Teach to monitor for warning signs of possible blood clots including the following (American Academy of Orthopaedic Surgeons, 2016): a. Swelling in the calf, ankle, or foot b. Tenderness or redness, which may extend above or below the knee c. Pain in the calf d. Warning signs of pulmonary embolism and call 911 if they occur e. Sudden chest pain f. Shortness of breath	5. These signs and symptoms may represent a venous thrombosis. These complications are most likely to occur during the first few weeks after surgery.
6. Teach to monitor incision site for signs of infection (American Academy of Orthopaedic Surgeons, 2016): a. Redness, tenderness, and swelling around the wound edges b. Drainage from the wound c. Increased pain or tenderness d. Shaking chills e. Elevated temperature, usually above 100° F if taken with an oral thermometer If these signs/symptoms of infection occur call the surgeon immediately.	
7. Ensure appointments are scheduled for home assessments (nursing, physical therapy, occupational therapy, social services) and surgeon.	7. For follow-up for any hospitalization, appointment-keeping behavior is enhanced when the inpatient team schedules outpatient medical follow-up before transition. Ideally, the inpatient care providers or case managers/transition planners will schedule follow-up visit(s) with the appropriate professionals, including primary care provider and surgeon (Barnsteiner, Disch, & Walton, 2014).
8. Initiate a discussion regarding a healthier lifestyle to prevent cardiovascular, pulmonary, and musculoskeletal complications. Emphasize the damaging effects of: a. Overweight/obesity on multiple body systems and occurrence of chronic diseases (e.g., diabetes mellitus). Refer to thePoint for a printout of "Getting Started to a healthy weight." b. Sedentary life style. Refer to thePoint for a printout of "Getting Started to moving more." c. Tobacco use. Refer to "Getting Started to Stop Smoking."	8. Motivation to improve a unhealthy lifestyle is often increased when individuals are experiencing a health problem, acutely (Barnsteiner et al., 2014).

> ***Clinical Alert Report***
>
> Before providing care, advise ancillary staff/student to report the following to the professional nurse assigned to the individual:
> - Vital signs (heart rate, temperature, respirations, and blood pressure)
> - Intake and output
> - Drain output
> - Decreased sensation in lower extremities, or any neurologic changes
> - Complaints of pain or discomfort

Documentation

Individual/family teaching

Thoracic Surgery

Thoracic surgery encompasses the operative, perioperative, and surgical critical care of individuals with acquired and congenital pathologic conditions within the chest. Included are the surgical repair of congenital and acquired conditions of the heart, including the pericardium, coronary arteries, valves, great vessels, and myocardium. It also includes pathologic conditions of the lung, esophagus, and chest wall; tumors of the mediastinum; and diseases of the diaphragm and pericardium. Management of the airway and injuries to the chest are also within the scope of the specialty.

Types of thoracic surgery (traditional or minimally invasive surgery):

- *Wedge resection:* Excision of a wedge of the lung that contains the malignant tissues along with a margin of the surrounding healthy tissue. Minimally invasive surgery wedge resections are performed for non–small cell lung cancer or pulmonary metastasis; for small (less than 3 cm) peripheral masses; and for individuals who are not appropriate candidates for lobectomy (e.g., those with pulmonary hypertension and severe medical illnesses).
- *Lobectomy:* Removal of an entire lobe of a cancerous lung. Most lobectomies can be *performed* by video-assisted thoracoscopy (VATS). A lobectomy performed by VATS should be a standard, anatomic resection, just as the procedure performed through a thoracotomy. The indications for VATS lobectomy include Stage I lung cancer; a tumor less than 6 cm in diameter; and benign disease (e.g., bronchiectasis). Relative contraindications include a tumor 5 to 8 cm in diameter, preoperative irradiation or chemotherapy, sleeve resections, and chest wall invasions. Contraindications are tumors greater than 8 cm in diameter, mediastinal invasion, and surgeon discomfort.
- *Pneumonectomy*: Removal of an entire lung in order to treat cancer. A pneumonectomy can be performed by VATS, and the specimen usually fits through the same size of incision that is used for a VATS-type lobectomy, depending on the size and location of the lesion. In general, a large central tumor is not appropriate for VATS owing to involvement of the mediastinal structures. The surgeon must ensure that the tumor is not amenable to a sleeve resection, which may be difficult to determine by the VATS approach. Therefore, rarely is pneumonectomy best handled by VATS.
- *Sleeve lobectomy*: A lung resection in which a section of bronchus or trachea is removed along with diseased lung tissue after which the proximal and distal ends are anastomosed. Surgeons with excellent video skills can perform a standard sleeve lobectomy by VATS.
- *Segmentectomy*: Removal of a segment of a lobe of the lung that contains malignant tissues. Segmentectomy is an option for small, anatomically well-situated lung cancer. The creation of a segmental fissure and dissecting out the segmental vessels can be done using a thoracoscopic technique.
- Mediastinal and esophageal procedures:
  - *Mediastinoscopy*: This is an important procedure for staging lung cancer. Video-assisted mediastinoscopy has greatly improved the quality and safety of the procedure. Node dissection can be performed with the standard video mediastinoscope.
  - *Mediastinal lymph node dissection (right- and left-sided):* This is a critical part of any lung cancer procedure. Lymph node dissection should be performed for all types of cancer resections (e.g., wedge, segmentectomy, lobectomy, pneumonectomy) to ensure proper staging and for possible therapeutic benefit. No additional incisions are made for mediastinal lymph node dissection; the procedure uses the existing incisions for video-assisted lobectomy, which usually precedes node dissection.

- *Esophageal mobilization:* Mobilization of the esophagus by VATS provides the advantage of a complete cancer operation performed by minimally invasive technique. Although most VATS procedures are performed with the individual in the lateral decubitus position, the prone position offers several advantages for surgery on structures in the posterior mediastinum. For example, in the prone position, lung retraction is not needed because gravity causes the lung to fall out of the way.
- *Thymectomy:* Using the VATS approach for this procedure is an excellent technique for individuals with myasthenia gravis and small (less than 4 cm) thymomas that do not appear to invade other structures.

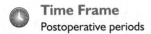 **Time Frame**
Postoperative periods

■■■ DIAGNOSTIC CLUSTER

Collaborative Problems

▲ Risk for Complications of Mediastinal Shift

▲ Risk for Complications of Subcutaneous Emphysema

▲ Risk for Complications of Acute Pulmonary Edema

▲ Risk for Complications of Arrhythmias

* Risk for Complications of Acute Lung Injury

* Risk for Complications of Bronchopleural Fistula

▲ Risk for Complications of Respiratory Insufficiency (refer to Unit II)

▲ Risk for Complications of Pulmonary Embolism (refer to Unit II)

△ Risk for Complications of Thrombophlebitis (refer to Unit II)

Nursing Diagnoses

▲ Ineffective Airway Clearance related to increased secretions and diminished cough secondary to pain and fatigue (refer to Unit II)

▲ Impaired Physical Mobility related to restricted arm and shoulder movement secondary to pain and muscle dissection and imposed position restrictions (refer to Unit II)

▲ Acute Pain related to surgical incision, chest tube sites, and immobility secondary to lengthy surgery (refer to Generic Surgical Care Plan)

Risk for Ineffective Health Management Related to Insufficient Knowledge of Activity Restrictions

Related Care Plans

Generic Surgery Care Plan

Cancer: Initial Diagnosis

Transition Criteria

Before transition, the individual or family will:

1. Describe at-home wound care.
2. Relate the need to continue exercises at home.
3. Verbalize precautions for activities.
4. State signs and symptoms that must be reported to a health-care professional.
5. Identify appropriate community resources and self-help groups.
6. Describe at-home pain management.

Transitional Risk Assessment Plan (TRAP)

Begin this plan on admission.

Implement the Transitional Risk Assessment Plan (TRAP):

* Refer to inside back cover.
* Add each validated risk diagnosis to individual's problem list with the risk code in ( ).
* Refer to the individual risk nursing diagnoses/collaborative problems for outcomes and interventions in Unit II.

  R: *"Close coordination of care in the post-acute period, early transition follow-up care, enhanced client education and self-management training, proactive end-of-life counseling, and extending the resources and clinical expertise over time via multidisciplinary team management" can lower readmission rates and improve health outcomes (Boutwell & Hwu, 2009, p. 14). Interventions are utilized to activate the individual and family to select changes in their everyday lifestyle choices to improve their health (Hibbard & Greene, 2013).*

Collaborative Problems

Risk for Complications of Acute Pulmonary Edema

Risk for Complications of Mediastinal Shift

Risk for Complications of Subcutaneous Emphysema

Risk for Complications of Arrhythmias

Risk for Complications of Acute Lung Injury

Risk for Complications of Bronchopleural Fistula

Collaborative Outcomes

The individual will be monitored for early signs and symptoms of (a) increased pneumothorax, (b) pulmonary edema, (c) mediastinal shift, (d) subcutaneous emphysema, and (e) arrhythmias and will receive collaborative interventions if indicated to restore physiologic stability.

Indicators of Physiologic Stability

* Respirations 16 to 20 breaths/min (a, b, c)
* Symmetrical, easy, rhythmic respirations (a, b, c)
* Breath sounds all lobes (a, b, c)
* No crackles or wheezing (a, b, c)
* Capillary refill <3 seconds (a, b, c)
* Oxygen saturation (Pao_2) >94% (a, b, c)
* pH 7.35 to 7.45 (a, b, c)
* Carbon dioxide ($Paco_2$) 35 to 45 mm Hg (a, b, c)
* Pulse 60 to 100 beats/min (a, b, c)
* BP >90/60, <140/90 mm Hg (a, b, c)
* Peripheral pulses equal full (a, b, c)
* Normal electrocardiogram (e)
* Larynx/trachea midline (c)
* No neck vein distention (c)
* Minimal subcutaneous air (d)

Carp's Cues

Please refer to the Generic Care Plan for the Surgical Client for detailed interventions for managing all surgical conditions. This care plan addresses specific additional interventions associated with the type of surgery performed.

Interventions	Rationales

> **CLINICAL ALERT:**
> • Thoracic surgery impairs postoperative respiratory function resulting in a relatively high risk of developing postoperative pulmonary complications (PPCs). The major respiratory complications are atelectasis, pneumonia, and respiratory failure. The most frequent risk factors include age, preoperative pulmonary function tests, cardiovascular comorbidity, smoking status, and chronic obstructive pulmonary disease (COPD). Individuals undergoing thoracic surgery are usually high-risk individuals with poor baseline pulmonary function (Agostini et al., 2010; Sengupta, 2015).

1. Follow institution protocols for chest drainage systems.

2. Assess chest tube function and insertion site every 2 hours:
   a. Evidence of bleeding
   b. Intact occlusive dressing

   c. Correct position of chest tubes
   d. Evidence of subcutaneous emphysema
   e. Presence of air leaks (expected or new onset)

2a. Recent bleeding can be detected early.
   b. An occlusive dressing is needed to prevent air from entering pleural space.
   c. Improper positioning of tubes can increase air and drainage in pleural space.
   e. An air leak is not uncommon immediately after tube placement.
      • Indicates that the lung has not fully reexpanded or that there is a leak in the system.
      • To prevent air leaks in the tubing or drainage system, ensure all connections are secure.
      • All new leaks should be investigated.

3. Document amount, consistency, and color of chest tube drainage every hour according to protocol. Notify the surgeon if drainage increases. Color and consistency of drainage in the chamber may be mixed and not appear accurately; assess drainage in the tubing for changes.

3. Increased drainage can indicate bleeding; no drainage can indicate a nonpatent tube that can cause an increase in intrapleural pressure.

4. Position:
   a. After lobectomy, turn the individual onto the NON-OPERATIVE side.
   b. After pneumonectomy, position supine or on the OPERATIVE side.
      • Promotes incision splinting and deep breathing
      • Positioning on the unaffected side can result in drainage of secretions to the unaffected lung

4a. This position will increase blood flow and oxygen to surgical area
   b. This position promotes drainage and inflation of the remaining lung.

5. Range of motion (ROM) to shoulder on operative side

6. Before removal of chest tubes (3 to 4 days post-op), assess for absence of chest tube drainage, no tidaling with respirations, and breath sounds in affected area (*Coughlin & Parchinsky, 2006).

6. These clinical findings indicate lung reexpansion.

7. Provide pain medication ½ to 1 hour before removal.

7. This reduces the pain during chest tube removal.

8. Chest tube dressing (American Association of Colleges of Nursing [AACN], 2015):
   a. Do not routinely change dressing unless it is compromised or a change in the individual's condition requires assessment of the wound.

8. Knots exposed to petroleum failed at significantly higher rate (Muffly et al., 2012).

Interventions	Rationales
b. Use a dry, sterile dressing. Avoid petroleum dressings. c. Secure the dressing with wide paper tape.	
9. Position tubing and use physics and gravity to facilitate fluid drainage. Avoid dependent loops (AACN, 2015; *Schmelz, Johnson, Norton, Andrews, Gordon, 1999).	9. Dependent loop can change pleural pressure from –18 cmH$_2$O to +8 cmH$_2$O and decrease fluid drained to zero in less than 30 minutes (AACN, 2015; *Schmelz et al., 1999).
10. Consult with surgeon regarding use of suction device.	10. In routine cases, chest tube duration and length of stay significantly reduced with minimal or no suction (i.e., gravity drainage) (AACN, 2014; Coughlin & Emmerton-Coughlin, 2012; Deng, Tan, Zhao, Wang, & Jiang, 2010; Morales, Mejia, Roldan, Saldarriaga, Duque, 2014). Without suction, the individual is not tethered to the wall; ambulation contributes to quicker recovery. Even when chest drain measures are equivalent, overall care favors gravity to allow ambulation.
11. Do not strip or milk chest tubes (AACN, 2015).	11. Stripping produces dangerously high pressures (–400 cmH$_2$O g) (*Duncan & Erickson, 1982).
12. Discuss the plan for chest tube removal (AACN, 2015).	12. Being aggressive with tube removal reduces length of stay and complications related to hospitalization. Chest tube duration is directly related to risk of hospital-acquired infection (Oldfield, El-Masri, & Fox-Wasylyshyn, 2009).
13. After tube removal, evaluate respiratory status: no distress, breath sounds present in all lobes, even chest movement, calm, and no arrhythmias instruct to: a. To use a spirometer at least 10 breaths an hour • Sit up as much as possible • Breathe in slowly and as deeply as possible • Breathe normally for a few breaths b. After using the spirometer, to cough properly. Instruct how to cough. Hold pillow to incision, apply gentle pressure, and cough.	13. Complications after tube removal can be pneumothorax, hemothorax, or mediastinal shift. Early detection in respiratory or cardiac function can prevent serious complications. a. Frequent use of spirometer increases lung volumes and prevents pneumonia.
14. Monitor vital signs, pulse oximetry, respiratory function (rate, rhythm, capillary refill, breath sounds, skin color) according to protocol.	14. Frequent respiratory assessments are needed to evaluate early signs and symptoms of atelectasis, pneumothorax, and hemothorax.
15. Provide oxygen as prescribed and position the individual in semi-Fowler's or full Fowler's.	15. The semi-Fowler's position aids in lung expansion. Oxygen may be needed until lungs are fully expanded.
16. Monitor for signs of acute pulmonary edema (severe dyspnea, tachycardia, adventitious breath sounds, persistent cough).	16. Circulatory overload can result from the reduced size of the pulmonary vascular bed caused by removal of pulmonary tissue and the yet-unexpanded lung postoperatively. Hypoxia produces increased capillary permeability, causing fluid to enter pulmonary tissue and triggering signs and symptoms.
17. Cautiously administer IV fluids as prescribed.	17. Caution is needed to prevent circulatory overload.
18. Monitor for signs of mediastinal shift: increased weak, irregular pulse rate, severe dyspnea, cyanosis, hypoxia, increased restlessness and agitation, deviation of larynx or trachea from midline, shift in the point of apical impulse, asymmetric chest excursion.	18. These changes in pressure provide a space for the contents of the mediastinum (heart, trachea, esophagus, pulmonary vessels) to shift. Constriction of vessels (aorta, vena cava) creates hypoxia and its resultant signs and symptoms (Sengupta, 2015).

CLINICAL ALERT:
• Activate Rapid Response Team.

Interventions	Rationales
19. If signs and symptoms of a mediastinal shift occur, do the following: a. Position the individual in a semi-Fowler's position. b. Maintain oxygen therapy.	19a. Sitting upright reduces mediastinal shifting. b. Oxygen therapy reduces hypoxia.

20. Monitor for signs of pneumothorax not resolving (Grossman & Porth, 2014):
a. Hypoxia/decreased cardiac output
 	
  • Increased heart rate and respiratory rate
  • Reduced or absent breath sounds in affected area
  • Jugular neck vein distention (decreased cardiac output)
  • Increasing dyspnea
  • Chest pain (pleuritic), usually increasing with respiratory effort
  • Air trapped in pleural space with displacement of respiratory structures.
  • Reduced chest wall movement on affected side
  • Asymmetry of chest
  • Clinical signs of mediastinal shift (e.g., tracheal deviation, subcutaneous emphysema (air in subcutaneous tissues of chest and neck)
	20. Pneumothorax is an expected outcome of surgery on the lung. Postoperatively, monitoring is focused on the pneumothorax resolving via chest tube use (Sengupta, 2015).
	a. Signs and symptoms result from air trapped in pleural cavity, hypoxia, and decreased cardiac output (Grossman & Porth, 2014).
	  • Subcutaneous emphysema can occur after thoracic surgery as air leaks out of incised pulmonary tissue.

> **CLINICAL ALERT:**
> • Activate Rapid Response Team.

Interventions	Rationales
21. Stay with individual and explain the situation and the treatments to expect.	21. Acute dyspnea is terrifying as is fear of the unknown.
22. Ensure appointments are scheduled for home assessments (nursing, physical therapy, occupational therapy, social services) (American Academy of Orthopaedic Surgeons, 2014).	
23. Ensure that supplies/prescriptions are provided as: a. Insulin (vials or pens), if needed b. Syringes or pen needles, if needed c. Oral medications, if needed d. Blood glucose meter and strips e. Lancets and lancing devices f. Urine ketone strips (type 1 diabetes) g. Glucagon emergency kit (insulin-treated individuals) h. Medical alert application/charms	

Clinical Alert Report

Before providing care, advise ancillary staff/student to report the following to the professional nurse assigned to the individual:
• Change in cognitive status
• New-onset chest pain or shortness of breath
• Oral temperature >100.5° F
• Systolic BP <90 mm Hg
• Resting pulse >100, <50
• Respiratory rate >28, <10/min
• Oxygen saturation <90%

Documentation

Vital signs
Intake and output records
Chest tube drainage (description, amount)

Nursing Diagnoses

Impaired Physical Mobility Related to Restricted Arm and Shoulder Movement Secondary to Pain and Muscle Dissection and Imposed Position Restrictions

NOC

Ambulation: Walking,
Joint Movement: Active,
Mobility Level

Goal

The individual will return or progress to preoperative arm and shoulder function.

NIC

Exercise Therapy:
Joint Mobility, Exercise
Promotion: Strength
Training, Exercise Therapy:
Ambulation, Positioning,
Teaching: Prescribed
Activity/Exercise

Indicators

- Demonstrate knowledge of the need to maintain certain positions.
- Demonstrate ROM exercises.

Interventions	Rationales
CLINICAL ALERT: • Thoracotomy can also lead to long-term restriction of shoulder function and ROM, reduced muscle strength, chronic pain, and reduced health-related quality of life (Reeve et al., 2010).	
1. Proceed with post-op protocol/consult with a physical therapist for early and frequent position changes in bed, sitting out of bed from the first postoperative day, early ambulation, and frequent pain assessment.	1. Postoperative pulmonary complications are a major cause of morbidity after thoracotomy, resulting in discomfort, prolonged length of hospital stay, and increased health care costs (Reeve et al., 2010). Reeve et al. (2010) reported "A physiotherapist-directed postoperative exercise program resulted in significant benefits in pain and shoulder function at discharge and at 3 months over usual care for individuals following open thoracotomy."
2. Explain the need for frequent position changes every 1 to 2 hours. Gently turn the individual: a. After lobectomy, turn the individual onto the NON-OPERATIVE side. b. After pneumonectomy, position supine or on the OPERATIVE side.	2. Turning mobilizes drainage of secretions, promotes circulation, inhibits thrombus formation, and aerates all parts of the remaining lung tissue. Lying on the operative side can be contraindicated after a wedge resection and pneumonectomy.
3. ROM to shoulder on operative side. Explain the need for frequent exercises of arms, shoulders, and trunk, even in the presence of some pain and discomfort.	3. The muscle groups transcended by a thoracotomy form the shoulder girdle and maintain the trunk's posture. Failure to perform exercises can result in muscle adhesions, contractures, and postural deformities. Active ROM exercises help to prevent adhesions of two incised muscle layers.
4. Initiate passive ROM exercises on the operative arm and shoulder within 4 hours per protocol after recovery from anesthesia. Begin with two times every 4 hours for the first 24 hours; progress to 10 to 20 times every 2 hours.	4. Reluctance to move the shoulder will cause "frozen shoulder" or adhesive capsulitis, which is a condition cause by immobility after a surgical intervention.
5. Encourage use of the affected arm in ADLs and stress the need to continue exercises at home.	5. Regular use increases ROM and decreases contractures.

Documentation

Limitations on performing activities
Frequency of therapeutic exercises performed
Turning, positioning, ambulation
Individual/family teaching

> **TRANSITION TO HOME/COMMUNITY CARE**
>
> If indicated, review the risk diagnoses identified for this individual on admission:
> * Is the person still at risk?
> * Can the family reduce the risks?
> * Is the person at higher risk at home?
> * Is a Home Health Nurse assessment needed?
> * Refer to transition planner/case manager/social service
> * When is this person scheduled for follow-up with primary provider? Specialists? Record dates of appointments.
> * Complete a medication reconciliation before transition. Refer to index.

STAR

Stop

Think Is this person at high risk for injury, falls, medical complications, and/or inability to care for self (activities of daily living)?

Is there a support person available?

Is the person competent to manage self-administration of medications, treatment procedures? Are additional resources needed?

Can the person explain how to monitor the condition (e.g., blood glucose, signs/symptoms of complications, dietary/mobility restrictions, and when to call his or her primary provider or specialist)?

Act Contact or provide the appropriate resource (e.g., contacting a support person, home health assessment, additional teaching, printed materials).

Review Has the problem been addressed? If not, use SBAR to communicate to the appropriate person.

Risk for Ineffective Health Therapeutic Regimen Management Related to Insufficient Knowledge of Activity Restrictions, Wound Care, Shoulder Exercises, Signs and Symptoms of Complications, and Follow-Up Care

NOC

Adherence Behavior, Knowledge: Treatment Regimen, Participation: Health Care Decisions, Treatment Behavior: Illness or Injury

NIC

Anticipatory Guidance, Risk Identification, Health Education, Learning Facilitation

Goals

The goals for this diagnosis represent those associated with transition planning. Refer to the transition criteria.

Interventions	Rationales

1. Instruct on activity/exercises:
  a. Walk every day. During inclement weather, walk indoors. Walk 3 to 4 times each day.
  b. Use your incentive spirometer 10 times every couple of hours (i.e., shopping mall, gymnasium, or at home). Explain they will tire easily at first, but to up strength and energy daily walking is required.
	1a. Walking is an excellent activity for increasing stamina.

(continued)

Interventions	*Rationales*
c. Instruct to breathe when especially lifting. Don't hold your breath. Breathe out when the work is hardest.	c. The deep breathing improves lung function and helps prevent postoperative complications with lung congestion.
d. Do ROM arm and shoulder exercises with your arms 10 times each 2 to 3 times daily for 3 weeks on the side where the thoracotomy incision was made. Advise may be helpful to do these in the shower, since warm water will loosen muscles.	d. It takes about three months for complete healing of your incision, muscles, and ribs. Do not lift more than 20 lb during this time. Active ROM exercises help to prevent adhesions of two incised muscle layers.
2. Advise to: a. Avoid crowds and bronchial irritants (smoke, fumes, aerosol sprays). b. Do not soak in a bathtub or hot tub or go swimming until evaluation by surgeon. c. Splinting with coughing (hold a pillow tight against the chest when coughing).	2. After major surgery, individuals should avoid exposure to possible sources of infection. c. Splinting will support the injured muscles reduce stretching and pain.
3. Explain wound care and engage a family member in the activity: a. Showering daily. Wash the incision and chest tube site(s) with soap and water. No dressing is necessary unless there is drainage. Do not apply ointments or cream directly on the incision unless instructed.	
4. Instruct to call the surgeon if any of the following occur: a. Increased drainage or change in color of drainage from your wound site b. Increased redness, swelling at the wound site c. Fever of 101.5° F or 38.5° C (or higher) d. Nausea, vomiting e. Pain that is not well controlled	4. These signs and symptoms can indicate infection, bleeding, and/or respiratory insufficiency.
5. Instruct to seek immediate emergency care or call 911 if: a. New-onset or increasing chest pain b. Increasing or severe shortness of breath when you can resume your usual act c. Cold, moist, and/or bluish-color skin	5. These signs and symptoms may indicate pulmonary embolism.
6. Initiate a discussion regarding tobacco use or exposure to second-hand smoke. a. Determine how important they think the behavior change is. Have they tried quitting? How long? Advise to access online sites for quitting, which are written by those who are successful. Refer to Getting Started to Quit Smoking on thePoint. Print and give to them. b. Diet high in fat or sodium. Refer to Getting Started to Better Nutrition on thePoint. Print and give to individual.	
7. Ensure appointments are scheduled for home assessments (nursing, physical therapy, occupational therapy, social services)	
8. Ensure that supplies/prescriptions are provided as (e.g., spirometer, dressing supplies)	8. Confirmations that supplies/prescriptions/follow-up appointments have been addressed and confirmed can reduce complications and readmission posttransition (Barnsteiner, Disch, & Walton, 2014).

Documentation

Individual/family teaching
Referrals (e.g., PT)
Exercises taught

Total Joint Replacement (Hip, Knee, Shoulder)

Joint replacement (arthroplasty) is the surgical replacement of all or part of a joint. This surgery is indicated for irreversibly damaged joints caused by osteoarthritis or rheumatoid arthritis, fractures of hip or femoral neck with avascular necrosis, trauma, and congenital deformity. Osteoarthritis remains the most common cause of arthroplasty. It is estimated that more than 300,000 total hip arthroplasties (THAs) are performed each year in the United States alone. More than 90% of THA individuals are working successfully, are pain-free, and are without complication 10 to 15 years postoperatively (Beswick, Wylde, Gooberman-Hill, Blom, & Dieppe, 2012). For hip replacements, a ball and socket prosthesis is implanted, either with cement or uncemented. Uncemented prostheses have porous surfaces that allow the individual's bone to grow into and stabilize the prosthesis.

For knee joint replacements, the prosthesis is tricompartmental, with femoral, tibial, and patellar components. As with hip prostheses, the knee prosthesis can be cemented or uncemented. Cemented fixation reduces blood loss because the cement seals open bone edges; it is therefore the most common fixation technique (American Association of Orthopedic Surgeons, 2016). Knee and hip arthroplasty can now be done with minimally invasive and small-incision techniques. These techniques reduce postoperative pain, length of hospital stay, rehabilitation requirements, and complications (American Association of Orthopedic Surgeons, 2016). Individuals are able to return to usual activities faster with fewer complications. The American Academy of Orthopaedic Surgeons (2016) reports more than 90% of modern total knee replacements are still functioning well 15 years after the surgery.

 Time Frame
Postoperative periods

■■■■■ DIAGNOSTIC CLUSTER

Postoperative Period

Collaborative Problems

▲ Risk for Complications of Hemorrhage/Hematoma Formation

▲ Risk for Complications of Dislocation/Subluxation of Joint

▲ Risk for Complications of Neurovascular Compromise (refer to Unit II)

▲ Risk for Complications of Fat Emboli (refer to Unit II)

▲ Risk for Complications of Sepsis/SIRS (refer to Unit II)

▲ Risk for Complications of Thromboemboli (refer to Unit II)

Nursing Diagnoses

▲ Impaired Physical Mobility related to pain, stiffness, fatigue, restrictive equipment, and prescribed activity restrictions (refer to Unit II)

▲ Risk for Impaired Skin Integrity related to pressure and decreased mobility secondary to pain and temporary restrictions (refer to Unit II)

▲ Risk for Injury related to altered gait and use of assistive devices (refer to Unit II)

Δ Risk for Ineffective Health Management related to insufficient knowledge of activity restrictions, use of assistive devices, signs of complications, and follow-up care (refer to Unit II)

(continued)

Related Care Plans
General Surgery Generic Care Plan
Anticoagulant Therapy
Amputation

Transition Criteria

Before transition, the individual and family will:

1. Describe activity restrictions.
2. Describe a plan for resuming ADLs.
3. Regain mobility while adhering to weight-bearing restrictions with the goal to ambulate without assistive devices within 6 weeks after surgery.
4. State signs and symptoms that must be reported to a health care professional.

> **Transitional Risk Assessment Plan (TRAP)**
>
> Begin this plan on admission.
> Implement the Transitional Risk Assessment Plan (TRAP):
> * Refer to inside back cover.
> * Add each validated risk diagnosis to individual's problem list with the risk code in ( ).
> * Refer to the individual risk nursing diagnoses/collaborative problems for outcomes and interventions in Unit II.
>
> > *R: "Close coordination of care in the post-acute period, early transition follow-up care, enhanced client education and self-management training, proactive end-of-life counseling, and extending the resources and clinical expertise over time via multidisciplinary team management" can lower readmission rates and improve health outcomes (Boutwell & Hwu, 2009, p. 14). Interventions are utilized to activate the individual and family to select changes in their everyday lifestyle choices to improve their health (Hibbard & Greene, 2013).*

Collaborative Problems

Risk for Complications of Hemorrhage/Hematoma

Risk for Complications of Dislocation of Joint (Hip, Knee)

Risk for Complications of Neurovascular Compromise

Collaborative Outcomes

The individual will be monitored for early signs and symptoms of (a) hemorrhage/hematoma, (b) dislocation (hip, knee), and (c) neurovascular compromise and will receive collaborative interventions if indicated to restore physiologic stability.

Indicators of Physiologic Stability

* Pulse 60 to 100 beats/min (a)
* Respirations 16 to 20 breaths/min (a)
* BP >90/60, <140/90 mm Hg (a)
* Capillary refill <3 seconds (a, c)
* Peripheral pulses full, bilateral (a, c)
* Warm, dry skin, no blanching (a, c)
* Urine output >0.5 mL/kg/hr (a)
* Hip in abduction or neutral rotation (b)
* Leg length even (b)
* Knee in neutral position (b)
* No complaints of tingling, numbness (c)

- Ability to move toes (c)
- Hemoglobin (a)
  - Male 13 to 18 g/dL
  - Female 12 to 16 g/dL
- Hematocrit (a)
  - Male 42% to 50%
  - Female 40% to 48%
- If on anticoagulant therapy:
- Partial thromboplastin time 1.5× control (a)
- Prothrombin time 1.5 to 2× normal (a)
- International normalized ratio (INR) 2 to 3 (a)

 ## Carp's Cues

Please refer to the Generic Care Plan for the Surgical Client for detailed interventions for managing all surgical conditions. This care plan addresses specific additional interventions associated with the type of surgery performed.

Interventions	Rationales
1. Identify individuals at risk for compromised wound healing: a. History of cardiac problems b. Poor nutritional status c. Obesity d. Diabetes mellitus e. History of deep vein thrombosis (DVT) or pulmonary embolism (PE) f. Blood dyscrasias g. Deconditioned state h. Older adults	1. Wound healing requires adequate stores of proteins, carbohydrates, fats, vitamins, and minerals and adequate blood flow/volume to supply nutrients and an inflammatory/immune response to initiate healing. Would healing is compromised by any condition that interferes with blood flow and oxygen transit as cardiovascular disorders, diabetes mellitus, obesity, chronic respiratory diseases, tobacco use that impairs the inflammatory/immune response needed for healing, diabetes mellitus, corticosteroid therapy (Grossman & Porth, 2014). Older adults, with associated comorbidities, are most vulnerable to postoperative complications and mortality. Preoperative identification of potential complications permits development of preventative strategies (Miller, 2015).
2. Ensure appropriate prophylaxis has been initiated to prevent DVTs. Refer to Risk for Complications of Deep Vein Thrombosis to determine this individual's risk in Unit II Section 2.	
3. Monitor drainage from suction device every hour.	3. The hip is a very vascular area and the use of anticoagulants creates a risk for bleeding.
4. Maintain pressure dressing and ice to surgical area as ordered.	4. Pressure can reduce bleeding at site, reducing hematoma formation.
5. Monitor for early signs and symptoms of bleeding and hypoxia: increased pulse rate, increased respirations, urinary output >0.5 mL/kg/hr. Promptly report change in clinical status.	5. Early signs and symptoms of bleeding and hypoxia can prompt rapid interventions to prevent hemorrhage.
6. Maintain correct positioning: a. Hip: Maintain hip in abduction, neutral rotation, or slight external rotation. b. Hip: Avoid hip flexion more than 60 degrees. c. Knee: Keep knees apart at all times and slightly elevated from hip; avoid gatching bed under knee or placing pillows under knee (to prevent flexion contractures); pillows should be placed under calf. d. Shoulder: Wear sling as directed Only move shoulder as instructed.	6. These positions prevent dislocation. c. The risk for dislocation is higher than other joint replacement because joint is shallow and the supporting structures are not as tight as the hip joint (Clarke & Santy-Tomilinson, 2014).

(continued)

Interventions	Rationales

7. Assess for signs of joint (hip, knee) dislocation:
  a. Hip:
    • Acute groin pain in operative hip
    • Shortening of leg and in external rotation
  b. Hip, knee:
    • "Popping" sound heard by individual
    • Inability to move
    • Bulge at surgical site
	7. Until the surrounding muscles and joint capsule heal, joint dislocation may occur if positioning exceeds the limits of the prosthesis, such as when flexing or hyperextending the knee or abducting the hip more than 45 degrees.

8. Keep affected joint in a neutral position with rolls, pillows, or specified devices.	8. This maintains alignment and prevents dislocation.
9. Individual may be turned toward either side, unless contraindicated by the surgeon. Always maintain abduction pillow when turning; limit use of Fowler's position.	9. If proper positioning is maintained including the abduction pillow, the individual may safely be turned toward operative and nonoperative sides. This promotes circulation and decreases the potential for pressure ulcer formation as a result of immobility. Prolonged Fowler's position can dislocate the prosthesis (*Graul, 2002; *Salmond, 1996).

10. Monitor for signs and symptoms of neurovascular compromise; compare findings with the unaffected limb:
  a. Diminished or absent pedal pulses
 	
  b. Capillary refill time >3 seconds
 	
  c. Pallor, blanching, cyanosis, coolness of extremity
  d. These symptoms may result from nerve compression
 	
  e. Increasing pain not controlled by medication
	10a. Surgical trauma causes swelling and edema that can compromise circulation and compress nerves.
	  b. Prolonged capillary refill time points to diminished capillary perfusion.
	  c. These signs may indicate compromised circulation.
	  d. Complaints of abnormal sensations (e.g., tingling and numbness).
	  e. Tissue and nerve ischemia produce a deep, throbbing, unrelenting pain.

11. Instruct the individual to report numbness, tingling, coolness, or change in skin color.
  a. Explain positions' precautions depending on the location of surgical site.
    • Posterior precautions: No hip flexion greater than 90 degrees, no hip adduction or internal rotation beyond neutral, and none of the above motions combined.
    • Anterior precautions: No lying flat, no prone lying, no bridging and no hip external rotation.
    • Lateral precautions: The individual will likely have hip abduction restrictions.
    • Global precautions: Global precautions are most often ordered for an individual after a hip resurfacing surgery. This set of precautions is a combination of both posterior and anterior dislocation precautions. This is owing to the large incision.
	11. Early detection of neurovascular compromise enables prompt intervention to prevent serious complications.

Clinical Alert Report

Before providing care, advise ancillary staff/student to report the following to the professional nurse assigned to the individual:
- Change in cognitive status
- Oral temperature >100.5° F
- Systolic BP <90 mm Hg
- Resting pulse >100, <50

- Respiratory rate >28, <10/min
- Oxygen saturation <90%
- Urine output <0.5 mL/kg/hr
- Prolonged capillary refill time points to diminished capillary perfusion.
- Pallor, blanching, cyanosis, coolness of extremity
- Increasing pain not controlled by medication
- Complaints of new-onset leg pain, chest pain

Documentation

Vital signs
Positioning
Peripheral circulation status

TRANSITION TO HOME/COMMUNITY CARE

If indicated, review the risk diagnoses identified for this individual on admission:

- Is the person still at risk?
- Can the family reduce the risks?
- Is the person at higher risk at home?
- Is a Home Health Nurse assessment needed?
- Refer to transition planner/case manager/social service
- When is this person scheduled for follow-up with primary provider? Specialists? Record dates of appointments.
- Complete a medication reconciliation before transition. Refer to index.

STAR   **Stop**

Think   Is this person at high risk for injury, falls, medical complications, and/or inability to care for self (activities of daily living)?

Is there a support person available?

Is the person competent to manage self-administration of medications, treatment procedures? Are additional resources needed?

Can the person explain how to monitor the condition (e.g., blood glucose, signs/symptoms of complications, dietary/mobility restrictions, and when to call his or her primary provider or specialist)?

Act   Contact or provide the appropriate resource (e.g., contacting a support person, home health assessment, additional teaching, printed materials).

Review   Has the problem been addressed? If not, use SBAR to communicate to the appropriate person.

Risk for Ineffective Health Management Related to Insufficient Knowledge of Activity Restrictions, Use of Assistive Devices, Signs of Complications, and Follow-Up Care

NOC

Compliance Behavior, Knowledge: Treatment Regimen, Participation: Health-Care Decisions, Treatment Behavior: Illness or Injury

NIC

Anticipatory Guidance, Risk Identification, Health Education, Learning Facilitation

Goals

The goals for this diagnosis represent those associated with transition planning. Refer to the transition criteria.

Interventions	*Rationales*

CLINICAL ALERT:
- On first post-op day individuals and their families/caregivers are educated on correct positioning of the operative LE, hip dislocation precautions, the importance of initiating early mobility, safety, weight-bearing precautions (if indicated), details of the PT intervention plan including independent exercises, wound care, DVT prevention, and the expected discharge goals and outcomes (Brigham and Women's Hospital, 2010).

Interventions	*Rationales*

1. Explain restrictions that typically include avoiding the following:
  a. Excessive bending and lifting
  b. Crossing the legs
  c. Jogging, jumping, and kneeling
	1. Some positions are contraindicated depending on the location of the surgical site.

2. Explain the need to continue prescribed exercises at home.	2. Exercises increase muscle strength and joint mobility.
3. Teach wound care and assessment techniques.	3. Instructions are needed to prevent infection and to detect early signs of infection.
4. Reinforce and encourage the safe use of assistive devices and therapeutic aids; request return demonstration of correct use.	4. Assistive devices may be needed. Return demonstration allows nurse to evaluate proper, safe use.
5. Explain the need to continue leg exercises (5 to 10 times an hour) and use of antiembolic hose at home.	5. The risk of thrombophlebitis continues after discharge.
6. For individuals on anticoagulant therapy, advise a. The importance of continuing medications at home and why laboratory tests are needed to prevent adverse effects.	6. At the time of transition, those who are at a high risk for deep vein thrombosis (DVT) will remain on anticoagulation therapy for 4 to 6 weeks. High-risk individuals include those who have undergone bilateral THA, have a history of prior DVT, are on estrogen therapy, and have a recent history of cancer (Brigham and Women's Hospital, 2010).

7. Monitor for signs and symptoms of wound infection and to report to surgeon.
  a. Increased swelling and redness
  b. Wound separation
  c. Increased serosanguineous or purulent drainage
  d. Prolonged subnormal temperature or significantly elevated temperature
  e. Unusual pain
	7. Tissue responds to pathogen infiltration with increased blood and lymph flow (manifested by edema, redness, and increased drainage) and reduced epithelialization (marked by wound separation). Circulating pathogens trigger the hypothalamus to elevate the body temperature; certain pathogens cannot survive at higher temperatures (Grossman & Porth, 2014).

8. Instruct to seek immediate emergency care or call 911 if:
  a. New-onset or increasing chest pain
  b. Increasing or severe shortness of breath when you can resume your usual act
  c. Cold, moist, and/or bluish-color skin
	8. These can represent a pulmonary embolism, which is fatal if treatment is delayed.

9. Explain the importance of continuing therapy program at home for at least 6 to 12 months.	9. Individuals with joint replacements should not be expected to regain full function for 6 to 12 months. Range of motion (ROM) should be assessed at 6 and 12 weeks after surgery. If ROM is not at the anticipated range, then manipulation under anesthesia may be required. With knees, most individuals resume all activities and are pain-free by the 12th week (*Branson & Goldstein, 2001).

Interventions	Rationales

10. Ensure that supplies/prescriptions/equipment are provided as (American Diabetes Association, 2015):
   a. Walker/crutches
   b. Commode chair
   c. Self-care assisted devices
	10. Adaptations may be needed (e.g., commode, eliminate scatter rugs). PT will start in home initially. Confirmation that supplies/prescriptions/follow-up appointments have been addressed can reduce complications and readmission posttransition (American Diabetes Association, 2015).

11. Ensure appointments have been scheduled for primary care provider, specialists, home nursing assessment as indicated.	
12. Consult with community nursing service to prepare home and physical therapy environment for discharge.	

Documentation

Individual/family teaching

Urinary Diversions

Urinary diversions, usually called urostomies or ileal conduits (Pullen, 2007), are performed when the bladder is bypassed or removed to divert urine from the ureters to a new exit site that is usually a stoma (opening in the skin). This procedure is most commonly performed because of bladder cancer, but may be necessary owing to birth defects, neurogenic bladder dysfunction, intractable interstitial cystitis, and refractory radiation cystitis.

Urinary diversion—Removal of the bladder requires that the urinary flow be redirected, which may take one of several forms (Shariat, Bochner, & Donahue, 2015):

- A noncontinent cutaneous diversion in which the urine flows from the ureters through a segment of bowel (usually ileum, termed an ileal conduit) to the skin surface as a stoma, where it is collected in an external appliance.
- A cutaneous continent reservoir may be constructed to avoid the need for an external appliance. The individual self-catheterizes at regular intervals to empty the reservoir.
- An orthotopic neobladder may be formed from a segment of bowel and attached to the urethra, enabling the individual to void through the urethra. Continent diversions may facilitate maintenance of individual perceptions of quality of life and self-image and increase their acceptance of radical cystectomy.

"Considerable variability exists in the reported early and long-term morbidity rates after urinary diversions. Morbidity rates 30 days after surgery range between 20 and 56%, while long-term morbidity >30 days ranges from 28 to 94%" (Lee et al., 2014, p. 18). Diversion-related complications are specific to the type of diversion and are generally categorized into those involving the bowel anastomosis, those related to the type of reservoir/conduit, and those associated with the ureteroenteric anastomosis (Lee et al., 2014).

"The primary goals in selecting a urinary diversion are to provide the lowest potential for complications and the highest health-related quality of life (HRQOL), while allowing for the timely completion of chemotherapy and therapeutic goals" (Lee et al., 2014, p. 15). The decision process is complex and involves consideration of issues related to cancer stage, comorbidities, treatment needs, and individual desires related to health-related quality of life (HRQOL). Individuals should be informed that intraoperative findings may dictate a change in the planned form of urinary diversion, e.g., positive urethral margin precluding orthotopic diversion (Lee et al., 2014, p. 15).

 Time Frame
Postoperative periods

 Carp's Cues

"The presence of a stoma is associated with significant psychological morbidity, including fears of bad hygiene, limitation in social or athletic activities, and elimination of intimate relationships."

Individuals and their significant others should have had at least one session with an ostomy/wound specialist to prepare for the surgery. Individuals and their significant others are "provided with real-life experiences and encouraged to engage in frank discussions regarding odor, leakage, diet, clothing and sexuality," teaching and reinforcement will continue postoperatively.

> **CLINICAL ALERT:**
>
> Before surgery to create an orthotopic diversion, the nurse should make every attempt to have soma site selection done. "A joint statement from the American 'Society of Colon & Rectal Surgeons and the Wound Ostomy Continence Nurses Society' stating that all clients undergoing intestinal ostomy surgery should have preoperative stoma site marking by an experienced, educated, competent clinician. These position statements caution that poor stoma placement can lead to unavoidable postoperative morbidity, including pain, leakage from the pouching system, peristomal skin irritation, fitting challenges, and impaired psychological health" (American Society of Colon and Rectal Surgeons Committee Members, & Wound Ostomy Continence Nurse Society Committee Members, 2007; Butler, 2009, p. 514).
>
> "For elective procedures, stoma site marking should be performed prior to surgery with the person supine, sitting, standing and bending forward." The site must be visible to the individual, and to improve adherence skin creases, bony prominences, scars, and drain sites should be avoided.

DIAGNOSTIC CLUSTER

Preoperative Period

Risk for Impaired Tissue Integrity related to anatomical barriers to precise placement of stoma during surgery.

Postoperative Period

Collaborative Problems

△ Risk for Complications of Anastomotic urinary leakage

▲ Risk for Complications of Urinary Tract Infection/Urinary Calculi/Peritonitis

▲ Risk for Complications of Peristomal Ulceration/Herniation

▲ Risk for Complications of Stomal Necrosis, Retraction, Prolapse, Stenosis, Obstruction (continent cutaneous urinary diversions)

Nursing Diagnoses

△ Anxiety related to possible leakage from appliance (refer to Ileostomy Care Plan)

△ Risk for Disturbed Self-Concept related to effects of ostomy on body image (refer to Ileostomy Care Plan)

▲ Risk for Ineffective Health Management related to insufficient knowledge of stoma pouching procedure, colostomy irrigation, peristomal skin care, perineal wound care, and incorporation of ostomy care into activity of daily living (ADL)

△ Risk for Ineffective Health Management related to insufficient knowledge of intermittent self-catheterization of continent urostomy (refer to intermittent self-catheterization in index)

Related Care Plans

Cancer: Initial Diagnosis

Ileostomy

▲ This diagnosis was reported to be monitored for or managed frequently (75% to 100%).
△ This diagnosis was reported to be monitored for or managed often (50% to 74%).

Transition Criteria

Before transition, the individual and family will:

1. Describe postsurgery care specific to type of urinary diversion preformed.
2. Demonstrate the proper stoma pouching procedure for orthotopic diversion.

3. State measures to help maintain peristomal skin integrity.
4. Demonstrate intermittent self-catheterization if indicated.
5. Discuss strategies for incorporating wound/ostomy management into ADLs.
6. Verbalize precautions for medication use, fluid intake, and prevention of UTI and stone formation.
7. State signs and symptoms that must be reported to a health care professional.
8. Verbalize an intent to share with significant others feelings and concerns related to surgical outcomes.

Transitional Risk Assessment Plan (TRAP)

Begin this plan on admission.
Implement the Transitional Risk Assessment Plan (TRAP):
- Refer to inside back cover.
- Add each validated risk diagnosis to individual's problem list with the risk code in ( ).
- Refer to the individual risk nursing diagnoses/collaborative problems for outcomes and interventions in Unit II.

R: "Close coordination of care in the post-acute period, early transition follow-up care, enhanced client education and self-management training, proactive end-of-life counseling, and extending the resources and clinical expertise over time via multidisciplinary team management" can lower readmission rates and improve health outcomes (Boutwell & Hwu, 2009, p. 14). Interventions are utilized to activate the individual and family to select changes in their everyday lifestyle choices to improve their health (Hibbard & Greene, 2013).

Nursing Diagnosis: Preoperative Period

Risk for Impaired Tissue Integrity related to anatomical barriers to precise placement of stoma during orthotopic diversion surgery

NOC
Tissue integrity: Skin and mucous membrane (stoma)

NIC
Teaching, Surveillance

Goal

The individual will have site selection and marking of stoma placement before surgery.

Indicators

- An ostomy nurse specialist will evaluate for site selection and will mark site
- If the situation is emergent, a nurse or physician, who has expertise in site selection, should be accessed.

Interventions	Rationales
1. When it is first known that an individual may have an ostomy, access the ostomy nurse specialist.	1. The sooner the specialist is activated the more likely that the expert will be available to do the site election. Multiple studies indicate that individuals who have their stoma site marked preoperatively by a trained clinician have fewer ostomy-related complications, e.g., peristomal dermatitis (Francone, 2015; Wound, Ostomy and Continence Nurses Society, 2014).
2. When it known that the specialist will not be available for site selection, notify the health professional known for competence in site selection.	2. "Stoma site marking should be performed by an Enterostomal Nurse (ETN), Rectal Surgeon or a health care professional who has been trained in the principles of stoma site marking and is aware of the implications of ostomy care and poor stoma site marking."

(continued)

Interventions   *Rationales*

> **CLINICAL ALERT:**
> • Site selection should never be done casually. Every attempt should be made to have the individual with the most expertise complete the site selection. The stoma site should be selected to avoid fat folds, scars, and bony prominences (Wound, Ostomy and Continence Nurses Society, 2014). The quality of life of this individual can be seriously impaired if incorrect placement results in leaking and peristomal dermatitis. "In retrospective reviews, proper site selection is essential for minimizing postoperative complications and achieving a good postoperative quality of life" (Francone, 2015).

3. Site selection should take place not in the operating room if at all possible. The following criteria may be useful in situation when an expert is not available (Wound, Ostomy and Continence Nurses Society, 2014, pp. 3, 4):

   a. Physical considerations: Large/protruding/pendulous abdomen, abdominal folds, wrinkles, scars/suture lines, other stomas, rectus abdominis muscle, waist line, iliac crest, braces, pendulous breasts, vision, dexterity, and the presence of a hernia.

   b. Examine the individual's exposed abdomen in various positions (e.g., standing, lying, sitting, and bending forward) to observe for creases, valleys, scars, folds, skin turgor, and contour.

   c. With the individual lying on his or her back, identify the rectus abdominis muscle. This can be done by having the individual do a modified sit-up (i.e., raise the head up and off the bed) or by having the individual cough. Palpate the edge of the rectus abdominis muscle. Expert opinion suggests that placement of the stoma within the rectus abdominis muscle may help prevent a peristomal hernia and/or a prolapse.

   d. The mark should initially be made with a sticker or ink pen that can be removed if this is not the optimal spot.

   e. It may be desirable to mark sites on the right and left sides of the abdomen to prepare for a change in the surgical outcome, and number the first choice as #1.

   f. Have the person assume sitting, bending, and lying positions to assess and confirm the best choice.

   g. It is important to have the individual confirm they can see the site. However, the critical consideration should be a flat pouching surface.

3. Principles of proper stoma site selection include placement of the stoma within the rectus abdominis muscle, use of multiple positions to identify appropriate stoma sites, avoidance of folds and scars, and consideration of the clothing/beltline. This could make the difference between an ostomy pouch leaking or not for the person's lifetime. Types of skin damage included erosion, maceration, erythema, and irritant dermatitis (Wound, Ostomy and Continence Nurses Society, 2014).

Collaborative Problems

Risk for Complications of Internal Urine Leakage

Risk for Complications of Urinary Tract Infection/Urinary Calculi, Peritonitis

Risk for Complications of Peristomal Skin Ulceration

Risk for Complications of Stomal Necrosis, Retraction, Prolapse, Stenosis, Obstruction

Collaborative Outcomes

The individual will be monitored for early signs and symptoms of (a) internal urine leakage, (b) urinary tract infection/urinary calculi, peritonitis, (c) peristomal skin ulceration, and (d) stomal necrosis/retraction and will receive collaborative interventions if indicated to restore physiologic stability.

Indicators of Physiologic Stability

- Temperature 98.5° F to 99° F (a)
- Urinary output >30 mL/hr (a)
- Pulse 60 to 100 beats/min (b)
- BP >90/60, <140/90 mm Hg (b)
- Respirations 16 to 20 breaths/min (b)
- Capillary refill <3 seconds (b)
- Oxygen saturation >94% (b)
- No sudden increase or decrease in drainage (a, b)
- Clear, light yellow urine (b)
- Urine pH 4.6 to 8.0 (b)
- No flank pain (b)
- No signs of peristomal ulceration or herniation (d)
- No abdominal distention (d)
- No complaints of nausea/vomiting (d)
- Stoma shrinking, with change in shape or color (d)

Carp's Cues

Please refer to the Generic Care Plan for the Surgical Client for detailed interventions for managing all surgical conditions. This care plan addresses specific additional interventions associated with the type of surgery performed.

Interventions	Rationales
1. Monitor drainage amount and color every hour for the first 24 hours from: a. Catheters and ureteric stents (originating in the renal pelvis). b. A suprapubic catheter may be present as a safety valve.	1. A sudden decrease in urine flow may indicate obstruction (edema, mucus) or dehydration. The ureteral stents prevent upper urinary tract obstruction owing to mechanical compression caused by postoperative edema. The urine output from the urethral catheter should preferably be >50 to 100 mL/hr and at least 0.5 mL/hr/kg a. Catheters and ureteric stents may be utilized to maintain adequate urinary drainage and to protect anastomoses.
2. Monitor every hour for the first 24 hours: a. Vital signs b. Capillary refill <3 seconds c. Oxygen saturation (pulse oximetry) d. Urine output e. Bowel sounds	2. Research shows that perioperative fluid therapy has a direct bearing on outcome. The goal of fluid therapy in the elective setting is to maintain the effective circulatory volume, while avoiding interstitial fluid overload, which may cause nausea and postoperative ileus (Geng et al., 2010, p. 30). Daily weighing is the best measure of fluid gain or loss.
3. Monitor for signs of anastomotic urinary leakage. Abdominal distention with decrease bowl motility: a. Fever b. Elevated serum creatinine level c. Decreased urine output despite adequate hydration	3. Urine leakage either from the ureteroileal anastomosis or from the base of the conduit occurs in as many as 8% of individuals with a urostomy. Leakage is confirmed through fluoroscopy. Small leaks may seal themselves with continuous drainage of the conduit via a stomal catheter.
4. Explain the reason for cloudy urine.	4. Because the intestine produces mucus, mucus in the diversion will cause urine to appear cloudy.
5. Monitor for signs and symptoms of urinary tract infection and urinary calculi. a. Fever b. Flank pain	5. The major cause of UTIs is poor urine flow through the conduit, leading to urinary stasis and bacterial contamination through the stoma.

(continued)

Interventions	*Rationales*
c. Malodorous, cloudy urine d. Alkaline urine pH **CLINICAL ALERT:** • Flank pain is a sensation of discomfort, distress, or agony in the part of the body below the rib and above the ileum, generally beginning posteriorly or in the midaxillary line and resulting from the stimulation of specialized nerve endings upon distention of the ureter or renal capsule from infection of renal calculi.	The physiological issues with the use of bowel in urinary diversion and its constant contact of urine with the intestinal surface encourages the exchange of chloride with bicarbonate. The loss of bicarbonate results in acidosis and hypercalciuria, resulting in calcium stones. The use of the ileum in urinary intestinal diversion may result in excess bile salts binding calcium and causing increased absorption of oxalate, increasing the risk of oxalate calculi (Vasdev, Moon, & Thorpe, 2013).
6. Monitor for stomal necrosis, prolapse, retraction, stenosis, and obstruction. Assess the following: a. Color, size, and shape of stoma b. Complaints of cramping abdominal pain, nausea and vomiting, abdominal distention	6. Daily assessment is necessary to detect early changes in stoma condition. a. Changes can indicate inflammation, retraction, prolapse, edema. b. These complaints may indicate obstruction.

 Clinical Alert Report

Before providing care, advise ancillary staff/student to report the following to the professional nurse assigned to the individual:

- Change in cognitive status
- Oral temperature >100.5° F
- Systolic BP <90 mm Hg
- Resting pulse >100, <50
- Respiratory rate >28, <10/min
- Decreased urine output despite adequate hydration
- Oxygen saturation <90%
- Changes in peristomal tissue
- Complaints of flank pain, cramping abdominal pain, nausea and vomiting, abdominal distention
- Abdominal distention with decreased bowel motility

Documentation

Vital signs
Intake and output
Abdomen (girth, bowel sounds)
Condition of peristomal area

Postoperative: Nursing Diagnoses

 TRANSITION TO HOME/COMMUNITY CARE

If indicated, review the risk diagnoses identified for this individual on admission:

- Is he person still at risk?
- Can the family reduce the risks?
- Is the person at higher risk at home?
- Is a Home Health Nurse assessment needed?
- Refer to transition planner/case manager/social service
- When is this person scheduled for follow-up with primary provider? Specialists? Record dates of appointments.
- Complete a medication reconciliation before transition. Refer to index.

S T A R   **Stop**

Think   Is this person at high risk for injury, falls, medical complications, and/or inability to care for self (activities of daily living)?

   Is there a support person available?

   Is the person competent to manage self-administration of medications, treatment procedures? Are additional resources needed?

   Can the person explain how to monitor the condition (e.g., blood glucose, signs/symptoms of complications, dietary/mobility restrictions, and when to call his or her primary provider or specialist)?

Act   Contact or provide the appropriate resource (e.g., contacting a support person, home health assessment, additional teaching, printed materials).

Review   Has the problem been addressed? If not, use SBAR to communicate to the appropriate person.

Risk for Ineffective Health Management Related to Insufficient Knowledge of Stomacare, Peristomal Skin Care, Perineal Wound Care, and Incorporation of Care into Activities of Daily Living (ADLs)

NOC

Compliance/ Engagement Behavior, Knowledge: Treatment Regimen, Participation: Health-Care Decisions, Treatment Behavior: Illness or Injury

NIC

Anticipatory Guidance, Risk Identification, Health Education, Learning Facilitation

Goals

The goals for this diagnosis represent those associated with transition planning. Refer to the transition criteria.

Interventions	Rationales
Carp's Cues Most clinical nurses are not responsible for the specific teaching of urinary diversion care and its implications on lifestyle and function. The wound care/ostomy specialist will provide an organized teaching plan. However, since nurses are responsible for care 24/7, each nurse needs to be confident in ostomy care that is their responsibility. A good method to learn this care is to watch the nurse specialist provide/teach ostomy care.	
1. When providing care, explore fears and concerns. Identify and dispel any misinformation or misconceptions the individual/significant others has regarding urinary diversion.	1. "Undergoing major surgery resulting in formation of a continent urinary diversion is very distressing for most patients. The threat of complications, helplessness, alteration in bodyimage and body-function concerning eliminating urine and impact of future sexual function contribute to anxiety and fear of the future" (*Geng et al., 2010, p. 22; White, 1998).
2. Explain why urine should be kept in an acid state and how: a. Drink cranberry juice. b. Avoid orange juice or other citrus juices. c. Sodium bicarbonate, sodium citrate (1 to 3 g four times a day) may be prescribed.	2. Acid urine reduces bacterial growth and prevents infections.

(continued)

Interventions	Rationales

3. Discuss signs and symptoms of fluid and electrolyte imbalances:
  a. Extreme thirst
  b. Dry skin and oral mucous membrane
  c. Dark yellow urine output
  d. Weakness, fatigue
  e. Muscle cramps
  f. Orthostatic hypotension (feeling faint when suddenly changing positions)	

4. Emphasize the importance of adequate fluid intake; explain also risk situations for dehydration such as:
  a. Hot weather
  b. Exercising in hot weather
  c. With episodes of diarrhea
  d. When intake is reduced (e.g., illness)
	4. Concentrated urine is more prone to bacterial growth

5. Teach signs and symptoms of infection including:
  a. Dark urine or urine containing excess mucus
  b. Strong-smelling urine
  c. Pain in the back
  d. Poor appetite
  e. Nausea
  f. Vomiting	

6. Explain to report any of these changes in their stoma or skin around it to surgeon, PCP, or ostomy nurse specialist:
  a. Is purple, gray, or black
  b. Has a bad odor
  c. Is dry
  d. Pulls away from the skin
  e. Opening gets big enough for your intestines to come through it
  f. Is at skin level or deeper
  g. Pushes farther out from the skin and gets longer
  h. Skin opening becomes narrower
  i. Skin irritations owing to leakage of urine or infection
  j. Incontinence and leakage
	6. These changes can indicate infection, ulceration, prolapse, and retraction.

7. Call your surgeon, PCP, or ostomy nurse specialist, if your stoma:
  a. Has a pale color
  b. Is dark red or purple
  c. Has moderate to severe swelling
  d. Has moderate to heavy bleeding
8. Call the surgeon or nurse specialist if:
  a. Fever for several days without cause
  b. Persisting difficulties when introducing the catheter
  c. Obstructed access to the neobladder
  d. Persisting lumbar pain
  e. Painful catheterization or urinating
  f. Low urine production although sufficient fluid intake
  g. Losing weight without possible explanation
  h. Nausea and vomiting
  i. Offensive urine odor or visible blood
	7, 8. The stoma is normally pink to red; changes can indicate necrosis, ischemia, infection.

9. Ensure that supplies/prescriptions are provided as:
  a. Supplies
  b. Gloves, dressing tape
	9. For follow-up for any hospitalization.

Interventions	Rationales
10. Refer interested individuals/families to online sources related to urinary diversion as: a. Leaving hospital after urostomy surgery, access at http://healthcareathome.ca/mh/en/Documents/Patient%20Edu.%20Book_Urostomy.PDF b. About Your Bladder Surgery with an Ileal Conduit (Urostomy), access at https://www.mskcc.org/cancer-care/patient-education/about-your-bladder-surgery-ileal-conduit-urostomy	
11. Ensure appointments have been scheduled for primary care provider, specialists, home nursing assessment, diagnostic tests.	11. The appointment behavior is enhanced when the inpatient team schedules outpatient medical follow-up before transition. Ideally, the inpatient care providers or case managers/transition planners will schedule follow-up visit(s) with the appropriate professionals, including primary care provider, specialist.

Documentation

Individual/family teaching

Outcome achievement or status

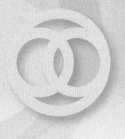

Section 3

Diagnostic and Therapeutic Procedures

Hemodialysis

Hemodialysis is the removal of metabolic wastes and excess electrolytes and fluids from the blood to treat acute or chronic kidney disease. The procedure uses the principles of diffusion, osmosis, and filtration. Blood is pumped into an artificial kidney through a semipermeable, cellophane-like membrane surrounded by a flow of dialysate, which is a solution composed of water, glucose, sodium, chloride, potassium, calcium, and acetate or bicarbonate. The amounts of these constituents vary depending on the amount of water, waste products, or electrolytes to be removed. Hemodialysis does not correct renal dysfunction; it only corrects metabolic waste, fluid, electrolyte, and acid–base imbalances (Castner, 2015).

 Time Frame
Predialysis, intradialysis, postdialysis

▪▪▪▪ DIAGNOSTIC CLUSTER

Collaborative Problems

▲ Risk for Complications of Electrolyte Imbalance (Potassium, Sodium, and Magnesium)

*   Risk for Complications of Hemolysis

△ Risk for Complications of Dialysis Disequilibrium Syndrome

▲ Risk for Complications of Clotting

▲ Risk for Complications of Air Embolism

▲ Risk for Complications of Pyrogen Reaction

▲ Risk for Complications of Fluid Imbalances (refer to Peritoneal Dialysis Care Plan)

*   Risk for Complications of Anaphylaxis/Allergies

Nursing Diagnoses

▲ Risk for Infection Transmission related to frequent contacts with blood and risk of hepatitis B and C

▲ Risk for Ineffective Health Management Related to Insufficient Knowledge of Condition, Dietary Restrictions, Daily Recording, Pharmacological Therapy, Signs/Symptoms of Complications, Follow-up Visits, and Community Resources

Related Care Plans

Chronic Kidney Disease or Acute Kidney Injury

External Arteriovenous Shunting

▲ This diagnosis was reported to be monitored for or managed frequently (75% to 100%).
Δ This diagnosis was reported to be monitored for or managed often (50% to 74%).
* This diagnosis was not included in the validation study.

Transitional Criteria

The individual and/or family will:

1. Describe the purpose of hemodialysis.
2. Discuss feelings and concerns regarding the effects of long-term therapy on self and family.
3. State signs and symptoms that must be reported to a health care professional.

> **Transitional Risk Assessment Plan (TRAP)**
>
> Begin this plan on admission
> Implement the Transitional Risk Assessment Plan (TRAP):
> * Refer to inside back cover.
> * Add each validated high-risk diagnosis to individual's problem list with the risk code in ( ).
> * Refer to Unit II to the individual high-risk nursing diagnoses/collaborative problems for outcomes and interventions.
>
> > *R:* *"Close coordination of care in the post-acute period, early discharge follow-up care, enhanced patient education and self-management training, proactive end-of-life counseling, and extending the resources and clinical expertise over time via multidisciplinary team management" can lower readmission rates and improve health outcomes (Boutwell & Hwu, 2009, p. 14). Interventions are utilized to activate the individual and family to select changes in their everyday lifestyle choices to improve their health (Hibbard & Greene, 2013).*
> >
> > Risk for Infection Transmission: Individual/family need education regarding good handwashing, avoidance of ill individuals, using appropriate bactericidal agent to clean up any blood spills, no sharing of personal items such as toothbrushes.
> >
> > If appropriate, individual/family should consider hepatitis B vaccine, annual influenza vaccine, and pneumonia vaccine.

Collaborative Problems

Risk for Complications of Electrolyte Imbalance (Potassium, Sodium, Magnesium)

Risk for Complications of Hemolysis

Risk for Complications of Dialysis Disequilibrium Syndrome

Risk for Complications of Clotting

Risk for Complications of Air Embolism

Risk for Complications of Anaphylaxis or Allergies

Collaborative Outcomes

The individual will be monitored to detect early signs and symptoms of (a) electrolyte imbalance, (b) hemolysis, (c) dialysis disequilibrium syndrome, (d) clotting, (e) air embolism, (f) fluid imbalances, (g) sepsis, and (h) anaphylaxis/allergies and will receive collaborative interventions if indicated to restore physiologic stability.

Indicators of Physiologic Stability

* No itching/hives (e, h, i)
* No or minimal edema (f)

- BP >90/60, <140/90 mm Hg (c, e, h, i)
- Pulse 60 to 100 beats/min with regular rate and rhythm (c, e, h, i)
- Respirations 16 to 20 breaths/min, relaxed, rhythmic, with no rales, or wheezing (e, h, i)
- Weight change of no more than 1 to 2 kg between dialysis treatment (f)
- No headache (c)
- No chest pain (e, i)
- No complaints of nausea/vomiting (c)
- Serum potassium 3.5 to 5 mEq/L (a)
- Serum sodium 135 to 148 mm/dL (a)
- Serum creatinine 0.6 to 1.2 mg/dL (a)
- Blood urea nitrogen 7 to 18 mg/dL (a)

Interventions	Rationales
1. Assess the following:	1. Predialysis assessment and documentation of individual's status are mandatory before initiation of the hemodialysis procedure to establish a baseline and to identify problems (Speranza-Reid, 2015a).
a. Skin (color, turgor, temperature, moisture, and edema)	a. Skin assessment can provide data to evaluate circulation, level of hydration, fluid retention, and uremia.
b. Blood pressure (lying, sitting, and standing, as appropriate for individual)	b. Low blood pressure may indicate intolerance to transmembrane pressure, hypovolemia, or the effects of antihypertensive medication given predialysis. High blood pressure may indicate overhydration, increased renin production, or dietary and fluid indiscretion.
c. Apical pulse (rhythm and rate and abnormalities)	c. Cardiac assessment evaluates the heart's ability to compensate for changes in fluid volume. Pericardial rub indicates uremia, gallops occur with fluid overload, arrhythmias can indicate volume changes, uremia, changes in cardiac function.
d. Respirations (rate, effort, and abnormal sounds)	d. Respiratory assessment evaluates compensatory ability of the system and presence of fluid or infection.
e. Weight (gain or loss)	e. Predialysis weight indicating gain or loss may necessitate a need to reevaluate dry weight.
f. Vascular access (site and patency and infection)	f. The vascular access site is assessed for signs of infection (warmth, redness, tenderness) or abnormal drainage. Patency is evaluated by assessment of bruits (swishing sound heard with a stethoscope) and thrills (vibration felt with light palpation) in fistulas and grafts. Notify the physician or advanced practice nurse before using a potentially compromised access (Deaver & Counts, 2015).
g. Pretreatment BUN, serum creatinine, sodium, and potassium levels	g. Pretreatment serum levels are used as a baseline for evaluation of the effectiveness of the dialysis.
2. Assess the individual's pretreatment condition (chest pain, shortness of breath, cramps, headache, dizziness, blurred vision, nausea and vomiting, change in mentation, or speech).	2. These assessment data help to determine if there has been a change in the individual's condition since last treatment or if a change in treatment is indicated. When an individual presents with problems predialysis, underlying etiology needs to be determined before initiation of treatment.
3. Intradialysis—Monitor for signs and symptoms of potassium and sodium imbalance. (Refer to the Peritoneal Dialysis Care Plan for more information.)	3. Dialysate fluid composition and rates of inflow and outflow determine electrolyte imbalances.
4. Monitor for manifestations of hemolysis: bright red and/or translucent blood in venous line, burning at the circulatory return site, pink- to red-tinged dialysate, abdominal or back pain, dyspnea, chest tightness, arrhythmias	4. Rupture of red blood cells can result from the hypotonic dialysate, high dialysate temperature, mechanical problems (e.g., pressure on RBCs from narrowed or occluded lines, or chloramines, nitrates, copper, zinc, or formaldehyde in the dialysate) (Speranza-Reid, 2015b).

Interventions	Rationales

> **CLINICAL ALERT:**
> - Hemolysis is a rare but ever-present potential complication of hemodialysis.
> - Symptoms may be subtle and similar to hypotension or may not manifest until after treatment.
> - Hemoglobin levels can drop dramatically so immediate care and investigation is necessary (Speranza-Reid, 2015b).

---

5. Monitor for signs and symptoms of dialysis disequilibrium syndrome (DDS): Headache, nausea, vomiting, restlessness, hypertension, increased pulse pressures, altered sensorium, arrhythmias, and blurred vision.

> **CLINICAL ALERT:**
> - DDS symptoms may be delayed for up to 24 hours after dialysis.
> - In addition to acute individuals with high BUNs, more susceptible populations are the elderly and pediatric, and chronic individuals who have missed several treatments (Speranza-Reid, 2015b).

5. As a result of hemodialysis, the concentration of BUN is reduced more rapidly than the urea nitrogen level in cerebrospinal fluid and brain tissue, because of the slow transport of urea across the blood–brain barrier. Urea acts as an osmotic agent, drawing water from the plasma and extracellular fluid into the cerebral cells and producing cerebral edema. Other factors, such as rapid pH changes and electrolyte shifts, also can cause cerebral edema. DDS more likely in acute dialysis with high pretreatment BUNs (Speranza-Reid, 2015b).

---

6. Monitor for clotting:
   a. Observe for clot formation in the dialyzer and drip chambers.
   b. Monitor pressure readings every 15 minutes.
   c. Observe for clots when aspirating fistula needles, arteriovenous access, or intravenous dialysis catheter.

   d. Provide anticoagulation therapy as ordered.

6. Blood contacting the nonvascular surface of the extracorporeal circuit activates the normal clotting mechanism. During dialysis, fibrin formation and a gradual increase in the circuit's venous pressure (resulting from clotting in the venous drip chamber or needle) may indicate inadequate heparinization. Clot formation elevates blood pressure readings (Speranza-Reid, 2015a).
   d. Increased clotting may indicate need for adjustments in anticoagulation therapy.

---

7. Monitor for signs and symptoms of air embolism: sudden onset of cyanosis, shortness of breath, chest pain, anxiety, persistent cough, loss of consciousness although symptoms may vary depending on position of individual at time of event (Speranza-Reid, 2015b).

7. As little as 10 mL of air introduced into the venous circulation is clinically significant. Large air bubbles are changed to foam as they enter the heart. Foam can decrease the volume of blood entering the lungs, decreasing left heart blood flow and cardiac output. Entry of air into the respiratory circulatory system causes a profound negative response.

---

8. If signs and symptoms of air embolism occur, take these steps (Speranza-Reid, 2015b):
   a. Clamp the venous line and stop the blood pump.

   b. Position individual on his or her left side with feet elevated for 30 minutes.

   c. Give 100% oxygen by mask.

8a. Clamping the line and stopping the pump can halt infusion of air.
   b. This prevents air from going to the head and traps air in the right atrium and in the right ventricle away from the pulmonic valve.
   c. Oxygen will aid in the reabsorption of the embolized air.

---

9. Monitor for signs and symptoms of anaphylaxis, which can include itching, hives, feeling of warmth, restlessness, feeling of impending doom, chest/back pain, shortness of breath, cough, cardiac arrest and death (Speranza-Reid, 2015b).
   a. Stop dialysis and do not return blood.
   b. Administer oxygen
   c. Per protocol and/or physician/nurse practitioner order administer intravenous antihistamines, steroids, and/or epinephrine.

9. This is due to an allergic response to the ingredients in the dialysate or dialysis membrane, which involves the interaction between immunoglobulin E (IgE) and mast cells. Anaphylaxis is a severe hypersensitivity response caused by a massive release of chemical mediators and other substances. The cardiovascular, respiratory, cutaneous, and gastrointestinal systems are generally involved in anaphylaxis. The IgE antibodies interact with mast cells, triggering the release of histamine, which, because of its potent

(continued)

Interventions	*Rationales*
	vasodilator effect, causes widespread edema and vascular congestion (Bellucci, 2015; Speranza-Reid, 2015b).
	a. This will prevent further contact with the offending agent.
	b. Oxygen will ease symptoms and provide additional oxygen for cardiac function.
	c. Medications will block allergic reaction.

Clinical Alert Report

Advise ancillary staff/student to report the following to the professional nurse assigned to the individual:

- Any new change or deterioration in behavior, cognition, or level of consciousness
- Change in systolic BP >200 mm Hg or <90 mm Hg; diastolic BP >90 mm Hg or outside of specifically prescribed parameters
- Resting pulse >120 or <55 beats/min or outside of specifically prescribed parameters
- Onset or changes in cardiac rhythm or heart sounds
- Change in respiratory rate >28 or <10/min
- Onset of new lung sounds (e.g., wheezes, rales, or increased respiratory effort)
- Changes in urinary output from usual baseline if applicable
- Temperature >100° F oral
- Bleeding from dialysis access
- Decrease in thrill or bruit of dialysis access
- New coolness, pain, or cyanosis in hand or foot below the dialysis access

Nursing Diagnoses

Risk for Infection Transmission Related to Frequent Contacts with Blood and People at Risk for Hepatitis B and C

NOC

Infection Status, Risk
Control, Risk Detection

NIC

Teaching: Disease
Process, Infection
Protection

Goal

The individual will relate the risks of hepatitis B virus (HBV) transmission.

Indicators

- Have antibodies to HBV.
- Take precautions to prevent transmission of HBV.

Interventions	*Rationales*
1. Follow universal precautions for all dialysis treatments:	
a. Wear personal protective equipment: face shield, impervious gown, and gloves for all individual or machine contact.	
b. All blood or dialysis effluent spills must be cleaned up immediately with antimicrobial soap and water.	
c. Do not permit staff and other personnel or visitors to eat or drink anything within the dialysis treatment area.	
d. Use individual supplies (e.g., thermometers, dressing change supplies, and individual medication vials for each individual).	

Interventions	Rationales

2. Observe strict isolation procedure for individuals who do not have the serologic marker for hepatitis B surface antibody:
  a. Wear an isolation gown and mask during dialysis treatment.
  b. Dialysis should be performed in individual's private room or a dialysis unit isolation area.
  c. All blood or dialysis effluent spills must be cleaned up immediately with antimicrobial soap and water.
  d. Observe isolation disposal procedure for all needles, syringes, and effluent.
  e. Do not permit staff and other personnel or visitors to eat or drink anything within the dialysis treatment area.
  f. Ensure that all specimens for laboratory analysis are labeled "Isolation" and placed in bags also labeled "Isolation."
  g. Use special disposable thermometers to assess temperature.
  h. Avoid contact with other dialysis individuals, if staffing level permits. If contact is necessary, change isolation gowns and wash hands carefully.
  i. Avoid any skin contact with the individual's blood.
  j. Follow isolation procedure for waste and linen disposal per institutional protocol.
  k. Follow the recommended sterilization procedure for the hemodialysis machine after use.
	2. Individuals who are hepatitis C positive dialyze with the general population using universal precautions. HBV/HCV is found in the blood, saliva, semen, and vaginal secretions. Transmission is usually through blood (percutaneous or permucosal). Hepatitis B virus is stable on and viable on environmental surfaces for 7 days. Regularly practicing certain precautions provides protection.

3. Administer hepatitis B immunizations, as appropriate, following facility policies.	3. High-risk individuals and others should be immunized.
4. Explain that there is no prophylaxis for hepatitis C virus (HCV) and that it can go unnoticed for years.	4. About 20% to 30% of people report an acute illness but symptoms often disappear. The disease becomes chronic in 75% to 85% of those who develop HCV (CDC, 2016c).
5. Minimize use of anticoagulants in individuals with liver disease. 6. Collaborate with physician and/or advanced practice nurse to adjust medications with potential hepatotoxicity, including immunosuppressants. 7. Reinforce to individual and family the serious nature of HBV/HCV, precautions, and risks.	5–7. Reiterating the seriousness of HBV/HCV and its possible sequelae may encourage compliance with instructions and precautions.

TRANSITIONAL CRITERIA TO HOME/COMMUNITY CARE

Review risk diagnoses identified on admission.

- Does the individual/family know how to follow-up the transition plan?
- If dialysis is to continue, ascertain that outpatient dialysis has been arranged, all necessary results have been obtained and transferred (labs, including hepatitis status, chest X-Ray, EKG, history and physical, medications, and dialysis prescription), time and location of next treatment have been confirmed.
- Discuss dietary changes and individual/family understanding.
- Medication reconciliation has been done and written list and instructions are provided.
- Does individual have contact information for questions and concerns?
- Use STAR (Stop, Think, Act, Review) to determine if transition plan is complete.
- Use SBAR (Situation, Background, Assessment, Recommendation) to relay necessary information to appropriate professional.

SBAR   *Situation:* Individual is being transition and next dialysis treatment is scheduled at outpatient facility 10 miles from individual's home.

Background: Individual does not drive and family member will be at work during dialysis treatment.

Action: Discuss with case manager/transition planner/social worker. (This potential problem may have already been addressed and resolved during hospitalization.)

Recommendation: Individual may be eligible for public assistance, car pool, or be considered for a different dialysis shift.

Risk for Ineffective Health Management Related to Insufficient Knowledge of Condition, Dietary Restrictions, Daily Recording, Pharmacological Therapy, Signs/Symptoms of Complications, Follow-up Visits, and Community Resources

NOC

Compliance Behavior, Knowledge: Treatment Regimen, Participation in Health Care Decisions, Treatment Behavior: Illness

NIC

Anticipatory Guidance, Learning Facilitation, Risk Identification, Health Education, Teaching: Procedure/ Treatment, Health System Guidance

Goals

The goals for this diagnosis represent those associated with transition planning. Refer to the transition criteria.

Interventions	Rationales

1. Review care of the dialysis access.
  a. Signs and symptoms of problems and who to contact for questions.
  b. No blood draws or blood pressure measurements on access arm.
 	
 CLINICAL ALERT:
 • A dialysis access should NEVER be used as an intravenous access or for phlebotomy, unless specified by the vascular access physician or nephrologist.
	1. An infected or poorly functioning access will not provide safe or adequate dialysis. Many problems can be dealt with quickly and without hospitalization. Drawing blood or taking blood pressures in the access arm increases the risk of thrombosis and infection (Deaver & Counts, 2015).

2. Review each medication, including dosing, purpose, and specific instructions (e.g., take the phosphate binders with the meal rather than between meals).	2. Kidney disease requires a large number of medications. Individuals will have more success with medication management if they understand why and how to take them (e.g., the antihypertensive regime may be different on dialysis vs. nondialysis days).
3. Discuss individual's choice of therapy.	3. The type of renal replacement therapy may change as the individual's health status or interests change. Ideally, all choices have been discussed but due to circumstances this may not have been possible during the hospitalization. Individuals can be directed to educational material as well as professionals for further information.
4. Reinforce importance of adhering to the prescribed dietary plan.	4. All individuals on dialysis have access to the professional dietitian who will review labs and adjust diet as needed. Individuals are encouraged to write down questions and participate in their diet plan.

Interventions	Rationales
5. If appropriate, individual/family should consider hepatitis B vaccine, annual influenza vaccine, and pneumonia vaccine.	5. Infectious diseases can further compromise the individual.
6. Provide opportunities for individual to voice concerns and questions regarding kidney disease and treatment.	6. Kidney disease and dialysis is a life-altering experience that depends on individuals being able to participate in their care. Additional support systems may be needed. Dialysis social workers can assist individuals with local or regional support groups. Accurate information and support are also available on the Internet through organization such as the American Association of Kidney Patients (AAKP) at www.aakp.org, the National Kidney Foundation (NKF) at www.kidney.org, and Life Options at http://lifeoptions.org

Documentation

Individual/family teaching
Monthly HBV screening results

Peritoneal Dialysis

Peritoneal dialysis (PD)—the repetitive instillation and drainage of dialysis solution into and from the peritoneal cavity—uses the processes of osmosis, ultrafiltration, and diffusion to remove wastes, toxins, and fluid from the blood. PD uses the individual's own peritoneal lining to serve as the semipermeable membrane through which diffusion, osmosis, and filtration occur (Blake & Daugirdas, 2015; Groenhoff, Ales, & Todd, 2015). The procedure is indicated for acute or chronic kidney disease and severe fluid or electrolyte imbalances unresponsive to other treatments.

Numerous techniques for instillation and drainage of dialysis fluid have been developed. These methods are both manual and automated. Therapy can be continuous or automated.

Continuous therapies include continuous ambulatory peritoneal dialysis (CAPD), carried out manually by the individual or caregiver, and automated peritoneal dialysis (APD) carried out by a PD machine. The variations of APD include continuous cycling peritoneal dialysis (CCPD), nocturnal intermittent peritoneal dialysis (NIPD), and tidal peritoneal dialysis (TPD). Other terms may be occasionally encountered (Groenhoff et al., 2015; Heimbürger & Blake, 2015). CAPD is most commonly used and provides dialysate inflow with a disposable bag and tubing, which is sterilely connected then covered with a sterile cap during dwell time. Exchanges are done four times/day with 2.0 to 2.5 L. CCPD uses an automated cycler to perform exchanges during sleep and the abdomen is left full during the day. IPD consists of treatment periods with dwell time and alternates with periods of peritoneal cavity draining. Intermittent techniques use multiple short dwell exchanges three or four times a week. Automated intermittent exchanges may occur with repeated small TPD or at night (NIPD). Manual IPD also may be done in hospitals for a prescribed number of cycles and length of time based on individual requirements. Manual peritoneal dialysis requires careful control of dialysate instillation (2 L), dwell time, and outflow.

 Time Frame
Pretherapy and intratherapy

▪▪▪■ DIAGNOSTIC CLUSTER

Collaborative Problems

▲ Risk for Complications of Fluid Imbalances

▲ Risk for Complications of Electrolyte Imbalances

▲ Risk for Complications of Uremia

(continued)

△ Risk for Complications of Hemorrhage

△ Risk for Complications of Hyperglycemia

△ Risk for Complications of Bladder/Bowel Perforation

▲ Risk for Complications of Inflow/Outflow Problems

* Risk for Complications of Sepsis

Nursing Diagnoses

▲ Risk for Infection related to access to peritoneal cavity

△ Risk for Ineffective Breathing Pattern related to immobility, pressure, and pain

△ Altered Comfort related to catheter insertion, instillation of dialysis solution, outflow, suction, and chemical irritation of peritoneum

△ Risk for Ineffective Health Management related to insufficient knowledge of rationale of treatment, medications, home dialysis procedure, signs and symptoms of complications, community resources, and follow-up care

△ Imbalanced Nutrition related to anorexia and loss of protein in peritoneal dialysis fluid (refer to Chronic Kidney Disease)

△ Interrupted Family Processes related to the effects of interruptions of the treatment schedule on role responsibilities (refer to Chronic Kidney Disease)

△ Powerlessness related to chronic illness and the need for continuous treatment (refer to Chronic Kidney Disease)

▲ This diagnosis was reported to be monitored for or managed frequently (75% to 100%).
△ This diagnosis was reported to be monitored for or managed often (50% to 74%).
* This diagnosis was not included in the validation study.

Transitional Criteria

Before transition, the individual or family will:

1. Be able to demonstrate home peritoneal dialysis procedures, if appropriate.
2. State signs and symptoms of infection.
3. Discuss the expected effects of long-term dialysis on the individual and family.
4. State signs and symptoms that must be reported to a health care professional.

Transitional Risk Assessment Plan (TRAP)

Begin this plan on admission.
Implement the Transitional Risk Assessment Plan (TRAP):
- Refer to inside back cover.
- Add each validated high-risk diagnosis to individual's problem list with the risk code in ( ).
- Refer to Unit II to the individual high-risk nursing diagnoses/collaborative problems for outcomes and interventions.

  R: "Close coordination of care in the post-acute period, early discharge follow-up care, enhanced patient education and self-management training, proactive end-of-life counseling, and extending the resources and clinical expertise over time via multidisciplinary team management" can lower readmission rates and improve health outcomes (Boutwell & Hwu, 2009, p. 14). Interventions are utilized to activate the individual and family to select changes in their everyday lifestyle choices to improve their health (Hibbard & Greene, 2013).

> **CLINICAL ALERT:**
> • If peritoneal dialysis is to be the ongoing treatment of choice, the individual/caregiver will be ultimately responsible for all aspects of the treatment procedure. Training may begin during the hospitalization and continue in a formal outpatient clinic setting. Arrangements need to be completed prior to transition.

Collaborative Problems

Risk for Complications of Fluid Imbalances

Risk for Complications of Electrolyte Imbalances

Risk for Complications of Uremia

Risk for Complications of Hemorrhage

Risk for Complications of Hyperglycemia

Risk for Complications of Bladder or Bowel Perforation

Risk for Complications of Inflow or Outflow Problems

Risk for Complications of Sepsis

Collaborative Outcomes

The nurse will detect early signs and symptoms of (a) fluid imbalances, (b) electrolyte imbalances, (c) uremia, (d) hemorrhage, (e) hyperglycemia, (f) bladder or bowel perforation, (g) inflow or outflow problems, and (h) sepsis, and will intervene collaboratively to stabilize the individual.

Indicators of Physiologic Stability

- Alert, oriented, calm (a, b, c, g)
- Skin warm, dry, usual color, no lesions (a, c, d, e, g)
- No or minimal edema (a)
- BP >90/60, <140/90 mm Hg (a, b, d, g)
- Pulse pressure (40 mm Hg difference in systolic or diastolic) (a, b, d, g)
- Pulse 60 to 100 beats/min (a, b, d, g)
- Respirations 16 to 20 breaths/min; relaxed, rhythmic; no rales or wheezing (a, g)
- No weight change (a)
- Flat neck veins (a)
- No headache (b, g)
- Bowel sounds present (b)
- No chest pain (c)
- No abdominal pain (b, e, g)
- Intact reflexes (b)
- No change in vision (c)
- No complaints of nausea/vomiting (c, g)
- Intact muscle strength (b, c)
- No seizures (b)
- Serum potassium 3.5 to 5 mEq/L (b, c)
- Fasting blood glucose 70 to 110 mg/dL (e)
- Hemoglobin (d)
  - Male 13.5 to 17.5 g/dL
  - Female 13 to 16 g/dL
- Hematocrit (d)
  - Male 40% to 54%
  - Female 37% to 47%
- Serum sodium 135 to 148 mm/dL (c)
- Patent inflow and outflow (g)

- Intact connections, no kinks (g)
- No urinary urgency (f)
- No glucose in urine (e, f)
- No bowel urgency (f)
- No diarrhea (c, f)
- No fecal material in dialysate (f)
- White blood cell count >4,000 cells/mms or <12,000 with bands <10% (g)
- Temperature >96.8° F or <100.4° F (g)

Interventions	Rationales

1. Monitor for signs and symptoms of hypervolemia:
  a. Edema
  b. Dyspnea or tachypnea
  c. Rales or frothy secretions
  d. Rapid, bounding pulse
  e. Hypertension
  f. Jugular vein distention
  g. S_3 heart sounds
	1. Hypervolemia may occur if dialysate does not drain freely or if excess IV or oral fluids have been infused or injected (Boudville & Blake, 2015). Excess fluid greater than 5% of body weight is needed to produce edema. Fluid in lungs produces signs and symptoms of hypoxia. Increasing flow rate will increase fluid removal with little change in clearance of solutes.

2. Monitor for signs and symptoms of hypovolemia:
  a. Dry skin and mucous membranes
  b. Poor skin turgor
  c. Thirst
  d. Tachycardia
  e. Tachypnea
  f. Hypotension with orthostatic changes
  g. Narrowed pulse pressure
  h. Altered level of consciousness
	2. Hypovolemia may occur from excessive or too-rapid removal of dialysate fluid, inadequate salt and fluid intake, increased insensible loss, or overuse of hypertonic solution. Decreasing dextrose concentration to 1.5% may remove solutes without fluid (Boudville & Blake, 2015).

3. Monitor intake and output.	3. Urine output varies depending on renal status.
4. Enforce fluid restrictions, as ordered.	4. Physician/nurse practitioner may restrict fluid intake to insensible losses or the previous day's urine output.
5. Weigh daily or before and after each dialysis treatment.	5. Daily weights help to evaluate fluid balance.
6. Add medications to dialysate, as ordered.	6. Heparin commonly is added to decrease fibrin clots in the catheter. Potassium is added to prevent hypokalemia.
7. Monitor peritoneal dialysis inflow, dwell time, and outflow.	7. *Inflow* (usually taking less than 15 minutes) is the infusion of dialysis solution by gravity into the peritoneal cavity. *Dwell time* is the length of time that the dialysis solution remains in the peritoneal cavity, which determines the amount of diffusion and osmosis that occurs. The time depends on the type of PD and can range from 0 minutes to hours. *Drain* (usually less than 20 minutes) is the emptying of the peritoneal cavity by gravity.

8. Monitor for signs and symptoms of hypernatremia with fluid overload:
  a. Thirst
  b. Agitation
  c. Convulsions
	8. Dialysate solution >4.25% or rapid outflow or no long swell can cause hypernatremia (Mehrotra, 2015; Satalowich & Prowant, 2008).

9. Monitor for signs and symptoms of hyponatremia:
  a. Lethargy or coma
  b. Weakness
  c. Abdominal pain
  d. Muscle twitching or convulsions
	9. Hyponatremia results from the dilutional effects of hypervolemia. Extracellular volume decrease lowers blood pressure and leads to hypoxia. It can also be an indication of malnutrition (Mehrotra, 2015).

Interventions	Rationales

10. Monitor for signs and symptoms of hyperkalemia:
  a. Weakness or paralysis
  b. Muscle irritability
  c. Paresthesias
  d. Nausea, vomiting, abdominal cramping, or diarrhea
  e. Irregular pulse
	10. Prolonged dwell time can increase potassium fluctuations that can affect neuromuscular transmission, reduce action of GI smooth muscles, and impair electrical conduction of the heart. Strategies to lower serum potassium include using dialysate without potassium, performing extra dialysis exchanges, and decreasing dietary potassium. Severe hyperkalemia may require emergency medical management (Groenhoff et al., 2015; Mehrotra, 2015).

11. Monitor for signs and symptoms of hypokalemia:
  a. Weakness or paralysis
  b. Leg cramps
  c. Decreased or absent tendon reflexes
  d. Hypoventilation
  e. Polyuria
  f. Hypotension
  g. Constipation or paralytic ileus
	11. Hypokalemia impairs neuromuscular transmission and reduces action of respiratory muscles and GI smooth muscles. Potassium can be repleted through diet, oral supplements, or as addition to dialysate (Groenhoff et al., 2015; Lambertson, 2015b; Mehrotra, 2015).

12. Monitor for signs and symptoms of uremia:
  a. Skin and mucous membrane lesions
  b. Pericardial friction rub
  c. Pleural friction rub
  d. GI disturbances
  e. Peripheral neuropathy
  f. Vision changes
  g. Central nervous system impairment
  h. Tachypnea
  i. Musculoskeletal changes
	12. A multisystem syndrome, uremia is a manifestation of end-stage renal disease resulting from waste products of protein metabolism, including urea, creatinine, and uric acid. To increase removal of wastes, the number of exchanges can be increased.

13. Monitor for blood in dialysate drainage:
  a. Trauma to bowel or blood vessel during catheter insertion
  b. Menstruation/ovulation
  c. Disease/illness (e.g., cyst, infection, neoplasm)
	13. Perforation of a blood vessel during catheter insertion can cause bloody dialysate, urine, or stool, or bleeding at insertion site. The fallopian tubes and ovaries open into the peritoneum, so blood effluent is common during ovulation and menses (Lambertson, 2015b).

14. If bleeding persists, apply a pressure dressing and carefully monitor vital signs. **CLINICAL ALERT:** • In addition to pressure and vital sign monitoring, rapid PD exchanges, ice packs, fluid/blood replacement, and surgery may be required (Lambertson, 2015b).	

15. Monitor for signs and symptoms of hyperglycemia:
  a. Elevated or depressed blood glucose level
  b. Polyuria
  c. Polyphagia
  d. Polydipsia
  e. Abdominal pain
  f. Diaphoresis
	15. The amount of dextrose absorbed from the dialysate varies with dextrose concentration and number of cycles. In two cycles of 1.5% solution, 41 kcal are absorbed. After dialysis is complete, hypoglycemia may occur because of increased insulin production during instillation of high dextrose concentrations.

16. Monitor for signs and symptoms of bladder or bowel perforation:
  a. Fecal material in dialysate
  b. Complaints of urgency
  c. Increased urine output with high glucose concentrations
	16. Catheter insertion may perforate bowel or bladder, allowing dialysate to infuse into bowel or bladder (Lambertson, 2015b).

(continued)

Interventions	Rationales
d. Complaints of pressure in the sensation to defecate e. Watery diarrhea **CLINICAL ALERT:** • Notify physician/nurse practitioner immediately.	
17. Have individual empty bladder and bowel before insertion of peritoneal dialysis catheter.	17. Emptying bladder and bowel decreases risk of perforation during catheter insertion (Lambertson, 2015a).
18. Monitor drug levels during dialysis to maintain therapeutic treatment.	18. Drugs may be added to the dialysate (Groenhoff et al., 2015).
19. If inflow or outflow problems occur, do the following: a. Increase height of the dialysate bag and lower the bed. b. Reposition individual and instruct him or her to cough. c. Check for kinks and closed clamps. d. Remove a nontransparent dressing to check for catheter obstruction. e. Check dressing for wetness. Dialysate leaking from exit site presents as a clear fluid testing strongly for glucose. **CLINICAL ALERT:** • Notify Physician/nurse practitioner if 50% of inflow is retained. f. Assess abdominal or shoulder pain on outflow. g. Assess amount of dialysate return. h. Ascertain if heparin has been added to dialysate. i. If ordered, irrigate with heparinized saline. j. If ordered, irrigate with fibrinolytic agents. k. Assess for constipation.	19. These measures can enhance the effectiveness of dialysis and prevent complications (Lambertson, 2015b) a. Raising the bag and lowering the bed can help to maximize gravity drainage. b. Repositioning and coughing may help to clear a blocked or kinked catheter. c. Dressing can obscure an external obstruction or kink. d. Leakage at site may be from poor insertion technique or delayed healing and infection. e. Abdominal pain may result from excessive suction on abdominal viscera or incorrect catheter position. Shoulder pain may indicate air in the abdomen. f. If catheter does not drain, omentum may be obstructing or fibrin may have formed in the catheter. h, i. Heparin can help to prevent catheter blockage from fibrin or blood clots. j. Fibrinolytic agents may be effective in removing blockage. k. Constipation may lead to shifting of catheter position, drainage failure, and catheter loss.
20. Calculate inflow and outflow volume at the end of each dialysis cycle. Report discrepancies in accordance with hospital protocol.	20. Accurate inflow and outflow records determine fluid loss or retention by individual (Groenhoff et al., 2015).

Clinical Alert Report

Advise ancillary staff/student to report the following to the professional nurse assigned to the individual:
- Any changes in mental status such as agitation, lethargy, confusion
- Blood pressure, pulse, or respirations outside of prescribed limits. See Indicators. Individual parameters may vary depending on individual's medications
- Temperature (oral) 1° F to 2° F over baseline. Uremia suppresses temperature so lower readings may still indicate fever
- Difficulty breathing or new onset of shortness of breath
- New onset of pain
- Inability of peritoneal dialysis fluid to drain
- Cloudy or blood tinged peritoneal dialysis fluid drainage
- Any redness, warmth, drainage, or tenderness at peritoneal catheter site
- Genital edema

Documentation

Vital signs
Intake and output
Weight and medications
Dialysate color
Abdominal girth
Serum glucose
Urine specific gravity
Other laboratory values
Changes in status
Inflow or outflow problems
Interventions

Nursing Diagnoses

Risk for Infection Related to Access to Peritoneal Cavity

NOC

Infection Status, Wound Healing: Primary Intention, Immune Status

NIC

Infection Control, Wound Care, Incision Site Care, Health Education

Goal

The individual will be infection free at catheter site and will not develop peritonitis or a systemic infection.

Indicators (Lambertson, 2015)

- Temperature >96.8° F or <100.4° F
- No edema or drainage at site

Interventions	Rationales
1. Ensure use of sterile technique when setting up equipment. 2. Ensure complete skin preparation before catheter insertion. 3. Use sterile technique when assisting with catheter insertion or removal and when performing dialysis. Wear gloves to examine exit site. 4. Apply masks to all staff/student and the individual during catheter insertion, removal, and dressing changes. 5. Minimize catheter movement at exit site (not to be used until site healed postinsertion, preferably 10 to 14 days).	1–5. Aseptic technique reduces microorganisms and helps prevent their introduction into the system (Lambertson, 2015).
6. Warm dialysate solution in a dedicated peritoneal dialysis microwave oven for the institution's recommended time frame. Agitate bag before infusing. Other heating methods include heating pad, laying bag in sunshine, or near other heat source. Avoid heating in water bath.	6. Because microwave ovens vary in rate, consistency, and method of heating, each institution needs to establish its own time frame and protocol. Heating in water may lead to possible contamination. High heat over a prolonged time can change the composition and clarity of the dialysate (Groenhoff et al., 2015).
7. Determine that dialysate is between 36.5° C and 37.5° C (97.7° F and 99.5° F) before infusing.	7. External temperature may be measured by folding the bag over an electronic thermometer. Bag should be tepid to touch (Groenhoff et al., 2015).
8. When performing manual peritoneal dialysis, prevent contamination of spikes when changing dialysate bags.	8. Peritoneal dialysate may be done manually with a manifold setup or by an automatic cycler. Use of bags allows the peritoneal dialysis system to remain closed except when connecting (Groenhoff et al., 2015).

(continued)

Interventions	Rationales
9. Monitor dialysate return for color and clarity. Obtain culture of any drainage.	9–13. Turbidity may indicate infection, noninfectious eosinophilia, or menstruation (Lambertson, 2015).
10. Perform routine exit site care using aseptic technique.	
11. Increase frequency of exit site care, as needed.	
12. Change cleansing agent for exit site care, as indicated.	
13. Teach alternative methods of exit site care.	

Documentation

Signs and symptoms of infection
Dressing changes

Risk for Ineffective Breathing Pattern Related to Immobility, Pressure, and Pain

NOC
Respiratory Status: Gas Exchange, Vital Sign Status, Anxiety Control

Goal

The individual will demonstrate optimal respiratory function.

Indicators

NIC
Respiratory Monitoring, Progressive Muscle Relaxation, Teaching, Anxiety Reduction

- Bilateral breath sounds, clear lung fields globally with no rales or crepitus
- Arterial blood gases

Interventions	Rationales
1. Encourage regular coughing and deep-breathing exercises.	1. Hypoventilation may result from increased pressure on the diaphragm as a result of dialysate instillation and position during cycle. Pulmonary edema, pleuritis, infection, or uremic lung also may contribute to respiratory distress (Bargman, 2015; Groenhoff et al., 2015).
2. Evaluate effect of smaller dialysate solution volumes on adequacy and initiate if appropriate. Evaluate potential for PD modality change to cycling therapy.	2. Stopping flow reduces pressure on the diaphragm, possibly relieving distress (Bargman, 2015; Lambertson, 2015b).

> **CLINICAL ALERT:**
> - If individual experiences respiratory distress, immediately stop inflow or begin outflow.
> - Respiratory distress can indicate an acute hydrothorax from a leak in the diaphragm.
> - The negative pressure in the thoracic cavity and the positive pressure in the intra-abdominal cavity moves the peritoneal fluid from the peritoneal to the pleural cavity (Bargman, 2015; Lambertson, 2015).

Documentation

Abnormal respiratory status

Impaired Comfort Related to Catheter Insertion, Instillation of Dialysis Solution, Outflow Suction, and Chemical Irritation of Peritoneum

NOC
Comfort Level, Pain Control

Goal

The individual will be as comfortable as possible during peritoneal dialysis.

NIC
Respiratory Monitoring, Progressive Muscle Relaxation, Pain Management, Anxiety Reduction (Lambertson, 2015b)

Indicators

Explain reason for discomforts

- No pressure or pain during the procedure
- Report measures used that reduced pain

Interventions	*Rationales*
1. Instruct individual to report excessive pain on catheter insertion or dialysate instillation. Have individual describe pain's severity on a scale of 0 to 10 (0 = no pain; 10 = most severe pain). **CLINICAL ALERT:** • Pain on catheter insertion calls for catheter repositioning; pain during dialysate instillation may result from various factors including too-rapid inflow rate, dialysate temperature too cool or too warm, and complications of treatment (Lambertson, 2015b).	
2. Position individual to minimize pain while maintaining good air exchange and free-flowing dialysate.	2. Certain positions can reduce abdominal discomfort during instillation.
3. Drain effluent to assess for cloudy or bloody fluid. Initiate protocol for peritonitis, if indicated.	3. Lidocaine may be used as an intraperitoneal analgesic.
4. As necessary, use nonpharmacologic pain-relief techniques such as distraction, massage, guided imagery, and relaxation exercises.	4. Nonpharmacologic pain-relief techniques can offer effective, safe alternatives to medication in some individuals.
5. Check temperature of dialysate before and during instillation. **CLINICAL ALERT:** • If individual reports extreme pain during dialysis, decrease inflow rate and consult with physician/nurse practitioner to decrease temporarily the amount of dialysate instilled.	5. A too-cool dialysate temperature can cause abdominal cramps; too warm a temperature can cause tissue damage. A slower instillation rate reduces intra-abdominal pressure and may decrease pain. A decrease in volume reduces degree of abdominal distention, especially on initiation of dialysis.
6. Investigate carefully any individual reports of pain in the shoulder blades.	6. Referred pain to the shoulders may be from diaphragmatic irritation or from air infused on insertion.

Documentation

Pain
Relief measures instituted
Individual's response

TRANSITION TO HOME/COMMUNITY CARE
- Review the risk diagnoses identified at admission.
- Review medications including purpose, dose, and schedule with individual. Provide written list including instructions.
- Ascertain that the follow-up plan for dialysis is in place and that the individual/family knows the schedule, time, and place of follow-up. Provide contact information for dialysis services.

- Discuss dietary changes. If individual is still uncertain, contact dietitian or refer to out-patient dietitian.
- Use STAR (Stop, Think, Act, Review) to determine if transition plan is complete.
- Use SBAR (Situation, Background, Assessment, Recommendation) to relay necessary information to appropriate professional.

SBAR   *Situation:* Individual is being transitioned on chronic dialysis but has not yet learned how to do own treatment. PD catheter was inserted 1 week ago.

Background: Individual is scheduled to start training in 1 week. Individual has been receiving hemodialysis with a temporary catheter.

Assessment: Verify with health team (a) is dialysis continuing? and (b) where will individual be receiving dialysis? (This potential problem may have already been addressed and resolved during hospitalization but individual and outpatient facility need clear plan.)

Recommendation: Individual may be eligible for public assistance, car pool, or be considered for a different dialysis shift.

Risk for Ineffective Heath Management Related to Insufficient Knowledge of Rationale of Treatment, Medications, Home Dialysis Procedure, Signs and Symptoms of Complications, Community Resources, and Follow-Up Care

NOC
Compliance (Engagement) Behavior, Knowledge: Treatment Regimen, Participation: Health Care Decisions, Treatment Behavior: Illness or Injury

NIC
Anticipatory Guidance, Learning Facilitation, Risk Identification, Health Education, Teaching: Procedure/ Treatment, Health System Guidance

Goals

The goals for this diagnosis represent those associated with transition planning. Refer to the transition criteria.

Interventions	Rationales
1. Reinforce physician's/nurse practitioner's explanations of renal disease and of peritoneal dialysis procedure and its effects. 2. Discuss all prescribed medications, covering purpose, dosage, and side effects.	1, 2. Individual's understanding can help to increase compliance and tolerance of treatment.

CLINICAL ALERT:
- In addition to general infection control education (handwashing, avoidance of sick individuals, maintenance of routine vaccinations), individual/family need instruction in peritoneal dialysis catheter care, avoidance of contamination during PD procedure, possible home risks (e.g., pets, swimming pool or pond/Jacuzzi, or lack of private space for procedure).

Interventions	*Rationales*
3. As appropriate, teach individual the following and ask individual to perform return demonstrations so nurse can evaluate individual's ability to do procedures safely and effectively: a. Aseptic technique b. Catheter care c. Dialysate preparation d. Positioning during treatment e. Instilling additives to dialysate f. Inflow and outflow procedure g. Obtain fluid sample for infection or peritoneal membrane characteristic study.	3. Many individuals can perform home peritoneal dialysis without assistance. Proper technique can help to prevent infection and inflow and outflow problems (Groenhoff et al., 2015).
4. Discuss how to manage inflow pain by ensuring proper temperature and flow rate of dialysate. **CLINICAL ALERT:** • Imbalance nutrition may change dramatically from predialysis diet. Current dietary habits, pain, abdominal distension from PD fluid, or anorexia may all impact nutritional intake. Dietary consult with reinforcement from nursing may be helpful.	4. Cold dialysate, too-rapid inflow, acid dialysate, and stretching of diaphragm can cause inflow pain.
5. Teach individual to maintain adequate protein and calorie intake.	5. Protein malnutrition is a major concern. Large protein losses occur with peritoneal dialysis. Low serum albumin levels are known to be associated with an increased risk of death. Because glucose is absorbed from the dialysate and weight gain may be a problem, high glucose solutions should be used sparingly and dietary intake of simple carbohydrates avoided (Groenhoff et al., 2015; Mehrotra, 2015).
6. Teach individual to prevent constipation through adequate diet, fluid intake, and physical activity.	6. Constipation or bowel distention impedes dialysate outflow (Lambertson, 2015b).
7. Teach individual to watch for and promptly report: a. Unresolved pain from inflow b. Outflow failure c. Low-grade fever, cloudy outflow, malaise, and catheter site changes (redness, inflammation, drainage, tenderness, warmth, and leaks). **CLINICAL ALERT:** • Advise to notify physician/nurse practitioner immediately.	7. Early detection of complications enables prompt intervention to minimize their seriousness (Lambertson, 2015b). a. This finding can indicate intraperitoneal infection. b. This finding may result from catheter obstruction, peritonitis, dislodged catheter, or a full colon. c. These signs can point to infection.
d. Signs of fluid/electrolyte imbalance (see Risk for Complications of Fluid Imbalance, Risk for Complications of Electrolyte Imbalances for specific signs and symptoms of various imbalances) e. Abdominal pain, stool changes, constipation **CLINICAL ALERT:** • Advise to call physician/nurse practitioner with symptoms.	d. Dialysis alters fluid and electrolyte levels, possibly resulting in imbalance. e. Bowel distention impedes outflow.
8. Ensure that individual knows how to order/obtain necessary supplies.	8. Knowledge of sources of supplies can prevent incorrect substitutions.

(continued)

Interventions	Rationales
9. Teach individual to record the following: a. Vital signs and weight before and after dialysis b. Percent of dialysate and amount of inflow c. Amount of outflow d. Number of exchanges required e. Medications taken f. Problems g. Urine output and number and character of stools	9. Accurate records aid in evaluating effectiveness of treatment.
10. Initiate referral to a home health care agency if indicated.	10. Home health referral may be needed for services such as medication management, physical and occupational therapy. Services managed by home dialysis are generally covered by that program.
11. Provide information on available community resources and self-help groups (e.g., National Kidney Foundation at www.kidney.org, American Association of Kidney Patients [AAKP] at www.aakp.org).	11. Access to resources and self-help groups may ease difficulties of home dialysis and help to minimize its effects on home life.

Documentation

Individual/family teaching
Outcome achievement or status
Referrals, if indicated

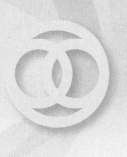

Section 4

Specialty Diagnostic Clusters

Section 4 contains five specialty care plans for Normal Newborn; Infants, Children, and Adolescents; the Family in the Prenatal and Postpartum periods; and Individuals with Mental Health Problems. Diagnostic clusters for each of these care plans are presented here. The reader can access the complete plan on thePoint, the website for additional supplements for this book.

Once the care plan is accessed on thePoint, it can be printed. Using the steps to create a care plan as outlined in Chapter 5, Eleven Steps to Care Planning, the student or nurse can also use additional nursing diagnoses or collaborative problems from Unit II. For example, for a child with diabetes mellitus, the nurse can access Risk for Complications of Hypo/Hyperglycemia (in Unit II) and add this to the specialty generic plan. Another example is an adolescent on a postsurgical unit, voicing suicide threats: the student or nurse can access Risk for Suicide in Unit II and add it to the care plan.

It is important to keep in mind that it is not possible to address all nursing diagnoses that an individual/family may have in addition to the generic plan. Therefore, if needed, review the criteria for priority diagnoses. Refer to the general index for the pages in Chapter 1.

Generic Newborn Care Plan

Transition from fetus to neonate requires profound physiologic adaptation. Key elements in the birth transition are (1) shift from maternally dependent oxygenation to continuous respiration; (2) change from fetal circulation to mature circulation with increase in pulmonary blood flow and loss of left-to-right shunting; (3) commencement of independent glucose homeostasis; (4) independent thermoregulation; and (5) oral feedings. Close observation of the infant's adaptation to extrauterine life is imperative to identify problems in transition and initiate interventions (Mattson & Smith, 2016). While most newborns achieve physiologic homeostasis without complications, assessment and monitoring of neonatal adaptation are essential for early identification of problems, including cold stress, hypoglycemia, infection, and hyperbilirubinemia. Vitamin K administration, eye prophylaxis, and routine screening for genetic and metabolic diseases help prevent and identify conditions that threaten the health and well-being of newborns. The perinatal history, including maternal, paternal, antepartal, and intrapartal data, gives perinatal and neonatal nurses important and baseline information regarding newborn risk. Nursing management during the early newborn period includes identification of risk factors, assessment, monitoring, intervention, and postdischarge follow-up.

Newborn Transition from Intrauterine to Extrauterine Life: Birth to 4 Hours of Life

■■■■■ DIAGNOSTIC CLUSTER

Collaborative Problems: Newborn Transition from Intrauterine to Extrauterine Life: Birth to 4 Hours of Life

Risk for Complications of Respiratory Dysfunction: Hypoxemia

Risk for Complications of Hypothermia

Risk for Complications of Hypoglycemia

Risk for Complications of Sepsis

Nursing Diagnoses: Newborn Transition from Intrauterine to Extrauterine Life: Birth to 4 Hours of Life

Risk for Ineffective Respiratory Function

　related to newborn transition to extrauterine life

　related to delayed clearance of fetal lung fluid

　related to persistent fetal circulatory pattern

　related to aspiration of blood, meconium, or amniotic fluid

Ineffective Thermoregulation

　related to newborn transition to extrauterine life

　related to immature temperature regulating mechanisms

　related to heat loss from exposure to cool temperature of birthing room, mother's room

Risk for Infection

　related to vulnerability of newborn secondary to immature immune system

　related to lack of normal flora

　related to exposure of eyes to vaginal secretions

　related to open wound (umbilical cord, spiral electrode lesion)

　related to colonization by/transmission of perinatal infection acquired in utero

　related to environmental hazards

Normal Newborn Care: 4 Hours to 4 Days of Life

■■■■■ DIAGNOSTIC CLUSTER

Collaborative Problems: Normal Newborn Care: 4 Hours to 4 Days of Life

Risk for Complications of Hypothermia

Risk for Complications of Hypoglycemia

Risk for Complications of Infection

Risk for Complications of Hyperbilirubinemia

Risk for Complications of Bleeding (Circumcision)

Risk for Complication of Sepsis

Nursing Diagnoses: Normal Newborn Care: 4 Hours to 4 Days of Life

Risk for Aspiration

   related to decreased muscle tone of the inferior esophageal sphincter

   related to secretions of the oropharynx

Ineffective Thermoregulation

   related to newborn transition to extrauterine life

   related to immature temperature regulating mechanisms

   related to heat loss from exposure to cool temperature of birthing room, mother's room

Risk for Infection

   related to vulnerability of newborn secondary to immature immune system

   related to lack of normal flora

   related to exposure of eyes to vaginal secretions

   related to open wound (umbilical cord, spiral electrode lesion, circumcision)

   related to colonization by/transmission of perinatal infection acquired in utero

   related to environmental hazards

Risk for Ineffective Breastfeeding

   related to incorrect positioning of newborn at the breast

   related to unsuccessful latch

   related to absence of regular and sustained suckling/swallowing at the breast

   related to maternal fatigue or anxiety due to inexperience with breastfeeding

Risk for Imbalanced Nutrition

   related to limited caloric intake during the first few days of life

   related to ineffective infant latch and sucking

   related to maternal nipple soreness

Risk for Impaired Skin Integrity

   related to diaper dermatitis, circumcision

Acute Pain

   related to injections, heel sticks, circumcision

Risk for Impaired Parent–Infant Attachment

   related to unwanted pregnancy

   related to prolonged or difficult labor and delivery

   related to postpartum pain or fatigue

(continued)

related to lack of positive support system

related to lack of positive role model

related to inability to prepare emotionally

Risk for Impaired Parenting

related to lack of access to resources

related to postpartum depression

related to adolescent parents

related to substance abuse

related to domestic violence

related to poor home environment

related to preterm birth

related to ineffective adaptation to stressors associated with parenting a new infant

related to impaired support system

Risk for Injury

related to parental lack of awareness of environmental hazards

Risk for Ineffective Infant Health Management

related to parents' insufficient knowledge of jaundice, adequate feeding, voiding and stooling, skin integrity, safe sleep measures, fall prevention, and when to call the infant's primary provider

Generic Medical Care Plan for Hospitalized Infants/Children/Adolescents

This care plan presents nursing diagnoses and collaborative problems that commonly apply to infants, children, and adolescents (and their significant others) undergoing hospitalization for any medical disorder. It represents a standard of care. For beginning students, it can represent the care that they are prepared to provide. As the student progresses in the curriculum, the care plans for specific medical conditions as pneumonia, diabetes mellitus, fractures, and those focusing on the care of individuals undergoing surgery or therapies as chemotherapy will be their focus of care.

By applying the principles of pediatric nursing, many of the care plans in the textbook can be adapted to children. For example, if a child has diabetes mellitus, one can also refer to the textbook in Section II Risk for Complications of Hypo/Hyperglycemia for specific interventions. If the child has had surgery, refer to Generic Surgical Care Plan in the textbook. If the child has asthma, refer to the care plan for adults with asthma and provide the interventions that are age-appropriate.

■■■■■ DIAGNOSTIC CLUSTER

Collaborative Problems

Risk for Complications of Cardiovascular Dysfunction

Risk for Complications of Respiratory Dysfunction

Risk for Complications of Dehydration/Hypovolemia

Risk for Complications of Infection/Sepsis

Nursing Diagnoses

Anxiety (child, caregivers) related to unfamiliar environment, routines, diagnostic tests, treatments, loss of control, and age-related fears

Parental Role Conflict related to effects of illness and/or hospitalization of a child on family unit secondary to fear of unknown, disruption of routines, change in role responsibilities, and fatigue associated with increased workload and visiting hour requirements.

Risk for Injury related to unfamiliar environment, developmental considerations, and physical and mental limitations secondary to condition, medications, therapies, and diagnostic tests

Risk for Infection related to increased microorganisms in environment, risk of person-to-person transmission, and invasive tests and therapies

(Specify) Self-Care Deficit related to developmental level, sensory, cognitive, mobility, endurance, or motivation problems

Acute Pain related to (specify)

   Gastrointestinal inflammation and infectious process

   Tissue trauma and reflex muscle spasms secondary to:

      Musculoskeletal disorders

         Spasms

         Fibromyalgia

         Fractures

      Visceral disorders

         Cardiac

         Renal

         Hepatic

      Pulmonary disorders

         Cancer

         Vasospasm

   Tissue trauma and reflex muscle spasms secondary to:

      Accidents

      Burns

      Diagnostic tests (venipuncture, invasive scanning, biopsy)

      Surgery

   Viscous blood and tissue hypoxia secondary to sickling

Chronic Pain related to (specify)

   Tissue trauma and reflex muscle spasms secondary to:

      Musculoskeletal Disorders

         Arthritis

         Fibromyalgia

         Spinal cord disorders

(continued)

Chronic visceral disorders

Cardiac

Intestinal

Pulmonary disorders

Renal

Hepatic

Cancer

Tissue trauma and reflex muscle spasms secondary to:

Burns

Motor vehicle trauma

Viscous blood and tissue hypoxia secondary to sickling

Risk for Imbalanced Nutrition related to developmental feeding issues; congenital or disease entities; altered route of nutrition (NG, ND, GT, central line/TPN); decreased appetite secondary to treatments, fatigue, environment, and changes in usual diet; and increased protein and vitamin requirements for healing

Risk for Deficient Fluid Volume

related insufficient intake secondary to fatigue, malaise, dyspnea, pain

related to fluid loss secondary to fever, diarrhea

related to difficult or painful swallowing

Risk for Impaired Skin Integrity

related to adhesive tape, dressings, monitoring devices, IV infiltrates

related to changes in stooling patterns, urinary/fecal incontinence

related to increased fragility of the skin associated with dependent edema

Risk for pressure ulcer (refer to Unit II Section 1 Risk for Pressure Ulcer)

related to prolonged pressure on tissues associated with decreased mobility

related to decreased tissue perfusion, malnutrition

Disturbed Sleep Pattern related to unfamiliar, noisy environment, change in bedtime ritual, emotional stress, and change in circadian rhythm

Interrupted Family Processes related to disruption of routines, change in role responsibilities, and fatigue associated with increased workload

Risk for Compromised Human Dignity related to multiple factors (intrusions, unfamiliar procedures and personnel, loss of privacy) associated with hospitalization

Risk for Ineffective Child Health Management related to complexity and cost of therapeutic regimen, complexity of health care system, insurance/financial issues, coordination of care, shortened length of stay, insufficient knowledge of treatment, and barriers to comprehension secondary to language barriers, cognitive deficits, hearing and/or visual impairment, anxiety, and lack of motivation

Generic Care Plan for Individuals With Mental Health Disorders

Individuals with mental disorders who require hospitalization do so because they are not functioning well or appropriately. Their compromised coping disrupts their ability to self-care, relate to others effectively, and problem-solve appropriately. They may, in addition, be at risk for harming themselves or others. This care plan focuses on functional health patterns that are disrupted, with an attempt to stabilize and comfort the individual and significant others.

Most individuals hospitalized for a mental disorder also have comorbidities as hypertension, diabetes mellitus, chronic obstructive pulmonary disease (COPD), and asthma. If indicated, refer to Unit II Section 2, Individual Collaborative Problems and select those that need monitoring, such as Risk for Complications of Hypertension, Risk for Complications of Respiratory Dysfunction, Risk for Complications of Hypo/Hyperglycemia.

If an individual with chronic mental health problems needs surgery, refer to the Generic Surgical Care Plan. Dysfunction related to a nursing diagnosis, such as Ineffective Coping related to faulty thinking secondary to (specify mental disorder), can be addressed by referring to this diagnosis in this plan.

When an individual is hospitalized for a mental disorder (in the diagnostic cluster below), the generic nursing diagnoses that relate to any individual in the hospital are applicable and can be found in under the Generic Medical Care Plan for the Hospitalized Adult found in the book.:

- Anxiety related to unfamiliar environment, routines, diagnostic tests, treatments, and loss of control
- Risk for Injury related to unfamiliar environment and physical and mental limitations secondary to condition, medications, therapies, and diagnostic tests
- Risk for Infection related to increased microorganisms in environment, risk of person-to-person transmission, and invasive tests and therapies
- (Specify) Self-Care Deficit related to sensory, cognitive, mobility, endurance, or motivation problems
- Risk for Imbalanced Nutrition related to decreased appetite secondary to treatments, fatigue, environment, and changes in usual diet and to increased protein and vitamin requirements for healing
- Risk for Constipation related to change in fluid and food intake, routine, and activity level; effects of medications; and emotional stress
- Risk for Pressure Ulcers related to prolonged pressure on tissues associated with decreased mobility, increased fragility of the skin associated with dependent edema, decreased tissue perfusion, malnutrition, and urinary/fecal incontinence
- Disturbed Sleep Pattern related to unfamiliar, noisy environment, change in bedtime ritual, emotional stress, and change in circadian rhythm
- Interrupted Family Processes related to disruption of routines, change in role responsibilities, and fatigue associated with increased workload and visiting hour requirements
- Risk for Compromised Human Dignity related to multiple factors (intrusions, unfamiliar procedures and personnel, loss of privacy) associated with hospitalization
- Risk for Ineffective Health Management related to complexity and cost of therapeutic regimen, complexity of health care system, shortened length of stay, insufficient knowledge of treatment, and barriers to comprehension secondary to language barriers, cognitive deficits, hearing and/or visual impairment, anxiety, and lack of motivation

Carp's Cues

Individuals with mental health conditions predominately live in the community and receive medical care in private offices or mental health centers. When an individual is hospitalized for a mental health condition, it is due to a deterioration in their ability to function in their home setting or in the community.

Their compromised functioning cannot be described using a psychiatric diagnosis as Depression, Affective Disorder, or Bipolar Disorder. Nursing Diagnosis provides the terminology of the compromised functioning that needs to be addressed for a successful transition back to living in the community. Describing an individual as depressed does not describe why the individual is having difficulty functioning in the community, but Risk for Suicide, Defensive Coping, Self-Care Deficits, Ineffective Denial, Noncompliance, and Impaired Home Maintenance Management do.

The following are examples of nursing diagnoses that represent dysfunction and ineffective coping in individuals with mental disorders. The nurse must focus on those problems that are most disruptive to the person's ability to function safely and effectively in the community. Students should seek the advice of their instructor or experienced nurse for selection of this individual's priority problems. It is not very helpful to focus on the psychiatric diagnosis because it will not help to determine nursing interventions. Instead focus on what Functional Health Patterns are disrupted that prevent him/her from functioning well in the community.

▪▪▪▪■■ DIAGNOSTIC CLUSTER

Nursing Diagnoses

Anxiety related to persistent ineffective coping and/or irrational thoughts

Risk for Disabled Family Coping

related to chronicity of illness

related to marital discord and role conflicts secondary to effects of chronic depression

related to effects of substance abuse on family members and relapses

Disturbed Self-Concept related to feelings of worthlessness and lack of ego boundaries

Chronic Low Self-Esteem related to feelings of worthlessness and failure secondary to (specify)

Ineffective Coping

related to internal conflicts (guilt, low self-esteem) or feelings of rejection

related to biochemical changes with faulty thinking secondary (specify mental disorder)

related to biochemical changes with poor impulse control and low frustration level

Defensive Coping related to unrealistic expectations secondary to exaggerated sense of self-importance and abilities

Impaired Social Interaction

related to alienation from others secondary to overt hostility, overconfidence, or manipulation of others

related to effects of behavior and actions on forming and maintaining relationships

related to feelings of mistrust and suspicion of others

Risk for Suicide related to feelings of hopelessness and loneliness

Risk for Other-Directed Violence

related to responding to delusional thoughts or hallucinations

related to impaired reality testing, impaired judgment, or compromised ability to control behavior

Disturbed Thought Processes

related to negative cognitive set (overgeneralizing, polarized thinking, selected abstraction, arbitrary inference)

related to unknown etiology (e.g., repressed fears, drug use, abuse)

related to biochemical disturbances

[1]Risk for Compromised Engagement related to feelings of no longer requiring medication, impaired judgment and thought disturbances

Ineffective Denial related to substance abuse

Impaired Social Interaction

related to unrealistic expectations of relationships and impaired ability to maintain enduring attachments

related to biochemical disturbances with preoccupation with egocentric and illogical ideas and extreme suspiciousness

Deficient Dimensional Activity

---

[1]This new nursing diagnosis has been developed by this author to replace noncompliance. Refer to Unit II Section 1 Compromised Engagement for more information.

related to a loss of interest or pleasure in usual activities and low energy levels

related to apathy, inability to initiate goal-directed activities, and loss of skills

Risk for Ineffective Health Management related to insufficient knowledge of condition, behavior modification, therapy options (pharmacologic, electroshock), and community resources

Impaired Home Maintenance related to impaired judgment, inability to self-initiate activity, and loss of skills over long course of illness

Generic Care Plan for Woman/Support Persons During Prenatal Period

This care plan focuses on the pregnant woman without a condition that complicates her pregnancy. If the mother also has a medical condition as diabetes mellitus or asthma, refer to Unit II Section 2 for the specific collaborative problem such as Risk for Complications (RC) of Hypo/Hyperglycemia, RC of Asthma Exacerbation and add it to the problem list.

Hemorrhagic complications during pregnancy are a significant causative factor of adverse maternal–fetal outcomes. Hemorrhage during pregnancy is one of the leading causes of maternal death in the United States, along with embolism and hypertensive disorders (Simpson & Creehan, 2014). Preterm labor resulting in preterm birth is estimated to be responsible for 70% of neonatal deaths and 36% of infant deaths as well as 25% to 50% of cases of long-term neurologic impairment in children in the United States (American College of Obstetricians and Gynecologists [ACOG], 2016a). Hypertension affects 12% to 22% of pregnancies in the United States and is one of the top three causes of maternal mortality (Lo, Mission, & Caughey, 2013). Pregnancy predisposes women to venous thromboembolism because of changes in the coagulation system that occur during pregnancy. If untreated, deep vein thrombosis (DVT) may progress to pulmonary embolism (PE) in about 15% to 25% of individuals (Troiano, Harvey, & Chez, 2013).

■■■■ DIAGNOSTIC CLUSTER

Collaborative Problems

Risk for Complications of Prenatal Bleeding

Risk for Complications of Preterm Labor

Risk for Complications of Gestational Hypertension

Risk for Complications of Deep Vein Thrombosis

Nursing Diagnoses

Nausea related to elevated estrogen and hCG levels, decreased blood sugar, or decreased gastric motility and pressure on cardiac sphincter from enlarged uterus (refer to Unit II Section 1).

Constipation related to elevated progesterone levels, relaxed GI tract, decreased gastric motility, and pressure of uterus on lower colon (refer to Unit II Section 1).

Activity Intolerance related to fatigue and dyspnea secondary to pressure of enlarging uterus on diaphragm and increased blood volume (refer to Unit II Section 1).

Risk for Impaired Oral Mucous Membranes related to hyperemic gums secondary to elevated estrogen and progesterone levels (refer to Unit II Section 1).

Risk for Falls related to syncope/hypotension secondary to peripheral venous pooling secondary to peripheral venous pooling (refer to Unit II Section).

(continued)

Risk for Ineffective Health Management related to insufficient knowledge of (examples) effects of pregnancy on body systems (cardiovascular, integumentary, gastrointestinal, urinary, pulmonary, musculoskeletal), psychosocial domain, sexuality/sexual function, family unit (spouse, children), fetal growth and development, nutritional requirements, hazards of smoking, excessive alcohol intake, drug abuse, excessive caffeine intake, excessive weight gain, signs and symptoms of complications (vaginal bleeding, cramping, gestational diabetes, excessive edema, preeclampsia), preparation for childbirth (classes, printed references).

Generic Care Plan for Woman/Support Persons During Postpartum Period

This care plan focuses on the care of the mother postdelivery and preparation of the family unit to transition to home. If the mother also has a medical condition as diabetes mellitus, asthma, or hypertension, refer to Section II for the specific collaborative problem as Risk for Complications (RC) of hypertension, RC of asthma exacerbation, or RC of hypo/hyperglycemia, and add it to the problem list. If a C-section is done, refer also to the Generic Surgical Care Plan.

The postpartum period (also known as the puerperium) begins at the time of delivery of the placenta and membranes and is complete when the woman's reproductive system returns to its prepregnant state at about 6 weeks. It is a time of physiologic and psychologic changes. The first 4 hours after birth is referred to as the fourth stage of labor and delivery. This is a time when physiologic complications may occur. While adapting to the maternal role, the mother may experience a great range of emotions as she is adjusting to the physical changes in her body.

The father's emotional status and interaction with the infant are particularly important because he usually serves as the mother's primary support person. Unrealistic expectations of the infant may lead to problems. A strong, consistent support system is a major factor in the adjustment of the new mother. Family members often provide a powerful support system, and their involvement is important to the adaptation of the family.

■■■ DIAGNOSTIC CLUSTER

Collaborative Problems

Risk for Complications of Bleeding/Postpartum Hemorrhage

Risk for Complications of Uterine Atony

Risk for Complications of Retained Placental Fragments

Risk for Complications of Lacerations

Risk for Complications of Hematomas

Risk for Complications of Urinary Retention

Risk for Complications of Deep Vein Thrombosis

Nursing Diagnoses

Risk for Infection related to bacterial invasion secondary to trauma during labor, delivery, episiotomy or cesarean surgical site, urinary catheterization, breasts (refer to Unit II Section 1)

Risk for Ineffective Breastfeeding related to inexperience or pain secondary to engorged breasts, sore nipples (refer to Unit II Section 1)

Acute Pain related to trauma to perineum during labor and delivery, hemorrhoids, engorged breasts, and involution of uterus (refer to Unit II Section 1)

Risk for Constipation related to food and fluid restrictions during labor, decreased intestinal peristalsis (postdelivery), decreased activity, and fear of pain with defecation due to perineal discomfort (refer to Unit II Section 1)

Risk for Impaired Parent–Infant Attachment related to (examples) inexperience, feelings of incompetence, powerlessness, unwanted child, disappointment with child, lack of role models, high-risk newborn

Stress Urinary Incontinence related to tissue trauma during delivery (refer to Unit II Section 1)

Risk for Falls related to orthostatic hypotension, blood loss, effect of epidural analgesia, fatigue (refer to Unit II Section 1)

Risk for Ineffective Infant Care Management related to insufficient knowledge and/or to primiparous status, inexperience with infant care (refer to Generic Newborn Care Plan)

Risk for Ineffective Coping related to history of anxiety or mood disorder, unmarried or not, cohabiting with partner, poor social support, low socioeconomic status, birth complications, smoking, multiparity, BMI >30, stressful life event during pregnancy and/or postpartum

Risk for Ineffective Health Management related to insufficient knowledge of perineal care and symptoms of complications and follow-up care

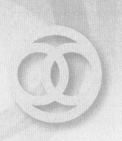

References

Abel, E. J., Wong, K., Sado, M., Leverson, G. E., Patel, S. R., Downs, T. M., & Jarrard, D. F. (2014). Surgical operative time increases the risk of deep venous thrombosis and pulmonary embolism in robotic prostatectomy. *Journal of the Society of Laparoendoscopic Surgeons, 18*(2), 282.

Adams, C., Bailey, D., Anderson, R., & Docherty, S. (2011). Nursing roles and strategies in end-of-life decisions: A systematic review of the literature. *Nursing Research and Practice.* doi:10.1155/2011/527834. Retrieved from http://www.hindawi.com/journals/nrp/2011/527834/

*Addams, S., & Clough, J. A. (1998). Modalities for mobilization. In A. B. Mahler, S. Salmond, & T. Pellino (Eds.), *Orthopedic nursing*. Philadelphia, PA: W. B. Saunders.

Adkins, E. S. (2015). Surgical treatment of ulcerative colitis. In *Medscape*. Retrieved from http://emedicine.medscape.com/article/937427-overview

Adler, J., & Malone, D. (2012). Early mobilization in the intensive care unit: A systematic review. *Cardiopulmonary Physical Therapy Journal, 23*(1), 5–13.

Adler, N. E., Page, A., & Institute of Medicine (U.S.). (2008). *Cancer care for the whole patient: Meeting psychosocial health needs*. Washington, DC: National Academies Press.

*Agency for Health Care Policy and Research. (1994). *Evaluation and management of early HIV infection. Clinical practice guideline* 7. Washington, DC: AHCPR, Public Health Service, U.S. Department of Health and Human Services.

Agency for Healthcare Research and Quality. (2010). *2009 National healthcare quality report* (AHRQ Publication No. 10-0003). Rockville, MD: Author. Retrieved from http://www.ahrq.gov/qual/nhqr09/nhqr09.pdf

Agostini, P., Cieslik, H., Rathinam, S., Bishay, E., Kalkat, M. S., Rajesh, P. B., . . . Naidu, B. (2010). Postoperative pulmonary complications following thoracic surgery: Are there any modifiable risk factors? *Thorax, 65*(9), 815–818.

*Agrawal, A., Ayantunde, A. A., & Cheung, K. L. (2006). Concepts of seroma formation and prevention in breast cancer surgery. *ANZ Journal of Surgery, 76*, 1088–1095.

AIDS.gov. (2015). *Newly diagnosed: What you need to know*. Retrieved from https://www.aids.gov/hiv-aids-basics/just-diagnosed-with-hiv-aids/overview/newly-diagnosed/index.html#manageable

AIDSinfo. (2014). *Limitations to treatment safety and efficacy. Guidelines for the use of antiretroviral agents in HIV-1-infected adults and adolescents*. Retrieved from https://aidsinfo.nih.gov/guidelines/html/1/adult-and-adolescent-arv-guidelines/30/adherence-to-art

Aiken, L. H., Sloane, D. M., Cimiotti, J. P., Clarke, S. P., Flynn, L., Seago, J. A., . . . Smith, H. L. (2010). *Implications of the California nurse staffing mandate for other states*. Retrieved from http://www.nationalnursesunited.org/assets/pdf/hsr_ratios_study_042010.pdf

*Akbari, C. M., Saouaf, R., Barnhill, D. F., Newman, P. A., LoGerfo, F. W., & Veves, A. (1998). Endothelium-dependent vasodilatation is impaired in both microcirculation and macrocirculation during acute hyperglycemia. *Journal of Vascular Surgery, 28*(4), 687–694.

*Albano, S. A., & Wallace, D. J. (2001). Managing fatigue in patients with SLE. *Journal of Musculoskelatal Medicine, 18*, 149–152.

*Alcee, D. (2000). The experience of a community hospital in quantifying and reducing patient falls. *Journal of Nursing Care Quality, 14*(3), 43–53.

Alcoholics Anonymous. (2008). *Welcome to alcoholics. A brief guide to Alcoholics Anonymous*. Retrieved from www.aa.org

Alexandraki, I., & Smetana, G. W. (2015). Acute viral gastroenteritis in adults. In *UpToDate*. Retrieved from http://www.uptodate.com/contents/acute-viral-gastroenteritis-in-adults

Alfaro-LeFevre, R. (2014). *Applying nursing process: The foundation for clinical reasoning* (8th ed.). Philadelphia, PA: Lippincott Williams & Wilkins.

Alguire, P. C., & Scovell, S. (2015). Overview and management of lower extremity chronic venous disease. In *UpToDate*. Retrieved from http://www.uptodate.com/contents/overview-and-management-of-lower-extremity-chronic-venous-disease

Alici, Y., & Levin, T. T. (2010). Anxiety disorders. In J. C. Holland (Ed.), *Psycho-oncology* (2nd ed.). New York, NY: Oxford University Press.

*Allen-Burge, R., Stevens, A., & Burgio, L. (1999). Effective behavioural interventions for decreasing dementia-related challenging behaviour in nursing homes. *International Journal of Geriatric Psychiatry, 14*, 213–228.

*ALLHAT Officers and Coordinators for the ALLHAT Collaborative Research Group. (2002). Major outcomes in high-risk hypertensive patients randomized to angiotensin-converting enzyme inhibitor or calcium channel blocker vs diuretic: The antihypertensive and lipid-lowering treatment to prevent heart attack trial (ALLHAT). *JAMA, 288*, 2981–2997.

*Altizer, L. (2004). Compartment syndrome. *Orthopedic Nursing, 23*(6), 391–396.

American Academy of Orthopaedic Surgeons, American Academy of Pediatrics. (2010). Fracture of the proximal femur. In L. Y. Griffin (Ed.), *Essentials of musculoskeletal care* (4th ed., pp. 563–567). Rosemont, IL: Author.

American Academy of Orthopedic Surgeons. (2012). *Lawn mower safety*. Retrieved from http://www.orthoinfo.org/topic.cfm?topic=A00670

American Academy of Orthopaedic Surgeons. (2014). *Management of hip fractures in the elderly evidence-based clinical practice guideline*. Retrieved from http://www.aaos.org/research/guidelines/HipFxGuideline.pdf

American Academy of Orthopaedic Surgeons. (2016a). *Neck and back*. Retrieved from http://orthoinfo.aaos.org/topic.cfm?topic=a00348

American Academy of Orthopedic Surgeons. (2016b). *Bicycle safety*. Retrieved from http://orthoinfo.aaos.org/topic.cfm?topic=A00711

American Academy of Orthopedic Surgeons. (2016c). *Total knee replacement*. Retrieved from http://orthoinfo.aaos.org/topic.cfm?topic=a00389

American Academy of Orthotists and Prosthetics. (2014). *Postoperative management of the lower extremity amputation*. Retrieved from http://www.oandp.org/olc/lessons/html/SSC_02/07stages.asp?frmCourseSectionId=514F4373-8EDF-434A-BA08-C221FA8ABD71

American Association of Critical Care Nurses. (2012). *Early progressive mobility protocol*. ACCNPearl. Retrieved from http://www.aacn.org/wd/practice/docs/tool%20kits/early-progressive-mobility-protocol.pdf

American Association of Critical Care Nurses. (2014). *Nurses removing chest tube*. Retrieved from http://www.atriummed.com/EN/chest_drainage/Clinical%20Updates/ClinicalUpdateFall2014.pdf

American Association of Critical Care Nurses. (2015). *Evidence-based care of patients with chest tubes evidence-based care of patients with chest tubes. 2015 National Teaching Institute ExpoEd*. Retrieved from http://www.atriummed.com/EN/chest_drainage/Documents/NTI2015Evidence-BasedCareofPatientswithChestTubes.pdf

American Association of Gynecologic Laparoscopists. (2011). Advancing minimally invasive gynecology worldwide. AAGL position statement: Route of hysterectomy to treat benign uterine disease. *Journal of Minimally Invasive Gynecology, 18*, 1.

*American Association of Hospice and Palliative Care Medicine. (2006). *Statement on palliative sedation*. Retrieved from http://aahpm.org/positions/palliative-sedation

American Association of Neuroscience Nurses. (2015). *Thoracolumbar spine surgery: A guide to preoperative and postoperative patient care*. Retrieved from http://www.aann.org/pubs/content/guidelines.html

American Cancer Society. (2007). *Breast reconstruction after mastectomy*. Retrieved from http://www.cancer.org/cancer/breastcancer/moreinformation/breastreconstructionaftermastectomy/breast-reconstruction-after-mastectomy-toc

American Cancer Society. (2011a). *Ileostomy: A guide*. Retrieved from http://www.cancer.org/acs/groups/cid/documents/webcontent/002870-pdf.pdf

American Cancer Society. (2011b). *Urostomy: A guide*. Retrieved from http://www.cancer.org/acs/groups/cid/documents/webcontent/002931-pdf.pdf

American Cancer Society. (2015). *Cancer facts & figures 2015*. Retrieved from http://www.cancer.org/acs/groups/content/@editorial/documents/document/acspc-044552.pdf

American Cancer Society. (2016a). *Key statistics for prostate cancer*. Retrieved from http://www.cancer.org/cancer/prostatecancer/detailedguide/prostate-cancer-key-statistics

American Cancer Society. (2016b). *Surgery for prostate cancer*. Retieved from http://www.cancer.org/cancer/prostatecancer/detailedguide/prostate-cancer-treating-surgery

American College of Chest Physicians. (2012). *Preventing DVT and PE in nonsurgical patients. ACCP Guidelines* (9th ed.). Northbrook, IL: Author.

American College of Obstetricians and Gynecologists. (2012). Prevention of deep vein thrombosis and pulmonary embolism (ACOG Practice Bulletin No. 84). *Obstetrics & Gynecology, 110*(2, Pt. 1), 429–440. Retrieved from http://www.acog.org/About-ACOG/News-Room/News-Releases/2007/ACOG-Issues-Recommendations-on-Prevention-of-Blood-Clots-in-Gynecologic-Surgery-Patients

American College of Obstetricians and Gynecologists Committee on Obstetric Practice; Society for Maternal–Fetal Medicine. (2010, March, Reaffirmed 2015). Committee Opinion No. 455: Magnesium sulfate before anticipated preterm birth for neuroprotection. *Obstetrics & Gynecology, 115*(3), 669–671.

American College of Sports Medicine. (2010). Exercise and type 2 diabetes: American College of Sports Medicine and the American Diabetes Association: Joint Position Statement. *Medicine and Science in Sports and Exercise, 42*(12), 2282–2303.

American Critical Care Association, ACCNPearl. (2012). *Early progressive mobility protocol.* http://www.aacn.org/wd/practice/docs/tool%20kits/early-progressive-mobility-protocol.pdf

American Diabetes Association. (2012a). Diagnosis and classification of diabetes mellitus. *Diabetes Care, 35*(Suppl. 1), S64–S71.

American Diabetes Association. (2012b). Executive summary: Standards of medical care in diabetes—2012. *Diabetes Care, 35*(Suppl. 1), S4–S10.

American Diabetes Association. (2015). Diabetes care in the hospital, nursing home, and skilled nursing facility. *Diabetes Care, 38*(Suppl. 1), S80–S85. Retrieved from http://care.diabetesjournals.org/content/38/Supplement_1/S80.full.pdf

American Diabetes Association. (2016). *Diagnosing diabetes and learning about prediabetes.* Retrieved from http://www.diabetes.org/diabetes-basics/diagnosis/?referrer=https://www.google.com/

American Foundation for Suicide Prevention. (2015). *Facts and figures.* Retrieved from www.afsp.org/understanding-suicide/facts-and-figures

*American Heart Association. (2003). *Let's talk about stroke and aphasia.* Retrieved from http://www.americanheart.org/downloadable/stroke/1079557856294500073%20ASA%20Strokeaphasia.pdf

*American Heart Association. (2004a). *Overview of stroke systems plans.* Retrieved from https://www.heart.org/idc/groups/heart-public/@wcm/@adv/documents/downloadable/ucm_466100.pdf

*American Heart Association. (2004b). *What is carotid endarectomy?* Retrieved from http://www.americanheart.org/downloadable/heart/110065676921546%20WhatIsCarotidEdarterect.pdf

*American Heart Association. (2005). *Heart disease and stroke statistics: 2005 update.* Dallas, TX: Author.

American Heart Association. (2007a). *Bypass surgery, coronary artery.* Retrieved from http://www.americanheart.org/presenter.jhtml?indentifier=4484

American Heart Association. (2007b). *Let's talk about complications after stroke.* Retrieved from http://www.americanheart.org/downloadable/stroke/1181161981749500068%20ASA%20ComplicationsStrk_4–07.pdf

American Heart Association. (2012). *About high blood pressure.* Retrieved from http://www. heart.org/HEARTORG/Conditions/HighBloodPressure/AboutHighBloodPressure/Understanding-Blood-Pressure-Readings_UCM_301764_Article.jsp

American Heart Association. (2012). *Prevention and treatment of heart failure.* Retrieved from http://www.heart.org/HEARTORG/Conditions/HeartFailure/PreventionTreatmentofHeartFailure/Heart-Failure-Medications_UCM_306342_Article.jsp

American Hospital Association, & USDHHS. (2014). *Health Research & Educational Trust, American Hospital Association, partnership for patients ventricular associated events (VAE) change package: Preventing harm from VAE—2014 Update.* Retrieved from www.hret-hen.org/index.php?option=com_content&view=article&id=10&Itemid=134

American Latex Allergy Association. (2010). *Statistics.* Retrieved from http://latexallergyresources.org/statistics

American Latex Allergy Association. (2016). *Cross reactive foods.* Retrieved from http://latexallergyresources.org/cross-reactive-food

American Lung Association. (2013). *Measuring your peak flow rate.* Retrieved from http://www.lung.org/lung-health-and-diseases/lung-disease-lookup/asthma/living-with-asthma/managing-asthma/measuring-your-peak-flow-rate.html?

*American Medical Association. (1999). Health Literacy: Report of the Council on Scientific Affairs. *JAMA, 28*(6), 552–557.

American Medical Association. (2007). *Health literacy and patient safety: Help patients understand: Manual for clinicians* (2nd ed.). Chicago IL: Author.

*American Nurses Association. (2001). *Code of ethics.* Retrieved from http://www.nursingworld.org/

American Nurses Association. (2010a). *Position Statement: Nurses' roles and responsibilities in providing care and support at the end of life.* Retrieved from http://www.nursingworld.org/MainMenuCategories/EthicsStandards/Ethics-Position-Statements/EndofLife-PositionStatement.pdf

American Nurses Association. (2010b). *Social policy statement.* Retrieved from http://nursingworld.org/Search?SearchMode=1&SearchPhrase=social+policy+statement

American Nurses Association. (2012). *ANA social policy statement.* Washington, DC: Author.

*American Pain Society. (2005). *Guideline for the management of cancer pain in adults and children.* Glenview, IL: Author.

American Psychiatric Association. (2014). *DSMV: Diagnostic and statistical manual of mental disorders* (4th ed., text revision). Washington, DC: Author.

American Society of Anethesiolgy. (2014). *ASA physical status classification system.* Retrieved from https://www.asahq.org/resources/clinical-information/asa-physical-status-classification-system

American Society of Colon and Rectal Surgeons Committee Members, Wound Ostomy Continence Nurse Society Committee Members. (2007). ASCRS and WOCN joint position statement on the value of preoperative stoma marking for patients undergoing fecal ostomy surgery. *Journal of Wound, Ostomy, and Continence Nursing, 34*(6), 627–628.

*American Speech-Language-Hearing Association. (2004). *Preferred practice patterns for the profession of speech-language pathology.* Rockville, MD: Author. Retrieved from http://www.asha.org/policy/PP2004-00191.htm

American Speech-Language-Hearing Association. (2007). *Laryngeal cancer.* Retrieved from http://www.asha.org

American Stroke Association. (2016a). *Impact of stroke (stroke statistics).* Retrieved from http://www.strokeassociation .org/STROKEORG/AboutStroke/Impact-of-Stroke-Stroke-statistics_UCM_310728_Article.jsp#.Vu65f_krK-9

American Stroke Association. (2016b). *What is a stroke?* Retrieved from http://www.strokeassociation.org /STROKEORG/AboutStroke/About-Stroke_UCM_308529_SubHomePage.jsp

Anand, B. S. (2012). *Peptic ulcer disease.* Retrieved from http://emedicine.medscape.com/article/181753-overview

Anastasi, J. K., Capili, B., & Chang, M. (2013). Managing irritable bowel syndrome. *The American Journal of Nursing, 113*(7), 42–52.

Andary, M. T., Oleszek, J. L., Maurelus, K., & White-McCrimmons, R. Y. (2016). *Guillain–Barré syndrome.* Retrieved from http://emedicine.medscape.com/article/315632-overview

Anderson, A., & West, S. G. (2011). Violence against mental health professionals: When the treater becomes the victim. *Innovations in Clinical Neuroscience, 8*(3), 34–39.

*Anderson, F., & Audet, A. (1998). *Best practices: Preventing deep vein thrombosis and pulmonary embolism.* Worcester, MA: Massachusetts Medical School/Center for Outcomes Research. Retrieved from http://www.outcomes-umassmed .org/dvt/best_practice/

Anderson, J. W., Baird, P., Davis, R. H., Ferreri, S., Knudtson, M., Koraym, A., . . . Williams, C. L. (2009). Health benefits of dietary fiber. *Nutrition Reviews, 67*(4), 188–205.

*Anderson, L. A. (2001). Abdominal aortic aneurysm. *Journal of Cardiovascular Nursing, 15*(4), 1–14.

Andersson, T., Lunde, O. C., Johnson, E., Moum, T., & Nesbakken, A. (2011). Long-term functional outcome and quality of life after restorative proctocolectomy with ileo-anal anastomosis for colitis. *Colorectal Disease, 13*(4), 431–437.

*Annon, J. S. (1976). The PLISSIT model: A proposed conceptual scheme for the behavioral treatment of sexual problems. *Journal of Sexual Education and Therapy, 2*, 211–215.

Annweiler, C., Montero-Odasso, M., Schott, A., Berrat, G., Fautino, B., & Beauchet, O. (2010). Fall prevention and vitamin D in the elderly: An overview of the key role of the non-bone effects. *Journal of Neuroengineering and Rehabilitation, 7*(1), 1.

Apfel, C. C., Heidrich, F. M., Jukar-Rao, S., Jalota, L., Hornuss, C., Whelan, R. P., . . . Cakmakkaya, O. S. (2012). Evidence-based analysis of risk factors for postoperative nausea and vomiting. *British Journal of Anaesthesia, 109*(5), 742–753.

*Apfel, C. C., Läärä, E., Koivuranta, M., Greim, C. A., & Roewer, N. (1999). A simplified risk score for predicting postoperative nausea and vomiting: Conclusions from cross-validations between two centers. *Anesthesiology, 91*(3), 693–700.

Araki, Y., Kumakura, H., Kanai, H., Kasama, S., Sumino, H., Ichikawa, A., . . . Kurabayashi, M. (2012). Prevalence and risk factors for cerebral infarction and carotid artery stenosis in peripheral arterial disease. *Atherosclerosis, 223*(2), 473–477.

Aranki, S., & Aroesty, J. M. (2015). Coronary artery bypass graft surgery: Long-term clinical outcomes. In *UpToDate.* Retrieved from http://www.uptodate.com/contents/coronary-artery-bypass-graft-surgery-long-term-clinical-outcomes

Aranki, S., & Aroesty, J. M. (2016). Coronary artery bypass graft surgery: Causes and rates of graft failure. In *UpToDate.* Retrieved from http://www.uptodate.com/contents/coronary-artery-bypass-graft-surgery-causes-and-rates-of-graft-failure

Aranki, S., Aroesty, J. M., & Suri, R. M. (2015). Early noncardiac complications of coronary artery bypass graft surgery. In *UpToDate.* Retrieved from http://www.uptodate.com/contents/early-noncardiac-complications-of-coronary-artery-bypass-graft-surgery

Arcangelo, V., & Peterson, A. (2016). *Pharmacotherapeutics for advanced practice* (6th ed.). Philadelphia, PA: Lippincott Williams & Wilkins.

Armstrong, D. G., & Meyr, P. M. (2014). Wound healing and risk factors for non-healing. In *UpToDate.* Retrieved from http://www.uptodate.com/contents/wound-healing-and-risk-factors-for-non-healing

Armstrong, D. G., & Meyr, P. M. (2016). Clinical assessment of wounds. In *UpToDate.* Retrieved from http://www .uptodate.com/contents/clinical-assessment-of-wounds?source=see_link

*Armstrong, J. A., & McCaffrey, R. (2006). The effects of mucositis on quality of life in patients with neck and head cancer. *Clinical Journal of Oncology Nursing, 10*(1), 53–56.

Arnaoutoglou, E., Kouvelos, G., Koutsoumpelis, A., Patelis, N., Lazaris, A., & Matsagkas, M. (2015). An update on the inflammatory response after endovascular repair for abdominal aortic aneurysm. In *Mediators of inflammation.* Retrieved from http://www.hindawi.com/journals/mi/2015/945035/

Aroesty, J. M. (2016). Patient information: Coronary artery bypass graft surgery (Beyond the basics). In *UpToDate.* Retrieved from http://www.uptodate.com/contents/coronary-artery-bypass-graft-surgery-beyond-the-basics

*Aronow, W. S. (2005). Management of peripheral arterial disease. *Cardiology in Review, 13*(2), 61–68.

Arsalaini-Zadeh, R., ElFadl, D., Yassin, N., & MacFie, J. (2011). Evidence-based review of enhancing postoperative recovery after breast surgery. *The British Journal of Surgery, 98*, 181–196.

Arthritis Foundation. (2008). *Take control; We can help.* Retrieved from http://www.arthritis.org/index.php

Arthritis Foundation. (2012). *Tips for improving your sleep.* Arthritis Today. Retrieved from www.arthritis.org/sleep-tips.php

Askin, D., & Wilson, D. (2007). The high risk newborn and family. In M. J. Hockenberry & D. Wilson (Eds.), *Wong's nursing care of infants and children* (8th ed., pp. 314–389). St. Louis, MO: Mosby Elsevier.

Association of Community Cancer Centers. (n.d.). *Cancer program guidelines* (Chapter 4). Retrieved from https://www.accc-cancer.org/publications/pdf/Cancer-Program-Guidelines-2012.pdf;section 6

Association of Women's Health Obstetric and Neonatal Nurses. (2011). Nursing support of laboring women. An official position statement of the Association of Women's Health, Obstetric & Neonatal Nursing. *Journal of Obstetric, Gynecologic, and Neonatal Nursing, 40*, 665–666.

*Astle, S. M. (2005). Restoring electrolyte balance. *RN, 68*(5), 34–39.

Atkinson, J., Cicardi, J., & Zuraw, B. (2014). Hereditary angioedema: Treatment of acute attacks. In *UpToDate*. Retrieved from http://www.uptodate.com/contents/hereditary-angioedema-treatment-of-acute-attacks

Auckland Allergy Clinic. (2012). *Idiopathic anaphylaxis: An update. Diagnosis and treatment of allergy.* Retrieved from http://www.allergyclinic.co.nz/idiopathic_anaphylaxis.aspx

*Aulivola, B., Hile, C. N., Hamdan, A. D., Sheahan, M. G., Veraldi, J. R., Skillman, J. J., . . . Pomposelli, F. B., Jr. (2004). Major lower extremity amputation: Outcome of a modern series. *Archives of Surgery, 139*(4), 395–399.

*Austin, J. K. (2003). Childhood epilepsy: Child adaptation and family resources. *Journal of Child and Adolescent Psychiatric Nursing, 1*(1), 8–24.

Austin, J., & Abdulla, A. (2012). Identifying and managing epilepsy in older adults. *Nursing Times, 109*(3), 20–23.

Australian Department of Health & Human Services. (2007a). *Clinical decision-making at end of life in palliative care. Care management guidelines.* Retrieved from http://www.dhhs.tas.gov.au/palliativecare/health_professionals/symptom_management_guidelines

Australian Department of Health & Human Services. (2007b). *Hypercalcemia in palliative care. Care management guidelines.* Retrieved from http://www.dhhs.tas.gov.au/palliativecare/health_professionals/symptom_management_guidelines

Australian Department of Health & Human Services. (2007c). *Breathlessness in palliative care. Care management guidelines.* Retrieved from http://www.dhhs.tas.gov.au/palliativecare/health_professionals/symptom_management_guidelines

Australian Department of Health & Human Services. (2007d). *Delirium in palliative care. Care management guidelines.* Retrieved from http://www.tas.gov.au/stds/codi.htm

Awaad, S., & Ma'Luf, R. (2015). *Opthalmologic manifestations of myasthenia gravis.* Retrieved from http://emedicine.medscape.com/article/1216417-overview

Axley, B. (2015). Hemodialysis in the acute care setting. In C. S. Counts (Ed.), *Core curriculum for nephrology nursing: Module 4. Acute kidney injury* (6th ed., pp. 55–106). Pitman, NJ: American Nephrology Nurses' Association.

Ayantunde, A. A., & Parsons, S. L. (2007). Pattern and prognostic factors in patients with malignant ascites: A retrospective study. *Annals of Oncology, 18*(5), 945–949. doi:10.1093/annonc/mdl499

Azer, S. A. (2011). *Intestinal perforation.* Retrieved from http://emedicine.medscape.com/article/195537-overview

Bach, V., Ploeg, J., & Black, M. (2009). Nursing roles in end-of-life decision making in critical care settings. *Western Journal of Nursing Research, 31*(4), 496–512.

Bader, M. K. (Speaker). (2009, May). *Different strokes for different folks: Assessment, interventions and outcomes* [Podcast]. Presentation of NTI 2009, New Orleans, LA. Retrieved from http://www.aacn.org

*Bader, M. K., & Lillejohns, L. R. (2004). *American Association of Neuroscience Nurses: Core curriculum for neuroscience nursing* (4th ed.). St. Louis, MO: Saunders.

*Badger, T., Braden, C. J., & Michel, M. (2001). Depression burden, self-help. Interventions and side effects experience in women receiving treatment for breast cancer. *Oncology Nursing Forum, 28*(3), 567–574.

Baer, A. N. (2016). Clinical manifestations of Sjögren's syndrome: Extraglandular disease. In *UpToDate*. Retrieved from http://www.uptodate.com/contents/clinical-manifestations-of-sjogrens-syndrome-extraglandular-disease?source=related_link

Baggs, J. (2007). Nurse–physician collaboration in intensive care units. *Critical Care Medicine, 35*(2), 641–642.

Bailey, P. P. (2008). Asthma. In T. M. Buttaro, J. Trybulski, P. P. Bailey, & J. Sandberg-Cook (Eds.), *Primary care: A collaborative practice* (3rd ed., pp. 398–422). St. Louis, MO: Mosby.

Bailey, P., Thomsen, G. E., Spuhler, V. J., Blair, R., Jewkes, J., Bezdjian, L., & Hopkins, R. O. (2007). Early activity is feasible and safe in respiratory failure patients. *Critical Care Medicine, 35*(1), 139–145.

Bailey, W., & Miller, R. (2016). Trigger control to enhance asthma management. In *UpToDate*. Retrieved from http://www.uptodate.com/contents/trigger-control-to-enhance-asthma-management?source=see_link

Baima, J., & Krivickas, L. (2008). Evaluation and treatment of peroneal neuropathy. *Current Review of Musculoskeletal Medicine, 1*(2), 147–153.

*Baird, M. S., Keen, J. H., & Swearingen, P. L. (2005). *Manual of critical care nursing: Nursing interventions and collaborative management* (5th ed.). St Louis, MO: Elsevier Mosby.

Balach, T. G., Scott Stacy, G., & Peabody, T. D. (2011). The clinical evaluation of bone tumors. *Journal Radiologic Clinics of North America, 49*(6), 1079–1093.

Balach, T., & Peabody, T. D. (2011). Management of skeletal metastases. In W. M. Stadler (Ed.), *Renal cancer.* New York, NY: Demos Medical.

Ball, C. G., Kirkpatrick, A. W., & McBeth, P. (2008). The secondary abdominal compartment syndrome: Not just another post-traumatic complication. *Canadian Journal of Surgery, 51*(5), 399–405.

Ball, C., deBeer, K., Gomm, A., Hickman, B., & Collins, P. (2007). Achieving tight glycaemic control. *Intensive and Critical Care Nurisng, 23*(3), 137–144.

Ball, J., Bindler, R., & Cowan, K. (2015). *Principles of pediatric nursing.* New York, NY: Pearson Education.

*Ballas, S., & Delengowski, A. (1993). Pain measurement in hospitalized adults with sickle cell painful episodes. *Annals of Clinical and Laboratory Science, 23*(5), 358–361.

*Bandura, A. (1982). Self efficacy mechanism in human agency. *American Psychologist*, *37*(2), 122–147.

Barbar, S., Noventa, F., Rossetto, V., Ferrari, A., Brandolin, B., Perlati, M., . . . Prandoni, P. (2010). A risk assessment model for the identification of hospitalized medical patients at risk for venous thromboembolism: The Padua Prediction Score. *Journal of Thrombosis and Haemostasis*, *8*, 2450–2457.

*Bard, M. R., Goettler, C. E., Toschlog, E. A., Sagraves, S. G., Schenarts, P. J., Newell, M. A., . . . Rotondo, M. F. (2006). Alcohol withdrawal syndrome: Turning minor injuries into a major problem. *Journal of Trauma Injury, Infection and Critical Care*, *61*(6), 1441–1446.

Bargman, J. M. (2015). Hernias, leaks, and encapsulating peritoneal sclerosis. In J. T. Daugirdas, P. G. Blake, & T. S. Ing (Eds.), *Handbook of dialysis* (5th ed., pp. 513–520). Philadelphia, PA: Wolters Kluwer.

*Barker, L. R., Burton, J., & Aieve, P. D. (Eds.). (2006). *Principles of ambulatory medicine* (6th ed.). Philadelphia, PA: Lippincott Williams & Wilkins.

Barkun, A., & Leontiadis, G. (2010). Systematic review of the symptom burden, quality of life impairment and costs associated with peptic ulcer disease. *The American Journal of Medicine*, *123*(4), 358–366.

*Barnason, S., Zimmerman, L., Nieveen, J., & Hertzog, M. (2006). Impact of a telehealth intervention to augment home health care on functional and recovery outcomes of elderly patients undergoing coronary artery bypass grafting. *Heart & Lung*, *35*(4), 225–233.

*Barner, C., Wylie-Rosett, J., & Gans, K. (2001). WAVE: A pocket guide for a brief nutrition dialogue in primary care. *The Diabetes Educator*, *27*(3), 352–362.

Barnsteiner, J., Disch, J., & Walton, M. K. (2014). *Person and family-centered care*. Indianapolis, IN: Sigma Theta Tau International.

Barrier, P. A., Li, J. T. C., & Jensen, N. M. (2003, February). Two words to improve physician-patient communication: What else? *Mayo Clinic Proceedings*, *78*(2), 211–214.

Barrisford, G. W., & Steele, G. S. (2015). Acute urinary retention. In *UpToDate*. Retrieved from http://www.uptodate.com/contents/acute-urinary-retention

*Barsevick, A. M., Much, J., & Sweeney, C. (2000). Psychosocial responses of cancer. In S. L. Groenwald, M. H. Frogge, M. Goodman, & C. Yarbro (Eds.), *Cancer nursing: Principles and practice* (5th ed.). Boston, MA: Jones & Bartlett.

Bartels, C. (2013). *Systemic lupus erythematosus (SLE) clinical presentation*. Retrieved from http://emedicine.medscape.com/article/332244-clinical

Bartick, M. (2009). *Small changes promote better sleep*. Today's Hospitalist. Retrieved from http://www.TodaysHospitalist.com/index.php?b=articles_read&cnt=899

Bartlett, J. G. (2014a). Diagnostic approach to community-acquired pneumonia in adults. In *UpToDate*. Retrieved from http://www.uptodate.com/contents/diagnostic-approach-to-community-acquired-pneumonia-in-adults

Bartlett, J. G. (2014b). Patient education: Preventing opportunistic infections in HIV (Beyond the Basics). In *UpToDate*. Retrieved from http://www.uptodate.com/contents/preventing- opportunistic-infections-in-hic-beyond-the-basics

Bartlett, J. G. (2015). Diagnostic approach to community-acquired pneumonia in adults. In *UpToDate*. Retrieved from http://www.uptodate.com/contents/diagnostic-approach-to-community-acquired-pneumonia-in-adults?source=search_result&search=community-acquired+pneumonia+in+adults&selectedTitle=2~150#H2

*Bartlett, J. G., & Finkbeiner, A. K. (2001). *The guide to living with HIV infection* (6th ed.). Baltimore, MD: The Johns Hopkins University Press.

Basile, J., & Bloch, M. J. (2016). Overview of hypertension in adults. In *UpToDate*. Retrieved from http://www.uptodate.com/contents/overview-of-hypertension-in-adults

Baskin, J. L., Ching-Hon Pui, C. H., Reiss, U., Wilimas, J. A., Metzger, M. L., Ribeiro, R. C., & Howard, S. C. (2009). Management of occlusion and thrombosis associated with long-term indwelling central venous catheters. *Lancet*, *374*(9684), 159. Retrieved from http://www.ncbi.nlm.nih.gov/pmc/articles/PMC2814365/

Baskin, J. L., Reiss, U., Wilimas, J. A., Metzger, M. L., Ribeiro, R. C., Pui, C. H., & Howard, S. C. (2012). Thrombolytic therapy for central venous catheter occlusion. *Haematologica*, *97*(5), 641–650.

Bassand, J.-P., Hamm, C. W., Ardissino, D., Boersma, E., Budaj, A., Fernández-Avilés, F., . . . Wijns, W. (2007). Guidelines for the diagnosis and treatment of non-ST-segment elevation acute coronary syndromes. *European Heart Journal*, *28*(13), 1598–1660.

*Bateman, A. L. (1999). Understanding the process of grieving and loss: A critical social thinking perspective. *Journal of American Psychiatric Nurses Association*, *5*(5), 139–149.

Bates, C. K. (2013). Patient information: Care after sexual assault (beyond the basics). In *UpToDate*. Retrieved from http://www.uptodate.com/contents/care-after-sexual-assault-beyond-the-basics

Bauer, K. A., & Lip, G. Y. (2015). Overview of the causes of venous thrombosis. In *UpToDate*. Retrieved from http://www.uptodate.com/contents/overview-of-the-causes-of-venous-thrombosis?source=search_result&search=as+Virchow+triad%2C&selectedTitle=1~150

Bauldoff, G. S. (2015). When breathing is a burden: How to help patients with COPD. *American Nurse Today*, *10*(2).

*Bauldoff, G., Hoffman, L., Sciurba, F., & Zullo, T. (1996). Home based upper arm exercises training for patients with chronic obstructive pulmonary disease. *Heart and Lung*, *25*(4), 288–294.

*Bauman, R. A., & Gell, G. (2000). The reality of picture archiving and communication systems (PACS): A survey. *Journal Digit Imaging, 13*(4), 157–169.

*Baumann, S. L. (1999). Defying gravity and fears: The prevention of falls in community-dwelling older adults. *Clinical Excellence for Nurse Practitioners, 3*(5), 254–261.

*Baumgarten, M., Margolis, D., van Doorn, C., Gruber-Baldini, A. L., Hebel, J. R., Zimmerman, S., & Magaziner, J. (2004). Black/White differences in pressure ulcer incidence in nursing home residents. *Journal of American Geriatric Society, 52*(8), 1293–1298.

Bautista, C., & Grossman, S. (2016). Disorders of motor function. In S. Grossman & C. M. Porth (Eds.). *Porth's pathophysiology: Concepts of altered health status* (9th ed., pp. 452–488). Philadelphia, PA: Wolters Kluwer.

Bautista, L., Cesar, J., & Sumpaico, M. (2007). Stevens-Johnson from hemodialysis-associated hypersensitivity reaction in a 61-year-old male. *World Allergy Organization Journal, 1*(6), 198–207.

Beattie, S. (2007). *Bedside emergency: Wound dehiscence modern medicine*. Retrieved at http://www.modernmedicine.com/content/bedside-emergency-wound-dehiscence

Becker, E., & Kamath, H. O. (2010). Neuroimaging of eye position reveals spatial neglect. *Brain, 133*, 909–914. Retrieved from http://brain.oxfordjournals.org/content/133/3/909

*Beckstrand, R. L., Callsiter, L. C., & Kirchhoff, K. T. (2006). Providing a "good death": Critical care nurse's suggestions for improving end-of-life care. *American Journal of Critical Care, 15*(1), 38–45.

Bednarski, D., Cahill, M. L., Castner, D., Counts, C. S., Groenhoff, C. L., Hall, L. M., . . . Witten, B. (2008). The individual with kidney disease. In C. S. Counts (Ed.), *Core curriculum for nephrology nursing* (5th ed.). Pitman, NJ: American Nephrology Nurses' Association.

*Beese-Bjurstrom, S. (2004). Hidden danger: Aortic aneurysms & dissections. *Nursing, 34*(2), 36–41.

Beling, J., & Roller, M. (2009). Multifactorial intervention with balance training as a core component among fall-prone older adults. *Journal of Geriatric Physical Therapy, 32*(3), 125–133.

Bellucci, A. (2015). Reactions to the hemodialysis membrane. In *UpToDate*. Retrieved from http://www.uptodate.com/contents/reactions-to-the-hemodialysis-membrane

*Bennett, M. A. (1995). Report of the Task Force on the implications for darkly pigmented intact skin in the prediction and prevention of pressure ulcers. *Advances in Wound Care, 8*(6).

*Bennett, R. (2000). Acute gastroenteritis and associated conditions. In L. R. Barker, J. Burton, & P. Zieve (Eds.), *Principles of ambulatory medicine*. Baltimore, MD: Williams & Wilkins.

*Bennett, S. J., Cordes, D., Westmoreland, G., Castro, R., & Donnelly, E. (2000). Self-care strategies for symptom management in patients with chronic heart failure. *Nursing Research, 49*(3), 139–145.

Benowitz, N. L. (2010). Nicotine addiction. *New England Journal of Medicine, 362*(24), 2295–2303. Retrieved from http://www.ncbi.nlm.nih.gov/pmc/articles/PMC2928221/

*Ben-Zacharia, A. B. (2001). Palliative care in patients with multiple sclerosis. *Neurologic Epilepsia, 51*(4), 676–685. doi:10.1111/j.1528-1167.2010.02522.x

Berg, A. T., Berkovic, S. F., Brodie, M. J., Buchhalter, J., Cross, J. H., van Emde Boas, W., & Scheffer, I. E. (2010). Revised terminology and concepts for organization of seizures and epilepsies: Report of the ILAE Commission on Classification and Terminology, 2005–2009. *Epilepsia, 19*(4), 801–827.

*Berger, M. F., Pross, R. D., Ilg, U. J., & Karnath, H. O. (2006). Deviation of eyes and head in acute cerebral stroke. *BMC Neurology, 6*(23), 1–8.

Berkani, K., Dimet, J., Breton, P., Bizieux-Thaminy, A., & Berruchon, J. (2012). Management of the sleep apnoea syndrome in a general hospital [in French]. *Revue des Maladies Respiratoires, 29*(7):871–877.

*Berkman, N. D., DeWalt, D. A., Pignone, M. P., Sheridan, S. L., Lohr, K. N., Lux, L., . . . Bonito, A. J. (2004). *Literacy and health outcomes*. (Evidence report/technology assessment #87.) (AHRQ Publication No. 04-E007-2). Rockville, MD: Agency for Healthcare Research and Quality.

Berlowitz, D. (2014a). Epidemiology, pathogenesis and risk assessment of pressure ulcers. In *UpToDate*. Retrieved from http://www.uptodate.com/contents/epidemiology-pathogenesis-and-risk-assessment-of-pressure-ulcers

Berlowitz, D. (2014b). Prevention of pressure ulcers. In *UpToDate*. Retrieved from http://www.uptodate.com/contents/prevention-of-pressure-ulcers

Bermas, B. L., & Smith, N. A. (2015). Pregnancy in women with systemic lupus erythematosus. In *UpToDate*. Retrieved from http://www.uptodate.com/contents/pregnancy-in-women-with-systemic-lupus-erythematosus?source=search_result&search=pregnancy+and+lupus&selectedTitle=1~150

Bernheisel, C. R., Schlauderecker, J. D., & Leopold, K. (2011). Subacute management of ischemic stroke. *American Family Physician, 84*(12), 1383–1388.

Berry, A. M., Davidson, P. M., & Masters, J. (2007). Systemic literature review of oral hygiene practices for intensive care patients receiving mechanical ventilation. *American Journal of Critical Care, 16*(4), 552–562.

Best, C., & Wilson, N. (2007). Administration of medication via a enteral tubing. *Nursing Times, 107*(41), 18–20.

Beswick, A. D., Wylde, V., Gooberman-Hill, R., Blom, A., & Dieppe, P. (2012). What proportion of patients report long-term pain after total hip or knee replacement for osteoarthritis? A systematic review of prospective studies in unselected patients. *BMJ Open, 2*(1), e000435.

*Bhardwaj, A., Mirskis, M. A., & Ulatowski, J. A. (2004). *Handbook of neurocritical care*. Totowa, NJ: Humana Press.

*Bhatt, D., Lee, L., Casterella, P., Pulsipher, M., Rogers, M., Cohen, M., . . . Lincoff, A. M. (2003). Coronary revascularization using integrilin and single bolus enoxaparin study. *Journal of the American College of Cardiology, 41*(1), 20–25.

Bhuvaneswar, C. G., Epstein, L. A., & Stern, T. A. (2007). Reactions to amputation: Recognition and treatment. *Journal of Clinical Psychiatry, 9*(4), 303–308.

*Bickley, B. (2003). *A guide to physical examination and history taking* (8th ed.). Philadelphia, PA: Lippincott Williams & Wilkins.

Bird, S. (2015). Treatment of myasthenia gravis. In *UpToDate*. Retrieved from http://www.uptodate.com/contents /treatment-of-myasthenia-gravis

Bischoff-Ferrari, H. A., Dawson-Hughes, B., Platz, A., Orav, E. J, Stähelin, H. B., Willett, W. C., . . . Theiler, R. (2010). Effect of high-dosage cholecalciferol and extended physiotherapy on complications after hip fracture: A randomized controlled trial. *Archives of Internal Medicine, 170*(9), 813–820.

*Black, P. K. (2004). Psychological, sexual and cultural issues for patients with a stoma. *British Journal of Nursing, 13*(12), 692–697.

Blake, P. G., & Daugirdas, J. T. (2015). Physiology of peritoneal dialysis. In J. T. Daugirdas, P. G. Blake, & S. I. Todd (Eds.), *Handbook of dialysis* (5th ed., pp. 392–407). Philadelphia, PA: Wolters Kluwer.

*Bliss, D. Z., Jung, H. J., Savik, K., Lowry, A., LeMoine, M., Jensen, L., . . . Schaffer, K. (2001). Supplementation with dietary fiber improves fecal incontinence. *Journal of Nursing Research, 50*(4), 203–213.

Block, A. (2007). *Chronic pain coping techniques. Pain management.* Retrieved from http://www.spine-health.com/conditions /chronic-pain/chronic-pain-coping-techniques-pain-management

Bluestein, D., & Javaheri, A. (2008). Pressure ulcers: Prevention, evaluation, and management. *American Family Physician, 78*(10), 1186–1194.

Boardman, M. B. (2008). Chronic obstructive pulmonary disease. In T. M. Buttaro, J. Trybulski, P. P. Bailey, & J. Sandberg-Cook (Eds.), *Primary care: A collaborative practice* (3rd ed., pp. 433–443). St. Louis, MO: Mosby.

*Bodenheimer, T., MacGregor, K., & Sharifi, C. (2005). *Helping patients manage their chronic conditions.* Retrieved from http://www.chcf.org/publications/2005/06/helping-patients-manage-their-chronic-conditions

Boggs, J. G. (2015). Treatment of seizures and epilepsy in the elderly patient. In *UpToDate*. Retrieved from http://www .uptodate.com/contents/treatment-of-seizures-and-epilepsy-in-the-elderly-patieretrieved

Bonanno, G. A., & Lilienfeld, S. O. (2008). Let's be realistic: When grief counseling is effective and when it's not. *Professional Psychology: Research and Practice, 39*(3), 377–378.

*Bone, R., Balk, R. C., Cerra, F. B., Dellinger, R. P., Fein, A. M., Knaus, W. A., . . . Sibbald, W. J. (1992). Definitions for sepsis and organ failure and guidelines for the use of innovative therapies in sepsis. *Chest, 101*(6), 1644–1655.

*Bonham, P. A. (2006). Get the LEAD out: Noninvasive assessment for lower extremity arterial disease using ankle brachial index and toe brachial index measurements. *Journal of Wound, Ostomy, Continence Nursing, 33*, 30–41.

*Boonpongmanee, S., Fleischer, D. E., Pezzullo, J. C., Collier, K., Mayoral, W., Al-Kawas, F., . . . Benjamin, S. B. (2004). The frequency of peptic ulcer as a cause of upper-GI bleeding is exaggerated. *Gastrointestinal Endoscopy, 59*(7), 788–794. Retrieved from http://emedicine.medscape.com/article/187857-overview

Boriaug, B. A. (2015). *Clinical manifestations and diagnosis of heart failure with preserved ejection fraction.* Retrieved from http://www.uptodate.com/contents/clinical-manifestations-and-diagnosis-of-heart-failure-with-preserved-ejection-fraction

Bosmans, J. C., Suurmeijer, T. P., Hulsink, M., van der Schans, C. P., Geertzen, J. H., & Dijkstra, P. U. (2007). Amputation, phantom pain and subjective well-being: A qualitative study. *International Journal of Rehabilitation Research, 30*, 1–8.

Boudville, N., & Blake, P. G. (2015). Volume status and fluid overload in peritoneal dialysis. In J. T. Daugirdas, P. G. Blake, & S. I. Todd (Eds.), *Handbook of dialysis* (5th ed., pp. 483–489). Philadelphia, PA: Wolters Kluwer.

*Boulware, L. E., Daumit, G. L., & Frick, K. D. (2001). An evidence-based review of patient-centered behavioral interventions for hypertension. *American Journal of Preventive Medicine, 21*, 221–232.

Boutwell, A., & Hwu, S. (2009). *Effective interventions to reduce rehospitalization: A survey of published evidence.* Cambridge, MA: Institute for Healthcare Improvement.

Boyd, M. A. (2012). *Psychiatric nursing: Contemporary practice* (5th ed.). Philadelphia, PA: Wolters Kluwer Health.

*Brandjes, D. P., Büller, H. R., Heijboer, H., Huisman, M. V., de Rijk, M., Jagt, H., & ten Cate, J. W. (1997). Randomised trial of effect of compression stockings in patients with symptomatic proximal-vein thrombosis. *The Lancet, 349*(9054), 759–762.

*Branson, J. J., & Goldstein, W. M. (2001). Sequential bilateral total knee arthroplasty. *AORN Journal, 73*(3), 608, 610, 613.

*Brant, J. M. (1998). The art of palliative care: Living with hope, dying with dignity. *Oncology Nursing Forum, 25*(6), 995–1004.

*Brauer, C., Morrison, R. S., & Silberzweig, S. B. (2000). The cause of delirium in patients with hip fracture. *Archives of Internal Medicine, 160*(12), 1856–1860.

The Breast Care site.com. (2011). *Spouses, partners, family.* Retrieved at http://www.thebreastcaresite.com/after-surgery /spouses-partners-family/

BreastCancer.org. (2007). *The role of surgery in breast cancer treatment.* Retrieved from http://www.breastcancer.org /treatment/surgery/index.jsp

Brem, H., Maggi, J., Nierman, D., Rolnitzky, L., Bell, D., Rennert, R., . . . Vladeck, B. (2010). High cost of stage IV pressure ulcers. *American Journal of Surgery, 200*(4), 473–477. Retrieved from www.ncbi.nlm.nih.gov/pmc/articels/PMC2950802/

*Breslin, E. H. (1992). Dyspnea-limited response in chronic obstructive pulmonary disease: Reduced unsupported arm activities. *Rehabilitation Nursing, 17,* 12–20.

Brienza, D., Kelsey, S., Karg, P., Allegretti, A., Olson, M., Schmeler, M., . . . Holm, M. (2010). A randomized clinical trial on preventing pressure ulcers with wheelchair seat cushions. *Journal of American Geriatrics Society, 58*(12), 2308–2314.

Brigham and Women's Hospital. (2010). *Standard of care: Total hip replacement.* Retrieved from http://www.brighamandwomens.org/Patients_Visitors/pcs/RehabilitationServices/Physical-Therapy-Standards-of-Care-and-Protocols/Hip-Total%20Hip%20Arthroplasty.pdf

Brommage, D., Cotton, A. B., Gonyea, J., Kent, P. S., & Stover, J. (2015). Foundations of nutrition and clinical applications in nephrology nursing: Special considerations in kidney disease. In C. S. Counts (Ed.), *Core curriculum for nephrology nursing: Module 2. Physiologic and psychosocial basis for nephrology nursing practice* (6th ed., pp. 268–279). Pitman, NJ: American Nephrology Nurses' Association.

Brown, C. J., Redden, D. T., Flood, K. L., & Allman, R. A. (2009). The under-recognized epidemic of low mobility during hospitalization of older adults. *Journal of American Geriatrics Society, 57*(9), 1660–1665.

*Brown, M. A., & Powell-Cope, G. (1991). AIDS family caregiving transitions through uncertainty. *Nursing Research, 40,* 338–345.

Bruera, E. (2012). Palliative sedation: When and how? *Journal of Clinical Oncology, 30,* 1258–1259.

*Bryant, R. A. (2000). *Acute and chronic wounds. Nursing management* (2nd ed.). Missouri, MO: Mosby.

*Bryson, K. A. (2004). Spirituality, meaning, and transcendence. *Palliative and Supportive Care, 2*(3), 321–328.

*Buchanan, R. J., Wang, S., & Ju, H. (2002). Analyses of the minimum data set: Comparisons of nursing home residents with multiple sclerosis to other nursing home residents. *Multiple Sclerosis, 8*(6), 512–522.

*Buchman, A. L. (2001). Side effects of corticosteroid therapy. *Journal of Clinical Gastroenterology, 33*(4), 289–294.

Buerhaus, P. I., & Kurtzman, A. (2008). New medicare payment rules: Danger or opportunity for nursing? *The American Journal of Nursing, 10*(6), 30–35.

Bulechek, G. M., Butcher, G. M., & Dochterman, J. M. (Eds.). (2013). *Nursing interventions: Treatments for nursing diagnoses* (5th ed.). Philadelphia, PA: W. B. Saunders.

*Bullock, B., & Henze, R. (2000). *Focus on pathophysiology.* Philadelphia, PA: Lippincott Williams & Wilkins.

Burakgazi, A. Z., Alsowaity, B., Burakgazi, Z. A., Unal, D., & Kelly, J. J. (2012). Bladder dysfunction in peripheral neuropathies. *Muscle & Nerve, 45*(1), 2–8.

*Burch, K., Todd, K., Crosby, F., Ventura, M., Lohr, G., & Grace, M. L. (1991). PVD: Nurse patient interventions. *Journal of Vascular Nursing, 9*(4), 13–16.

Bureau of Justice. (2010). *Female victims of sexual violence, 1994–2010.* Retrieved from http://www.bjs.gov/content/pub/pdf/fvsv9410.pdf

Burke-Galloway, L. (2014). Pain management during labor. In *Women's Health Resource Library.* Retrieved from http://www.whrl.org/

*Burkhart, L., & Solari-Twadell, A. (2001). Spirituality and religiousness: Differentiating the diagnoses through review of the literature. *International Journal of Nursing Terminologies and Classification, 12*(2), 45–54.

Burks, W. (2015). Clinical manifestations of food allergy: An overview. In *UpToDate.* Retrieved from http://www.uptodate.com/contents/clinical-manifestations-of-food-allergy-an-overview

Burneo, J. G., Fang, J., & Saposnik, G; Investigators of the Registry of the Canadian Stroke Network. (2010). Impact of seizures on morbidity and mortality after stroke: A Canadian multi-centre cohort study. *European Journal of Neurology, 17*(1), 52–58.

Burns, S. (2014). *AACN Chula's essentials of critical care nursing* (3rd ed.). New York, NY: McGraw-Hill.

Bushkin, E. (1993). Signposts of survivorship. *Oncology Nursing Forum, 20*(6), 869–875.

Butler, D. (2009). Early postoperative complications following ostomy surgery: A review. *Journal of Wound, Ostomy, and Continence Nursing, 36*(5), 513–519.

*Butler, D. J., Turkal, N. W., & Seidl, J. J. (1992). Amputation: preoperative psychological preparation. *The Journal of the American Board of Family Practice, 5*(1), 69–73.

Cagir, B. (Ed.). (2015). *Short-bowel syndrome.* Retrieved from http://emedicine.medscape.com/article/193391-overview

Cagir, B. (Ed.). (2016). *Lower gastrointestinal bleeding.* Retrieved from http://emedicine.medscape.com/article/188478-overview

Cahill, M., & Groenhoff, C. L. (2015a). Individualizing the care of those with kidney disease: Cultural diversity. In C. S. Counts (Ed.), *Core curriculum for nephrology nursing: Module 2—Physiologic and psychosocial basis for nephrology nursing practice* (6th ed., pp. 200–211). Pitman, NJ: American Nephrology Nurses' Association.

Cahill, M., & Groenhoff, C. L. (2015b). Individualizing the care of those with kidney disease: Patient and family education. In C. S. Counts (Ed.), *Core curriculum for nephrology nursing: Module 2—Physiologic and psychosocial basis for nephrology nursing practice* (6th ed., pp. 211–219). Pitman, NJ: American Nephrology Nurses' Association.

Calvert, E., Penner, M., Younger, A., & Wing, K. (2007). Transmetatarsal amputations. *Techniques in Foot and Ankle Surgery, 6*(3), 140–146.

Campbell, K. E. (2009). A new model to identify shared risk factors for pressure ulcers and frailty in older adults. *Rehabilitation Nursing, 34*(6), 242–247.

Camp-Sorrell, D. (2007). Chemotherapy: Toxicity management. In C. Yarbro, M. H. Frogge, M. Goodman, & S. Groenwald (Eds.), *Cancer nursing: Principles and practice*. Boston, MA: Jones & Barlett.

*Canadian Association of Endostomal Therapy. (2005). *A guide to living with an ileostomy*. Retrieved from https://caet .ca/wp-content/uploads/2015/02/caet-guide-to-living-with-an-ileostomy.pdf

Caplan, L. R. (2015). Overview of the evaluation of stroke. In *UpToDate*. Retrieved from http://www.uptodate.com /contents/overview-of-the-evaluation-of-stroke

*Carek, P. J., Dickerson, L. M., & Sack, J. L. (2001). Diagnosis and management of osteomyelitis. *American Family Physician*, *63*(12), 2413–2420.

Carlson, D. S., & Pfadt, E. (2012). Preventing deep vein thrombosis in perioperative patients. *OR Nursing*, *6*(5), 14–20.

*Carosella, C. (1995). *Who's afraid of the dark?* New York, NY: HarperCollins.

*Carpenito. L. J. (1986). *Nursing diagnosis: Application to clinical practice*. Philadelphia, PA: Lippincott Williams & Wilkins.

*Carpenito, L. J. (1987). *Nursing diagnosis: Application to clinical practice* (3rd ed.). Philadelphia, PA: J. B. Lippincott.

*Carpenito, L. J. (1997). *Nursing diagnosis: Application to clinical practice* (7th ed.). Philadelphia, PA: J. B. Lippincott.

*Carpenito, L. J. (1999). *Nursing diagnosis: Application to clinical practice* (8th ed.). Philadelphia, PA: Lippincott Williams & Wilkins.

Carpenito-Moyet, L. J. (2016a). *Nursing diagnoses: Application to clinical practice* (15th ed.). Philadelphia, PA: Lippincott Williams & Wilkins.

Carpenito-Moyet, L. J. (2016b). *Handbook of nursing diagnoses* (15th ed.). Philadelphia, PA: Lippincott Williams & Wilkins.

*Carr, E. (2005). Head and neck malignancies. In C. H. Yarbo, M. H. Frogge, & M. Goodman (Eds.), *Cancer nursing: Principles and practice* (6th ed.). Boston, MA: Jones & Bartlett.

Carson, A. P., Howard, G., Burke, G. L., Shea, S., Levitan, E. B., & Muntner, P. (2011). Ethnic differences in hypertension incidence among middle-aged and older adults the multi-ethnic study of atherosclerosis. *Hypertension*, *57*(6), 1101–1107.

*Carson, V. B. (1999). *Mental health nursing: The nurse–patient journey* (2nd ed.). Philadelphia, PA: W. B. Saunders.

*Carson, V. B., & Green, H. (1992). Spiritual well-being: A predictor of hardiness in patients with acquired immunodeficiency syndrome. *Journal of Professional Nursing*, *8*, 209–220.

*Carson, V. M., & Smith-DiJulio, K. (2006). Family violence. In E. M. Varcarolis, V. M. Carson, & N. C. Shoemaker (Eds.), *Foundations of psychiatric mental health nursing* (5th ed.). Philadelphia, PA: W. B. Saunders.

Carvalho, C. R., Deheinzelin, D., & Kairalla, R. A. (2016). Interstitial lung disease associated with Sjögren's syndrome: Clinical manifestations, evaluation, and diagnosis. In *UpToDate*. Retrieved from http://www.uptodate.com/ contents/interstitial-lung-disease-associated-with-sjogrens-syndrome-clinical-manifestations-evaluation-and-diagnosis?source=see_link

*Casey, K. (1997). Malnutrition associated with HIV/AIDS. Part two: Assessment and interventions. *Journal of the Association of Nurses in AIDS Care*, *8*(5), 39–48.

*Cassells, J. M., & Redman, B. K. (1989). Preparing students to be moral agents in clinical nursing practice. *Nursing Clinics of North America*, *24*, 463–473.

*Casswell, D., & Cryer, H. G. (1995). When the nurse and the doctor don't agree. *Journal of Cardiovascular Nursing*, *9*, 30–42.

Castillo-Bueno, M., Moreno-Pina, J. P., Martínez-Puente, M. V., Artiles-Suárez, M. M., Company-Sancho, M. C., García-Andrés, M. C., . . . Hernández-Pérez, R. (2010). Effectiveness of nursing intervention for adult patients experiencing chronic pain: A systematic review. *JBI Library of Systematic Reviews*, *28*(8), 1112–1168.

Castner, D. (2015). Hemodialysis: Principles of hemodialysis. In C. S. Counts (Ed.), *Core curriculum for nephrology nursing: Module 3. Treatment options for patients with chronic kidney failure* (6th ed., pp. 74–100). Pitman, NJ: American Nephrology Nurses' Association.

*Centers for Disease Control and Prevention. (2002). *Guideline for hand hygiene in health-care settings*. Retrieved from https://www.premierinc.com/safety/topics/guidelines/downloads/03_cdchandhygfinal02.pdf

Centers for Disease Control and Prevention. (2010). *Hip fractures among older adults*. Retrieved from http://www.cdc .gov/homeandrecreationalsafety/falls/adulthipfx.html

Centers for Disease Control and Prevention. (2011). Sexual identity, sex of sexual contacts, and health-risk behaviors among students in grades 9–12—Youth Risk Behavior Surveillance, selected sites, United States, 2001-2009. *Morbidity and Mortality Weekly Report. Surveillance Summaries*, *60*(7), 1–133.

Centers for Disease Control and Prevention. (2012). *Respiratory hygiene/cough etiquette in healthcare settings*. Retrieved from www.cdc.gov/flu/professionals/infectioncontrol/resphygiene.htm

Centers for Disease Control and Prevention. (2013a). *Frequently asked questions—Personal protective equipment (masks, protective eyewear, protective apparel, gloves)*. Retrieved from https://www.cdc.gov/oralhealth/infectioncontrol/faq /protective_equipment.htm

Centers for Disease Control and Prevention. (2013b). *Stigma of mental illness*. Retrieved from https://www.cdc.gov/ mentalhealth/data_stats/mental-illness.htm

Centers for Disease Control and Prevention. (2014a). *COPD: Data and statistics*. Retrieved from http://www.cdc.gov /copd/data.htm

Centers for Disease Control and Prevention. (2014b). *2014 surgeon general's report: The health consequences of smoking—50 years of progress*. Retrieved from http://www.cdc.gov/tobacco/data_statistics/sgr/50th-anniversary/

Centers for Disease Control and Prevention. (2015a). *Healthcare-associated Infections (HAIs)*. Retrieved from http://www.cdc.gov/HAI/surveillance/

Centers for Disease Control and Prevention. (2015b). *Tobacco-related mortality*. Retrieved from https://www.cdc.gov/tobacco/data_statistics/fact_sheets/health_effects/tobacco_related_mortality

Centers for Disease Control and Prevention. (2015c). *Sexual assault and abuse and STD*. Retrieved from http://www.cdc.gov/std/tg2015/sexual-assault.htm

Centers for Disease Control and Prevention. (2016a). *Older adult falls*. Retrieved from http://www.cdc.gov/homeandrecreationalsafety/falls/

Centers for Disease Control and Prevention. (2016b). *Hand hygiene guideline*. Retrieved from https://www.cdc.gov/handhygiene/providers/guideline.html

Centers for Disease Control and Prevention. (2016c). *Bloodstream infection event (central line-associated bloodstream infection and non-central line-associated bloodstream infection)*. Retrieved from http://www.cdc.gov/nhsn/pdfs/pscmanual/4psc_clabscurrent.pdf

Centers for Disease Control and Prevention. (2016d). *Peripheral arterial disease (PAD) fact sheet*. Retrieved from http://www.cdc.gov/dhdsp/data_statistics/fact_sheets/fs_pad.htm

Centers for Disease Control and Prevention. (2016e). *Asthma: Data, statistics, and surveillance*. Retrieved at http://www.cdc.gov/asthma/

Centers for Disease Control and Prevention. (2016f). *Adults: Protect yourself with pneumococcal vaccines*. Retrieved from https://www.cdc.gov/features/adult-pneumococcal/

Centers for Disease Control and Prevention. (2016g). *Respiratory hygiene/cough etiquette in healthcare settings*. Retrieved from https://www.cdc.gov/flu/professionals/infectioncontrol/resphygiene.htm.

Centers for Disease Control and Prevention. (2016h). *Pre-exposure prophylaxis (PrEP)*. Retrieved from http://www.cdc.gov/hiv/research/index.html

Centers for Disease Control and Prevention. (2016i). *HIV in the United States: At a glance*. Retrieved from http://www.cdc.gov/hiv/statistics/overview/ataglance.html

Centers for Disease Control and Prevention. (2016j). *Smoking and tobacco use*. Retrieved from https://www.cdc.gov/tobacco/

Centers for Disease Control and Prevention. (2016k) *National vital statistics reports: Deaths—Final data for 2013*. Retrieved from http://www.cdc.gov/nchs/data/nvsr/nvsr64/nvsr64_02.pdf

*Centers for Medicare & Medicaid Services. (2005). *Survey and certification (S & C) group. Delay in effective date for revisions of appendix PP, state operations manual (SOM), surveyor guidance for urinary incontinence and catheters (Tag F315)*. CMS S & C Publication No. S&C-05-23. Retrieved from www.cms.hhs.gov/medicaid/survey-cert/sc0523.pdf

Centers for Medicare & Medicaid Services. (2008a). *Proposed changes to the hospital inpatient prospective payment systems and fiscal year 2009*. Retrieved from https://www.cms.gov/Medicare/Medicare-Fee-for-Service-Payment/AcuteInpatientPPS/IPPS-Regulations-and-Notices-Items/CMS1227598.html

Centers for Medicare & Medicaid Services. (2008b). *Roadmap for implementing value driven healthcare in the traditional Medicare fee-for-service program*. Retrieved from https://www.cms.gov/Medicare/Quality-Initiatives-Patient-Assessment-Instruments/QualityInitiativesGenInfo/downloads/vbproadmap_oea_1-16_508.pdf

Centers of Medicare & Medicaid Services. (2012). *Acute inpatient PPS*. Retrieved from http://www.cms.gov/Medicare/Medicare-Fee-for-Service-Payment/AcuteInpatientPPS/index.html?redirect=/acuteinpatientpps

Centers for Medicare & Medicaid Services. (2015a). *Catheter-associated urinary tract infections (CAUTI)*. Retrieved from https://partnershipforpatients.cms.gov/p4p_resources/tsp-catheterassociatedurinarytractinfections/toolcatheterassociatedurinarytractinfectionscauti.html/

Centers for Medicare & Medicaid Services. (2015b). *Hospital-acquired conditions and present on admission indicator reporting provision*. Retrieved from https://www.cms.gov/Outreach-and-Education/Medicare-Learning-Network-MLN/MLNProducts/Downloads/wPOA-Fact-Sheet.pdf

Cesario, K. R., Choure, A., & Carey, W. D. (2010). *Complications of cirrhosis: Ascites, hepatic encephalopathy, and variceal hemorrhage*. Retrieved from http://www.clevelandclinicmeded.com/medicalpubs/diseasemanagement/hepatology/complications-of-cirrhosis-ascites

Chaer, R. A. (2015). Complications of endovascular abdominal aortic repair. In *UpToDate*. Retrieved from http://www.uptodate.com/contents/complications-of-endovascular-abdominal-aortic-repair?source=see_link

Chaisson, K., Sanford, M., Boss, R. A., Jr, Leavitt, B. J., Hearne, M. J., Ross, C. S., . . . Malenka, D. J. (2014). Improving patients' readiness for coronary artery bypass graft surgery. *Critical Care Nurse, 34*(6), 29–38.

Chait, M. (2007). Lower gastrointestinal bleeding in the elderly. *Annals of Long-Term Care, 15*(4), 40–46.

Challacombe, B., & Dasgupta, P. (2007). Reconstitution of the lower urinary tract by laparoscopic robotic surgery. *Current Opinion in Urology, 17*, 390–395.

Chan, D., & Man, D. (2013). Unilateral neglect in stroke: A comparative study. *Topics in Geriatric Rehabilitation, 29*(2), 126–134.

*Chang, J. Y., & Tsai, P. F. (2004). Assessment of pain in elders with dementia. *MEDSURG Nursing, 13*(6), 364–369, 390.

*Chapman, D., & Moore, S. (2005). Breast cancer. In C. Yarbo, M. H. Frogge, & M. Goodman (Eds.), *Cancer nursing: Principles and practice* (6th ed.). Boston, MA: Jones & Bartlett.

Chasens, E. R., & Umlauf, M. G. (2012). *Nursing standard practice protocol: Excessive sleepiness*. Retrieved from http://consultgerirn.org/topics/sleep/want_to_know_more

*Cheadle, W. G. (2006). Risk factors for surgical site infection. *Surgical Infections, 7*(Suppl. 1), S7–S11.

*Cheng, D., Allen, K., Cohn W., Connolly, M., Edgerton, J., Falk, V., . . . Vitali, R. (2005). Endoscopic vascular harvest in coronary artery bypass grafting surgery: A meta-analysis of randomized trials and controlled trials. *Innovations (Phila), 1*(2), 61–74.

Cheng, S. (2011). Mineral and bone disorders. In J. T. Daugirdas (Ed.), *Handbook of chronic kidney disease management.* Philadelphia, PA: Lippincott Williams & Wilkins.

*Cherny, N., Ripamonti, N., Pereira, J., Davis, C., Fallon, M., McQuay, H., . . . Vittorio Ventafridda, V. (2001). Strategies to manage the adverse effects of oral morphine: An evidence-based report. *Journal of Clinical Oncology, 19*(9), 2542–2554.

Chester, M., Wasko, M., Hubert, H., Lingala, V., Elliot, J., Luggen, M., . . . Ward, M. M. (2007). Hydroxychloroquine and risk of diabetes in patients with rheumatoid arthritis. *JAMA, 298*(2), 187–193.

*Cheville, A., & Gergich, N. (2004). Lymphedema: Implications for wound care. In P. J. Sheffield, A. P. S. Smith, & C. Fife (Eds.), *Wound care practice* (pp. 285–303). Flagstaff, AZ: Best.

*Chin, T., Sawamura, S., & Shiba, R. (2006). Effect of physical fitness on prosthetic ambulation in elderly amputees. *American Journal of Physical Medicine & Rehabilitation, 85*(12), 992–996.

Chmielowski, B., Casciato, D. A., & Wagner, R. F. (2009). Cutaneous complications. In D. A. Casciato & M. C. Territo (Eds.), *Manual of clinical oncology* (pp. 585–605). Philadelphia, PA: Lippincott Williams & Wilkins.

Choi, H., & Menditatta, A. (2014). Seizures and epilepsy in the elderly patient: Etiology, clinical presentation, and diagnosis. In *UpToDate.* Retrieved from http://www.uptodate.com/contents/seizures-and-epilepsy-in-the-elderly-patient-etiology-clinical-presentation-and-diagnosis?source=see_link

Chou, K. L. (2016a). Diagnosis and differential diagnosis of Parkinson disease. In *UpToDate.* Retrieved from http://www.uptodate.com/contents/diagnosis-and-differential-diagnosis-of-parkinson-disease

Chou, R. (2016b). Subacute and chronic low back pain: Surgical treatment. In *UpToDate.* Retrieved from http://www.uptodate.com/contents/subacute-and-chronic-low-back-pain-surgical-treatment

Chou, R., Dana, T., Bougatsos, C., Blazina, I., Starmer, A., Reitel, K., & Buckley, D. (2013). *Pressure ulcer risk assessment and prevention: Comparative effectiveness* (Comparative Effectiveness Review No. 87). Prepared by Oregon Evidence-based Practice Center under Agency for Healthcare Research and Quality, Rockville, MD. Retrieved from http://www.effectivehealthcare.ahrq.gov/ehc/products/309/1489/pressure-ulcer-prevention-report-130528.pdf

*Christman, N., & Kirchhoff, K. (1992). Preparatory sensory information. In G. Bulechek & J. McCloskey (Eds.), *Nursing interventions.* Philadelphia, PA: W. B. Saunders.

Chronic pain: What psychosocial interventions work? (2011). In *Critical Science.* Retrieved from http://criticalscience.com/chronic-pain-psychosocial-interventions.html

Chu, Y.-F., Jiang, Y., Meng, M., Jiang, J.-J., Zhang, J.-C., Ren, H.-S., & Wang, C.-T. (2010). Incidence and risk factors of gastrointestinal bleeding in mechanically ventilated patients. *World Journal of Emergency Medicine, 1*(1), 32–36.

*Cicirelli, V., & MacLean, A. P. (2000). Hastening death: A comparison of two end-of-life decisions. *Death Studies, 24*(3), 401–419.

*Cimprich, B. (1992). Attentional fatigue following breast cancer surgery. *Research in Nursing and Health, 15,* 199–207.

Cirelli, C., & Tononi, G. (2015). Sleep and synaptic homeostasis. *Sleep, 38*(1), 161–162.

Ciucci, M., & Busch, J. (2014). *Parkinson's: Swallowing and dental challenges.* Parkinson's Disease Foundation. Retrieved from http://www.pdf.org/pdf/parkinson_briefing_swallowing_slides_011414.pdf

*Clanet, M., & Brassat D. (2000). The management of multiple sclerosis patients. *Current Opinion in Neurology, 13*(3), 263–270.

*Clark, J. (2006). *Ileostomy guide.* Retrieved from www.ostomy.org/uploaded/files/ostomy_info/IleostomyGuide.pdf

*Clark, J., & Dubois, H. (2004). *Urostomy guide.* United Ostomy Associations of America (UOAA). Retrieved from www.ostomy.org/uploaded/files/ostomy_info/UrostomyGuide.pdf

Clark, M. (2010). Skin assessment in dark pigmented skin: A challenge in pressure ulcer prevention. *Nursing Times, 106*(30), 16–17.

Clarke, S., & Santy-Tomilinson, J. (2014). *Orthopedic and trauma nursing.* Hoboken, NJ: Wiley-Blackwell.

*Clemen-Stone, E., Eigasti, D. G., & McGuire, S. L. (2001). *Comprehensive family and community health nursing* (6th ed.). St. Louis, MO: Mosby–Year Book.

Clement, L., & Kent, P. S. (2015). Foundations of nutrition and clinical applications in nephrology nursing: Nutritional intervention. In C.S. Counts (Ed.), *Core curriculum for nephrology nursing: Module 2. Physiologic and psychosocial basis for nephrology nursing practice* (6th ed., pp. 279–289). Pitman, NJ: American Nephrology Nurses' Association.

*Clover, K., Carter, G. L., & Whyte, I. M. (2004). Posttraumatic stress disorder among deliberate self-poisoning patients. *Journal of Traumatic Stress, 17*(6), 509–517.

Cohen, M. S., Chen, Y. Q., McCauley, M., Gamble, T., Hosseinipour, M. C., Kumarasamy, N., . . . Godbole, S. V. (2011). Prevention of HIV-1 infection with early antiretroviral therapy. *New England Journal of Medicine, 365*(6), 493–505.

Cohen, S. M., Linenberger, H. K., Wehry, L. E., & Welz, H. K. (2011). Recovery after hysterectomy: A year-long look. *WebmedCentral Obstetrics and Gynaecology, 2*(3). Retrieved from http://www.webmedcentral.com/article_view/1761

*Cohen-Mansfield, J. (2000). Use of patient characteristics to determine non-pharmacologic interventions for behavioural and psychological symptoms of dementia. *International Psychogeriatrics, 12*(Suppl. 1), 373–380.

Cole, C., & Richards, K. (2007). Sleep disruption in older adults. *The American Journal of Nursing, 107*(5), 40–49.

Coleman-Jensen, A., Gregory, C., & Singh, A. (2013). *Household food security in the United States*. Washington, DC: U.S. Department of Agriculture/Economic Research Service.

Coleman-Jensen, A., Rabbitt, M. P., Gregory, C., & Singh, A. (2015). *Household food security in the United States*. Washi Cngton, DC: U.S. Department of Agriculture/Economic Research Service. Retrieved from http://www.ers.usda.gov /media/1896841/err194.pdf

*Collett, K. (2002). Practical aspects of stoma management. *Nursing Standard, 17*(8), 45–52.

*Collier, J. D., Ninkovic, M. J., & Compston, E. (2002). Guidelines on the management of osteoporosis associated with chronic liver disease. *Gut, 50*, i1–i9.

Collins, K. A. (2015). Overview of abdominal aortic aneurysm. In *UpToDate*. Retrieved from http://www.uptodate.com /contents/overview-of-abdominal-aortic-aneurysm

*Collins, R. L., Leonard, K., & Searles, J. (1990). *Alcohol and the family: Research and clinical perspectives*. New York, NY: Guilford.

*Colten, H. R., & Altevogt, B. M. (Eds.). (2006). *Sleep disorders and sleep deprivation. An unmet public health problem*. Washington, DC: National Academies Press. Retrieved from http://www.ncbi.nlm.nih.gov/books/NBK19960/

Colucci, W. S. (2016). Overview of the therapy of heart failure with reduced ejection fraction. In *UpToDate*. Retrieve from http://www.uptodate.com/contents/overview-of-the-therapy-of-heart-failure-with-reduced-ejection-fraction

Colwell, J. C., & Beitz, J. (2007). Survey of wound, ostomy and continence (WOC) nurse clinicians on stomal and peristomal complications. *Journal of Wound, Ostomy, and Continence Nursing, 34*(1), 57–69.

*Colwell, J. C., Goldberg, M. T., & Carmel, J. E. (2004). *Fecal and urinary diversions: Management principles*. St. Louis, MO: Mosby.

*Conn, V. S., Hafdahl, A. R., Porock, D. C., McDaniel, R., & Nielsen, P. J. (2006). A meta-analysis of exercise interventions among people treated for cancer. *Support Care Cancer, 14*(7), 699–712.

*Connors, A. F., Dawson, N. V., Desbiens, N. A., Fulkerson, W. J., Goldman, L., Knaus, W. A., . . . Oye, R. K. (1995). The SUPPORT study: A controlled trial to improve care for seriously ill hospitalized patients: The study to understand prognoses and preferences for outcomes and risks of treatments (SUPPORT). *JAMA, 274*(20), 1591–1598.

Conte, M. S., & Farber, A. (2015). Revascularization for chronic limb-threatening ischaemia. *The British Journal of Surgery, 102*(9), 1007–1009.

*Conti, R. C. (2009). Myocardial revascularization: PCI/stent or coronary artery bypass graft—What is best for our patients? *Clinical Cardiology, 32*(11), 606–607.

*Convertino, V. A., Previc, F. H., Ludwig, D. A., & Engelken, E. J. (1997). Effects of vestibular and oculomotor stimulation on responsiveness of the carotid-cardiac baroreflex. *American Journal of Physiology-Regulatory, Integrative and Comparative Physiology, 273*(2), R615–R622.

Conwell, Y., Van Orden, K., & Caine, E. D. (2011). Suicide in older adults. *Psychiatric Clinics of North America, 34*(2), 451–468.

*Cook, D. J., Fuller, H. D., Guyatt, G. H., Marshall, J. C., Leasa, D., Hall, R., . . . Roy, P; Canadian Critical Care Trials Group. (1994). Risk factors for gastrointestinal bleeding in critically ill patients. *New England Journal of Medicine, 330*(6), 377–381.

Cook, S., & Lloyd, A. (2010). *Guidelines for the diagnosis, management and prevention of delirium (acute confusion) in adults age 18 years and older*. Retrieved from https://www.nice.org.uk/guidance/cg103?unlid=81238245320166715 1246

Cooke, H. (2015). *CAM-cancer consortium. Progressive muscle relaxation* [Online document]. http://www.cam-cancer.org /CAM-Summaries/Mind-body-interventions/Progressive-Muscle-Relaxation

*Coombs-Lee, B. (2004). A model that integrates assisted dying with excellent end of life care. In T. E. Quill & M. P. Battin (Eds.), *Physician-assisted dying. The case for palliative care and patient choice* (pp. 190–201). Baltimore/London: The John Hopkins University Press.

Coombs Lee, B. (2014). Oregon's experience with aid in dying: Findings from the death with dignity laboratory. *Annals of the New York Academy of Sciences, 1330*(1), 94–100.

COPD Foundation. (2015). *Breathing techniques*. Washington, DC: Author. Retrieved from http://www.copdfoundation. org/What-is-COPD/Living-with-COPD/Breathing-Techniques.aspx

*Corley, M., Minick, P., Elswick, R., & Jacobs, M. (2005). Nurse moral distress and ethical work environments. *Nursing Ethics, 12*(4), 381–389.

Cornett, P. A., & Dea, T. O. (2012). Cancer. In S. J. McPhee & M. A. Papadakis (Eds.), *Current medical diagnosis and treatment*. New York, NY: McGraw-Hill Lange.

*Cornish, P., Knowles, S., Tam, V., Shadowitz, S., Juurlink, D., & Etchells, E. (2005). Unintended medication discrepancies at the time of hospital admission. *Archives of Internal Medicine, 165*(4), 424–429.

Correia de Sa, J., Airas, L., Bartholome, E., Grigoriadis, N., Mattle, H., Oreja-Guevara, C., . . . Walczak, A. (2011). Symptomatic therapy in multiple sclerosis: A review for a multimodal approach in clinical practice. *Therapeutic Advances in Neurological Disorders, 4*(3), 139–168.

Cotton, A. B. (2008). Kidney disease and kidney replacement therapies in nutrition in kidney disease, dialysis, and transplantation. In C. S. Counts (Ed.), *Core curriculum for nephrology nursing* (5th ed.). Pitman, NJ: American Nephrology Nurses' Association.

Cotton, P., & Heisters, D. (2012). How to care for people with Parkinson's disease. *Nursing Times, 108*(16), 12–14.

*Cotton, S., Puchalski, C. M., Sherman, S. N., Mrus, J. M., Peterman, A. H., Feinberg, J., . . . Tsevat, J. (2006). Spirituality and religion in patients with HIV/AIDS. *Journal of General Internal Medicine, 21*(Suppl. 5), S5–S13.

*Coughlin, A. M., & Parchinsky, C. (2006). Go with the flow of chest tube therapy. *Nursing, 36*(3), 36–42.

Coughlin, S. M., & Emmerton-Coughlin, H. M. (2012). Management of chest tubes after pulmonary resection: A systematic review and meta-analysis. *Canadian Journal of Surgery, 55*(4), 264.

Coulter, A. (2012). Patient engagement—What works? *Journal of Ambulatory Care Management, 35*(2), 80–89.

Counts, C. S., Benavente, G., McCarley, P. B., Pelfrey, N. J., Petroff, S., & Stackiewicz, L. (2008a). Chronic kidney disease: Deterring chronic kidney disease. In C. S. Counts (Ed.), *Core curriculum for nephrology nursing* (5th ed.). Pitman, NJ: American Nephrology Nurses' Association.

Counts, C. S., Benavente, G., McCarley, P. B., Pelfrey, N. J., Petroff, S., & Stackiewicz, L. (2008b). Chronic kidney disease: Empowering strategies and the introduction to kidney replacement therapies. In C. S. Counts (Ed.), *Core curriculum for nephrology nursing* (5th ed.). Pitman, NJ: American Nephrology Nurses' Association.

Courtney, A., Nemcek, A. A., Rosenberg, S., Tutton, S., Darcy, M., & Gordon, G. (2008). Prospective evaluation of the PleurX catheter when used to treat recurrent ascites associated with malignancy. *Journal of Vascular and Interventional Radiology, 19*(12), 1723–1731. doi: 10.1016/j.jvir.2008.09.002

*Cowin, L. S., Davies, R., Estall, G., Berlin, T., Fitzgerald, M., & Hoot, S. (2003). De-escalating aggression and violence in the mental health setting. *International Journal of Mental Health Nursing, 12*, 64–73.

Coyne, D. W. (2007). Use of epoetin in chronic renal failure. *JAMA, 297*(15), 1713–1716.

Creager, M. A., & Libby, P. (2007). Peripheral arterial disease. In P. Libby, R. O. Bonow, D. L. Mann, & D. P. Zipes (Eds.), *Braunwald's heart disease: A textbook of cardiovascular medicine* (8th ed., Chapter 57). Philadelphia, PA: Saunders.

*The Criteria Committee of the New York Heart Association. (1994). *Nomenclature and criteria for diagnosis of diseases of the heart and great vessels* (9th ed., pp. 253–256). Boston, MA: Little, Brown and Company.

Crowe, S. E. (2015). Treatment regimens for *Helicobacter pylori*. In *UpToDate*. Retrieved from http://www.uptodate.com /contents/treatment-regimens-for-helicobacter-pylori?source=search_result&search=management+of+H+Pylori+ +of+peptic+ulcer&selectedTitle=2~150

*Cukierman, T., Gatt, M. E., Hiller, N., & Chajek-Shaul, T. (2005). Fracture diagnosis. *New England Journal of Medicine, 353*, 509–514.

*Cunningham, M., Bunn, F., & Handscomb, K. (2006). Prophylactic antibiotics to prevent surgical site infection after breast cancer surgery. *Cochrane Database of Systematic Reviews*, (2), CD005360.

Cunningham, R. S., & Huhmann, M. B. (2011). Nutritional disturbances. In C. H. Yarbro, D. Wujcik, & B. H. Gobel (Eds.), *Cancer nursing: Principles and practice* (7th ed.). Boston, MA: Jones & Bartlett.

Curhan, G. C., Aronson, M. D., & Preminger, G. M. (2015). Diagnosis and acute management of suspected nephrolithiasis in adults. In *UpToDate*. Retrieved from http://www.uptodate.com/contents/diagnosis-and-acute-management-of-suspected-nephrolithiasis-in-adults

*Currie, S. R., & Wang, J. (2004). Chronic back pain and major depression in the general Canadian population. *Pain, 107*(1), 54–60.

*Currie, S. R., & Wang, J. (2005). More data on major depression as an antecedent risk factor for first onset of chronic back pain. *Psychological Medicine, 35*, 1275–1282.

*Cutilli, C. C. (2005). Health literacy: What you need to know. *Orthopedic Nursing, 24*(3), 227–231.

*Cutler, C. J., & Davis, N. (2005). Improving oral care in patients receiving mechanical ventilation. *American Journal of Care, 14*(5), 389–394.

Czogala, J., Goniewicz, M. L., Fidelus, B., Zielinska-Danch, W., Travers, M. J., & Sobczak, A. (2014). Secondhand exposure to vapors from electronic cigarettes. *Nicotine & Tobacco Research, 16*(6), 655–662.

Da Vinci Hysterectomy. (2007). *Da Vinci hysterectomy*. Retrieved from http://www.davincisurgery.com/da-vinci-gynecology//-da-vincihysterectomy/index.aspx

*Dadd, M. (1983). Self-care for side effects. *Cancer Nursing, 6*, 63–66.

Dahlin, C. (2013). *Clinical practice guidelines for quality palliative care* (3rd ed.). Pittsburgh, PA: National Consensus Project for Quality Palliative Care.

Damron, T. A., Bogart, J., & Bilsky, M. (2015). Evaluation and management of complete and impending pathologic fractures in patients with metastatic bone disease, multiple myeloma, and lymphoma. In *UpToDate*. Retrieved from http://www.uptodate.com/contents/evaluation-and-management-of-complete-and-impending-pathologic-fractures-in-patients-with-metastatic-bone-disease-multiple-myeloma-and-lymphoma

Danila, M. I., Pons-Estel, G. J., Zhang, J., Vilá, L. M., Reveille, J. D., & Alarcón, G. S. (2009). Renal damage is the most important predictor of mortality within the damage index: Data from LUMINA LXIV, a multiethnic US cohort. *Rheumatology, 48*(5), 542–545.

Davies, E. T., Moxham, T., Rees, K. S., Singh, S., Coats, A., Ebrahim, S., ... Taylor, R. (2010). Exercise training for systolic heart failure: Cochrane systematic review and meta-analysis. *European Journal of Heart, 12*(7), 706–715.

*Davis, A. J. (1989). Clinical nurses' ethical decision making in situations of informed consent. *Advanced Nursing Science, 11*(3), 63–69.

*Davis, C. (1998). *ABCs of palliative care. Breathlessness, cough, and other respiratory problems*. Retrieved from http://www .ncbi.nlm.nih.gov/pmc/articles/PMC2127624/pdf/9361545.pdf

Davis, C. J., Sowa, D., Keim, K. S., Kinnare, K., & Peterson, S. (2012). The use of prealbumin and C-reactive protein for monitoring nutrition support in adult patients receiving enteral nutrition in an urban medical center. *Journal of Parenteral and Enteral Nutrition, 36*(2), 197–204.

*Davis, C. L. (1997). *ABCs of palliative care. Breathlessness, cough, and other respiratory problems. BMJ, 315*(7113), 931–934. Retrieved from http://www.ncbi.nlm.nih.gov/pmc/articles/PMC2127624/pdf/9361545.pdf

Davis, C. P. (n.d.). *Hepatitis A*. Retrieved from http://emedicinehealth.com/hepatitis_a-health/article_em.htm

Davis, C., Chrisman, J., & Walden, P. (2012). To scan or not to scan? Detecting urinary retention. *Nursing made incredibly easy! 10*(4), 53–54. doi:10.1097/01.NME.0000415016.88696.9d

*Davis, J. (2003). *One-side neglect: Improving awareness to speedy recovery; Life after stroke*. Retrieved from http://www.strokeassociation.org/STROKEORG/LifeAfterStroke/RegainingIndependence/EmotionalBehavioral-Challenges/One-side-Neglect-Improving-Awareness-to-Speed-Recovery_UCM_309735_Article.jsp

Davis, N. J., Vaughan, C. P., Johnson, T. M., Goode, P. S., Burgio, K. L., Redden, D. T., & Markland, A. D. (2013). Caffeine intake and its association with urinary incontinence in United States men: Results from National Health and Nutrition Examination Surveys 2005–2006 and 2007–2008. *The Journal of Urology, 189*(6), 2170–2174.

Davis, Y., Perham, M., Hurd, A. M., Jagersky, R., Gorman, W. J., Lynch-Carlson, D., & Senseney, D. (2014). Patient and family member needs during the perioperative period. *Journal of PeriAnesthesia Nursing, 29*(2), 119–128.

de Feiter, P. W., van Hooft, M. A., Beets-Tan, R. G., & Brink, P. R. (2007). Fat embolism syndrome: Yes or no? *Journal of Trauma and Acute Care Surgery, 63*(2), 429–431.

*De Ridder, D. J., Everaert, K., Fernández, L. G., Valero, J. V., Durán, A. B., Abrisqueta, M. L., & Ventura, M. G. (2005). Intermittent catheterisation with hydrophilic-coated catheters (SpeediCath) reduces the risk of clinical urinary tract infection in spinal cord injured patients: A prospective randomised parallel comparative trial. *European Urology, 48*(6), 991–995.

de Souza, D. M. S. T., & de Gouveia Santos, V. L. C. (2010). Incidence of pressure ulcers in the institutionalized elderly. *Journal of Wound, Ostomy, and Continence Nursing, 37*(3), 272–276.

Deandrea, S., Montanari, M., Moja, L., & Apolone, G. (2008). Prevalence of undertreatment in cancer pain. A review of published literature. *Annals of Oncology, 19*(12), 1985–1991.

DeAngelis, L. M. (2009). Cutaneous complications. In D. A. Casciato & M. C. Territo (Eds.), *Manual of clinical oncology* (pp. 639–640). Philadelphia, PA: Lippincott Williams & Wilkins.

Deaver, K., & Counts, C. S. (2015). Hemodialysis: Vascular access for hemodialysis. In C. S. Counts (Ed.), *Core curriculum for nephrology nursing: Module 3. Treatment options for patients with chronic kidney failure* (6th ed., pp. 172–225). Pitman, NJ: American Nephrology Nurses' Association.

DeBaun, M. R., & Vichinsky, M. (2015). Vasoocclusive pain management in sickle cell disease. In *UpToDate*. Retrieved from http://www.uptodate.com/contents/vasoocclusive-pain-management-in-sickle-cell-disease?source=machineLearning&search=pain+in+sickle+cell&selectedTitle=1~150&sectionRank=1&anchor=H34#H34

Gavin-Dreschnack, D., Nelson, A., Fitzgerald, S., Harrow, J., Sanchez-Anguiano, A., Ahmed, S., & Powell-Cope, G. Development of a Screening Tool for Safe Wheelchair Seating. In D. Gavin-Dreschnack, L. Schonfeld, A. Nelson, & S. Luther (Eds.), *Advances in patient safety: From research to implementation* (Volume 4: Programs, Tools, and Products). Rockville: MD: Agency for Healthcare Research and Quality.

Deegens, J. K., & Wetzels, J. F. M. (2011). Nephrotic range proteinuria. In J. T. Daugirdas (Ed.), *Handbook of chronic kidney disease management*. Philadelphia, PA: Lippincott Williams & Wilkins.

*Defloor, T., & Grypdonck, M. F. (2005). Pressure ulcers: Validation of two risk assessment scales. *Journal of Nursing, 14*(3), 373–382.

*Defloor, T., & Schoonhoven, L. (2004). Inter-rater reliability of the EPUAP pressure ulcer classification system using photographs. *Journal of Clinical Nursing, 13*, 952–959.

DeJong, N. W., Patiwael, J. A., de Groot, H., Burdorf, A., & Gerth van Wijk, R. (2011). Natural rubber latex allergy among healthcare workers: Significant reduction of sensitization and clinical relevant latex allergy after introduction of powder-free latex gloves. *Journal of Allergy and Clinical Immunology, 127*(2), AB70.

Dellaripa, P. F., & Danoff, S. (2016). Pulmonary manifestations of systemic lupus erythematosus in adults. In *UpToDate*. Retrieved from http://www.uptodate.com/contents/pulmonary-?source=see_link

Deng, B., Tan, Q. Y., Zhao, Y. P., Wang, R. W., & Jiang, Y. G. (2010). Suction or non-suction to the underwater seal drains following pulmonary operation: Meta-analysis of randomised controlled trials. *European Journal of Cardio-Thoracic Surgery, 38*(2), 210–215.

Denny, D. L., & Guido, G. W. (2012). Undertreatment of pain in older adults: An application of beneficence. *Nursing Ethics, 19*(6), 800–809.

*Denys, P., Schurch, B., & Fraczek, S. (2005). Poster 59: Management of neurologic bladder with focal administration of botulinum toxin A: Minimizing risks associated with increased detrusor pressure. *Journal of Pelvic Medicine & Surgery, 11*(Suppl. 1), S52–S53.

Department of Health. (2010). *NHS surveys: Adult Inpatient Survey 2010*. Retrieved from http://www.nhssurveys.org/surveys/497

*DePippo, K. L., Holas, M. A., & Reding, M. J. (1992). Validation of the 3-oz water swallow test for aspiration following stroke. *Archives of Neurology, 49*, 1259–1261.

Derrer, D. (2014). *Diet, drugs, and urinary incontinence*. WebMD. Retrieved from www.webmd.com/urinary-incontinence-oab/urinary-incontinence-diet-medications-chart?page=2

DeWalt, D. A., Callahan, L. F., Hawk, V. H., Broucksou, K. A., Hink, A., Rudd, R., & Brach, C. (2010, April). *Health literacy universal precautions toolkit* (Prepared by North Carolina Network Consortium, The Cecil G. Sheps Center for Health Services Research, The University of North Carolina at Chapel Hill, under Contract No. HHSA290200710014.) (AHRQ Publication No. 10-0046-EF). Rockville, MD: Agency for Healthcare Research and Quality.

*Dewey, R., Delley, R., & Shulman, L. (2002). A better life for patients with Parkinson's disease. *Patient Care*, *36*(7), 8–14.

Diaz, V., & Newman, J. (2015). Surgical site infection and prevention guidelines: A primer for Certified Registered Nurse Anesthetists. *Journal of the American Association of Nurse Anesthetists*, *83*(1), 63–68.

Dillavou, E. D. (2015). Surgical and endovascular repair of ruptured abdominal aortic aneurysm. In *UpToDate*. Retrieved from http://www.uptodate.com/contents/surgical-and-endovascular-repair-of-ruptured-abdominal-aortic-aneurysm

Dillingham, T. (2007). Musculoskeletal rehabilitation: Current understandings and future directions. *American Journal of Physical Medicine and Rehabilitation*, *86*, S19–S28.

Dillion, P. M. (2007). Assessing the respiratory system. In P. M. Dillion (Ed.), *Nursing health assessment: A critical thinking case studies approach* (2nd ed., pp. 393–436). Philadelphia, PA: F. A. Davis.

*Dinwiddie, L., Burrows-Hudson, S., & Peacock, E. (2006). Stage 4 chronic kidney disease: Preserving kidney function and preparing patients for stage 5 kidney disease. *The American Journal of Nursing*, *106*(9), 40–51.

Ditillo, B. A. (2002). Should there be a choice for cardiopulmonary resuscitation when death is expected? Revisiting an old idea whose time is yet to come. *Journal of Palliative Medicine*, *5*(1), 107–116.

*Dodd, M. J., Dibble, S. L., & Miaskowski, C. (2000). Randomized clinical trial of the effectiveness of 3 commonly used mouthwashes to treat chemotherapy-induced mucositis. *Oral Surgery, Oral Medicine, Oral Pathology, Oral Radiology, and Endodontics*, *90*(1), 39–47.

Dodd, M., Miaskowski, C., Dibble, S., Paul, S., MacPhail, L., Greenspan, D., & Shiba, G. (2008). Factors influencing oral mucositis in patients receiving chemotherapy. *Cancer Practice*, *8*(6), 291–297.

Does, A., Rhudy, L., Holland, D. E., & Olson, M. E. (2011). The experience of transition from hospital to home hospice. *Journal of Hospice & Palliative Nursing*, *13*(6), 394–402.

Doley, J. (2010). Nutrition management of pressure ulcers. *Nutrition in Clinical Practice*, *25*, 50–60.

*Dolin, R., Masur, H., & Saag, M. (2003). *AIDS therapy* (2nd ed.). Philadelphia, PA: Churchill Livingston.

Donovan, N. J., Daniels, S. K., Edmiaston, J., Weinhardt, J., Summers, D., & Mitchell, P. H. (2013). Dysphagia screening: state of the art: Invitational conference proceeding from the State-of-the-Art Nursing Symposium, International Stroke Conference 2012. *Stroke*, *44*, e24–e31.

Doran, K., & Halm, M. A. (2010). Integrating acupressure to alleviate postoperative nausea and vomiting. *American Journal of Critical Care*, *19*(6), 553–556.

Doran, M. (2007). Rheumatoid arthritis and diabetes mellitus: Evidence for an association? *Journal of Rheumatology*, *34*, 469–473.

Dorner, B., Posthauer, M. E., & Thomas, D. (2009). The role of nutrition in pressure ulcer prevention and treatment: National Pressure Ulcer Advisory Panel white paper. *Advances Skin and Wound Care*, *22*(5), 212–221.

Dorsher, P. T., & McIntosh, P. M. (2012). Neurogenic bladder. *Advances in Urology*. doi:10.1155/2012/816274. Retrieved from http://www.hindawi.com/journals/au/2012/816274/ref/

*Dougherty, M. (1998). Current status of research on pelvic muscles strengthening techniques. *Journal of Wound, Ostomy, and Continence*, *25*(3), 75–83.

*Douglas, S., & James, S. C. B. (2004). Non-pharmacological interventions in dementia. *Advances in Psychiatric Treatment*, *10*, 171–177.

Drews, R. E. (2007). Superior vena cava syndrome. In *UpToDate*. Retrieved from http://www.uptodate.com/contents/malignancy-related-superior-vena-cava-syndrome

Droogh, J. M., Smit, M., Absalom, A. R., Ligtenberg, J., & Zijlstra, J. (2015). Transferring the critically ill patient: are we there yet? *Critical Care*, *19*(1), 62.

Drossman, D. A. (2006a). Appendix A: Rome III diagnostic criteria for functional gastrointestinal disorders. *Gastroenterology*, *130*(5). Retrieved from http://www.romecriteria.org/assets/pdf/19_RomeIII_apA_885-898.pdf

Drossman, D. A. (2006b). The functional gastrointestinal disorders and the Rome III process. *Gastroenterology*, *130*(5), 1377–1390. Retrieved from http://www.gastrojournal.org/article/S0016-5085(06)00503-8/fulltext?refuid=S0002-8223(09)00461-1&refissn=0002-8223

Drulovic, J., Basic⊠Kes, V., Grgic, S., Vojinovic, S., Dincic, E., Toncev, G., . . . Miletic⊠Drakulic, S. (2015). The prevalence of pain in adults with multiple sclerosis: A Multicenter Cross⊠Sectional Survey. *Pain Medicine*, *16*(8), 1597–1602.

*Dudas, S. (1997). Altered body image and sexuality. In S. L. Groenwald, M. H. Frogge, M. Goodman, & C. Yarbro (Eds.), *Cancer nursing: Principles and practice* (4th ed.). Boston, MA: Jones & Bartlett.

Dudek, S. (2014). *Nutrition essentials for nursing practice* (7th ed.). Philadelphia, PA: Wolters Kluwer.

Dumoulin, C., Hay-Smith, E., & Mac Habee-Segui, G. (2014). Pelvic floor muscle training versus no treatment, or inactive control treatments, for urinary incontinence in women. *Cochrane Database of Systematic Reviews*, *5*, CD005654. doi:10.1002/14651858.CD005654.pub3

Dumoulin, C., Hay-Smith, J., Frawley, H., McClurg, D., Alewijnse, D., Bo, K., . . . Van Kampen, M. (2015). 2014 consensus statement on improving pelvic floor muscle training adherence: International Continence Society 2011 state-of-the-science seminar. *Neurourology and Urodynamics*, *34*(7), 600–605.

*Duncan, C., & Erickson, R. (1982). Pressures associated with chest tube stripping. *Heart & Lung, 11*(2), 166–171.

*Duncan, D. G., Beck, S. J., Hood, K., & Johansen, A. (2006). Using dietetic assistants to improve the outcome of hip fracture: a randomised controlled trial of nutritional support in an acute trauma ward. *Age Ageing, 35*(2), 148–153.

Duncan, J. W., & Bailey, R. A. (2011). Cauda equina syndrome following decompression for spinal stenosis. *Global Spine Journal, 1*(1), 15–18.

Dunne, S., Coffey, L., Gallagher, P., & Desmond, D. (2014). "If I can do it I will do it, if I can't, I can't": A study of adaptive self-regulatory strategies following lower limb amputation. *Disability and Rehabilitation, 36*(23), 1990–1997.

Dutka, P. (2008). Journal club discussion: Guarding against hidden hemolysis during dialysis: An overview. *Nephrology Nursing Journal, 35*(1), 45–50.

Dutka, P., & Szromba, C. (2015). The kidney in health and injury: Pathophysiology. In C.S. Counts (Ed.), *Core curriculum for nephrology nursing: Module 2. Physiologic and psychosocial basis for nephrology nursing practice* (6th ed., pp. 52–90). Pitman, NJ: American Nephrology Nurses' Association.

Eachempati, S., Wang, J., Hydo, L., Shou, J., & Barie, P. (2007). Acute renal failure in critically ill surgical patients: Persistent lethality despite new modes of renal replacement therapy. *Journal of Trauma, 63*(50), 987–993.

*Early, L. M., & Poquette, R. (2000). Bladder and kidney cancer. In S. L. Groenwald, M. H. Frogge, M. Goodman, & C. H. Yarbro (Eds.), *Cancer nursing: Principles and practice* (5th ed.). Boston, MA: Jones & Bartlett.

*Ebihara, S., Saito, H., Kanda, A., Nakajoh, M., Takahashi, H., Arai, H., & Sasaki, H. (2003). Impaired efficacy of cough in patients with Parkinson disease. *Chest Journal, 124*(3), 1009–1015.

Edelman, C., & Mandle, C. (2010). *Health promotion throughout the lifespan.* St. Louis, MO: Mosby.

Edelman, C., Kudszma, E., & Mandel, C. (2013). *Health promotion through the life span* (8th ed.). St. Louis, MO: Elsevier

Edelman, S., & Henry, R. (2011). *Diagnosis and management of type 2 diabetes* (4th ed.). New York, NY: Professional Communications.

*Edwards, R., Abullarade, C., & Turnbull, N. (1996). Nursing management and follow-up of the postoperative vascular patient in a clinic setting. *Journal Vascular Nursing, 14*(3), 62–67.

Eidt, J. F. (2015). Open surgical repair of abdominal aortic aneurysm. In *UpToDate.* Retrieved from http://www.uptodate.com/contents/open-surgical-repair-of-abdominal-aortic-aneurysm?source=machineLearning&search=Mortality++of+AAA&selectedTitle=2~150&sectionRank=1&anchor=H365977583#H365977583

Eilers, J., Harris, D., Henry, K., & Johnson, L. A. (2014). Evidence-based interventions for cancer treatment-related mucositis: Putting evidence into practice. *Clinical Journal of Oncology Nursing, 18*(6), 80–96.

*Eisenberg, P. (1990). Monitoring gastric pH to prevent stress ulcer. *Focus on Critical Care, 17*(4), 316–322.

*Ellerhorst-Ryan, J. M. (2000). Infection. In S. Groenwald, M. Frogge, M. Goodman, & C. Yarbro (Eds.), *Cancer nursing: Principles and practice* (5th ed.). Boston, MA: Jones & Bartlett.

*Ellershaw, J. E., & Wilkinson, S. (2003). *Care of the dying: A pathway to excellence.* Oxford, NY: Oxford University Press.

*Elliot, D. (2002). The treatment of peptic ulcers. *Nursing Standards, 16*(23), 37–42.

Elliott, D. Y., Geyer, C., Lionetti, T., & Doty, L. (2012). Managing alcohol withdrawal in hospitalized patients. *Nursing, 42*(4), 22–30.

*Ellstrom, K. (2006). The pulmonary system. In J. Grif-Alspach (Ed.), *Core curriculum for critical care nursing* (6th ed., pp. 45–183). St. Louis, MO: Saunders-Elsevier.

Elmets, C. A. (2015). Overview of cutaneous photosensitivity: Photobiology, patient evaluation, and photoprotection. In *UpToDate.* Retrieved from http://www.uptodate.com/contents/overview-of-cutaneous-photosensitivity-photobiology-patient-evaluation-and-photoprotection?source=see_link

*Elpern, E., Covert, B., & Kleinpell, R. (2005). Moral distress of staff nurses in a medical intensive care unit. *American Journal Critical Care, 14*(6), 523–530.

El-Salhy, M., Lillebø, E., Reinemo, A., Salmelid, L., & Hausken, T. (2010). Effects of a health program comprising reassurance, diet management, probiotics administration and regular exercise on symptoms and quality of life in patients with irritable bowel syndrome. *Gastroenterology Insights, 2*(1), 21–26.

Forsh, D. A. (n.d.). Deep venous thrombosis prophylaxis in orthopedic surgery. In *Medscape.* Retrieved from http://emedicine.medscape.com/article/1268573-overview

Entwistle, V. A., McCaughan, D., Watt, I. S., Birks, Y., Hall, J., Peat, M., . . . Wright, J. (2010). Speaking up about safety concerns: multi-setting qualitative study of patient's views and experiences. *Quality and Safety in Health Care, 19*(6), e33.

Epilepsy Foundation. (2007). *What is epilepsy? Frequently asked questions.* Retrieved from http://www.epilepsyfoundation.org/about/faq/index.cfm

Epstein, R. M., & Street, R. L., Jr. (2011). The values and value of patient-centered care. *Annals of Family Medicine, 9*(2), 100–103.

Erens, G. A., Thornhill, T. S., & Katz, J. N. (2015). Total hip arthroplasty. In *UpToDate.* Retrieved from http://www.uptodate.com/contents/total-hip-arthroplast

Erichsén, E., Milberg, A., Jaarsma, T., & Friedrichsen, M. (2015). Constipation in specialized palliative care: Prevalence, definition, and patient-perceived symptom distress. *Journal of Palliative Medicine, 18*(7), 585–592.

Eriksson, B. I., Quinlan, D. J., & Eikelboom, J. W. (2011). Novel oral factor Xa and thrombin inhibitors in the management of thromboembolism. *Annual Review of Medicine, 62*, 41–57.

*Errsser, S. J., Getliffe, K., Voegeli, D., & Regan, S. (2005). A critical review of the inter-relationship between skin vulnerability and urinary incontinence and related nursing intervention. *International Journal of Nursing Studies, 2*, 823–835.

Ertl, J. P. (2012). Amputations of the lower extremity treatment & management. In *Medscape*. Retrieved from http://emedicine.medscape.com/article/1232102-treatment

*Esche, C. A. (2005). Resiliency: A factor to consider when facilitating the transition from the hospital to home in older adults. *Geriatric Nursing, 26*(4), 218–222.

*Eslinger, P. (2002). Empathy and social-emotional factors in recovery from stroke. *Current Opinion in Neurology, 15*(1), 91–97.

European Commission. (2010). *Choice and control: The right to independent living*. Retrieved from http://fra.europa.eu/sites/default/files/choice_and_control_en_13.pdf

European Pressure Ulcer Advisory Panel and National Pressure Ulcer Advisory Panel. (2009). *Prevention and treatment of pressure ulcers: Quick reference guide*. Washington, DC: National Pressure Ulcer Advisory Panel.

Evan, A. P., Lingeman, J. E., & Coe, F. L. (2009). Intra-tubular deposits, urine and stone composition are divergent in patients with ileostomy. *Kidney International, 76*(10), 1081–1088.

*Evans, B. (2005). Best practice protocols: VAP prevention. *Nursing Management, 36*(12), 10–15.

*Ewing, J. A. (1984). Detecting alcoholism: The CAGE questionnaire. *Journal of American Medical Association, 252*, 1905–1907.

*Ezzone, S., Baker, C., Rosselet, R., & Terepka, E. (1998). Music as an adjunct to antiemetic therapy. *Oncology Nursing Forum, 25*(9), 1551–1556.

Fairman, R. M. (2016). Carotid endarterectomy. In *UpToDate*. Retrieved from https://www.uptodate.com/contents/carotid-endarterectomy

Falck-Ytter, Y., Francis, C. W., Johanson, N. A, Curley, C., Dahl, O. E., Pauker, S. G., . . . American College of Chest Physicians. (2012). Prevention of VTE in orthopedic surgery patients: Antithrombotic Therapy and Prevention of Thrombosis (9th ed.). American College of Chest Physicians Evidence-Based Clinical Practice Guidelines. *Chest, 141*, e278S.

Fallone, S., & Cotton, A. B. (2015). Acute kidney injury. In C. S. Counts (Ed.), *Core curriculum for nephrology nursing: Module 4. Acute kidney injury* (6th ed., pp. 19–54). Pitman, NJ: American Nephrology Nurses' Association.

Fanta, C. H. (2014a). Patient information: Asthma treatment in adolescents and adults (Beyond the Basics). In *UpToDate*. Retrieved from http://www.uptodate.com/contents/asthma-treatment-in-adolescents-and-adults-beyond-the-basics

Fanta, C. H. (2014b). Diagnosis of asthma in adolescents and adults. In *UpToDate*. Retrieved from http://www.uptodate.com/contents/diagnosis-of-asthma-in-adolescents-and-adults

Fanta, C. H. (2014c). An overview of asthma management. In *UpToDate*. Retrieved from http://www.uptodate.com/contents/an-overview-of-asthma-management

Fanta, C. H. (2014d). Treatment of acute exacerbations of asthma in adults. In *UpToDate*. Retrieved from http://www.uptodate.com/contents/treatment-of-acute-exacerbations-of-asthma-in-adults?source=search_result&search=asthma+adult&selectedTitle=3~150

Faraklas, I., Holt, B., Tran, S., Lin, H., Saffle, J., & Cochran, A. (2013). Impact of a nursing-driven sleep hygiene protocol on sleep quality. *Journal of Burn Care & Research, 34*(2), 249–254.

*Farrell, S., Harmon, R., & Hastings, S. (1998). Nursing management of acute psychotic episodes. *Nursing Clinics of North America, 33*(1), 187–200.

Fazia, A., Lin, J., & Staros, E. (2012). Urine sodium. In *Medscape*. Retrieved from http://emedicine.medscape.com/article/2088449-overview

Feigelson, H. S., James, T. A., Single, R. M., Onitilo, A. A., Aiello Bowles, E. J., Barney, T., . . . McCahill, L. E. (2013). Factors associated with the frequency of initial total mastectomy: Results of a multi-institutional study. *Journal of the American College of Surgeons, 216*(5), 966–975.

Feller-Kopman, D. J., & Schwartzstein, R. M. (2015). Mechanisms, causes, and effects of hypercapnia. In *UpToDate*. Retrieved from http://www.uptodate.com/contents/mechanisms-causes-and-effects-of-hypercapnia

*Fellowes, D., Barnes, K., & Wilkinson, S. (2004). Aromatherapy and massage for symptom relief in patients with cancer. *Cochrane Database of Systematic Reviews, 2*(6), CD002287.

Ferenci, P. (2013). Hepatic encephalopathy in adults: Clinical manifestations and diagnosis. In *UpToDate*. Retrieved from http://www.uptodate.com/contents/hepatic-encephalopathy-in-adults-clinical-manifestations-and-diagnosis?source=search_result&search=hepatic+encephalopathy.&selectedTitle=2~150

*Ferrell, B. R. (1995). The impact of pain on quality of life. *Nursing Clinics of North America, 30*(4), 609–624.

Ferucci, E. D., Johnston, J. M., Gaddy, J. R., Sumner, L., Posever, J. O., Choromanski, T. L., . . . Helmick, C. G. (2014). Prevalence and incidence of systemic lupus erythematosus in a population-based registry of American Indian and Alaska Native people, 2007–2009. *Arthritis & Rheumatology, 66*(9), 2494–2502.

*Fetterman, L. G., & Lemburg, L. (2004). A silent killer—Often preventable. *American Journal of Critical Care, 13*(5), 431–436.

*Field, J. B. (1989). *Hypoglycemia: Definition, clinical presentations, classification, and laboratory tests*. Retrieved from http://www.ncbi.nlm.nih.gov/pubmed/2645129

Field, J. J., & DeBaun, M. R. (2015). Acute chest syndrome in adults with sickle cell disease. In *UpToDate*. Retrieved from http://www.uptodate.com/contents/acute-chest-syndrome-in-adults-with-sickle-cell-disease?source=see_link

Field, J. J., Vemulakonda, V. M., & DeBaun, M. R. (2014). Diagnosis and management of priapism in sickle cell disease. In *UpToDate*. Retrieved from http://www.uptodate.com/contents/diagnosis-and-management-of-priapism-in-sickle-cell-disease?source=see_link

Field, J. J., Vichinsky, E. P., & DeBaun, M. R. (2016). Overdrive of the management and prognosis of sickle cell disease. In *UpToDate*. Retrieved at http://www.uptodate.com/contents/overview-of-the-management-and-prognosis-of-sickle-cell-disease?source=search_result&search=sickle+cell+crisis&selectedTitle=2~39

Fields, L. (2008). Oral care intervention to reduce incidence of ventilator-associated pneumonia in the neurologic intensive care unit. *American Association of Neuroscience Nurses*, 40(5), 291–298.

Fil, T. M. (2015). Prognosis of community-acquired pneumonia in adults. In *UpToDate*. Retrieved from http://www.uptodate.com/contents/prognosis-of-community-acquired-pneumonia-in-adults?source=see_link

Filho, J. O. (2015). Initial assessment and management of acute stroke. In *UpToDate*. Retrieved from http://www.uptodate.com/contents/initial-assessment-and-management-of-acute-stroke

*Fineman, L. D., LaBrecque, M. A., Shih, M., & Curley, M. A. Q. (2006). Prone positioning can be safely performed in critically ill infants and children. *Pediatric Critical Care Medicine*, 7(5), 413–422.

*Finkelman, A. W. (2000). Self-management for psychiatric patient at home. *Home Care Provider*, 5(6), 95–101.

Firestein, G. S. (2016). Pathogenesis of rheumatoid arthritis. In *UpToDate*. Retrieved from http://www.uptodate.com/contents/pathogenesis-of-rheumatoid-arthritis

Fisher, R. S. (2014). *The 2014 definition of epilepsy: A perspective for patients and caregivers*. International League Against Epilepsy. Retrieved from http://www.ilae.org/visitors/centre/Definition-2014-Perspective.cfm

Fisher, R. S., Acevedo, C., Arzimanoglou, A., Bogacz, A., Cross, J. H., Elger, C. E., . . . Wiebe, S. (2014). ILAE official report: a practical clinical definition of epilepsy. *Epilepsia*, 55(4), 475–482.

*Fitch, M. I. (2006). Programmatic approaches to psychological support. In R. M. Carroll Johnson, L. M. Gorman, & N. J. Bush (Eds.), *Psychosocial nursing care along the cancer continuum* (2nd ed., pp. 419–438). Pittsburgh, PA: Oncology Nursing Society.

*Fitzmaurice, D., Blann, A., & Lip, G. (2002). Bleeding risks of antithrombotic therapy. *BMJ*, 12(325)(7368), 828–831. Retrieved from http://www.ncbi.nlm.nih.gov/pmc/articles/PMC1124331/

Fleming, N. D., Alvarez-Secord, A., Von Gruenigen, V., Miller, M. J., & Abernethy, A. P. (2009). Indwelling catheters for the management of refractory malignant ascites: A systematic literature overview and retrospective chart review. *Journal of Pain and Symptom Management*, 38(3), 341–349. doi:10.1016/j.jpainsymman.2008.09.008

*Fletcher, L. (2006). Management of patients with intermittent claudication. *Nursing Standard*, 20(31), 59–65.

Fletcher, M. J., & Dahl, B. H. (2013). Expanding nurse practice in COPD: Is it key to providing high quality, effective and safe patient care? *Primary Care Respiratory Journal*, 22, 230–233.

*Flor, H. (2002). Phantom-limb pain: Characteristics, causes, and treatment. *The Lancet. Neurology*, 1(3), 182–189.

*Flor, H., Nikolajsen, L., & Jensen, T. S. (2006). Phantom limb pain: A case of maladaptive CNS plasticity? *Nature Reviews Neuroscience*, 7(11), 873–881.

*Foltz, A. (2000). Nutritional disturbances. In S. Groenwald, M. Frogge, M. Goodman, & C. Yarbro (Eds.), *Cancer nursing: Principles and practice* (5th ed.). Boston, MA: Jones & Bartlett.

Fontana G. A., & Widdicombe, J. (2007). What is cough and what should be measured? *Pulmonary Pharmacology Therapy*, 20(4), 307–312.

*Fore, J. (2006). A review of skin and the effects of aging on skin structure and function. *Ostomy Wound Management*, 52(9), 24–35.

*Forsythe, B., & Faulkner, K. (2004). Overview of the tolerability of gefitinib (IRESSA) monotherapy: Clinical experience in non-small-cell-lung cancer [Electronic version]. *Drug Safety*, 27(14), 1081–1092. Retrieved from http://www.ebsco.waldenu.edu/ehost/pdf?vid=144&hid=102&sid=781c7c0c-696c-44ec-9c5d-f6382763aca4%40sessionmgr106

Foster, K. W. (2015). Hip fractures in adults. In *UpToDate*. Retrieved at http://www.uptodate.com/contents/hip-fractures-in-adults

Foulks, G. N., Forsstot, S. L., Dinshik, P. C., Forstot, J. Z., Goldstein, M. H., Lemp, M. A., . . . Jacobs, D. S. (2015). Clinical guidelines for management of dry eye associated with sjögren disease. *The Ocular Surface*, 13(2), 118–132.

Fouque, D., & Juillard, L. (2011). Protein intake. In J. T. Daugirdas (Ed.), *Handbook of chronic kidney disease management*. Philadelphia, PA: Lippincott Williams & Wilkins.

Francis, J. (2015). Delirium and acute confusional states: Prevention, treatment, and prognosis. In *UpToDate*. Retrieved from http://www.uptodate.com/contents/delirium-and-acute-confusional-states-prevention-treatment-and-prognosis

Francone, T. D. (2015). Overview of surgical ostomy for fecal diversion. In *UpToDate*. Retrieved from http://www.uptodate.com/contents/overview-of-surgical-ostomy-for-fecal-diversion

Franz, M. G., Steed, D. L., & Robson, M. C. (2007). Optimizing healing of the acute wound by minimizing complications. *Current Problems in Surgery*, 44(11), 691–763.

French, K., Beynon, C., & Delaforce, J. (2007). Alcohol is the true "rape drug." *Nursing Standard*, 21(29), 26–27.

*Fried, L. P., Ferrucci, L., Darer, J., Williamson, J. D., & Anderson, G. (2004). Untangling the concepts of disability, frailty, and comorbidity: Implications for improved targeting and care. *Journals of Gerontology—Series A Biological Sciences and Medical Sciences, 59*(3), 255–263.

*Fried, L. P., Tangen, C. M., Walston, J., Newman, A. B., Hirsch, C., Gottdiener, J., . . . Cardiovascular Health Study Collaborative Research Group. (2001). Frailty in older adults: Evidence for a phenotype. *Journals of Gerontology— Series A Biological Sciences and Medical Sciences, 56*(3), M146–M156.

Friesen, M. A., White, S. V., & Byers, J. F. (2008). Handoffs: Implications for nurses. In R. G. Hughes (Ed.), *Patient safety and quality: An evidence-based handbook for nurses* (Chapter 34). Rockville, MD: Agency for Healthcare Research and Quality (US). Retrieved from http://www.ncbi.nlm.nih.gov/books/NBK2649/

Frosch, D. L., & Elwyn, G. (2014). Don't blame patients, engage them: Transforming health systems to address health literacy. *Journal of Health Communication: International Perspectives, 19*(2), 10–14. Retrieved from http://dx.doi.org /10.1080/10810730.2014.950548

Frosch, D. L., May, S. G., Rendle, K. A., Tietbohl, C., & Elwyn, G. (2012). Authoritarian physicians and patients' fear of being labeled 'difficult' among key obstacles to shared decision making. *Health Affairs, 31*(5), 1030–1038.

*Funnell, M. M., Kruger, D. F., & Spencer, M. (2004). Self-management support for insulin therapy in type 2 diabetes. *Diabetes Educator, 30*(2), 274–280.

Furie, K., Kasner, S., Adams, R., Albers, G., Bush, R., Fagan, S., . . . Wentworth, D. (2011). *Guidelines for the prevention of stroke in patients with stroke or transient ischemic attack. A Guideline for Healthcare Professionals From the American Heart Association/American Stroke Association.* Retrieved from http://www.stroke.ahajournals.org/content/early/2010/10/21 /STR.0b013e3181f7d043.full.pdf+html

Gabriel, S. E., & Crowson, C. S. (2015). Epidemiology of, risk factors for, and possible causes of rheumatoid arthritis. In *UpToDate.* Retrieved from http://www.uptodate.com/contents/epidemiology-of-risk-factors-for-and-possible-causes-of-rheumatoid-arthritis

Gallagher, P., Horgan, O., Franchignoni, F., Giordano, A., & MacLachlan, M. (2007). Body image in people with lower-limb amputation: A Rasch analysis of the amputee body image scale. *American Journal of Physical Medicine and Rehabilitation, 86*(3), 205–215.

Gallanagh, S., Quinn, T. J., Alexander, J., & Walters, M. R. (2011). Physical activity in the prevention and treatment of stroke. *ISRN Neurology, 2011.* Retrieved from https://www.hindawi.com/journals/isrn/2011/953818/

Ganio, M. S., Armstrong, L. E., Casa, D. J., McDermott, B. P., Lee, E. C., Yamamoto, L. M., . . . Chevillotte, E. (2011). Mild dehydration impairs cognitive performance and mood of men. *British Journal of Nutrition, 106*(10), 1535–1543. Retrieved from http://www.journals.cambridge.org/action/displayAbstract?fromPage=online&aid=8425835&fileI d=S0007114511002005

*Gans, K. M., Ross, E., Barner, C. W., Wylie-Rosett, J., McMurray, J., & Eaton, C. (2003). REAP and WAVE: New tools to rapidly assess/discuss nutrition with patients. *The Journal of Nutrition, 133*(2), 556S–562S.

Garcia-Albea, V., & Limaye, K. (2012). The clinical conundrum of pruritus. *Journal of the Dermatology Nurses, 4*(2), 97–105.

Garcia-Tsao, G. (2011). Cirrhosis and its sequelae. In L. Goldman & A. I. Schafer (Eds.), *Cecil medicine* (24th ed., Chapter 156). Philadelphia, PA: Saunders Elsevier.

Garcia-Tsao, G., Sanyal, A. J., Grace, N. D., Carey, W. D., Practice Guidelines Committee of American Association for Study of Liver Diseases, & Practice Parameters Committee of American College of Gastroenterology. (2007). Prevention and management of gastroesophageal varices and variceal hemorrhage in cirrhosis. *American Journal of Gastroenterology, 102*(12), 2086–2102.

*Gary, R., & Fleury, J. (2002). Nutritional status: Key to preventing functional decline in hospitalized older adults. *Topics in Geriatric Rehabilitation, 17*(3), 40–71.

Garzon, D. L., Kempker, T., & Piel, P. (2011). Primary care management of food allergy and food intolerance. *Nurse Practitioner, 36*(12), 34–40.

*Gavin-Dreschnack, D., Nelson, A., Fitzgerald, S., Harrow, J., Sanchez-Anguiano, A., Ahmed, S., . . . Powell-Cope, G. (2005). Wheelchair-related falls: Current evidence and directions for improved quality care. *Journal of Nursing Care Quality, 20*(2), 119–127.

*Geary, C. M. B. (1987). Nursing grand rounds: The patient with viral cardiomyopathy. *Journal of Cardiovascular Nursing, 2*(1), 48–52.

*Geerlings, S. E., & Hoepelman, A. I. (1999). Immune dysfunction in patients with diabetes mellitus (DM). *FEMS Immunology and Medical Microbiology, 26*(3–4), 259–265.

*Geerts, W. H., Pineo, G. F., Heit, J. A., Bergqvist, D., Lassen, M. R., Colwell, C. W., . . . Ray, J. G. (2004). Prevention of venous thromboembolism: The Seventh ACCP Conference on Antithrombotic and Thrombolytic Therapy. *CHEST Journal, 126*(3, Suppl.), 338S–400S.

Geng, V., Eelen, P. S., Fillingham, S., Holroyd, S., Kiesbye, B., Pearce, I., . . . Vahr, S. (2010). Continent urinary diver- sions good practice in health care. *European Association of Urology Nurses (EAUN).* Retrieved at http://nurses.uroweb .org/guideline/continent-urinary-diversion/

George, A., & DeBaun, M. R. (2016). Bone and joint complications in sickle cell disease. In *UpToDate.* Retrieved from http://www.uptodate.com/contents/bone-and-joint-complications-in-sickle-cell-disease?source=search_result&se arch=osteonecrosis+sickle+cell&selectedTitle=1~15

Gestring, M. (2015). Abdominal compartment syndrome. In *UpToDate*. Retrieved from http://www.uptodate.com/contents/abdominal-compartment-syndrome

*Ghotkar, S. V., Grayson, A. D., Fabri, B. M., Dihmis, W. C., & Pullan, D. M. (2006). Preoperative calculation of risk for prolonged intensive care unit stay following coronary artery bypass grafting. *Journal of Cardiothoracic Surgery*, *1*(14), 8090–8091.

*Giardina, E. (1999). Cardiovascular effects of nicotine. In *UpToDate*. Retrieved from http://www.uptodate.com/contents/cardiovascular-effects-of-nicotine

*Gil, K., Carson, J., Sedway, J., Porter, L., Schaeffer, J., & Orringer, E. (2000). Follow-up of coping skills training in adults with sickle cell disease. *Health Psychology*, *19*(1), 85–90.

*Gillenwater, J. Y., Grayhack, J. T., Howards, S. S., & Duckett, J. W. (1996). *Adult and pediatric urology* (3rd ed.). St. Louis, MO: Mosby-Year Book.

Gillis, A., MacDonald, B., & MacIssac, A. (2008). Nurses' knowledge, attitudes, and confidence regrading preventing and treating deconditioning in older adults. *The Journal of Continuing Education in Nursing*, *39*(12), 547–554.

*Ginzler, E., & Tayar, J. (2004). *Systemic lupus erythematosus*. Retrieved from http://www.rheumatolgy.org/public/factsheets/sle_new.asp

Giuliano, A. E., & Hurvitz, S. A. (2012). Breast disorders. In S. McPhee & M. Papadakis (Eds.), *2012 Current medical diagnosis & treatment* (pp. 699–726). New York, NY: McGraw-Hill Lange.

Givertz, M. (2015). Noncardiogenic pulmonary edema. In *UpToDate*. Retrieved from http://www.uptodate.com/contents/noncardiogenic-pulmonary-edema

Gladman, D. D. (2015). Overview of the clinical manifestations of systemic lupus erythematosus in adults. In *UpToDate*. Retrieved from http://www.uptodate.com/contents/overview-of-the-clinical-manifestations-of-systemic-lupus-erythematosus-in-adults?source=search_result&search=cardiac++complications+with+lupus&selectedTitle=1~t

Glantz, M., Chamberlain, M., Liu, Q., Hsieh, C., Edwards, K., VanHorn, A., . . . Recht, L. (2009). Gender disparity in the rate of partner abandonment in patients with serious medical illness. *Cancer*, *115*(22), 5237–5242.

*Glaser, V. (2000). Topics in geriatrics: Effective approaches to depression in older patients. *Patient Care*, *17*, 65–80.

Gleason, J. L., Richter, H. E., Redden, D. T., Goode, P. S., Burgio, K. L., & Markland, A. D. (2013). Caffeine and urinary incontinence in US women. *International Urogynecology Journal*, *24*(2), 295–302.

Global Strategy for The Diagnosis, Management, and Prevention of COPD: Updated 2015. *Global Initiative for Chronic Obstructive Lung Disease (GOLD)*. Retrieved from http://www.goldcopd.org

*Gobel, B. H. (2005). Bleeding disorder. In S. Groenwald, M. Frogge, M. Goodman, & C. Yarbro (Eds.), *Cancer nursing: Principles and practice* (6th ed.). Boston, MA: Jones & Bartlett.

Goldberg, M., Aukett, L. K., Carmel, J., Fellows, J., Folkedahl, B., Pittman, J., . . . Palmer R. (2010). Management of the patient with a fecal ostomy: Best practice guideline for clinicians. *Journal of Wound, Ostomy, and Continence Nursing*, *37*(6), 596–598.

Goldberg, E. G., & Chopra, S. (2015a). Cirrhosis in adults: Overview of complications, general management, and prognosis. In *UpToDate*. Retrieved from http://www.uptodate.com/contents/cirrhosis-in-adults-overview-of-complications-general-management-and-prognosis

Goldberg, E. G., & Chopra, S. (2015b). Cirrhosis in adults: Etiologies, clinical manifestations, and diagnosis. In *UpToDate*. Retrieved from http://www.uptodate.com/contents/cirrhosis-in-adults-etiologies-clinical-manifestations-and-diagnosis

Goldenberg, D. L., & Sexton, D. J. (2015). Septic arthritis in adults. In *UpToDate*. Retrieved from http://www.uptodate.com/contents/septic-arthritis-in-adults

Gonzalez, E. L., Patrignani, P., Tacconelli, S., & Rodriquez, L. A. (2010). Variablity among nonsteriodial antiinflammatory drugs in risk for upper GI bleeding. *Arthritis & Rheumatism*, *62*(6), 1592–1601.

*Goodman, M., & Hayden, B. K. (2000). Chemotherapy: Principles of administration. In C. H. Yarbo, M. H. Frogge, & M. Goodman (Eds.), *Comprehensive cancer nursing review* (6th ed.). Boston, MA: Jones & Bartlett.

*Gooszen, A. W., Geelkerken, R. H., Hermans, J., Lagaay, M. B., & Gooszen, H. G. (2000). Quality of life with a temporary stoma: Ileostomy vs. colostomy. *Diseases of Colon and Rectum*, *43*(5), 650–655.

Gor, H. (2012). Hysterectomy. In *Medscape*. Retrieved from http://emedicine.medscape.com/article/267273-overview

*Gordon, A. J. (2006). Identification and treatment of alcohol-use disorders in the perioperative period. *Post Graduate Medicine*, *199*(2), 46–55.

Gordon, A. J. (2016). Identification and management of unhealthy alcohol use in the perioperative period. In *UpToDate*. Retrieved from http://www.uptodate.com/contents/identification-and-management-of-unhealthy-alcohol-use-in-the-perioperative-period

*Gordon, M. (1994). *Nursing diagnosis: Process and application*. New York, NY: McGraw-Hill.

*Gorski, L. A. (2002, October). Effective teaching of home IV therapy [Electronic version]. *Home Healthcare Nurse*, *20*(10), 666–674. Retrieved from http://www.gateway.tx.ovid.com.library.gcu.edu:2048/gw2/ovidweb.cgi

*Goshorn, J. (2000). Management of patients with urinary and renal dysfunction. In S. Smeltzer & B. Bare (Eds.), *Brunner & Suddarth's textbook of medical-surgical nursing* (9th ed.). Philadelphia, PA: Lippincott Williams & Wilkins.

Goss, L., Coty, M. B., & Myers, J. A. (2011). A review of documented oral care practices in an intensive care unit. *Clinical Nursing Research*, *20*(2), 181–196.

Graf, J., & Janssens, U. (2007). Recognizing shock: Who cares, and when? *Critical Care Medicine*, *35*(11), 2651–2652.

*Grainger, R. (1990). Anxiety interrupters. *The American Journal of Nursing, 90*(2), 14–15.

Grant, J. E. (2011). *Neurobiology and pathological gambling in national center for responsible gaming. Gambling and the brain: Why neuroscience research is vital to gambling research.* Retrieved from http://www.ncrg.org/sites/default/files/uploads/docs/monographs/ncrgmonograph6final.pdf

Grattagliano, I., Ubaldi, E., Bonfrate, L., & Portinc, P. (2011). Management of liver cirrhosis between primary care and specialists. *World Journal Gastroenterology, 17*(18), 2273–2282.

*Graul, T. (2002). Total joint replacement: Baseline benchmark data for interdisciplinary outcomes management. *Orthopaedic Nursing, 21*(3), 57–67.

Graves, N. S. (2013). Acute gastroenteritis. *Primary Care, 40*(3), 727–741.

*Gray-Miceli, D., Johnson, J. C., & Strumpf, N. E. (2005). A step-wise approach to a comprehensive post-fall assessment. *Annals of Long-Term Care: Clinical Care and Aging, 13*(12), 16–24.

Gray-Miceli, D., Ratcliffe, S. J., & Johnson, J. (2010). Use of a postfall assessment tool to prevent falls. *Western Journal of Nursing Research, 32*(7), 932–948.

Greco, M. T., Roberto, A., Corli, O., Deandrea, S., Bandieri, E., Cavuto, S., & Apolone, G. (2014). Quality of cancer pain management: an update of a systematic review of undertreatment of patients with cancer. *Journal of Clinical Oncology, 32*(36), 4149–4154.

*Greelish, J., Mohler, E., & Fairman, R. (2006a). Carotid endarectomy in asymptomatic patients. In *UpToDate*. Retrieved from http://www.uptodate.com

*Greelish, J., Mohler, E., & Fairman, R. (2006b). Carotid endarectomy: Preoperative evaluation; surgical technique; and complications. In *UpToDate*. Retrieved from http://www.uptodate.com

*Greenberger, P. A. (2002). Anaphylaxis. In *Manual of Allergy & Immunology* (p. 10). Retrieved from Ovid database.

Greenberger, P. A. (2007). Idiopathic anaphylaxis. *Immunology Allergy Clinician North America, 27*(2), 273.

Greene, J. H. (2011). Restricting dietary sodium and potassium: A dietitian's perspective. In J. T. Daugirdas (Ed.), *Handbook of chronic kidney disease management.* Philadelphia, PA: Lippincott Williams & Wilkins.

Griebling, T. L. (2009). Urinary incontinence in the elderly. *Clinics in Geriatric Medicine, 25*(3), 445–457.

*Griffin-Broan, J. (2000). Diagnostic evaluation, classification, and staging. In C. Yarbo, M. H. Frogge, M. Goodman, & S. Groenwald (Eds.), *Cancer nursing: Principles and practice* (5th ed.). Boston, MA: Jones & Bartlett.

Grise, E. M., & Adeoye, O. (2012). Blood pressure control for acute ischemic and hemorrhagic stroke. *Current Opinion Critical Care, 18*(2), 132.

*Grisham, K., & Estes, N. (1982). Dynamics of alcoholic families. In N. Estes & M. E. Heinemann (Eds.), *Alcoholism: Development, consequences and interventions.* St. Louis, MO: Mosby-Year Book.

Gröber, U., & Kisters, K., (2007). Influence of drugs on vitamin D and calcium metabolism. *Dermatoendocrinology, 4*(2), 158–166.

Groenhoff, C. L., Ales, L., & Todd, L. B. (2015). Peritoneal dialysis: Peritoneal dialysis therapy. In C. S. Counts (Ed.). *Core curriculum for nephrology nursing: Module 3. Treatment options for patients with chronic kidney disease* (6th ed., pp. 240–267). Pitman, NJ: American Nephrology Nurses Association.

Grossbach, I., Stranberg, S., & Chlan, L. (2011). Promoting effective communication for patients receiving mechanical ventilation. *Critical Care Nurse, 31*(3), 46–60.

Grossman, S., & Porth, C. A. (2014). *Porth's pathophysiology: Concepts of altered health states* (9th ed.). Philadelphia, PA: Wolters Kluwer.

Gruman, J. (2011). *Engagement does not mean compliance.* Center for Advancing Health. Retrieved from www.cfah.org/blog/2011/engagement-does-not-mean-compliance

Guagnozzi, D., & Lucendo, A. J. (2014). Anemia in inflammatory bowel disease: A neglected issue with relevant effects. *World Journal Gastroenterology, 20*(13), 3542–3551.

Guillain-Barre syndrome fact sheet. (n.d.). Retrieved from http://www.ninds.nih.gov/disorders/gbs/detail_gbs.htm

Gulati, M., Shaw, L. S., & Merz, N. B., (2012). Myocardial ischemia in women: Lessons from the NHLBI WISE Study. *Clinical Cardiology, 35*(3), 141–148.

Guo, S., & DiPietro, L. A. (2010). Factors affecting wound healing. *Journal of Dental Research, 89*(3), 219–229.

Gupta, A., & Reilly, C. (2007). Fat embolism. *Continuing Education in Anaesthesia, Critical Care & Pain, 7*(5), 148–151. Retrieved from http://www.ceaccp.oxfordjournals.org/content/7/5/148.full

Gutekunst, L. (2011). Restricting protein and phosphorus: A dietitian's perspective. In J. T. Daugirdas (Ed.), *Handbook of chronic kidney disease management.* Philadelphia, PA: Lippincott Williams & Wilkins.

Gutman, N. (Ed.). (2011). *ILEOSTOMY GUIDE. United Ostomy Association (UOA).* Retrieved from http://www.ostomy.org/uploaded/files/ostomy_info/IleostomyGuide.pdf?direct=1

Gysels, M. H., & Higginson, I. J. (2011). The lived experience of breathlessness and its implications for care: A qualitative comparison in cancer, COPD, heart failure and MND. *BMC Palliative Care, 10*, 15.

Haber, J. R., Bucholz, K. K., Jacob, T., Grant, J. D., Scherrer, J. F., Sartor, C. E., . . . Heath, A. (2010). Effect of paternal alcohol and drug dependence on offspring conduct disorder: Gene–environment interplay*. *Journal of Studies on Alcohol and Drugs, 71*(5), 652–663.

*Haddock, J. (1994). Towards further clarification of the concept "dignity." *Journal of Advanced Nursing, 24*(5), 924–931.

*Hadley, S. K., & Gaarder, S. M. (2005). Treatment of irritable bowel syndrome. *American Family Physician*, 72(12), 2501–2506.

Häggström, M., & Bäckström, B. (2014). Organizing safe transitions from intensive care. *Nursing Research and Practice*, *2014*. doi:10.1155/2014/175314

Hahn, B. H., McMahon, M. A., Wilkinson, A., Wallace, W. D., Daikh, D., Fitzgerald, J. D., . . . American College of Rheumatology. (2012). American College of Rheumatology guidelines for screening, treatment, and management of lupus nephritis. *Arthritis Care & Research*, *64*(6), 797–808.

Hain, D. J., & Haras, M. S. (2015). Chronic kidney disease. In C. S. Counts (Ed.), *Core curriculum for nephrology nursing: Module 2. Physiologic and psychosocial basis for nephrology nursing practice* (6th ed., pp. 153–188). Pitman, NJ: American Nephrology Nurses' Association.

Haire, W. D. (2007). Catheter-induced upper extremity venous thrombosis. In *UpToDate*. Retrieved from http://www .uptodate.com

*Hall, B. (1990). The struggle of the diagnosed terminally ill person to maintain hope. *Nursing Science Quarterly*, *3*(4), 177–184.

*Hall, G. R. (1991). Altered thought processes: Dementia. In M. Maas, K. Buckwalter, & M. Hardy (Eds.), *Nursing diagnoses and interventions for the elderly*. Menlo Park, CA: Addison-Wesley.

*Hall, G. R. (1994). Caring for people with Alzheimer's disease using the conceptual model of progressively lowered stress threshold in the clinical setting. *Nursing Clinics of North America*, *29*(1), 129–141.

*Hall, G. R., & Buckwalter, K. C. (1987). Progressively lowered stress threshold: A conceptual model for care of adults with Alzheimer's disease. *Archives of Psychiatric Nursing*, *1*(6), 399–406.

Halloran, R. (2009). Caring for the patient with inflammatory response, shock, and severe sepsis. In K. Osborn (Ed.), *Medical surgical nursing: Preparation for practice* (Vol. 1, Chapter 61). Upper Saddle River, NJ: Prentice Hall.

Halm, M. A., & Krisko-Hagel, K. (2008). Instilling normal saline with suctioning: Beneficial technique or potentially harmful sacred cow? *American Journal of Critical Care*, *17*(5), 469–472.

Halpert, A., & Godena, E. (2011). Irritable bowel syndrome patients' perspectives on their relationships with healthcare providers. *Scandandian Journal of Gastroenterology*, *46*(7–8), 823–830.

Halstead, J. A., & Stoten, S. S. (2010). *Orthopedic nursing: Caring for patients with musculoskeletal disorders*. Brockton, MA: Western Schools.

Halter, M. J. (2014). *Varcolaris foundations of psychiatric mental health nursing* (7th ed.). Philadelphia, PA: W. B. Saunders.

Halter, M. J., & Carson, V. B. (2010). Sexual assault. In E. Varcarolis (Ed.), *Foundations of psychiatric mental health nursing* (6th ed.). Philadelphia, PA: Saunders.

Halyard, M., & Ferrans, C. (2008). Quality of life assessment for routine clinical practice. *Journal of Supportive Oncology*, *6*(5), 221–229, 233.

Hamdy, O. (2016). Hypoglycemia. In *Medscape*. Retrieved from http://emedicine.medscape.com/article/122122-overview

*Hamilton, H. (2006). Complications associated with venous access devices: Part one. *Nursing Standard*, *20*(26), 43–50. Retrieved from http://web.b.ebscohost.com/abstract?direct=true&profile=ehost&scope=site&authtype=crawler&j rnl=00296570&AN=20092656&h=MRPUxJ2HV5xQq%2fVXstxmvGr2vyyr2tebRYgMIi%2f4rGgeMcn50NhT1 RYiXkbsOG0mN6RZBOczPMexkhnjdylDAg%3d%3d&crl=f&resultNs=AdminWebAuth&resultLocal=ErrCrlN otAuth&crlhashurl=login.aspx%3fdirect%3dtrue%26profile%3dehost%26scope%3dsite%26authtype%3dcrawler %26jrnl%3d00296570%26AN%3d20092656

Hamilton, R. G. (2015). Latex allergy: Epidemiology, clinical manifestations, and diagnosis. In *UpToDate*. Retrieved from http://www.uptodate.com/contents/latex-allergy-epidemiology-clinical-manifestations-and-diagnosis

*Hampton, S. (2005). Importance of the appropriate selection and use of continence pads. *British Journal of Nursing*, *14*(5), 265–269.

*Hamric, A. B. (2000). Moral distress in everyday ethics. *Nursing Outlook*, *49*(2), 199–201.

Han, M. L. K., Dransfield, M. T., & Martinez, F. J. (2015). Chronic obstructive pulmonary disease: Definition, clinical manifestations, diagnosis, and staging. In *UpToDate*. Retrieved from http://www.uptodate.com/contents /chronic-obstructive-pulmonary-disease-definition-clinical-manifestations-diagnosis-and-staging?source=see_link

Hanly, J. G., Su, L., Farewell, V., McCurdy, G., Fougere, L., & Thompson, K. (2009). Prospective study of neuropsychiatric events in systemic lupus erythematosus. *Journal of Rheumatology*, *36*(7), 1449.

*Hanna, D. (2004). Moral distress: The state of the science. *Research and Theory for Nursing Practice: An International Journal*, *18*(1), 73–79.

*Hansen, L. B., & Vondracek, S. F. (2004). Prevention and treatment of nonpostmenapausal osteoporosis. *American Journal of Health-System Pharmacy*, *61*(24), 2637–2654.

Happ, M. B., Swigert, V. A., Tate, J. A., Arnold, R. M., Serelka, S. M., & Hoffman, L. A. (2007). Family presence and surveillance during weaning from prolonged mechanical ventilation. *Heart & Lung*, *36*(1), 47–57.

*Harari, D., Coshall, C., Rudd, A., & Wolfe, C. (2003). New-onset fecal incontinence after stroke. *Prevalence, Natural History, Risk Factors, and Impact Stroke*, *34*, 144–150.

Harding, S. M. (2015). Gastroesophageal reflux and asthma. In *UpToDate*. Retrieved from http://www.uptodate.com /contents/gastroesophageal-reflux-and-asthma

Hardt, J., Jacobsen, C., Goldberg, J., Nickel, R., & Buchwald, D. (2008). Prevalence of chronic pain in a representative sample in the United States. *Pain Medicine Pain Medicine*, *9*(7), 803–812.

*Harker, J. (2006). Wound healing complications associated with lower limb amputation. *World wide wounds*. Retrieved from http://www.worldwidewounds.com/2006/september/Harker/Wound-Healing-Complications-Limb-Amputation.html

Harman, E., & Dutka, P. (2007). Hemolysis: A hidden danger. *Nephrology Nursing Journal, 34*(2), 219–224.

*Harmanli, O. H., Khilnani, R., Dandolu, V., & Chatwani, A. J. (2004). Narrow pubic arch and increased risk of failure for vaginal hysterectomy. *Obstetrics & Gynecology, 104*(4), 697–700.

*Harrington, K. D. (1985). Metastatic disease of the spine. *Clinical Orthopaedics, 192*, 222–228.

Harris, L., & Dryjski, M. (2015). Epidemiology, risk factors, and natural history of peripheral artery disease. In *UpToDate*. Retrieved from http://www.uptodate.com/contents/epidemiology-risk-factors-and-natural-history-of-peripheral-artery-disease

Harsha, G. A., & Bray, G. A. (2008). Controversies in hypertension weight loss and blood pressure control (Pro). *Hypertension, 51*(6), 1420–1425.

Hartley, J. (2007). *Compartment syndrome*. Retrieved from http://www.ceufast.com

Harvey, S., & Whelan, C. A. (2008). Pneumonia. In T. M. Buttaro, J. Trybulski, P. P. Bailey, & J. Sandberg-Cook (Eds.), *Primary care: A collaborative practice* (3rd ed., pp. 466–475). St. Louis, MO: Mosby.

*Harwood, R. H., Sahota, O., Gaynor, K., Masud, T., & Hosking, D. J. (2004). A randomised, controlled comparison of different calcium and vitamin D supplementation regimens in elderly women after hip fracture: The Nottingham Neck of Femur (NONOF) Study. *Age Ageing, 33*(1), 45–51.

*Hashemi, E., Kaviani, A., Najafi, M., Ebrahimi, M., Hooshmand, H., & Montazeri, A. (2004). Seroma formation after surgery for breast cancer. *World Journal of Surgical Oncology, 2*(1), 1.

Haas, J., Frese, K. S., Park, Y. J., Keller, A., Vogel, B., Lindroth, A. M., ... & Marquart, S. (2013). Alterations in cardiac DNA methylation in human dilated cardiomyopathy. *EMBO Molecular Medicine, 5*(3), 413–429. doi:10.1002/emmm.201201553

*Haugen, V., Bliss D. Z., & Savik, K. (2006). Perioperative factor that affect long-term adjustment to an incontinent ostomy. *Journal of Wound, Ostomy, and Continence Nursing, 33*(5), 525–535.

*Haughney, A. (2004). Nausea and vomiting in end-stage cancer: These symptoms can be treated most effectively if the underlying cause is known. *The American Journal of Nursing, 104*(11), 40–48.

Havemann, B. D., Henderson, C. A., & El-Serag, H. B. (2007). The association between gastro-oesophageal reflux disease and asthma: A systematic review. *Gut, 56*(12), 1654.

Headley, C. M., & Wall, B. M. (2007). Flash pulmonary edema in patients with chronic kidney disease and end stage renal disease. *Nephrology Nursing Journal, 34*(1), 15–26, 37; quiz 27–28.

Hegarty, M. (2007). Care of the spirit that transcends religious, ideological and philosophical boundaries. *Indian Journal of Palliative Care, 13*(2), 42–47.

*Heard, L., & Buhrer, R. (2005). How do we prevent UTI in people who perform intermittent catheterization? *Rehabilitation Nursing, 30*(2), 44–45.

Heaven, A., Cheater, F., Clegg, A., Collinson, M., Farrin, A., Forster, A., . . . Hulme, C. (2014). Pilot trial of Stop Delirium!(PiTStop)—A complex intervention to prevent delirium in care homes for older people: study protocol for a cluster randomised controlled trial. *Trials, 15*(1), 1.

*Heidelbaugh, J. J., & Sherbondy, M. (2006). Cirrhosis and chronic liver failure: Part II. Complications and treatment. *American Family Physician, 74*(5), 767–776. Retrieved from http://www.aafp.org/afp/2006/0901/p767.html

Heidenreich, P. A., Trogdon, J. G., Khavjou, O. A., Butler, J., Dracup, K., Ezekowitz, M. D., . . . Council on Cardiovascular Surgery and Anesthesia, and Interdisciplinary Council on Quality of Care and Outcomes Research. (2011). Forecasting the future of cardiovascular disease in the United States: A policy statement from the American Heart Association. *Circulation, 123*(8), 933–944.

Heimbürger, O., & Blake, P. G. (2015). Apparatus for peritoneal dialysis. In J. T. Daugirdas, P. G. Blake, & S. I. Todd (Eds.), *Handbook of dialysis* (5th ed., pp. 408–424). Philadelphia, PA: Wolters Kluwer.

*Heinrich, L. (1987). Care of the female rape victim. *Nurse Practitioner, 12*(11), 9–27.

Heist, K., &. Ruskin, J. N. (2010). Drug induced arrythmis. *Circulation, 122*, 1426–1435.

Heisters, D. (2011). Parkinson's: Symptoms, treatments and research. *British Journal of Nursing, 20*(9), 548–544.

Heitman, J. (2012). Acute ischemic stroke management. In *RN.com*. Retrieved from http://www.rn.com/getpdf.php/1739.pdf?Main_Session=3025b55ccecb8a9bf3bfa10ece7f06ce

*Held-Warmkessel, J. (2005). Prostate cancer. In C. Yarbo, M. Frogge, & M. Goodman (Eds.), *Cancer nursing: Principles and practice* (5th ed.). Boston, MA: Jones & Bartlett.

*Heller, L., Levin, S. L., & Butler, C. E. (2006). Management of abdominal wound dehiscence using vacuum assisted closure in patients with compromised healing. *The American Journal of Surgery, 191*(2), 165.

Hemphill, R. (2012). Hyperosmolar hyperglycemic state. In *Medscape*. Retrieved from http://www.emedicine.medscape.com/article/1914705-overview

Hensley, M., & McCarthy, M. P. (2015). Foundations of nutrition and clinical applications in nephrology nursing: Chronic kidney disease. In C. S. Counts (Ed.), *Core curriculum for nephrology nursing: Module 2. Physiologic and psychosocial basis for nephrology nursing practice* (6th ed., pp. 261–267). Pitman, NJ: American Nephrology Nurses' Association.

*Hernán, M. A., Jick, S. S., Logroscino, G., Olek, M. J., Ascherio, A., & Jick, H. (2005). Cigarette smoking and the progression of multiple sclerosis. *Brain, 128*(Pt. 6), 1461–1465.

*Hernigou, P., Bachir, D., & Galacteros, F. (2003). The national history of symptomatic osteonecrosis in adults with sickle cell disease. *Journal of Bone and Joint Surgery, 85*(3), 500–504.

Hesketh, P. J. (2015). Prevention and treatment of chemotherapy-induced nausea and vomiting. In *UpToDate*. Retrieved from http://www.uptodate.com/contents/prevention-and-treatment-of-chemotherapy-induced-nausea-and-vomiting

Hess, C. (2011). Checklist for factors affecting wound healing. *Advances in Skin & Wound Care, 24*(4), 192.

*Hess, J. A., Woollacott, M., & Shivitz, N. (2006). Ankle force and rate of force production increase following high intensity strength training in frail older adults. *Aging Clinical Experimental Research, 18*(2), 107–115.

Hibbard, J. H., & Cunningham, P. J. (2008). *How engaged are consumers in their health and health care, and why does it matter? Findings from HSC No. 8:Providing insights that contribute to better health policy*. Washington, DC: HSC.

Hibbard, J. H., & Greene, J. (2013). What the evidence shows about patient activation: Better health outcomes and care experiences; Fewer data on costs. *Health Affairs, 32*(2), 207–214.

Hibbard, J., & Gilburt, H. (2014). Supporting people to manage their health: An introduction to patient activation. In *The Kings Funds*. Retrieved from https://www.kingsfund.org.uk/sites/files/kf/field/field_publication_file/supporting-people-manage-health-patient-activation-may14.pdf

Hickey, J. V. (2014). *The clinical practice of neurosurgical nursing* (7th ed.). Philadelphia, PA: Lippincott Williams & Wilkins.

Hickey, J. V., & Livesay, S. (2016). *The continuum of stroke care: An interprofessional approach to evidence-based*. Philadelphia, PA: Lippincott Williams & Wilkins.

*Hickman, A., Bell, D., & Preston, J. (2005). Acupressure and postoperative nausea and vomiting. *AANA Journal, 73*(5), 379–385.

Hill, L. (2015). Individualizing the care of those with kidney disease: Psychosocial impact and spirituality. In C. S. Counts (Ed.), *Core curriculum for nephrology nursing: Module 2. Physiologic and psychosocial basis for nephrology nursing practice* (6th ed., pp. 192–200). Pitman, NJ: American Nephrology Nurses' Association.

Hillis, L. D., Smith, P. K., Anderson, J. L., Bittl, J. A., Bridges, C. R., Byrne, J. G., . . . American Heart Association Task Force on Practice Guidelines. (2011). 2011 ACCF/AHA guideline for coronary artery bypass graft surgery. A report of the American College of Cardiology Foundation/American Heart Association Task Force on Practice Guidelines. *Circulation, 124*, e652–e735. Retrieved from http://www.circ.ahajournals.org/content/124/23/e652

Himiak, L. (2007). The amputee community continues to face undue hardships and discrimination. Retrieved from http://www.nursing.advanceweb.com/Editorial/Content/Editorial.aspx?CC=100852&CP=2

*Hirsch, A. T., Haskal, Z. J., Hertzer, N. R., Bakal, C. W., Creager, M. A., Halperin, J. L., . . . Vascular Disease Foundation. (2006). ACC/AHA guidelines for the management of patients with peripheral arterial disease (lower extremity, renal mesenteric, and abdominal aortic). *Journal of Vascular Interventional Radiology, 113*(11), e463–e654.

Hlebovy, D. (2008). Hemodialyis: Fluid removal: Obtaining estimated dry weight during hemodialysis. In C. S. Counts (Ed.), *Core curriculum for nephrology nursing* (5th ed.). Pitman NJ: American Nephrology Nurses' Association.

Hockenberry, M. J., & Wilson, D. (2015). *Wong's essentials of pediatric nursing* (10th ed.). St. Louis, MO: Elsevier.

Hoffman, R. S., & Weinhouse, G. L. (2015). Management of moderate and severe alcohol withdrawal syndromes. In *UpToDate*. Retrieved from http://www.uptodate.com/contents/management-of-moderate-and-severe-alcohol-withdrawal-syndromes?source=search_result&search=alcohol+withdrawal&selectedTitle=1~68#H23

Holditch-Davis, D., & Blackburn, S. (2007). Neurobehavioral development. In C. Kenner & J W. Lott (Eds.), *Comprehension neonatal care: A interdisciplinary approach* (pp. 448–479). St Louis, MO: Saunders.

*Holland, J. C., & Reznik, I. (2005). Pathways for psychosocial care of cancer survivors. *Cancer, 104*(Suppl. 11), 2524–2637. doi:10.1002/cncr.21252

*Holman, J. S., & Shwed, J. A. (1992). Influence of sucralfate on the detection of occult blood in simulated gastric fluid by two screening tests. *Clinical Pharmacology, 11*(7), 625–627.

*Holt, P. R. (2001). Diarrhea and malabsorption in the elderly. *Gastroenterology Clinics of North America, 30*(2), 427–444.

Holzer, L. A., Sevelda, F., Fraberger, G., Bluder, O., Kickinger, W., & Holzer, G. (2014). Body image and self-esteem in lower-limb amputees. *PloS One, 9*(3), e92943.

*Hooyman, N. R., & Kramer, B. J. (2006). *Living through loss: Interventions across the life span*. New York, NY: Columbia University Press.

Hopkins R. O., & Spuhler V. J. (2009). Strategies for promoting early activity in critically ill mechanically ventilated patients. *AACN Advanced Critical Care, 20*(3), 277–289.

Horowitz, D., Katzap, E., Horowitz, S., & Barilla-LaBarca, M. (2011). Approach to septic arthritis. *American Family Physician, 84*(6), 653–660.

Horwitz, M. (2012). Hypercalcemia of malignancy. In *UpToDate*. Retrieved from http://uptodate.com/contents/hypercalcemia-of-malignancy

*Hoskins, C. N., & Budin, W. C. (2000). Measurement of psychosocial adjustment to breast cancer: A unidimensional or multidimensional construct? *Psychological Reports, 87*(2), 649–663.

*Hoskins, C. N., & Haber, J. (2000). Adjusting to breast cancer. *The American Journal of Nursing, 100*(4), 26–33.

Hoskin, T. L., Hieken, T. J., Degnim, A. C., Jakub, J. W., Jacobson, S. R., & Boughey, J. C. (2016). Use of immediate breast reconstruction and choice for contralateral prophylactic mastectomy. *Surgery, 159*(4), 1199–1209.

Hospice and Palliative Nurses Association. (2013). *Final days (patient/family teaching sheet)*. Retrieved from http://www.stjosephhomehealth.org/documents/Final-Days-(English).pdf

Hospice and Palliative Nurse's Association. (2016). *Final days*. Retrieved from http://hpna.advancingexpertcare.org/education/patient-family-teaching-sheets/

Houle, L. (2010). *Language barriers in health care* (Unpublished paper). Retrieved from http://www.digitalcommons.uri.edu/srhonorsprog/175/

*Howard, J. F. (2006). *Clinical overview of MG. Myasthenia gravis: A summary*. Retrieved from http://www.myasthenia.org/HealthProfessionals/ClinicalOverviewofMG.aspx

Howe, A. S. (2016). General principles of fracture management: Early and late complications. In *UpToDate*. Retrieved from http://www.uptodate.com/contents/general-principles-of-fracture-management-early-and-late-complications

Hsiu-Feng, H., Monica, J. E., Cain, K. C., Burr, R. L., Deechakawan, W., & Heitkemper, M. M. (2011). Does a self-management program change dietary intake in adults with irritable bowel syndrome? *Gastroenterology Nursing, 34*(2), 108–116.

Huang, H. W., Zheng, B. L., Jiang, L., Lin, Z. T., Zhang, G. B., Shen, L., & Xi, X. M. (2015). Effect of oral melatonin and wearing earplugs and eye masks on nocturnal sleep in healthy subjects in a simulated intensive care unit environment: Which might be a more promising strategy for ICU sleep deprivation? *Critical Care, 19*(1), 124.

Hudman, L., & Bodenham, A. (2013). Practical aspects of long-term venous access. *Continuing Education in Anaesthesia, Critical Care & Pain, 13*(1), 6–11. Retrieved from http://www.medscape.com/viewarticle/782389_4

*Huffman, G. B. (2002). Evaluating and treating unintentional weight loss in the elderly [Electronic Version]. *American Family Physician, 65*(4). Retrieved from http://www.aafp.org/afp/2002/0215/p640.html

Huffman, J. L. (2015). Chronic pancreatitis. In *Medscape*. Retrieved from http://emedicine.medscape.com/article/181554-overview

*Hull, R. D., Pineo, G. F., Stein, P. D., Mah, A. F., MacIsaac, S. M., Dahl, O. E., . . . Raskob, G. E. (2001). Timing of initial administration of low-molecular-weight heparin prophylaxis against deep vein thrombosis in patients following elective hip arthroplasty: A systematic review. *Archives of Internal Medicine, 161*(16), 1952–1960.

*Hunter, J. H., & Cason, K. L. (2006). *Nutrient density Clemson University Cooperative Extension Service*. Retrieved at http://www.clemson.edu/extension/hgic/food/nutrition/nutrition/dietary_guide/hgic4062.html

Hunter, K. F., Moore, K. N., & Glazner, C. M. A. (2007). Conservative management for postprostatectomy urinary incontinence [Systematic review]. *Cochrane Database of Systematic Reviews, 3*(2), CD001843.

*Hunter, M., & King, D. (2001). COPD: Management of acute exacerbations and chronic stable disease. *American Family Physician, 64*(4), 603–612.

Hurkmans, E., van der Giesen, F. J., Vliet Vlieland, T. P. M., Schoones, J., & Van den Ende, E. C. H. M. (2009). Dynamic exercise programs (aerobic capacity and/or muscle strength training) in patients with rheumatoid arthritis. *Cochrane Database of Systematic Reviews*. Retrieved from http://www.summaries.cochrane.org/CD006853/dynamic-exercise-programs-aerobic-capacity-andor-muscle-strength-training-in-patients-with-rheumatoid-arthritis

Huskamp, H., Keating, N., Malin, J., Zaslavsky, A., Weeks, J. C., Earle, C. C., . . . Ayanian, J. Z. (2009). Discussions with physicians about hospice among patients with metastatic lung cancer. *Archives of Internal Medicine, 169*(10), 954–962.

Hussain, S. F., Irfan, M., Waheed, Z., Mansoor, N. A. S., & Islam, M. (2014). Compliance with continuous positive airway pressure (CPAP) therapy for obstructive sleep apnea among privately paying patients—A cross sectional study. *BMC Pulmonary Medicine, 14*, 188. doi:10.1186/1471-2466-14-188

*Hyland, J. (2002). The basics of ostomies. *Gastroenterology Nursing, 25*(6), 241–244.

Hyzy, R. C. (2015). Physiologic and pathophysiologic consequences of mechanical ventilation. In *UpToDate*. Retrievded from http://www.uptodate.com/contents/physiologic-and-pathophysiologic-consequences-of-mechanical-ventilation

*Iezzoni, L. I., O'Day, B., Keleen, M. A., & Harker, H. (2004). Improving patient care: Communicating about health care: Observations from persons who are deaf or hard of hearing. *Annals of Internal Medicine, 140*(5), 356–362.

Institute for Clinical Systems Improvement. (2008). *Healthcare guidelines: Venous thromboembolism prophylaxis* (5th ed.). Bloomington, MN: Author. Retrieved from www.icsi.org

Institute for Healthcare Improvement. (2008). *Implement the ventilator bundle: Elevation of the head of the bed*. Retrieved from http://www.ihi.org/IHI/Topics/CriticalCare/IntensiveCare/Changes/IndividualChanges/Elevationofthehead-ofthebed.htm

*Institute for Safe Medication Practices: Intimidation. (2004, March 11). Practitioners speak up about this unresolved problem (Part 1). *ISMP Medical Safety Alert!*. Retrieved from http://www.ismp.org/Newsletters/acutecare/articles/20040311_2.asp

*Institute of Medicine. (2006, October 9). *Medication errors injure 1.5 million people and cost billions of dollars annually*. Retrieved from http://www8.nationalacademies.org/onpinews/newsitem.aspx?RecordID=11623

Institute of Medicine. (2007). *Cancer care for the whole patient: Meeting psychosocial health needs*. Washington, DC: National Academies Press.

Institute of Medicine. (2009). Sleep disorders and sleep deprivation: An unmet public health problem. *Gerontology, 55*(2), 162–168.

International Association of the Study of Pain. (2011). Part III: Pain terms, a current list with definitions and notes on Usage. In *Classification of chronic pain* (2nd ed.). Washington, DC: Author.

International League Against Epilepsy. (2007). *Classifications of seizures*. Retrieved from http://www.ilae-epilepsy.org

International Osteoporosis Foundation. (2015). *Facts and statistics.* Retrieved from http://www.iofbonehealth.org/facts-statistics#category

Inzucchi, S. (2012). *Diabetes facts and guidelines.* New Haven, CT: Yale Diabetes Center.

Inzucchi, S., Bergenstal, R., Buse, J., Diamant, M., Ferrannini, E., Nauck, M., . . . Mathews, D. (2012). Management of hyperglycemia in type 2 diabetes: a patient-centered approach: *Position statement of the American Diabetes Association (ADA) and the European Association for the Study of Diabetes (EASD).* Retrieved from http://care.diabetesjournals.org/content/36/2/490

Ioannidis, O., Lavrentieva, A., & Botsios, D. (2008). Nutrition support in acute pancreatitis. *Journal of Periodontology, 9*(4), 375–390.

Irwin, M. L., McTiernan, A., Manson, J. E., Thomson, C. A., Sternfeld, B., Stefanick, M. L., . . . Chlebowski, R. (2011). Physical activity and survival in postmenopausal women with breast cancer: results from the women's health initiative. *Cancer Prevention Research, 4*(4), 522–529.

Ishida, K. (2015). Medical complications of stroke. In *UpToDate.* Retrieved from http://www.uptodate.com/contents/medical-complications-of-stroke?source=see_link

Iuga, A. O., & McGuire, M. J. (2014). Adherence and health care costs. *Risk Management and Healthcare Policy, 7,* 35–44. doi:10.2147/RMHP.S19801

*Jablonski, R. (2001). Discovering asthma in the older adult. *Nurse Practitioner, 25*(1), 14, 24–25, 29–32.

Jacobson, R. (2014). Epidemic of violence against health care workers plagues hospitals. In *Scientific American.* Retrieved from http://www.scientificamerican.com/article/epidemic-of-violence-against-health-care-workers-plagues-hospitals/

Jain, S., Mittal, M., Kansal, A., Singh, Y., Kolar, P. R., & Saigal, R. (2008). Fat embolism syndrome. *JAPI, 56,* 245–249. Retrieved from http://www.japi.org/april2008/R-245.pdf

James, M. L. (2007). Prostate cancer (early). BMJ Clinical Evidence, 2007.

James, P. A., Oparil, S., Carter, B. L., Cushman, W. C., Dennison-Himmelfarb, C., Handler, J., . . . Ortiz, E. (2014). 2014 evidence-based guideline for the management of high blood pressure in adults report from the panel members appointed to the Eighth Joint National Committee (JNC 8). *JAMA, 311*(5), 507–520.

James, W. D., Berger T. G., & Elston D. M. (Eds.). (2011). *Andrews' diseases of the skin: Clinical dermatology* (11th ed.). Philadephia, PA: Elsevier.

*Jamison, K., Wellisch, D. K., Katz, R. L., & Pasnau, R. O. (1979). Phantom breast syndrome. *Archives of Surgery, 114*(1), 93.

Jauch, E. C., Cucchiara, B., Adeoye, O., Meurer, W., Brice, J., Chan, Y., . . . Hazinski, M. (2010). American Heart Association guidelines for cardiopulmonary resuscitation and emergency cardiovascular care. *Circulation, 122*(Suppl. 3), S818–S828.

Jauch, E. C., Saver, J. L., Adams, H. P., Jr., Bruno, A., Connors, J. J., Demaerschalk, B. M., . . . Yonas, H. (2013). AHA/ASA Guideline: Guidelines for the early management of patients with acute ischemic stroke: A guideline for healthcare professionals from the American Heart Association. *Stroke, 44*(3), 870–947.

*Jenkins, T. (2002). Sickle cell anemia in pediatric intensive care unit. *AACN Clinical Issues, 13*(2), 154–168.

Jennings-Ingle, S. (2007). The sobering facts of alcohol withdrawal. *Nursing Made Incredibly Easy, 5*(1), 50–60.

Jepson, R. G., & Craig, J. C. (2008). Cranberries for preventing urinary tract infections. *Cochrane Database of Systematic Reviews, 2,* CD00132. doi:10.1002/14651858.CD001321.pub4

Johns Hopkins Breast Cancer Center. (2007). *Johns Hopkins decision of plastic and reconstructive surgery: Breast reconstruction.* Retrieved from http://www.hopkinsmedicine.org/breast_center/treatments_services/reconstructive_breast_surgery/

*Johnson, J. E., Rice, V., Fuller, S., & Endress, P. (1978). Sensory information instruction in coping strategy and recovery from surgery. *Research in Nursing and Health, 1*(1), 4–17.

Johnson, K., Peereboom, K., Hejal, R., & Rowbottom, J. (2009). *Feasibility of a protocol to implement early progressive mobility among ICU patients with prolonged critical illness* [Abstract]. Retrieved from http://www.meeting.chestpubs.org/cgi/content/abstract/136/4/58S-g?maxtoshow=&hits=10[Context Link]

*The Joint Commission. (2004). *Sentinel event statistics.* Retrieved from http://www.jacho.org/accredited+organizations/ambulatory+care/sentinel+events/sentinel+events+statistics

*The Joint Commission. (2006). *Using medication reconciliation to prevent errors.* Retrieved from https://www.jointcommission.org/assets/1/18/SEA_35.PDF

The Joint Commission. (2008a). *Improving America's hospitals. (The Joint Commission's Annual Report on Quality and Safety).* Retrieved from http://www.jointcommission.org/assets/1/6/2008_Annual_Report.pdf

The Joint Commission. (2008b). *Patient safety goals.* Retrieved from http://assistedlivingconsult.com/issues/03-06/alc1112-JCAHO-1130.pdf

The Joint Commission. (2010). *Achieving effective communication, cultural competence, and patient-centered care: A roadmap for hospitals.* Oakland Terrace, IL: Author.

The Joint Commission. (2012a). *Hot topics in health care. Transitions of care: The need for a more effective approach to continuing patient care.* Retrieved from http://www.jointcommission.org/assets/1/18/hot_topics_transitions_of_care.pdf

The Joint Commission. (2012b). *Improving America's hospitals. The Joint Commission's Annual Report on Quality and Safety.* Retrieved from https://www.jointcommission.org/assets/1/18/TJC_Annual_Report_2015_EMBARGOED_11_9_15.pdf

The Joint Commission. (2015a). *A crosswalk of the national standards for culturally and linguistically appropriate services (CLAS) in health and health care to the joint commission hospital accreditation standards.* Retrieved from http://www.jointcommission.org/assets/1/6/crosswalk-_clas_-20140718.pdf

The Joint Commission. (2015b). *Hospital accreditation program national patient safety goals*. Retrieved from http://www .jointcommission.org/assets/1/6/2015_npsg_hap.pdf

The Joint Commission. (2015c). *National patient safety. Hospital Accreditation Program*. Retrieved from http://www .jointcommission.org/topics/hai_standards_and_npsgs.aspx

The Joint Commission. (2016). *Sentinel event policy and procedures*. Retrieved from http://www.jointcommission.org /sentinel_event_policy_and_procedures/

*Joyce, N. (2002). *Eye care for intensive care patients. A systematic review* (No. 21). Adelaide, Australia: The Joanna Briggs Institute for Evidence-Based Nursing and Midwifery. Retrieved from http://graphics.ovid.com/db/cinahl /pdfs/2002044923.pdf

*Junkin, J., & Beitz, J. M. (2005). Sexuality and the person with a stoma: Implications for comprehensive WOC nursing practice. *Journal of Wound, Ostomy, and Continence Nursing, 32*(2), 121–128.

Kaakinen, J. R., Coelho, D. P., Steele, R., Tabacco, A., & Hanson, S. M. (2015). *Family health care nursing: Theory, practice & research* (5th ed.). Philadelphia: F.A. Davis.

Kaakinen, J. R., Gedaly-Duff, V., & Hanson, S. M. (2010). *Family health care nursing : Theory, practice, and research* (4th ed.). Philadelphia, PA: F.A. Davis.

Kahn, S. R. (2013). Elastic compression stockings failed to prevent post-thrombotic syndrome. *HemOnc Today, 14*(3), 31.

Kahn, S. R., Lim, W., Dunn, A. S., Cushman, M., Dentali, F., Akl, E. A., . . . American College of Chest Physicians. (2012). Prevention of VTE in nonsurgical patients. American college of chest physicians evidence-based clinical practice guidelines. *CHEST, 141*(2), e195S–e226S.

Kain, C. (2016). *Multiple loss and aids-related bereavement*. Retrieved from http://www.apa.org/pi/aids/resources /education/bereavement.aspx

Kalapatapu, V. (2016). Lower extremity amputation. In *UpToDate*. Retrieved from https://www.uptodate.com/contents /lower-extremity-amputation

Kalf, J. G., de Swart, B. J., Bloem, B. R., & Munneke, M. (2012). Prevalence of oropharyngeal dysphagia in Parkinson's disease: A meta-analysis. *Parkinsonism Related Disorders, 18*(4), 311–315.

Kalfas, I. A., Lobo, B., & McCormack, B. M. (2012). *Cerebrospinal fluid fistula and pseudomeningocele after spine surgery in spine surgery* (3rd ed., Chapter 200, pp. 1905–1909). Retrieved from http://www.clinicalgate.com /cerebrospinal-fluid-fistula-and-pseudomeningocele-after-spine-surgery/

Kalff, J. C., Wehner, S., & Litkouhi, B. (2015). Postoperative ileus. In *UpToDate*. Retrieved from http://www.uptodate .com/contents/postoperative-ileus

*Kalichman, S. C., Cain, D., Fuhel, A., Eaton, L., Di Fonzo, K., & Ertl, T. (2005). Assessing medication adherence self-efficacy among low-literacy patients: Development of a pictographic visual analogue scale. *Health Education Research, 20*(1), 24–35.

Kalisch, B. J., Lee, S., & Dabney, B. W. (2014). Outcomes of inpatient mobilization: A literature review. *Journal of Clinical Nursing, 23*(11/12), 1486–1501.

Kane, R. L., Shamliyan, T., Mueller, C., Duval, S., & Wilt, T. (2007). *Nurse staffing and quality of patient care*. (Evidence report/technology assessment #151.) (Prepared by the Minnesota Evidence-based Practice Center under Contract No. 290-02-0009.) (AHRQ Publication No. 07-E005). Rockville, MD: Agency for Healthcare Research and Quality. Retrieved from https://archive.ahrq.gov/downloads/pub/evidence/pdf/nursestaff/nursestaff.pdf

*Kannel, W. B., & Belanger, A. J. (1991). Epidemiology of heart failure. *American Heart Journal, 121*(3), 951–957.

*Kantaff, P., Carroll, P., D'Amico, A., Isaacs, J., Ross, R., & Schertt, C. (2001). *Prostate cancer: Principles and practice*. Philadelphia, PA: Lippincott Williams & Wilkins.

*Kaplan, J. E., Masur, H., & Holmes, K. K. (2002). USPHS infectious disease society of America: Guidelines for preventing opportunistic infections in HIV infected groups. *MMWR, 51*(RR8), 1–52.

Kaplan, N. M. (2016). Cardiovascular risks of hypertension. In *UpToDate*. Retrieved from http://www.uptodate.com /contents/cardiovascular-risks-of-hypertension

*Kappas-Larson, P., & Lathrop, L. (1993). Early detection and intervention for hazardous ethanol use. *Nurse Practitioner, 18*(7), 50–55.

Karagozoglu, S., Tekyasar, F., & Yilmaz, F. A. (2013). Effects of music therapy and guided visual imagery on chemotherapy-induced anxiety and nausea-vomiting. *Journal of Clinical Nursing, 22*(1–2), 39–50.

Karalis, M. (2008), Nutrition intervention. In C. S. Counts (Ed.), *Core curriculum for nephrology nursing* (5th ed.). Pitman, NJ: American Nephrology Nurses' Association.

*Katz, A. (2005). Sexually speaking: Sexuality and hysterectomy: Finding the right words: Responding to patients' concerns about the potential effects of surgery. *The American Journal of Nursing, 105*(12), 65–68.

*Katz, A. (2006). What have my kidneys got to do with my sex life? The impact of late stage chronic kidney disease on sexual function. *The American Journal of Nursing, 106*(9), 81–83.

*Katz, P. (2003). Peptic ulcer disease. In L. R. Baker, J. Burton, & P. Zieve. *Principles of ambulatory medicine* (6th ed.). Philadelphia, PA: Lippincott Williams & Wilkins.

Kaufmann, H., & Kaplan, N. M. (2015). *Mechanisms, causes, and evaluation of orthostatic hypotension*. In *UpToDate*. Retrieved from http://www.uptodate.com/contents/mechanisms-causes-and-evaluation-of-orthostatic-hypotension

*Kawada, E., Moridaira, K., Itoh, K., Hoshino, A., Tamura, J., & Morita, T. (2006). Long-term bedridden elderly patients [Electronic version]. *Annals of Nutrition & Metabolism, 50*(5), 420–424. Retrieved from http://www.ebsco.waldenu .edu/ehost/pdf?vid=11&hid=102&sid=b2fae363-688a-4e54-96d6-e87f0fde711c%40ses sionmgr103

*Kee, J. L. (2004). *Handbook of laboratory & diagnostic tests with nursing implications* (5th ed.). Upper Saddle River, NJ: Pearson Education, Prentice Hall.

*Keenan, G. (1997). Management of complications of glucocorticoid therapy. *Clinics in Chest Medicine, 18*(3), 507–520.

Kelley, L., & Bednarski, D. (2015). Individualizing the care of those with kidney disease: The financial impact. In C. S. Counts (Ed.), *Core curriculum for nephrology nursing: Module 2. Physiologic and psychosocial basis for nephrology nursing practice* (6th ed., pp. 225–233). Pitman, NJ: American Nephrology Nurses' Association.

*Kelly, K. J., Kurup, V. P., Reijula, K. E., & Fink, J. N. (1994). The diagnosis of natural rubber latex allergy. *Journal of Allergy and Clinical Immunology, 93*(5), 813–816.

*Kemler, M. A., de Vries, M., & van der Tol, A. (2006). Duration of preoperative traction associated with sciatic neuropathy after hip fracture surgery. *Clinical Orthopedic Related Research, 445,* 230–232.

*Kemp, C. (2006). Spiritual care interventions. In B. Ferrell & N. Coyle (Eds.), *Textbook of palliative nursing* (2nd ed., pp. 440–455). New York, NY: Oxford University Press.

*Kendrick, D., Elkan, R., Hewitt, M., Dewey, M., Blair, M., Robinson, J., ... & Brummell, K. (2000). Does home visiting improve parenting and the quality of the home environment? A systematic review and meta analysis. *Archives of Disease in Childhood, 82*(6), 443–451.

*Kenney, W. M., & Chin, P. (2001). Influence of age on thirst and fluid intake. *Official Journal of the American College of Sports Medicine, 33*(9), 1524–1532.

Kersting, A., Brähler, E., Glaesmer, H., & Wagner, B. (2011). Prevalence of complicated grief in a representative population-based sample. *Journal of Affective Disorders, 131*(1), 339–343.

Kersting, A., & Wagner, B. (2012). Complicated grief after perinatal loss. *Dialogues in Clinical Neuroscience, 14*(2), 187–194.

Khalaila, R., Zbidat, W., Anwar, K., Bayya, A., Linton, D. M., & Sviri, S. (2011). Communication difficulties and psychoemotional distress in patients receiving mechanical ventilation. *American Journal of Critical Care, 20*(6), 470–479.

Khardori, R. (Ed.). (n.d.). Infection in patients with diabetes mellitus. In *Medscape.* Retrieved from http://emedicine .medscape.com/article/2122072-overview

Khayyat, Y., & Attar, S. (2015). Vitamin D deficiency in patients with irritable bowel syndrome: Does it exist? *Oman Medical Journal, 30*(2), 115–118.

Khraim, F. M. (2007). The wider scope of video-assisted thoracoscopic surgery. *AORN Journal, 85*(6), 1199–1208.

Kibel, S, Adams, K., & Barlow, G. (2011). Diagnostic and prognostic biomarkers of sepsis in critical care. *Journal of Antimicrobial Chemotherapy, 66*(Suppl. 2), ii33–ii40.

*Killey, B., & Watt, E. (2006). The effect of extra walking on the mobility, independence and exercise self-efficacy of elderly hospital in-patients: A pilot study. *Contemporary Nurse, 22*(1), 120–133.

King, L. (2012). Developing a progressive mobility activity protocol. *Orthopaedic Nursing, 31*(5), 253–262.

*Kirkeby-Garstad, I., Wisloff, U., Skogvoll, E., Stolen, T., Tjonna, A. E., Stenseth, R., . . . Sellevold, O. F. (2006). The marked reduction in mixed venous oxygen saturation during early mobilization after cardiac surgery: The effect of posture or exercise? *Anesthesia & Analgesia, 102*(6), 1609–1616.

Kitabchi, A., Hirsch, I. B., & Emmett, M. (2015). Diabetic ketoacidosis and hyperosmolar hyperglycemic state in adults: Clinical features, evaluation. In *UpToDate.* Retrieved from http://www.uptodate.com/contents/diabetic-ketoacidosis-and-hyperosmolar-hyperglycemic-state-in-adults-clinical-features-evaluation-and-diagnosis?source=see_link&sect ionName=DIAGNOSTIC+CRITERIA&anchor=H5509770#H5509770

Kwon, S., & Hirst, J. (2014). Overview of anxiety in palliative care. In *UpToDate.* Retrieved from http://www.uptodate .com/contents/overview-of-anxiety-in-palliative-care

Klein, E. A. (2016). Radical prostatectomy for localized prostate cancer. In *UpToDate.* Retrieved from http://www .uptodate.com/contents/radical-prostatectomy-for-localized-prostate-cancer

*Knodrup, J., Allison, S. P., Elia, M., Vellas, B., & Plauth, M. (2003). ESPEN guidelines for nutrition screening 2002. *Clinical Nutrition, 22*(4), 415–442.

*Koch, A. (2003). Angiogenesis as a target in rheumatoid arthritis. *Annals of Rheumatic Diseases, 62*(Suppl. 2), ii60–ii67.

Kohtz, C., & Thompson, M. (2007). Preventing contrast medium-induced nephrology. *The American Journal of Nursing, 107*(9), 40–49.

*Kok, N., Alwayn, I., Tran, K., Hop, W., Weimar, W., & Ijzermans, J. (2006). Psychosocial and physical impairment after mini-incision open and laparoscopic donor nephrectomy: A positive study [Electronic version]. *Transplantation, 82*(10), 1291–1297. Retrieved http://www.academia.edu/27793511/Psychosocial_and_Physical_Impairment_After_Mini-Incision_Open_and_Laparoscopic_Donor_Nephrectomy_A_Prospective_Study

Kotlinska-Lemieszek, A., Klepstad, P., & Haugen, D. F. (2015). Clinically significant drug-drug interactions involving opioid analgesics used for pain treatment in patients with cancer: A systematic review. *Drug Design, Development and Therapy, 9,* 5255–5267. doi:10.2147/DDDT.S86983

Koul, R., Dufan, T., Russell, C., Guenther, W., Nugent, Z., Sun, X., . . . Cookie, A. L. (2007). Efficacy of complete decongestive therapy and manual lymphatic drainage on treatment-related lymphedema in breast cancer. *International Journal of Radiation Oncology, Biology, Physics, 67*(3), 841–846.

Kovesdy, C. P., Kopple, J. D., & Kalantar-Zadeh, K. (2015). Inflammation in renal insufficiency. In *UpToDate*. Retrieved from http://www.uptodate.com/contents/inflammation-in-renal-insufficiency

Krause, J. S., Reed, K. S., & McArdle, J. J. (2010). A structural analysis of health outcomes after spinal cord injury. *The Journal of Spinal Cord Medicine, 33*(1), 22–32.

Krauss, M. J., Nguyen, S. L., Dunagan, W. C., Birge, S., Costantinou, E., Johnson, S., . . . Fraser, V. J. (2007). Circumstances of patient falls and injuries in 9 hospitals in a midwestern healthcare system. *Infection Control and Hospital Epidemiology, 28*(5), 544–555.

*Krebs, L. U. (2000). Sexual and reproductive dysfunction. In S. L. Groenwald, M. H. Frogge, M. Goodman, & C. Yarbro (Eds.), *Cancer nursing: Principles and practice* (5th ed.). Boston, MA: Jones & Bartlett.

*Kumar, N., Van Gerpen, J. A., Bower, J. H., & Ahlskog, J. E. (2005). Levodopa-dyskinesia incidence by age of Parkinson's disease onset. *Movement Disorders, 20*(3), 342.

Kuntzsch, T., & Voge, C. (2009). Hypersensitivity reactions to chemotherapy in acute care oncology. In C. Chernecky & K. Murphy-Ende (Eds.), *Nursing* (2nd ed.). St. Louis, MO: Saunders.

*Kutner, M., Greenberg, E., Jin, Y., & Paulsen, C. (2006). *The health literacy of America's adults: Results from 2003 National Assessment of Adult's Literacy*. Washington, DC: U.S. Department of Education, National Center for Education Statistics.

Kwon, S., Thompson, R., & Dellinger, P. I. (2013). Importance of perioperative glycemic control in general surgery a report from the surgical care and outcomes assessment program. *Annals of Surgery, 257*(1), 8–14.

Kwong, A., & Sabel, M. S. (2016). Mastectomy: Indications, types, and concurrent axillary lymph node management. In *UpToDate*. Retrieved from http://www.uptodate.com/contents/mastectomy-indications-types-and-concurrent- axillary-lymph-node-management

Kynoch, K., Wu, C. J., & Chang, A. M. (2011). Interventions for preventing and managing aggressive patients admitted to an acute hospital setting: A systematic review. *Worldviews on Evidence-Based Nursing, 8*(2), 76–86.

*Ladd, A., Jones, H. H., & Otanez, O. (2003). *Osteomyelitis*. Retrieved from http://www.osteomyelitis.stanford.edu

Lalani, T. (2015). Overview of osteomyelitis in adults. In *UpToDate*. Retrieved from http://www.uptodate.com/contents /overview-of-osteomyelitis-in-adults

Lambertson, K. (2015). Peritoneal dialysis: Peritoneal dialysis access. In C. S. Counts (Ed.). *Core curriculum for nephrology nursing: Module 3. Treatment options for patients with chronic kidney disease* (6th ed., pp. 227–278). Pitman, NJ: American Nephrology Nurses Association.

Lancaster, A. D., Ayers, A., Belbot, B., Goldner, V., Kress, L., Stanton, D., . . . Sparkman, L. (2007). Preventing falls and eliminating injury at Ascension Health. *Joint Commission Journal on Quality and Patient Safety, 33*(7), 367–375.

Lander, L., Howsare, J., & Byrne, M. (2013). The impact of substance use disorders on families and children: From theory to practice. *Social Work in Public Health, 28*(3–4), 194–205.

Landmann, R. G. (2015). Routine care of patients with an ileostomy or colostomy and management of ostomy complications. In *UpToDate*. Retrieved from http://www.uptodate.com/contents/routine-care-of-patients-with-an-ileostomy-or-colostomy-and-management-of-ostomy-complications

Langemo, D. K., & Black, J. (2010). Pressure ulcers in individuals receiving palliative care: A National Pressure Ulcer Advisory Panel White Paper. *Advances in Skin & Wound Care, 23*(2), 59–72.

Lankshear, A., Harden, J., & Simms, J. (2010). Safe practice for patients receiving anticoagulant therapy. *Nursing Standard, 24*(20), 47–55.

Lanza, F. L., Chan, F. M., & Quigley, E. M. (2009). Practice parameters committee of the American College of Gastroenterology. Prevention of NSAID-related ulcer complications. *American Journal of Gastroenterology, 104*(3), 728–738.

LaReau, R., Bensen, L., Watcharotone, K., & Manguba, G. (2008). Examining the feasibility of implementing specific nursing interventions to promote sleep in hospitalized elderly patients. *Geriatric Nursing, 29*(3), 197–206.

*Larsson, G. U., Johannesson, A., & Oberg, T. (2004). From major amputation to prosthetic outcome: A prospective study of 190 patients in a defined population. *Prosthetics and Orthotics International, 28*(1), 9–21.

LaSala, C. A., & Bjarnason, D. (2010). Creating workplace environments that support moral courage. *Online Journal of Issues in Nursing, 15*(3), 1–11. Retrieved from http://www.nursingworld.org/OJIN

Lawes, C. M., Vander Hoorn, S., & Rodgers, A. (2008). International society of hypertension. Global burden of blood-pressure-related disease, 2001. *Lancet, 371*(9623), 1513–1518.

Lawn, N., Kelly, A., Dunne, J., Lee, J., & Wesseldine, A. (2013). First seizure in the older patient: Clinical features and prognosis. *Epilepsy Research, 107*(1–2), 109–114.

*Lazarus, R. (1985). The costs and benefits of denial. In A. Monat & R. Lazarus (Eds.), *Stress and coping: An anthology* (2nd ed.). New York, NY: Columbia University Press.

Leadingham, C. (2014). *Maintaining the vision in the intensive care unit* (Doctoral dissertation). Retrieved from http://www.core-scholar.libraries.wright.edu/nursing_dnp/1

Liebeskind, D. A. (2016). *Hemorrhagic stroke*. Retrieved from http://emedicine.medscape.com/article/1916662-overview

*Ledford, D. K. (1998). Immunologic aspects of vasculitis and cardiovascular disease. *International Journal of Cardiology, 66*(1), 101–105.

*Ledray, L. E. (2001). *Evidence collection and care of the sexually assault survivor: SANE-SART response*. Retrieved from http://www.vaw.umn.edu/documents/commissioned/2forensicvidence.htlm

Lee, I. M., Haskell, W. L., Pate, R. R., Powell, K. E., Blair, S. N., Franklin, B. A., . . . Bauman, A. (2007). Physical activity and public health: Updated recommendation for adults from the American College of Sports Medicine and the American Heart Association. *Medicine and Science in Sports and Exercise, 39*(8), 1423–1434.

Lee, R. K. (2012a). Compartment syndrome: A comprehensive overview. *Critical Care Nurse, 32*(1), 19–31.

Lee, R. K. (2012b). Intra-abdominal hypertension and abdominal compartment syndrome a comprehensive overview cover. *Critical Care Nurse, 32*(1), 19–31.

Lee, M., & Moorhead, S. (2014). Nursing care patterns for patients receiving total hip replacements. *Orthopedic Nursing, 33*(3), 149–158.

Lee, R. K., Abol-Enein, H., Artibani, W, Bochner, B., Dalbagni, G., Daneshmand, S., . . . Shariat, S. F. (2014). Urinary diversion after radical cystectomy for bladder cancer: Options, patient selection, and outcomes. *British Journal of Urology International, 113(1)*, 11–23.

*Leenerts, M. H., Teel, C. S., & Pendelton, M. K. (2002). Building a model of self-care for health promotion in aging [Electronic version]. *Journal of Nursing Scholarship, 34*(4), 355–361. Retrieved from http://www.web.ebscohost.com /ehost/detail?vid=21&hid=106&sid=c7e5d2b4-3-4480-a27f-fdf75c59b820%40session mgr106

LeFevre, M. L., & U.S. Preventive Services Task Force. (2014). Screening for abdominal aortic aneurysm: U.S. Preventive Services Task Force recommendation statement. *Annals of Internal Medicine, 161*(4), 281–290.

*Lehne, R. A. (2004). *Pharmacology for nursing care* (5th ed.). St. Louis, MO: W. B. Saunders.

*Lehrner, J., Marwinski, G., Lehr, S., Johren, P., & Deecke, L. (2005). Ambient odors of orange and lavender reduce anxiety and improve mood in a dental office. *Physiology and Behaviour, 86*(1–2), 92–95.

Lemming, M. R., & Dickinson, G. E. (2010). *Understanding dying, death, and bereavement* (7th ed.). Belmont, CA: Wadsworth.

Lemone, P., Burke, K., Dwyer, T., , Levett-Jones, T., Moxham, L., Reid-Searl, K., . . . Luxford, Y. (2011). *Medical-surgical nursing: Critical thinking in client care.* Frenchs Forest, New South Wales, Australia: Pearson Australia.

*Leng, G., Fowler, B., & Ernst, E. (2000). Exercise for intermittent claudication. *Cochrane Database of Systematic Reviews,* (7), CD000990. doi:10.002/14651858.CD000990.pub3

*Leonard, M., Graham, S., & Bonacum, D. (2004). The human factor: The critical importance of effective teamwork and communication in providing safe care. *Quality and Safety in Health Care, 13*(Suppl. 1), i85–i90.

Leonardi, B. C., Faller, M., & Siroky, K. (2011). *Preventing never events/evidence-based practice* (White paper). San Diego, CA: AMN Healthcare. Retrieved from http://www.amnhealthcare.com/uploadedFiles/MainSite/Content/Healthcare_Industry_Insights/Healthcare_News/Never_Events_white_paper_06.16.11.pdf

Lerner, S. P., & Raghavan, D. (2015). Overview of the initial approach and management of urothelial bladder cancer. In *UpToDate.* Retrieved from http://www.uptodate.com/contents/overview-of-the-initial-approach-and-management-of-urothelial-bladder-cancer?source=see_link#H13

Lethbridge, E, Johnston, G. M., & Turnbull, G. (2013). Co-morbidities of persons dying of Parkinson's disease. *Progress in Palliative Care, 21*(3), 140–145.

Leukemia & Lymphoma Society. (2007a). *Hairy cell leukemia.* Retrieved from http://www.leukemia-lymphoma.org/all_page?itemid=8507

Leukemia & Lymphoma Society. (2007b). *Leukemia.* Retrieved from http://www.leukemia-lymphoma.org/all_page?itemid=7026

Leuttel, D., Beaumont, K., & Healey, F. (2007). *Recognizing and responding appropriately to early signs of deterioration in hospitalized patients: National Patient Safety Agency.* Retrieved from http://www.nrls.npsa.nhs.uk/EasySiteWeb /getresource.axd?AssetID=60151

*Levin, R. F., Krainovitch, B. C., Bahrenburg, E., & Mitchell, C. A. (1989). Diagnostic content validity of nursing diagnoses. *Image: The Journal of Nursing Scholarship, 21*(1), 40–44.

*Lew, D. P., & Waldvogel, F. A. (2004). Osteomyelitis. *Lancet, 364*(9431), 369–379.

Lewington, A., & Kanagasundaram, S. (2013). Acute renal injury. In *The Renal Association.* Retrieved from http://www.renal.org/guidelines/modules/acute-kidney-injury#sthash.n0tMLU45.dpbs

*Lewis, S. M., Heitkemper, M. M., Dirksen, S. R., O'Brien, P. G., Giddens, J. F., & Bucher, L. (2004). *Medical-surgical nursing: Assessment and management of clinical problems* (6th ed.). St. Louis, MO: Mosby.

Lewis, S. M., Heitkemper, M. M., Dirksen, S. R., O'Brien, P. G., Giddens, J. F., & Bucher, L. (2011). *Medical-surgical nursing: Assessment and management of clinical problems* (7th ed.). St. Louis, MO: Mosby.

*Licker, M., de Perrot, M., Spiliopoulos, A., Robert, J., Diaper, J., Chevalley, C., . . . Tschopp, J. M. (2003). Risk factors for acute lung injury after thoracic surgery for lung cancer. *Anesthesia & Analgesia, 97*(6), 1558–1565.

*Lieberman, P., Kemp, S. F., Oppenheimer, J., Lang, D. M., Bernstein, I. L., & Nicklas, R. A. (2005). The diagnosis and management of anaphylaxis: An updated practice parameter. *Journal of Allergy and Clinical Immunology, 115*(3), 483–523.

Lilly, M. B., Robinson, C. A., Holtzman, S., & Bottorff, J. L. (2012). Can we move beyond burden and burnout to support the health and wellness of family caregivers to persons with dementia? Evidence from British Columbia, Canada. *Health & Social Care in the Community, 20*(1), 103–112.

*Lim, W. S., van der Eerden, M. M., Laing, R., Boersma, W. G., Karalus, N., Town, G. I., . . . Macfarlane, J. T. (2003). Defining community acquired pneumonia severity on presentation to hospital: An international derivation and validation study. *Thorax, 58*(5), 377–382.

Lindahl, D. A. (2011). Parkinson's: Treating the symptoms. *British Journal of Nursing, 20*(14), 852–857.

*Lindemann, E. (1941). Observations of psychiatric sequelae to surgical operations in women. *American Journal of Psychiatry, 98*(1), 132–139.

*Lindqvist, O., Widmark, A., & Rasmussen, B. H. (2006). Reclaiming wellness—Living with bodily problems, as narrated by men with advanced prostate cancer. *Cancer Nursing: An International Journal for Cancer Care, 24*(9), 327–337.

Ling, S. M., & Mandl, S. (2013). *Pressure ulcers: Update & perspectives.* Centers for Medicare & Medicaid Services. Retrieved from http://www.npuap.org/wp-content/uploads/2012/01/NPUAP2013-LingMandl-FINAL2-25-131.pdf

Lip, G. Y., & Hull, R. D. (2016a). Overview of the treatment of lower extremity deep vein thrombosis (DVT). In *UpToDate*. Retrieved from http://www.uptodate.com/contents/overview-of-the-treatment-of-lower-extremity-deep-vein-thrombosis-dvt

Lip, G. Y., & Hull, R. D. (2016b). Rationale and indications for indefinite anticoagulation in patients with venous thromboembolism. In *UpToDate*. Retrieved from http://www.uptodate.com/contents/rationale-and-indications-for-indefinite-anticoagulation-in-patients-with-venous-thromboembolism?source=see_link&sectionName=Assessing+the+risk+of+bleeding&anchor=H380273132#H380273132

Little, B. P., Gilman, M. D., Humphrey, K. L., Alkasab, T. K., Gibbons, F. K., Shepard, J. O., . . . Wu, C. C. (2014). Outcome of recommendations for radiographic follow-up of pneumonia on outpatient chest radiography. *Cardiopulmonary Imaging, 202*(1). Retrieved from http://www.ajronline.org/doi/abs/10.2214/AJR.13.10888

Lloyd-Jones, D., Adams, R. J., Brown T. M., Carnethon, M., Dai, S., De Simone, G., . . . American Heart Association Statistics Committee and Stroke Statistics Subcommittee. (2010). Heart disease and stroke statistics—2010 update: A report from the American Heart Association. *Circulation, 121*(7), e46–e215.

Lo, J. O., Mission, J. F., & Caughey, A. B. (2013). Hypertensive disease of pregnancy and maternal mortality. *Current Opinion in Obstetrics and Gynecology, 25*(2), 124–132.

Longdon, S. (2015). Individualizing the care of those with kidney disease: Patient and family engagement. In C. S. Counts (Ed.), *Core curriculum for nephrology nursing: Module 2. Physiologic and psychosocial basis for nephrology nursing practice* (6th ed., pp. 219–223). Pitman, NJ: American Nephrology Nurses' Association.

*Longino, C. F., & Kart, C. S. (1982). Explicating activity theory: A formal replication. *Journal of Gerontology, 37*(6), 713–722.

*Lopez-Bushnell, K., Gary, G., Mitchell, P., & Reil, E. (2004). Joint replacement and case management in indigent hospitalized patients. *Orthopaedic Nursing, 23*(2), 113–117.

*Lord, R., & Dayhew, J. (2001). Visual risks factors for falls in older people. *American Journal of Geriatric Society, 49*(5), 58–64.

Lowitz, M., & Casciato, D. (2009). *Manual of clinical oncology* (5th ed.). Philadelphia, PA: Lippincott Williams & Wilkins.

Luettel, D., Beaumont, K., & Healey, F. (2007). *Recognising and responding appropriately to early signs of deterioration in hospitalised patients*. National Patient Safety Agency. Retrieved from http://www.nrls.npsa.nhs.uk/EasySiteWeb/getresource.axd?AssetID=60151

Lukacz, E. (2015). Treatment of urinary incontinence in women. In *UpToDate*. Retrieved from www.uptodate.com/contents/treatment-of-urinary-incontinence-in-women

Lukacz, E. S., Segall, M. M., & Wexner, S. D. (2015). Evaluation of an anal insert device for the conservative management of fecal incontinence. *Diseases of the Colon & Rectum, 58*(9), 892–898.

Lupus Foundation of America. (2013). *What is lupus?* Retrieved from http://www.lupus.org/webmodules/-webarticlesnet/templates/new_learnunderstanding.aspx?articleid=2232&zoneid=523

Lusardi, P., Jodka, P., Stambovsky, M., Stadnicki, B., Babb, B., Plouffe, D., . . . Montonye, M. (2011). The going home initiative: Getting critical care patients home with hospice. *Critical Care Nurse, 31*(5), 46–57.

Lussier-Cushing, M., Repper-Del, J., Mitchell, M. T., Lakatos, B. E., Mahoud, F., & Lipkis-Oralando, R. (2007). Is your medical/surgical patient withdrawing from alcohol? *Nursing, 37*(10), 50–55.

Lutz, C. A., Mazur, E., & Litch, N. (2015). *Nutrition and diet therapy* (6th ed.). Philadelphia, PA: F. A. Davis.

*Lynch, C. S., & Phillips, M. W. (1989). Nursing diagnosis: Ineffective denial. In R. M. Carroll-Johnson (Ed.), *Classification of nursing diagnosis: Proceedings of the eighth conference*. Philadelphia, PA: J. B. Lippincott.

Lynch, M., Sriprasad, S., Subramonian, K, & Thompson, P. (2010). Postoperative haemorrhage following transurethral resection of the prostate (TURP) and photoselective vaporisation of the prostate (PVP). *Annals of The Royal College of Surgeons of England, 92*(7), 555–558.

Lyndon, A., & Ali, L. U. (Eds.). (2015). *Fetal heart monitoring principles & practices* (5th ed.). Dubuque, IA: Kendall-Hunt.

Lyndon, A., Sexton, J. B., Simpson, K. R., Rosenstein, A., Lee, K. A., & Wachter, R. M. (2012). Predictors of likelihood of speaking up about safety concerns in labour and delivery. *BMJ Quality and Safety, 21*(9), 791–799.

Lynn, S. (2012). Caring for patients with Parkinson's disease. *American Nurse Today, 7*(12). Retrieved from https://www.americannursetoday.com/caring-for-patients-with-parkinsons-disease/

Lyon, B. L. (2002). Cognitive self-care skills: A model for managing stressful lifestyles. *Nursing Clinics of North America, 37*(2), 285–294.

Maakaron, J. (2013). Sickle cell anemia. In *Medscape*. Retrieved from http://emedicine.medscape.com/article/205926-overview

Mabvuure, N. T., Malahias, M., Hindocha, S., Khan, W., & Juma, A. (2012). Acute compartment syndrome of the limbs: Current concepts and management. *The Open Orthopaedics Journal, 6*(1), 535–543.

Macdougall, I. C. (2011). Anemia. In J. T. Daugirdas (Ed.), *Handbook of chronic kidney disease management*. Philadelphia, PA: Lippincott Williams & Wilkins.

*MacFie, J. (2004). Current status of bacterial translocation as a cause of surgical sepsis. *British Medical Bulletin*, *71*(1), 1–11.

MacGregor, M. S., & Methven, S. (2011). Assessing kidney function. In J. T. Daugirdas (Ed.), *Handbook of chronic kidney disease management* (pp. 1–18). Philadelphia, PA: Lippincott Williams & Wilkins.

Mack, J. W., & Smith, T. J. (2012). Reasons why physicians do not have discussions about poor prognosis, why it matters, and what can be improved. *Journal of Clinical Oncology*, *30*(22), 2715–2717.

Mackowaik, P. (2007). Diagnosis of osteomyelitis in adults. In *UpToDate*. Retrieved from http://www.uptodate.com

*Maclean, C., Louie, R., Leake, B., McCaffery, D., Paulus, H., Brook, R., & Shekelle, P. G. (2000). Quality of care for patients with rheumatoid arthritis. *Journal of the American Medical Association*, *284*(8), 984–992.

Macon Vascular Institute. (2014). *Discharge instructions lower extremity bypass surgery*. Retrieved from https://www.navicenthealth.org/js/tinymce/plugins/filemanager/files/macon-cardiovascular-institute/pdfs/MCVI-DI-Lower-Extremity-Bypass.pdf

*Maher, A. B., Salmond, S. W., & Pellino, T. (1998). *Orthopedic nursing* (2nd ed.). Philadelphia, PA: W. B. Saunders.

*Maher, K. (2005). Radiation therapy: Toxicities and management. In C. H. Yarbro, M. H. Frogge, & M. Goodman (Eds.), *Cancer nursing: Principle and practice* (6th ed.). Boston, MA: Jones & Bartlett.

*Mairis, E. (1994). Concept clarification of professional practice—Dignity. *Journal of Advanced Nursing*, *19*(5), 947–953.

*Maklebust, J., & Sieggreen, M. (2006). *Pressure ulcers: Guidelines for prevention and nursing management* (3rd ed.). Springhouse, PA: Springhouse.

*Maliski, S., Heilemann, M. S., & McCorkle, R. (2001). Mastery of postprostatectomy incontinence and impotence: His work, her work, our work. *Oncology Nursing Forum*, *28*(6), 985–992.

*Mallinson, R. K. (1999). The lived experience of AIDS-related multiple losses by HIV-negative gay men. *Journal of Association of Nurses in AIDS Care*, *10*(5), 22–31.

Maloni, H. (2012). *Pain in multiple sclerosis clinical bulletin information for health professionals*. Retrieved from http://www.nationalmssociety.org/NationalMSSociety/media/MSNationalFiles/Brochures/Clinical-Bulletin-Maloni-Pain.pdf

Maltoni, M., Scarpi, E., Rosati, M., Derni, S., & Fabbri, L. (2012). Palliative sedation in end-of-life care and survival: A systematic review. *Journal of Clinical Oncology*, *30*(12), 1378–1383.

Manack, A., Motsko, S. P., Haag-molkenteller, C., Dmochowski, R. R., Goehring, E. L., Jr., Nguyen-Khoa, B. A., . . . Jones, J. K. (2011). Epidemiology and healthcare utilization of neurogenic bladder patients in a U.S. claims database. *Neurourology and Urodynamics*, *30*(3), 395–401.

Mangera, Z., Panesar, G., & Makker, H. (2012). Practical approach to management of respiratory complications in neurological disorders. *International Journal of General Medicine*, *5*, 255–263. doi:10.2147/IJGM.S26333

Mangusan, R. F., Hooper, V., Denslow, S. A., & Travis, L. (2015). Outcomes associated with postoperative delirium after cardiac surgery. *American Journal of Critical Care*, *24*(2), 156–163.

Mann, W. J. (2015). Complications of gynecologic surgery. In *UpToDate*. Retrieved from http://www.uptodate.com/contents/complications-of-gynecologic-surgery?source=related_link

Margaretten, M., Kohlwes, J., Moore, D., & Bent, S. (2007). Synovial lactic acid and septic arthritis. *Journal of the American Medical Association*, *298*(1), 40.

Mariano, E. R. (2015). Management of acute perioperative pain. In *UpToDate*. Retrieved from http://www.uptodate.com

Marinell, M. A. (2008). Refeeding syndrome in cancer patients. *International Journal of Clinical Practice*, *62*(3), 460–465.

*Markey, D. W., & Brown, R. J. (2002). An interdisciplinary approach to addressing patient activity and mobility in the medical-surgical patient. *Journal of Nursing Care Quarterly*, *16*(4), 1–12.

Markland, A. D. (2013). Caffeine intake and its association with urinary incontinence in United States men: Results from National Health and Nutrition Examination Surveys 2005-2006 and 2007-2008. *The Journal of Urology*, *189*(6), 2170–2174.

Marrie, R. A., Reider, N., Cohen, J., Trojano, M., Sorensen, P. S., Cutter, G., . . . Stuve, O. (2014). A systematic review of the incidence and prevalence of sleep disorders and seizure disorders in multiple sclerosis. *Multiple Sclerosis Journal*, *21*(3), 342–349.

Marshall, K. (2011). Acute coronary syndrome: Diagnosis, risk assessment and management. *Nursing Standard*, *25*(23), 47–57.

*Martin, C. G., & Turkelson, S. L. (2006). Nursing care of the patient undergoing coronary artery bypass grafting. *Journal of Cardiovascular Nursing*, *21*(2), 109–117.

Martin, L. R., Haskard-Zolnierek, K. B., & DiMatteo, M. R. (2010). *Health behavior change and treatment adherence evidence-based guidelines for improving healthcare*. New York, NY: Oxford University Press.

*Martin, L. R., Williams, S. L., Haskard, K. B., & DiMatteo, M. R. (2005). The challenge of patient adherence. *Therapeutic Clinical Risk Management*, *1*(3), 189–199. Retrieved from www.ncbi.nlm.nih.gov/pmc/articles/PMC1661624/

Marui, A., Okabayashi, H., Komiya, T., Tanaka, S., Furukawa, Y., Kita, T., . . . Sakata, R. (2012). Benefits of off-pump coronary artery bypass grafting in high-risk patients. *Circulation*, *126*(11, Suppl. 1), S151–S157.

Massey, R., & Jedlicka, D. (2002). The Massey bedside swallowing screen. *Journal of Neuroscience Nursing*, *34*(5), 252–253, 257–260.

Massó González, E. L., Patrignani, P., Tacconelli, S., & García Rodríguez, L. A. (2010). Variability among nonsteroidal antiinflammatory drugs in risk of upper gastrointestinal bleeding. *Arthritis & Rheumatism*, *62*(6), 1592–1601.

*Mathew, J. P., Fontes, M. L., Tudor, I. C., Ramsay, J., Duke, P., Mazer, C. D., . . . Mangano, D. T. (2004). Multicenter study of perioperative ischemia research group. *JAMA, 291*(14), 1720–1729.

Matsuda, P. N., Shumway-Cook, A., Ciol, M. A., Bombardier, C. H., & Kartin, D. A. (2012). Understanding falls in multiple sclerosis: Association of mobility status, concerns about falling, and accumulated impairments. *Physical Therapy, 92*(3), 407–415.

Mattar, K., & Finelli, A. (2007). Expanding the indications of laparoscopic radical nephrectomy [Electronic version]. *Current Opinion in Urology, 17*(2), 88–92. Retrieved from http://www.kidney.org

Mattson, S., & Smith, J. E. (2016). *Core curriculum for maternal-newborn nursing* (5th ed.). St. Louis, MO: Saunders Elsevier.

*Matzo, M., & Sherman, D. (Eds.). (2001). *Palliative care nursing: Quality care to the end of life* (3rd ed.). New York, NY: Springer Publishing Company.

*Mauer, K. A., Abrahams, E. B., Arslanian, C., Schoenly, L., & Taggart, H. M. (2002). National practice patterns for the care of the patient with total joint replacement. *Orthopedic Nursing, 21*(3), 37–47.

*Mauk, K. L., & Schmidt, N. A. (2004). *Spiritual care in nursing practice*. Philadelphia, PA: Lippincott Williams & Wilkins.

Mayo Clinic. (2012). Kegel exercises: A how-to guide for women. In *Healthy lifestyle/women's health*. Retrieved from http://www.mayoclinic.org/healthy-lifestyle/womens-health/in-depth/kegel-exercises/art-20045283?pg=1

Mayo Clinic. (2014). *DLMP critical values/critical results list summary*. Retrieved at http://www.mayomedicallaboratories.com/articles/criticalvalues/view.php?name=Critical+Values%2FCritical+Results+List.

Mayo Clinic. (2016). *Kegel exercises for men: Understand the benefits*. Retrieved from http://www.mayoclinic.org/healthy-lifestyle/mens-health/in-depth/kegel-exercises-for-men/art-20045074

Mayor, S. (2007). Breathing and relaxation technique cut asthma symptoms by one third. *British Medical Journal, 335*(7611), 119.

*McCafferty, M. (2003). *Pain: Clinical manual for nursing practice*. St. Louis, MO: Mosby.

McCafferty, M., & Pasero, C. (2011). *Pain assessment and pharmacological management*. New York, NY: Mosby.

*McClave, S. A., DeMeo, M. T., DeLegge, M. H., DiSario, J. A., Heyland, D. K., Maloney, J. P., . . . Zaloga, G. P. (2002). North American summit on aspiration in the critically ill patient: Consensus statement. *Journal of Parenteral and Enteral Nutrition, 26*(Suppl. 6), S80–S85.

*McCullough, J., & Ownby, D. (1993). A comparison of three in vitro tests for latex specific IgE [Abstract]. *Journal of Allergy Clinical Immunology, 91*, 242.

McCutcheon, T. (2013). The ileus and oddities after colorectal surgery. *Gastroenterology Nursing, 36*(5), 368–375.

McDermott, M. M., Guralnik, J. M., Criqui, M. H., Liu, K., Kibbe, M. R., & Ferrucci, L. (2014). Six-minute walk is a better outcome measure than treadmill walking tests in therapeutic trials of patients with peripheral artery disease. *Circulation, 130*(1), 61–68.

*McDermott, M. M., Mehta, S., & Greenland, P. (1999). Exertional leg symptoms other than intermittent claudication are common in peripheral arterial disease. *Archives of Internal Medicine, 159*(4), 387–392.

*McDermott, M. M., Tiukinhoy, S., Greenland, P., Liu, K., Pearce, W. H., Guralnik, J. M., . . . Ferrucci, L. (2004). A pilot exercise intervention to improve lower extremity functioning in peripheral arterial disease unaccompanied by intermittent claudication. *Journal of Cardiopulmonary Rehabilitation, 24*(3), 187–196.

*McGrory, B., Callaghan, J., Kraay, M., Jacobs, J., Robb, W., Brand, R. A., . . . Wasielewski, R. (2005). Editorial: Minimally invasive and small-incision joint replacement surgery—What surgeons should you consider. *Clinical Orthopaedics and Related Research, 440*, 251–254.

*McGuire, D., Sheidler, V., & Polomano, R. C. (2000). Pain. In S. Groenwald, M. Frogge, M. Goodman, & C. Yarbo (Eds.), *Cancer nursing: Principles and practice* (5th ed.). Boston, MA: Jones & Bartlett.

*McKinley, M. (2005). Alcohol withdrawal syndrome: Overlooked and mismanaged? *Critical Care Nurse, 25*(3), 40–49.

McKinney, E. S., James, S. R., Murray, S. S., Nelson, K. A., & Ashwill, J. W. (2013). *Maternal child nursing* (4th ed.). St. Louis, MO: Saunders Elsevier.

McMenamin, E. (2011). Pain management principles. *Current Problems in Cancer, 35*(6), 317–323.

*McQuellon, R. P., Wells, M., Hoffman, S., Craven, B., Russell, G., Cruz, J., . . . Savage, P. (1998). Reducing distress in cancer patients with an orientation program. *Psycho-Oncology, 7*(3), 207–217.

Mechem, C., & Zafren, K. (2014). Accidental hypothermia in adults. In *UpToDate*. Retrieved from http://www.uptodate.com/contents/accidental-hypothermia-in-adults

Mehrotra, R. (2015). Metabolic, acid-base, and electrolyte aspects of peritoneal dialysis. In J. T. Daugirdas, P. G. Blake, & S. I. Todd (Eds.), *Handbook of dialysis* (5th ed., pp. 521–526). Philadelphia, PA: Wolters Kluwer.

*Melody, G. (1962). Depressive reactions following hysterectomy. *American Journal of Obstetrics and Gynecology, 83*, 413.

Melsom, H., & Danjoux, G. (2011). Perioperative care for lower limb amputation in vascular disease. *Continuing Education in Anaesthesia, Critical Care & Pain*. Retrieved from http://ceaccp.oxfordjournals.org/content/early/2011/07/12/bjaceaccp.mkr024.full.pdf

Meltzer, L., Davis, K. F., Jodi, A., & Mindell, J. A. (2012). Patient and parent sleep in a children's hospital. *Pediatric Nursing, 38*(2), 64–71.

Menon, M., Shrivastava, A., Kaul, S., Badani, K. K., Bhandani, M., & Peabody, J. O. (2007). Vattikuti Institute prostatectomy: Contemporary technique and analysis of results. *European Urology, 51*(3), 648–657.

Mercadante, S., Intravaia, G., Ferrera, P., Villari, P., & David, F. (2008). Peritoneal catheter for continuous drainage of ascites in advanced cancer patients. *Supportive Care in Cancer, 16*(8), 975–978.

Mercadante, S., Intravaia, G., Villari, P., Ferrera, P., David, F., & Casuccio, A. (2009). Controlled sedation for refractory symptoms in dying patients. *Journal of Pain Symptom Management, 37*(5), 771–779.

Mercandetti, M. (2013). Wound healing and repair. In *Medscape*. Retrieved from http://emedicine.medscape.com /article/1298129-overview

*Merck Manual Online Library. (2005). *Osteomyelitis*. Retrieved from http://www.merck.com/mmpe/sec04/ch039 /ch039d.html

Metheny, N. A., Mueller, C., Robbins, S., Wessel, J., & The A.S.P.E.N. Board of Directors. (2009). A.S.P.E.N. enteral nutrition practice recommendations. *Journal of Parenteral Enteral Nutrition, 33*(2), 122–167.

*Meurman, J., Odont, D., Sorvari, R., Pelttari, A., Rytömaa, I., Odont, R., . . . Kroon, L. (1996). Hospital mouth—Cleaning aids may cause dental erosion. *Special Care in Dentistry, 16*(6), 247–250.

Miller, C. (2015). *Nursing for wellness in older adults* (7th ed.). Philadelphia, PA: Wolters Kluwer.

Miller, E. T. (2015). Nursing best practices to prevent stroke in women. *Stroke, 46*(4), e75–e77.

Miller, E., Murray, L., Richards, L., Zorowitz, R., Bakas, T., Clark, P., . . . Billinger, S. (2010). Comprehensive overview of nursing and interdisciplinary rehabilitation care of the stroke patient: A scientific statement from the American Heart Association. *Stroke, 41*(10), 2402–2448.

Miller, J., & Mink, J. (2009). Acute ischemic stroke: Not a moment to lose. *Nursing, 39*(5), 37–42.

*Miller, M., & Kearney, N. (2004). Chemotherapy-related nausea and vomiting—Past reflections, present practice and future management. *European Journal of Cancer Care (England), 13*(1), 71–81.

Miller, N. C., & Askew, A. E. (2007). Tibia fractures: An overview of evaluation and treatment. *Orthopaedic Nursing, 26*(4), 216–223.

Miller, N., Allcock, L., Hildreth, A. J., Jones, D., Noble, E., & Burn, D. J. (2009). Swallowing problems in Parkinson disease: Frequency and clinical correlates. *Journal of Neurological Neurosurgical Psychiatry, 80*(9), 1047–1049.

Mink, J., & Miller, J. (2011). Opening the window of opportunity. *Nursing, 41*(1), 24–33.

Minkes, R. (2013). Stomas of the small and large intestine treatment & management. In *Medscape*. Retrieved from http://emedicine.medscape.com/article/939455-treatment

Minkes, R. K. (2015). Stomas of the small and large intestine. In *Medscape*. Retrieved from http://emedicine .medscape.com/article/939455-overview

Minniti, C. P., Eckman, J., Sebastiani, P., Steinberg, M. H., & Ballas, S. K. (2010). Leg ulcers in sickle cell disease. *American Journal of Hematology, 85*(10), 831–833.

Mitchell, A. J. (2007). Pooled results from 38 analyses of the accuracy of distress thermometer and other ultra-short methods of detecting cancer-related mood disorder. *Journal of Clinical Oncology, 25*(29), 4670–4681.

Mitchell, M., Mohler, E., & Carpenter, J. (2007). Acute arterial occlusion of the lower extremity. In *UpToDate*. Retrieved from http://www.uptodate.com

Miura, H. (2012). An exercise program for improving and/or maintaining arterial function in middle-aged to older individuals. *Advanced Exercise Sports Physiology, 18*(3), 47–51.

Mizell, J. S. (2014). Complications of abdominal surgical incisions. In *UpToDate*. Retrieved from http://www.uptodate.com

Mizuno, K., Tsuji, T., Takebavashi, T., Fujiwara, T., Hase, K., & Liu, M. (2011). Prism adaptation therapy enhances rehabilitation of stroke patients with unilateral spatial neglect: A randomized, controlled trial. *Neurorehabilitation Neural Repair, 25*(8), 711–720.

Mohler, E. P., 3rd. (2015). Patient education: Peripheral artery disease and claudication (Beyond the Basics). In *UpToDate*. Retrieved from http://www.uptodate.com/contents/peripheral-artery-disease-and-claudication-beyond-the-basics

Mohler, E. R., 3rd, & Fairman, R. M. (2015). Complications of carotid endarterectomy. In *UpToDate*. Retrieved from http://www.uptodate.com/contents/complications-of-carotid-endarterectomy?source=see_link&sectionName=HY PERPERFUSION+SYNDROME&anchor=H101624751#H101624751

Mohler, E. R., 3rd. (2016). Screening for abdominal aortic aneurysm. In *UpToDate*. Retrieved from http://www.uptodate .com/contents/screening-for-abdominal-aortic-aneurysm?source=search_result&search=Monitoring++of+AAA& selectedTitle=5~132

Mohler, E. R., 3rd, & Mehrara, B. (2016). Clinical staging and conservative management of peripheral lymphedema. In *UpToDate*. Retrieved from http://www.uptodate.com/contents/clinical-staging-and-conservative-management-of-peripheral-lymphedema?source=see_link

Mokdad, A., Balluz, L. S., & Okoro, C. A. (2008). Association between selected unhealthy lifestyle factors, body mass index, and chronic health conditions among individuals 50 years of age or older, by race/ethnicity. *Ethnicity and Disease, 18*(4), 450–457.

Mokry, L. E., Ross, S., Ahmad, O. S., Forgetta, V., Smith, G. D., Goltzman, D., . . . Richards, J. B. (2015). Vitamin D and risk of multiple sclerosis: A Mendelian randomization study. *PLoS Medicine, 12*(8), e1001866.

Monczewski, L. (2013). Managing bone metastasis in the patient with advanced cancer. *Orthopaedic Nursing, 32*(4), 209–214.

*Montgomery, G. H., & Bovbjerg, D. H. (2004). Presurgery distress and specific response expectations predict postsurgery outcomes in surgery patients confronting breast cancer. *Health Psychology, 23*(4):381–387.

Moore, L. J., Moore, F. A., Todd, S. R., Jones, S. L., Turner, K. L., & Bass, B. L. (2010). Sepsis in general surgery. The 2005–2007 National Surgical Quality Improvement Program perspective. *Archives of Surgery, 145*(7), 695–700.

Morales, C. H., Mejia, C., Roldan, L. A., Saldarriaga, M. F., & Duque, A. F. (2014). Negative pleural suction in thoracic trauma patients: A randomized controlled trial. *Journal of Trauma and Acute Care Surgery, 77*(2), 251–255.

More, K. N., Truong, V., Estey, E., & Voaklander, D. C. (2007). Urinary incontinence after prostatectomy: Can men at risk be indentified preoperatively? *Journal of Wound, Ostomy, and Continence, 34*(3), 270–279; quiz 280–281.

Morgenstern, L. B., Hemphill, J. C., 3rd, Anderson, C., Becker, K., Broderick, J. P., Connolly, E. S., Jr., . . . on behalf of the American Heart Association Stroke Council and Council on Cardiovascular Nursing. (2010). Guidelines for the management of spontaneous intracerebral hemorrhage: A guideline for healthcare professionals from the American Heart Association/American Stroke Association. *Stroke, 41*(9), 2108–2129.

Morrison, R. S., & Siu, A. L. (2015). Medical consultation for patients with hip fracture. In *UpToDate*. Retrieved from http://www.uptodate.com/contents/medical-consultation-for-patients-with-hip-fracture?source=see_link

Morse, J. (2007). Enhancing the safety of hospitalization by reducing patient falls. *American Journal of Infection Control, 30*(6), 376–380.

Morse, J. (2009). *Preventing patient falls: Establishing a fall intervention program* (2nd ed.). New York, NY. Springer Publishing Company.

*Morton, K., & Gambier, E. (2000). *Guidelines for prescribing nutritional supplements in primary care*. Retrieved from http://www.bolton.nhs.uk/Library/Leaflets/patient/nutrition/guidelines.pdf

The MS Socitey. (2014). *When a parent has MS: A teenager's guide*. Retrieved from http://www.nationalmssociety.org/NationalMSSociety/media/MSNationalFiles/Brochures/Brochure-When-a-Parent-Has-MS-A-Teenagers-Guide.pdf

Mueller, A. C., & Bell, A. E. (2008). Electrolye update: Potassium, chloride, and magnesium. *Nursing Critical Care, 3*(1), 5–7.

Mueller, E. R. (2016). Postoperative urinary retention in women. In *UpToDate*. Retrieved from http://www.uptodate.com

Muffly, T. M., Couri, B., Edwards, A., Kow, N., Bonham, A. J., & Paraíso, M. F. R. (2012). Effect of petroleum gauze packing on the mechanical properties of suture materials. *Journal of Surgical Education, 69*(1), 37–40.

*Mukherjee, D. (2003). Perioperative cardiac assessment for noncardiac surgery: Eight steps to the best possible outcome. *Circulation, 107*, 2771–2774. doi:10.1161/Circulation

Mulhauser, G. (2007). *Welcome to the CAGE questionnaire, a screening test for alcohol dependence*. Retrieved from http://www.counsellingresource.com/quizzes/alcohol-cage/index.html

Multiple Sclerosis Foundation. (2016). *Multiple sclerosis by the numbers: Facts, statistics, and you*. Retrieved from http://www.healthline.com/health/multiple-sclerosis/facts-statistics-infographic

The Multiple Sclerosis Society. (2014). *Pediatric MS*. Retrieved from http://www.nationalmssociety.org/For-Professionals/Clinical-Care/Managing-MS/Pediatric-MS

Multiple Sclerosis.Net. (2016). *Therapy for swallowing problems*. Retrieved from https://www.multiplesclerosis.net/treatment/swallowing-problems-therapy/

*Munoz, A., & Katerndahl, D. (2000). Diagnosis and management of acute pancreatitis. *American Family Physician, 62*(1), 164–174.

*Murphy, S. A. (1993). Coping strategies of abstainer from alcohol up to three years post-treatment. *Journal of Nursing Scholarship, 25*(2), 87.

*Murray, J. (2001). Loss as a universal concept: A review of the literature to identify common aspects of loss in diverse situations. *Journal of Loss and Trauma: International Perspectives on Stress & Coping, 6*(3), 2179–241.

Murray, R. B., Zentner, J. P., & Yakimo, R. (2009). *Health promotion strategies through the life span* (8th ed.). Upper Saddle River, NJ: Pearson Prentice Hall.

*Murray, S. A., Boyd, K., & Sheikh, A. (2005). Palliative care in chronic illness. *BMJ, 330*(7492), 611–612.

*Mutlu, G. M., Mutlu, E. A., & Factor, P. (2001). GI complications in patients receiving mechanical ventilation. *CHEST, 119*(4), 1222–1241. Retrieved from http://www.journal.publications.chestnet.org/data/Journals/CHEST/21961/1222.pdf

Myasthenia Gravis Foundation of America. (2010a). *Myasthnai gravis: A manual for health care providers*. New York, NY: Author.

Myasthenia Gravis Foundation of America. (2010b). *Ocular myasthenia gravis* [Brochure]. New York, NY: Author.

Myers-Glower, M. (2013). Preventing complications in patients receiving opioids. *American Nurse Today, 8*(12), 1–9.

Nahabedia, M. (2015). Overview of breast reconstruction. In *UpToDate*. Retrieved from http://www.uptodate.com/contents/overview-of-breast-reconstruction

Nair, S. (2010). Vitamin D deficiency and liver disease. *Gastroenterology & Hepatology, 6*(8), 491.

NANDA International. (2009). *Nursing diagnoses: Definitions and classification*. Philadelphia, PA: Author.

Nardin, R., & Freeman, R. (2015). Epidemiology, clinical manifestations, diagnosis, and treatment of HIV-associated peripheral neuropathy. In *UpToDate*. Retrieved from http://www.uptodate.com/contents/epidemiology-clinical-manifestations-diagnosis-and-treatment-of-hiv-associated-peripheral-neuropathy

*National Cancer Institute. (2003). *Types of leukemia*. Retrieved from http://www.cancer.gov/cancertopics/wyntk/leukemia/page5

National Cancer Institute. (2007). *Lymphedema management*. Retrieved from http://www.cancer.gov/cancertopics/pdq/supportivecare/lymphedema/HealthProfessional/page2

National Cancer Institute. (2008). *Support and resources*. Retrieved from http://www.cancer.gov/cancertopics/support

National Cancer Institute. (2010). *Palliative care in cancer*. Retrieved from http://www.cancer.gov/cancertopics/factsheet/Support/palliative-care

National Cancer Institute. (2013). *Adjustment to cancer: Anxiety and distress (PDQ) [Comprehensive cancer information]*. Bethesda, MD: Author. Retrieved from http://www.cancer.gov/cancertopics/pdq/supportivecare/adjustment/HealthProfessional/page3#Reference3

National Cancer Institute. (2014, January 31). *Oral complications of chemotherapy and head-neck radiation*. Retrieved from http://www.cancer.gov/cancertopics/pdq/supportivecare/oralcomplications/HealthProfessional/page5

National Cancer Institute. (2015). Adjustment to cancer: Anxiety and distress. In *PubMed Health*. Retrieved from https://www.ncbi.nlm.nih.gov/pubmedhealth/PMH0032514/

*National Cholesterol Education Program. (2004). *Third report of the national cholesterol education program (NCEP). Expert panel on detection, evaluation and treatment of high blood cholesterol in adults (Adult treatment panel III)*. Retrieved from http://www.scymed.com/en/smnxdj/edzr/edzr9610.htm

National Comprehensive Cancer Network. (2008). *Oral mucositis is often underrecognized and undertreated*. Retrieved from http://www.bestpractice.bmj.com/best-practice/monograph/1135/treatment/guidelines.html

National Comprehensive Cancer Network. (2014). *NCCN guidelines for patients*. Retrieved from http://www.nccn.org/patients/guidelines/stage_i_ii_breast/files/assets/common/downloads/files/stageiiibreast.pdf

The National Council on Alcoholism and Drug Dependence. (2016). *Family disease*. Retrieved from https://www.ncadd.org/family-friends/there-is-help/family-disease

National Database of Nursing Quality Indicators. (2016). *Pressure ulcer survey guide*. Retrieved from https://www.members.nursingquality.org/NDNQIPressureUlcerTraining/Module3/PressureUlcerTeamTraining_2.aspx

National Digestive Diseases Information Clearinghouse. (n.d.). *Viral gastroenteritis*. Retrieved from http://www.digestive.niddk.nih.gov/ddiseases/pubs/viralgastroenteritis/

National Guideline Clearinghouse. (2009). *Guideline for prevention of catheter-associated urinary tract infections*. Retrieved from http://www.guideline.gov/content.aspx?id=15519

National Heart, Lung, and Blood Institute. (2015). *How can atherosclerosis be prevented or delayed?* Retrieved from https://www.nhlbi.nih.gov/health/health-topics/topics/atherosclerosis/prevention

National Institute for Health and Clinical Excellence. (2016). *Heart failure*. Retrieved from https://www.nice.org.uk/guidance/conditions-and-diseases/cardiovascular-conditions/heart-failure

National Institute of Allergy and Infectious Diseases. (2011). *Guidelines for the diagnosis and management of food allergy in the United States*. Retrieved from http://www.allergywatch.org/niaid/patients.pdf

*National Institute of Arthritis and Musculoskeletal and Skin Diseases. (2003). *Lupus*. Retrieved from http://www.niams.nih.gov/Health_Info/Lupus/default.asp

National Institute of Arthritis and Musculoskeletal and Skin Diseases. (2008). *Health information page*. Retrieved from http://www.naims.nih.gov/Health_Info/Fibromyalgia/fibrmyalgia_ff.asp

National Institute of Clinical Excellence. (2005). *Clinical practice guidelines for violence: The short-term management of disturbed/violent behavior in psychiatric in-patient and emergency departments*. Retrieved from http://www.rcpsych.ac.uk/PDF/NICE%20Guideline%202005.pdf

National Institute of Health. (2012). *Urostomy and continent urinary diversion*. Retrieved from http://www.kidney.niddk.nih.gov/kudiseases/pubs/urostomy/

National Institute of Health. (2013). *Parkinson's disease*. Retrieved from http://www.nlm.nih.gov/medlineplus/parkinsonsdisease.html

National Institute of Health. (2015). *Guidelines for the prevention and treatment of opportunistic infections in HIV-infected adults and adolescents*. Retrieved from https://www.aidsinfo.nih.gov/contentfiles/lvguidelines/adult_oi.pdf

National Institute of Neurological Disorders and Stroke. (2007). *Multiple sclerosis*. Retrieved from http://www.commondataelements.ninds.nih.gov/ms.aspx#tab=Data_Standards

National Institute of Neurological Disorders and Stroke. (2011, August 19). *Guillain-Barre syndrome fact sheet*. Retrieved from http://www.ninds.nih.gov/disorders/gbs/detail_gbs.htm

National Institute of Neurological Disorders and Stroke. (2012). *NINDS deep brain stimulation for Parkinson's disease information*. Retrieved from http://www.ninds.nih.gov/disorders/deep_brain_stimulation/deep_brain_stimulation.htm#What_is

National Institute of Neurologic Disorders and Stroke. (2016a). *Guillain-Barre syndrome fact sheet*. Retrieved from http://www.ninds.nih.gov/disorders/myasthenia_gravis/myasthenia_gravis.htm

National Institute of Neurologic Disorders and Stroke. (2016b). *Myasthenia gravis fact sheet*. Retrieved from http://www.ninds.nih.gov/disorders/myasthenia_gravis/myasthenia_gravis.htm

The National Institute on Alcohol Abuse and Alcoholism. (2007). *Alcohol and tobacco*. Retrieved from http://pubs.niaaa.nih.gov/publications/AA71/AA71.htm

National Institute on Deafness and Other Communication Disorders. (2013). *American sign language*. Retrieved from http://www.nidcd.nih.gov/health/hearing/pages/asl.aspx

National Institutes of Health. (2007). *Asthma action plan*. Retrieved from https://www.nhlbi.nih.gov/files/docs/public/lung/asthma_actplan.pdf

National Institutes of Health. (2011). *Who is at risk for deep vein thrombosis?* Retrieved from http://www.nhlbi.nih.gov/health/health-topics/topics/dvt/atrisk

National Institutes of Health. (2015a). *Sickle cell disease*. National Heart, Lung and Blood Institute. Retrieved at http://www.nhlbi.nih.gov/health/health-topics/topics/sca

National Institutes of Health. (2015b). *Guidelines for the prevention and treatment of opportunistic infections in HIV-infected adults and adolescents*. Retrieved from https: //aidsinfo.nih.gov/contentfiles/lvguidelines/adult_oi.pdf

National Kidney Foundation. (2007). *Facts about chronic kidney disease*. Retrieved from http://www.kidney.org

National Kidney Foundation. (2015). *Nephrectomy*. Retrieved from https://www.kidney.org/atoz/content/nephrectomy

*National Library of Medicine. (2006). *Leukemia*. Retrieved from https://medlineplus.gov/leukemia.html

National Parkinson Foundation. (2016). *Exercise*. Retrieved from http://www.parkinson.org/understanding-parkinsons/treatment/Exercise

National Pressure Ulcer Advisory Panel. (2007). National Pressure Ulcer Advisory Panel's updated pressure ulcer staging system. *Urology Nursing, 27*(2), 144–150, 156.

National Pressure Ulcer Advisory Panel, European Pressure Ulcer Advisory Panel. (2014). *Clinical practice guideline*. Retrieved from http://www.npuap.org/resources/educational-and-clinical-resources/prevention-and-treatment-of-pressure-ulcers-clinical-practice-guideline/

*National Quality Forum. (2006). *Practices for better healthcare*. Retrieved from https://www.qualityforum.org/News_And_Resources/Press_Kits/Safe_Practices_for_Better_Healthcare.aspx

National Sleep Foundation. (2015). *National sleep foundation recommends new sleep times*. Retrieved from https://www.sleepfoundation.org/media-center/press-release/national-sleep-foundation-recommends-new-sleep-times

National Spinal Cord Injury Association. (2007). *More about spinal cord injury*. Retrieved from http://www.spinalcord.org

National Stroke Association. (2013a). *Recovery & rehabilitation*. Retrieved from http://www.stroke.org/site/PageServer?pagename=rehabt

National Stroke Association. (2013b). *Stroke 101 and prevention*. Retrieved from http://www.stroke.org/site/PageServer?pagename=factsheets

NCCN Clinical Practice Guidelines in Oncology. (2013). *NCCN—Evidence-based cancer guidelines, oncology drug compendium, oncology continuing medical education: Distress management*. Retrieved from http://www.nccn.org

*Nead, K. G., Halterman, J. S., Kaczorowski, J. M., Auinger, P., & Weitzman, M. (2004). Overweight children and adolescents: A risk group for iron deficiency. *Pediatrics, 114*(1), 104–108.

*Nelson, K. A., Walsh, D., Behrens, C., Zhukovsky, D. S., Lipnickey, V., & Brady, D. (2000). The dying cancer patient. *Seminars in Oncology, 27*(1), 84–89.

Neschis, D. G., & Golden, M. A. (2014). Treatment of chronic lower extremity critical limb ischemia. In *UpToDate*. Retrieved at http://www.uptodate.com/contents/clinical-features-and-diagnosis-of-lower-extremity-peripheral-artery-disease

Neschis, D. G., Mohler, E. R., & Golden, M. A. (2012). Surgical management of claudication. In *UpToDate*. Retrieved from http://www.uptodate.com/contents/surgical-management-of-claudication

NeSmith, E., Weinrich, S., Andrews, J., Medeiros, S., Hawkins, M., & Weinrich, M. (2009). Systemic inflammatory response syndrome score and race as predictors of length of stay in the intensive care unit. *American Journal of Critical Care, 18*(4), 339–345.

*Ness, J., Aronow, W. S., Newkirk, E., & McDanel, D. (2005). Prevalence of symptomatic peripheral arterial disease, modifiable risk factors, and appropriate use of drugs in the treatment of peripheral arterial disease in older persons seen in a university general medicine clinic. *Journals of Gerontology Series A: Biological Sciences and Medical Sciences, 60*(2), 255–257.

*Nettina, S. M. (2006). *Lippincott manual of nursing practice* (8th ed.). Ambler, PA: Lippincott Williams & Wilkins.

Neubauer, A. C., & Fink, A. (2009). Intelligence and neural efficiency. *Neuroscience and Biobehavioral Reviews, 33*(7), 1004–1023.

Neubauer, D. N. (2009). Current and new thinking in the management of comorbid insomnia. *The American Journal of Managed Care, 15*(Suppl.), S24–S32.

Neviere, R. (2016). Sepsis syndromes in adults: Epidemiology, definitions, clinical presentation, diagnosis, and prognosis. In *UpToDate*. Retrieved from http://www.uptodate.com/contents/sepsis-syndromes-in-adults-epidemiology-definitions-clinical-presentation-diagnosis-and-prognosis

*Newcombe, P. (2002). Pathophysiology of sickle cell disease crisis. *Emergency Nurse, 9*(9), 9–22.

*Newman, D. K. (2005, June). Urinary incontinence and indwelling catheters: CMS guidance for long-term care. *ECPN*, 50–56. Retrieved from http://www.health.state.mn.us/divs/fpc/profinfo/urinconcath/p50_54_ecpn06_newmance.pdf

Newman, D. K., & Willson, M. M. (2011). Review of intermittent catheterization and current best practices. *Urologic Nursing, 31*(1), 12–28, 48; quiz 29.

*Newswanger, D. L., & Warren, C. R. (2004). Guillain-Barre syndrome. *American Family Physician, 69*(10), 2405–2410.

Ng, B. L., & Anpalahan, M. (2011). Management of chronic kidney disease in the elderly. *Internal Medicine Journal*, *41*(11), 761–768.

Nguyen, T., Gwynn, R., Kellerman, S., Begier, E., Garg, R., Konty, K., . . . Thorpe, L. (2008). Population prevalence of reported and unreported HIV and related behaviors among the household adult population in New York City, 2004. *AIDS: Official Journal of the International AIDS Society*, *22*(2), 281–287.

*Nichols, R. I. (1991). Surgical wound infections. *American Journal of Medicine*, *91*(Suppl. 3B), 54–64.

Nickloes, T. A. (2012). Superior vena cava syndrome treatment & management. In *Medscape*. Retrieved from http://emedicine.medscape.com/article/460865-treatment

Nicolini, D., Mengis, J., & Swan, J. (2012). Understanding the role of objects in cross-disciplinary collaboration. *Organization Science*, *23*(3), 612–629.

*Nighorn, S. (1988). Narcissistic deficits in drug abusers: A self-psychological approach. *Journal of Psychosocial Nursing & Mental Health Services*, *26*(9), 22–26.

North American Nursing Diagnosis Association. (2009). *Nursing diagnoses: Definitions and classifications 2009–2010*. Ames, IA: Wiley-Blackwell.

Northouse, L., Williams, A. L., Given, B., & McCorkle, R. (2012). Psychosocial care for family caregivers of patients wih cancer. *Journal of Clinical Oncology*, *30*(11), 1227–1234.

Northrop, D. E., & Frankel, D. (2010). *Nursing home care of individuals with multiple sclerosis*. National Multiple Sclerosis Society. Retrieved at http://www.nationalmssociety.org/NationalMSSociety/media/MSNationalFiles/Brochures/Nursing-Home-Care-of-Individuals-with-MS.pdf

*Norton, B., Homer-Ward, M., Donnelly, M. T., Long, R. G., & Holmes, G. K. (1996). A randomized prospective comparison of percutaneous endoscopic gastrostomy and nasogastric tube feeding after acute dysphagic stroke. *BMJ*, *3*(12), 13–16.

Nostrant, T. T. (2012). Clinical features, diagnosis, and treatment of radiation proctitis. In L. Friedman & C. Willett (Eds.), *UpToDate*. Retrieved from http://www.uptodateonline.com

Nucifora, G., Hysko, F., Vit, A., & Vasciaveo, A. (2007). Pulmonary fat embolism: Common and unusual computed tomography findings. *Journal of Computer Assisted Tomography*, *31*(5), 806–807.

*Nygaard, I. E., Thompson, F. L., Svengalis, S. L., & Albright, J. P. (1994). Urinary incontinence in elite nulliparous athletes. *Obstetrics & Gynecology*, *84*(2), 183–187.

O'Brien, M. E. (2010). *Spirituality in nursing: Standing on holy ground* (4th ed.). Boston, MA: Jones & Bartlett.

O'Donnell, P. (2012). *Impending fracture & prophylactic fixation*. Retrieved from http://www.orthobullets.com/pathology/8002/impending-fracture-and-prophylactic-fixation

O'Dowd, L. C., & Kelley, M. A. (2015). Air embolism. In *UpToDate*. Retrieved from http://www.uptodate.com/contents/air-embolism?source=search_result&search=air+embolism&selectedTitle=1~114

O'Grady, N. P., Alexander, M., Burns, L. A., Dellinger, P. E., Garland, J., Heard, S. O., . . . The Healthcare Infection Control Practices Advisory Committee (HICPAC). (2011). *Guidelines for the prevention of intravascular catheter-related infections*. Atlanta, GA: Centers for Disease Control and Prevention. Retrieved from www.cdc.gov/hicpac/pdf/guidelines/bsi-guidelines-2011.pdf

O'Mallon, M. (2009). Vulnerable populations: Exploring a family perspective of grief. *Journal of Hospice & Palliative Nursing*, *11*(2), 91–98.

*O'Neill, M. J., Weissleder, R., Gervais, D. A., Hahn, P. F., & Mueller, P. R. (2001). Tunneled peritoneal catheter placement under sonographic and fluoroscopic guidance in the palliative treatment of malignant ascites. *American Journal of Roentgenology*, *177*(3), 615–618.

Occupational Safety & Health Administration. (2010). *Blood borne pathogens and needle stick prevention*. Retrieved from https://www.osha.gov/SLTC/bloodbornepathogens/

Office of Student Disabilities Services, & University of Chicago. (2014). *Teaching students with disabilities resources for instructors 2014-2015*. Chicago, IL: Author. Retrieved from https://www.disabilities.uchicago.edu/sites/disabilities.uchicago.edu/files/uploads/docs/Teaching%20Students%20with%20Disabilities%20201415.pdf

Ogata, T., Kamouchi, M., Matsuo, R., Hata, J., Kuroda, J., Ago, T., . . . Fukuoka Stroke Registry. (2014). Gastrointestinal bleeding in acute ischemic stroke: Recent trends from the fukuoka stroke registry. *Cerebrovascular Disease Extra*, *4*(2), 156–164.

*Oka, R. K. (2006). Peripheral arterial disease in older adults: Management of cardiovascular disease risk factors. *Journal of Cardiovascular Nursing*, *21*(Suppl. 5), S15–S20.

Okorie, C. O. (2015). Is continuous bladder irrigation after prostate surgery still needed? *World Journal of Clinical Urology*, *4*(3), 108–114.

Oldfield, M. M., El-Masri, M. M., & Fox-Wasylyshyn, S. M. (2009). Examining the association between chest tube-related factors and the risk of developing healthcare-associated infections in the ICU of a community hospital: A retrospective case-control study. *Intensive and Critical Care Nursing*, *25*(1), 38–44.

Olek, M. J. (2015). Clinical course and classification of multiple sclerosis. In *UpToDate*. Retrieved from http://www.uptodate.com/contents/clinical-course-and-classification-of-multiple-sclerosis?source=see_link

Olek, M. J. (2016). Diagnosis of multiple sclerosis in adults. In *UpToDate*. Retrieved from http://www.uptodate.com/contents/diagnosis-of-multiple-sclerosis-in-adults

Olek, M. J., & Mowry, E. (2016). Pathogenesis and epidemiology of multiple sclerosis. In *UpToDate*. Retrieved from http://www.uptodate.com/contents/pathogenesis-and-epidemiology-of-multiple-sclerosis

Olek, M. J., Narayan, R. N., & Frohma, E. M. (2016). Clinical features of multiple sclerosis in adults. In *UpToDate*. Retrieved at http://www.uptodate.com/contents/clinical-features-of-multiple-sclerosis-in-adults

Olin, J. W., & Sealove, B. A. (2010). Peripheral artery disease: Current insight into the disease and its diagnosis and management. *Mayo Clinical Proceedings*, *85*(7), 678–692.

Oliver, M. J. (2007). Chronic hemodialysis vascular access: Types and placement. In *UpToDate*. Retrieved from http://www.uptodate.com

Olujohungbe, A., & Burnett, A. L. (2013). How I manage priapism due to sickle cell disease. *British Journal of Haematology*, *160*(6), 754.

Omar, M. I., & Alexander, C. E. (2013). Drug treatment for faecal incontinence in adults. *Cochrane Database Systematic Reviews*, (6), CD002116. doi:10.1002/14651858.CD002116.pub2

Oncology Nursing Society. (2007). *Mucositis: What interventions are effective for managing oral mucositis in people receiving treatment for cancer* [ONS PEP Cards]. Pittsburgh, PA: Author.

*Onizuka, Y., Mizuta, Y., Isomoto, H., Takeshima, F., Murase, K., Miyazaki, M., . . . Kohno, S. (2001). Sludge and stone formation in the gallbladder in bedridden elderly patients with cerebrovascular disease: Influence of feeding method [Electronic version]. *Journal of Gastroenterology*, *36*(5), 330–337. Retrieved from http://www.web.ebscohost.com /ehost/pdf?vid=132&hid=106&sid=c7e5d2b4-a3-4480-a27f-fdf75c59b820%40session mgr106

Osborn, K. S., Wraa, C. E., & Watson, A. (2010). *Medical-surgical nursing: Preparation for practice*. Upper Saddle River, NJ: Pearson.

Osinbowale, O. O., & Milani, R. V. (2011). Benefits of exercise therapy in peripheral arterial disease. *Progress in Cardiovascular Diseases*, *53*(6), 447–453.

Oxman, A. D., Lavis, J. N., Lewin, S., & Fretheim, A. (2009). SUPPORT Tools for evidence-informed health Policymaking (STP) 10: Taking equity into consideration when assessing the findings of a systematic review. *Health Research Policy and Systems*, *7*(Suppl. 1), S10.

Pace, R. C. (2007). Fluid management in patients on hemodialysis. *Nephrology Nursing Journal*, *34*(5), 557–559.

Pai, M., & Douketis, J. D. (2015). Prevention of venous thromboembolism in adult travellers. In *UpToDate*. Retrieved from http://www.uptodate.com/contents/prevention-of-venous-thromboembolism-in-adult-travelers?source=search_res ult&search=prolonged+travel&selectedTitle=2~21

Pai, M., & Douketis, J. D. (2016). Prevention of venous thromboembolic disease in surgical patients. In *UpToDate*. Retrieved from http://www.uptodate.com/contents/prevention-of-venous-thromboembolic-disease-in-surgical-patients? source=see_link

*Paice, J. A., Noskin, G. A., & Vanagunas, A. (2005). Efficacy and safety of scheduled dosing opioid analgesics: A quality improvement study. *Journal of Pain*, *6*(10), 639–643.

Panula, J., Pihlajamäki, H., Mattila, V. M., Jaatinen, P., Vahlberg, T., Aarnio, P., . . . Kivelä, S. L. (2011). Mortality and cause of death in hip fracture patients aged 65 or older: a population-based study. *BMC Journal of Musculoskeletal Disorders*, *12*, 105. doi:10.1186/1471-2474-12-105

*Paparella, P., Sizzi, O., De Benedittis, F., Rossetti, A., & Paparella, R. (2004). Vaginal hysterectomy in generally considered contraindications to vaginal surgery. *Archives of Gynecological Obstetrics*, *270*(2), 104–109.

*Parekattil, S. J., Gill, I. S., Castle, E. P., Burgess, S. V., Walls, M. M., Thomas, R., . . . Andrews, P. E. (2005). Multi-institutional validation study of neural networks to predict duration of stay after laparoscopic radical/simple or partial nephrectomy. *Journal of Urology*, *174*(4, Pt. 1), 1380–1384.

Parikh, S., Koch, M., & Narayan, R. (2007). Traumatic brain injury. *International Anesthesiology Clinics*, *45*(3), 119–135.

*Park, J. J., Del Pino, A., Orsay, C. P., Nelson, R. L., Pearl, R. K., Cintron, J. R., . . . Abcarian, H. (1999). Stoma complications: The Cook County Hospital experience. *Diseases of the Colon and Rectum*, *42*(12), 1575–1580.

*Park, R. H. R., Allison, M. C., Lang, J., Spence, E., Morris, A. J., Danesh, B. J., . . . Mills, P. R. (1992). Randomised comparison of percutaneous endoscopic gastrostomy and nasogastric tube feeding in patients with persisting neurological dysphagia. *BMJ*, *304*(6839), 1406–1409.

Parkinson's Disease Foundation. (2007). *Parkinson's disease: An overview. What is Parkinson's disease?* Retrieved from http://www.pdf.org/about_pd

*Pasacreta, J. V., & Massie, M. J. (1990). Nurses' reports of psychiatric complications in patients with cancer. *Oncology Nursing Forum*, *17*(3), 347–353.

Pasacreta, J. V., Kenefick, A. L., & McCorkle, R. (2008). Managing distress in oncology patients. *Cancer Nursing*, *31*(6), 485–490.

Pasero, C. (2010). Pain care around-the-clock (ATC) dosing of analgesics. *Journal of PeriAnesthesia Nursing*, *25*(1), 36–39.

*Pasero, C., & McCaffery, M. (2002). Monitoring sedation: It's the key to preventing opioid-induced respiratory depression. *The American Journal of Nursing*, *102*(2), 67–69.

*Pasero, C., & McCaffery, M. (2004). Comfort–function goals: A way to establish accountability for pain relief. *The American Journal of Nursing*, *104*(9), 77–81.

Pasero, C., & McCaffery, M. (2011). *Pain assessment and pharmaceutical management*. New York, NY: Mosby.

Pasquel, F., Spiegelman, R., Smiley, D., Umpierrez, D., Johnson, R., . . . Umpierrez, G. (2010). Hyperglycemia during total parenteral nutrition. *Diabetes Care*, *33*(4), 739–741.

Patel, A., Lall, C. G., Jennings, S. G., & Sandrasegaran, K. (2007). Abdominal compartment syndrome. *American Journal of Roentgenology, 189*(5), 1037–1043.

Patel, V., Romano, M., Corkins, M. R. (2010). Nutrition screening and assessment in hospitalized patients: A survey of current practice in the United States. *Nutrition in Clinical Practice, 29*(4), 483–490.

Payne, A. B., Miller, C. H., Hooper, W. C., Lally, C., & Austin, H. D. (2014). High factor VIII, von Willebrand factor, and fibrinogen levels and risk of venous thromboembolism in blacks and whites. *Ethnicity & disease, 24*(2), 169.

Peacock, E. J., Counts, C. S., German, S., Holloway, K., Howard, L., & Wiseman, K. (2015). Foundations of infection prevention, control, and clinical application in nephrology nursing. In C. S. Counts (Ed.), *Core curriculum for nephrology nursing: Module 2. Physiologic and psychosocial basis for nephrology nursing practice* (6th ed., pp. 331–396). Pitman, NJ: American Nephrology Nurses' Association.

Pear, S. (2007). Patient risk factors and best practices. *Managing Infection Control*, 56–64. Retrieved from www.halyardhealth.com/media/1515/patient_risk_factors_best_practices_ssi.pdf

Pearce, H. (2011). Abdominal aortic aneurysms. In *Medscape*. Retrieved from http://emedicine.medscape.com/article/1979501-overview

Pearce, J. M. (2007). Documenting peritoneal dialysis. *Nursing, 37*(10), 28.

*Pearson, L., & Hutton, J. (2002). A controlled trial to compare the ability of foam swabs and toothbrushes to remove dental plaque. *Journal of Advanced Nursing, 39*(5), 480–489.

*Pellino, T., Polacek, L. P., Preston, A., Bell, N., & Evans, R. (1998). Complications of orthopedic disorders and orthopedic surgery. In A. Maher, S. Salomond, & T. Pellino (Eds.), *Orthopaedic nursing* (2nd ed.). Philadelphia, PA: W. B. Saunders.

Pelzang, R. (2010). Time to learn: Understanding patient-centered care. *British Journal of Nursing, 19*(14), 912–917.

Pennsylvania Patient Safety Advisory. (2012). Analysis of the multiple risks involving the use of IV Fentanyl. *Pennsylvania Patient Safety Advisory, 9*(4), 122–129.

*Pepine, C, Balaban, R. S., Bonow, R. O., Diamond, G. A., Johnson, B. D., Johnson, P. A., . . . American College of Cardiology Foundation. (2004). Women's ischemic syndrome evaluation. Current status and future research directions: Report of the National Heart, Lung and Blood Institute Workshop: October 2–4, 2002: Section 1: Diagnosis of stable ischemia and ischemic heart disease. *Circulation, 109*(6), e44–e46.

Peppercorn, M. A., & Cheifetz, A. S. (2015). Definition, epidemiology, and risk factors in inflammatory bowel disease. In *UpToDate*. Retrieved from http://www.uptodate.com/contents/definition-epidemiology-and-risk-factors-in-inflammatory-bowel-disease

*Pepys, M. B., & Hirschfield, G. M. (2003, June). C-reactive protein: A critical update. *Journal of Clinical Investigation, 111*(12), 1805–1812.

Pereira, J. M. V., Cavalcanti, A. C. D., Santana, R. F., Cassiano, K. M., Queluci, G. D. C., & Guimarães, T. C. F. (2011). Nursing diagnoses for inpatients with cardiovascular diseases. *Escola Anna Nery [Online], 15*(4), 737–745.

Peretto, G., Durante, A., Limite, L. R., & Cianflone, D. (2014). Postoperative arrhythmias after cardiac surgery: Incidence, risk factors, and therapeutic management. *Cardiology Research and Practice, 2014*, 615987. doi:10.1155/2014/615987

Peripheral Artery Disease. This increasingly common disorder often goes undetected in women until serious problems arise. (2012). *Harvard Women's Health Watch, 19*(8), 4–6.

Perry, D., Borchert, K., Burke, S., Chick, K., Johnson, K., Kraft, W., . . . Thompson, S. (2012). *Institute for clinical systems improvement. Pressure ulcer prevention and treatment protocol*. Retrieved from https://www.icsi.org/_asset/6t7kxy/

*Persson, E., & Hellström, A. L. (2002). Experiences of Swedish men and women 6 to 12 weeks after ostomy surgery. *Journal of Wound, Ostomy, and Continence Nursing, 29*(2), 103–108.

*Persson, E., & Larsson, B. (2005). Quality of care after ostomy surgery: A perspective study of patients. *Ostomy Wound Management, 51*(8), 40–48.

Peterson, M. J., Gravenstein, N., Schwab, W. K., van Oostrom, J. H., & Caruso, L. J. (2013). Patient repositioning and pressure ulcer risk—Monitoring interface pressures of at-risk patients. *Journal of Rehabilitation Research and Development, 50*(4), 477–488.

Petterson, R., Haig, Y., Nakstad, P. H., & Wyller, T. B. (2008). Subtypes of urinary incontinence after stroke: Relation to size and location of cerebrovascular damage. *Age and Ageing, 37*(3), 324–327.

Pezzilli, R., Corinaldesi, R., & Morselli-Labate, A. (2010). Pancreatic cancer and cancer screening programs: From nihilism to hope. *Journal of the Pancreas, 11*(6), 654–655.

Philbin, T. M., DeLuccia, D. M., Nitsch, R. F., & Maurus, P. B. (2007). Syme amputation and prosthetic fitting challenges. *Techniques in Foot and Ankle Surgery, 6*(3), 147–155.

*Piasecki, P. A. (2000). Bone and soft tissue sarcoma. In S. Groenwald, M. Frogge, M. Goodman, & C. Yarbro (Eds.), *Cancer nursing: Principles and practice* (5th ed.). Boston, MA: Jones & Bartlett.

*Picard, K., Donoghue, S., Young-Kershaw, D., & Russell, K. (2006). Development and implementation of a multidisciplinary sepsis protocol. *Critical Care Nurse, 26*(3), 42–54.

*Pieper, B., & Mikols, C. (1996). Predischarge and postdischarge concerns of persons with an ostomy. *Journal of WOCN, 23*(2), 105–109.

Pierpont, Y. N., Dinh, T. P., Salas, R. E., Johnson, E. L., Wright, T. G., Robson, M. C., . . . Payne, W. G. (2014). Obesity and surgical wound healing: a current review. *ISRN Obesity, 2014*. Retrieved from http://www.hindawi.com/journals/isrn/2014/638936/

*Piette, J. D. (2005). *Using telephone support to manage chronic disease.* Retrieved from http://www.chef.org/topics /chronicdisease/index.cfm

*Pike, N. A., & Gundry, S. R. (2003). Robotically assisted cardiac: Minimally invasive technology to totally endoscopic heart surgery. *Journal of Cardiovascular Nursing, 18*(5), 238–388.

Pillitteri, A. (2014). *Maternal & child health nursing: Care of the childbearing & childrearing family* (7th ed.). Philadelphia, PA: Lippincott Williams & Wilkins.

Pinto, D., & Kociol, R. (2015). Pathophysiology of cardiogenic pulmonary edema. In *UpToDate*. Retrieved from http://www.uptodate.com/contents/pathophysiology-of-cardiogenic-pulmonary-edema

Pinto, D. S., Kohli, P., Fan, W., Kirtane, A. J., Kociol, R. D., Meduri, C., . . . Michael Gibson, C. (2016). Bivalirudin is associated with improved clinical and economic outcomes in heart failure patients undergoing percutaneous coronary intervention: Results from an observational database. *Catheterization and Cardiovascular Interventions, 87*(3), 363–373.

*Pirraglia, P. A., Bishop, D., Herman, D. S., Trisvan, E., Lopez, R. A., Torgersen, C. S., . . . Stein, M. D. (2005). Caregiver burden and depression among informal caregivers of HIV-infected individuals. *Journal of General Internal Medicine, 20*(6), 510–514.

Pitts, T., Bolser, D., Rosenbek, J., Troche M., Okun, M. S., & Sapienza C. (2009). Impact of expiratory muscle strength training on voluntary cough and swallow function in Parkinson disease. *CHEST, 135*(5), 1301–1308.

Plummer, M. P., Blaser, A. R., & Deane, A. M. (2014). Stress ulceration: prevalence, pathology and association with adverse outcomes. *Critical Care, 18*(2), 213

*Podsiadlo, D., & Richardson, S. (1991). The timed "Up and Go" test: A test of basic functional mobility for frail elderly persons. *Journal of American Geriatric Society, 39*, 142–148. Retrieved from http://www.fallrventiontaskforce.orgpdf. TimedUpandGoTest.pdf

Politis, M., Wu, K., Molloy, S., Bain, P. G., Chaudhuri, K. R., & Piccini, P. (2010). Parkinson's disease symptoms: The patient's perspective. *Movement Disorders, 25*(11), 1646–1651.

Pollack, A. (2010). *Radiation therapy for prostate cancer.* Retrieved from http://www.cancer.org/cancer/prostatecancer /detailedguide/prostate-cancer-treating-radiation-therapy

Ponferrada, L. P., & Prowant, B. F. (2008). Peritoneal dialysis: Peritoneal dialysis therapy. In C. S. Counts (Ed.), *Core curriculum for nephrology nursing* (5th ed.). Pitman, NJ: American Nephrology Nurses' Association.

*Pontieri-Lewis, V. (2006). Basics of ostomy care. *Medical and Surgical Nursing, 15*(4), 199–202.

Pope, B. B., Rodzen, L., & Spross, G. (2008). Raising the SBAR: How better communication improves patient outcomes. *Nursing, 38*(3), 41–43.

Porat, R., & Dinarello, C. A. (2015). Pathophysiology and treatment of fever in adults. In *UpToDate*. Retrieved from http://www.uptodate.com

*Powars, D. R. (1975). Natural history of sickle cell disease—The first ten years. *Seminars in Hematology, 12*(3), 267.

Powers M. A., Bardsley, J., Cypress, M., Duker, P., Funnell M. M., Hess Fisch, A., . . . Vivian, E. (2015). Diabetes self-management education and support in type 2 diabetes: A joint position statement of the American Diabetes Association, the American Association of Diabetes Educators, and the Academy of Nutrition and Dietetics. *Diabetes Care, 38*, 1372–1382.

*Powell-Cope, G., & Brown, M. A. (1992). Going public as an AIDS family caregiver. *Social Science & Medicine, 34*(5), 571–580.

*Prandoni, P., Lensing, A. W., Prins, M. H., Frulla, M., Marchiori, A., Bernardi, E., . . . Girolami, A. (2004). Below-knee elastic compression stockings to prevent the post-thrombotic syndrome: a randomized, controlled trial. *Annals of Internal Medicine, 141*(4), 249–256.

Price, C. S., Williams, A., Philips, G., Dayton, M., Smith, W., & Morgan, S. (2008). Staphylococcus aureus nasal colonization in preoperative orthopaedic outpatients. *Clinical Orthopedic Related Research, 466*(11), 2842–2847.

Priftis, K., Passarini, L., Pilosio, C., Meneghello, F., & Pitteri, M. (2013). Visual scanning training, limb activation treatment, and prism adaptation for rehabilitation left neglect: Who is the winner? *Frontiers in Human Neuroscience, 7*, 360. doi:10.3389/fnhum.2013.00360

Procter, N., Hamer, H., McGarry, D., Wilson, R., & Froggatt, T. (2014). *Mental health: A person-centered approach.* Port Melbourne, VIC: Cambridge Press.

Prommer, E. (2009). Talking with cancer patients and their families. In D. A. Casciato, & M. C. Territo (Eds.), *Manual of clinical oncology* (6th ed.). Philadelphia, PA: Lippincott Williams & Wilkins.

Puchalski, C. M., & Ferrell, B. (2010). *Making health care whole: Integrating spirituality into patient care.* West Conshohocken, PA: Templeton Press.

*Puchalski, C. M., & McSkimming, S. (2006). Creating healing environments. *Health Progress, 87*(3), 30–35.

Pugh, S., Mathiesen, C., Meighan, M., Summers, D., & Zrelak, P. (2009). Guide to the care of the hospitalized patient with ischemic stroke. In *AANN Clinical Practice Guideline Series* (2nd ed.). Retrieved from http://www.aann.org/pdf /cpg/aannischemicstroke.pdf

Pullen, R. L., Jr. (2007). Replacing a urostomy drainage pouch. *Nursing, 37*(6), 14.

Purkayastha, S., Zhang, G., & Cai, D. (2011). Uncoupling the mechanisms of obesity and hypertension by targeting hypothalamic IKK-β and NF-B. *National Medicine, 17*(7), 883–887.

Quinn, B., Baker, D. L., Cohen, S., Stewart, J. L., Lima, C. A., & Parise, C. (2014). Basic nursing care to prevent non-ventilator hospital-acquired pneumonia. *Journal of Nursing Scholarship, 46*(1), 11–17.

Rackley, R. (2011, November). Neurogenic bladder. In *Medscape*. Retrieved from http://emedicine.medscape.com/article/453539-overview

Raghavan, V. A., & Hamdy, O. (2012). Diabetic ketoacidosis treatment & management. In *Medscape*. Retrieved from http://emedicine.medscape.com/article/118361-treatment

Ramthun, M., Mocelin, A. J., & Delfino, V. D. (2011). Hypernatremia secondary to post-stroke hypodipsia: Just add water! *Clinical Kidney Journal*. Retrieved from http://www.ckj.oxfordjournals.org/content/early/2011/05/12/ndtplus.sfr057.full

*Rando, T. A. (1984). *Grief, dying, and death: Clinical interventions for caregivers*. Champaign, IL: Research Press.

Rangel-Castillo, L., Gopinath, S., & Robertson, C. S. (2008). Management of intracranial hypertension. *Neurologic Clinics, 26*(2), 521–541.

Rantanen, T. (2013). Promoting mobility in older people. *Journal of Preventive Medicine and Public Health, 46*(Suppl. 1), S50–S54. Retrieved from http://www.ncbi.nlm.nih.gov/pmc/articles/PMC3567319/

Rape, Abuse and Incest National Network. (2016). *About sexual assault*. Retrieved at https://www.rainn.org/about-sexual-assault

*Ratzan, S. C., & Parker, R. M. (2000). Introduction. In C. R. Selden, M. Zorn, S. C. Ratzan, & R. M. Parker (Eds.), *National library of medicine, current bibliographies in medicine: Health literacy* (NLM Publication No. CBM 2000-1). Bethesda, MD: National Institutes of Health, U.S. Department of Health and Human Services.

*Ray, R. I. (2000). Complications of lower extremity amputations. *Topics in Emergency Medicine, 22*(3), 35–42.

Reeder, G. S., & Awtry, E. (2016). Initial evaluation and management of suspected acute coronary syndrome (myocardial infarction, unstable angina) in the emergency department. In *UpToDate*. Retrieved from http://www.uptodate.com/contents/initial-evaluation-and-management-of-suspected-acute-coronary-syndrome-myocardial-infarction-unstable-angina-in-the-emergency-department

Reeve, J., Stiller, K., Nicol, K., McPherson, K. M., Birch, P., Gordon, I. R., & Denehy, L. (2010). A postoperative shoulder exercise program improves function and decreases pain following open thoracotomy: A randomised trial. *Journal of Physiotherapy, 56*(4), 245–252.

*Registered Nurses' Association of Ontario. (2005, March). *Risk assessment and prevention of pressure ulcers*. Toronto, ON: Author.

Registered Nurses' Association of Ontario. (2009). *Ostomy care and management*. Toronto, ON: Author.

*Richardson, C., Glenn, S., Nurmikko, T., & Horgan, M. (2006). Incidence of phantom phenomena including phantom limb pain 6 months after major lower limb amputation in patients with peripheral vascular disease. *Clinical Journal of Pain, 22*(4), 353–358.

Richbourg, L., Thorpe, J. M., & Rapp, C. G. (2007). Difficulties experienced by the ostomate after hospital discharge. *Journal of Wound, Ostomy, and Continence Nursing, 34*(1), 70–79.

*Riefkohl, E. Z., Heather, L., Bieber, H. L., Burlingame, M. B., & Lowenthal, D. T. (2003). Medications and falls in the elderly: A review of the evidence and practical considerations. *Pharmacy & Therapeutics, 28*(11), 724–733.

Riestra, A. R., & Barrett, A. M. (2013). Rehabilitation of spatial neglect. *Handbook of Clinical Neurology, 110*, 347–355. Retrieved from http://www.ncbi.nlm.nih.gov/entrez/eutils/elink.fcgi?dbfrom=pubmed&retmode=ref&cmd=prlinks&id=23312654

*Rigdon, J. L. (2006). Robotic-assisted laparoscopic radical prostatectomy. *AORN, 84*(5), 759–762, 764, 766–770.

Rigotti, N. A., Clair, C., Munafò, M. R., & Stead, L. F. (2012). Interventions for smoking cessation in hospitalised patients. *Cochrane Database of Systematic Reviews*, (5), CD001837. Retrieved from http://www.ncbi.nlm.nih.gov/pmc/articles/PMC4498489

*Rindfleisch, J., & Muller, D. (2005). Diagnosis and management of rheumatoid arthritis. *American Family Physician, 72*(6), 1037–1047.

Roberts, I. (2012). *Diagnosis and management of chronic radiation enteritis*. Retrieved from http://www.aboutcancer.com/radiation_enteritis_utd_807.htm

Robinson, A. (2008). Review article: Improving adherence to medication in patients with inflammatory bowel disease. *Alimentary Pharmacology & Therapeutics, 27*(Suppl. 1), 9–14.

Robinson, J. H., Callister, L. C., Berry, J. A., & Dearing, K. A. (2008). Patient⬚centered care and adherence: Definitions and applications to improve outcomes. *Journal of the American Academy of Nurse Practitioners, 20*(12), 600–607.

Robson, K. M., & Lombo, A. J. (2015). Fecal incontinence in adults: Etiology and evaluation. In *UpToDate*. Retrieved from http://www.uptodate.com/contents/fecal-incontinence-in-adults-etiology-and-evaluation

*Rockman, C. B., Cappadona, C., Riles, T. S., Lamparello, P. J., Giangola, G., Adelman, M. A., & Landis, R. (1997). Causes of the increased stroke rate after carotid endarterectomy in patients with previous strokes. *Annals of Vascular Surgery, 11*(1), 28–34.

Roe, B., Flanagan, L. B., Barrett, J., Chung, A., Shaw, C., & Williams, K. (2011). Systematic review of the management of incontinence and promotion of continence in older people in care homes: Descriptive studies with urinary incontinence as primary focus. *Journal of Advanced Nursing, 67*(2), 228–250.

Rolim de Moura, C., Paranhos, A., Jr., & Wormald, R. (2007). Laser trabeculoplasty for open angle glaucoma [Systematic review]. *Cochrane Database of Systematic Reviews*, (4), CD003919. doi:10.1002/14651858.CD003919.pub2

*Rollnick, S., Mason, P., & Butler, C. (2000). *Health behavior change: A guide for practitioners*. Edinburgh, UK: Churchill Livingstone.

*Roman, M., Weinstein, A., & Macaluso, S. (2003). Primary spontaneous pneumothorax. *Medical and Surgical Nursing, 12*(3), 161–169.

Rooke, T. W., Hirsch, A. T., Misra, S., Sidawy, A. N., Beckman, J. A., Findeiss, L. K., . . . Society for Vascular Surgery. (2011). 2011 ACCF/AHA focused update of the guideline for the management of patients with peripheral artery disease (Updating the 2005 Guideline): A report of the American College of Cardiology Foundation/American Heart Association Task Force on practice guidelines. *Journal of the American College of Cardiology, 58*(19), 2020–2045.

*Rosen, J., Mittal, V., Degenholtz, H., Castle, N., Mulsant, B. H., Hulland, S., ... Rubin, F. (2006). Ability, incentives, and management feedback: organizational change to reduce pressure ulcers in a nursing home. *Journal of the American Medical Directors Association, 7*(3), 141–146.

Rosenberg, M. (2015). Overview of the management of chronic kidney disease in adults. In *UpToDate*. Retrieved from http://www.uptodate.com/contents/overview-of-the-management-of-chronic-kidney-disease-in-adults

*Rosenberg, S. M. (2006). Palliation of malignant ascites. *Gastroenterology Clinics of North America, 35*(1), 189–199. doi:10.1016/j.gtc.2005.12.006

Rosenberg, J. B., & Eisen, L. A. (2008). Eye care in the intensive care unit: narrative review and meta-analysis. *Critical Care Medicine, 36*(12), 3151–3155.

*Rost, K., & Roter, D. (1987). Predictors of recall of medication regimens and recommendations for lifestyle changes in elderly patients. *Gerontologist, 27*(4), 510–515.

*Roter, D. L., Rude, R. E., & Comings, J. (1998). Patient literacy: A barrier to quality of care. *Journal of General Internal Medicine, 13*(12), 850–851.

*Rowley, H. A. (2005). Extending the time window for thrombolysis: Evidence from acute stroke trials. *Neuroimaging Clinics of North America, 15*(3), 575–587, x.

Roy, P. (2011). Hepatitis D. In *Medscape*. Retrieved from http://emedicine.medscape.com/article/178038-overview

Royal College of Psychiatrists. (1998). *National audit of violence standards for in-patient mental health services*. Retrieved from http://www.rcpsych.ac.uk/pdf/Standards_Final_version_with_foreword_for%20website.pdf

Runyon, B. A. (2009). *Management of adult patients with ascites due to cirrhosis: An update*. Retrieved from https://www.aasld.org/sites/default/files/guideline_documents/adultascitesenhanced.pdf

Runyon, B. A. (2015). Hepatorenal syndrome. In *UpToDate*. Retrieved from http://www.uptodate.com/contents/hepatorenal-syndrome?source=search_result&search=hepatorenal+syndrome&selectedTitle=1~150

*Russo, C. A., & Elixhauser, A. (2006). *Hospitalizations related to pressure sores, 2003* (HCUP Statistical Brief #3). Retrieved from http://www.hcup-us.ahrq.gov/reports/statbriefs/sb3.pdf

*Russo, C. A., Steiner, C., & Spector, W. (2006). *Hospitalizations related to pressure ulcers among adults 18 years and older*. Retrieved from http://www.hcup-us.ahrq.gov/reports/statbriefs/sb64.pdf

Saberi A., & Pouresmail, Z. (2007). The effect of acupressure on phantom pain in client with extremities amputation. *European Journal of Pain, 11*(S1), 127–128.

Saberi, O. B. (2012). *Coping with aging and amputation: How changing the way you think could change your health*. Retrieved from http://www.amputee-coalition.org/senior_step/coping_aging.html

Sabia, S., Elbaz, A., Dugravot, A., Head, J., Shipley, M., Hagger-Johnson, G., . . . Singh-Manoux, A. (2010). Impact of smoking on cognitive decline in early old age. The Whitehall II Cohort Study. *Archives of General Psychiatry, 69*(6), 627–635.

*Sacco, R. L., Adams, R., Albers, G., Alberts, M., Benavente, O., Furie, K., . . . Tomsick, T. (2006). Guidelines for prevention of stroke in patients with ischemic stroke or ransient ischemic attack. *Stroke, 37*(2), 577–617.

Sacco, R. L., Kasner, S. E., Broderick, J. P., Caplan, L. R., Connors, J. J., Culebras, A., . . . Council on Nutrition, Physical Activity and Metabolism. (2013). An updated definition of stroke for the 21st century: A statement for healthcare professionals from the American Heart Association/American Stroke Association. *Stroke, 44*(7), 2064–2089.

Sadr-Azodi, O., Andrén-Sandberg, Å., Orsini, N., & Wolk, A. (2012). Cigarette smoking, smoking cessation and acute pancreatitis: A prospective population-based study *Gut, 61*(2), 262.

Saewyc, E. M., Skay, C. L., Hynds, P., Pettingell, S., Bearinger, L. H., Resnick, M. D., . . . Reis, E. (2007). Suicidal ideation and attempts among adolescents in North American school-based surveys: Are bisexual youth at increasing risk? *Journal of LGBT Health Research, 3*(2), 25–36.

Sahjian, M., & Frakes, M. (2007). Crush injuries: Pathophysiology and current treatment. *Nurse Practitioner: The American Journal of Primary Health Care, 32*(9), 13–18.

Saito, Y. A. (2011). The role of genetics in IBS. *Gastroenterol Clinics of North America, 40*(1), 45–67.

Saito, Y. A., Petersen, G. M., Larson, J. J., Atkinson, E. J., Fridley, B. L., de Andrade, M., . . . Talley, N. J. (2010). Familial aggregation of irritable bowel syndrome: A family case-control study. *The American Journal of Gastroenterology, 105*(4), 833–841.

Saitz, R. (2015). Alcohol: no ordinary health risk. *Addiction, 110*(8), 1228–1229.

Salai, P. B. (2008). Patient management: The dialysis procedure. In C. S. Counts (Ed.), *Core curriculum for nephrology nursing* (5th ed.). Pitman, NJ: American Nephrology Nurses' Association.

Salcido, R. (2012). Pressure ulcers and wound care. In *Medscape*. Retrieved from http://emedicine.medscape.com /article/319284-overview

*Salmond, S. (Ed.). (1996). Core curriculum for orthopedic nursing (3rd ed.). Pitman, NJ: National Association of Orthopedic Nurses.

Salomé, G. M., Almeida, S. A. D., & Silveira, M. M. (2014). Quality of life and self-esteem of patients with intestinal stoma. *Journal of Coloproctology (Rio de Janeiro)*, *34*(4), 231–239.

Salzer, J., Hallmans, G., Nyström, M., Stenlund, H., Wadell, G., & Sundström, P. (2012). Vitamin D as a protective factor in multiple sclerosis. *Neurology*, *79*(21), 2140.

Samet, J. M. (2015). Secondhand smoke exposure: Effects in adults. In *UpToDate*. Retrieved from http://www.uptodate. com/contents/secondhand-smoke-exposure-effects-in-adults?source=search_result&search=second+hand+smoke &selectedTitle=2~92

*Sampselle, C. M., Miller, J. M., Mims, B. L., Delancey, J. O., Ashton-Miller, J. A., & Antonakos, C. L. (1998). Effect of pelvic muscle exercise on transient incontinence during pregnancy and after birth. *Obstetrics & Gynecology*, *91*(3), 406–412.

*Sampson, H. W. (2002). Alcohol and other factors affecting osteoporosis risk in women [Electronic version]. *Alcohol Research and Health*, *26*(4), 292–298. Retrieved from http://www.ebsco.waldenu.edu/ehost /pdf?vid=6&hid=102&sid=55fdd3ae-a6d5-4629-8fa9-fd330627fcf%40sessionmgr103

Sanofi-Aventis U.S. (2011). *Lovenox (enoxaparin sodium) injection prescribing information*. Bridgewater, NJ: Author.

*Santoni-Reddy, L. (2006, Spring). Heads up on cerebral bleeds. *ED Insider*, *36*(5), 4–9.

Santucci, R. A. (2015). *Radical nephrectomy treatment and management*. In *Medscape*. Retrieved at http://emedicine .medscape.com/article/448878

Satalowich, R. J., & Prowant, B. F. (2008). Peritoneal dialysis: Peritoneal dialysis access. In C. S. Counts (Ed.), *Core curriculum for nephrology nursing* (5th ed.). Pitman, NJ: American Nephrology Nurses' Association.

Satin, J. R., Linden, W., & Phillips, M. J. (2009). Depression as a predictor of disease progression and mortality in cancer patients. *Cancer*, *115*(22), 5349–5361. doi:10.1002/cncr.24561

*Savitz, L. A., Jones, C. B., & Bernard, S. (2005). Quality indicators sensitive to nurse staffing in acute care settings. In K. Henriksen, J. B. Battles, E. S. Marks, & D. I. Lewin (Eds.), *Advances in patient safety: From research to implementation* (Vol. 4: Programs, Tools, and Products). Rockville, MD: Agency for Healthcare Research and Quality.

Sax, P., Cohen, C., & Kuritzkes, D. (2012). *HIV essentials*. Boston, MA: Jones & Bartlett.

*Scardillo, J., & Aronovitch, S. A. (1999). Successfully managing incontinence-related irritant dermatitis across the lifespan. *Ostomy Wound Management*, *45*(4), 36–44.

Schachter, S. (2015). Evaluation of the first seizure in adults. In *UpToDate*. Retrieved from http://www.uptodate.com /contents/evaluation-of-the-first-seizure-in-adults

Schachter, S. C. (2016). Overview of the management of epilepsy in adults. In *UpToDate*. Retrieved from http://www .uptodate.com/contents/overview-of-the-management-of-epilepsy-in-adults

Schira, M. (2008a). The kidney: Anatomy and physiology. In C. S. Counts (Ed.), *Core curriculum for nephrology nursing* (5th ed., pp. 4–32). Pitman, NJ: American Nephrology Nurses' Association.

Schira, M. (2008b). The kidney: Pathophysiology. In C. S. Counts (Ed.), *Core curriculum for nephrology nursing* (5th ed., pp. 33–62). Pitman, NJ: American Nephrology Nurses' Association.

*Schmelz, J. O., Johnson, D., Norton, J. M., Andrews, M., & Gordon, P. A. (1999). Effects of position of chest drainage tube on volume drained and pressure. *American Journal Of Critical Care*, *8*(5), 319–323.

Schmidt, A., & Mandel, J. (2012). Management of severe sepsis and septic shock in adults. In *UpToDate*. Retrieved from http://www.uptodate.com/contents/management-of-severe-sepsis-and-septic-shock-in-adults

*Schmidt, L. M. (2004). Herbal remedies: The other drugs your patients take [Electronic version]. *Home Healthcare Nurse*, *22*(3), 169–175. Retrieved from http://www.gateway.tx.ovid.com.library.geu.edu:2048/gw2/ovidweb.cgi

Schmitt, S. K. (2015). Treatment and prevention of osteomyelitis following trauma in adults. In *UpToDate*. Retrieved from http: //www.uptodate.com/contents/treatment-and-prevention-of-osteomyelitis-following-trauma-in-adults?source=related_link

*Schmulson, M. J., Ortiz-Garrido, O. M., Hinojosa, C., & Arcila, D. (2006). A single session of reassurance can acutely improve the self-perception of impairment in patients with IBS. *Journal of Psychosomatic Research*, *61*(4), 461–467.

Schneidman, A., Reinke, L., Donesky, D., & Carrieri-Kohlman, V. (2014). Patient information series. Sudden breathlessness crisis. *American Journal of Respiratory and Critical Care Medicine*, *189*(5), P9–P10.

*Schoenfelder, D. P., & Crowell, C. M. (1999). From risk for trauma to unintentional injury risk: Falls—A concept analysis. *International Journal of Nursing Terminologies and Classifications*, *10*(4), 149–157. Retrieved from http://www.nanda.org

Schonder, K., & Cincotta, E. (2008). Pharmacologic aspects of chronic kidney disease. In C. Counts (Ed.), *Core curriculum for nephrology nursing* (5th ed.). American Nephrology Nurses' Association.

*Schulman, M., Lowe, L. H., Johnson, J., Neblett, W. W., Polk, D. B., Perez, R., Jr., . . . Cywes, R. (2001). In vivo visualization of pyloric mucosal hypertrophy in infants with hypertrophic pyloric stenosis: Is there an etiologic role? *American Journal of Roentgenology*, *177*(4), 843–848.

*Schummer, W., Schummer, C., & Schelenz, C. (2003). Case report: The malfunctioning implanted venous access device [Electronic version]. *British Journal of Nursing*, *12*(4), 210–214. Retrieved from http://www.web.ebscohost.com/ehost /pdf?vid=139&hid=106&sid=c7e5d2b4-a693-4480-a27f-fdf75c59b820%40session mgr106

Schur, P. H. (2015). Neurologic manifestations of systemic lupus erythematosus. In *UpToDate*. Retrieved from http://www.uptodate.com/contents/neurologic-manifestations-of-systemic-lupus-erythematosus?source=search_result&search=neurological++complications+with+lupus&selectedTitle=1~150

Schur, P. H., Ravinder, N., Maini, R. N., & Gibofsky, A. (2014). Nonpharmacologic therapies and preventive measures for patients with rheumatoid arthritis. In *UpToDate*. Retrieved from http://www.uptodate.com/contents/nonpharmacologic-therapies-and-preventive-measures-for-patients-with-rheumatoid-arthritis?source=see_link

*Schwamm, L. H., Pancioli, A., Acker, J. E., Goldstein, L. B., Zorowitz, R. D., Shephard, T. J., . . . American Stroke Association's Task Force on the Development of Stroke Systems. (2005). Recommendations for the establishment of stroke systems of care: Recommendations from the American Stroke Association's Task Force on the development of stroke systems. *Stroke, 36*, 690–703.

Schweickert, W. D., Pohlman, M. C., Pohlman, A. S., Nigos, C., Pawlik, A. J., Esbrook, C. L., . . . & Schmidt, G. A. (2009). Early physical and occupational therapy in mechanically ventilated, critically ill patients: A randomised controlled trial. *Lancet (London, England), 373*(9678), 1874–1882.

Schyve, P. M. (2007). Language differences as a barrier to quality and safety in health care: the Joint Commission perspective. *Journal of General Internal Medicine, 22*(2), 360–361.

Seamon, M. J., Wobb, J., Gaughan, J. P., Kulp, H., Kamel, I., & Dempsey, D. T. (2012). The effects of intraoperative hypothermia on surgical site infection: An analysis of 524 trauma laparotomies. *Annals of Surgery, 255*(4), 789–795.

Selius, B. A., & Subedi, R. (2008). Urinary retention in adults: Diagnosis and initial management. *American Family Physician, 77*(5), 643–650. Retrieved from http://www.aafp.org/afp/2008/0301/p643.html

Sengupta, S. (2015). Post-operative pulmonary complications after thoracotomy. *Indian Journal of Anaesthesia, 59*(9), 618–626.

Sesler, J. M. (2007). Stress-related mucosal disease in the intensive care unit: An update on prophylaxis. *AACN Advanced Critical Care, 18*(2), 119–128.

Seymour, C. W., Liu, V. X., Theodore J., Iwashyna, T. J., Brunkhorst, F. M., Rea, T. D., . . . Angus, D. C. (2016). Assessment of clinical criteria for sepsis for the third international consensus definitions for sepsis and septic shock (Sepsis-3). *JAMA, 315*(8), 762–774. Retrieved from http://www.jama.jamanetwork.com/article.aspx?articleid=2492875#Results

Shadgan, B., Menon, M., Sanders, D., Berry, G., Martin, C., Jr., Duffy, P., . . . Stephen D. (2010). Current thinking about acute compartment syndrome of the lower extremity. *Canadian Journal of Surgery, 53*(5), 329–334.

Shafir, A., & Rosenthal, J. (2012). *Shared decision making: Advancing patient-centered care through state and federal implementation*. Informed Medical Decisions Foundation. Retrieved from http://www.nashp.org/sites/default/files/shared.decision.making.report.pdf

Shah, A. K., & Goldenberg, W. D. (2016). Myasthenia gravis. In *Medscape*. Retrieved from http://emedicine.medscape.com/article/1171206-overview

Shaikh, N. (2009). Emergency management of fat embolism syndrome. *Journal of Emergency Trauma and Shock, 2*(1), 29–33.

Shariat, S. F., Bochner, B. H., & Donahue, T. F. (2015). Urinary diversion and reconstruction following cystectomy. In *UpToDate*. Retrieved from http://www.uptodate.com/contents/urinary-diversion-and-reconstruction-following-cystectomy

Shatzer, M. B., George, E. L., & Wei, L. (2007). To pump or not to pump? *Critical Care Nursing Quarterly, 30*(1), 67–73.

Shaughnessy, K. (2007). Massive pulmonary embolism. *Critical Care Nurse, 27*(1), 39–51.

*Sheahan, S. L. (2002). How to help older adults quit smoking [Electronic version]. *Nurse Practitioner, 27*(12), 27–34. Retrieved from http://www.web.ebscohost.com/ehost/results?vid=14&hid=106&sid=c7e5d2b4-a3-4480-a27f-fdf75c59b820%40sessionmgr106

Shear, M. K. (2012). Grief and mourning gone awry: Pathway and course of complicated grief *Dialogues in Clinical Neuroscience, 14*(2), 119–128.

*Shelton, B. K. (2005). Infection. In C. H. Yarbo, M. H. Frogge, & M. Goodman (Eds.), *Cancer nursing: Principles and practice* (6th ed.). Boston, MA: Jones & Bartlett.

Shepherd, A. (2011). Practical care: Feeding and assisting residents to eat. *Nursing and Residential Care, 13*(10), 487–489.

*Sheppard, C. M., & Brenner, P. S. (2000). The effects of bathing and skin care practices on skin quality and satisfaction with an innovative product. *Journal of Gerontological Nursing, 26*(10), 36–45.

Sheth, K. (2007). *Increased intracranial pressure*. Retrieved from http://www.nlm.nih.gov/medlineplus/ency/-article/000793.htm

*Shigehiko, U., Kellum, J., Bellomo, R., Doig, G., Morimatsu, H., Morgera, S., . . . Ronco, C. (2005). Acute renal failure in critically ill patients. *Journal of the American Medical Association, 294*(7), 813–818.

*Shipes, E. (1987). Psychosocial issues: The person with an ostomy. *Nursing Clinics of North America, 22*(2), 291–302.

*Shirato, S. (2005). How CAM helps systemic lupus erythematosus. *Holistic Nursing Practice, 19*(1), 36–39.

Shreve, J., Van Den Bos, J., Gray, T., Halford, M., Rustagi, K., & Ziemkiewicz, E. (2010). *The economic measurement of medical errors*. (Published by Society of Actuaries' Health Section and sponsored by Milliman, Inc). Retrieved from https://www.soa.org/files/research/projects/research-econ-measurement.pdf

Sickle Cell Disease Association of America. (2016). *Fact sheet*. Retrieved from https://www.cdc.gov/ncbddd/sicklecell/index.html

*Siedliecki, S. L., & Good, M. (2006). Effect of music on power, pain, depression and disability. *Journal of Advanced Nursing, 54*(5), 553–562.

Siegel, J. D., Rhinehart, E., Jackson, M., Chiarello, L., & The Healthcare Infection Control Practices Advisory Committee. (2007, June). *2007 guideline for isolation precautions: Preventing transmission of infectious agents in healthcare settings.* Retrieved from http://www.cdc.gov/ncidod/dhqp/pdf/isolation2007.pdf

Siegel, R., Ward, E., Brawley, O., & Jemal, A. (2011). The impact of eliminating socioeconomic and racial disparities on premature cancer deaths. *Cancer Journal for Clinicians, 61*(4), 212–236.

*Sieggreen, M. (2006). A contemporary approach to peripheral arterial disease. *Nurse Practitioner, 31*(7), 14–25.

Sieggreen, M. (2007). Recognize acute arterial occlusion. *Nursing Critical Care, 2*(5), 50–59.

Silvestry, F. E. (2016). Postoperative complications among patients undergoing cardiac surgery. In *UpToDate*. Retrieved from http://www.uptodate.com/contents/postoperative-complications-among-patients-undergoing-cardiac-surgery

Simkin, P., & Ancheta, R. (2011). *The labor progress book: Early interventions to prevent and treat dystocia* (3rd ed.). New York, NY: Wiley-Blackwell.

*Simkin, P., & Bolding, A. (2004). Update on nonpharmacologic approaches to relive labor pain and prevent suffering. *Journal of Midwifery & Women's Health, 49*(6), 489–504.

*Simmons, S. F., & Levy-Storms, L. (2005). The effect of dining location on nutritional care quality in nursing homes. *Journal of Nutrition Health and Aging, 9*(6), 434–439.

Simons, F. E. (2015). Patient education: Anaphylaxis symptoms and diagnosis (Beyond the Basics). In *UpToDate*. Retrieved from http://www.uptodate.com/contents/anaphylaxis-symptoms-and-diagnosis-beyond-the-basics#H1

Simpson, K. R., & Creehan, P. A. (2014). *Perinatal nursing* (4th ed.). Philadelphia, PA: Lippincott Williams & Wilkins.

*Sims, J. M. (2006). An overview of asthma [Electronic version]. *Dimensions of Critical Care Nursing, 25*(6), 264–268. Retrieved from http://www.gateway.tx.ovid.com.library.gcu.edu:2048/gw2/ovidweb.cgi

*Singer, L. T., Salvator, A., Guo, S., Collin, M., Lilien, L., & Baley, J. (1999). Maternal psychological distress and parenting stress after the birth of a very low-birth-weight infant. *JAMA, 281*(9), 799–805.

*Singer, P., & Martin, D. (1999). Quality of life care patient's perspectives. *The Journal of the American Medical Association, 281*(2), 166–168.

Sjogren's Syndrome Foundation. (2008). *Home page*. Retrieved from http://www.sjogrens.org

*Skillman, J. J., Bushnell, L. S., Goldman, H., & Silen, W. (1969). Respiratory failure, hypotension, sepsis, and jaundice: A clinical syndrome associated with lethal hemorrhage from acute stress ulceration of the stomach. *American Journal of Surgery, 117*(4), 523–530.

*Slater, J. E. (1989). Rubber anaphylaxis. *New England Journal of Medicine, 320*(17), 1126–1130.

Slavin, J. (2008). Position of the American Dietetic Association: Health implications of dietary fiber. *Journal of American Dietetic Association, 108*, 1716–1731.

Smeltzer, S., & Bares, B. (2008). *Textbook of medical-surgical nursing* (10th ed.). Philadelphia, PA: Lippincott Williams & Wilkins.

Smith, E. R., & Amin-Hanjani, S. (2013). Evaluation and management of elevated intracranial pressure in adults. In *UpToDate*. Retrieved from http://www.uptodate.com/contents/evaluation-and-management-of-elevated-intracranial-pressure-in-adults

Smith, M. (2007). Intensive care management of patients with subarachnoid hemorrhage. *Current Opinion in Anesthesiology, 20*(5), 400–407.

Smith, M., Robinson, L., & Segal, R. M. A. (2012). *Memory loss and aging: Causes, treatment, and help for memory problems*. Retrieved from http://www.helpguide.org/articles/memory/age-related-memory-loss.htm

Smith, P. P., McCrery, R. J., & Appell, R. A. (2006). Current trends in the evaluation and management of female urinary incontinence. *Canadian Medical Association Journal, 175*(10), 1233–1240.

Smith, W. R., & Scherer, M. (2010). Sickle-cell pain: Advances in epidemiology and etiology. *American Society of Hematolgy: Education Book*, (1), 409–415. doi:10.1182/asheducation-2010.1.409

Smith, W. R., McClish, D. K., Dahman, B. A., Levenson, J. L., Aisiku, I. P., de A Citero, V., . . . Roseff, S. D. (2015). Daily home opioid use in adults with sickle cell disease: The PiSCES project. *Journal of Opioid Management, 11*(3), 243.

*Smith-DiJulio, K. (2001). Rape. In E. Varcarolis (Ed.), *Foundations of psychiatric mental health nursing* (4th ed.). Philadelphia, PA: W. B. Saunders.

Smith-DiJulio, K. (2006). Care of the Chemically Impaired. In E. M. Varcarolis, V. B. Carson, & N. C. Shoemaker (Eds.), *Foundations of psychiatric mental health nursing* (5th ed.). New York, NY: Elsevier.

*Snyder, M. (1983). Relation of nursing activities to increases in intracranial pressure. *Journal of Advanced Nursing, 8*(4), 273–279. Retrieved from http://www.onlinelibrary.wiley.com/doi/10.1111/j.1365-2648.1983.tb00326.x/abstract

Society for Vascular Nursing. (2014). *Circulating the facts about peripheral arterial disease: Lower extremity amputations*. Menomonee Falls WI: Society for Vascular Nursing.

*Söderberg, A., Gilje, F., & Norberg, A. (1998). Dignity in situations of ethical difficulty in ICU. *Intensive Critical Care Nursing Journal Palliative Care, 14*(1), 36–42.

Sofaer, S., & Schumann, M. J. (2013). *Fostering successful patient and family engagement Nursing's critical role*. This white paper was prepared for the nursing alliance for quality care with grant support from the agency for healthcare research and quality (AHRQ). Retrieved from http://www.naqc.org/WhitePaper-PatientEngagement

*Soholt, D. (1990). *A life experience: Making a health care treatment decision* (Unpublished master's thesis). Brookings, SD: South Dakota State University.

*Solomon, J., Yee, N., & Soulen, M. (2000). Aortic stent grafts: An overview of devices, indications and results. *Applied Radiology Supplement*, *29*(7, Suppl. 1), 43–51.

Sørensen, L. T. (2012). Wound healing and infection in surgery: The pathophysiological impact of smoking, smoking cessation, and nicotine replacement therapy: A systematic review. *Annals of Surgery*, *255*(6), 1069–1079.

*Sotir, M. J., Lewis, C., Bisher, E. W., Ray, S. M., Soucie, M., & Blumberg, H. M. (1999). Epidemiology of device—Associated infections related to a long-term implantable vascular access device. *Infection Control and Hospital Epidemiology*, *20*(3), 187–191.

*South Carolina Department of Disabilities and Special Needs. (2006). *Nursing management of seizures*. Retrieved from http://nursingpub.com/nursing-care-for-seizures

Speaar, M. (2008). Wound care management: Risk factors for surgical site infections. *Plastic Surgical Nursing*, *28*(4), 201–204.

Speranza-Reid, J. E. (2015a). Hemodialysis: The hemodialysis treatment. In C. S. Counts (Ed.), *Core curriculum for nephrology nursing: Module 3. Treatment options for patients with chronic kidney failure* (6th ed., pp. 114–122). Pitman, NJ: American Nephrology Nurses' Association.

Speranza-Reid, J. E. (2015b). Hemodialysis: Complications of hemodialysis: Prevention and management. In C. S. Counts (Ed.), *Core curriculum for nephrology nursing: Module 3. Treatment options for patients with chronic kidney failure* (6th ed., pp. 136–155). Pitman, NJ: American Nephrology Nurses' Association

*Speros, C. (2004). Health literacy: Concept and analysis. *Journal of Advanced Nursing*, *50*(6), 633–640.

Spies, L. (2009). Diarrhea A to Z: America to Zimbabwe. *Journal of the American Academy of Nurse Practitioners*, *21*(6), 307–313.

Spiller, R. (2008). Review article: Probiotics and prebiotics in irritable bowel syndrome. *Alimentary Pharmacology & Therapeutics*, *28*, 385–396.

Spiller, R., & Garsed, K. (2009). Postinfectious irritable bowel syndrome. *Gastroenterology*, *136*(6), 1979–1988.

Stajduhar, K. I., Martin, W. L., & Barwich, D. (2008). Factors influencing family caregivers ability to cope with providing end-of-life cancer at home. *Cancer Nursing: An International Journal for Cancer Care*, *31*(1), 77–85.

Stanbridge, R., Hon, J. K. F., Bateman, E., & Roberts, S. (2007). Minimally invasive anterior thoracotomy for routine lung cancer resection. *Innovations*, *2*(2), 76–83.

Stanford Medicine. (2009). *Laboratory critical/panic value list*. Pathology & Laboratory Medicine. Retrieved from http://www.stanfordlab.com/pages/panicvalues.htm

*Stanley, M. M., Ochi, S., Lee, K. K., Nemchausky, B. A., Greenlee, H. B., Allen, J. I., . . . Camara, D. S. (1989). Peritoneovenous shunting as compared with medical treatment in patients with alcoholic cirrhosis and massive ascites. *New England Journal of Medicine*, *321*(24), 1632–1638.

*Starling, B. P., & Martin, A. C. (1990). Adult survivors of parental alcoholism: Implications for primary care. *Nursing Practice*, *15*(7), 16–24.

*Starnes, D. N., & Sims, T. W. (2006). Care of the patient undergoing robotic-assisted prostatectomy. *Urology Nursing*, *26*(2), 129–136.

*Starnes, D. N., & Sims, T. W. (2006). Robotic prostatectomy surgery. *Urologic Nursing*, *26*(2), 138–140.

Starr, S. P., & Raines, D. (2011). Cirrhosis: Diagnosis, management, and prevention. *American Family Physician*, *84*(12), 1353–1359.

Stawski, R. S., Mogle, J. A., & Sliwinski, M. J. (2013). Daily stressors and self-reported changes in memory in old age: The mediating effects of daily negative affect and cognitive interference. *Aging & Mental Health*, *17*(2), 168–172. Retrieved from http://www.ncbi.nlm.nih.gov/pmc/articles/PMC3652656/

*Steeves, R. H. (1992). Patients who have undergone bone marrow transplantation: Their quest for meaning. *Oncology Nursing Forum*, *19*(6), 899–905.

Stein, J. (2008). Stroke. In W. R. Frontera, J. K. Silver, & T. D. Rizzo, Jr. (Eds.), *Essentials of physical medicine and rehabilitation* (2nd ed., Chapter 149). Philadelphia, PA: Saunders.

Stein, P. D., Beemath, A., Matta, F., Weg, J. G., Yusen, R. D., Hales, C. A., . . . & Buckley, J. D. (2007). Clinical characteristics of patients with acute pulmonary embolism: data from PIOPED II. *The American Journal of Medicine*, *120*(10), 871–879.

Stephany, K., & Murkowski, P. (2015). *The ethic of care: A moral compass for Canadian nursing practice*. Oak Park, IL: Bentham Science Publishers.

Sterns, R. H. (2015). Disorders of plasma sodium—Causes, consequences, and correction. *The England Journal of Medicine*, *372*(1), 55–65.

Stoller, J. K. (2015). Management of exacerbations of chronic obstructive pulmonary disease. In *UpToDate*. Retrieved from http://www.uptodate.com/contents/management-of-exacerbations-of-chronic-obstructive-pulmonary-disease

*Stone, M. S., Bronkesh, S. J., Gerbarg, Z. B., & Wood, S. D. (1998). Improving patient compliance. *Strategic Medicine*. Retrieved from https://novoed.com/mhealth/reports/50424

*Story, K. T. (2006). Malignant pleural effusion. In M. Kaplin (Ed.), *Understanding and managing oncologic emergencies: A resource for nurses* (pp. 123–155). Pittsburgh, PA: Oncology Nursing Society.

Stracciolini, A., & Hammerberg, E. M. (2014). Acute compartment syndrome of the extremities. In *UpToDate*. Retrieved from http://www.uptodate.com/contents/acute-compartment-syndrome-of-the-extremities

Strate, L. (2015a). Etiology of lower gastrointestinal bleeding in adults. In *UpToDate*. Retrieved from http://www.uptodate.com/contents/etiology-of-lower-gastrointestinal-bleeding-in-adults

Strate, L. (2015b). Approach to acute lower gastrointestinal bleeding in adults. In *UpToDate*. Retrieved from http://www.uptodate.com/contents/approach-to-acute-lower-gastrointestinal-bleeding-in-adults?source=see_link

*Streitberger, K., Diefenbacher, M., Bauer, A., Conradi, R., Bardenheuer, H., Martin, E., . . . Unnebrink, K. (2004). Acupuncture compared to placebo-acupuncture for postoperative nausea and vomiting prophylaxis: A randomised placebo-controlled patient and observer blind trial. *Anaesthesia*, *59*(2), 142–149.

*Streitberger, K., Witte, S., Mansmann, U., Knauer, C., Krämer, J., Scharf, H. P., . . . Victor, N. (2004). Efficacy and safety of acupuncture for chronic pain caused by gonarthrosis: a study protocol of an ongoing multi-centre randomized controlled clinical trial [ISRCTN27450856]. *BMC Complementary and Alternative Medicine*, *4*(1), 1.

Strobik, Y. (2007). Protocols, practice and patients: The case of alcohol withdrawal. *Critical Care Medicine*, *35*(3), 955.

Strobl, R. A. (2009). Radiation therapy. In S. Newton, M. Hickey, & J. Marrs (Eds.), *Mosby's oncology nursing advisor: A comprehensive guide to clinical practice* (p. 141). St. Louis, MO: Mosby Elsevier.

Stroke Association. (2012). *Communication problems after a stroke*. Retrieved from http://www.stroke.org.uk/sites/default/files/Communication%20problems%20after%20stroke.pdf

*Stuart, G. W., & Sundeen, S. (2002). *Principles and practice of psychiatric nursing* (6th ed.). St. Louis, MO: Mosby-Year Book.

Stubbs, B., & Dickens, B. (2008). Prevention and management of aggression in mental health: An interdisciplinary discussion. *International Journal of Therapy and Rehabilitation*, *15*(8), 351–357.

Su, Y. H., & Ryan-Wenger, N. A. (2007). Children's adjustment to parental cancer: A theoretical model development. *Cancer Nursing*, *30*(5), 362–381.

Subedi, B., & Grossberg, G. T. (2011). Phantom limb pain: Mechanisms and treatment approaches. *Pain Research and Treatment*, *2011*, 864605. doi:10.1155/2011/864605

Sublett, C. M. (2007). Critique of "Effects of advanced practice nursing on patient and spouse depressive symptoms, sexual function, and marital interaction after radical prostatectomy." *Urology Nursing*, *27*(1), 78–80.

Substance Abuse and Mental Health Services Administration. (2014). *Alcohol facts and statistics*. Retrieved from https://www.niaaa.nih.gov/alcohol-health/overview-alcohol-consumption/alcohol-facts-and-statistics

Such, J., & Runyon, B. A. (2016). Ascites in adults with cirrhosis: Diuretic-resistant ascites. In *UpToDate*. Retrieved from http://www.uptodate.com/contents/ascites-in-adults-with-cirrhosis-diuretic-resistant-ascites?source=machineLearning&search=%E2%80%9CRefractory+ascites&selectedTitle=3~150&sectionRank=1&anchor=H5#H5

*Sullivan, M. J., & Hawthorne, M. H. (1996). Nonpharmacologic interventions in the treatment of heart failure. *Journal of Cardiovascular Nursing*, *10*(2), 47–57.

*Sullivan, J. T., Sykora, K., Schneiderman, J., Naranjo, C. A., & Sellers, E. M. (1989). Assessment of alcohol withdrawal: the revised clinical institute withdrawal assessment for alcohol scale (CIWA☒Ar). *British Journal of Addiction*, *84*(11), 1353–1357.

*Sullivan, M. J., Reesor, K., Mikail, S., & Fisher, R. (1992). The treatment of depression in chronic low back pain: Review and recommendations. *Pain*, *50*(1), 5–13. Retrieved from http://www.ncbi.nlm.nih.gov/pubmed/1387469

*Support Study. (1995). The SUPPORT prognostic model. Objective estimates of survival for seriously ill hospitalized adults. Study to understand prognoses and preferences for outcomes and risks of treatments. *Annals of Internal Medicine*, *122*(3), 191–203.

Susan, B., & Komen for the Cure. (2007a). *Lymphedema*. Retrieved from http://www.cms.komen.org/komen/aboutbreastcancer/aftertreatment/3-6-3?ssSourceNodeld=301&ssSourceSiteld=Komen

Susan, B., & Komen for the Cure. (2007b). *Sex and sexuality*. Retrieved from http://www.cms.komen.org/komen/aboutbreastcancer/aftertreatment/3-3-4?ssSourceNodeld=301&ssSourceSiteld=Komen

*Sussman, G., & Gold, M. (1996). *Guidelines for the management of latex allergies and safe latex use in health care facilities*. Arlington Heights, IL: American College of Allergy, Asthma & Immunology. http://acaai.org/allergies/types/skin-allergies/latex-allergy

Sutton, E. J., Davidson, J. E., & Bruce, I. N. (2013). The systemic lupus international collaborating clinics (SLICC) damage index: a systematic literature review. *Seminars in Arthritis and Rheumatism*, *43*(3), 352.

Suzuki, K., Miyamoto, M., Miyamoto, T., Iwanami, M., & Hirata, K. (2011). Sleep disturbances associated with Parkinson's disease. *Parkinson's Disease*, *2011*, 219056. doi:10.4061/2011/219056

Swadener-Culpepper, L. (2010). Continuous lateral rotation therapy. *Critical Care Nurse*, *30*(2), S5–S7. Retrieved from Medline Database.

Swanson, J., & Koch, L. (2010). The role of the oncology nurse navigator in distress management of adult in patients with cancer: A retrospective study. *Oncology Nursing Forum*, *37*(1), 69–76.

*Swanson, K. M. (1991). Empirical development of a middle range theory of caring. *Nursing Research*, *40*, 161–166.

*Swanson, M. C. (2004). Encouraging adherence to treatment regimen in a CCPD patient. *Nephrology Nursing Journal*, *31*(1), 80.

*Symes, L. (2000). Arriving at readiness to recover emotionally after sexual assault. *Archives of Psychiatric Nursing*, *14*(1), 30–38.

Tang, N. K. Y., Wright, K., & Salkovskis, P. M. (2007). Prevalence and correlates of clinical insomnia co-occurring with chronic pain. *Journal of Sleep Research*, *16*(1), 85–95.

Tanner, D., & Culbertson, W. (2014). Avoiding negative dysphagia outcomes. *OJIN: The Online Journal of Issues in Nursing*, *19*(2).

Tapasi, S., & Harmeet, S. (2007). Noninfectious complications of peritoneal dialysis. *Southern Medical Journal*, *100*(1), 54–58.

Tarr, J. M., Kaul, K., Chopra, M., Kohner, E. M., & Chibber, R. (2013). Pathophysiology of diabetic retinopathy. *ISRN Ophthalmology*, *2013*, 343560.

Tarsy, D. (2015a). Patient education: Parkinson disease treatment options — education, support, and therapy (Beyond the Basics). In *UpToDate*. Retrieved from http://www.uptodate.com/contents/parkinson-disease-treatment-options-education-support-and-therapy-beyond-the-basics?source=search_result&search=exercise++and+parkinson%27s&selectedTitle=4~150

Tarsy, D. (2015b). Pharmacologic treatment of Parkinson disease. In *UpToDate*. Retrieved from http://www.uptodate.com/contents/pharmacologic-treatment-of-parkinson-disease?source=machineLearning&search=Long-Term+Levodopa+Treatment+Syndrome&selectedTitle=1~150&sectionRank=3&anchor=H4#H4

Tattersall, J. E., & Daugirdas, J. T. (2011). Preparing for dialysis. In J. T. Daugirdas (Ed.), *Handbook of chronic kidney disease management*. Philadelphia, PA: Lippincott Williams & Wilkins.

*Taylor, J. (1993). *Discretion versus policy rules in practice*. Retrieved from http://web.stanford.edu/~johntayl/Papers/Discretion.PDF

*Tewari, A., Peabody, J., Sarle, R., Balakrishnan, G., Hemal, A., Shrivastava, A., . . . Menon, M. (2002). Technique of Da Vinci robot-assisted anatomic radical prostatectomy. *Urology*, *60*(4), 569–572.

*Thakar, R., Ayers, S., Clarkson, P., Stanton, S., & Manyonda, I. (2002). Outcomes after total versus subtotal abdominal hysterectomy. *New England Journal of Medicine*, *347*(17), 1318–1325.

Thomas, M., Corbin, R., & Leung, L. (2014, January-February). Effects of ginger for nausea and vomiting in early pregnancy: A meta-analysis. *Journal of American Board Family Medicine*, *27*(1), 115–122.

Thompson, B. T. (2015). Clinical presentation, evaluation, and diagnosis of the adult with suspected acute pulmonary embolism. In *UpToDate*. Retrieved from http://www.uptodate.com/contents/clinical-presentation-evaluation-and-diagnosis-of-the-adult-with-suspected-acute-pulmonary-embolism

*Thompson, C., & Fuhrman, M. P. (2005). Nutrients and wound healing: Still searching for the magic bullet. *Nutrition in Clinical Practice*, *20*(3), 331–347.

Thompson, C., Aitken, L., Doran, D., & Dowding, D. (2013). An agenda for clinical decision making ad judgement in nursing research and education. *Nursing Studies*, *50*(12), 1720–1726.

*Thompson, F. E., Midthune, D., Subar, A. F., McNeel, T., Berrigan, D., & Kipnis, V. (2005). Dietary intake estimates in the National Health Interview Survey, 2000: methodology, results, and interpretation. *Journal of the American Dietetic Association*, *105*(3), 352–363.

Thompson, H. J., & Maui, K. L. (Eds). (2012). *Nursing management of the patient with multiple sclerosis AANN, ARN, and IOMSN clinical practice guideline series*. Retrieved from http://www.rehabnurse.org/uploads/cpgms.pdf

Thompson, M. A., Mugavero, M. J., Amico, K. R., Cargill, V. A., Chang, L. W., Gross, R., . . . Nachega, J. B. (2012). Guidelines for improving entry into and retention in care and antiretroviral adherence for persons with HIV: Evidence-based recommendations from an International Association of Physicians in AIDS Care panel. *Annals of Internal Medicine*, *156*(11), 817–833. Retrieved from http://www.ncbi.nlm.nih.gov/pubmed/22393036

*Thompson, P., Langemo, D., Anderson, J., Hanson, D., & Hunter, S. (2005). Skin care protocols for pressure ulcers and incontinence in long-term care: a quasi-experimental study. *Advances in Skin & Wound Care*, *18*(8), 422–429.

Thompson, V. L. (2013). Making decisions in a complex information environment: Evidential preference and information we trust BMC. *Medical Informatics and Decision*, *13*(Suppl. 3), S7.

*Tilden, V. P., & Weinert, C. (1987). Social support and the chronically ill individual. *Nursing Clinics of North America*, *22*(3), 613–620.

Timmerman, R. A. (2007). A mobility protocol for critically ill adults. *Dimensions of Critical Care Nursing*, *26*(5), 175–179. Retrieved from http://www0.sun.ac.za/Physiotherapy_ICU_algorithm/Documentation/Rehabilitation/References/Timmerman_2007.pdf

*Timoney, J. P., Eagan, M. M., & Sklarin, N. T. (2003). Establishing clinical guidelines for the management of acute hypersensitivity reactions secondary to the administration of chemotherapy/biologic therapy. *Journal of Nursing Care Quality*, *18*(1), 80–86.

Tinkham, M. R. (2015). Care of the endovascular aneurysm repair patient with an endoleak. *OR Nurse*, *7*(3), 32–40. Retrieved from http://www.nursingcenter.com/cearticle?an=01271211-201305000-00009

Tisminetzky, M., Bray, B. C., Miozzo, R., Aupont, O., & McLaughlin, T. (2012). Classes of depression, anxiety, and functioning in acute coronary syndrome patients. *American Journal of Health Behavior*, *36*(1), 20–30.

*Titler, M., Dochterman, J., Xie, X., Kanak, M., Fei, Q., Picone, D., . . . Shever, L. (2006). Nursing interventions and other factors associated with discharge disposition in elderly patients after hip surgery. *Nursing Research*, *55*(4), 231–242.

*Torpy, J., Glass, T. J., & Glass, R. M. (2005). Myasthenia gravis. *Journal of the American Medical Association*, *293*(15), 1940.

Townsend, C. M., Beauchamp, R. D., Evers, B. M., & Mattox, K. L. (Eds.). (2012). *Sabiston textbook of surgery* (19th ed.). St. Louis, MO: W. B. Saunders.

Toy, P. C. (2012). General principles of amputations. In S. T. Canale & J. H. Beaty, (Eds.), *Campbell's operative orthopaedics* (12th ed., Chapter 14). Philadelphia, PA: Mosby Elsevier.

Treadwell, M. J., Barreda, F., Kaur, K., & Gildengorin, G. (2015). Emotional distress, barriers to care, and health-related quality of life in sickle cell disease. *Journal of Clinical Outcomes Management, 22*(1), 10–21.

Trinka, E., Cock, H., Hesdorffer, D., Rossetti, A. O., Scheffer, I. E., Shinnar, S., . . . Lowenstein, D. H. (2015). A definition and classification of status epilepticus—Report of the ILAE task force on classification of status epilepticus. *Epilepsia. 56*(10), 1515–1523.

Troiano, N. H., Harvey, C. J., & Chez, B. F. (2013). *High-risk & critical care obstetrics* (3rd ed.). Philadelphia, PA: Lippincott Williams & Wilkins.

*Truscott, W. (1995). The industry perspective on latex. *Immunology and Allergy Clinics of North America, 15*(1), 89–115.

*Tucker, D., Molsberger, S. C., & Clark, A. (2004). Walking for wellness: A collaborative program to maintain mobility in hospitalized older adults. *Geriatric Nursing, 25*(4), 242–245.

Turban, S., & Miller, E. R., 3rd. (2011). Sodium and potassium intake. In J. T. Daugirdas (Ed.), *Handbook of chronic kidney disease management*. Philadelphia, PA: Lippincott Williams & Wilkins.

Turner, J. R. (2010). The gastrointestinal tract. In V. Kumar, A. K. Abbas, & N. Fausto (Eds.), *Robbins and Cotran pathologic basis of disease* (8th ed., pp. 763–831). Philadelphia, PA: Saunders Elsevier.

Tzeng, H. M. (2010). Understanding the prevalence of inpatient falls associated with toileting in adult acute care settings. *Journal of Nursing Care Quality, 25*(1), 22–30.

*U.S. Department of Health and Human Services. (1992). *Management and therapy of sickle cell disease* (NIH Publication No. 92-2117). Washington, DC: Author.

U.S. Department of Justice. (2014). *Rape and sexual assault*. Retrieved from www.bjs.gov/index.cfm?ty=tp&tid=317

*U.S. National Library of Medicine. (2006). *Osteomyelitis*. Retrieved from http://www.nlm.nih.gov/medlineplus/ency/article/000437.htm

*Underwood, C. (2004). How can we best deliver an inclusive health service? *Primary Health Care, 14*(9), 20–21.

*United Ostomy Association. (2006). *Urostomy: A guide*. Retrieved from http://www.cancer.org/docroot/CRI/content/CRI_2_6x_Urostomy.asp

University of Michigan Health System. (2007). *Instructions for care following conventional prostatectomy/Robotic prostatectomy*. Retrieved from http://www.med.umich.edu/1libr/urology/postcare/rprostatectomy.htm

*Unruh, L. Y., & Fottler, M. D. (2006). Patient turnover and nursing staff adequacy. *Health Services Research, 41*(2), 599–612.

*Urbano, F. (2001). Homans' sign in the diagnosis of deep venous thrombosis. *Hospital Physician, 3*, 22–24. Retrieved from http://www.turner-white.com

Uren, S. A., & Graham, T. M. (2013). Subjective experiences of coping among caregivers in palliative care. *Online journal of issues in nursing, 18*(1), 88.

Urinary Retention. (2012, June). Retrieved from http://www.kidney.niddk.nih.gov/kudiseases/pubs/UrinaryRetention/

*Vacco v. Quill–521 U.S. 793. (1997). *Assisted suicide*. Retrieved from http://www.supreme.justia.com/cases/federal/us/521/793/

Vakil, N. B. (2014). Epidemiology and etiology of peptic ulcer disease. In *UpToDate*. Retrieved from http://www.uptodate.com/contents/epidemiology-and-etiology-of-peptic-ulcer-disease?source=search_result&search=peptic+ulcer+etiology&selectedTitle=1~150

Vakil, N. B. (2015a). Peptic ulcer disease: Management. In *UpToDate*. Retrieved from http://www.uptodate.com/contents/peptic-ulcer-disease-management

Vakil, N. B. (2015b). Peptic ulcer disease: Clinical manifestations and diagnosis. In *UpToDate*. Retrieved from http://www.uptodate.com/contents/peptic-ulcer-disease-clinical-manifestations-and-diagnosis

*Valente, S. (2004). End-of-life challenges: Honoring autonomy. *Cancer Nursing: An International Journal for Cancer Care, 27*(4), 314–319.

*van Goor, H., & Boontje, A. H. (1995). Results of vascular reconstructions for atherosclerotic arterial occlusive disease of the lower limbs in young adults. *European Journal Vascular and Endovascular Surgery, 10*(3), 323–326.

van Kimmenade, R. R. J., & Januzzi, J. L., Jr. (2011). Heart failure. In J. T. Daugirdas (Ed.), *Handbook of chronic kidney disease management*. Philadelphia, PA: Lippincott Williams & Wilkins.

van Ramshorst, G. H., Nieuwenhuizen, J., Hop, W. C. J., Arends, P., Broom, J., Jeekel, J., . . . Lange, J. H. (2010). Abdominal wound dehiscence in adults: Development and validation of a risk model. *World Journal of Surgery, 34*(1), 20–27.

*Vanezis, M., & McGee, A. (1999). Mediating factors in the grieving process of the suddenly bereaved. *British Journal of Nursing, 8*(14), 932–937.

Varcarolis, E. M. (2011). *Manual of psychiatric nursing care planning* (4th ed.). St. Louis, MO: Saunders.

*Varcarolis, E. M., Carson, V. B., & Shoemaker, N. C. (2006). *Foundations of psychiatric mental health nursing: A clinical approach* (5th ed.). St. Louis, MO: Elsevier.

Vasavada, S. (2013). Urinary incontinence. In *Medscape*. Retrieved from http://emedicine.medscape.com/article/452289-overview

Vasdev, N., Moon, A., & Thorpe, A. C. (2013). Metabolic complications of urinary intestinal diversion. *Indian Journal of Urology, 29*(4), 310.

Vassar, T., Batenjany, M., Kooman, W., & Ricci, M. (2008). Nursing issues. In J. F. Howard (Ed.), *Myasthenia gravis: A manual for health care providers* (pp. 32–53). St. Paul, MN: Myasthenia Gravis Foundation of America.

*Vasterling, J., Jenkins, R. A., Tope, D. M., & Burish, T. G. (1993). Cognitive distraction and relaxation training for the control of side effects due to cancer chemotherapy. *Journal of Behavioral Medicine, 16*(1), 65–80.

Vasudevan, J. M., Baheti, N. D., Naber, R. I., & Fredericson, M. (2012). Physiotherapy, pain management, and surgical interventions for low back pain: Initial review. *Current Sports Medicine Reports, 11*(1), 35–42.

Vege, S. S. (2014a). Predicting the severity of acute pancreatitis. In *UpToDate*. Retrieved from http://www.uptodate.com/contents/predicting-the-severity-of-acute-pancreatitis

Vege, S. S. (2014b). Pathogenesis of acute pancreatitis. In *UpToDate*. Retrieved from http://www.uptodate.com/contents/pathogenesis-of-acute-pancreatitis?source=machineLearning&search=respiratory+complications+of+pancreatitis&selectedTitle=2~150&sectionRank=2&anchor=H8#H8

Vege, S. S. (2015). Etiology of acute pancreatitis. In *UpToDate*. Retrieved from http://www.uptodate.com/contents/etiology-of-acute-pancreatitis

Venables, P. J. W., & Maini, R. N. (2016). Disease outcome and functional capacity in rheumatoid arthritis. In *UpToDate*. Retrieved from http://www.uptodate.com/contents/disease-outcome-and-functional-capacity-in-rheumatoid-arthritis?source=machineLearning&search=prognosis+in+RA&selectedTitle=1~150&sectionRank=2&anchor=H7#H7

Vere-Jones, E. (2007). Nursing the survivors of sexual assault. *Nursing Times, 103*(35), 18–19.

*Vermeer, S., Hollander, M., van Dijk, E., Hofman, A., Koudstaal, P., Breteler, M., . . . The Rotterdam Scan Study. (2001). Silent brain infarcts and white matter lesions increase stroke risk in the general population. *Stroke, 34*, 1126–1129.

*Vernava, A. M., 3rd, Moore, B. A., Longo, W. E., & Johnson, F. E. (1997). Lower gastrointestinal bleeding. *Diseases of the Colon & Rectum, 40*(7), 846–858.

Vichinsky, E. P. (2014). Overview of the clinical manifestations of sickle cell disease. In *UpToDate*. Retrieved from http://www.uptodate.com/contents/overview-of-the-clinical-manifestations-of-sickle-cell-disease?source=search_result&search=sickle+cell+disease+adult&selectedTitle=2~150

Vichinsky, E. P., & Mahoney, D. H. (2014). Diagnosis of sickle cell disorders. In *UpToDate*. Retrieved from http://www.uptodate.com/contents/diagnosis-of-sickle-cell-disorders

Vinik, A. I., Erbas, T., & Casellini, C. M. (2013). Diabetic cardiac autonomic neuropathy, inflammation and cardiovascular disease. *Journal of Diabetes Investigation, 4*(1), 4–18.

*Vinik, A. I., Maser, R. E., Mitchell, B. D., & Freeman, R. (2003). Diabetic autonomic neuropathy. *Diabetes Care, 26*(5), 1553–1579.

Virani, A., Werunga, J., Ewashen, C., & Green, T. (2015). Caring for patients with limb amputation. *Nursing Standard, 30*(6), 51–60.

*Volker, D. (2000). Palliative sedation and terminal weaning are ethical and realistic interventions in a percentage of dying patients whose symptoms remain unbearable despite aggressive palliative. *Clinical Journal of Oncology Nursing, 7*, 653–667, 668.

Volland, J., & Fisher, A. (2014). Best practices for engaging patients with dementia. *Nursing, 44*(11), 44–50.

Vollman, K. M. (2012). Hemodynamic instability: Is it really a barrier to turning critically ill patients? *Critical Care Nurse, 32*(1), 70–75.

van der Ploeg, E. S., Walker, H., & O'Connor, D. W. (2014). The feasibility of volunteers facilitating personalized activities for nursing home residents with dementia and agitation. *Geriatric Nursing, 35*(2), 142–146.

van Rompaey, B., Elseviers, M. M., Van Drom, W., Fromont, V., & Jorens, P. G. (2012). The effect of earplugs during the night on the onset of delirium and sleep perception: a randomized controlled trial in intensive care patients. *Critical Care, 16*(3), R73.

von Jürgensonn, S. (2010). Prevention and management of air in an IV infusion system. *British Journal of Nursing (Intravenous supplement), 19*(10), S28–S30.

*Wagner, K. D., Johnson, K., & Kidd, P. S. (2006). *High acuity nursing* (4th ed.). Upper Saddle River, NJ: Prentice Hall.

Wald, A. (2014). Pathophysiology of irritable bowel syndrome. In *UpToDate*. Retrieved from http://www.uptodate.com/contents/pathophysiology-of-irritable-bowel-syndrome

Wald, A. (2015). Patient information: Constipation in adults (Beyond the Basics). In *UpToDate*. Retrieved from http://www.uptodate.com/contents/constipation-in-adults-beyond-the-basics#H1

Walker, C., Hogstel, M. O., & Curry, L. (2007). Hospital discharge of older adults: How nurses can ease the transition. *The American Journal of Nursing, 107*(6), 60–70.

Walker, T. G., Kalva, S. P., Yeddula, K., Wicky, S., Kundu, S., Drescher, P., . . . Canadian Interventional Radiology Association. (2010). Clinical practice guidelines for endovascular abdominal aortic aneurysm repair. Written by the Standards of Practice Committee for the Society of Interventional Radiology and Endorsed by the Cardiovascular and Interventional Radiological Society of Europe and the Canadian Interventional Radiology Association. *Journal of Vascular International Radiology, 21*(11), 1632–1655.

Wallace, D. J. (2015). Overview of the management and prognosis of systemic lupus erythematosus in adults. In *UpToDate*. Retrieved from http://www.uptodate.com/contents/overview-of-the-management-and-prognosis-of-systemic-lupus-erythematosus-in-adults

*Walsh, K., & Kowanko, I. (2002). Nurses' and patients' perceptions of dignity. *International Journal of Nursing Practice*, 8(3), 143–151.

*Walsh, P. C., Marschke, P., Ricker, D., & Burnett, A. L. (2000). Patient-reported urinary continence and sexual function after anatomic radical prostatectomy. *Urology*, 55(1), 58–61.

Walshe, M. (2014). Oropharyngeal dysphagia in neurodegenerative disease. *Journal of Gastroenterology and Hepatology Research*, 3(10), 1265–1271. Retrieved from http://www.ghrnet.org/index.php/joghr/article/view/883

Walters, M. D. (2016). Choosing a route of hysterectomy for benign disease. In *UpToDate*. Retrieved from http://www.uptodate.com/contents/choosing-a-route-of-hysterectomy-for-benign-disease

Walton, J. (2015). The kidney in health and injury: Chronic kidney disease. In C. S. Counts (Ed.), *Core curriculum for nephrology nursing: Module 2. Physiologic and psychosocial basis for nephrology nursing practice* (6th ed., pp. 117–152). Pitman, NJ: American Nephrology Nurses' Association.

Walton, L., & Nottingham, J. M. (2007). Palliation of malignant ascites. *Journal of Surgical Education*, 64(1), 4–9.

Wanke, C. (2015). Approach to the adult with acute diarrhea in resource-rich countries. In *UpToDate*. Retrieved from http://www.uptodate.com/contents/approach-to-the-adult-with-acute-diarrhea-in-resource-rich-countries

Warnick, A. L. (2015). Supporting youth grieving the dying or death of a sibling or parent: considerations for parents, professionals, and communities. *Current Opinion in Supportive and Palliative Care*, 9(1), 58–63.

*Warrington, T., & Bostwick, M. (2006). Psychiatric adverse effects of corticosteroids. *Mayo Clinic Proceedings*, 81(10), 1361–1367.

*Washington v. Glucksberg. (1997). Legatal Information Institute. Retrieved from http://www.law.cornell.edu/supct/html/historics/USSC_CR_0521_0702_ZO.html

Wasserman, A. M. (2011). Diagnosis and management of rheumatoid arthritis. *American Family Physician*, 84(11), 1245–1252.

Weathers, E., McCarthy, G., & Coffey, A. (2016). Concept analysis of spirituality: an evolutionary approach. *Nursing Forum*, 51(2), 79–96.

*Weaver, T., & Narsavage, G. (1992). Physiological and psychological variables related to functional status in chronic obstructive pulmonary disease. *Nursing Research*, 41(5), 286–291.

Webb, D. (2015). The latest on lactose intolerance: What it is, how it's diagnosed, and tips for counselling clients. *Today's Dietitian*, 17(5), 38.

Weeks, J. C., Catalano, P. J., Cronin, A., Finkelman, M. D., Mack, J. W., Keating, N. L., & Schrag, D. (2012). Patients' expectations about effects of chemotherapy for advanced cancer. *New England Journal of Medicine*, 367, 1616–1625.

Weeks, S. R., Anderson-Barnes, V. C., & Tsao, J. W. (2010). Phantom limb pain: Theories and therapies. *The Neurologist*, 16(5), 277–286.

Weinhouse, G. L. (2015). Stress ulcer prophylaxis in the intensive care unit. In *UpToDate*. Retrieved from http://www.uptodate.com/contents/stress-ulcer-prophylaxis-in-the-intensive-care-unit

Weinhouse, G. L. (2016). Fat embolism syndrome. In *UpToDate*. Retrieved from http://www.uptodate.com/contents/fat-embolism-syndrome?source=search_result&search=fat+embolism&selectedTitle=1~58

Weinstein, J. N., Tosteson, T. D., Lurie, J. D., Tosteson, A. N., Hanscom, B., Skinner, J. S., . . . Deyo, R. A. (2006). Surgical vs nonoperative treatment for lumbar disk herniation: The Spine Patient Outcomes Research Trial (SPORT): A randomized trial. *JAMA*, 296(20), 2441–2450.

Weisberg, J. N., & Boatwright, B. A. (2007). Mood, anxiety and personality traits and states in chronic pain. *Pain*, 133(1–3), 1–2.

Weissman, D. (2009). *What is palliative care?* Retrieved from http://www.getpalliativecare.org

*Welch, P., Porter, J., & Endres, J. (2003). Efficacy of a medication pass supplement program in the long term-care compared to a traditional system. *Journal of Nutrition in Elderly*, 22(3), 19–29.

Wendell, L. C, & Levine, J. M. (2011). Myasthenic crisis. *Neurohospitalist*, 1(1), 16–22.

*Whelton, S. P., Chin, A., Xin, X., & He, J. (2002). Effect of aerobic exercise on blood pressure: A meta-analysis of randomized, controlled trials. *Annals of Intern Medicine*, 136(7), 493–503.

*White, C. (1998). Psychological management of stoma related concerns. *Nursing Standard*, 12(36), 35–38. Retrieved from http://www.ncbi.nlm.nih.gov/pubmed/9732612

*White, S. (2003). *Assessing the Nation's Health Literacy: Key concepts and findings of the National Assessment of Adult Literacy (NAAL).* Retrieved July 26, 2013, from http://s3.amazonaws.com/zanran_storage/www.ama-assn.org/ContentPages/11339828.pdf

Wilde, M. H., Bliss, D. Z., Booth, J., Cheater, F. M., & Tannenbaum, C. (2014). Self-management of urinary and fecal incontinence. *The American Journal of Nursing*, 114(1), 38–45.

*Wilkins, K. L., McGrath, P. J., Finley, G. A., & Katz, J. (2004). Prospective diary study of nonpainful and painful phantom sensations in a preselected sample of child and adolescent amputees reporting phantom limbs. *The Clinical Journal of Pain*, 20(5), 293–301.

Wilkinson, J., & Van Leuven, K. (2007). *Fundamentals of nursing: Theory, concepts & applications*. Philadelphia, PA: F. A. Davis.

Willett, C. (Ed.). (n.d.). *UpToDate*. Retrieved from http://www.uptodateonline.com

Williams, H. F. (2015). Continuous renal replacement therapies. In C. S. Counts (Ed.), *Core curriculum for nephrology nursing: Module 4. Continuous renal replacement therapies* (6th ed., pp. 161–210). Pitman, NJ: American Nephrology Nurses' Association.

Williams, H. F., Bogle, J. L., & Davey-Tresemer, J. (2008). Acute kidney injury and acute renal failure. In C. S. Counts (Ed.), *Core curriculum for nephrology nursing* (5th ed., pp. 144–175). Pitman, NJ: American Nephrology Nurses' Association.

Williams, J. Z., & Barbul, A. (2003). Nutrition and wound healing. *Surgical Clinics of North America, 83*(3), 571–596.

Williams, L. S., Brizendine, E. J., Plue, L., Bakas, T., Tu, W., Hendrie, H., . . . Kroenke, K. (2005). Performance of the PHQ-9 as a screening tool for depression after stroke. *Stroke, 36*(3), 635–638.

*Williams, M. V., Parker, R. M., Baker, D. W., Parikh, N. S., Pitkin, K., Coates, W. C., & Nurss, J. R. (1995). Inadequate functional health literacy among patients at two public hospitals. *JAMA, 274*(21), 1677–1682.

Williamson, M. A., Snyder, L. M., & Wallach, J. B. (2011). *Wallach's interpretation of diagnostic tests* (9th ed.). Philadelphia, PA: Lippincott Williams & Wilkins.

Williamson, M. T., & Snyder, L. M. (2014). *Wallach's interpretation of diagnostic tests: Pathways to arriving at a clinical diagnosis* (10th ed.). Philadelphia, PA: Lippincott Williams & Wilkins.

*Wilson, J. A., & Clark, J. J. (2004). Obesity: Impediment to postsurgical wound healing. *Advances in Skin & Wound Care, 17*(8), 426–435.

*Wilson, K. G., Eriksson, M. Y., D'Eon, J. L., Mikail, S. F., & Emery, P. C. (2002). Major depression and insomnia in chronic pain. *Clinical Journal of Pain, 18*(2), 77–83.

Wilson, L. D., Detterbeck, F. C., & Yahalom, J. (2007). Clinical practice: Superior vena cava syndrome with malignant causes. *New England Journal of Medicine, 356*(18), 1862–1869.

Wilson, P. W. (2015). Overview of the risk equivalents and established risk factors for cardiovascular disease. In *UpToDate*. Retrieved from http://www.uptodate.com/contents/overview-of-the-risk-equivalents-and-established-risk-factors-for-cardiovascular-disease

*Wilson, P., Berghmans, B., Hagen, S., Hay-Smith, J., Moore, K., Nygaard, I., . . . Wyman, J. (2005). *Adult conservative management in incontinence. Incontinence, volume 2: Management*. Paris: International Continence Society Health Publication.

Wingerchuk, D. M. (2012). Smoking: effects on multiple sclerosis susceptibility and disease progression. *Therapeutic Advances in Neurological Disorders, 5*(1), 13–22.

Winkelman C., & Peereboom K. (2010). Staff-perceived barriers and facilitators. *Critical Care Nurse, 30*(2), 13–16.

*Witting, M. D., Magder, L., Heins, A. E., Mattu, A., Granja, C. A., & Baumgarten, M. (2006). Usefulness and validity of diagnostic nasogastric aspiration in patients without hematemesis. *Annals of Emergency Medicine, 43*(4), 280–285. Retrieved from http://www.ncbi.nlm.nih.gov/pubmed/16635697

Wolf, M., Bäumer, P., Pedro, M., Dombert, T., Staub, F., Heiland, S., . . . Pham, M. (2014). Sciatic nerve injury related to hip replacement surgery: Imaging detection by MR neurography despite susceptibility artifacts. *PloS One, 9*(2), e89154.

*Women's Health. (2005). *Women's support center for rape victims*. Retrieved from http://www.womenshealth.gov

Woodbury, M. G., Hayes, K. C., & Askes, H. K. (2008). Intermittent catheterization practices following spinal cord injury: A national survey. *Canadian Journal Urology, 15*(3), 4065–4071.

*Worden, W. (2002). *Grief counseling and grief therapy* (3rd ed.). New York, NY: Springer Publishing Company.

World Health Organization. (2011). *World Health Statistics 2011*. Retrieved from http://www.who.int/whosis/whostat/2011

World Health Organization. (2013). *Asthma*. Retrieved from http://www.who.int/mediacentre/factsheets/fs307/en/

World Health Organization. (2014). *Mental health: A state of well-being*. Retrieved from http://www.who.int/features/factfiles/mental_health/en/

World Health Organization. (2016). *WHO definition of palliative care*. Retrieved from http://www.who.int/cancer/palliative/definition/en/

The World Society of the Abdominal Compartment Syndrome. (2013). *Intra-abdominal hypertension and the abdominal compartment syndrome: Updated consensus definitions and clinical practice guidelines from the World Society of the Abdominal Compartment Syndrome*. Retrieved from http://www.wsacs.org/images/2013%20Guidelines%20slide%20set.pdf

*Wound Ostomy Continence Nursing. (2003). *Guideline for prevention and management of pressure ulcers*. Glenview, IL: Author.

Wound, Ostomy, and Continence Nurses Society. (2010). *Guideline for prevention and management of pressure ulcers* (p. 96, WOCN Clinical Practice Guideline No. 2). Mt. Laurel, NJ: Author.

Wound, Ostomy and Continence Nurses Society. (2014). *WOCN society and ASCRS position statement on preoperative stoma site marking for patients undergoing colostomy or ileostomy surgery*. Mt. Laurel, NJ: Author.

*Wright, L. M. (2004). *Spirituality, suffering, and illness: Ideas for healing*. Philadelphia, PA: F. A. Davis.

Wright, J. D., Hughes, J. P., Ostchega, Y., Yoon, S. S., & Nwankwo, T. (2011). *Mean systolic and diastolic blood pressure in adults aged 18 and over in the United States, 2001–2008* (National health statistics reports no 35). Hyattsville, MD: National Center for Health Statistics.

Wright, M., Wood, J., Lynch, T., & Clark, D. (2008). Mapping levels of palliative care development: A global view. *Journal of Pain and Symptom Management, 35*(5), 469–485.

Wright, P. M., & Hogan, N. S. (2008). Grief theories and models: Applications to hospice nursing practice. *Journal of Hospice & Palliative Nursing, 10*(6), 350–355.

Wu, L., Li, W., Hu, Z., Rao, N. Y., Song, C. G., Zhang, B., . . . Shao, Z. M. (2008). The prevalence of BRCA1 and BRCA2 germline mutations in high-risk breast cancer patients of Chinese Han nationality: Two recurrent mutations were identified. *Breast Cancer Research and Treatment, 110*(1), 99–109.

Xu, J., Murphy, S. L., Kochanek, K. D., & Bastian, B. A. (2016). Deaths: Final data for 2013. *National Vital Statistics Reports, 64*(2), 1–119.

*Yakimo, R., (2006). Perspectives on psychiatric consultation liaison nursing. *Perspectives in Psychiatric Care, 42*(1), 59–62.

*Yakimo, R., Kurlowicz, L. H., & Murray, R. B. (2004). Evaluation of outcomes in psychiatric consultation-liaison nursing practice. *Archives of Psychiatric Nursing, 18*(6), 215–227.

Yaklin, K. M. (2011). Acute kidney injury: An overview of pathophysiology and treatments. *Nephrology Nursing Journal, 38*(1), 13–18.

Yang, N. Y., Zhou, D. R., Li-Tsang, C., & Fong, K. (2013). Rehabilitation interventions for unilateral neglect after stroke: A systematic review from 1997 through 2012. *Frontiers in Human Neuroscience, 7*, 187. doi:10.3389/fnhum.2013.00187

Yanoff, J., & Duker, M. (2009). *Ophthalmology* (3rd ed.). New York, NY: Mosby.

Yarbro, C., Wujeck, D., & Gobel, B. (2011). *Cancer nursing: Principles and practice* (7th ed.). Boston, MA: Jones & Bartlett.

*Yates, J. K., Sawczuk, I. S., & Munver, R. (2003). Complications of laparoscopic and robotic radical prostatectomy prevention & management (Chapter 71). *In Prevention and management of laparoendoscopic surgical complications* (3rd ed.). Maimi, FL: Society of Laparoendoscopic Surgeons

*Yates, P. C. (1993). Toward a reconceptualization of hope for patients with a diagnosis of cancer. *Journal of Advanced Nursing, 18*(4), 701–708.

Yazicioglu, K., Taskaynatan, M. A., Guzelkucuk, U., & Tugcu, I. (2007). Effect of playing football (soccer) on balance, strength, and quality of life in unilateral below-knee amputees. *American Journal of Physical Medicine and Rehabilitation, 86*(10), 800–805.

Yealy, D. M., & Fine, M. J. (2015). Community-acquired pneumonia in adults: Risk stratification and the decision to admit. In *UpToDate*. Retrieved from http://www.uptodate.com/contents/community-acquired-pneumonia-in-adults-risk-stratification-and-the-decision-to-admit

*Yetzer, E. A. (1996). Helping the patient through the experience of an amputation. *Orthopaedic Nursing, 15*(6), 45–49.

*Yosipovitch, G., & Hundley, J. L. (2004). Practical guidelines for relief of itch. *Dermatology Nursing, 16*(4), 325–328.

*Young, M. G. (2001). Providing care for the caregiver. *Patient Care for the Nurse Practitioner, 2*, 36–47.

Young, M. P. (2015). Complications of central venous catheters and their prevention. In *UpToDate*. Retrieved from http://www.uptodate.com/contents/complications-of-central-venous-catheters-and-their-prevention?source=see_link&sectionName=Venous+air+embolism&anchor=H15#H15

*Yount, S., & Schoessler, M. (1991). A description of patient and nurse perceptions of preoperative teaching. *Journal of Post Anesthesia Nursing, 6*(1), 17–25.

Yun, Y. H., Kwon, Y. C., Lee, M. K., Lee, W. J., Jung, K. H., Do, Y. R., . . . Park, S. Y. (2010). Experiences and attitudes of patients with terminal cancer and their family caregivers toward the disclosure of terminal illness. *Journal of Clinical Oncology, 28*(11), 1950–1957.

Zagaria, M. E. (2011). Acute pancreatitis: Risks, causes, and mortality in older adults. *US Pharmacist, 36*(12), 24–27.

*Zalon, M. (2004). Correlates of recovery among older adults after major abdominal surgery. *Nursing Research, 53*(2), 99–106.

Zeller, J., Lynm, C., & Glass, R. M. (2007). Septic arthritis. *Journal of the American Medical Association, 297*(13), 1510.

Zero, D. T., Brennan, M. T., Daniels, T. E., Papas, A., Stewart, C., Pinto, A., . . . Sjögren's Syndrome Foundation Clinical Practice Guidelines Committee. (2016). Clinical practice guidelines for oral management of Sjögren disease. *Journal of the American Dental Association, 147*(4), 295–305.

Zia, J. K., Barney, P., Cain, K. C., Jarrett, M. E., & Heitkemper, M. M. (2016). Comprehensive self-management irritable bowel syndrome program produces sustainable changes in behavior after 1 year. *Clinical Gastroenterology and Hepatology, 14*(2), 212.e2–219.e2.

Zidan, J., Hussein, O., Abzah, A., Tamam, S., & Farraj, Z. (2008). Oral premedication for the prevention of hypersensitivity reactions to paclitaxel. *Medical Oncology, 25*(3), 274–278.

Zijdenbos I. L., de Wit, N. J., van der Heijden, G. J., Rubin, G., & Quartero, A. O. (2009). Psychological treatments for the management of irritable bowel syndrome. *Cochrane Database Systematic Reviews*, (1), CD006442. doi:10.1002/14651858.CD006442.pub2

Zisman, A. L., Worcester, E. M., & Coe, F. L. (2011). Evaluation and management of stone disease. In J. T. Daugirdas (Ed.), *Handbook of chronic kidney disease management* (pp. 482–492). Philadelphia, PA: Lippincott Williams & Wilkins.

Zomorodi, M., Topley, D., & McAnaw, M. (2012). Developing a mobility protocol for early mobilization of patients in a surgical/trauma ICU. *Critical Care Research and Practice, 2012*. Retrieved from http://www.hindawi.com/journals/ccrp/2012/964547/

*Zozula, R., & Rosen, R. (2001). Compliance with continuous positive airway pressure therapy: assessing and improving treatment outcomes. *Current Opinion Pulmonary Medicine, 7*(6), 391–398.

Appendix A

Nursing Diagnoses Grouped by Functional Health Pattern[1]

1. Health Perception–Health Management

[2,3]Engagement, Compromised
[2,3]Engagement, Risk for Compromised
Falls, Risk for
[3]Corneal Injury, Risk for
[3]Obesity
   [3]Overweight
   [3]Overweight, Risk for
Health Management, Ineffective

2. Nutritional–Metabolic

Adverse Reaction to Iodinated Contrast
   Media, Risk for
Fluid Volume, Deficient
Fluid Volume, Excess
Infection, Risk for
[2]Infection Transmission, Risk for
Latex Allergy Response
   Latex Allergy Response, Risk for
Nutrition, Imbalanced
Oral Mucous Membrane, Impaired
   [3]Oral Mucous Membrane, Risk for
     Impaired
[3]Pressure Ulcer, Risk for

3. Elimination

Bowel Incontinence
Constipation
Diarrhea
Urinary Elimination, Impaired
  [2]Continuous Urinary Incontinence

Functional Urinary Incontinence
Overflow Urinary Incontinence
Stress Urinary Incontinence

4. Activity–Exercise

Activity Intolerance
Disuse Syndrome, Risk for
Mobility, Impaired Physical
[2]Respiratory Function, Risk for
  Ineffective
[2]Self-Care Deficit Syndrome
  Feeding Self-Care Deficit
  Bathing Self-Care Deficit
  Dressing Self-Care Deficit
  [2]Instrumental Self-Care Deficit
  Toileting Self-Care Deficit
Sudden Infant Death Syndrome, Risk for
Tissue Perfusion, Ineffective (Specify
  Type)
  Cardiac Tissue Perfusion, Risk for
   Decreased
  Cerebral Tissue Perfusion, Risk for
   Ineffective
  Gastrointestinal Tissue Perfusion,
   Risk for Ineffective

5. Sleep–Rest

Sleep Pattern, Disturbed

6. Cognitive–Perceptual

Nausea
Pain, Acute

Pain, Chronic
[3]Pain, Labor
Decisional Conflict
Neglect, Unilateral

7. Self-Perception

Anxiety
  Anxiety, Death
Human Dignity, Risk for Compromised

8. Role–Relationship

[2]Communication, Impaired
  Communication, Impaired Verbal

9. Sexuality–Reproductive

10. Coping–Stress Tolerance

Coping, Compromised Family
Coping, Ineffective
  Denial, Ineffective
  Suicide, Risk for
Violence, Risk for Other-Directed

11. Value–Belief

Spiritual Distress
  Spiritual Distress, Risk for

---

[1]The Functional Health Patterns were identified in Gordon, M. (1994). *Nursing diagnosis: Process and application*. New York: McGraw-Hill, with minor changes by the author.
[2]These diagnoses are not currently in the NANDA-I taxonomy. They have been developed by the author.
[3]New NANDA-I Nursing Diagnoses 2015–2017

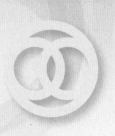

Appendix B

Nursing Admission Data Base

Nursing Admission Data Base

Date _____ Arrival Time _____ Contact Person _____ Phone _____

ADMITTED FROM: _____ Home alone   _____ Home with relative   _____ Long-term care facility

_____ Homeless   _____ Home with _____ (Specify)

_____ ER   _____ Other _____

MODE OF ARRIVAL: _____ Ambulatory _____ Wheelchair _____ Ambulance _____ Stretcher

REASON FOR HOSPITALIZATION:_____

_____

_____

Analysis: Does the individual understand why he is in the hospital?

LAST HOSPITAL ADMISSION: Date_____ Reason _____

_____

Analysis: Was this hospitalization related to the last admission?

PAST MEDICAL HISTORY:_____

_____

MEDICATION

(Prescription/Over-the-Counter)	DOSAGE	LAST DOSE	FREQUENCY

Analysis: Ask if taking the med and if missing doses? Why?

Health Maintenance–Perception Pattern

USE OF:

Tobacco: _____ None _____ Quit (date) _____ Smokeless _____ Pipe _____ Cigar _____ <1 pk/day

_____ 1–2 pks/day _____ >2 pks/day pks/year history _____

Want to quit? Have you tried to quit? When? How long?

Alcohol: _____ Date of last drink _____ Amount/Type

_____ No. of days in a month when alcohol is consumed

Should you cut down?

Drug Use: _____ No _____ Yes Type _____ Use _____

Would you like help?

Allergies (drugs, food, tape, dyes): _____ Reaction _____

_____

Side One

Activity–Exercise Pattern

SELF-CARE ABILITY:

0 = Independent   1 = Assistive device   2 = Assistance from others

3 = Assistance from person and equipment   4 = Dependent/Unable

	0	1	2	3	4
Eating/Drinking					
Bathing					
Dressing/Grooming					
Toileting					
Bed Mobility					
Transferring					
Ambulating					
Stair Climbing					
Shopping					
Cooking					
Home Maintenance					

ASSISTIVE DEVICES: ____ None ____ Crutches ____ Bedside commode ____ Walker
____ Cane ____ Splint/Brace ____ Wheelchair ____ Other

CODE: (1) Not applicable (2) Unable to acquire (3) Not a priority at this time
(4) Other (specify in notes)

Is it this person at risk for a complex transition?

Nutrition–Metabolic Pattern

Special Diet/Supplements _____

Previous Dietary Instruction: ____ Yes ____ No

Appetite: ____ Normal ____ Increased ____ Decreased ____ Decreased taste sensation
____ Nausea ____ Vomiting

Weight Fluctuations Last 6 Months: ____ None _____ lbs. Gained/Lost

Swallowing difficulty: ____ None ____ Solids ____ Liquids

Dentures: ____ Upper (___ Partial ___ Full) ____ Lower (___ Partial ___ Full)
With Person ____ Yes ____ No

History of Skin/Healing Problems: ____ None ____ Abnormal Healing ____ Rash
____ Dryness ____ Excess Perspiration

Elimination Pattern

Bowel Habits: ____ # BMs q ___/day ____ Date of last BM ____ Within normal limits
____ Constipation ____ Diarrhea ____ Incontinence
____ Ostomy: Type: ____ Appliance ____ Self-care ____ Yes ____ No

Bladder Habits: ____ WNL ____ Frequency ____ Dysuria ____ Nocturia ____ Urgency
____ Hematuria ____ Retention

Incontinence: ____ No ____ Yes ____ Total ____ Daytime ____ Nighttime
____ Occasional ____ Difficulty delaying voiding
____ Difficulty reaching toilet ____ Difficulty perceiving cues

Assistive Devices: ____ Intermittent catheterization
____ Indwelling catheter ____ External catheter
____ Incontinent briefs

Side Two

Sleep–Rest Pattern

Habits: ____ hrs/night ____ AM nap ____ PM nap
        Feel rested after sleep ____ Yes ____ No
Problems: ____ None ____ Early waking ____ Difficulty falling asleep ____ Nightmares

Cognitive–Perceptual Pattern

Mental Status: ____ Alert ____ Receptive aphasia ____ Poor historian
               ____ Oriented ____ Confused ____ Combative ____ Unresponsive
Speech: ____ Normal ____ Slurred ____ Garbled ____ Expressive aphasia
        Spoken language _____ Interpreter _____
Language Spoken: ____ English ____ Spanish ____ Other _____
Ability to Read English: ____ Yes ____ No _____
Ability to Communicate: ____ Yes ____ No ____ Verbally ____ Written ____ Interpreter_____
Ability to Comprehend: ____ Yes ____ No Memory intact ____ Yes ____ No____
Level of Anxiety: ____ Appropriate ____ Mild ____ Moderate ____ Severe ____ Panic
Interactive Skills: ____ Appropriate ____ Other _____
Hearing: ____ WNL ____ Impaired (____ Right ____ Left) ____ Deaf (____ Right ____ Left)
         _____ Hearing Aid

Is this individual capable to learning and performing self-care?

Vision: ____ WNL ____ Eyeglasses ____ Contact lens
        ____ Impaired ____ Right ____ Left
        ____ Blind ____ Right ____ Left
        ____ Prosthesis ____ Right ____ Left
Vertigo: ____ Yes ____ No
Discomfort/Pain: ____ None ____ Acute ____ Chronic ____ Description_____
_____
Pain Management: Meds, other therapies _____

Coping–Stress Tolerance/Self-Perception/Self-Concept Pattern

Major concerns regarding hospitalization or illness (financial, self-care): _____
Does the person need a referral to social servic-
es?_____
Major loss/change in past year: ____ No ____ Yes   Specify_____
Do you feel safe? ____ Yes ____ No Why? _____
CODE: (1) Not applicable (2) Unable to acquire (3) Not a priority at this time
      (4) Other (specify in notes)

Sexuality–Reproductive Pattern

LMP: _____ Gravida ____ Para_____ Birth Control _____
Menstrual/Hormonal Problems: ____ Yes ____ No _____
Last Pap Smear: _____ Hx of Abnormal PAP_____
Last Mammogram: _____ Last colonoscopy_____
Sexual Concerns: _____
_____

Role–Relationship Pattern

Single____ Married ____ Widowed ____ Divorced _____ Separated _____ Lives with _____
Occupation:_____
Employment Status: ____ Employed ____ Short-term disability ____ Long-term disability
                   ____ Unemployed

Side Three

Support System: _____ Spouse _____ Neighbors/Friends _____ None
_____ Support in same residence _____ Support in separate residence_____ Other
Will the person need assistance at home? How much? 24/7
Family concerns regarding hospitalization: _____
_____

Value–Belief Pattern

Religion: _____
Religious Restrictions: _____ No _____ Yes (Specify)_____
Request Chaplain Visitation at This Time: _____ Yes _____ No

PHYSICAL ASSESSMENT (Objective)

1. CLINICAL DATA
Age _____ Height _____ Weight _____ BMI Temperature_____
Pulse: _____ Strong _____ Weak _____ Regular _____ Irregular_____
Blood Pressure: Right Arm _____ Left Arm _____ Sitting _____ Lying _____

2. RESPIRATORY/CIRCULATORY
Rate_____
Quality: _____ WNL _____ Shallow _____ Rapid _____ Labored _____ Other_____
Cough: _____ No _____ Yes/Describe_____
Auscultation:
  Upper rt lobes _____ WNL _____ Decreased _____ Absent _____ Abnormal sounds _____
  Upper lt lobes _____ WNL _____ Decreased _____ Absent _____ Abnormal sounds _____
  Lower rt lobes _____ WNL _____ Decreased _____ Absent _____ Abnormal sounds _____
  Lower lt lobes _____ WNL _____ Decreased _____ Absent _____ Abnormal sounds _____
Right Pedal Pulse: _____ Strong _____ Weak _____ Absent
Left Pedal Pulse: _____ Strong _____ Weak _____ Absent

3. METABOLIC–INTEGUMENTARY
SKIN:
  Color: _____ WNL _____ Pale _____ Cyanotic _____ Ashen _____ Jaundice _____ Other _____
  Temperature: _____ WNL _____ Warm _____ Cool
  Edema: _____ No _____ Yes/Description/location_____
  Lesions: _____ None _____ Yes/Description/location_____
  Bruises: _____ None _____ Yes/Description/location_____
  Reddened: _____ No _____ Yes/Description/location_____
  Pruritus: _____ No _____ Yes/Description/location_____
  Is the person at risk for pressure ulcer?
MOUTH:
  Gums: _____ WNL _____ White plaque _____ Lesions _____ Other_____
  Teeth: _____ WNL _____ Other_____
ABDOMEN:
  Bowel Sounds: _____ Present _____ Absent

4. NEURO/SENSORY
Pupils: _____ Equal _____ Unequal describe
Reactive to light:
  Left: _____ Yes _____ No/Specify _____
  Right: _____ Yes _____ No/Specify _____
Eyes: _____ Clear _____ Draining _____ Reddened _____ Other_____

Side Four

5. MUSCULAR–SKELETAL

Range of Motion: _____ Full _____ Other Balance and Gait: _____ Steady _____ Unsteady

Hand Grasps: ____ Equal ____ Strong ____ Weakness/Paralysis (____ Right ____ Left)

Leg Strength: ____ Equal ____ Strong ____ Weakness/Paralysis (____ Right ____ Left)

6. OTHER SIGNIFICANT OBSERVATIONS

TRANSITION PLANNING

Intended Destination Posttransition: ____ Home ____ Undetermined ____ Other ____

Previous Utilization of Community Resources:

_____ Home care/Hospice ____ Adult day care ____ Church groups ____ Other _____

_____ Meals on Wheels ____ Homemaker/Home health aide ____ Community support group

Postdischarge Transportation:

____ Car ____ Ambulance ____ Bus/Taxi

____ Unable to determine at this time

Anticipated Financial Assistance Postdischarge?:____ No ____ Yes_____

Anticipated Problems with Self-care Postdischarge?: ____ No ____ Yes_____

Assistive Devices Needed Postdischarge?: ____ No ____ Yes_____

Referrals: (record date)

Discharge Coordinator_____Home Health_____

Social Service_____

SIGNATURE/TITLE _____ Date_____

Side Five

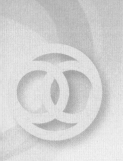

Appendix C

Strategies to Increase Motivation and Engagement in Individuals/Families

"Clinicians must recognize that the extent to which individual's and family members are able to engage or choose to engage may vary greatly based on individual circumstances, cultural beliefs and other factors" (Sofaer & Schumann, 2013).

"Activation refers to a person's ability and willingness to take on the role of managing their health and health care" (Hibbard & Cunningham, 2008).

 Carp's Cues

Health care professionals must quiet themselves regarding what they THINK a person or family needs to know. The goal is to find what information the individual wants to know; otherwise even the best teaching techniques will "fall on deaf ears."

Use Individual-Centered Practices
(Robinson, Callister, Berry, & Dearing, 2008)

R: "Strategies are needed to ensure that individuals/families are supported to become engaged, at the level they desire, instead of the status quo, in which they are rarely actively empowered and encouraged to engage in health care decisions, where preferences are rarely elicited, and where there is a lack of interest in how their life circumstances shape their priorities" (Frosch & Elwyn, 2014).

* Communication (direct information or sharing)
    * Direct information style to address simple complaints (e.g., take diuretic in morning to prevent sleep interruptions)
    * Sharing style to discuss chronic illness, life-style changes, or stressors (e.g., exploration of pattern of tobacco use and the specific harmful effects present now)

    R: A directing style is appropriate in communicating simple instructions for management but will be perceived as controlling when sharing discussions are warranted (Robinson et al., 2008).

    * Shared decision making

Personalized Information (Paper and Electronic) Reinforced by Professional or Lay Support (Coulter, 2012)

R: "Making the suggestion to lose 20 pounds, start going to the gym, and regularly take their hypertension medication to a person who has little understanding that they even have a chronic illness, the nature of that illness, or that they must play a part in managing it, is unlikely to result in the desired outcome" (Hibbard & Gilburt, 2014).

- Determines person's goal in treatment.
- Serves to identify barriers to adherence and solutions.

    R: "Starting with appropriate goals that fit the person's level of activation, and working toward increasing activation step by step, he/she can experience small successes and steadily build up the confidence and skill for effective self-management" (Hibbard & Gilburt, 2014).

- Support for self-management.
- Face-to-face: timely follow-up visits, progress reports, positive feedback
- Non face-to-face: print, intranet, telephone calls
- Low literacy: visual displays of information

    R: Positive outcomes have been reported when a variety of education interventions are utilized (Robinson et al., 2008).

- Accept that the person/family may appear resistant or not interested

    R: The potential for individuals to contribute to their safety by speaking up about their concerns depends heavily on the quality of patient–professional interactions and relationships (Entwistle et al., 2010).

- Offer praise for honesty about problems with compliance and for sharing reasons. For example:
  - "I'm glad you told me that you stopped taking Motrin because it made your stomach hurt. Now I understand why your hands still ache. Let's talk about other ways we can get you some comfort."
  - "It's good that you told me about your stopping the blood pressure pills. That explains your headaches and higher pressure today. Let's discuss how those pills made you feel."

    R: Individuals /Families "will only be successful in taking greater responsibility for their health care decisions and actions if they are well-nurtured in this process, consistently protected from making profoundly negative decisions along the way, and kept safe" (Sofaer & Schumann, 2013, p. 19).

- Self-monitoring is useful to determine positive and negative influences on compliance.
  - Daily records
  - Charts
  - Diary of progress or symptoms, clinical values (e.g., blood pressure), or dietary intake

    R: Involving the individual/family in decision-making places some responsibility on him or her to make sure the plan works, promoting engagement with treatment plan.

    R: Fostering successful engagement goes beyond information exchange to include skill- and capacity-building on the one hand, and embracing the engagement of individuals on the other. Some individuals and family members are pioneers—that is, they may be proactive even if no one encourages them—but most are not. Many persons who are ready to engage believe that they will engage at their peril, which clinicians and others will react negatively if they ask probing questions, disagree, suggest an alternative approach, ask for a second opinion, question an insurance company decision, or indicate dissatisfaction (Frosch, May, Rendle, Tietbohl, & Elwyn, 2012; Sofaer & Schumann, 2013).

    R: Further, the public and other health care team members may lack understanding of the knowledge and skills nurses possess, resulting in an undervaluing of the nurse's role. Even though patient-centered care and individual engagement are central to nursing theory and practice, for nurses to foster successful engagement effectively, nurses must often challenge other health professionals directly, requiring nurses to be viewed as fully credible as they exert their influence in the work environment on behalf of individuals. (Sofaer & Schumann, 2013)

Medication Reconciliation and Barriers to Adherence

Medication errors occur 46% of the time during transitions, admission, transfer, or discharge from a clinical unit/hospital. Almost 60% of individuals have at least one discrepancy in their medication history completed on admission. "The most common error (46.4%) was omission of a regularly used medication. Most (61.4%) of the discrepancies were judged to have no potential to cause serious harm. However, 38.6% of the discrepancies had the potential to cause moderate to severe discomfort or clinical deterioration" (*Cornish et al., 2005, p. 424).

Medication reconciliation on admission to the health care facilities often entails:

- Name of medication (prescribed, over the counter)
- Prescribed dose
- Frequency (daily, b.i.d., t.i.d., as needed)

A list of medications that have been prescribed by a provider does not represent a process of medication reconciliation. A family member recently took an older relative to the ER with chest pain. A typed list of her medications was given to the ER nurse. No discussion occurred about her medication.

Unfortunately, one of two hypertension medications she regularly took was not entered in the electronic health record. Since her blood pressure was elevated on admission and persisted, another antihypertensive medication was ordered. After two deep, another medication was added with good results.

The first medication that was added was the medication she was already taking prior to admission. So essentially, no new medication was added as a result of the error. She spent three unnecessary days in the hospital with increased costs to Medicare and would have definitely rather been home eating her own food and having a good night's sleep in her own bed.

According to the Joint Commission (2006, p. 1),

> Medication reconciliation is the process of comparing an individual's medication orders to all of the medications that the individual has been taking. This reconciliation is done to avoid medication errors such as omissions, duplications, dosing errors, or drug interactions. It should be done at every transition of care in which new medications are ordered or existing orders are rewritten. Transitions in care include changes in setting, service, practitioner, or level of care. The process comprises five steps: (1) develop a list of current medications; (2) develop a list of medications to be prescribed; (3) compare the medications on the two lists; (4) make clinical decisions based on the comparison; and (5) communicate the new list to appropriate caregivers to the individual.

Critical to acquiring a list of medications from credible sources PCP Office, Pharmacy, medication bottles, are the additional assessment questions, which are the defining elements for medication reconciliation: *"versus a list of medications reported to be taking."*

The individual/family member is asked the following:

For each medication reported ask:

- What is the reason you are taking each medication?
- Are you taking the medication as prescribed? Specify once a day, twice a day, etc.
- Are you skipping any doses? Do you sometimes run out of medications?
- How often are you taking the medication prescribed "if needed as a pain medication"?
- Have you stopped taking any of these medications?
- How much does it cost you to take your medications?
- Are you taking anybody else's medication?

Carp's Cues

Do not assume an individual can read and understand health literature even if translated.

Types of Literacy

Functional Illiteracy

- When someone who has minimal reading and writing skills does not have the capacity for health literacy to manage ordinary everyday needs and requirements of most employments.

Individuals who are illiterate (who cannot read or write) are easier to identify than someone who is functionally illiterate.

Health Literacy

Health literacy is the capacity to obtain, process, and understand basic health information and services needed to

- Make appropriate health decisions (*Ratzan & Parker, 2000)
- Follow instructions for treatments, medications (*White, 2003)
- Sign a consent form
- Make appointments

The National Assessment of Adult Literacy (NAAL) (*2003) reported that 9 out of 10 English-speaking adults in the United States do not have health literacy (*Kutner, Greenberg, Jiny, & Paulsen, 2006). A large study on the scope of health literacy at two public hospitals found (*Williams et al., 1995):

- Half of English-speaking individuals could not read and understand basic health education material
- 60% could not understand a routine consent form
- 26% could not understand the appointment card
- 42% failed to understand directions for taking their medications

The American Medical Association's (AMA) (*1999) committee of Health Literacy found inadequate health literacy was most prevalent in the elderly and individuals who report poor overall health. The report concluded that individuals who reported "the worst health status have less understanding about their medical conditions and treatment" (*AMA, 1999, p. 57).

Carp's Cues

"Social and educational levels have little relationship to health literacy" (*Speros, 2004, p. 638). Individuals will hide the literacy problems if allowed. Many individuals are at risk of understanding, but it is hard to identify them (DeWalt et al., 2010).

Table 1   Red Flags for Low Literacy
• Frequently missed appointments
• Incomplete registration forms
• Noncompliance with medication
• Unable to name medications, explain purpose, or dosing
• Identifies pills by looking at them, not reading label
• Unable to give coherent, sequential history
• Asks fewer questions
• Lack of follow-through on tests or referrals

Source: DeWalt, D. A., Callahan, L. F., Hawk, V. H., Broucksou, K. A., Hink, A., Rudd, R., & Brach, C. (2010, April). *Health literacy universal precautions toolkit* (Prepared by North Carolina Network Consortium, The Cecil G. Sheps Center for Health Services Research, The University of North Carolina at Chapel Hill, under Contract No. HHSA290200710014.) (AHRQ Publication No. 10-0046-EF). Rockville, MD: Agency for Healthcare Research and Quality.

The Complexity of the Health Care System

The health care system increasing the expectations of individuals to self-manage their conditions continues to increase in areas of (DeWalt et al., 2010):
- Self-assessment of health status (e.g., peak flow meters, glucose testing)
- Self-treatment (act on information) (e.g., insulin adjustments, wound care)
- Prevention (e.g., nutrition, exercise, dental care, cancer screenings)
- Access health care system (e.g., decisions to go to ER, when to call primary care, referral process, follow-up instructions, navigation of insurance/Medicare coverage)

Strategies to Improve Comprehension

Research shows that individuals remember and understand less than half of what clinicians explain to them (*Roter, Rune, & Comings, 1998; *Williams et al., 1995). Testing general reading levels do not ensure individual understanding in the clinical setting (*AMA, 2007).

Principles of Health Care Teaching

For comprehension to occur, the nurse must accept that there is limited time and that the use of this time is enhanced by:
- Using every contact time to teach something
- Creating a relaxed encounter
- Using eye contact
- Slowing down—break it down into short statements
- Limited content—focus on two or three concepts
- Using plain language (refer to Box 1)

Box 1 REPLACING MEDICAL JARGON/WORDS WITH PLAIN WORDS	
Medical Jargon/Words	Plain Words
Hepatic	Livers
Pulmonary function	Lungs
Medications	Pills
Nutrition	Food
Beverages	Drinks
Dermatologist	Skin doctor
Opthalmology	Eye doctor
Dermatitis	Rash

- Engaging individual/family in discussion
- Using graphics
- Explaining what you are doing to the individual/family and why
- Asking them to tell you about what you taught. Tell them to use their own words.

Use the Teach-Back Method

Refer to Chapter 4—Preparation of Individual/Family for Care at Home.

- Explain/Demonstrate
  - Explain one concept (e.g., medication, condition, when to call PCP)
  - Demonstrate one procedure (e.g., dressing charge, use of inhaler)
- Assess
  - I want to make sure, I explained _____ clearly, can you tell me _____
  - Tell me what I told you
  - Show me how to _____
  - Avoid asking: Do you understand?
- Clarify
  - Add more explanation if you are not satisfied the person understands or can perform the activity
  - If the person cannot report the information, don't repeat the same explanation; rephrase it

Carp's Cues

Be careful the person/family does not think you are testing him or her. Assure them it is important that you help them to understand that the teaching method can help you teach and also diagnose educational needs.

- Teach-Back Questions (Examples)
  - When should you call your PCP?
  - How do you know your incision is healing?
  - What foods should you avoid?
  - How often should you test your blood sugar?
  - What should you do for low blood sugar?
  - What weight gain should you report to your PCP?
  - Which inhaler is your rescue inhaler?
  - Is there something you have been told to do that you do not understand?
  - What should you bring to your PCP office?
  - Is there something you have a question about?

Carp's Cues

Use every opportunity to explain a treatment, a medication, the condition, and/or restrictions. For example, as you change a dressing:
- Explain and ask the individual/family member to redress the wound.
- Point out how the wound is healing and what would indicate signs of infection.

Teach-Back Method: A Strategy to Improve Understanding
- Reminder Card
  - Who—*me*
  - What—*anything important I want them to understand*

- When—*every time*
- Why—*I need to know they understand*
- How—Focus on "need to know" and "need to do"
- Demonstrate/draw pictures
- Provide simple written education materials
- Break content into short sentences
- Go slow
- Use Teach-Back every day with all assigned individuals who are capable of recall
- Practice with and improve one's Teach-Back skills
- Understanding
  - Based on the person's response or demonstration, there is confidence that the person/family can apply the teaching to safe self-care at home.

 Carp's Cues

When individual/family do not understand what was said or demonstrated, the teach-back needs to be revised in a manner that will improve understanding. Teach-Back has the potential to improve health outcomes because if done correctly, it forces the nurse to limit the information to need to know. The likelihood of success is increased when the individual is not overwhelmed.

Elements to Teach for Optional Self-Care or Care at Home

The Condition

- Medical Conditions
  - What do you know about your condition?
  - How do you think this condition will affect you after you leave the hospital?
  - What do you want to know about your condition?
- Surgical Procedure
  - What do you know about the surgery you had?
  - Do you have any questions about your surgery?
  - How will surgery affect you after you leave the hospital?

Medications

- Renew all the medications that the individual will continue to take at home
- Explain what OTC not to take
- Finish all the meds like antibiotics
- Do not take any medications that are at home unless approved by PCP
- Ask individual to bring all his or her medications to next visit to PCP (e.g., prescribed, OTC, vitamins, herbal medicines)
- Depending on the literacy level of the individual/family, provide
  - A list of each medication, what used for, times to take, with food or without food
  - Create a pill card with columns
    - Pictures of pill
    - Simple terms for used for
    - Time using symbols with pictures of pills in spaces

Refer to Chapter 4—Preparation of Individual/Family for Care at Home for an example of a pill card
- Warn an individual that if a pill looks different, check with pharmacy.
- Emphasize not to take any other medications except those on list unless approved by PCP.
- In the author's primary care practice, hospitalized individuals may be given a different medication in the same class due to formulary restrictions. When the individual has a follow-up used in the office, during medication reconciliation, it is discovered he or she is taking two β-blockers, one prescribed in the hospital and the one previously taken.

Financial Implications of Prescribed Medication

- Does the person have insured medication coverage? If yes, does it cover the medication ordered? If yes, what is the co-pay? Can the person afford this?
- If there is no insurance or no medication coverage, how will the person access these medications?

- Is there an inexpensive generic available?
- Which medications are critical?
- Most pharmaceutical companies provide free branded medications (not generic) through individual-assisted programs.
- Applications can be accessed via the pharmaceutical website. Social service departments can also assist with this process.
- Some medications can be acquired free (e.g., oral diabetic medications, antibiotics), or low cost (e.g., Target).
- Advise individual/family to call PCP office if they do not want to continue a medication before they stop taking it, to discuss why (e.g., side effects).

Diet

- Ask individual/family to report if there are any dietary limitations
- Ensure there are written directions
- Explain why some foods/beverages are to be avoided (e.g., avoid olives, pickles on a low-salt diet)

Activities

- Provide instructions on activities permitted and restrictions
- When they can drive
- Return to work; what kind of job do they have?

Treatments

- Explain each treatment to be continued at home
- Equipment needed, frequency of treatment
- Write down what signs and symptoms should be reported (e.g., decrease in output for catheter)

Evaluation

- Can this treatment be provided safely by the individual or caregiver?
- If not, consult with the transition specialist in the health care agency.

If a home health agency is referred to, validate that their arrival will be timely in order to begin the treatment on time.

Summary

The positive outcomes achieved in the acute care setting will quickly evaporate if the individual/family is not prepared to continue care at home. Teach-Back is an effective strategy to focus on "need to know" rather than overwhelming everyone, leading them to be confused and stressed. Fear and uncertainty are a very common reason individuals return to the emergency room and are often readmitted.

Nursing Diagnoses Index

Collaborative Problems Index

General Index

Note: Page numbers followed by *f*, *t*, and *b* indicate figures, tables and boxes, respectively.

A

Abdominal aortic aneurysm repair, 620–627
  endovascular, 621
  open, 621
Abdominal hysterectomy, 680
Abscess, bone, in osteomyelitis, 525
Acid–base balance
  in asthma, 347
  in Guillain–Barré Syndrome, 457
Acidosis
  diabetic ketoacidosis, in diabetes mellitus, 379–383
  metabolic
    in acute kidney injury, 420–426
    in chronic kidney disease, 430–436
Acquired immunodeficiency syndrome (AIDS), 537–547. *See also* **Human immunodeficiency virus (HIV)**
Acute arterial thrombosis, in peripheral arterial disease (atherosclerosis), 339–340
Acute chest syndrome, in sickle cell disease, 499–503
Acute coronary syndrome (ACS), 328–337
  recurrent, 330–333
Acute kidney injury (AKI), 419–428
  intrarenal, 419
  postrenal, 419
  prerenal, 419
Acute lung injury (ALI), in thoracic surgery, 720–724
Acute pulmonary edema, in thoracic surgery, 720–724
Acute renal injury/failure, after coronary artery bypass grafting, 669
Acute respiratory distress syndrome, in pancreatitis, 390–393
Acute respiratory failure (ARF), in Guillain–Barré Syndrome, 457–459
Addendum diagnoses, in care plan, 279
Adherence, barriers to, 17–19
Adult respiratory distress syndrome, in cerebrovascular accident (stroke), 443–447
Adverse events, prevented by communication, 11–16
AIDS. *See* **Acquired immunodeficiency syndrome**
Air embolism, in hemodialysis, 743–746
Airway obstruction, in carotid endarterectomy, 653–655
Albumin, serum, in chronic renal failure, 434
Alcohol
  abuse, and pancreatitis, 393, 395–396
  dependency, 562–571

hallucinosis, in alcohol dependency, 564–568
withdrawal, in pancreatitis, 390–393
Alcohol withdrawal syndrome, 566
ALI. *See* **Acute lung injury**
Alkalosis, in acute renal failure, 422
Allergies, in hemodialysis, 743–746
Amputation, 627–638
Anaphylaxis, in hemodialysis, 743–746
Anastomosis disruption, in arterial bypass grafting in lower extremity, 639–641
Anemia
  in chronic kidney disease, 430–436
  in inflammatory bowel syndrome, 404–406
  in sickle cell disease, 499–503
Aneurysm, abdominal aortic, repair, 620–627
Angina, unstable, 355–365
Antacid therapy, 417
Antiseptic hand hygiene, 287
Aortoenteric fistula, in abdominal aortic aneurysm repair, 623–625
Aphasia, stroke and, 448
Aplastic crisis, in sickle cell disease, 501
Apraxia, stroke and, 448
ARF. *See* **Acute respiratory failure**
Arrhythmias
  in acute coronary syndrome, 330–333
  in acute kidney injury, 420–426
  in thoracic surgery, 720–724
Arterial bypass grafting
  coronary artery, 665–674
  in lower extremity, 638–644
Arterial thrombosis, acute, in peripheral arterial disease, 339–340
Arthritis
  infectious, 528–536
  rheumatoid, 528–536
  septic
    in inflammatory joint disease, 528–536
    in systemic lupus erythematosus, 549–552
Arthroplasty, 788–794
Artificial disc replacement, 611
Ascites
  in cirrhosis, 369–372
  in palliative care, 576–581
Aspiration
  in myasthenia gravis, 475–477
  in Parkinson's disease, 483–484
Assessment
  for care planning, 30–31
  same day, 31
Asthma, 345–353. *See also* **Chronic obstructive pulmonary disease (COPD)**

Atelectasis, in cerebrovascular accident (stroke), 443–447
Atherosclerosis, 337–344
  and carotid endarterectomy, 656
Automated peritoneal dialysis, 749
Autonomic hyperactivity, in alcohol dependency, 564–568
Autonomic nervous system failure, in Guillain–Barré Syndrome, 457–459
Avascular necrosis, in inflammatory joint disease, 530–532

B

Barriers
  to adherence, 17–19
  to caring, 39
  home environment, 19–20
  personal, 19
  and stressors, 37
  support system, 19
Benzodiazepines, adverse effects and side effects, 566
Bifocal Clinical Practice Model, 5–10, 6*f*
Biliary cirrhosis, 367
Bladder
  perforation, in peritoneal dialysis, 751–755
  in peritoneal dialysis, 751–755
  trauma, in hysterectomy, 682–684
Bleeding. *See also* **Hemorrhage**
  gastrointestinal
    in acute kidney injury, 420–426
    in inflammatory bowel syndrome, 404–406
  intra-abdominal, 625
  retroperitoneal, 625
  vaginal, in hysterectomy, 682–684
  variceal, in cirrhosis, 369–372
Blood clot. *See* **Clotting**
Blood pressure. *See also* **Hypertension**
  control, in diabetes, 382
  normal, 321
  prehypertension, 321
Blood sugar. *See* **Glucose, plasma/blood**
Bone abscess, in osteomyelitis, 525
Bowel
  function, lumbar spinal surgery, 714
  obstruction, in palliative care, 576–581
  perforation, in peritoneal dialysis, 751–755
  trauma, in hysterectomy, 682–684
Brain attack. *See* **Stroke**
Breast cancer, 644–651
Breast surgery, 644–651
Bronchiectasis bronchitis, chronic, 353–360
Bronchopleural fistula, in thoracic surgery, 720–724

High Risk for Falls

Fall Risk Assessment

Assess for the following risk factors. Record the number of checks in the Fall assessment scores in the ( ) as High Risk for Falls (score) or add the risk factors for example as High Risk for Falls related to instability, postural hypotension and IV equipment.

Assess all individuals for risk factors for falls, using the assessment tool in the institution. The following represents one assessment tool:

Variables Score

History of falling
No (score as 0).
Yes (score as 25).

Secondary diagnosis
No (score as 0).
Yes (score as 15).

Ambulatory aid
Bed rest/nurse assist (score as 0).
Crutches/cane/walker (score as 15).
Furniture (score as 30).

IV or IV access
No (score as 0).
Yes (score as 20).

Gait
Normal/bed rest/immobile (score as 0).
Weak (score as 10).
Impaired (score as 20).

Mental status
Knows own limits (score as 0).
Overestimates or forgets limits (score as 15).

Total Score _____

Risk Level MFS Score Action

No risk
0–24 Good basic nursing care

Low to moderate risk
25–45 Implement standard fall prevention interventions

High risk
46 + Implement high-risk fall prevention interventions

Morse Fall Scale (Morse, 2009). Used with permission

Republished with permission of Springer Publishing Company, Inc, from *Preventing Patient Falls*, Janice Morse, Second Edition, 2008; permission conveyed through Copyright Clearance Center, Inc.

For individuals who are independent and ambulatory but frail, fatigued and/or with possible compromised ambulation, assess the person's ability to Timed Up and Go (TUG):

- Have the person wear their usual footwear and use any assistive device they normally use.
- Have the person sit in the chair with their back to the chair and their arms resting on the arm rests.
- Ask the person to stand up from a standard chair and walk a distance of 10 ft (3m).
- Have the person turn around, walk back to the chair, and sit down again.
- Timing begins when the person starts to rise from the chair and ends when he or she returns to the chair and sits down.

The person should be given one practice trial and then three actual trials if needed. The times from the three actual trials are averaged.

Predictive Results

Seconds Rating
<10 Freely mobile
10–19 Mostly independent
20–29 Variable mobility
>29 Impaired mobility

Risk Factors for Surgical Site Infection

The Risk of Surgical Site Infection is influenced by the amount and virulence of the microorganism and the ability of the individual to resist it (Pear, 2007).

Assess for the following risk factors. Record the number of Risk Factors in the ( ) as High Risk for Surgical Site Infection (1–10) or add the risk factors for example as as High Risk for Surgical Site Infection related to obesity, diabetes mellitus, and tobacco use.

Infection colonization of microorganisms (1)
Pre-Existing Remote Body Site Infection (1)
Pre-operative contaminated or dirty wound (e.g., post trauma) (1)
Glucocorticoid Steroids (2)
Tobacco Use (3)
Malnutrition (4)
Obesity (5)
Perioperative Hyperglycemia (6)
Diabetes Mellitus (7)
Altered immune response (8)
Chronic alcohol use/acute alcohol intoxication (9)

1. Preoperative nares colonization with *Staphylococcus aureus* noted in 30% of most healthy populations, and especially methicillin-resistant *staph aureus* (MRSA), predisposes individuals to have higher risk of SSI (Price et al., 2008).
2. Systemic glucocorticoids (GC), which are frequently used as anti-inflammatory agents, are well-known to inhibit wound repair *via* global anti-inflammatory effects and suppression of cellular wound responses, including fibroblast proliferation and collagen synthesis. Systemic steroids cause wounds to heal with incomplete granulation tissue and reduced wound contraction (Franz *et al.*, 2007).
3. "Smoking has a transient effect on the tissue microenvironment and a prolonged effect on inflammatory and reparative cell functions leading to delayed healing and complications" (Sørensen, 2012). Quit smoking four weeks before surgery "restores tissue oxygenation and metabolism rapidly" (Ibid).
4. Malnourished individuals have been found to have less competent immune response to infection and decreased nutritional stores which will impair wound healing (Speaar, 2008).
5. An obese individuals may experience a compromise in wound healing due to poor blood supply to adipose tissue. In addition, antibiotics are a not absorbed well by adipose tissue. Despite excessive food intake, many obese individuals have protein malnutrition, which further impedes the healing (Cheadle, 2006).
6. There are two primary mechanisms that place individuals experiencing acute perioperative hyperglycemia at increased risk for SSI. The first mechanism is the decreased vascular circulation that occurs, reducing tissue perfusion and impairing cellular-level functions. A clinical study by Akbari et al. noted that when healthy, non-diabetic subjects ingested a glucose load, the endothelial-dependent vasodilatation in both the micro and macro circulations were impaired similar to that seen in diabetic patients (1998). The second affected mechanism is the reduced activity of the cellular immunity functions of chemotaxis, phagocytosis, and killing of polymorphonuclear cells as well as monocytes/macrophages that have been shown to occur in the acute hyperglycemic state (Akbari et al., 1998).
7. Postsurgical adverse outcomes related to DM are believed to be related to the pre-existing complications of chronic hyperglycemia, which include vascular atherosclerotic disease and peripheral as well as autonomic neuropathies (Geerlings et al., 1999).
8. Suppression of the immune system by disease, medication, or age can delay wound healing (Cheadle, 2006).
9. Chronic alcohol exposure causes impaired wound healing and enhanced host susceptibility to infections. Wounds from trauma in the presence of acute alcohol exposure have a higher rate of post-injury infection due to decreased neutrophil recruitment and phagocytic function (Guo & DiPietro, 2010).